Thomson Delmar Learning's

MEDICAL-SURGICAL

NURSING CARE PLANS

Thomson Delmar Learning's
MEDICAL-SURGICAL
NURSING CARE PLANS

SHIELDA GLOVER RODGERS, RN, PhD

Clinical Associate Professor
The University of North Carolina at Chapel Hill
School of Nursing
Chapel Hill, North Carolina

THOMSON

DELMAR LEARNING™

Australia   Brazil   Canada   Mexico   Singapore   Spain   United Kingdom   United States

8/07

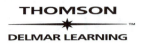

THOMSON
DELMAR LEARNING

Thomson Delmar Learning's Medical-Surgical Nursing Care Plans
Shielda Glover Rodgers, RN, PhD

Vice President, Health Care Business Unit:
William Brottmiller

Director of Learning Solutions:
Matthew Kane

Acquisitions Editor:
Tamara Caruso

Senior Product Manager:
Elisabeth F. Williams

Editorial Assistant:
Jennifer Waters

Marketing Director:
Jennifer McAvey

Marketing Manager:
Michelle McTighe

Marketing Coordinator:
Danielle Pacella

Technology Director:
Laurie K. Davis

Production Director:
Carolyn Miller

Senior Content Project Manager:
James Zayicek

Library of Congress Cataloging-in-Publication Data

Rodgers, Shielda.
  Thomson Delmar Learning's Medical-Surgical Nursing Care Plans / Shielda Rodgers.
       p. ; cm.
  Includes bibliographical references and index.
  ISBN-13: 978-0-7668-5997-5
  ISBN-10: 0-7668-5997-5
  1. Nursing care plans. I. Title. II. Title: Medical-surgical nursing care plans.
  [DNLM: 1. Patient Care Planning. 2. Nursing Care—methods. 3. Nursing Process.
4. Perioperative Nursing—methods. WY 100 R691d 2008]
  RT49.R63 2008
  610.73—dc22

                                    2006035031

NOTICE TO THE READER

DEDICATION

This book is dedicated to my wonderful mother Clara Glover
and to the memory of my father Joseph Glover.

CONTENTS

AN INTRODUCTION TO THE USE OF THE NURSING CARE PLANS

The benchmarks towards excellence in nursing practice are encompassed in the nursing diagnostic processes of assessment, diagnosis, planning, intervention, and evaluation. The nursing process provides a strong framework that gives direction to the practice of nursing. Nursing care planning is the application of the nursing process in the practice environment with individual patients, families, or communities. Without the planning process, quality and consistency in patient care would most likely be compromised. Nursing care plans provide a means of communication among nurses, nursing students, patients, and other health care providers as they endeavor to achieve optimum health care outcomes.

Nursing diagnoses are useful in labeling the patient problems that the nurse will address in the provision of care and provide a basis for selection of appropriate therapeutic interventions. Now more than ever, the nurse is relied upon to make judgments and clinical decisions that are significantly complex and that may result not only in positive outcomes but in far-reaching negative consequences for the patient as well. Having a foundation in nursing process and critical thinking prepares the nurse clinician to make these decisions based on scientific and nursing principles. In the health care arena of today with limited resources (human and material), priorities must be set forth to distinguish between what is critical for the patient's optimal health or survival and what is simply a desirable intervention. The primary purpose of the nursing process is to allow nurses to develop a plan of care for and in conjunction with the patient that results in resolution of health problems, prevention of new problems or illness, health promotion, and education of the patient to be an active participant in his or her care or in activities to promote health.

In the current health care environment, specifically the thrust into an interdisciplinary care model, nurses are positioned for a level of accountability not seen in prior health care practice climates. In addition to requiring more independent decision making by the nurse, health care institutions are seeking to engage various disciplines in working together and jointly sharing responsibility for achievement of positive patient outcomes. The changes that are occurring offer nursing a renewed opportunity to define its boundaries and to use the nursing process to deliver care. Nurses, especially beginning nurses and student nurses, need tools that can assist them in accurately predicting achievable patient outcomes for a given primary condition, and in tailoring interventions to the individual patient and his or her unique circumstances. This text is designed to provide that guidance.

STANDARDIZED NURSING CARE PLANS AND INDIVIDUAL PATIENT CARE NEEDS

This book is intended to facilitate the care planning process for nurses working with adult patients experiencing medical-surgical problems as their primary condition. The nursing diagnoses that are used throughout this book are taken from the North American Nursing Diagnosis Association's Taxonomy II (NANDA, 2005). On occasion, patient problems are suggested in the care plan that are not NANDA-approved, and these are marked by an asterisk. The outcome statements may be made in two ways: using the nursing outcome classification (NOC) or writing an outcome statement. Both are included for use. This text also contains two sources of interventions for each diagnosis: a list of recommended nursing interventions, and suggested nursing intervention classifications (NIC), to assist the reader in selecting interventions for application to the clinical setting.

For each primary condition, the care plan provides general information about the primary condition with common clinical manifestations. In addition, each plan includes the following:

1. Nursing diagnoses with their etiological (related) factors and defining characteristics

2. Broad patient goal

3. Outcome criteria that are patient-focused and measurable

4. Nursing interventions that are comprehensive

5. Rationales for the nursing interventions to assist in building a knowledge base to apply the information, to make clinical decisions, and to think how best to respond to the patient's needs

6. Evaluation criteria for each diagnosis

7. Community/home care considerations for each diagnosis in the care plan

8. Documentation guidelines for each diagnosis

The nursing care plans provided in this text are intended to serve as a catalyst for reflection and critical thinking. In order for the nurse or student nurse to apply them to a patient situation, they must think critically about what is known about the patient based on the patient's history and/or a physical examination. Nurses must actively pursue all parts of the patient information database, examining the evidence the patient has brought forth to define specific problems, and then establish specific goals and outcomes that need to be accomplished in relationship to those problems.

The next step in the process is to determine how to actualize these goals and outcomes by selecting interventions from those provided that are realistic and specific to the patient that will assist the patient in resolution of the problem. Standardized care plans do not provide a "cookie-cutter" approach to provision of nursing care that can be used without consideration of the patient's unique situation. Rather, they provide the clinician with a sample of what might be an acceptable plan of care with minimum expectations and predictable patterns of responses against which the nurse can compare the patient's presentation. At this point, the nurse or student can move forward in designing a plan of care based on selected aspects of the standardized plan that is individualized and responsive to a specific patient and that also reflects current management modalities.

The process for planning individualized care involves the same steps as the nursing process.

1. Collect and review the patient assessment data.

Typically the information will be found in the standardized facility assessment sheet or nurse's notes, the patient's medication administration record, laboratory reports, and the progress notes from other disciplines such as nutrition, physical therapy, respiratory therapy, social work, chaplains, or physicians. Interview the patient and complete an assessment record that can be the focused assessment tool provided by the facility, or for students, an assessment documentation form from a specific class at school. After studying the health record, organize the information into a summary of patient issues.

2. Identify applicable nursing diagnoses and potential "risk for" situations.

Review the nursing diagnoses provided by the standardized care plan. Choose those that fit the patient database that has been collected. The diagnostic process is individualized by identifying "related to" factors and "defining characteristics" that have been identified in the assessment process. Consider the following example of a nursing diagnosis: "acute pain r/t surgical incision as evidenced by patient verbalizing pain at a 9 on a scale of 1 to 10." The patient's own words and pain rating allow the nurse to match the defining characteristics and interventions in the standardized plan to the patient's own perceptions.

3. Develop goals and outcome criteria.

The goals should pertain to the specific patient interventions and move the patient toward resolution of the problem. The outcomes provided in the text will support this and allow for timeframes or target times to be added to allow for evaluation of outcome achievement and individualization of the plan. "The patient verbalizes pain at a level 3 or less" would be a standardized outcome. The outcome becomes individualized when the nurse determines a timeframe for achievement of the goal, such as "within the next 24 hours."

4. Design interventions to meet the goal and resolve the nursing diagnosis.

Choose interventions that are relevant or significant for the patient, that are congruent with cultural values, and that are consistent with the medical orders. Placing the patient in a position of comfort or encouraging deep breathing would be examples of independent nursing interventions, and the administration of pain medications would be an example of collaborative nursing interventions that would achieve the outcome and resolve the "acute pain" diagnosis.

5. Evaluate the effectiveness of the plan.

By setting target dates or times, the plan communicates the need for ongoing evaluation and updating. The user returns to the outcome criteria to determine if the target outcome criteria have been achieved by the target dates or time. When outcomes have been achieved, the nurse indicates resolution of the problem. If the patient is making progress towards achievement of the outcomes but has not achieved them, the nurse or student reviews the plan to determine which interventions are working and how much additional time may be needed for resolution of the problem. The plan of care is then revised with attention to setting new goals and outcome criteria, revising the nursing interventions required for resolution of the problem, and adding additional interventions or deleting others.

CRITICAL THINKING, THE NURSING PROCESS, AND CARE PLAN DEVELOPMENT

Critical thinking and decision-making skills are used in identifying nursing diagnoses. Critical thinking entails purposeful, goal-directed thinking, with attention to analysis of large amounts of patient data. The nurse uses critical thinking to analyze and synthesize the information from the data collection (assessment, history, patient records), and then makes judgments about how to utilize the information to identify nursing diagnoses and develop a plan of care in the clinical setting. The standardized nursing care plans in this book provide the clinician with a starting point for the nursing process, allowing the nurse to review the patient's data, compare it with the information on the standardized care plan, and then develop an individualized plan of care.

The following situation illustrates how to apply the standardized care plan to an evolving patient situation. The case study analysis provides an example of how to use the steps in the nursing process and the current standardized care plans in this text, differentiating among the possible nursing diagnoses for the patient. As part of the individualization process, organize diagnostic statements according to their presenting priority.

CASE STUDY

A 32-year-old female is admitted to the hospital from the physician's office this morning because of increasing shortness of breath and wheezing unrelieved with usual treatments over the past 48 hours. The patient is employed in an office as an administrative assistant, is married, has one 8-year-old child, and has health insurance with prescription coverage for medications. The initial assessment reveals wheezing bilaterally on expiration, coughing, skin warm to touch, temperature 98 degrees F, blood pressure 118/70, pulse 88, respiratory rate 28, and the expectoration of thick mucous when coughing. History from the patient includes a feeling of anxiety, reports that "I just can't catch my breath," "my chest feels tight," "they changed the ceiling tiles in my office and cleaned the carpet, I think they stirred up something," and "I haven't had an asthmatic attack for almost a year." Laboratory results reveal white blood cell (WBC) count—eosinophil of $375/mm^3$, initial arterial blood gases (ABGs) with a ph of 7.33, pO_2 of 88, and pCO_2 of 48.

NURSING DIAGNOSIS 1

 ### INEFFECTIVE AIRWAY CLEARANCE

Related to:

Thick mucous

Exposure to allergens

Defining Characteristics:

Expiratory wheezes

Respiratory rate of 28 (tachypnea)

$PO_2 = 88$

$PCO_2 = 48$

$Ph = 7.33$

Goal:

The patient's airway remains patent.

Outcome Criteria

✔ The patient's breath sounds will be clear (no wheezing) in 24 hours.

✔ The patient will expectorate mucous when coughing.

✔ Arterial blood gases will be within normal range (no acidosis) within 48 hours.

NOC *Asthma control*

Allergic response: Systemic

INTERVENTIONS	RATIONALES
Assess respiratory status: breath sounds, respiratory rate, oxygen saturation; note abnormalities such as dyspnea, presence of cyanosis, retractions, use of accessory muscles, and flaring of nostrils.	Abnormal breathing patterns may signal worsening of condition; retractions and flaring of nostrils indicate a significant decline in respiratory status; establishes a baseline and allows monitoring of response to interventions.
Monitor the patient for signs of occluded airway: cyanosis, cessation of wheezing, absence of breath sounds over lungs, holding throat, and continuous coughing.	If bronchospasm is severe, there may be no air movement, and therefore no wheezing. Be very careful when auscultating the chest to pay particular attention to the sound of any air movement, as focusing on wheezing may cause one to miss the fact that there is no air movement; patient may cough almost continuously in an attempt to open the airway.
Assess ABGs, as ordered.	ABGs provide data for treatment regarding the lungs' ability to oxygenate tissues; initially ABG analysis will reveal respiratory alkalosis as the tachypnea blows off more carbon dioxide, but as the airway narrows the lungs are unable to blow off carbon dioxide and acidosis is noted.
Assess for anxiety and reassure patient with presence.	Being unable to breathe causes anxiety and fear; the patient needs a calming presence, as anxiety increases the demand for oxygen.
Establish intravenous (IV) access.	Helps to ensure a route for rapid-acting medications.
Place the patient in a high Fowler's position and support with overbed table as needed.	Maximizes chest excursion and subsequent movement of air.
Assist respiratory therapist with administration of beta-adrenergic agonists (such as albuterol, metaproterenol) via nebulizer or metered dose inhaler, as ordered, and monitor for side effects.	Stimulates $beta_2$-adrenergic receptor sites in the pulmonary system to increase levels of cAMP, which relaxes smooth muscles, causing bronchodilation, reducing bronchospasm; common side effects include tremors, tachycardia, and anxiety.
Encourage expectoration of secretions and assess the viscosity, amount, and color of secretions.	Thickened secretions of asthma are more likely to occlude the airway; making this observation would allow for implementation of measures to thin and loosen the secretions; the color of secretions allows for early detection of color changes due to infection.
Monitor for signs and symptoms of respiratory infection: fever, rales, increased mucous production, elevated WBC count, and chest x-ray reports.	The presence of infection can worsen asthma; monitoring for signs of infection allows for early treatment that can prevent complications.
Provide humidified oxygen, as ordered, to maintain oxygen saturation at > 90 percent.	Loosens secretions making them easier to expectorate with coughing and improves oxygenation.
Reinforce teaching about prevention of acute exacerbations.	Knowledge increases the chance that the patient can engage in health-promoting behaviors and take control of disease.

NIC *Asthma management*

Cough enhancement

Presence

Respiratory monitoring

Oxygen therapy

The above diagnosis is individualized by using the underlying factors (etiologies/"related to" statement) of the patient's reported subjective information and the objective data. It is important to review the assessment data to assure the related factors and defining characteristics are present in the patient at the time the care plan is being designed, using the text as a reference. This is done by comparing the patient assessment findings with those in the text's "related to" statements and "defining characteristics." The patient's assessment data need to match this information, or a new diagnosis may need to be considered.

CLINICAL PATHWAYS: A METHOD OF ACHIEVING OUTCOMES, CONSUMER SATISFACTION, AND A CONTINUUM OF CARE

Health care consumers are becoming more sophisticated when they encounter the health care system. As a result, they expect to be satisfied with the health care services they are consuming. Health care organizations publish their outcomes and report them to state, federal, and independent agencies as a method of maintaining practice standards and of attracting consumers and health care providers. In addition, the rapid rise in health care costs has caused third-party payers to play a role in what services are needed or eligible for reimbursement and to scrutinize their patients' health outcomes. The demand for the most effective and cost-efficient manner of restoring patients to health has led to the clinical pathway or care map collaborative patient care model.

Clinical pathways, also known as "critical paths" and "care maps," are tools used by nursing that outline the expected clinical course, patient response to interventions, and outcomes for a specific diagnosis on each day that the patient is hospitalized. The manner in which a pathway is constructed is usually agency-specific, but typically they follow the patient's length of stay on a day-to-day basis for the specific disease process or surgical intervention. Critical pathways or care maps are interdisciplinary in nature and are intended to enhance cost-effective, high-quality care, ensure provision of needed services, and eliminate unnecessary extended hospital stays. The pathway guides the care providers along a sequence of interdisciplinary interventions that incorporate standardized aspects such as patient and family teaching, nutrition, medications, activities, diagnostic studies, and treatments. Ideally, the tool is developed collaboratively by all health team members and includes predictable and established timeframes. A care map assists the provider to deliver consistent, competent care, not just on a shift-by-shift basis, but throughout the entire hospital stay across all disciplines involved in the patient's care. Because of the standardization of practice, clinical pathways also allow for measuring performance improvement within an agency and between similar agencies over time.

The task here is to appreciate that clinical pathways guide rather than dictate the course of care for an individual. They do not take into account coexistent patient problems that may have an impact on the patient's recovery process. Therefore, the process of incorporating clinical pathways and the use of this text is the same as in individualizing standard care plans. The nurse must incorporate the individualized needs that exist in conjunction with the clinical pathway. When the patient is unable to meet the outcome achievement timeframe, the nurse must reassess, report, and address the variance in order to help the patient achieve the desired outcomes. The manner of reporting variances is also agency specific. At times, the variances are documented on the clinical pathway; other times the nursing care plan format is incorporated into the document, or an individualized care plan is initiated and documentation about the variance is continued until it is resolved. Not all patient care can be planned using a clinical pathway, and in some instances applying the various standardized nursing diagnoses in this text may be more appropriate.

Well-designed nursing care plans and/or care maps move the patient from one level of care on the health care continuum to another. They help the nurse to monitor and guide the progress of the patient from an acutely ill phase of illness to restoration of an optimal state of health with attention to disease prevention, health promotion, and/or end-of-life care. Care planning organizes and coordinates the patient care with attention to providing quality nursing care as defined by professional standards in a manner that promotes consistency and communication across disciplines and that incorporates a problem-solving process that integrates responsiveness to patient needs and cost efficiency.

ACKNOWLEDGMENTS

I give loving appreciation to my wonderful husband, Kenneth, who has encouraged me throughout this process, especially when I doubted my ability to complete the project; and to my wonderful and lovely children, Nia and Shaun, who expressed great excitement and unrelenting faith in their mom's ability to write a book.

I also acknowledge the love and encouragement of my three sisters, Sharon, Sylvia, and Setonya, who anxiously await the arrival of the book.

Grateful acknowledgement is given to the hundreds of nursing students who have written care plans for me during 24 years of clinical experiences. I truly understand now the agony you experienced on the night before clinical!

REVIEWERS

Catherine Andrews, RN, PhD
Associate Professor
Department of Nursing
Edgewood College
Madison, Wisconsin

Susan Baltrus, RNC, BSPA, MSN
Central Maine General Hospital School of Nursing
Lewiston, Maine
St. Joseph's College
Standish, Maine
University of Southern Maine
Portland, Maine

Patricia Campbell, RN, MSN
Faculty
Carolinas College of Health Sciences
Charlotte, North Carolina

Yvonne Garner, RN, EDS
Faculty
School of Nursing
Miami Dade College
Miami, Florida

Rebecca Gesler, RN, MSN
Assistant Professor
School of Nursing
Spalding University
Louisville, Kentucky

Donna Headrick, RN, MSN, FNP
Instructor
Bakersfield College
Bakersfield, California

Joanna Hill, ARNP-BC, LHRM, PhD
Faculty
College of Nursing
St. Petersburg College
St. Petersburg, Florida

Yvonne Johnston, RN, MS, FNP
Clinical Assistant Professor
The Decker School of Nursing
Binghamton University
Binghamton, New York

Bonnie Kirpatrick, RN, MS, CNS
Assistant Professor
College of Nursing
The Ohio State University
Columbus, Ohio

Karen March, RN, PhD
Assistant Professor
College of Nursing
York College
York, Pennsylvania

Kathleen Upham, RN, MSN, ONC
Associate Professor of Nursing
Coastal Georgia Community College
Brunswick, Georgia

UNIT 1

CARDIOVASCULAR SYSTEM

CHAPTER 1.1

ABDOMINAL AORTIC ANEURYSM (AAA) OR DISSECTION

GENERAL INFORMATION

An abdominal aortic aneurysm is a weakening of one or two of the layers of the wall of the aorta, causing either a "ballooning" area to form (aneurysm) or the layers of the abdominal wall to separate (dissection). It usually results from atherosclerosis in the presence of hypertension, post-trauma, or from congenital causes, where extraordinary pressure is placed on non-elastic tissue. Seventy-five percent of all aortic aneurysms are abdominal; they occur more often in men, increasing in incidence with age (Lewis, Heitkemper, and Dirksen, 2004). Abdominal aneurysms are usually asymptomatic and detected when an individual has x-rays, examinations, or scans for some other reason. Patient complaints, when present, include abdominal or back pain. When the aneurysm is discovered, care should be directed at reducing the pressure in the aorta to prevent aortic rupture/dissection and at preparing the patient for surgery to repair the aneurysm. Repair is accomplished by replacing the aneurysm area with a graft. If the aneurysm is not large (smaller than 6 cm), medical treatment may be an option. This includes decreasing blood pressure and monitoring the aneurysm for early detection of increasing size every 6 months.

NURSING DIAGNOSIS 1

 INEFFECTIVE TISSUE PERFUSION (DISSECTION/RUPTURE)

Related to:

Possibility of rupture of the aneurysm

Increased pressure in the aorta secondary to increased blood pressure

Defining Characteristics:

Pulsating abdominal mass

Hypertension

Tachycardia

Goal:

Adequate tissue perfusion will be maintained.

Outcome Criteria

✔ The patient's blood pressure decreases and is maintained at ≤ 120 systolic and ≤ 80 diastolic.

✔ The patient has no signs and symptoms of dissection/rupture.

NOC *Circulation status*

Tissue perfusion: Cardiac

Vital signs

Tissue perfusion: Abdominal organs

INTERVENTIONS	RATIONALES
Assess abdomen for pulsating abdominal mass, but do not palpate.	An AAA pulsates and sudden disappearance indicates a problem; palpation may cause rupture.
Assess for pain location, intensity, and characteristic.	The presence of pain may indicate worsening of aneurysm; as most are asymptomatic, pain may mimic other disorders or be the result of other causes.
Administer pain medications as ordered based on assessment.	Relieving pain will decrease cardiac demand, and continued pain indicates dissection or rupture.

INTERVENTIONS	RATIONALES
Assess vital signs, particularly blood pressure and pulse.	Allows early treatment of elevated blood pressure in order to decrease pressure on aorta that could cause rupture; changes in vital signs may indicate change in status of aneurysm.
Administer vasodilator (sodium nitroprusside [Nipride]), as ordered.	Reduces systolic blood pressure to < 120 mm Hg and decreases pressure on aortic wall through vasodilation.
Administer beta blockers, as ordered.	Slows heart rate and lowers blood pressure; decreases myocardial contractility and thus decreases pressure on aortic wall.
Establish a quiet environment.	Noise and other stimuli will increase blood pressure.
Assess for peripheral pulses, especially femoral arteries (bilateral); pain; pallor; and cool, clammy extremities.	These indicate decreased peripheral tissue perfusion secondary to acute rupture or progression of dissection.
Assess for change in mental status, decreased urine output, and increased respirations.	These may be indicators of shock caused by dissection or rupture.
Monitor ordered laboratory and diagnostic studies (angiography, abdominal x-rays, CT scans, abdominal ultrasounds, CBC, PT, Ptt).	Results of these tests are used to confirm the diagnosis.
For aneurysms > 6 mm, prepare the patient for emergency surgery.	These aneurysms require surgical intervention to prevent or treat rupture or dissection and to decrease chances of mortality.
For the patient treated medically, teach the importance of follow-up care to monitor blood pressure and monitor for increase in size of aneurysm.	Increased size would indicate a need for surgical intervention, and elevated blood pressure would require changes in medications to prevent rupture or dissection.

NIC   *Vital signs monitoring*
Surveillance
Cardiac care: Acute
Pain management
Medication administration: IV

Evaluation

The nurse should evaluate the degree to which the patient understands the disease process and required regimens (surgical versus medical). Blood pressure monitoring is critical in order to decrease the risk of rupture or dissection. A positive outcome is for the blood pressure to remain close to the recommended normal range of < 120 systolic and < 80 diastolic. Evaluate whether the patient's pulse has decreased since initiation of beta blockers. The patient should exhibit no signs of decreased peripheral tissue perfusion, shock, or indicators that the aneurysm has ruptured.

Community/Home Care

Patients who do not undergo surgery will need to take precautions to reduce risk of rupture/dissection. This includes controlling stress (physiological and psychological) in the environment that may elevate the blood pressure and pulse. It should be stressed that adhering to medication regimens to control blood pressure is crucial in decreasing risk of rupture and subsequent mortality. The nurse should investigate the possibility of the patient doing self-monitoring of blood pressure at home. Consider the patient's motivation, dexterity, and finances; if self-monitoring is not feasible, a referral to a home health nurse is warranted. Extension or growth of a small aneurysm needs to be monitored by a health care provider and the importance of this follow-up should be emphasized to the client.

Documentation

Document both blood pressure and pulse as ordered, but at least every 4 hours. Include in the documentation any teaching, as well as the patient's understanding of content. Assessment findings pertinent to the AAA, such as presence of pulsating mass, peripheral pulses, responses to medications, and mental status, are important data that should be indicated in the patient record.

NURSING DIAGNOSIS 2

   ## ACUTE PAIN

Related to:

Dissection or rupture of aortic wall

Decreased tissue perfusion secondary to occlusion of arteries

Surgical intervention

Defining characteristics:

Severe abdominal pain radiating into flank, back, groin

Pain in surgical site

Goals:

The patient experiences reduced pain.

Adequate tissue perfusion is re-established.

Outcome Criteria

✔ The patient verbalizes that pain is alleviated.

NOC *Pain level*

Pain control

Medication response

INTERVENTIONS	RATIONALES
Assess patient for complaints of pain that radiates into back, groin, flank, and genitals, or pain at surgical site for those patients who have had surgical repair and for intensity and characteristic.	Assists in accurate diagnosis and treatment, severe pain or increasing intensity of pain could indicate a leak or rupture.
Administer pain medications (narcotics are drug of choice), as ordered.	Reduces pain and anxiety, which will lead to reduced blood pressure.
Administer nitroglycerin and morphine sulfate, as ordered.	Decreased blood pressure will reduce pressure on aneurysm and reduce pain.
Encourage positions of comfort and splint abdomen if patient has had surgical repair.	Positioning to patient's comfort level will enhance effects of medications; side-lying positions relieve pressure on back and abdomen.
Utilize guided imagery and relaxation.	Enhances the effectiveness of pharmacological measures.
Remain in the room if the patient is anxious.	Staying with the patient calms the patient and decreases anxiety that adds to pain.
Assess response to pain medications and other interventions.	Provides evaluation of the effectiveness of interventions and determines whether further interventions are required.

NIC *Pain management*

Medication management

Analgesic administration

Presence

Evaluation

Assess the degree to which the pain has been relieved or has increased in severity. Pain status may be used as an indicator of stability of the aneurysm and should be evaluated frequently.

Community/Home Care

For patients who have undergone surgical repair, pain from abdominal aneurysms should be alleviated. Post-operative care is the same as that for coronary artery bypass surgery. Post-operatively, patients should be visited by a nurse once at home to be sure that the patient is able to manage care independently or with family assistance. Areas for examination include activity restrictions, comfort, and incisional care. The patient at home may find that energy levels are decreased, necessitating frequent rest periods during the day. Increased activity may increase pain. (For more specific information on home care for post-op patients see nursing care plan "Coronary Artery Bypass Graft/Valve Replacement Surgery.") Aneurysms < 6 mm are treated conservatively, and patients will need to be taught signs of problems. When at home, the patient should make note of pain in the abdomen that increases or becomes severe, which would indicate a leak or rupture, and which requires immediate emergency treatment. Also of concern should be increasing size of any pulsating area. The need for frequent follow-up with a physician is required to monitor the status of the aneurysm.

Documentation

Using a pain-rating scale, document severity of the pain and nursing interventions implemented. Be sure to include both pharmacological and non-pharmacological interventions. The effectiveness of strategies employed should be included. Document whether the pain has increased in severity, and indicate new strategies implemented.

NURSING DIAGNOSIS 3

 ### DECREASED CARDIAC OUTPUT

Related to:

Dissection or rupture of aneurysm

Defining Characteristics:

Decreased level of consciousness

Decreased blood pressure

Rapid pulse

Weak, thready pulses

Capillary refill > 2 seconds

Restlessness and anxiety

Goal:

Patient's cardiac output is maximized to the greatest extent possible.

Outcomes

✔ The patient's oxygen saturation is 90–100 percent.

✔ The patient's pulse is > 60, systolic blood pressure is > 120, and urine output is > 30 ml/hour.

NOC *Cardiac pump effectiveness*

INTERVENTIONS	RATIONALES
Insert two large bore IVs, and infuse Ringer's Lactate or packed red cells, as ordered.	Replaces lost fluid volume.
Prepare patient for emergency surgery by anticipating type and cross-match for blood, by implementing pre-operative activities according to hospital protocols, and by educating the patient.	Repairs the rupture or dissection.
Administer high-flow oxygen via non-rebreather mask.	Ensures maximum oxygen saturation and adequate tissue perfusion.
Monitor vital signs for decreased blood pressure and increased pulse.	These changes would indicate impending shock.
Monitor cardiac rhythm strips for abnormalities such as ST segment and T wave changes.	These changes indicate an alteration in cardiac output due to ischemia and are precursors of complications secondary to rupture/dissection.
Assess for changes in mental status and level of consciousness.	Restlessness or changes in level of consciousness indicates a decrease in cerebral tissue perfusion secondary to decreased cardiac output.
Assess renal function by monitoring output hourly.	In the presence of impending shock, the body selectively slows perfusion to other organs such as the kidneys, which is manifested in decreasing output (< 30 ml/hour).
Inform family and patient of impending emergency surgery and what to expect in the post-operative course.	Allays fears and anxiety; pre-operative knowledge enhances the likelihood of positive post-operative outcomes.
Stay with patient and explain all procedures.	Allays fears and keeps patient calm.

NIC *Presence*
Vital signs monitoring
Hemodynamic regulation

Evaluation

Note changes in patient status that may indicate problems with cardiac output or hemodynamic stability. Parameters to be noted include blood pressure, pulse, renal function, and mental status. Evaluate the patient's understanding of the disease process and the possibility of emergency surgical interventions.

Community/Home Care

For the patient who has had surgery, follow-up at home by a home nurse is required. The patient will need to follow an activity regimen of gradual progression. Wound care, including recognition of signs and symptoms of infection, will need to be taught to the family and the patient. Maintenance of blood pressure and pulse within recommended parameters will continue at home. For the patient who has not undergone surgery, it will be crucial that the patient and family understand signs and symptoms that would indicate decreased cardiac output and require medical attention. Of crucial importance is the presence of increased severity of pain or size of the abdominal mass. Adherence/compliance with medications to control blood pressure is critical, and health care workers should be sure the patient and family understands the rationale for this.

Documentation

Document findings from a cardiac assessment, including vital signs, oxygen saturation, and any change in mentation, such as lethargy, restlessness, or confusion. If surgery is planned, the nurse should document all pre-operative procedures according to hospital protocol. An assessment of the patient's psychological state should be made and documented. All teaching, including pre-operative teaching, should be documented thoroughly in the patient record.

NURSING DIAGNOSIS 4

 ### DEFICIENT KNOWLEDGE

Related to:

No previous history of the disease/new onset of disease

Lack of information about the disease and its treatment and prevention

Defining Characteristics:

Ask no questions

Have many questions/concerns

Is anxious

Goal:

The patient and family understand the disease process and treatments.

Outcome Criteria

✔ The patient verbalizes an understanding of the AAA.

✔ The patient expresses an understanding of the available treatment options.

✔ The patient is able to identify any medications prescribed, including actions, side effects, and expected therapeutic responses.

✔ Patient verbalizes an understanding of the symptomatology that would indicate a need to seek medical intervention.

NOC *Knowledge: Disease process*
Knowledge: Prescribed activity
Knowledge: Medication

INTERVENTIONS	RATIONALES
Assess patient's current knowledge, ability to learn, and readiness to learn.	Any instruction should build on what the patient already knows; teachings need to be tailored to the patient's ability and willingness to learn for maximum effectiveness.
Instruct patient/family about the disease: — Definition of aneurysms and information on causes — Treatments available—medical and surgical — Medications used to control blood pressure — Pre-operative activities and anticipated post-operative interventions — When to seek emergency health care attention — Importance of blood pressure control to prevent recurrence and other complications	Knowledge of disease, prevention, and treatment options improves patient outcomes and provides the patient and family with realistic expectations. When the patient and family understand the patient's disease process, medication regime, and possible surgical interventions, controllable aspects of the disease process occur; complications of the disease and of surgery decrease and/or repeat hospitalizations are reduced.
Teach incrementally—simple to complex	The patient will learn and retain knowledge better when information is presented in small segments starting with simple concepts.
Ask the patient and family members to repeat the information and ask questions. If the patient is going for emergency surgery, provide the most important information only.	This allows the nurse to hear in the patient's words what he or she understood. Due to stress and anxiety, the patient cannot retain great amounts of information during an emergency situation.
Offer printed materials and other audiovisual aides.	Printed and audiovisual aides enhance learning.
Provide family members with literature about the disease and inform them of opportunities for increased learning.	When a patient's family understands the disease process, they will be better able to assist the patient.
Establish that the patient has the resources required to be compliant when discharged.	If needed resources such as finances for medication, transportation, and psychosocial support are not available the patient cannot be compliant.

NIC *Learning readiness enhancement*
Learning facilitation
Teaching: Prescribed medication
Teaching: Disease process
Teaching: Preoperative

Evaluation

Evaluate the degree to which the patient has achieved the expected outcomes. The patient and family verbalize an understanding of the disease and treatment options (medical and surgical), and state that their questions have been answered. Prior to discharge, the nurse should determine whether the patient has the necessary resources to be compliant with follow-up care.

Community/Home Care

Upon discharge home, the patient who is to be treated conservatively with medications will need to understand the disease process thoroughly and the role of controlling blood pressure in the treatment process with the use of pharmacological and non-pharmacological measures. Success is dependent upon the patient being able to monitor blood pressure on a regular basis at home. In addition, the patient or family should monitor the abdominal mass if visible to note any increase in size. For the patient who has surgery, post-operative care at home will include attention to wound healing and recognition of signs and symptoms of infection by the patient or family. Follow-up care for either treatment type is critical, and the availability of transportation to appointments should be investigated. Determine if the patient has the means to monitor blood pressure (has equipment and knows the psychomotor skill).

Documentation

Document the specific content taught and the titles of any printed materials given to the family or patient. After the teaching session, document the degree to which the patient and/or family members verbalize understanding. The nurse should indicate any areas that will require further instruction and note any referrals that have been made.

CHAPTER 1.2

ANGINA PECTORIS (STABLE ANGINA)

GENERAL INFORMATION

Angina pectoris, also known as stable angina, is the first phase of a three-phase continuum of Coronary Artery Disease (CAD) that includes stable angina, unstable angina, and myocardial infarction (Phipps, Monahan, Sands, Marek, and Neighbors, 2003). It is a substernal pain that occurs as a result of myocardial ischemia due to an inadequate oxygen supply secondary to a vascular obstruction (usually atherosclerotic plaques that reduce blood flow to the coronary arteries) or narrowing of one or more of the arteries supplying the myocardium. When the myo- cardium's demand for oxygen exceeds the supply available, angina will occur. This may result from increased physical activity, a large meal, or emotional stress. Stable angina is described as chest pain lasting < 5 minutes. The pain is usually self-limiting once the patient rests or takes a vasodilating medication, such as nitroglycerin. According to the American Heart Association (2004), significantly more women than men have angina in terms of both total numbers of cases and percentages by age. The incidence per 1000 population of new and recurrent episodes of angina reflect a higher incidence in African American women (29.4 for ages 65–74) versus other women (18.8 for the same age group) (AHA, 2004).

NURSING DIAGNOSIS 1

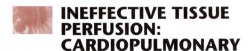

INEFFECTIVE TISSUE PERFUSION: CARDIOPULMONARY

Related to:

Obstructed flow of blood to myocardium

Myocardial ischemia when oxygen demand exceeds supply

Defining Characteristics:

Tachycardia

Chest pain with activity

Dyspnea

Pain lasts < 5 minutes; relieved with rest or nitroglycerin

Goal:

Adequate cardiac perfusion will be re-established.

Outcome Criteria

✔ The patient's blood pressure and heart rate return to baseline.

✔ The patient verbalizes that pain has been alleviated with nitroglycerin and/or rest.

✔ The patient verbalizes an understanding of the difference in signs and symptoms of angina versus myocardial infarction.

✔ The patient verbalizes ways to reduce stress and relax.

NOC *Pain level*
Pain control
Medication response

INTERVENTIONS	RATIONALES
Assess patient pain for intensity using a pain rating scale, for precise location, and for precipitating factors.	Identifying intensity, precipitating factors, and location will assist in accurate diagnosis.
Administer or assist with self-administration of vasodilators (usually nitroglycerin sublinqual), as ordered.	The vasodilator nitroglycerin enhances blood flow to the myocardium. It reduces the amount of blood returning to the heart, decreasing preload, which in turn decreases workload of the heart and the demand of the myocardium for oxygen.

INTERVENTIONS	RATIONALES
Assess response to medications (nitroglycerin) every 5 minutes.	Assessing response determines effectiveness of medication and whether further interventions are required. Chest pain not relieved by three nitroglycerin tablets taken 5 minutes apart may represent a more serious acute cardiac event.
Give beta blockers as ordered (Atenolol, Toprol).	Beta blockers decrease oxygen consumption by the myocardium and are given to prevent subsequent angina episodes.
Give aspirin as ordered.	Aspirin inhibits platelet aggregation.
Establish a quiet environment.	A quiet environment reduces the energy demands on the patient.
Elevate head of bed.	Elevation improves chest expansion and oxygenation.
Monitor vital signs, especially pulse and blood pressure, every 5 minutes until pain subsides.	Tachycardia and elevated blood pressure usually occur with angina and reflect compensatory mechanisms secondary to sympathetic nervous system stimulation. Medications given to treat angina have as a side effect a decrease in blood pressure (nitroglycerin) and a decrease in pulse (beta blockers).
Provide oxygen and monitor oxygen saturation via pulse oximetry, as ordered.	Oxygenation increases the amount of circulating oxygen in the blood and, therefore, increases the amount of available oxygen to the myocardium, decreasing myocardial ischemia and pain.
Assess results of serum cardiac markers—total creatine phosphokinase (CPK), CK-MB, total LDH, LDH-1, LDH-2, troponin, and myoglobin ordered by physician.	These enzymes elevate in the presence of myocardial infarction at differing times and assist in ruling out a myocardial infarctionas the cause of the chest pain.
Assess cardiac and circulatory status: heart sounds, pulse, blood pressure, peripheral pulses, skin temperature, and skin color.	Assessment establishes a baseline and detects changes that may indicate a change in cardiac output or perfusion.
Monitor cardiac rhythms on patient monitor and the results of 12 lead EKG.	Notes abnormal tracings that would indicate ischemia.

Teach the patient relaxation techniques (guided imagery, controlled breathing, etc.) and how to use them to reduce stress.	Anginal pain is often precipitated by emotional stress that can be relieved by non-pharmacological measures such as relaxation.
Teach the patient how to distinguish between angina pain and signs and symptoms of myocardial infarction.	In some cases, the chest pain may be more serious than stable angina. Myocardial infarction pain is described as crushing, severe, accompanied by shortness of breath and radiation to jaw or arm, and is unrelieved by nitroglycerin. The patient needs to understand the differences in order to seek emergency care in a timely fashion.
Instruct the patient or collaborate with a cardiac nurse educator who will teach the patient: — The role of diet in cardiac health — The role of exercise in cardiac health — How to take nitroglycerin tablets and side effects of the medicine — The names and actions of all prescribed medications — When to activate the EMS/911 system	The patient will need to understand how to modify his or her lifestyle to reduce risk for heart disease.

NIC *Pain management*
Oxygen therapy
Vital signs monitoring

Evaluation

The patient is able to report what caused the pain and to what degree relief has been achieved. In addition, both pulse and blood pressure will be at the patient's baseline. Following instruction by the nurse, the patient is able to distinguish between the signs and symptoms of angina versus myocardial infarction. The patient verbalizes an understanding of needed changes to lifestyle to control heart disease risk factors.

Community/Home Care

Patients diagnosed with angina will be required to be cognizant of activities that precipitate the onset of pain when at home. When at home, many patients may be anxious about the possibility of pain and engage in extreme self-limiting of activities. Climbing stairs, doing household or outdoor chores, or engaging in sexual activity may precipitate chest pain. The patient should be instructed to take nitroglycerin before engaging in activities that are likely to cause pain. By trial and error, the patient will be able to identify those activities that should be avoided. It is important to teach the patient what to do when pain occurs and when to seek medical attention. Written instructions that outline the protocol for nitroglycerin administration as ordered are reviewed with the patient, and the patient is asked to repeat the information for the nurse. The patient can keep a pain diary in which he or she records episodes of pain, activity at the time of onset, how the pain was relieved, and how long it took for pain to subside. This record can be taken to the health care provider when returning for follow-up visits. The patient should be made aware that a change in lifestyle to improve cardiac health may be required, such as regular exercise, stress reduction, and a heart-healthy diet. The nurse or dietitian should assure that the patient understands which foods are necessary and which foods should be avoided. When making dietary recommendations, consider the patient's culture and any religious preferences, as well as his or her ability to purchase special foods or foods that others in the family may not eat. Prior to discharge, have the patient plan menus for several days as a means of evaluating the patient's understanding. The physician can prescribe an activity regimen for the patient that is in keeping with the patient's capabilities and his or her motivation to engage in the activity. Many malls open early in the morning allowing patrons to enter to walk, and some even have organized walking clubs. The nurse can make a cardiac folder for the patient that contains all literature and written instructions given to the patient.

Documentation

Include in the documentation the patient's report of what may have precipitated the chest pain. Document the results of all descriptors of pain and interventions implemented for relief. Chart the patient's response to interventions including time for pain relief, pulse, and blood pressure. Document in the patient's record all teaching done relevant to angina including medications, diet, and lifestyle changes required.

NURSING DIAGNOSIS 2

ACTIVITY INTOLERANCE

Related to:

> Increased oxygen demands when activity increases, causing myocardial ischemia

Defining Characteristics:

> Chest pain or other chest discomfort with exertion
>
> Dypsnea

Goal:

> The patient is able to tolerate activities.

Outcome Criteria

✔ The patient is able to perform activities of daily living free of anginal pain.

✔ The patient states that anginal pain is relieved 5 minutes after taking nitroglycerin.

✔ Pain is relieved with rest.

NOC *Activity tolerance*
Energy conservation

INTERVENTIONS	RATIONALES
Obtain subjective data from patient regarding normal activities prior to onset of diagnosis of angina and current activity status.	Determines the effect the angina has had on the patient's ability to be active and allows for an individualized realistic plan for future activity regimens.
Reduce level of activity as required in response to chest pain.	If anginal pain is caused by increased physical activity, activity should be reduced until oxygenation is adequate (saturation >90 percent) and pain control has been achieved.
Encourage periods of rest and activity during the day.	Conserves oxygen.
Monitor vital signs and oxygen saturation before and after activity.	Use the results to indicate when activity may be increased or decreased.
Gradually increase activity as tolerated and share guidelines for progression with patient.	Activities should be increased gradually, as tolerated, to avoid overtaxing the patient.

INTERVENTIONS	RATIONALES
Teach patient about a home walking program that is within patient's activity tolerance.	Walking is a suggested activity for cardiac patients; knowledge of a specific program of activity will provide a guideline to follow and enhance compliance.
Teach patient about appropriate expectations for sexual activity and use of nitroglycerin.	Patient may have concern about future sexual activity; nitroglycerin taken before sexual activity can decrease the chance of angina by increasing the supply of oxygen to the myocardium.
Teach patient how to organize activities once at home and what to do if pain occurs.	Gives patient a sense of control and helps decrease anxiety.
Teach patient about possible need for Exercise Stress Test in the future if ordered.	Exercise Stress Test is a diagnostic tool used to diagnose angina and may be scheduled as an outpatient once pain is controlled.

NIC *Cardiac precautions*
Energy management
Teaching: Prescribed activity/exercise

Evaluation

Evaluate whether the patient has achieved the stated desired outcomes. The patient verbalizes that he or she is able to carry out desired activities without chest pain. After engaging in activity the patient's pulse, blood pressure, and respirations return to baseline values following rest. The patient verbalizes a willingness to continue exercise to promote cardiac health.

Community/Home Care

Ensure that patient has all of his or her questions answered related to activities allowed and how to increase endurance. Participation in prescribed activities is crucial to maintaining heart health and preventing complications. The patient should start gradually and progress as directed. A journal or diary should be kept by the patient to record the type of exercise attempted, the duration of the activity, the response to the activity (heart racing, shortness of breath or chest pain, fatigue), and if symptoms occurred, how relief was obtained. If walking, the patient should estimate

the distance or use a pedometer, record this, and then progress gradually until the walking maintenance goal is achieved. This record can then be taken to the physician for a more accurate history of activity rather than relying on memory. It is important that the patient is at ease asking and getting answers from nurses or physicians to concerns about the ability to engage in sexual activity. Some cardiologists recommend that the patient can take a nitroglycerin prior to engaging in sexual intercourse, but this assumes that all sexual activity is planned and not spontaneous. The patient, however, should understand that the onset of action for nitroglycerin is rapid (2 minutes), which would make the medication available to the body if chest pain should occur once engaged in sexual intercourse. The proper protocol for nitroglycerin administration prn for chest pain or anticipated exertion should be discussed. A health care provider should follow up with the patient initially to ensure that the patient is adapting to changes in health status.

Documentation

The nurse should chart the patient's tolerance for activity to include vital signs and the presence/absence of chest pain or dyspnea. Referrals to physical therapists or cardiac rehabilitation programs for assistance with activity is documented. Be specific in the record about the type of activity the patient is able to perform, the duration of the activity, and in the case of walking, the distance walked. Document any questions or concerns of the patient, and the need for further teaching.

NURSING DIAGNOSIS 3

 ANXIETY

Related to:
Chest pain
Threat to self-image
Fear of dying
Deficient knowledge

Defining Characteristics:
Restlessness
Denial
Anger

Diaphoresis

Tachycardia

Verbalization of anxiety

Goal:

Anxiety is relieved

Outcome Criteria

✔ The patient verbalizes that anxiety has been reduced.

✔ The patient states that he or she is relaxed.

✔ The patient has no physiological signs of anxiety such as nervousness, hyperventilation, or increased pulse.

✔ The patient asks questions about angina.

NOC *Anxiety level*

Anxiety self-control

Acceptance: Health status

INTERVENTIONS	RATIONALES
Have patient rate anxiety on a numerical scale.	Allows for a more objective measure of anxiety level.
Provide oxygen, as ordered.	Supplemental oxygen improves oxygenation reserves and during physical activity decreases the likelihood of shortness of breath and chest pain that should decrease anxiety. In addition, anxiety increases the demand for oxygen.
Control pain, as appropriate and as ordered.	Reduction of pain will help to reduce anxiety level.
Reassure patient by explaining the process of angina and treatment modalities.	Fear of the unknown contributes to higher levels of anxiety; knowing what to expect helps the patient maintain control of environment; an educated patient/family can be more proactive in helping the patient prevent/control pain and anxiety.
Encourage patient to verbalize concerns about health status.	Verbalizing concerns can help patient deal with issues and avoid negative feelings.
Stay with patient during episodes of pain and use a calm manner.	Makes the nurse available to offer comfort, care, and assurances to reduce anxiety and fear.
Teach patient relaxation techniques (such as slow, purposeful breathing) and encourage their use.	Reduces anxiety and creates a feeling of comfort.

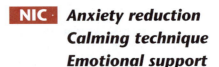

NIC *Anxiety reduction*

Calming technique

Emotional support

Evaluation

The patient should verbalize that anxiety is reduced and that he or she feels comfortable. Assess the patient for physiological signs of anxiety such as increased pulse and sweating. During evaluation be sure to inquire about the use of relaxation techniques. The patient is able to verbalize that he or she understands angina.

Community/Home Care

The patient will need to know how to control anxiety in the home setting. It is crucial that health care providers provide the patient knowledge to make the patient feel in control of his or her health. A patient who knows how to treat the pain of angina and modify his or her lifestyle accordingly will have fewer incidences of anxiety and fear. Prior to exiting the health care system, the nurse should help the patient explore ways to reduce anxiety at home. Suggestions may include reading a good book, listening to soothing music, meditating, using guided imagery, or watching a favorite television program. A short walk in the yard, if the patient is able, or engaging in computer games may also work. If the patient has practiced an organized religion, reading religious books or talking to a religious leader may also help reduce anxiety and calm any fears. By ensuring that the patient understands the health care regimen and knows what to do if acute symptoms develop, the health care provider may prevent unnecessary emergency room visits.

Documentation

Document the degree of anxiety experienced by the patient. Using some type of numerical rating scale similar to the pain scale will give health care providers a more objective measure of the degree of anxiety the patient is experiencing. Document any physiological or observable signs of anxiety such as restlessness, tachycardia, or diaphoresis. Interventions implemented to treat these should be documented along with subsequent assessments to determine their effectiveness.

NURSING DIAGNOSIS 4

 ## DEFICIENT KNOWLEDGE

Related to:

>   Insufficient knowledge of angina and medication regimen
>
>   Need for lifestyle changes

Defining Characteristics:

>   Asks questions/has concerns
>
>   Repeated episodes of angina
>
>   Repeated visits to emergency room for chest pain

Goal:

>   The patient verbalizes an understanding of treatments and changes in lifestyle required.

Outcome Criteria

✔ The patient verbalizes a desire to learn necessary information.

✔ The patient verbalizes a willingness to keep appointments and follow prescribed regimen.

✔ The patient demonstrates knowledge of disease.

✔ The patient demonstrates knowledge of medications and changes in lifestyle such as diet, activity restrictions, and stress reduction required to promote health.

NOC   *Knowledge: Disease process*
Knowledge: Treatment regimen
Compliance behavior

INTERVENTIONS	RATIONALES
Assess patient's current knowledge as well as his or her ability to learn and readiness to learn.	Teachings need to be tailored to the patient's ability and willingness to learn for maximum effectiveness.
Teach patient and family/ significant others about: — Cardiac disease: pathophysiology, symptoms — Cardiac risk factors: smoking, high fat and high sodium diet, sedentary lifestyle, stress — Medications: nitroglycerin, beta blockers, aspirin, calcium channel blockers as ordered (rationale for use, side effects, dosage, frequency) — One should not chew or swallow nitroglycerin; if angina unrelieved after 3 tablets (or in accordance with physician recommendations) activate the EMS through 911 — Diet: low sodium, low fat, low cholesterol as ordered — Relaxation techniques — Activity regimen and restrictions with attention to prevention of chest pain — Methods for smoking cessation if patient smokes — Weight reduction strategies if overweight — Control of hypertension (medications, exercise, weight loss, stress reduction) — When to seek emergency health care attention	Knowledge of disease, prevention, and treatment may improve compliance and awareness of the patient's ability to control disease.
Be attuned to the patient's religious and cultural practices when teaching.	Culturally competent care that also considers religious practices is a holistic individualized approach that will enhance compliance.
Give printed material of information covered in teaching session to patient and family.	Patient and family may be more comfortable at home knowing that there is printed material for future reference.
Ask patient to repeat information and ask questions as needed.	This allows the nurse to hear in the patient's own words what was taught, and reveals what information may need to be reinforced.
Establish that the patient has the resources required to be compliant.	If needed resources such as finances, transportation, and psychosocial support are not available, the patient cannot be compliant.

NIC *Learning readiness enhancement*
Learning facilitation
Teaching: Prescribed medication
Teaching: Prescribed activity/exercise
Teaching: Disease process
Teaching: Prescribed diet
Exercise promotion

Evaluation

Evaluate the degree to which the patient has achieved the expected outcomes. The patient verbalizes an understanding of the medical regimen, including change in lifestyle behaviors that are modifiable risk factors for heart disease. The nurse must determine that the patient is capable of being compliant and should also ascertain whether the patient expresses a willingness to comply. Once this is established, it is crucial to determine that the patient has the necessary information to manage angina effectively including episodes of chest pain, stress reduction, and administration of medications.

Community/Home Care

Once at home, the patient may be anxious or unsure about the medical regimen. Successful management will depend on the patient's understanding of the information provided in teaching sessions and the internal motivation to implement health-promoting behaviors. Changes in lifestyle may be difficult at first, and reinforcement through follow-up home visits or telephone consultation may be required. The patient will need to establish a routine that includes activity and rest, medication scheduling, and meals. Special diets that are heart-healthy generally require more thought, planning, and preparation, so the person who prepares meals will need to plan for this additional time. The patient is more likely to adhere to the diet if all members of the household eat the same food. Family members can make a concerted effort to focus on the entire family's health by incorporating everyone into the lifestyle changes the patient needs to make. Exercising can be a routine part of family/significant other time together. The patient needs clear-cut instructions for progression of activity such as guidelines for a home walking program. Frequently, the patient has questions regarding resumption of sexual activities but feels uncomfortable initiating the topic, so the nurse or other health care provider who follows the patient should breach the subject. Be sure that the patient understands how to store nitroglycerin (keep away from light or heat in closed dark container) and the protocol for its use. Remind the patient to keep the nitroglycerin with him or her when traveling and not in suitcases, so that it is available for immediate use. In addition, if the patient is a smoker, information on smoking cessation strategies should be provided to the patient and the use of at least one strategy implemented. Cardiac support groups may provide social support and allay anxiety, but may not be available in rural areas. At follow-up appointments, the health care provider can ascertain if additional teaching is required.

Documentation

Document the specific content taught and the titles of printed materials given to the patient or family. Chart the patient's understanding of the content and the methods used to evaluate learning. The nurse must clearly indicate areas that need to be reinforced. After the teaching session is complete, the nurse should determine if the patient indicates a willingness to comply with health care recommendations. If the teaching included a significant other, indicate this in the documentation. In addition, if referrals are made, these should be documented in the patient record.

CHAPTER 1.3

AORTIC VALVE STENOSIS/REGURGITATION

GENERAL INFORMATION

In aortic valve stenosis, the leaflets of the valve become thick, calcified, rigid, and scarred. Because the aortic valve is proximal to the electrical conduction system of the heart, the conduction system may also become calcified, scarred, and dysfunctional. Causes of aortic valve stenosis and/or regurgitation are rheumatic fever, congenital defects, connective tissue disorders (such as Marfan syndrome), and bacterial or viral endocarditis. Aortic stenosis can also occur as a result of a congenital bicuspid (rather than tricuspid) valve. When aortic stenosis occurs and the valve opening progressively becomes smaller, blood is "trapped" in the left ventricle, and pressure increases within the left ventricle as it tries to produce an adequate stroke volume by ejecting its volume through a narrowed valve into the aorta. When this occurs, pressure cannot equalize between the aorta and the left ventricle during systole. The ventricular wall muscle will hypertrophy and become thickened as it works to try to overcome the pressure gradient. The muscle will eventually reach its maximum thickness and cardiac output will become fixed at a certain amount. Left atrial pressures also increase, affecting the pulmonary circulation. When demand for increased cardiac output occurs (i.e., during increased activity periods), the heart can no longer accommodate the demand and coronary artery perfusion and cerebral perfusion will not be adequate. The patient will develop myocardial ischemia and syncope.

Aortic stenosis may be asymptomatic for years, but with disease progression clinical manifestations of left heart failure (lung crackles, shortness of breath, and orthopnea) become evident. Classic manifestations include dyspnea on exertion, exertional syncope, and angina pectoris (Lemone and Burke, 2004). Later in the disease, the patient also demonstrates signs of right-sided failure (peripheral edema, jugular vein distention). Aortic stenosis is more common in men than in women and symptoms of heart failure usually occur between the ages of 50 and 70.

In aortic regurgitation, the valve is unable to close properly, which allows blood to leak back into the left ventricle during diastole, causing a volume overload to occur. This also causes the muscle of the left ventricle to thicken as it works harder to produce an adequate stroke volume. Over time, this reaches a point of maximum muscle thickening and hypertrophy, leading to cardiac failure. In addition, because of the failure of the aortic valve to close, blood flow to the coronary arteries (which usually occurs in diastole) decreases and results in myocardial ischemia. It is more common in men; when it exists in women, it is correlated with coexisting mitral valve disease. Most cases of aortic regurgitation result from rheumatic heart disease. The patient complains of persistent palpitations, dizziness, dyspnea, angina, and fatigue. Characteristic/classic findings include a head bob with each heart beat (Musset's sign), a murmur heard during diastole at the third left intercostal space, and a widened pulse pressure. The point of maximal impulse is often displaced to the left.

NURSING DIAGNOSIS 1

 ### DECREASED CARDIAC OUTPUT

Related to:

Stenosis of valves impairing ventricular filling affecting cardiac output (preload and afterload)

Regurgitation of blood into the atria during systole

Decreased pump effectiveness of left ventricle

Defining Characteristics:

Tachycardia

Syncope

Anginal pain

Decreased SaO_2

Pulmonary edema

Lung crackles

Peripheral edema

Jugular vein distention

Shortness of breath

Murmurs

Narrowing pulse pressure (stenosis)

Widening pulse pressure (regurgitation)

Goal:

Adequate cardiac output is achieved.

Outcome Criteria

✔ The patient achieves adequate cardiac output as evidenced by urine output of 30 ml/hour or greater; breath sounds are clear; edema is absent or decreased; pulse rate is < 100.

✔ The patient reports no angina pain.

✔ The patient reports decreased shortness of breath, and a return of pulse to baseline 10 minutes after cessation of activity.

✔ The patient reports no syncope and has no injuries secondary to syncope.

NOC *Cardiac pump effectiveness*
Cardiac disease: Self-management
Medication response

INTERVENTIONS	RATIONALES
Assess cardiac status: blood pressure (note decreases or changes in pulse pressure), pulse (tachycardia), respirations (increased rate), heart sounds (noting presence of S_3, S_4, murmurs, palpitations), presence of dysrhythmias on cardiac monitor (atrial fibrillation), palpable systolic thrill, peripheral pulses, skin temperature.	These are all symptoms of disease progression and indicators of the heart's inability to maintain adequate output and perfusion to vital organs.
Assess breath sounds for crackles along with rate, rhythm, and quality of respirations.	Helps to detect any early symptoms of left ventricular failure.
Assess urine output for quantity.	As the disease progresses and cardiac output decreases, perfusion to kidneys may decrease and be manifested as decreased output.
Monitor for change in mental status, noting confusion, restlessness, or agitation.	These indicate decreased cerebral tissue perfusion.
Monitor results of diagnostic and laboratory tests: — EKG: for ST depression and T wave inversion indicative of ischemia — Echocardiography: for defects in valve leaflet and thickening of ventricle wall — Chest x-ray: for ventricular hypertrophy and pulmonary congestion as well as aortic calcification — Cardiac catherization: for definite diagnosis and severity of the disease — Cardiac enzymes: for indication of damage to the myocardial tissue — Electrolytes, bun, serum creatinine: for increases that are indicative of renal dysfunction	Results of these tests provide definitive diagnosis as well as clues to status of disease, damage to the myocardium, renal function, and response to treatments.
Monitor oxygen saturation and arterial blood gases.	Provides information regarding the heart's ability to perfuse distal tissues with oxygenated blood.
Give supplemental oxygen if signs of left ventricular failure are present.	Makes oxygen available for gas exchange.
Encourage physical and mental rest.	Resting decreases myocardial oxygen demand, reducing the workload of the heart.
Administer diuretics as ordered for the patient with signs of heart failure.	Reduces vascular sodium and reduces vascular fluid load.
Administer digitalis preparations as ordered for the patient with signs of heart failure.	Digitalis has a positive inotrophic effect on the myocardium, which strengthens contractility, thus improving cardiac output.
Administer angiotensin converting enzyme inhibitors as ordered.	Reduces peripheral arterial resistance (afterload) and pulmonary vascular resistance, and improves cardiac output.

INTERVENTIONS	RATIONALES
Assist with activities, particularly ambulation.	Patients with aortic stenosis and regurgitation often have syncope and dizziness, which predisposes them to falls.
Give anticoagulants as ordered if the patient is experiencing atrial fibrillation.	Atrial fibrillation often produces emboli, and prophylactic treatment is required to prevent emboli from reaching other organs.
Restrict sodium in diet.	Decreases fluid retention and the workload of the heart.
Collaborate with surgeons to prepare the patient for surgery (balloon valvuloplasty or prosthetic valve replacement) and implement pre-operative teaching for surgical intervention.	For aortic valve stenosis, the treatment of choice is aortic valve replacement (surgically separate thickened valve leaflets or the fused commissures) or valvuloplasty (to dilate stenosed valve without surgical risk); for aortic regurgitation surgery is required if the patient is symptomatic; pre-operative teaching reduces anxiety and enhances post-operative recovery.
Teach the patient about disease process, required activity restrictions, medical regimens, and surgical options.	Informing the patient about disease process and possible treatments increases the likelihood of compliance with prescribed regimen.

NIC *Oxygen therapy*
Cardiac care: Acute
Hemodynamic regulation
Vital signs monitoring
Circulatory care

Evaluation

Determine if the patient's cardiac output has improved. Evidence for a positive outcome include clear breath sounds, absence of edema, urine output of a least 30 ml/hour, and pulse and blood pressure returned to patient's baseline. In addition, the patient should have no chest pain and be able to tolerate activities without extreme fatigue. Evaluate for the presence of syncope and ascertain whether the patient has had any injuries as a result.

Community/Home Care

Patients with asymptomatic aortic stenosis and regurgitation are monitored closely for disease progression, making compliance with follow-up appointments extremely important. For patients with aortic stenosis and symptomatic aortic regurgitation, surgery is the treatment of choice, but the patient may have a period of time at home prior to surgical intervention. For all patients, there is a need to implement strategies at home to prevent fatigue. This includes understanding how to balance activity and rest in order to conserve energy. A gradual increase in activities is required so as not to overtax the cardiac system. The patient needs to be able to monitor self for signs of heart failure, including weight gain, difficulty breathing, and edema. It is crucial that the patient learns how to check his or her pulse and note irregularities. The patient, home health nurse, or other health care provider should monitor blood pressure regularly. If the patient has had surgery, attention should be given to wound care, prevention of infection at site of replacement valve or external wound, monitoring of cardiac status, and a gradual return to normal activities. Whether the patient has had valve replacement surgery or is being treated medically, the nurse should determine the availability of resources needed for positive patient outcomes.

Documentation

In the patient record, document the status of achievement of the stated outcome criteria. Findings during cardiac assessment should be included, such as the presence of any signs and symptoms of heart failure. Pulse and blood pressure should be noted, as well as peripheral pulses. Any teaching that has been done regarding the disease process, pre-operative teaching, and the patient's understanding of teaching should be documented in the patient record.

NURSING DIAGNOSIS 2

ACTIVITY INTOLERANCE

Related to:

Decreased cardiac output secondary to valvular disease

Defining Characteristics:

Tachycardia that persists > 3 minutes after activity ends

Shortness of breath

Tachypnea

Syncope

Rhythm changes with activity

Goal:

The patient will tolerate selected activities.

Outcome Criteria

✔ The patient will perform activities of daily living without shortness of breath.

✔ The patient will identify activities that cause fatigue and shortness of breath.

✔ The patient's pulse rate and respirations will return to baseline in 3 minutes or fewer following cessation of activity.

NOC *Activity tolerance*

Energy conservation

Endurance

INTERVENTIONS	RATIONALES
Ensure rest; create a rest schedule.	Decreases cardiac workload.
Assist with activities as needed.	Conserves energy and reduces myocardial oxygen demand; patient lacks enough oxygen reserves to perform activities independently.
Progress activities gradually from getting out of bed to taking short walks.	Allows the patient opportunity to develop tolerance for activity over time.
Have oxygen available for use if patient becomes short of breath.	Initial activity may produce shortness of breath; having oxygen readily available allows nurse to intervene quickly to restore respiratory status.
Pace activities and provide for rest periods before and after activity.	Reduces workload of the heart by conserving energy and decreasing oxygen demands.
Inform patient to cease any activity that causes shortness of breath, chest pain, or dizziness.	These are indicators of intolerance to activity, and the level of activity should be evaluated.
Monitor response to activity (increased pulse, increased respiratory rate and dyspnea, lightheadedness, pallor, palpitations).	Increased pulse and respirations, along with dyspnea, indicate an intolerance to the activity; in addition if lightheadedness, pallor, and palpitations occur, it may indicate cardiac decompensation.
Rearrange the room so that there is minimal movement required to gain access to the toilet, phone, chair, and other needed items.	Helps to provide easy access with a minimum of effort and to decrease fatigue/exhaustion.
Collaborate with other disciplines, such as physical and respiratory therapy, as ordered to assist with activities.	Respiratory therapy may need to provide oxygen when the patient first starts activity, and physical therapy can assist with monitoring activity.
Teach the patient and family needed information about diet, energy conservation, and prescribed activity limitations, as well as reportable signs and symptoms indicative of cardiac decompensation.	Education will assist the patient to be compliant with therapeutic regimen.

NIC *Activity therapy*

Energy management

Evaluation

Examine the degree to which the patient has achieved the outcome criteria as stated. The patient should be able to walk short distances to the bathroom without experiencing shortness of breath or tachycardia, and if present should return to baseline within 3 minutes. The patient should verbalize his or her understanding of activity limitations and be able to identify those activities that cause symptoms. With time and gradual increase in activity, the patient should report better tolerance.

Community/Home Care

The home environment should be discussed with the patient to identify layout of the home (stairs, distance to bathroom and kitchen) and furniture placement to determine what changes may be necessary in order for the patient to maneuver with the least amount of energy expenditure. The patient should be taught how to progress activities at home as well as how to prioritize which activities should be done and which may require higher energy. An occupational therapist may be helpful in this endeavor by also presenting information on work/task simplification. The dietitian could be useful in assisting the patient and family in selecting foods that provide sources of energy. The patient can start an activity journal to record all activities along with the response, including length of time of the activity.

Documentation

Document the patient's specific activity goals and progress towards the established outcome criteria. Include in the patient record specific patient behaviors in terms of response to activity. Always document the specific activities that the patient has attempted. If other disciplines are involved in the patient's care, document their visits in the chart.

NURSING DIAGNOSIS 3

 ANXIETY

Related to:

    Fear of disease, surgery, unknown outcome

Defining Characteristics:

    Restlessness

    Anxiety

    Decreased attention span

    Expressed fear

    Numerous questions

Goal:

    Anxiety is decreased or relieved.

Outcome Criteria

✔ The patient verbalizes that anxiety has been relieved.

✔ The patient has no physiological symptoms of anxiety.

✔ The patient appears relaxed.

NOC *Anxiety self-control*
Acceptance: Health status
Coping enhancement

INTERVENTIONS	RATIONALES
Assess for verbal and nonverbal signs of anxiety and fear.	Helps to detect the presence of anxiety and allows for early intervention to prevent physiological alterations.
Monitor the intensity of anxiety/ fear by having the patient rate on a numerical scale.	Allows for a more objective measure of anxiety and fear levels.
Encourage the patient to verbalize fears and anxiety regarding diagnosis, needed interventions, and health status.	Recognition of fear and anxiety is the first step to coping with issues and to avoidance of negative feelings.
Teach the patient relaxation techniques (such as slow, purposeful breathing) and encourage their use.	Reduces anxiety and creates a feeling of comfort.
Reassure the patient by explaining disease process, all procedures, treatment options, and required lifestyle changes.	Fear of the unknown contributes to anxiety; knowing what to expect helps the patient maintain a sense of control.
Stay with patient during acute episodes of shortness of breath or pain, or if fear and anxiety are evident.	Offers comfort, care, and assurances to reduce anxiety and fear.
Administer anti-anxiety medications, as ordered.	Helps decrease the patient's anxiety level.

NIC *Anxiety reduction*
Calming technique
Presence

Evaluation

Assess the patient for the degree that fear/anxiety has been controlled. The patient should verbalize his or her feelings and indicate whether interventions have produced a comfortable state of anxiety and fear. Determine if the patient understands aortic stenosis and regurgitation and the impact they may have on health status. During evaluation, be sure to inquire about the use of coping strategies and relaxation techniques. Determine if patient understands disease process and prescribed treatment regimens.

Community/Home Care

The patient will need to develop coping strategies and relaxation techniques to utilize in the home setting. The nurse must adequately equip the patient with knowledge necessary to make him or her feel in control. An understanding of what to expect from physiological alterations will assist the patient to control the disease and prevent complications. In the home the patient may be able to reduce anxiety more quickly through use of common everyday activities such as a short walk, reading, meditating, listening to the radio, and spending time with emotionally supportive family and friends. For the patient who is awaiting surgery, it is important to control anxiety before time of surgery through pre-operative teaching regarding post-operative expectations.

Documentation

Using the numerical scale, document the degree of fear or anxiety the patient is experiencing. In addition, include any verbal, nonverbal, or physiological clues that could be indicators of anxiety or fear such as restlessness, tachycardia, or diaphoresis. Interventions that the nurse implements to treat anxiety or fear should be documented along with the patient responses. Teaching regarding relaxation techniques, coping strategies, and disease process, and any preoperative teaching should be documented in the patient record.

CHAPTER 1.4

CARDIAC CATHETERIZATION

GENERAL INFORMATION

Cardiac catheterization is an invasive diagnostic procedure utilized to assess and diagnose anatomical alterations of the cardiac system. The procedure, which can be either right-sided or left-sided, is performed in a special cardiac catheterization laboratory by a cardiologist. Guided by fluoroscopy, the cardiologist threads catheters through the designated vessels to reach the heart and measures a variety of pressures that provide information regarding cardiac function in addition to function of valves. A contrast medium/dye is injected to outline the anatomical structures, circulatory patterns, and left ventricle motion. Cardiac catheterization plays a crucial role in the diagnosis and evaluation of coronary artery disease, valvular disease, angina, myocardial disease, and status of treatments such as coronary artery bypass graft and angioplasty.

NURSING DIAGNOSIS 1

 DEFICIENT KNOWLEDGE

Related to:

New diagnostic test

Defining Characteristics:

Has not had test performed before

Asks questions

Asks no questions

Verbalizes lack of knowledge

Goal:

Patient will understand cardiac catheterization.

Outcome Criteria

✔ The patient will verbalize an understanding of the planned procedure.

✔ The patient will verbalize an understanding of complications of the procedure.

✔ The patient will verbalize an understanding of the required interventions post-procedure.

NOC *Knowledge: Treatment procedures*

INTERVENTIONS	RATIONALES
Assess patient's current knowledge regarding cardiac disease and cardiac catheterization, as well as his or her ability and readiness to learn.	Any instruction should build on what the patient already knows; teachings need to be tailored to the patient's ability and willingness to learn for maximum effectiveness.
Instruct patient/family about the cardiac catheterization procedure: — Purpose of the procedure — How the procedure is performed — What to expect during the procedure (will be awake; will experience warm flushing feeling and metallic taste in mouth caused by dye, nausea, pressure in chest, abnormal heartbeats; may be asked to cough or change position) — Possible complications of the procedure (bleeding at catheter insertion site, hematoma, infection at site, loss of peripheral pulses, cool extremities) — Pre-operative care requirements (voiding before procedure, liquid breakfast or nothing by mouth as ordered, cardiac drugs not taken, intravenous lines, premedications that may make the patient drowsy)	Knowledge of procedure improves patient compliance with requirements during and after procedure.

(continues)

(continued)

INTERVENTIONS	RATIONALES
— Post-operative care requirements (pressure to catheter insertion site, monitoring of vital signs and of affected extremity frequently by agency protocol, increased fluid intake, frequent diuresis, activity limitations)	
Teach incrementally: simple to complex.	The patient will learn and retain knowledge better when information is presented in small segments starting with simple concepts.
Ask the patient and family to repeat the information regarding the procedure and ask questions.	This allows the nurse to hear in the patient's own words what he or she understood.
Offer printed materials about cardiac catheterization (preferably with pictures) and other audiovisual aides such as videotapes.	Printed and audiovisual aides enhance learning.
Check patient record for consent and allergies, particularly to iodine.	Consents must be signed prior to pre-medication and allergies to iodine should be treated before the procedure with Benadryl to avert an allergic reaction during procedure.

NIC   *Learning readiness enhancement*
        Learning facilitation
        Teaching: Procedure/treatment
        Preparatory sensory information

Evaluation

Evaluate the degree to which the patient has achieved the expected outcomes. The patient and family verbalize an understanding of all aspects of cardiac catheterization, and state that their questions have been answered. Prior to discharge, the nurse should determine whether the patient has understood the discharge instructions regarding care of the site and activity limitations.

Community/Home Care

The patient who has had a cardiac catheterization will generally go home the same day or within 24 hours. Teaching should be done thoroughly at some point during the pre-procedure phase and again post-procedure. Upon discharge home, the patient will need to continue to monitor the extremity for any signs of a thromboembolic event (cool, absent pulses and pain). Be sure that the patient understands activity limitations, diet requirements, and follow-up required. This is particularly crucial if significant cardiac disease has been validated.

Documentation

Document the specific content taught and the titles of any printed materials given to the family or patient. After the teaching session, document the degree to which the patient and/or family verbalizes understanding of the cardiac catheterization procedure. If the patient continues to have questions before the procedure, this should be documented in the chart. Use agency pre-procedure checklists for teaching as indicated.

NURSING DIAGNOSIS 2

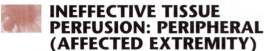

INEFFECTIVE TISSUE PERFUSION: PERIPHERAL (AFFECTED EXTREMITY)

Related to:

Utilization of extremity for invasive procedure (cardiac catheterization)

Defining Characteristics:

Diminished or absent pulses

Skin color changes (pallor)

Skin temperature changes (cool)

Goal:

Tissue perfusion is adequate.

Outcome Criteria

✔ The patient's extremity will remain warm.

✔ Pulses in affected extremity will remain strong at 4+ or at patient's baseline.

✔ The affected extremity will have normal color.

✔ Vital signs are within patient's baseline.

NOC   *Tissue perfusion: Peripheral*
        Circulation status
        Vital signs

INTERVENTIONS	RATIONALES
Establish a baseline assessment of the extremity to be used for the procedure to include temperature, color, presence, and quality of pulses. If pulses are difficult to find, use a Doppler and mark locations with black marker.	This allows the nurse to have data for comparison during post-procedure, pulses that are difficult to find pre-procedure may be even more difficult to palpate after the cardiac catheterization.
Following the procedure, assess pulses, color, sensation, and temperature of the extremity every 15 minutes × 4, every 30 minutes × 2, and every hour × 2 or according to agency protocol.	Pallor, decreased or absent pulse, decreased sensation, and coolness in the extremity indicate ineffective perfusion.
Assess dressing covering puncture site for active bleeding (if noted notify physician, reinforce dressing, and apply pressure with sandbag). Palpate around puncture site for formation of hematoma (if present, notify physican and implement strategies as directed by physician).	Bleeding may occur following the procedure due to invasion into high flow vessel (artery) as well as hematoma formation. Early detection allows for prevention of complications such as arterial occlusion due to hematoma and decreased vascular volume due to bleeding.
Encourage intake of fluid.	Helps kidneys to rid body of dye.
Keep patient on bedrest, maintaining head of bed no higher than 30 degrees with extremity straight and pressure dressing intact as ordered by physician.	Helps to prevent bleeding and hematoma formation; elevating the HOB higher will put pressure on site.
Implement discharge teaching to include: — Activity restrictions: no driving or climbing stairs for 24 hours (or as directed by physician), no strenuous activity for 3 days — Wound care: do not take tub baths until wound is healed or as directed by physician; monitor site for swelling, bruising, or increased pain; may remove or change dressing and shower after 24 hours or as directed by physician — Comfort: take mild analgesics as directed — Follow-up: return to physician as directed or when any untoward symptoms are noted	Discharge teaching assists the patient to be compliant with recommended therapeutic regimen and prevent complications.

NIC *Bleeding precautions*
Discharge planning
Peripheral sensation management
Vital signs monitoring
Circulatory precautions
Bleeding reduction: Wound

Evaluation

The nurse should evaluate whether the patient has met the outcome criteria. The extremity should remain warm to touch and with peripheral pulses within the patient's baseline. Assess the extremity for skin color and sensation and note any pain at site. There should be no bleeding from the puncture site and no hematoma, even though minimal bruising may be present. Vital signs should return to the patient's baseline.

Community/Home Care

The patient undergoing cardiac catheterization has a very short hospital stay, usually fewer than 24 hours, but the risk for complications remains for several days. The patient and family will need to know signs and symptoms that may indicate complications such as pain in extremity, change in sensation, and coolness of extremity. In addition, if the dressing has not been removed prior to discharge, the patient should remove dressing 24 hours after the procedure and inspect the site for swelling and bruising. At home the patient should restrict strenuous activities such as heavy lifting and heavy housework for several days or as directed by the physician. The patient should not climb stairs or drive for at least 24 hours. The nurse should stress to the patient the importance of returning for any follow-up care. If the patient has validated cardiac disease the nurse or physician will need to institute teaching to address the specific condition. In many instances, the cardiac catherization identifies previously undiagnosed disease that will require surgery, as well as serving as a definitive diagnostic tool prior to scheduled open heart surgery. In both instances, extensive preoperative teaching should be undertaken. If major blockages are discovered, the patient may not be allowed to go home until surgical repair has been achieved.

Documentation

Prior to cardiac catheterization, findings from a thorough assessment of the extremity to be used should be charted. Document vital signs and status of extremity, including pulses, temperature, sensation, and status of dressing. Assess the catheterization site for bleeding or hematoma and document findings in the chart. The amount of urine output from the first voiding following the procedure should also be documented. In the patient's record document teaching that has been implemented and the patient's verbalization of understanding. If the patient voices any complaints, document these along with interventions implemented and the patient's response.

CHAPTER 1.5

CARDIOMYOPATHY

GENERAL INFORMATION

Cardiomyopathy is a disease of the myocardial muscle of the heart. There are three categories of cardiomyopathy: hypertrophic cardiomyopathy, dilated cardiomyopathy, and restrictive cardiomyopathy. The most common form of cardiomyopathy is dilated or congestive cardiomyopathy, which accounts for 87 percent of all cases (AHA, 2004). In this condition, the entire myocardium is dilated, but left ventricular dilation is prominent with resulting ineffective systole. Because the myocardium becomes inelastic, resistance is increased and subsequently causes elevated filling pressures. Both end diastolic and end systolic volumes increase, and the left ventricular ejection fraction is substantially reduced, decreasing cardiac output (Lemone and Burke, 2004). The cause of dilated cardiomyopathy is unknown, but it has been linked to alcohol and cocaine abuse, chemotherapeutic drugs, pregnancy, and systemic hypertension, and in some cases a genetic predisposition exists. Clinical manifestations of the disease include those of heart failure and include shortness of breath, weakness, fatigue, peripheral edema, abnormal heart sounds, and dysrhythmias. Hypertrophic cardiomyopathy involves the thickening of the interventricular septum (as compared to the free wall of the left ventricle). This thickening makes the ventricular walls inelastic (noncompliant), which causes increased resistance as blood enters the left ventricle from the left atrium, contributing to greatly reduced end diastolic volumes and a decrease in cardiac output. In addition, this condition is often marked by the obstruction of outflow from the left ventricle. Hypertrophic cardiomyopathy is genetically transmitted and may be asymptomatic for years. It is estimated that 36 percent of all deaths in young athletes who die suddenly are due to hypertrophic cardiomyopathy (Lemone and Burke, 2004). Clinical manifestations of hypertrophic cardiomyopathy include dyspnea, angina, syncope, fatigue, dysrhythmias, and a characteristic crescendo-descendo systolic murmur heard at the lower left sternal border (Lemone and Burke, 2004). In restrictive cardiomyopathy, the rarest form of the disease, the ventricular walls are normal in size but are very rigid, causing the heart to have an abnormal diastolic (filling) function. Causes of restrictive cardiomyopathy include myocardial fibrosis, amyloidosis, or other infiltrative diseases. Clinical manifestations of restrictive cardiomyopathy mimic those of a patient with heart failure-dyspnea on exertion, fatigue, and abnormal heart sounds (S_3 and S_4) are most common.

NURSING DIAGNOSIS 1

DECREASED CARDIAC OUTPUT

Related to:

Ventricular dilation

Poor ventricular contractility with decreased pump effectiveness

Decreased ventricular filling

Inelastic myocardium/intraventricular septum

Defining Characteristics:

Fatigue

Edema

Dyspnea

Tachycardia

Dysrhythmias

Abnormal heart sounds

Goal:

The patient exhibits improved cardiac output, and signs and symptoms of cardiomyopathy are alleviated.

Outcome Criteria

✔ Pulse rate is < 100 but > 60; blood pressure is at patient's baseline and no dysrhythmias are noted.

✔ The patient will have clear breath sounds, no shortness of breath, and no peripheral edema.

✔ Urine output will be > 30 ml/hour.

NOC *Cardiac pump effectiveness*
Circulation status
Respiratory status: Gas exchange
Tissue perfusion: Cerebral
Tissue perfusion: Peripheral
Vital signs
Medication response

INTERVENTIONS	RATIONALES
Monitor for tachycardia, dysrhythmias, abnormal heart sounds (murmur, S_3, S_4), and blood pressure.	Assessment of cardiac status gives early clues to disease and response to interventions and establishes baseline.
Assess for signs of heart failure (cyanosis; jugular venous distention; dependent edema; cool, pale extremities; diminished peripheral pulses; capillary refill > 2 seconds; dyspnea on exertion).	To detect severity of disease and progression, as the ventricles lose ability to pump pulmonary congestion and peripheral blood flow becomes worse.
Monitor for changes in mental status (confusion, restlessness, agitation).	These changes indicate decreased cerebral tissue perfusion.
Monitor arterial blood gases and oxygen saturation level.	These are measures of the ability of the heart to perfuse tissues with oxygenated blood.
Monitor results of any ordered diagnostic tests such as EKG, echocardiogram, and chest x-ray.	These tests reveal definitive diagnosis and aid in monitoring response to interventions (EKG will show any dysrhythmias or cardiac enlargement; echocardiogram will show chamber size and thickness as well as systolic and diastolic function; chest x-ray will show heart enlargement and any pulmonary congestion).
Monitor urine output.	Decreased urine output < 30 ml/hour may indicate decreased tissue perfusion to the kidneys.
Administer supplemental oxygen, as ordered based on results of ABGs and oxygen saturation.	Helps to maximize amount of oxygen available for gas exchange, alleviate signs of hypoxia, and to decrease the workload of the myocardium.
Administer vasodilator, as ordered for dilated or restrictive cardiomyopathy.	Helps to improve myocardial blood flow by dilating arteries.
Administer inotropic agents/cardiac glycosides (digoxin), as ordered for dilated or restrictive cardiomyopathy.	Inotropic agents increase the force of myocardial cardiac contractility and, therefore, increase cardiac output.
Administer beta blockers as ordered for hypertrophic cardiomyopathy.	Reduces risk of anginal episodes.
Administer diuretics, as ordered for restrictive or dilated cardiomyopathy.	Reduces vascular fluid load through prevention of the reabsorption of sodium and chloride, enhancing urinary fluid excretion, which reduces pulmonary congestion and peripheral edema.
Encourage patient to rest; provide assistance with activities and monitor for fatigue.	Patients with cardiomyopathy are often fatigued easily, and rest and assistance will reduce myocardial oxygen demand and myocardial workload.
Monitor serum electrolytes, BUN, digoxin levels, and liver enzymes as ordered.	These tests may be abnormal as a result of the disease process or as an effect of medication regimens.

NIC *Cardiac care: Acute*
Oxygen therapy
Vital signs monitoring
Energy management
Medication management

Evaluation

The patient has no signs of decreased cardiac output. Breath sounds are clear, the patient experiences minimal shortness of breath at rest, and edema is absent. Urinary output has been maintained at or above 30 ml/hour. The patient's pulse and blood pressure have returned to baseline/normal. In addition, the patient reports decreased or absence of fatigue.

Community/Home Care

The patient with cardiomyopathy will need to be educated thoroughly about the prescribed regimen. Adaptations will need to be made to accommodate changes in health status that may impact their work, social activities, and self-care ability. Because of the fatigue that patients with cardiomyopathy experience, strategies for energy conservation should be discussed with the patient. The patient will need to understand all aspects of their medication regimen, including side effects especially with diuretics, beta blockers, and digoxin. The loss of fluid from diuretics and the side effect of fatigue from beta blockers could compound the feeling of tiredness that is a part of cardiomyopathy. The in-home nurse or other health care provider needs to question the patient regarding the ability to remain functional. Psychomotor skills required for management of the regimen include knowing how to monitor pulse and weight. The nurse will have an integral part in the patient's achievement of positive outcomes through teaching and in home follow-up (see diagnoses "Deficient Knowledge" and "Activity Intolerance").

Documentation

Chart the status of achievement of outcomes with specific patient behaviors. Include pulse, blood pressure, oxygen saturation, heart sounds, and breath sounds. Document all indicators of cardiac output and tissue perfusion. Include in the chart the patient's understanding of the disease process, interventions employed, and the patient's response to the interventions. The patient's response to activity should be included in the chart.

NURSING DIAGNOSIS 2

EXCESS FLUID VOLUME

Related to:

Decreased ability of heart for effective contractility

Decreased cardiac output affecting renal perfusion

Defining Characteristics:

Crackles in lung

Jugular vein distention

Increased weight

Increased peripheral edema

Pulmonary congestion due to excess fluid accumulation

Increased respirations

Increased blood pressure

Goal:

Fluid volume excess is decreased.

Outcome Criteria

✔ The patient will demonstrate weight loss.

✔ The patient's lung sounds will be clear.

✔ Edema will be absent or decreased.

NOC *Fluid balance*
Electrolyte and acid/base balance

INTERVENTIONS	RATIONALES
Assess location and extent of edema.	Helps to assess severity of the fluid excess and guides treatment.
Assess breath sounds for crackles.	Crackles are an indicator of fluid in the lungs and should be monitored for worsening or improvement as an indicator of disease status and response to interventions.
Place patient in high Fowler's position.	Minimizes cardiac workload and decreases fluid return to the heart.
Administer oxygen as ordered.	Improves oxygenation and peripheral perfusion.
Administer diuretics, such as Lasix®, as ordered.	Inhibits the reabsorption of sodium and chloride, thereby causing an increased fluid output by the kidneys.
Weigh patient daily at the same time on the same scale, in the morning before breakfast.	The most accurate method of determining fluid volume loss is through daily weighing; 1 kilogram of weight loss = 1 liter of fluid lost. Morning weights are a better reflection of true weights because most people accumulate fluid as the day progresses.

(continues)

(continued)

INTERVENTIONS	RATIONALES
Implement a diet low in sodium.	Sodium increases fluid retention; thus, decreasing the amount of dietary sodium intake will decrease the amount of retained fluid.
Implement fluid restrictions as ordered if respiratory symptoms are pronounced.	Restricting the fluid intake can assist in decreasing circulating volume, thereby decreasing cardiac workload.
Obtain accurate intake and output.	Helps to monitor balance between fluid consumed and urinary output; output also gives an indicator of renal perfusion.
Monitor electrolytes (especially potassium).	Diuretics cause an abnormal excretion of electrolytes.
Provide potassium supplements as ordered.	Replaces urinary potassium loss caused by diuretics.
Protect edematous skin in extremities and sacrum.	Fluid in tissue inhibits adequate circulation to the tissue predisposing the patient to skin breakdown.
Monitor blood pressure and pulse.	Blood pressure and pulse may be elevated during the initial phase of fluid volume excess in the patient with cardiomyopathy, but after therapy is implemented, the patient may become hypotensive secondary to diuretic therapy.

NIC *Fluid management*
Electrolyte monitoring

Evaluation

The patient has weight loss and output > intake. Edema is absent or decreasing, with no pitting edema. Blood pressure returns to baseline and breath sounds are clear. Abnormal laboratory results return to normal levels. The patient reports the absence of shortness of breath.

Community/Home Care

Ensure that the patient at home understands the importance of monitoring fluid status. Weighing daily at home will allow the patient to notice subtle changes in fluid retention. Patients should be

instructed to take note of clothing that becomes too tight in a short period of time, which is an indicator of fluid retention. At home, the patient needs to limit the intake of salt and sodium-rich foods. Teach the patient how to read food labels for sodium content. Diet instructions for home should consider the patient's normal diet and any cultural or religious preferences and restrictions. Have the patient keep a log of food and fluid intake, as well as weights. Assist the client to develop a schedule for taking prescribed diuretics that is mindful of his or her lifestyle and daily routines, specifically avoiding late evening administrations that would interrupt sleep patterns. Adequate sleep is required for the patient with cardiomyopathy, who almost always experience fatigue, in order to restore the body for increased physiological demands of daily activities. Stress the need for follow-up care.

Documentation

Always document the extent to which the outcome criteria have been achieved. Chart the presence of edema and an assessment of affected skin over edematous areas. Record the patient's response to all therapies, including intake and output, blood pressure, pulse, respiratory rate, weights, breath sounds, and the patient's understanding of the therapies for eliminating fluid excess.

NURSING DIAGNOSIS 3

ACTIVITY INTOLERANCE

Related to:

Impaired oxygen transport secondary to heart failure caused by cardiomyopathy

Low cardiac output

Decreased cardiac reserve

Defining Characteristics:

Dyspnea/Shortness of breath with exercise

Tachypnea

Increased pulse

Reports of fatigue

Goal:

The patient's activity tolerance gradually increases.

Outcome Criteria

✔ The patient will perform activities of daily living without shortness of breath.

✔ The patient will report improved ability to engage in activities such as ambulation.

NOC *Activity tolerance*
Energy conservation
Endurance

INTERVENTIONS	RATIONALES
Administer oxygen as ordered.	Improves oxygenation, decreases myocardial hypoxia, and thus allows an increased activity level.
Assist with activities as needed, and provide bedrest if extreme fatigue occurs.	Conserves energy and reduces myocardial oxygen demand; patient lacks enough oxygen reserves to perform activities independently. Bedrest reduces cardiac output demand and myocardial oxygen demand, as well as conserves needed energy.
Progress activities gradually from getting out of bed to taking short walks.	Allows the patient the opportunity to develop a tolerance for activity over time.
Pace activities and provide rest periods before and after activity.	Helps to reduce workload of the heart.
Monitor response to activity (pulse, respiratory rate, any dyspnea).	Increased pulse and respirations, along with dyspnea, indicate an intolerance to the activity.
Monitor electrolytes.	Treatment of heart failure with diuretics often causes electrolyte imbalance that can cause muscle weakness and fatigue, which may prevent a patient from participating in activity.
Inform patient to stop any activity that causes shortness of breath, chest pain, or dizziness.	These indicate intolerance to activity and the level of activity being performed should be evaluated.
Collaborate with other disciplines such as physical therapy and respiratory therapy as ordered to assist with ambulation.	Respiratory therapy may need to provide oxygen when the patient first starts an activity program, and physical therapy can assist with monitoring activity progression.

Plan and review activity schedule with patient; allow the patient to participate in planning his/her activity schedule.	Helps to promote as much independence as possible. Planning will help to set realistic expectations.

NIC *Activity therapy*
Energy management

Evaluation

The patient is able to tolerate performance of self-care activities. The patient is able to walk short distances without fatigue or shortness of breath. The patient verbalizes an understanding of the need to progress activities gradually, restrict activity as needed, conserve energy, and monitor response to activity.

Community/Home Care

At home, the patient must understand how to continue progression of activities. Instructions should include specific activity goals, monitoring response to activity, and energy conservation. Home maintenance will require that the patient evaluate which of his or her usual activities or routines can be continued. The home environment is assessed for factors such as stairs and distance to bathroom from patient's usual resting place. Returning to the usual state of activity for the patient with cardiomyopathy may not be a possibility due to the progressive decreasing function of the myocardium. If this is true, the patient will need to adjust to this change and adapt his or her lifestyle accordingly. The fatigue and activity intolerance can become a source of frustration and anxiety for the patient as he or she realizes that dependence on others for assistance is a possibility. Dietary initiatives should include the inclusion of energy-rich foods that are high in iron such as organ meats (if not contraindicated due to culture or religion), green leafy vegetables, and whole grain cereals. The nurse or other health care provider should monitor the patient closely for reports of excessive fatigue, depression, or extreme self-limiting of activities, and intervene appropriately.

Documentation

Document the specific activity goals prescribed for the patient. When the patient attempts activity, document the exact activity and the patient's response to the activity (cardiac or respiratory symptoms).

Include in the record any assistance required of the patient for ambulation or activities of daily living.

NURSING DIAGNOSIS 4

 ## DEFICIENT KNOWLEDGE

Related to:

No previous history of the disease/new onset of disease

Lack of information about the disease and its treatment

Defining Characteristics:

Ask no questions

Have many questions/concerns

Is anxious

Goal:

The patient and family understand cardiomyopathy and its treatments.

Outcome Criteria

✔ The patient verbalizes an understanding of the disease process of cardiomyopathy.

✔ The patient expresses an understanding of the prescribed treatment regimen.

✔ The patient is able to identify medications prescribed including actions, side effects, and expected therapeutic responses.

✔ The patient verbalizes an understanding of the symptoms that would indicate a need to seek medical intervention.

NOC   *Knowledge: Disease process*
        Knowledge: Prescribed activity
        Knowledge: Medication

INTERVENTIONS	RATIONALES ·
Assess patient's current knowledge as well as his or her ability to learn and readiness to learn.	Any instruction should build on what the patient already knows; teachings need to be tailored to the patient's ability and willingness to learn for maximum effectiveness.
Instruct patient/family about the disease: — Definition of cardiomyopathy and information on causes — Treatments available — Medications ordered to control the disease (vasodilators, beta blockers, cardiac glycosides, diuretics, calcium channel blockers) — When to seek emergency health care attention — Importance of activity restrictions and energy conservation	Knowledge of the disease, as well as of prevention and treatment options, improves patient outcomes and provides the patient and family with realistic expectations. When the patient/family understands the patient's disease process and medication regime, the patient is able to manage controllable aspects of the disease process, and complications of the disease decrease and/or repeat hospitalizations are reduced.
Teach incrementally: simple to complex.	The patient will learn and retain knowledge better when information is presented in small segments starting with simple concepts.
Ask the patient and family to repeat the information and ask questions.	This allows the nurse to hear in the patient's own words what he or she understood.
Offer printed materials and other audiovisual aides.	Printed and audiovisual aides enhance learning.
Provide family members with literature about the disease and inform them of opportunities for increased learning.	When a patient's family members understand the disease process, they will be better able to assist the patient.
Establish that the patient has the resources required to be compliant when discharged.	If needed resources such as finances for medication, transportation, and psychosocial support are not available, the patient cannot be compliant.

NIC   *Learning readiness enhancement*
        Learning facilitation
        Teaching: Prescribed medication
        Teaching: Disease process

Evaluation

Evaluate the degree to which the patient has achieved the expected outcomes. The patient and family verbalize an understanding of the disease and treatment options, and states that their questions have been answered. Prior to discharge, the nurse should determine whether the patient has the necessary resources to be compliant with follow-up care.

Community/Home Care

Compliance with the prescribed regimen can only occur if the nurse takes the responsibility to educate the patient thoroughly about all aspects of the plan. Upon discharge home, the patient will need to understand the disease process thoroughly and the role of medications in the treatment. The patient will need to balance work, activity, and rest, and may be required to make major adaptations in lifestyle. Teaching should incorporate any religious, cultural, or socioeconomic factors that may impact compliance. Success is dependent upon the patient being able to monitor pulse and identify signs and symptoms that would indicate a need to see a health care provider, such as rapid weight gain, elevated pulse and blood pressure, increasing shortness of breath and chest pain. The nurse should inquire about availability of a scale in the home and the patient's ability to weigh self. Investigations should be made to determine if the patient has the necessary resources to carry out the prescribed instructions.

Documentation

Document the specific content taught and the titles of any printed materials given to the family or patient. After the teaching session document the degree to which the patient and family verbalize understanding. The nurse should indicate any areas that will require further instruction and note any referrals that have been made.

NURSING DIAGNOSIS 5

 FEAR

Related to:
New diagnosis of heart disease
Deficient knowledge regarding disease process
Threat to health
Increasing fatigue
Inability to perform normal activities

Defining Characteristics:
Verbalizes fear and anxiety
Restlessness

Goal:
Fear and anxiety are relieved.

Outcome Criteria

✔ The patient expresses concerns and fears.
✔ The patient verbalizes that fear and anxiety have been alleviated or reduced.
✔ The patient appears relaxed.
✔ The patient requests information regarding disease.

NOC *Anxiety self-control*
Fear self-control

INTERVENTIONS	RATIONALES
Assess for verbal and nonverbal signs of anxiety and fear.	Helps to detect the presence of anxiety and for early intervention to prevent physiological alterations.
Monitor the intensity of anxiety/fear by having patient rate on a numerical scale.	Allows for a more objective measure of anxiety and fear levels.
Encourage patient to verbalize fears and anxiety regarding health status.	Recognition of fears and anxiety is the first step to coping with issues and avoiding negative feelings.
Teach patient relaxation techniques (such as slow, purposeful breathing) and encourage their use.	Reduces anxiety and creates a feeling of comfort.
Reassure the patient by explaining procedures, treatments, and disease process or by having physician discuss.	Fear of the unknown contributes to anxiety; knowing what to expect helps the patient maintain a sense of control.
Stay with patient if fear and anxiety are evident.	Offers comfort, care, and assurances to reduce anxiety and fear.
Recognize that a significant change in lifestyle such as the inability to perform usual activities may cause anger, denial, frustration, and anxiety, and assist the patient to utilize acceptable coping strategies.	Accepting the patient's feelings and supporting him or her in efforts to cope will assist the patient to be realistic in his or her approach to managing the disease.

NIC *Anxiety reduction*
Calming technique
Presence

Evaluation

Assess the patient for the degree that fear and anxiety have been controlled. The patient should verbalize his or her feelings and indicate whether interventions have produced a comfortable state of anxiety and fear. Determine if the patient understands cardiomyopathy and the impact on health. During evaluation, be sure to inquire about the use of coping strategies and relaxation techniques.

Community/Home Care

The patient will need to develop coping strategies and relaxation techniques to utilize in the home setting. The nurse must adequately equip the patient with knowledge necessary to make him or her feel in control. An understanding of what to expect from physiological alterations due to cardiomyopathy will assist the patient to control the disease and prevent complications. In the home, the patient may be able to reduce anxiety more quickly through use of common everyday activities such as short walks, reading, meditating, listening to the radio, and spending time with emotionally supportive family and friends.

Documentation

Using the numerical scale, document the degree of fear or anxiety the patient is experiencing. In addition, include any verbal, nonverbal, or physiological clues that could be indicators of anxiety or fear, such as restlessness, tachycardia, or diaphoresis. Interventions that the nurse implements to treat anxiety or fear should be documented along with the patient responses. Teaching regarding relaxation techniques, coping strategies, and the disease process should be documented in the patient's record.

CHAPTER 1.6

CORONARY ARTERY BYPASS GRAFT/VALVE REPLACEMENT (POST-OPERATIVE)

GENERAL INFORMATION

Coronary artery bypass graft (CABG) is done to improve myocardial circulations by grafting sections of veins (usually taken from the saphenous vein) or arteries (usually taken from the internal mammary artery) above and below the obstruction in one or multiple vessels of the coronary arteries so that blood flow to the myocardial muscle distal to the obstruction can be enhanced. Diagnosis and confirmation of the need for the CABG is accomplished by cardiac catheterization. Following this procedure, perfusion to the area of the myocardium that has been ischemic is re-established. Coronary artery disease is the most common reason for the surgery. Specific indicators include angina pectoris caused by multiple vessel disease, diseased left ventricle, or serious obstructions of the left main coronary artery (Lemone and Burke, 2004). In valve replacement surgery, valves of the heart are replaced due to stenosis, regurgitation, or loss of function. The valves may be mechanical, human, or animal. A CABG or valve replacement generally involves a median sternotomy to allow access to the cardiac vessels and structures. During the actual placement of the bypass vessels or the valve, the heart is temporarily stopped while blood is diverted from both the heart and lungs through a cardiopulmonary bypass pump (heart-lung machine). The heart-lung machine will oxygenate the patient's blood and keep it at an acceptable temperature and circulating, etc., while the bypass surgery is being accomplished. Hypothermia is induced to decrease metabolic rate, thereby decreasing the demand for oxygen. In recent years, advances have led to the development of a minimally invasive direct coronary artery bypass (MIDCAB) for people who only need one vessel replaced. The MIDCAB involves a small incision at the left sternal border of the anterior thorax, but does not require the use of the heart-lung machine or induction of hypothermia (Phipps, Monahan, Sands, Marek, and Neighbors, 2003).

NURSING DIAGNOSIS 1

 DECREASED CARDIAC OUTPUT

Related to:

Myocardial ischemia and myocardial dysfunction

Defining Characteristics:

Tachycardia

Hypotension

Narrowing pulse pressure

Dyspnea

ECG changes (ischemia/MI)

Dysrhythmias

Increased pulmonary pressure

Weak, thready pulses

Tachypnea

Cyanosis

Decreased urine output

Decreased peripheral pulses

Mental status changes

Goal:

Cardiac output is adequate and tissue perfusion is restored.

Outcome Criteria

✔ Pulse is strong and regular.

✔ Blood pressure returns to patient's baseline or set parameters.

✔ Urine output is 30 ml/hour or more.

✔ There is no cyanosis.

✔ The patient has no signs or symptoms of cardiac tamponade (pulse that decreases in amplitude during inspiration, muffled heart sounds, narrowed pulse pressure, tachycardia, and distended neck veins).

NOC   *Cardiac pump effectiveness*
Tissue perfusion: Cardiac
Circulatory status

INTERVENTIONS	RATIONALES
Assess vital signs: noting particularly temperature, decreasing blood pressure, increasing pulse, and the quality of the beats.	During the immediate post-operative period, the patient is expected to have a slow heart rate and to be hypothermic. However, as intraoperative hypothermia is corrected through warming, the heart rate should increase and the temperature should rise. Hypothermia also produces vasoconstriction that could lead to elevations in blood pressure. Low blood pressure with a narrow pulse pressure and increased heart rate, as well as a weak and thready pulse, indicate decreased volume with an inability to perfuse vital organs and would indicate complications following surgery. Monitoring of pulse and blood pressure in the early post-operative period is achieved via invasive monitoring.
Assess peripheral pulses.	Absent or severely diminished peripheral pulses indicate impaired perfusion to cells in distal parts of the body.
Assess breath sounds along with rate, rhythm, and quality of respirations, noting any areas of diminished sounds or crackles.	Detects pulmonary complications following CABG or valve replacement. Atelectasis, especially of the left lower lobe, is a common finding among CABG patients.
Assess heart sounds for rate, rhythm, and quality; note monitor pacing strips and	Detects early the presence of dysrthymias, ischemia, and other parameters that indicate
results of 12 lead EKG; notify physician if dysrhythmias occur or follow agency protocol.	ineffective cardiac function. A diminished S_1 and S_2 may be auscultated due to decreased contractility, the presence of an S_3 may indicate heart failure, and S_4 could indicate decreased ventricular compliance. Atrial fibrillation is the most common dysrhythmia occurring post-operatively.
Monitor the patient for signs and symptoms of cardiac tamponade: decreased blood pressure, increased pulse, muffled heart sounds, jugular vein distention, a paradoxical pulse (a significant decrease in the amplitude of the pulse when the patient breathes in, a decrease in systolic pressure of more than 10 mm/hg during inspiration), narrowed pulse pressure, weak peripheral pulses, cool mottled skin, tachypnea. If signs of cardiac tamponade are detected, notify physician immediately as this could lead to cardiogenic shock or death and assist as directed; pericardiocentesis may be indicated.	Following cardiac surgery, cardiac tamponade can be caused by the accumulation of blood or fluid in the pericardium or thoracic cavity that impedes effective filling of the ventricle and contraction of the myo-cardium, thus impairing output that manifests itself in changes in blood pressure and pulse, as well as signs of ineffective perfusion (cool, mottled skin, weak peripheral pulses). The excess fluid causes an increase of fluid in the neck veins (JVD) and makes heart sounds difficult to auscultate with a muffled sound. Pericardiocentesis is performed to remove excess fluid from the pericardial sac to allow maximum contractibility of myocardial muscle.
Assess mental status.	Detects changes caused by decreased cerebral blood flow.
Monitor arterial blood gases.	Blood gases provide information on homeostasis and oxygenation status.
Administer high-flow oxygen to keep $SaO_2 > 90$ percent via non-rebreather mask, as ordered.	Maximizes oxygen saturation and reduces the risk of hypoxemia.
Maintain two IV access lines with large bore needles or central line, as ordered.	Provides easy administration of medications and fluids.
Administer intravenous fluids, crystalloids, or colloids as ordered (see nursing diagnosis "Deficient fluid volume").	Replaces volume loss due to blood loss during surgery.
Position patient with head of bed elevated 30 degrees and legs slightly elevated.	This position promotes venous return and improves cardiac output.
Maintain all invasive lines as required by agency protocol: central venous line, arterial	These lines allow for invasive monitoring of cardiac status, especially cardiac output and

INTERVENTIONS	RATIONALES
line, temporary pacing wires, and pulmonary artery catheter. Keep a temporary pacemaker by the patient's bedside.	fluid status; pacing wires are in place in case of an emergency. Particularly in the early post-operative period, temporary pacing may be required if the patient is unable to achieve adequate cardiac output, especially if the patient has bradycardia.
Monitor chest tube drainage every hour or according to agency protocol.	During the first two post-operative hours, the amount should be approximately 100 cc/hr and for the first 24 hours should not exceed 500 cc/hr. Observe for frank bleeding (bright red) or increasing amounts of bloody drainage that could indicate bleeding from internal surgical site, which could lead to hypovolemic shock. Decreased amounts of drainage that occur over a very short period of time may indicate a clot or malfunctioning of the system, which if not corrected could lead to accumulation of fluids in the chest cavity leading to compression of heart and great vessels (cardiac tamponade).
Administer vasodilating agents, as ordered: nitroglycerin, sodium nitroprusside (Nipride).	Nitroglycerin dilates coronary arteries, reduces pain, improves coronary artery perfusion, and reduces preload and afterload; Sodium nitroprusside decreases afterload, causes vasodilation, and improves coronary artery circulation. Sodium nitroprusside (Vasodilator) also improves hypothermia.
Administer inotropic medications—dopamine, dobutamine, and low doses of epinephrine—as ordered.	Improves myocardial contractility and increase systolic pressure, thereby improving cardiac output.
Administer morphine sulfate, as ordered.	Reduces pain and anxiety, decreases afterload, and causes vasodilation.
Obtain pulmonary artery wedge pressure (PAWP).	PAWP is a direct reflection of left ventricular pressure and can be used to assess cardiac function and guide fluid volume replacement.

Keep patient warm: use warming blankets or warmed IV fluids as ordered.	Hypothermia is common following CABG and in most cases attempts to warm the patient occur intraoperatively; however, in some cases hypothermia persists in the early post-operative period. For some patients shivering occurs, which increases myocardial workload. Warming is needed to decrease metabolic demands for oxygen.
Monitor intake and output every hour, maintain indwelling urinary catheter as ordered; monitor renal function studies—BUN and creatinine.	Monitors fluid balance as an indicator of renal perfusion. Approximately 25 percent of CABG patients have some degree of renal failure following surgery. Creatinine is a direct measure of kidney nephron function; BUN may fluctuate in response to fluid status, but an elevated BUN with an elevated creatinine signals renal impairment.

NIC *Vital signs monitoring*
Invasive hemodynamic monitoring
Hemodynamic regulation
Circulatory care
Cardiac care: Acute
Oxygen therapy

Evaluation

Evaluation is made by examining the extent to which the patient has achieved the stated outcomes. Cardiac output is increased as evidenced by blood pressure and pulse returning to patient's baseline. Pulse is strong and regular, and peripheral pulses are present. The patient's skin is warm and has returned to its normal color. Renal output of ≥ 30 cc/hour reflects adequate perfusion to kidneys and renal studies (BUN, creatinine) are within normal range. The patient had no complications, such as cardiac tamponade.

Community/Home Care

Patients with decreased cardiac output due to CABG surgery are seriously ill and the period of time required for full recovery may be extensive even though hospitalization is of short duration, approximately 5 days. Following CABG surgery, patients may be overcautious about being active because of the fear of chest pain or shortness of breath. The patient should be taught how to take his or her pulse and monitor his or her responses to activity, such as shortness of breath and increased heart rate. At home, the patient will need to be encouraged to attempt the activities that are allowed post-operatively and to know what to do if they are not tolerated. The patient should immediately cease any activity that causes chest pain because cardiac output is not sufficient to meet the oxygen demands. The patient will need to gradually increase activities as tolerated and ensure adequate periods of rest throughout the day. Of particular concern may be resumption of sexual activities, especially for younger patients. Discussion of fears and concerns regarding engaging in sexual intercourse and what to expect should be discussed openly and honestly. The patient can keep a diary of activity attempted and record his or her pulse rate as well as general feelings following completion of the activity. The diary can be shared with the health care provider on follow-up visits. Understanding the proper storage and use of nitroglycerin and guidelines for decisions regarding activating the EMS system should be clear to the patient. The patient may require the services of a home health nurse who can reinforce teaching and monitor response to continued therapies such as medications, prescribed activity, healing of wounds, oxygen, and rest. Assessment should be made of factors in the patient's environment and usual routine that enhance or inhibit compliance. It is crucial that the patient and home care providers understand the prescribed medical regimen and verbalize a willingness to comply. The nurse should make sure that the patient knows what to do if problems arise, and the importance of follow-up appointments. Referrals to cardiac rehabilitation programs or cardiac support groups may be beneficial to the patient in order to implement changes in lifestlye.

Documentation

Document the status of achievement of goals and outcome criteria. All interventions employed to address the patient's cardiac status (fluid administration, medications, oxygen, assessments, monitoring) should be specifically documented in the record. Include in the patient chart objective indicators such as pulse, blood pressure, readings from invasive monitoring devices, and specific responses to activity. Prior to discharge from the hospital, documentation should be made of education provided and the patient's or family's understanding of the prescribed regimen. Referrals made to such entities as cardiac support groups, cardiac rehabilitation programs, and home health services should be noted.

NURSING DIAGNOSIS 2

 ## DEFICIENT FLUID VOLUME

Related to:
  Blood/fluid loss

Defining Characteristics:
  Restlessness, agitation
  Tachycardia
  Hypotension
  Delayed capillary refill (> 2 seconds)
  Cool, clammy skin
  Decreased urinary output

Goal:
  Fluid volume will be restored.

Outcome Criteria

✔ The patient's skin will be warm and dry.
✔ Mucous membranes will be moist.
✔ The patient's blood pressure and pulse will return to baseline.
✔ Urinary output will be ≥ 30 ml/hour.
✔ Electrolytes will be within normal limits.

NOC *Fluid balance*

INTERVENTIONS	RATIONALES
Assess surgical sites for bleeding and monitor chest tube drainage for increasing amounts of drainage, particularly frank red drainage.	Increasing amounts of bright red drainage in the chest tube drainage device indicates internal bleeding from the surgical site, which could lead to hypovolemia.
Establish IV access with large bore catheters (16 gauge or larger) as ordered and maintain central lines according to agency guidelines.	Post-operatively, the patient will have central lines and peripheral lines for fluid and medication administration. IV access is crucial to treatment;

INTERVENTIONS	RATIONALES
	large gauge catheters allow for fluids to be given quickly, and blood products will run best in large catheters.
Administer intravenous fluids, as ordered.	Restores circulating volume and maintains cardiac output.
Prepare to administer blood as ordered.	Blood may be ordered to increase oxygen-carrying capacity particularly if hemoglobin is <12.
Warm all solutions administered for fluid replacement.	Rapid infusion of large amounts of cool or room temperature solutions can cause a drop in core body temperature; during the immediate post-operative period, this would compound surgically induced hypothermia, which could produce life-threatening dysrhythmias and a drop in blood pressure. Hypothermia also increases the body's demand for oxygen due to increased metabolic rate.
Maintain indwelling urinary catheter to measure urinary output accurately.	Following cardiac surgery, strict output measurements are warranted to detect alterations that would indicate decreased cardiac output. Decreased urinary output may signal that the kidneys are hypoperfused as a compensatory mechanism.
Monitor cardiac status: blood pressure, pulse (quality and rate), pulse pressure and capillary refill, pulmonary artery wedge pressure, and central venous pressure as required.	Changes in blood pressure and pulse give information relevant to cardiac output and impending shock. Capillary refill is an indicator of perfusion. Pulmonary artery wedge pressure and pulmonary artery pressure both give clues to fluid status and ventricular function; the PAWP and central venous pressure will be decreased in hypovolemia.
Monitor skin temperature and color for baseline and during treatment for improvement.	Pale, cool, clammy skin indicates decreased perfusion. As treatment progresses, skin should be warm and return to normal color.
Monitor oxygen saturation using pulse oximetry. It may be necessary to use the ear or nose.	Oxygen saturation indicates ability to perfuse tissues; in the presence of decreased cardiac output, perfusion to the fingers
	or toes may not be sufficient to obtain readings in these sites.
Monitor results of laboratory studies: hemoglobin and hematocrit, BUN, electrolytes.	Hematocrit and hemoglobin fluctuate in response to fluid status, absolute losses from volume results in a decrease in hematocrit and further drops are noted during aggressive fluid resuscitation due to hemodilution; the hemoglobin may be decreased. BUN and electrolytes would give indicators of renal function; BUN may be elevated initially, but decrease due to hemodilution of fluid replacement. Electrolyte imbalances (especially calcium and potassium) result from fluid volume losses and can be a cause of post-operative dysrhythmias; early detection allows for early treatment.
Treat the cause of the fluid loss as ordered.	Correction of underlying cause controls and corrects the fluid deficit.
If blood is administered, monitor for transfusion reaction (see nursing care plan "Transfusion").	Transfusion reactions may occur due to allergenic response or immune response and need to be treated promptly.
During treatment, monitor the patient for signs of fluid overload.	Aggressive fluid administration measures place the patient at risk for fluid overload, especially in the elderly and those with chronic left ventricular disease.

NIC *Fluid management*
Fluid monitoring
Hypovolemia management
Intravenous insertion
Intravenous therapy

Evaluation

Assess the patient for return of normal fluid volume. The patient's blood pressure should return to baseline or be > 70 systolic. The pulse should be strong and regular and at the patient's baseline or only slightly increased. Skin should be warm and color should return to the patient's normal appearance. Renal function should sufficient, with an hourly output on the average of 30 ml/hour. Following fluid replacement, the patient should be assessed for fluid overload that may occur in the elderly and those with chronic left ventricular disease.

Community/Home Care

Patients treated for deficient fluid volume secondary to CABG/valve replacement have normal fluid status restored prior to discharge home. At home, the patient may not require any follow-up because this is an acute situation that for the most part has no long-term complications. Fatigue may be an issue and should be addressed at home; it can be handled simply by informing the patient to perform activities as tolerated until stamina/endurance is reestablished. The health care provider may want the patient to return for a follow-up appointment to ensure that parameters such as hemoglobin, hematocrit, and renal function studies have returned to normal.

Documentation

In this situation, document initial assessment findings such as blood pressure, pulse, respirations, temperature, breath sounds, skin status, weight, and mental status. If there is an obvious bleeding source, document site, an estimate of blood loss, and measures implemented to stop bleeding. Document all interventions such as intravenous catheter insertion, fluids initiated (type, rate), and insertion of indwelling urinary catheter. Chart urinary output and intake according to agency protocol. Be specific when charting patient responses to treatment so that other health care providers can clearly determine improvement or deterioration. If hemodynamic monitoring is initiated, document readings (PAWP, CVP) as required by agency/unit specific protocols.

NURSING DIAGNOSIS 3

 ## ACUTE PAIN

Related to:

    Surgical intervention

    Multiple incisions

    Presence of chest tubes

Defining Characteristics:

    Verbalizations of pain

    Facial expressions demonstrate being uncomfortable: grimacing

    Moaning

    Holding areas that are painful

    Slow movement

    Tachycardia

    Tachypnea

    Restlessness

Goal:

    Pain will be relieved.

Outcome Criteria

✔ The patient will verbalize that pain has been relieved.

✔ Nonverbal signs of pain are absent.

✔ Vital signs are at baseline.

NOC *Pain level*

    Pain control

    Medication response

INTERVENTIONS	RATIONALES
Assess for location, intensity, and quality of pain; use a pain rating scale.	A thorough pain assessment will assist in accurate diagnosis and treatment of the pain. Because of the extensive surgical procedure, with two surgical sites (CABG), pain is an expected occurrence. Having the patient rate the pain provides a more objective description of the level of pain.
Administer narcotic analgesics as ordered on a regular dosing schedule and maintain patient-controlled analgesia (PCA) as ordered.	Pain increases myocardial oxygen demand; alleviating pain will decrease workload of the heart. Pain with inspiration causes the patient to breathe shallowly, which increases the risk for respiratory infection.
Administer medications prior to patient activity.	Less pain will encourage patient mobility.
Instruct patient in techniques to reduce pain, such as splinting with a pillow while coughing or moving.	This provides support to the chest incision and can help reduce pain.
Assist patient with positioning.	Correct positioning can help to relieve stress on incision site.

INTERVENTIONS	RATIONALES
Implement relaxation techniques (deep breathing, guided imagery, soft music) and comfort measures (back rub, massage).	Relaxation techniques and comfort measures enhance the effects of medications, and help to diminish pain impact and alter perception of pain.
Encourage appropriate rest between activity periods.	Fatigue decreases the body's ability to tolerate pain.
Assess the effectiveness of interventions to treat pain, particularly medications.	Determines if new interventions are required.

NIC *Pain management*
Analgesic administration
Anxiety reduction

Evaluation

The patient reports that the pain has been relieved or reduced by the nursing interventions. The degree to which the patient is able to assist in the management of the pain through use of relaxation techniques is assessed. The patient should appear calm and relaxed, and is able to participate in self-care activities as allowed without pain.

Community/Home Care

The surgical incisions of CABG/valve replacement are extensive and the pain will require treatment following discharge from the hospital to home. Postoperative recovery time has been shown to be shorter for patients who engage in recommended physical activities, but for some patients this is not done because of pain. For this reason, the patient should take pain medications before engaging in prescribed activity. Incorporating relaxation techniques into the daily routine should be done by the patient at home to assist with pain control. In addition, if pain is not controlled, the patient may tend to have weak inspiratory efforts that predispose him or her to the development of atelectasis and pneumonia. At home, pain is managed with oral analgesics that are used for mild to moderate pain. Have the patient keep a pain diary to document the onset of any pain, precipitating factors, and relief measures. If the pain worsens at home, the patient should contact the health care provider to determine other causes of the pain; most often increased pain signals a wound infection. Because the threshold for pain varies among patients, if the recommended analgesics and non-pharmacological measures do not control the pain, the patient should seek follow-up care for a different regimen.

Documentation

Include in the documentation assessments made relevant to the pain. Document in the patient's own words the intensity, quality, location, and description of the pain. Use a pain assessment tool to document a specific level of pain. Chart all interventions employed for pain including non-pharmacological measures and the patient's response to the interventions. All teaching should be indicated in the patient record with an indication of the patient's level of understanding.

NURSING DIAGNOSIS 4

 IMPAIRED GAS EXCHANGE

Related to:

Decreased availability of oxygenated blood for exchange of gases at the capillary membrane level

Decreased cardiac output

Defining Characteristics:

Hypoxia

Tachycardia

Tachypnea

Dyspnea

Cyanosis

Pale skin

Goal:

Adequate oxygenation will be achieved.

Outcome Criteria

✔ Arterial blood gases will be within normal ranges.

✔ Oxygen saturation will reach 90–100 percent.

✔ Skin color will be normal.

✔ Respirations will be unlabored.

✔ Vital signs will return to patient's baseline range.

NOC *Respiratory status: Gas exchange*

INTERVENTIONS	RATIONALES
Assess respiratory status to include rate, rhythm, depth, and breath sounds.	Increased pulmonary vascular pressures cause fluid to accumulate in the alveolar spaces, causing congestion. This in turn translates into crackles and increased rate and depth of respiration in an effort to improve gas exchange.
Monitor arterial blood gases and oxygen saturation as ordered.	Following cardiac surgery, the lungs may not be able to return to pre-operative level of functioning immediately. Because of the incisions on the chest wall, chest tubes, and pain, breathing patterns may not be effective. Arterial blood gases and oxygen saturation will detect these changes and provide a means for monitoring for hypoxemia.
Assess skin for cyanosis, pallor, and temperature, being sure to check mucous membranes for darker skinned patients.	Due to peripheral vasoconstriction and decreased peripheral tissue perfusion, the skin becomes cool and cyanotic or pale. Changes in color are more easily detected in mucous membranes in darker skinned patients.
Position patient with head slightly elevated.	Improves chest expansion.
Administer high-flow supplemental oxygen by non-rebreather mask.	Maximizes oxygen saturation in the circulating blood volume.
Monitor and assist with maintenance of mechanical ventilation, as ordered (see nursing care plan "Mechanical ventilation").	Ensures delivery of a specified amount and percentage of oxygen at predetermined intervals. Patients who have cardiac surgery will be on a ventilator in the early post-operative period.
Ensure proper functioning of chest tube drainage system.	If chest tubes are not functioning properly, fluids may accumulate in the pleural space, which can impair gas exchange.
Following removal of endotracheal tube/mechanical ventilation, teach patient to turn, cough, and deep breathe, as well as correct use of the incentive spirometer, and encourage use of both techniques.	Turn-cough-deep breathing and incentive spirometer allow for airway opening and full lung expansion that increase oxygenation, improve tissue perfusion, and decrease risk of lung infections secondary to atelectasis.

NIC *Oxygen therapy*
Respiratory monitoring
Ventilation assistance

Evaluation

Examine specific patient responses to interventions that would indicate that the patient's oxygenation status has stabilized or improved. Arterial blood gas and oxygen saturation level will be in normal ranges, indicating an absence of hypoxia and hypoxemia. Respirations will be unlabored and return to patient's baseline rate. Cyanosis, if present, should be absent following institution of measures to correct decreased gas exchange.

Community/Home Care

For most patients who have had cardiac surgery, respiratory status returns to baseline and is not an issue when discharged to home. However, if home oxygen is required, appropriate referrals should be made. Some intolerance to activity is expected in the early recovery phase following cardiac surgery. The patient needs to understand the concept of oxygen supply and demand as it relates to activity. Methods to improve endurance should be taught to the patient prior to discharge home to include gradual increase in activities with a balance of rest and activity. Any shortness of breath not relieved by rest may signal a problem that needs to be reported to the health care provider. An undisturbed afternoon rest may need to be scheduled for the patient at home. Short rest or nap periods serve to restore the body and provide energy for the remainder of the day. Follow-up is needed to monitor the patient for return to an optimal level of function and for compliance with the prescribed activity regimen. Home health nurses or personal care assistants may be needed for a period of time to assist with personal care and household chores if family is not available. Assessment of the ability to follow all prescribed recommendations should be made, taking into consideration normal diet, religion, cultural practices, health beliefs, and availability of financial resources.

Documentation

Documentation includes extent to which outcomes have been achieved. Document arterial blood gases and oxygen saturation to determine adequate gas exchange. Results of a respiratory assessment should be made with documentation of skin/mucous membrane color, breath sounds, respiratory rate, depth, and rhythm. The patient's response to activity should be clearly charted in the patient record, and all interventions employed to address gas exchange are included. During the time the patient is on a ventilator, document assessments and settings as required by agency protocol.

NURSING DIAGNOSIS 5

IMPAIRED SKIN INTEGRITY

Related to:

Surgical interventions

Insertion of chest tube

Invasive monitoring devices

Defining Characteristics:

Surgical incision on chest wall and/or leg

Stab wounds on side of chest for chest tube insertion sites

Staples or sutures present

Drainage device insertion sites

Intravenous sites

Central line access sites

Goal:

Wounds will heal by primary intention.

Outcome Criteria

✔ Incision will be well approximated.

✔ Incisions or chest tube insertion sites will have no redness/discoloration, purulent drainage, heat, or edema at site.

✔ The patient will remain afebrile.

✔ White blood cell count will be within normal limits.

NOC *Wound healing: Primary intention*

INTERVENTIONS	RATIONALES
Assess surgical sites, chest tube insertion sites, central line insertion sites, and drainage tube insertion sites for signs and symptoms of infection-redness/discoloration, swelling, purulent drainage, and odor.	Early identification of infection can expedite treatment.
Maintain patency of chest tube drainage system and assess drainage for amount, color, and consistency.	The chest tube drainage system allows drainage of fluid and blood from surgical area; if not draining properly the drainage can accumulate at the site and lead to cardiac tamponade.
Take temperature every 4 hours.	Detects elevations that may signal infection.
Change dressings (chest and/or leg) as ordered and clean area using sterile technique, cleansing site of drainage devices last.	Maintenance of a clean incisional site decreases number of organisms and reduces risk of infection.
Administer antipyretics (such as acetaminophen [Tylenol®]) as ordered.	Reduces fever.
Administer antibiotics, as ordered IV (intravenously) or PO (by mouth).	Reduces number of infective organisms and eliminates or prevents infection.
Restrict visitors with colds or other upper respiratory infections.	Reduces likelihood of patient exposure to infective agents.
Encourage adequate nutritional intake orally, with intake of protein, vitamin C, and iron; or provide nutrition parenterally or enterally.	Adequate nutrient intake, especially of vitamin C, protein, and iron, is required for healing and tissue repair.
Monitor white blood cell count.	White blood cells increase in the presence of infections.
Practice good hand hygiene.	Effective hand washing is the first-line prevention measure. Most hospital-acquired infections can be prevented by adequately washing hands.
Teach the patient and family post-operative care required at home.	The patient and family will need to continue interventions for skin care and preventing infection in the home because incision sites will not be healed at time of discharge (see nursing diagnosis "Deficient Knowledge").

NIC *Incision site care*
Infection control
Nutrition management
Wound care
Wound care: Closed drainage

Evaluation

Evaluate the degree to which the outcome criteria have been met. The surgical site, chest tube insertion sites, and central line sites are intact healing by primary intention with incision well approximated. Redness, swelling, purulent drainage, and heat should be absent from the site. Drainage from the drainage devices should be serosanguineous and should be decreasing in amount. The patient should be afebrile and white blood cell counts should return to normal.

Community/Home Care

The status of the surgical sites may remain a problem after the patient has been discharged home. For the patient who has valve surgery, only one incision requires care but for the patient who has had CABG, there are two incisions: chest wall and the donor site. The risk for infection remains once the patient is discharged, and the family will need to know what symptoms may signal the onset of infection (redness/discoloration, drainage, heat, increased pain at site). Care of the incisions may include dressing changes, but in most instances the incision is left open to air with staples intact. It is crucial that the patient and/or family realize the importance of refraining from touching the surgical wounds unless hands have been thoroughly washed. Irritation of the incision by clothing and bed covers needs to be prevented, possibly through the application of clean dressings. In addition, for incisions on the lower extremities, the risk of bumping the leg on household items is great, and a dressing may protect the incision, especially for patients whose clothing expose the incision. The patient will need to understand the importance of good nutrition in complete wound healing and include foods rich in vitamin C, protein, and zinc in the diet. The nurse completing discharge teaching should provide the patient a list of foods that meet this requirement. The importance of completing any ordered medications such as antibiotics once at home should be stressed. The patient should be instructed to contact his or her health care provider if the wound opens, shows any evidence of infection, or is injured.

Documentation

Document assessment findings from the incisions to include color, approximation, and drainage, being sure to note any signs of infection. Chart the status of drainage devices or tubes indicating the color, amount, and consistency of drainage. Vital signs are documented according to agency protocol as ordered for post-operative patients.

NURSING DIAGNOSIS 6

ANXIETY

Related to:

Strange environment (critical care unit)

Serious illness

Fear

Defining Characteristics:

Restlessness

Agitation

Verbalizations of anxiety

Tachycardia

Goal:

Anxiety is decreased or alleviated.

Outcome Criteria

✔ The patient reports being less anxious.

✔ The patient demonstrates no outward signs of anxiety, such as restlessness or agitation.

✔ The patient's pulse is at baseline.

NOC *Anxiety control*
      Comfort level
      Coping

INTERVENTIONS	RATIONALES
Assess level of anxiety (mild, moderate, severe); have patient rate on a scale of 1–10 with 10 being the greatest.	Gives the nurse an objective measure of the extent of the anxiety.
Use a calm and reassuring manner keep patient informed of all that is going on, including information about therapeutic interventions and numerous invasive lines and equipment.	Communication about interventions in a reassuring, calm, and straightforward manner may help to relieve anxiety and gives the patient a sense of well-being.
Stay with the patient as possible and allow family to visit.	Provides emotional support and promotes a sense of comfort.

INTERVENTIONS	RATIONALES
Encourage patient to verbalize fears and concerns.	Verbalization of fears contributes to dealing with concerns.
To the extent possible, control multiple sources of stimuli that could cause sensory overload and explain the setting to the patient.	Overstimulation can worsen anxiety.
Seek spiritual consult as needed or requested by the patient and/or family.	Meeting spiritual needs of the patient helps the patient to deal with fears through use of spiritual or religious rituals.
Administer anti-anxiety medications as ordered.	Reduces anxiety uncontrolled by non-pharmacological measures.

NIC   *Anxiety reduction*
        Coping enhancement
        Emotional support

Evaluation

The patient will verbalize a decrease in anxiety and fear. Physiological signs of anxiety such as tachycardia and elevated blood pressure will be absent. Restlessness and agitation are not noted.

Community/Home Care

Anxiety is common during the post-operative period for patients following cardiac surgery. The relationship between anxiety and increasing oxygen demands by the myocardium should be explained to the patient so that he or she can understand the importance of controlling fears and anxiety. At home, the patient will need to practice relaxation techniques that can reduce anxiety and promote a sense of calm or peace. Nurses should discuss usual successful coping mechanisms with the patient and encourage their use by the patient at home. Methods of controlling the anxiety could be reading, music, backrubs, favorite television shows, and guided imagery. The patient will need to experiment with several to determine what works. If the patient practices an organized religion, in-home visits by the religious/spiritual counselor should be planned. This provides an avenue for expression of concerns and fears. If questions should arise at home regarding the patient's health status or prescribed regimen, the patient should have a means of contact with a health care provider for answers.

Documentation

The degree to which the patient has decreased anxiety should be documented in the patient record. A rating system provides an objective way to relay to others the extent of the anxiety. Document whether the patient is able to verbalize a feeling of decreased anxiety and whether there are outward signs of anxiety. Blood pressure and pulse rates should be documented because anxiety often causes an increase in both vital signs. Document methods the patient uses to decrease anxiety.

NURSING DIAGNOSIS 7

 DEFICIENT KNOWLEDGE

Related to:
> Misunderstanding
> No prior experience with post-operative coronary artery bypass graft/valve replacement
> Post-operative care
> Lack of information
> Anxiety

Defining Characteristics:
> Ask many questions
> Verbalizes misunderstanding

Goal:
> The patient verbalizes an understanding of the operative procedure and prescribed post-operative regimens.

Outcome Criteria

✔ The patient verbalizes a willingness and desire to learn the necessary information.
✔ The patient verbalizes an understanding of the operative procedure and post-operative interventions required.
✔ The patient verbalizes an understanding of activity restrictions required during convalescence.
✔ The patient will be able to identify signs and symptoms of wound infection.
✔ The patient verbalizes an understanding of medications (dose, schedule, action, side effects).

NOC *Knowledge: Disease process*
Knowledge: Health behavior
Treatment behavior: Illness or injury

INTERVENTIONS	RATIONALES
Assess readiness of client to learn (motivation, cognitive level, physiological status).	Patient must be motivated to learn, have the capability to learn the content, and be free of distractions from learning, such as pain and emotional distress.
Assess what the patient already knows.	The patient may have some knowledge about CABG/valve replacement and its sequelae, and teaching should begin with what the patient already knows.
Create a quiet environment conducive to learning.	Environmental noise can prevent the learner from focusing on what is being taught.
Teach the learners about the pathophysiology of coronary artery disease (blockage) and/or valve disease and the specific surgical procedure.	Understanding of pathophysiology and the surgical procedure assists with rationale for therapeutic interventions.
Teach patient deep-breathing exercises and how to splint chest incision.	Maximizes ventilatory excursion and reduces likelihood of atelectasis and pneumonia.
Teach patient activity recommendations and restrictions as ordered: — Perform prescribed activities 3–5 times daily or as ordered. — Do not lift any objects heavier than 5–10 pounds. — Refrain from strenuous activities or any activity that places strain on breastbone. — No driving for at least 4–6 weeks, or as prescribed by physician. — No stair-climbing for 1 month. — Avoid sexual activity for 4 weeks or as directed. — Ambulate as tolerated or recommended by cardiac rehabilitation protocols. — Splint incision when ambulating.	Knowledge enhances compliance and prevents complications. The activity restrictions are intended to protect the surgical site, allow for healing, and to limit cardiac demands on a compromised cardiac system.
Teach patient wound care and infection control measures: — Keep incision clean and dry. — Use unscented soap. — Do not apply any creams or lotions to incisions. — Change dressings using aseptic technique. — Monitor for signs of wound infection: warmth, redness/discoloration, purulent drainage, odor, increased pain, elevated temperature. — Report signs and symptoms of infection to health care provider. — Take all antibiotics as ordered.	The patient needs to understand incisional care. The patient may be at home when post-operative infections occur, so it is crucial that the patient know what to look for that would signal onset of infection to allow for early treatment.
Provide patient with information related to sexuality: — No sexual activity for 4 weeks or as prescribed by physician. — If pain occurs with sexual, activity report to the physician; take nitroglycerin as ordered.	The period of time it takes to establish enough stamina for sexual activity varies from patient to patient, but generally sexual activity is allowed after 4 weeks. The patient may express apprehension about the possibility of pain with intercourse and this should be discussed openly.
Teach the patient signs and symptoms of thrombophlebitis to report to a health care provider: pain in calf, swollen calf or lower leg, warmth over calf, pain with ambulation.	Immobility or limited activity predisposes the patient to pooling and stasis of blood in the lower extremities that place the patient at risk for development of thrombus; the patient needs to be aware of the indicators of thrombophlebitis to allow for early intervention.
Teach the patient regarding anticoagulant therapy: — For mechanical valve replacement, anticoagulation therapy is required for life. — For tissue valves, anticoagulant therapy is needed for a short time only. — Teach method of action, side effects. — Need to monitor body fluids for blood and report any nosebleeds, bruising, or bleeding gums. — Need to have follow-up blood studies. — Do not take aspirin products. — Safety precautions to prevent bleeding.	Clots may form on mechanical valves and in the early post-operative period, clot formation may occur on tissue valves. The patient needs to know how to monitor self for bleeding and how to prevent bleeding.

INTERVENTIONS	RATIONALES
Talk to patient about short- and long-term expectations.	Frequently the patient may not have a clear understanding of what to expect following surgery in terms of symptom control; to avoid frustration and disappointment, the patient needs to be aware of what can be expected and the limitations that may be experienced.
Discuss heart-healthy diets (low salt, low fat, low cholesterol) with patient, or reinforce teaching by dietitian; assess patient for cultural and religious restrictions or preferences that impact dietary practices.	Encouraging healthy eating habits that consider the patient's religion and culture as well as likes, dislikes, and the ability to purchase special foods enhances compliance.
Refer to cardiac rehabilitation as required.	Support provided by cardiac rehabilitation programs will help patient in long-term goal achievement.
Evaluate the patient's understanding of all content covered by asking questions.	Identifies areas that require more teaching and ensures that the patient has enough information to ensure compliance.
Give the patient written information.	Patient will have information for reference at a later time, and for review.

 NIC *Teaching: Disease process*
Teaching: Individual
Positioning

Evaluation

The patient is able to repeat all information for the nurse and asks questions about the operative procedure (CABG/valve replacement) and possible outcomes. Prior to discharge, the patient verbalizes an understanding of all prescribed therapeutic interventions. Activity recommendations and restrictions, including sexual activity, are understood by the patient, who agrees to comply. The patient is able to demonstrate to the nurse how to splint the incision when breathing and moving and how to perform deep breathing exercises, and is able to identify measures to relieve pain. Signs and symptoms of

infection can be accurately stated, as can signs and symptoms of thrombophlebitis. The patient should be able to verbalize when to seek health care assistance, specifically with respect to indicators of worsening cardiac or respiratory status and signs and symptoms of infection.

Community/Home Care

For patients who have had a CABG/valve replacement, the hospital stay is relatively short, which dictates that knowledge deficits be identified early in order to improve the likelihood that the patient will be prepared for self-care and self-monitoring. Whether the patient requires in-home visits by a nurse will depend upon the availability of support persons and the patient's willingness to perform self-care. Several aspects of the teaching plan are emphasized here. The patient will need to monitor self for onset of wound infections, respiratory complications such as pneumonia, and thrombophlebitis. Follow-up care with a health care provider focuses on assurance that no complications have occurred and any wounds are healing as expected. An additional priority of the health care provider who visits is to determine the patient's tolerance for physical activity and his or her willingness to perform activity as ordered. The patient may have a tendency to become dependent in the sick role and refrain from engaging in any activity because of the fear of experiencing pain. The patient should understand that any activity that causes chest pain or pressure, dizziness, or shortness of breath should be stopped. When assessing for home care issues, it is critical that the health care provider broach the topic of sexual activity rather than relying on the patient to express concerns. As the patient resumes more of his or her normal activity, he or she may discover that fatigue persists for up to 2–3 months but should resolve with time. Periods of rest are incorporated into the daily routine to prevent fatigue. Family members can place needed items within easy reach of the patient. It is important that the patient understand safety precautions needed for anticoagulant therapy. Encourage the use of electric razors for all shaving and the need to refrain from using over-the-counter products that contain aspirin. Often, when teaching is done in the early post-operative period or during periods of anxiety, the learner may not comprehend or even hear the information, making it necessary for a thorough assessment of what the patient knows prior to discharge. Booklets that contain the necessary information or other written instructions can be placed in a folder or a three-ring binder for the patient with dividers for sections on different topics. All discharge instructions should be made with consideration given to the patient's normal diet, religion, cultural practices, health beliefs, and availability of resources (both human and financial).

Documentation

Document all content taught and the patient's verbalization of understanding. Specific attention should be given to documentation of any specific concerns that the patient or his or her significant other expresses. If a significant other was included in the teaching sessions, chart this information. Include in the documentation the patient's willingness to comply with all recommendations and prescribed regimens regarding activity, medications, and wound care. Any area that requires further teaching should be clearly indicated in the record. Chart any questions or concerns that the patient has verbalized. Always include the names of any printed literature given to the patient for reinforcement.

CHAPTER 1.7

DEEP VEIN THROMBOSIS/ THROMBOPHLEBITIS

GENERAL INFORMATION

Deep vein thrombosis (DVT) is the formation of a venous blood clot that occurs due to stasis of blood in the veins, defects in the endothelial lining of the walls of the veins, or blood clotting defects.

Thrombophlebitis is vein-wall inflammation that may cause a blood clot to form and can occur in both superficial and deep veins. Deep vein thrombosis and thrombophlebitis occur most commonly in the lower extremities. The most serious areas are especially in larger veins and deeper veins, such as those in the groin areas or the pelvic area. Most patients (80 percent) who experience DVT are asymptomatic. When present, clinical manifestations include pain in the extremities, unilateral edema, and redness or warmth in the presence of thrombophlebitis. DVT poses a threat to circulatory integrity due to the risk for occlusion of blood flow and the possibility of breaking loose and becoming an embolus. The most serious complication of DVT is pulmonary embolus, which may prove to be life threatening. Emphasis should be placed on prevention of deep vein thrombosis and thrombophlebitis by identifying those patients who are at high risk. Risk factors include prolonged immobility, dehydration, orthopedic surgery, pelvic surgery, sickle cell anemia, drug irritants, polycythemia, smoking, oral contraceptive use, prolonged sitting, and long-term presence of intravenous lines or central lines.

NURSING DIAGNOSIS 1

INEFFECTIVE TISSUE PERFUSION: PERIPHERAL

Related to:

Diminished/absent peripheral blood flow secondary to thrombus

Defining Characteristics:

Pain

Tenderness

Redness

Warmth

Edema

Positive Homan's sign (only 20 percent of patients)

Palpable cordlike vein for superficial thrombophlebitis

Goal:

Adequate perfusion is re-established.

Outcome Criteria

✔ The patient verbalizes diminished pain.

✔ The patient has no redness, warmth, or edema in affected extremity.

✔ The patient has no signs or symptoms of pulmonary emboli as evidenced by absence of chest pain; respirations are regular, equal, and unlabored.

NOC *Circulation status*

Tissue perfusion: Peripheral

INTERVENTIONS	RATIONALES
Assess for signs and symptoms of DVT or thrombophlebitis (warmth, tenderness, edema, redness, pain).	Establishes a baseline and assists in distinguishing between deep vein involvement and superficial vein involvement.
Assess patient for contributing factors such as immobility, dehydration, etc.	Identification and elimination of causes will assist in preventing future episodes through education of the patient.

(continues)

(continued)

INTERVENTIONS	RATIONALES
Monitor results of any diagnostic tests such as the venogram, impedence plethysmography, doppler studies, ultrasounds, duplex scans, and radiolabeled fibrinogen scans.	These specialized studies validate the diagnosis, give information on extent of the thrombus, and offer information regarding effect on blood flow allowing for accurate treatment.
Measure circumference of the leg or calf at time of diagnosis and daily.	Provides an accurate measure of edema and establishes a baseline for comparison during treatment.
Encourage bedrest.	Activity increases the likelihood that the thrombus will break loose and become an emboli.
Elevate limb as ordered (slightly above the level of the heart).	Helps to avoid venous stasis and promotes venous return to the central circulation and to reduce limb edema.
Apply moist heat packs to the affected area of the limb.	Moist heat causes vasodilation, which will increase the vascular space around the thrombus and result in improved circulation. It has the added benefit of muscle relaxation, which may reduce pain.
Administer mild analgesics (NSAIDs) as ordered for complaints of pain.	Promotes comfort and also decreases inflammation.
Encourage isometric exercises and active or passive range of motion exercises, the avoidance of leg crossing, and the massaging of affected extremities.	Isometric exercises help to maintain muscle tone and improve circulation; crossing legs restricts venous return and promotes venous stasis; massaging of legs may dislodge the thrombus.
Maintain or increase fluid intake.	Helps to decrease viscosity of blood.
Administer anticoagulants as ordered: low molecular weight Heparin® (lovenox) subcutaneously, regular infractionated Heparin intravenously using an infusion device maintaining a continuous infusion without interruption, and Coumadin by mouth after initial treatment phase with Heparin.	Heparin deactivates clotting factors IX, X, XI, and XII to prevent further clot formation. Coumadin diminishes the formation of prothrombin by the liver. It also disrupts formation of extrinsic clotting factors VII, IX, and X. Coumadin is initiated prior to discharge, and the patient receives both Heparin and Coumadin for several days because of the time required to

	achieve sufficient therapeutic blood levels of the Coumadin.
Anticipate administration of thrombolytic agents (streptokinase, urokinase, tissue plasminogen activator), as ordered.	Thrombolytics may be given to dissolve larger clots in the very early stage and act by activating the conversion of plasminogen to plasmin, the enzyme that degrades fibrin, fibrinogen, and other proteins into soluble fragments.
Monitor patient for signs of bleeding (bleeding gums, blood in urine, blood in feces, easy bruising, bleeding from IV sites or venipuncture sites); for patients on Heparin, monitor bleeding studies (APTT), noting levels above the agency's therapeutic range and adjust dosing as ordered; for patients on Coumadin, monitor INR or PT and note elevations above the agency's therapeutic range.	Patients on anticoagulants often experience abnormal bleeding from body orifices, this requires adjustments in dosing; monitoring of coagulation studies and early detection can prevent massive hemorrhage.
Have the patient brush teeth with soft toothbrush to avoid gum bleeding; apply pressure to simple sticks such as venipunctures for blood and intravenous access.	Helps to decrease risk for bleeding due to anticoagulation medications; even simple procedures such as these can cause abnormal bleeding.
Monitor the patient's bleeding studies for levels that are lower than the agency's therapeutic range; if noted, adjust anticoagulant dose per agency protocol or as ordered to achieve therapeutic blood levels.	Levels that are lower than the therapeutic range prolong treatment and predispose the patient to complications.
Assess the patient for response to treatment by re-evaluating the signs and symptoms of DVT.	Decrease in initial symptoms such as redness/discoloration, edema, and tenderness indicate beginning resolution of the clot.

NIC *Embolus care: Peripheral Embolus precautions*

Evaluation

Evaluate the degree to which the interventions have alleviated the patient's symptoms. The patient should be free of pain and the extremity should be assessed for the absence of or decrease in redness and warmth. The circumference of the extremity or calf should decrease after several days of treatment. Assess the patient for chest pain and respiratory alterations that may indicate pulmonary emboli.

Community/Home Care

The patient needs to practice health promotion behaviors that include preventing the development of subsequent clots. At home, the patient needs to continue with ambulation and avoidance of positions that cause stasis or pooling of blood. It will be important for the nurse to question the patient regarding availability of resources to purchase long-term anticoagulants. Follow-up home health care will include blood draws for anticoagulation studies. The patient will need methodical, well-planned teaching relevant to disease prevention, complications of the disease, and medications (see diagnosis "Deficient Knowledge").

Documentation

Document a thorough assessment of the affected extremity, noting the presence or absence of signs and symptoms of deep vein thrombosis/thrombophlebitis. It is crucial to document precise indicators, such as circumference of the calf or leg, skin color, and temperature. Chart all interventions implemented and the patient's response. If protocols are revised, be sure to include this in the documentation, and if possible, also include the data that supports the need for change. Be sure to include any patient complaints precisely as the patient states them.

NURSING DIAGNOSIS 2

DEFICIENT KNOWLEDGE

Related to:

New onset of disease

Complex treatment protocol

Misunderstanding of information

Defining Characteristics:

Ask many questions

Ask no questions

Verbalize a lack of knowledge/understanding

Goal:

The patient will understand the condition and the steps necessary to prevent complications.

Outcome Criteria

✔ The patient verbalizes a desire to learn necessary information.

✔ The patient verbalizes an understanding of deep vein thrombosis: causes, prevention, and complications.

✔ The patient expresses an understanding of the treatment regimen for deep vein thrombosis, including activity restrictions, medications, and untoward effects of treatment.

✔ The patient verbalizes an understanding of follow-up care required and expresses a willingness to comply.

NOC *Knowledge: Disease process*
Knowledge: Treatment regimen
Compliance behavior

INTERVENTIONS	RATIONALES
Assess patient's current knowledge, as well as his or her ability to learn and readiness to learn.	The teacher needs to ascertain what the patient already knows and build on this; if the patient is not capable of learning or is not ready to learn, teaching will not be effective due to disinterest or inability to understand.
Start with the simplest information and move to complex information.	Patients can understand simple concepts easily and then can build on those to understand more complex concepts.
Teach patient and significant others: — Disease process of deep vein thrombus — Risk factors for deep vein thrombosis (sitting for prolonged periods, crossing legs, dehydration, obesity, immobility, smoking, etc.) — Medications (anticoagulants) used to treat DVT, including rationale for use, dosage, frequency, side effects, scheduling, and interactions with other medications — Importance of wearing a medic alert bracelet and carrying a wallet card stating that he or she is taking anticoagulants — Signs and symptoms of complications that would indicate a need to seek health care (abnormal bleeding, new	Knowledge of disease, treatments required, and prevention of complications empowers the patient to take control and be compliant.

(continues)

(continued)

INTERVENTIONS	RATIONALES
onset of shortness of breath, sudden sharp chest pain, restlessness, worsening signs, and symptoms of DVT)	
Instruct patient on the correct use of anti-embolic or compression stockings. Have patient demonstrate application of these devices.	Anti-embolic stockings are difficult to apply, and the nurse needs to know that the patient can correctly perform this activity prior to discharge.
Teach patient and family about activity and position requirements: bedrest and avoidance of crossing legs.	Even though some physicians allow limited ambulation, bedrest may be required in the early stages until inflammation and swelling subsides. Bedrest prevents dislodging of emboli. Crossing of legs causes constriction of blood flow.
Assess the patient and family's understanding of all teaching by encouraging them to repeat information and ask questions as needed.	This allows the nurse to hear in the patient's own words what was taught and makes it easier to know what information may need to be reinforced.
Establish that the patient has the resources required to be compliant.	If needed resources such as finances and transportation to follow-up appointments are not available, the patient cannot be compliant; the nurse will need to make necessary referrals.

NIC *Learning readiness enhancement*
Learning facilitation
Teaching: Disease process
Teaching: Prescribed medication

Evaluation

Evaluate the degree to which the patient has achieved the outcome criteria relevant to the teaching sessions. The patient should verbalize an understanding of the content presented by repeating the information, particularly the risk factors for deep vein thrombosis and anticoagulation medications. The patient must understand the need to monitor self for bleeding and when to report symptoms to the health care provider. The nurse must determine if the patient is capable of being compliant with the recommended regimen. If further teaching is required at time of discharge, the appropriate referrals should be made to continue education.

Community/Home Care

The patient will need to implement the medical regimen in the home setting over an extended period of time. The success of this implementation will be dependent upon the degree to which the patient has received adequate teaching and has subsequently understood and internalized it. The patient will need to follow a routine that includes administration of anticoagulants and self-assessment of bleeding. If coagulation studies are to be done by the home nurse or at an outpatient center, the patient should understand when or if he or she should take the medication on that day. It is crucial that the patient understands that the medication regimen will continue past the time that symptoms dissipate and the importance of continuing the therapy until discontinued by the health care provider. The interaction of other medications with anticoagulants—especially especially commonly used over-the-counter products, such as aspirin— should be discussed. The patient should avoid dangerous activities that would predispose him or her to cuts or bruises until anticoagulation therapy is completed. The nurse and patient should discuss risk factors for DVT development and ascertain if any risk factors continue to exist for the patient and the feasibility of their elimination.

Documentation

Document the specific content taught and the titles of any printed documents given to the patient. Include in the chart the patient's degree of understanding of the content and the methods used to evaluate learning. Document the patient's ability to perform the psychomotor skill of applying anti-embolism stockings. Any areas that need to be reinforced should be documented to ensure appropriate follow-up. If family members are present for the teaching sessions, document this in the chart, and always document any referrals made.

CHAPTER 1.8

DYSRHYTHMIAS

GENERAL INFORMATION

The term *dysrhythmia* is applied to abnormal cardiac rhythms, electric conduction patterns, and abnormally fast or slow heart rates. Dysrhythmias are classified according to the location of the dysrhythmia and the resulting rate or electrical conduction pattern disturbance. Normal sinus rhythm is a normal conduction pattern with a rate of 60–100 beats per minute (BPM). Rates < 60 are considered bradycardia, and rates > 100 are referred to as tachycardia. Supraventricular dysrhythmias originate above the ventricle and include sinus tachycardia, sick sinus syndrome, sinus bradycardia, premature atrial contractions, atrial fibrillation, atrial flutter, and paroxysmal supraventricular tachycardia. Ventricular dysrhythmias originate in the ventricle and include premature ventricular contractions, ventricular tachycardia, and ventricular fibrillation. Conduction dysrhythmias can be ventricular or atrioventricular and include first-, second-, or third-degree blocks; AV dissociation; and bundle branch blocks. There are many causes of dysrhythmias, including electrolyte imbalance, myocardial infarction, medications, pain, hypothermia, excitement, shock, heart failure, caffeine, and other heart diseases. Some dysrhythmias, such as ventricular tachycardia, ventricular fibrillation, third-degree block, and electrical mechanical dissociation, may be incompatible with life. Immediate therapeutic interventions are required to convert the dysrhythmia to a rhythm that is life sustaining. Interventions may include electrical intervention (cardioversion, defibrillation, pacemaker), medications to correct the dysrhythmia, or correction of the underlying cause of the dysrhythmia. Clinical manifestations vary depending upon the type of dysrhythmia with many patients having no reportable symptoms. When present, clinical manifestations may include dizziness/syncope, palpitations, fatigue, exercise intolerance, hypotension, changes in level of consciousness, decreased output, and notable changes in the normal sinus rhythm on cardiac monitor.

NURSING DIAGNOSIS 1

 DECREASED CARDIAC OUTPUT

Related to:
Altered cardiac rate and rhythm
Dysfunctional electrical conductivity of cardiac cells
Ineffective/decreased myocardial function

Defining Characteristics:
Cardiac dysryhthmias
Tachycardia/bradycardia
Hypotension
Decreased capillary refill
Pale, cool skin
Decreased urine output
Altered mental status
Thready peripheral pulses
Abnormal heart sounds

Goal:
The patient exhibits improved cardiac output and dysrhythmias are alleviated.

Outcome Criteria

✔ Pulse rate is < 100 but > 60.
✔ Blood pressure is at patient's baseline.
✔ Heart sounds are normal.
✔ The patient will have a normal sinus rhythm.
✔ The patient is alert and oriented.
✔ Urine output will be > 30 ml/hour.

NOC *Cardiac pump effectiveness*
Circulation status
Tissue perfusion: Cerebral
Tissue perfusion: Peripheral
Vital signs
Medication response

INTERVENTIONS	RATIONALES
Monitor for tachycardia, dysrhythmias, abnormal heart sounds (murmur, S_3, S_4), and changes in blood pressure; take both apical and radial pulse noting rate rhythm, quality, and any pulse deficit.	Assessment of cardiac status gives early clues to disease and response to interventions and establishes a baseline; hypotension and pulse deficits may result from decreased cardiac output.
Assess peripheral perfusion: skin color, temperature, peripheral pulses, capillary refill.	Monitors for decreased perfusion secondary to decreased cardiac output: decreased peripheral pulses and increased capillary refill > 2 seconds are indicators of poor perfusion.
Monitor for changes in mental status (confusion, restlessness, agitation).	These indicate decreased cerebral tissue perfusion.
Assist with obtaining 12 lead EKG and any other ordered diagnostic tests, such as echocardiogram and chest x-ray, and monitor results. Twelve lead EKGs offer more data than other tests.	These tests reveal definitive diagnosis and aid in monitoring response to interventions: EKG will show any dysrhythmias or cardiac enlargement; echocardiogram will show chamber size and thickness as well as systolic and diastolic function that may be contributing to the dysrhythmias; chest x-ray will give information regarding cardiac diseases such as heart failure that can be a causative factor.
Place the patient on continuous cardiac monitoring, monitor cardiac monitor strips, and document rhythm according to agency protocol.	The nurse is responsible for monitoring for dysrhythmia and intervening according to protocol or notifying physician for prompt treatment.
Monitor arterial blood gases and oxygen saturation level.	These are measures of the ability of the heart to perfuse tissues with oxygenated blood.
Monitor urine output.	Decreased urine output < 30 ml/hour may indicate decreased tissue perfusion to the

kidneys as a result of decreased cardiac output.

Assist in identification of causative factors.	Correcting the causative factor will correct the dysrhythmia.
Administer supplemental oxygen as ordered based on results of ABGs and oxygen saturation.	Helps to maximize amount of oxygen available for gas exchange, assists to alleviate signs of hypoxia; hypoxia can be a cause of dysrhythmia.
Establish intravenous access.	Provides medications as ordered and in case of emergency.
Administer antidysrhythmic medications as ordered based on type of dysrhythmia (examples: lidocaine, amiodarone, epinephrine, procainamide, atropine).	Helps to correct the abnormality before complications occur.
Prepare for electrical intervention according to agency protocols.	Some patients require synchronized cardioversion, defibrillation, or a pacemaker to correct dysrhythmia. These medical interventions performed by qualified cardiologists restore normal electrical activity and conduction in the heart tissue.
If the patient is bradycardic, be sure to avoid any activities that stimulate the vagal nerve (the Valsalva maneuver), such as straining to have a bowel movement or administration of enemas.	Vagal stimulation decreases the heart rate.
For patients who are tachycardic, encourage the Valsalva maneuver as directed.	These maneuvers (vagal nerve stimulation) stimulate the parasympathetic nervous system and decrease heart rate.
Encourage patient to rest, provide assistance with activities, and monitor for fatigue.	Patients with dysrhythmias are often fatigued easily, and rest and assistance will promote conservation of energy.
Monitor serum electrolytes and correct as needed; monitor BUN, Digoxin levels, and liver enzymes as ordered.	These tests may be abnormal as a result of decreased cardiac output or as an effect of medication regimens; digoxin toxicity causes dysrhythmias; electrolyte imbalances alter depolarization and repolarization and are a common cause of dysrhythmias
For life-threatening dysrhythmias, prepare to initiate advanced cardiac life support as needed.	ACLS implementation is the definitive treatment for certain dysrhythmias.

NIC *Dysrhythmia management*
Cardiac care: Acute
Electrolyte monitoring
Oxygen therapy
Vital signs monitoring
Medication management
Code management

Evaluation

The patient has no signs of decreased cardiac output. Dysrhythmias have been alleviated with a return to normal sinus rhythm as evidenced by the cardiac monitor readings. Urinary output has been maintained at or above 30 ml/hour. The patient's pulse and blood pressure have returned to baseline/ normal.

Community/Home Care

The patient with dysrythmias will need to be educated thoroughly about the prescribed regimen. Adaptations will need to be made to accommodate changes in health status that may have an impact on his or her work, social activities, and self-care ability. Particularly for patients whose dysrhythmias were caused by cardiac disease or other chronic illnesses, concern at home centers on functional ability and some degree of anxiety about health status. The patient will need to understand all aspects of his or her medication regimen, including side effects of antidysrhythmic medications. If devices such as pacemakers or implantable defibrillators have been inserted the patient needs specific instruction on these devices including indicators of malfunctioning. Psychomotor skills required for management of the regimen include knowing how to monitor pulse for rate and rhythm and recognizing when a finding should be reported to the health care provider. Family members or significant others should be encouraged to learn how to perform Cardiopulmonary Resuscitation (CPR) in case of sudden cardiac death. Giving family members appropriate information on where they can enroll in a CPR course will be beneficial. The nurse will play an integral part in the patient's achievement of positive outcomes through teaching and in-home follow-up.

Documentation

Chart the status of achievement of outcomes with specific patient behaviors. Include pulse, blood pressure, oxygen saturation, heart sounds, and type of rhythm noted on cardiac monitor. Document all indicators of cardiac output and tissue perfusion. Include in the chart the patient's understanding of dysrhythmias, interventions employed, and patient response to the interventions.

NURSING DIAGNOSIS 2

 FEAR

Related to:
Unknown
Deficient knowledge regarding dysrhythmia
Threat to health with fear of death

Defining Characteristics:
Verbalizes fear and anxiety
Restlessness

Goal:
Fear and anxiety are relieved.

Outcome Criteria

✔ The patient expresses concerns and fears.
✔ The patient verbalizes that fear and anxiety have been alleviated or reduced.
✔ The patient requests information regarding disease.

NOC *Anxiety self-control*
Fear self-control

INTERVENTIONS	RATIONALES
Assess for verbal and nonverbal signs of anxiety and fear.	Helps to detect the presence of anxiety and allows for early intervention to prevent physiological alterations.
Monitor the intensity of anxiety/ fear by having patient rate on a numerical scale.	Allows for a more objective measure of anxiety and fear levels; helps determine how the patient is coping with the stressors of dysrhythmias.

(continues)

(continued)

INTERVENTIONS	RATIONALES
Encourage patient to verbalize fears and anxiety regarding health status.	Recognition of fears and anxiety is the first step to coping with issues and avoiding negative feelings.
Teach patient relaxation techniques (such as slow, purposeful breathing) and encourage their use.	Reduces anxiety and creates a feeling of comfort.
Reassure the patient by explaining procedures, treatments, and the disease process.	Fear of the unknown contributes to anxiety; knowing what to expect helps the patient maintain a sense of control.
Stay with patient if fear and anxiety are evident.	Offers comfort, care, and assurances to reduce anxiety and fear.
Teach the patient about dysrhythmias: pathophysiology, treatment, outcomes, prognosis (see nursing diagnosis "Deficient Knowledge").	Information can often reduce the patient's anxiety level.

NIC *Anxiety reduction*
Calming technique
Presence

Evaluation

Assess the patient to determine the degree to which fear and anxiety have been controlled. The patient should verbalize his or her feelings and indicate whether interventions have produced a comfortable state of anxiety and fear. Determine if the patient understands dysrhythmias and their impact on health. During evaluation, be sure to inquire about the use of coping strategies and relaxation techniques.

Community/Home Care

The patient will need to develop coping strategies and relaxation techniques to use in the home setting. The nurse must adequately equip the patient with the knowledge necessary to make him or her feel in control. An understanding of what to expect from physiological alterations will assist the patient to control the disease and prevent complications. In the home, the patient may be able to reduce anxiety more quickly through the use of common everyday activities such as walking, reading, meditating, listening to the radio, and spending time with

emotionally supportive family and friends. Knowing that someone close by knows how to perform CPR may also decrease anxiety regarding the possibility of sudden cardiac death.

Documentation

Using the numerical scale, document the degree of fear or anxiety the patient is experiencing. In addition, include any verbal, nonverbal, or physiological clues that could indicate anxiety or fear, such as restlessness, tachycardia, or diaphoresis. Interventions that the nurse implements to treat anxiety or fear should be documented along with the patient's responses. Instruction on relaxation techniques and the disease process should be documented in the patient record.

NURSING DIAGNOSIS 3

 DEFICIENT KNOWLEDGE

Related to:

> No previous history of the disease/new onset of disease

> Lack of information about the disease and its treatment

Defining Characteristics:

> Asks no questions

> Has many questions

> Is anxious

Goal:

> The patient and family members understand the disease process and its treatments.

Outcomes

✔ The patient verbalizes an understanding of dysrhythmias.

✔ The patient expresses an understanding of the prescribed treatment regimen.

✔ The patient is able to identify medications prescribed including actions, side effects, and expected therapeutic responses.

✔ The patient verbalizes an understanding of the symptoms that would indicate a need to seek medical intervention.

NOC **NOC** *Knowledge: Disease process*
Knowledge: Prescribed activity
Knowledge: Medication

NIC *Learning readiness enhancement*
Learning facilitation
Teaching: Prescribed medication
Teaching: Disease process

INTERVENTIONS	RATIONALES
Assess patient's current knowledge as well as his or her ability to learn and readiness to learn.	Any instruction should build on what the patient already knows; teachings need to be tailored to the patient's ability and willingness to learn for maximum effectiveness.
Instruct patient/family about the disease: — Definition of dysrhythmias and information on causes — Treatments available (cardioversion, defibrillation, medications, pacemakers) — Medications ordered to control the disease (lidocaine, amiodarone, procainamide, digoxin, Cardizem, or others) — When to seek emergency health care attention	Knowledge of disease, prevention of complications, and treatment options improve patient outcomes and provides the patient and family with realistic expectations. When the patient and family members understand the disease process and the medical regimen, the patient takes hold of controllable aspects of the disease process, and complications of the disease decrease and/or repeat hospitalizations are reduced.
Teach incrementally: simple to complex.	The patient will learn and retain knowledge better when information is presented in small segments, starting with simple concepts.
Ask the patient and family to repeat the information and ask questions.	This allows the nurse to hear in the patient's own words what was understood.
Offer printed materials and other audiovisual aids.	Printed and audiovisual aids enhance learning.
Provide family members with literature about the disease and inform them of opportunities for increased learning.	When a patient's family understands the disease process, they will be better able to assist the patient with implementation of the regimen and provide support.
Establish that the patient has the resources required to be compliant when discharged.	If needed resources, such as finances for medication, transportation, and psychosocial support are not available, the patient cannot be compliant.

Evaluation

Evaluate the degree to which the patient has achieved the expected outcomes. The patient and family verbalize an understanding of the disease and treatment options, and state that their questions have been answered. Prior to discharge, the nurse should determine whether the patient has the necessary resources to be compliant with follow-up care.

Community/Home Care

Compliance with the prescribed regimen can only occur if the nurse takes the responsibility to thoroughly educate the patient about all aspects of the plan. Upon discharge home, the patient will need to understand the process of dysrhythmias thoroughly and the role of medications in the treatment. If the patient's dysrhythmia is caused by cardiac disease, he or she may need to balance work, activity, and rest, as well as make adaptations in lifestyle. Teaching should incorporate any religious, cultural, or socioeconomic factors that may affect compliance. Success depends upon the patient being able to monitor pulse and identify signs and symptoms that would indicate a need to see a health care provider, such as elevated pulse, irregular pulse, blood pressure, and chest pain.

Documentation

Document the specific content taught and the titles of any printed materials given to the family or patient. After the teaching session, document the degree to which the patient and/or family members verbalize understanding. The nurse should indicate any areas that will require further instruction and note any referrals that have been made.

CHAPTER 1.9

EPISTAXIS (NOSE BLEED)

GENERAL INFORMATION

Epistaxis is bleeding from the nose that may be caused by blunt or penetrating trauma; rupture of a vessel due to increased pressure, as occurs in hypertension; vessel erosion, as occurs in cocaine use; or drying of the mucous membrane of the nose such as what occurs with oxygen use via nasal cannula. Nosebleeds may also be related to diseases such as acute leukemia, liver disease, thrombocytopenia, and aplastic anemia. Steroidal nasal sprays and inhalants may also predispose a patient to nosebleed. Anterior epistaxis usually results from rupture of the anterior and/or inferior turbinates in the area of the anterior nasal septum known as the area of Kiesselbach and accounts for 90 percent of all nosebleeds (Lemone and Burke, 2004). Chronic hypertension, arteriosclerotic heart disease, blood dyscrasias, and tumors are the most frequent causes of posterior epistaxis. Posterior nosebleeds tend to be more severe, may result in hypovolemia, and are seen more often in the older adult. In general, epistaxis most frequently occurs in children and in adults between the ages of 50 and 70. It can also occur in patients on anticoagulant therapy, patients with allergies, chronic alcohol users, and patients with Rendu-Osler-Weber disease (a hereditary hemorrhagic telangiectasia).

NURSING DIAGNOSIS 1

INEFFECTIVE AIRWAY CLEARANCE

Related to:

Bleeding and aspiration of or potential aspiration of blood

Defining Characteristics:

Vomits large amounts of swallowed blood

Chokes on bloody drainage

Has difficulty removing airway secretions (blood)

Goal:

Bleeding is controlled and the patient maintains an open airway.

Outcome Criteria

✔ Bleeding will stop 10 minutes after interventions are implemented.

✔ The patient will not experience aspiration of blood, as evidenced by clear breath sounds, no shortness of breath, and patient will verbalize absence of choking sensations.

✔ The patient's vitals signs (blood pressure and pulse) are within patient's normal baseline values.

NOC *Aspiration prevention*
Respiratory status: Airway patency
Symptom control

INTERVENTIONS	RATIONALES
Place patient in upright position leaning forward, tilting head down.	Helps to decrease flow of blood to the nose and backflow to nasopharynx; decreases chance of swallowing blood and decreases venous pressure.
Apply pressure to nostrils for 5–10 minutes by pinching the nose towards the septum.	Pressure causes venous stasis and the bleeding area clots.
Apply ice or cold compress to nose.	Cold causes vasoconstriction of blood vessels.
If bleeding continues, collaborate with physician for medical	Vasoconstriction causes decreased bleeding; cauterization will cause

INTERVENTIONS	RATIONALES
interventions: For anterior bleed: Apply cotton pledgets soaked in vasoconstrictor solution (such as cocaine or phenyleprine), as ordered; cauterize bleeding sites with silver nitrate sticks or anterior packing. For posterior bleed: Apply posterior packing.	vessel opening to contract and bleeding to cease; pressure from packing causes blood vessels to clot.
Monitor patient for airway clearance, especially those with posterior packing.	Blood draining into throat and packing can occlude the airway, causing symptoms of respiratory distress.
Inform patient not to swallow blood during bleeding and not to blow nose.	Swallowed blood often causes nausea and vomiting that would further increase risk for aspiration; blowing of the nose could cause disruption of forming clots, which would cause bleeding to resume.
Monitor patient for respiratory and cardiovascular complications (tachycardia, tachypnea, decreased blood pressure, decreased oxygen saturation, signs of ineffective airway clearance).	Tachycardia, tachypnea, decreasing blood pressure, crackles, and decreased oxygen saturation may be signs of cardiac and respiratory alterations.
Monitor for signs of fluid volume deficit: tachycardia, decreased blood pressure, and change in mental status (see care nursing care plan "Hypovolemic Shock"), and report to physician.	If bleeding is profuse, the patient may show signs of cardiac compensation to maintain perfusion to vital organs by increasing heart rate; blood pressure drops as a result of decreased circulating volume; changes in mental status indicate decreased perfusion to cerebral tissue.
For the patient with packing, administer oxygen as ordered based on oxygen saturation readings.	Posterior packing often inhibits effective inspiration of atmospheric oxygen, and the presence of packing causes patient to take shallow breaths.
Monitor for: — Posterior nasal packing in proper place — Blood collecting in posterior pharynx area — Posterior pack dislodged and is in posterior pharyngeal area — Feeling of choking on blood — Feeling of posterior packing slipping — Ability to swallow liquids and food	Helps to detect untoward effects of bleeding and of treatments; packing can slip and occlude the airway, and often makes eating and drinking uncomfortable.
Monitor patient for hypotension; tachycardia; decreased hematocrit and hemoglobin; pale, cool, clammy skin.	If blood loss is serious, the patient shows these indicators of decreased volume and subsequent decrease in perfusion.
Educate the patient on the etiology of epistaxis, treatments, and complications.	Knowledge enhances reduction of anxiety and allows the patient to understand health status.

Evaluation

Assess the degree to which outcome criteria has been achieved. The patient should have a clear airway and bleeding should stop. For the patient with packing it should be ascertained that the packing is still in place. Vital signs should be within the patient's baseline and skin should be pink, warm, and dry.

Community/Home Care

Most patients with epistaxis are treated in the emergency department unless there is a need for posterior packing. For the patient without packing, the health care provider should teach the patient and family how to stop the bleeding through positioning, pinching of the nares, and application of ice. In addition, the patient should be informed not to blow the nose, which could dislodge clotting and begin bleeding again. Provide the patient with an emesis basin to take home and encourage expectoration of blood rather than swallowing. The patient will need to avoid any type of strenuous activities as directed by the physician. A humidifier placed by the bedside, especially at night, will prevent excess nasal drying that could contribute to bleeding. The patient discharged home with packing in place should fully understand instructions involving care and complications. Signs and symptoms of airway obstruction and cardiovascular impairments should be taught to the patient and family. Those treating the patient for epistaxis should review the patient's medications, such as steroidal inhalers or aspirin that many people take for cardiovascular prophylaxis or arthritis, to ascertain if these could be contributing to the bleeding. It is important for the patient to understand the importance of seeking further health care if spontaneous bleeding should occur.

Documentation

Chart the presence or absence of bleeding with an estimation of amount. Interventions and patient responses should be included in the patient record. Blood pressure and pulse readings that indicate cardiac response to bleeding should be documented.

Findings from a respiratory assessment are documented per protocol. Subjective data regarding airway status and packing fit should also be included in the record.

NURSING DIAGNOSIS 2

 ANXIETY

Related to:

> Blood loss
>
> Fear of airway obstruction
>
> Unknown health status
>
> Discomfort

Defining Characteristics:

> Tachycardia
>
> Restlessness
>
> Verbalization of anxiety, concern, fear

Goal:

> Anxiety is relieved.

Outcome Criteria

✔ The patient appears calm and relaxed.

✔ The patient verbalizes that anxiety has been reduced or alleviated.

✔ The patient asks appropriate questions regarding epistaxis.

NOC *Anxiety self-control*
Symptom control

INTERVENTIONS	RATIONALES
Assess for verbal and nonverbal signs of anxiety and fear, including increased heart rate.	Helps to detect the presence of anxiety and allows for early intervention to prevent physiological alterations.
Monitor the intensity of anxiety/fear by having patient rate on a numerical scale.	Allows for a more objective measure of anxiety and fear levels.
Encourage patient to verbalize fears and anxiety regarding health status (nosebleed).	Recognition of fears and anxiety is the first step to coping with issues and avoiding negative feelings.
Teach patient relaxation techniques (such as slow, purposeful breathing) and encourage their use.	Reduces anxiety and creates a feeling of comfort.
Reassure the patient by explaining procedures, treatments, and etiology of nosebleed.	Fear of the unknown contributes to anxiety; knowing what to expect helps the patient maintain a sense of control.
Stay with patient during active bleeding and during periods when fear and anxiety are evident.	Offers comfort, care, and assurances to reduce anxiety and fear.

NIC *Anxiety reduction*
Calming technique
Presence

Evaluation

Assess the patient for the degree that fear and anxiety has been controlled. The patient should verbalize his or her feelings and indicate whether interventions have produced a comfortable state of anxiety and fear. Determine if the patient understands epistaxis and interventions required for treatment by the health care provider and the patient. During evaluation, be sure to inquire about the use of coping strategies and relaxation techniques.

Community/Home Care

The patient will need to develop coping strategies and relaxation techniques to use in the home setting. The nurse must adequately equip the patient with knowledge necessary to make him or her feel in control. An understanding of what to expect if epistaxis occurs at home will assist the patient in controlling anxiety if it should occur again and in prompt treatment to prevent complications. At home, the patient may be able to reduce anxiety more quickly through use of common everyday activities such as walking, reading, meditating, listening to the radio, and spending time with emotionally supportive family and friends.

Documentation

Using the numerical scale, document the degree of fear or anxiety the patient is experiencing. In addition, include any verbal, nonverbal, or physiological clues that could indicate anxiety or fear, such as restlessness, tachycardia, or diaphoresis. Interventions that the nurse implements to treat anxiety or fear should be documented, along with the patient responses. Document instruction on relaxation techniques and the disease process.

CHAPTER 1.10

HEART FAILURE

GENERAL INFORMATION

Heart failure is the inability of the heart to pump adequate amounts of blood to supply the needs of the body. It can result from a variety of cardiac disorders such as myocardial infarction, hypertension, and coronary artery disease. The most common underlying pathophysiological process is an impairment of myocardial contraction, frequently the left ventricle, which results in decreased cardiac output. Left ventricular failure (LVF) can also result from impaired filling of the left ventricle due to ventricular noncompliance. Right ventricular failure (RVF) occurs when blood flow to the lung is impaired. The most common causes are left ventricular failure and chronic pulmonary disease. In left ventricular failure, client manifestations include feeling tired and, in the early stages, activity limitations. Later, the patient manifests symptoms of pulmonary congestion, such as lung crackles, shortness of breath,' and orthopnea. If untreated, acute pulmonary edema occurs with significant impairment of respiratory function due to the pronounced congestion in the lung. Right ventricular failure follows left ventricular failure, but when it occurs without LVF, it is usually caused by lung disease such as Chronic Obstructive Pulmonary Disease. The right ventricle is unable to pump blood into the lungs, causing blood to back up in the venous system. This creates clinical manifestations of peripheral edema—legs, feet, sacrum—and in some cases engorgement of abdominal organs such as the liver and jugular vein distention. Heart failure is the only major cardiovascular disease that has demonstrated an increase in incidence, prevalence, and mortality rates. According to recent statistics from the American Heart Association, there are 550,000 new cases of heart failure annually. The incidence of heart failure increases as a person ages, and it is estimated that treatment of heart failure is the most common reason for admission to hospitals for people older than 65 years (Lewis, Heitkemper, Dirksen, 2004). The death rate for heart failure is greatest for African American males (21.7). White females and African American females have similar death rates at 18.1 and 18.8, respectively.

NURSING DIAGNOSIS 1

DECREASED CARDIAC OUTPUT

Related to:

Decreased contractility of myocardium

Failure of heart to provide enough blood to meet patient's metabolic needs

Defining Characteristics:

Increased heart rate

Dyspnea

Orthopnea

Decreased urine output

Diminished peripheral pulses

Adventitious breath sounds: crackles

Peripheral edema

Jugular vein distention

Shortness of breath with activity

Goal:

The patient achieves adequate cardiac output.

Outcome Criteria

✔ Breath sounds will be clear.

✔ Urine output will be 30 ml/hour or greater.

✔ Edema will be absent or decreased.

✔ Pulse rate is < 100 but > 60.

NOC *Cardiac pump effectiveness*
Circulation status
Respiratory status: Gas exchange

INTERVENTIONS	RATIONALES
Perform assessment of the cardiac system, including heart sounds, peripheral pulses, pulse, blood pressure, and presence of edema.	A third heart sound develops as the heart tries to fill a distended ventricle and the left ventricle becomes less compliant; peripheral pulses may be difficult to palpate due to edema or decreased peripheral perfusion; edema in the periphery is a finding consistent with right ventricular failure and can occur in feet, legs, sacrum, and other dependent areas of the body as well, as abdominal organs. Tachycardia occurs as a compensatory mechanism to increase cardiac output; blood pressure readings show a decreased systolic pressure but an increased diastolic pressure. These assessments are needed to monitor patient response to treatment and to detect worsening condition.
Assess respiratory status to include breath sounds, rate, rhythm, and depth, and note shortness of breath.	Detects severity and progression of disease; as the left ventricle loses the ability to pump, pulmonary congestion worsens.
Assess urine output for quantity.	Decreased urine output indicates decreased perfusion to kidneys; urine output is also used to monitor effectiveness of diuretics.
Monitor for change in mental status (restlessness, confusion, agitation, decreased level of consciousness).	These are indicators of decreased perfusion/oxygenation of cerebral tissues.
Monitor results of laboratory and diagnostic tests (chest x-ray, electrocardiogram, blood urea nitrogen, electrolytes, creatinine, oxygen saturation, arterial blood gases).	Results of these tests provide data to validate the disease and give clues to status of disease. Chest x-rays will demonstrate whether there is pulmonary congestion or cardiac enlargement; EKG may be normal or in significant LVF the tracings may demonstrate ischemia, dysrhythmias, or hypertrophy; BUN is elevated due to decreased renal perfusion; creatinine is increased due to impaired renal function; electrolytes will reveal a decreased sodium level due to increased total body water; oxygen saturation is decreased

	due to inadequate perfusion; arterial blood gases reveal a decreased oxygen level due to pulmonary congestion that impairs gas exchange, and carbon dioxide levels are often decreased due to increased respiratory rate.
Assist patient in assuming a high Fowler's position.	Allows for better chest expansion, thereby improving pulmonary capacity.
Give high-flow oxygen if indicated by oxygen saturation and arterial blood gases.	Makes more oxygen available for gas exchange, assisting to alleviate signs of hypoxia.
Administer diuretics, such as Lasix, as ordered.	Diuretics reduce vascular sodium, and thereby, reduce vascular fluid load; diuretics also prevent the reabsorption of sodium and chloride in the loop of Henle.
Administer inoptropic/cardiac glycoside agents (digitalis preparations) as ordered, and monitor for toxicity. Take apical pulse for one full minute before administration and if below 60 withhold medication and notify physician.	Digitalis has a positive inoptropic effect on the myocardium, which strengthens contractility, thus improving cardiac output. Common signs of toxicity include visual changes such as halos or yellow lights, nausea, and vomiting. Hypokalemia (a common side effect of diuretics) increases the chance of digoxin toxicity and thus the concurrent use of diuretics and digitalis medications predispose the patient to toxicity.
Administer angiotensin converting enzyme inhibitors as ordered (such as Vasotec).	These enzyme inhibitors reduce peripheral arterial resistance (afterload), pulmonary vascular resistance, and improve cardiac output as well as exercise tolerance.
Encourage periods of rest, and assist with all activities.	Reduces cardiac workload and minimizes myocardial oxygen consumption.
Weigh patient daily.	Weight is a good reflection of fluid lost in response to diuretic therapy (see nursing diagnosis "Excess Fluid Volume").

NIC   ***Oxygen therapy***
Cardiac care: Acute
Hemodynamic regulation
Vital signs monitoring

Evaluation

Examine the extent to which the stated outcome criteria have been achieved. The patient's cardiac output is improved. Evaluate the patient's response to medications by noting an improvement in symptoms. The patient's lungs are clear to auscultation, and blood pressure and pulse have returned to the patient's baseline/normal. No shortness of breath is noted and the patient tolerates activity within limitations. The patient should have no edema in extremities or sacral area.

Community/Home Care

The patient with heart failure will need to receive structured education prior to exiting the health care system in order to monitor his or her cardiac status at home and reduce the number of hospitalization readmissions. Patients with decreased cardiac output should be taught how to take their pulse rate and if possible their blood pressure when at home. Many drugstores and some retail stores, such as Wal-Mart, have blood pressure stations that are easy to use. In addition, there are many free clinics at a variety of sites. The patient can keep a medical diary that records daily pulses, blood pressure readings, and activity with any problems related to tolerance. Following an episode of acute heart failure, the patient should have a gradual increase in activity with monitoring of response in terms of shortness of breath, increased respiratory rate, and increased pulse. Monitoring self for fluid retention is a mainstay of in-home self-care and requires some education by the nurse (see nursing diagnosis "Excess Fluid Volume"). Home care follow-up is required by a health care professional to ensure understanding and compliance with medical regimen. This is particularly crucial for medications because most heart failure patients require a polypharmacy approach to treatment. A written schedule for the patient may enhance compliance and prevent interactions or decreased absorption. Follow-up by a visiting nurse should be recommended to ensure that the patient is able to implement the plan at home and to monitor response to therapy in the early post-hospital phase. Such things as work schedules, diets, religion, social support systems, and beliefs about health influence adherence to the regimen.

Documentation

Always document the status of achievement of outcome criteria with specific patient behaviors.

Documentation should focus on responses to the therapeutic interventions, particularly to medications such as Lasix. Chart the oxygenation saturation results, blood pressure, pulse, breath sounds, output, daily weight, presence of edema, and the patient's tolerance for activity. Include in the patient record the patient's understanding of the disease process.

NURSING DIAGNOSIS 2

 EXCESS FLUID VOLUME

Related to:
> Increased preload
> Decreased ability of the heart for effective contractility
> Decreased cardiac output

Defining Characteristics:
> Crackles in lung
> Jugular vein distention
> Increased respirations
> Nocturnal dyspnea
> Increased blood pressure
> Tachycardia
> Peripheral edema
> Weight gain

Goal:
> Fluid volume excess is decreased.

Outcome Criteria

✔ The patient will demonstrate weight loss.
✔ The patient's lung sounds will be clear.
✔ Edema will be absent or decreased.
✔ Output will be > intake.
✔ Jugular vein distention will be decreased or absent.
✔ Blood pressure and pulse will return to the patient's baseline.

NOC *Fluid balance*
Fluid overload severity
Electrolyte and acid/base balance

INTERVENTIONS	RATIONALES
Assess location and extent of edema.	Assessment reveals severity of the fluid excess.
Assess respiratory system: respiratory rate, effort, depth and quality, skin color, breath sounds, and oxygen saturation; breath sounds for crackles.	The patient may demonstrate dyspnea, tachypnea, orthopnea, and nocturnal dyspnea. Monitor for cyanosis due to decreased ability for gas exchange and for oxygenation to tissues. Crackles may be heard on auscultation; crackles are an indicator of fluid in the lungs and should be monitored for worsening. Oxygen saturation may be decreased as the lungs fill with fluid that impairs ability for gas exchange.
Place patient in high Fowler's position.	Minimizes cardiac workload and decreases fluid return to the heart.
Administer diuretics, such as Lasix, as ordered.	Relieves symptoms of volume overload by increasing fluid output by the kidneys, thereby decreasing circulating volume.
Administer oxygen as ordered.	Improves oxygenation and peripheral perfusion.
Weigh patient daily at the same time, in similar clothing, on the same scale, in the morning before breakfast and after voiding.	The most accurate method of determining fluid volume loss is through daily weighing; 1 kilogram of weight loss = 1 liter of fluid lost. Morning weights are a better reflection of true weights because most people accumulate fluid as the day progresses.
Implement a diet low in sodium.	A low-sodium diet decreases fluid retention.
Implement fluid restrictions as ordered if respiratory symptoms are pronounced.	Restricting the fluid intake can assist in decreasing circulating volume and cardiac workload, thereby decreasing fluid in lungs, which leads to improvement in respiratory status.
Obtain accurate intake and output.	Output gives an indicator of renal perfusion and effectiveness of diuretics in decreasing fluid volume; it is also used to monitor balance between fluid consumed and urinary output.
Monitor electrolytes (especially potassium).	Diuretics cause an abnormal excretion of electrolytes;

	decreased levels of potassium can lead to serious dysrhythmias.
Provide potassium supplements as ordered.	Corrects potassium loss caused by diuretics.
Protect edematous skin in extremities and sacrum.	Fluid in tissue inhibits adequate circulation to the tissue, predisposing the patient to skin breakdown.
Monitor blood pressure and pulse.	Blood pressure and pulse may be elevated during the acute phase of heart failure, but after therapy is implemented, the patient may become hypotensive secondary to diuretic therapy.

NIC *Fluid management*
Fluid monitoring
Electrolyte monitoring

Evaluation

Patient has weight loss and output is > intake. Jugular vein distention does not occur, and edema is absent or decreasing (if pitting edema was present, it has been relieved or is decreasing). The patient reports the absence of shortness of breath and breath sounds are clear. Blood pressure and pulse return to baseline. Abnormal laboratory results return to normal levels, or are at the patient's baseline.

Community/Home Care

Ensure that the patient at home understands the importance of monitoring fluid status. The patient should have a reliable scale that is calibrated and easily accessible. Weighing daily at home will allow the patient to notice subtle changes in fluid retention that may be an early sign of increasing fluid volume and a recurrence of the problem. If the patient notices a weight gain of 3 or more pounds in 2–5 days, he or she should notify the health care provider for more aggressive interventions. Patients should be instructed to take note of clothing that becomes too tight in a short period of time, which is an indicator of fluid retention. The patient needs to limit the intake of salt and sodium-rich foods. The patient should be taught to read food labels for sodium content. The dietitian or nurse can give the patient printed lists of foods that are high in sodium. Diet instructions for home should consider the patient's normal diet and any cultural or religious preferences and restrictions. Have the patient keep a log of food and fluid intake as well as weights. This information can be shared with the health care provider at follow-up visits. Assist the client to develop a schedule for taking prescribed diuretics that is mindful of his or her lifestyle and daily routines. Stress the need for follow-up care.

Documentation

Always document the extent to which the outcome criteria have been achieved. Record intake and output, blood pressure, pulse, weights, breath sounds, and the patient's understanding of the therapies for eliminating fluid excess. If fluid restrictions have been implemented, include this in the record with specifications for amounts to be administered each shift. Medications that are administered for excess fluid volume (diuretics) should be documented on the medication administration record and the nurse should indicate the amount of fluid the patient lost in response.

NURSING DIAGNOSIS 3

ACTIVITY INTOLERANCE

Related to:

Impaired oxygen transport secondary to heart failure

Pulmonary congestion

Defining Characteristics:

Dyspnea

Shortness of breath with activity

Tachypnea

Increased pulse

Reports of fatigue

Goal:

The patient's activity level increases.

Outcome Criteria

✔ The patient will perform activities of daily living without shortness of breath.

✔ The patient will report improved ability to engage in activities such as ambulation.

NOC *Activity tolerance*
Energy conservation
Endurance

INTERVENTIONS	RATIONALES
Administer oxygen as ordered.	Improves oxygenation and thus allows an increased activity level.
Assist with activities as needed.	Helps to conserve energy and reduce myocardial oxygen demand; patient lacks enough oxygen reserves to perform activities independently.
Progress activities gradually from getting out of bed to taking short walks.	Allows the patient the opportunity to develop a tolerance for activity over time.
Pace activities and provide rest periods before and after activity.	Reduces workload of the heart.
Monitor response to activity (pulse, respiratory rate, and dyspnea).	Increased pulse and respirations, along with dyspnea, indicate an intolerance to the activity.
Monitor electrolytes.	Treatment of heart failure with diuretics often causes electrolyte imbalances that can result in muscle weakness and fatigue, which may prevent a patient from participating in activity.
Inform patient to stop any activity that causes shortness of breath, chest pain, or dizziness.	The occurrence of these symptoms indicates intolerance to activity, and the level of activity being performed should be evaluated.
Collaborate with other disciplines such as physical therapy and respiratory therapy as ordered to assist with ambulation.	Respiratory therapy may need to provide oxygen when patient first starts an activity program, and physical therapy can assist with monitoring activity progression.

NIC *Activity therapy*
Energy management

Evaluation

The patient is able to tolerate performance of self-care activities. The patient is able to walk short distances without fatigue or shortness of breath. The patient verbalizes an understanding of the need to progress activities gradually, restrict activity as needed, conserve energy, and monitor response to activity.

Community/Home Care

The patient may continue to experience some fatigue and intolerance to activity after discharge. At home, the patient must understand how to continue progression of activities and how to adjust his or her activity in response to feelings of fatigue or shortness of breath. Instructions should include specific activity goals, monitoring response to activity, and energy conservation. Home maintenance will require the patient to evaluate which of his or her usual activities or routines can be continued. The home environment is assessed for factors, such as stairs and distance to bathroom from patient's usual resting place. In the early stages of recovery, the patient may need to alter the environment and shorten the distance to his or her favorite places in the home by rearranging furniture and placing more needed items (eyeglasses, tissues, remote control, medicines, etc.) close to his or her resting place. In order to increase stamina and energy, the patient needs to increase foods that are good sources of iron, vitamin C, and protein in the diet. If the patient is unable to gradually increase his or her activity, he or she should notify a health care provider.

Documentation

Document the specific activity goals prescribed for the patient. When the patient attempts activity, document the exact activity and the patient's response to the activity. Chart vital signs and record pulse, respirations, and oxygen saturation before and after activity. If the patient verbalizes any complaints of fatigue or shortness of breath, document these in the patient's own words, along with interventions carried out to obtain relief.

NURSING DIAGNOSIS 4

DEFICIENT KNOWLEDGE

Related to:

Complexity of therapeutic regimen

New onset of disease

Insufficient knowledge

Defining Characteristics:

Verbalizes a desire to manage the prescribed regimen

Verbalizes difficulty with integrating one or more aspects of the prescribed treatment regimen

Repeated hospital admissions or visits to emergency room

Asks many questions

Asks no questions

Goal:

The patient understands the therapeutic regimen as prescribed.

Outcome Criteria

✔ The patient demonstrates knowledge of the disease, signs, and symptoms, and verbalizes the need for follow-up health care.

✔ The patient verbalizes an understanding of medications prescribed to include purpose/action, side effects, and dosing schedule.

✔ The patient verbalizes an understanding of the need to incorporate activity into lifestyle as prescribed by health care provider and verbalizes a willingness to follow activity as prescribed.

✔ The patient verbalizes an understanding of a low sodium diet and is able to identify high sodium foods from a list.

NOC *Knowledge: Disease process*
Knowledge: Diet
Knowledge: Medication
Knowledge: Energy conservation

INTERVENTIONS	RATIONALES
Assess readiness of patient to learn (motivation, cognitive level, physiological status).	Patient must be motivated to learn, have the capability to learn the content, and be free of distractions from learning, such as pain and shortness of breath.
Identify a family member or significant other who will also learn the content and assist the patient with compliance.	This person can reinforce the teaching and assist with implementation if the patient becomes incapable of follow-through.

INTERVENTIONS	RATIONALES
Create a quiet environment conducive to learning.	Environmental noise can prevent the learner from focusing on what is being taught.
Teach the learners about the pathophysiology of heart disease, including complications, in the initial teaching session.	Patient must understand what the disease is and how it affects the body before understanding the rationale for treatments.
Teach the learners about the prescribed diet, including sodium and fluid restriction and possible potassium replacement if on diuretics, taking into consideration the patient's normal diet and any cultural/religious needs.	Understanding the rationale for these interventions will enhance compliance and considering cultural/religious preferences will increase the likelihood that the prescribed changes will be assimilated into the patient's routine.
Teach the learners about prescribed medications (diuretics, digitalis preparations, beta blockers, etc.) to include action, side effects, and dosing schedule; teach how to monitor the heart rate.	Knowledge of why the medication is needed and how it works will focus on the importance of the medication. Identification of side effects will minimize anxiety if these untoward effects should occur. When taking beta blockers and digitalis preparations, the patient needs to monitor pulse rate due to the side pulse rate due to effect of bradycardia.
Teach learners about the required activity restrictions, including how to progress exercise gradually while monitoring responses, understanding that some preferred activities may need to be eliminated. Inform patient to eliminate any activity that produces chest pain or dizziness.	Teach that incorporation of exercise into daily routine is needed to strengthen cardiac muscle and improve endurance.
Teach the patient which signs and symptoms to report to a health care provider, such as increased shortness of breath, weight gain, and edema.	Monitoring for signs and symptoms early can prevent a crisis that requires hospitalization.
Evaluate the patient's understanding of all content covered by asking questions.	Identifies areas that require more teaching and ensures that the patient has enough information to ensure compliance.
Give the patient written information.	So that the patient will have information for reference at a later time, and for review.

NIC *Teaching: Prescribed activity/exercise*
Teaching: Prescribed diet
Teaching: Disease process
Teaching: Prescribed medication

Evaluation

The patient is able to repeat all information for the nurse and asks questions about the prescribed regimen (activity, diet, medications). The patient can identify all medications by name, the purpose of the medications, and report the common side effects, as well as the dosing schedule. The patient should be able to discuss knowledge of the disease process and verbalize when health care assistance should be sought. There is a commitment from the patient to comply with all recommendations.

Community/Home Care

For patients with heart failure, home care is crucial to prevent crisis situations. A visiting nurse or a health care provider within an office setting must evaluate the effectiveness of teaching by asking specific questions related to the disease, the medication regimen, activity performance, and diet and fluid restrictions. The nurse should also be attuned to patient concerns that may indicate that he or she is experiencing difficulties with the regimen or with adaptation to the illness. Vital signs and cardio/respiratory status need to be monitored in the home to detect early signs of decompensation. If teaching has been successful, the patient is able to take pulse, monitor activity progression, weigh self, and record all of this information in a log to share with health care providers. As the patient resumes more of his or her normal activity following an acute episode of heart failure, he or she may discover that some activities cannot be resumed. The health care provider must work with the patient to determine a realistic activity regimen. Printed information given to the patient at time of discharge can be placed in a bright colored folder or notebook for handy reference. Separating the notebook into sections for each aspect of the regimen (diet instructions, medication information, activity prescriptions) and a section for recording vital signs and weights will make it easier to use for the patient and family. Determine if the patient has the needed resources (transportation, financial, psychosocial) to be compliant with the medical regimen. The polypharmacy approach to treating heart disease may require significant financial resources, especially if the patient has no health insurance.

Documentation

Chart the content of all teaching sessions. The nurse should document who was present for the teaching sessions. Include in the patient record the patient's verbalization of understanding of the content and whether he or she can demonstrate the skills of taking a pulse, counting respirations, and reading food labels. Specifically document the patient's willingness and ability to comply with the prescribed regimen. If there are areas that need to be reinforced, these should be included in the patient record.

CHAPTER 1.11

HYPERTENSION: ESSENTIAL

GENERAL INFORMATION

Essential hypertension (also known as benign, primary, or idiopathic hypertension) is described as three consecutive readings at different times of a systolic blood pressure of 140 mm Hg or more and/or a diastolic blood pressure of 90 mm Hg or more. Blood pressure is classified into four categories: normal-systolic < 120 and diastolic < 80; prehypertensive-systolic 120–139 or diastolic 80–89; stage 1 hypertension systolic 140–159 or diastolic 90–99; stage 2 hypertension systolic > 160 or diastolic > 100 (Seventh Report of the Joint National Committee on Prevention, Detection, Evaluation, and Treatment of High Blood Pressure, National Institutes of Health, 2003). It has an insidious onset, producing no symptoms for the majority of people. Specific causes of hypertension are unclear, but the two underlying changes that contribute to the development of hypertension are increases in cardiac output, total peripheral resistance, or both. Hypertension (HBP) may cause changes in the vascular system in both large and small vessels. Vascular hypertrophy occurs, followed by decreased vascular compliance, and vascular resistance due to noncompliant vessels. Atherosclerotic plaque contributes to increased pressure in the vessels as the lumina of the vessels become narrow with resulting decreased blood flow to the heart, extremities, kidneys, and brain. As the damage progresses, symptoms of organ damage appear and this is generally when patients may begin to have noticeable symptoms such as headache, dizziness, and nosebleeds; however, a majority of patients who are diagnosed have no symptoms, hence the name "the silent killer." Hypertensive crisis, a diastolic blood pressure > 120, is life threatening and must be treated immediately with antihypertensive agents, frequently intravenously. Essential hypertension accounts for 90 percent of all cases and has no known cause. For patients in the prehypertensive stage, lifestyle modifications are the recommended strategy for treatment. For stage 1 and stage 2 hypertension treatment, medications are added to the lifestyle modifications. Common risk factors for development of the disease include high sodium intake, family history, obesity, gender, ethnicity, sedentary lifestyle, elevated serum lipids, and age. Hypertension is more prevalent in men than women up to the age of 55, but after age 55 hypertension occurs in a slightly higher percentage of women than men. The prevalence of high blood pressure among African Americans and whites is higher in the southeastern United States than in other regions. According to the American Heart Association (Heart Disease and Stroke Statistics: 2004 Update, 2004) the death rate from HBP for African American males was 47.8 compared to 13.7 for white males; 38.9 for African American females versus 13.4 for white females.

NURSING DIAGNOSES 1

 INEFFECTIVE TISSUE PERFUSION

Related to:

Vasoconstriction

Decreased coronary artery perfusion

Myocardial ischemia

Peripheral vascular resistance

Defining Characteristics:

Systolic blood pressure > 140

Diastolic Blood pressure > 90

Ischemic changes on ECG

Complaints of headache

Goal:

Blood pressure will decrease.

Outcome Criteria

✔ Blood pressure decreases to an acceptable level: systolic blood pressure is < 140, diastolic blood pressure is < 90.

✔ The patient reports absence of headache or dizziness.

NOC   *Circulation status*
        Vital signs

INTERVENTIONS	RATIONALES
Take blood pressure and pulse every 4 hours or more often as ordered.	Helps to determine the patient's baseline and to monitor response to treatments, for prevention and early detection of hypertensive crisis. If the patient is hospitalized, blood pressure readings may be taken every hour.
Assess patient for subjective complaints such as headache, dizziness, and palpitations.	Helps to monitor for progression of disease and need for further interventions.
Monitor laboratory studies (BUN, creatinine, electrolytes, urine for catecholamines, 17 ketosteroids).	Helps to detect changes in kidney perfusion/function caused by hypertension and to detect other causes for elevated blood pressure, such as adrenal gland disorders.
Monitor electrocardiogram results.	Monitors cardiac status that may be compromised due to sustained elevated blood pressure; elevated blood pressure may cause myocardial ischemia.
Assess vision and eye structure.	Changes in vision may occur due to damage to the retina caused by elevated blood pressure.
Administer beta blockers as ordered.	Blocks beta adrenergic receptors in cardiac muscle, reduces rate, and force of cardiac contractions; decreases peripheral vascular resistance and increases tissue perfusion.
Administer angiotensin-converting enzyme inhibitors as ordered.	Inhibits conversion of angiotensin I to angiotensin II; decreases peripheral vascular resistance.
Administer calcium channel blockers as ordered.	Causes vasodilation of peripheral arteries/arterioles, which decreases peripheral vascular resistance; protects against stroke.
Give diuretics as ordered.	Decreases absorption of sodium by the kidneys, which enhances excretion of water leading to decreased intravascular volume and a drop in blood pressure.
Monitor for side effects of medications (tiredness, impaired sexual function, dizziness, weakness, decreased pulse).	Helps to determine if medication needs adjustment.
Implement dietary restrictions (low sodium).	Sodium content in foods causes fluid retention and increases peripheral vascular resistance that in turn raises the blood pressure.
Encourage regular exercise.	Facilitates cardiovascular fitness and reduction of heart disease risk; decreases blood pressure.
Encourage rest periods when blood pressure is elevated.	Rest will decrease oxygen demand and workload on the heart.
Assess for stress in life; teach patient relaxation techniques and encourage their use.	Stress has been associated with elevated blood pressure.
Teach patient all aspects of therapeutic regimen (see nursing diagnosis "Ineffective Management of Therapeutic Regimen: Individual").	Informing the patient will enhance ability to comply with recommendations for health promotion.

NIC   *Vital signs monitoring*
       Electrolyte monitoring

Evaluation

Assess the patient's blood pressure on a regular schedule (at least every 4 hours in the hospital setting and at least weekly when at home) to detect changes and trends. Look for a decrease that would indicate a therapeutic response to interventions. Evaluate the patient for other signs of elevated blood pressure such as nosebleed, headache, or dizziness.

Community/Home Care

The patient at home should be aware of the dangers of elevated blood pressure and implement strategies to reduce the blood pressure. These strategies include lifestyle modifications to prevent long-term complications such as stroke and kidney disease. The patient should have a way of checking the blood pressure, either by purchasing a monitor for home use or by going to a local health department, retail store, drugstore, or clinic. If the patient purchases blood pressure monitoring equipment, the nurse will need to be sure that the patient can use it correctly. The patient can record the readings and take the log to his or her health care provider when he or she returns for follow-up. Exercise has been proven to assist with lowering the blood pressure, and exercise can be added to the patient's routine by implementing a simple walking routine for 3 times a week. If the patient lives close to a mall, he or she can go there to walk, regardless of weather conditions such as rain, cold, or excess heat. Most malls open early, some have organized walking clubs, and some even have distances marked off so that the patient can determine the distance walked. A dosing schedule for medications that is compatible with the patient's normal routine/work schedule needs to be established; this is of particular concern if diuretics are a part of the regimen. The importance of adherence to the regimen should be stressed. Health care providers should assess the patient's understanding of and compliance with the regimen at each visit, including any issues that prevent the patient from being compliant, such as side effects of medications or resources. (See nursing diagnosis "Ineffective Management of Therapeutic Regimen: Individual.")

Documentation

Document the extent to which outcomes were achieved including actual blood pressure readings. If the patient voices any complaints, such as headaches, this is documented along with interventions carried out to address them. Include in the patient's record his or her understanding of the disease process, the prescribed medications, and verbalizations of an intent to follow recommendation. Changes to the therapeutic regimen and the patient's response should always be documented. All interventions are documented, including any teaching.

NURSING DIAGNOSIS 2

INEFFECTIVE MANAGEMENT OF THERAPEUTIC REGIMEN: INDIVIDUAL

Related to:

New onset hypertension

Side effects of therapy

Disinterest

Misinformation

Insufficient information on previous contact with health care system

Defining Characteristics:

Patient or family members state that they do not understand information.

Patient or family members request information about disease

Patient's or family members' discussion about disease contains incorrect or incomplete information.

Patient's therapeutic regimen is multifaceted.

Goal:

The patient verbalizes an understanding of the disease process and the prescribed regimen.

Outcome Criteria

✔ The patient verbalizes a desire to learn the necessary information.

✔ The patient verbalizes an understanding of the disease process and interventions required to manage high blood pressure.

✔ The patient demonstrates knowledge of medications and changes in lifestyle, such as exercise, diet, and stress reduction required to promote health.

✔ The patient verbalizes that he or she has resources to manage the regimen.

✔ The patient verbalizes a willingness to keep appointments and follow the prescribed regimen.

NOC *Knowledge: Disease process*
Knowledge: Medications
Knowledge: Diet
Compliance behavior

INTERVENTIONS	RATIONALES
Assess the patient's current knowledge regarding hypertension.	The patient may have some knowledge about elevated blood pressure and teaching should begin with what the patient already knows.
Assess patient for readiness and willingness to learn.	Various factors, including denial, can affect a patient's desire to learn. If the patient is not ready or willing to learn, he or she is not likely to incorporate necessary changes into his or her lifestyle.

(continues)

(continued)

INTERVENTIONS	RATIONALES
Teach information that is simple first and only as much as the patient feels he or she can handle in a given session.	Patient will learn and retain knowledge better when information is segmented into smaller components, and simple information must be understood before the patient can understand more complex information.
Teach patient and family/ significant others: — Hypertension disease process — Cardiac risk factors — Medications: beta blockers, calcium channel blockers, diuretics, ace inhibitors (rationale for use, side effects, dosage, frequency, scheduling) — Diet: low sodium, low fat, low cholesterol, as ordered — When to seek health care follow-up: persistent elevated readings with self-monitoring, onset of any new symptoms such as headaches, chest pain, impaired vision, numbness in extremities, sexual dysfunction, extreme fatigue — Exercise methods and role of exercise in cardiac health — Strategies to reduce stress and relaxation techniques	Knowledge of the disease and all aspects of the recommended regimen (diet, medications, lifestyle changes) and signs of complications provides the patient with the information needed to be compliant and gives the patient a sense of control.
Consider the patient's religious and cultural practices when teaching.	Teaching that considers religious and cultural practices is a holistic approach that will enhance compliance.
Have the patient or family repeat the information and encourage them to ask questions.	Allows the nurse to hear in the patient's own words what was taught and makes it easier to know what information may need to be reinforced.
Assess the patient's financial resources.	Helps to ensure that the patient has the needed resources to be compliant, especially with respect to medications and blood pressure monitoring.
Evaluate if the patient has a means to purchase a blood pressure monitor, and if not, locate local drugstores or free clinics offering blood pressure monitoring.	Allows the patient to monitor blood pressure on a regular basis.
Offer printed materials and other audiovisual learning aides. Obtain brochures and booklets from the American Heart Association or the local health department on hypertension.	Printed and audiovisual learning aides enhance the learning process. These agencies offer free publications in simple language that provide excellent information on the disease and how to control it.

NIC *Learning readiness enhancement*
Learning facilitation
Teaching: Prescribed medication
Teaching: Disease process
Teaching: Prescribed diet
Exercise promotion

Evaluation

Evaluate whether the outcomes have been achieved. The patient should verbalize an understanding of the medical regimen, including medications and lifestyle changes that are required to reduce the risk factors for heart disease. The nurse must determine if the client is willing to be compliant and if the patient has the resources to be compliant.

Community/Home Care

The patient with hypertension often presents a challenge to health care providers because this disease is treated on an outpatient basis. Successful management of hypertension is dependent upon the patient's willingness to follow the prescribed regimen, most importantly the medications. Because many of the medications may cause side effects that are annoying, patients may discontinue them without consulting their health care provider. Of particular concern may be the side effects of fatigue and sexual alterations (impotence and decreased libido). It is crucial to provide information relevant to side effects so that when these side effects occur, the patient understands that it is acceptable to contact the health care provider to discuss a revision or change in the regimen. Part of the ideal regimen for home management is the inclusion of exercise in life routines. The patient should understand the role of exercise in maintaining cardiac health. Walking is a simple activity for the patient and can be accomplished in many local malls that open early for this purpose. It is important that the patient has his or her blood pressure checked on a regular basis. The patient can be taught how to monitor his or her blood pressure with some of the simpler digital blood pressure machines, if the patient can afford one. A nurse or other health care provider should teach the patient this skill and be sure that the patient is performing it correctly. If this is not an option, the nurse should locate free clinics or drugstores that have machines and give the patient a list of available options. The patient should be shown how to document the readings and keep a log with dates and times; the patient should be told to bring the documentation to each appointment.

Documentation

Document the content taught and the learner's understanding of the content. Include in the documentation the titles of any printed materials given and the methods used to evaluate learning. The areas that may require further teaching or reinforcement should also be documented. Document questions and concerns the patient may have so that subsequent health care providers can follow up. Always include whether the patient has verbalized a willingness to comply with recommendations and whether there is a need for financial assistance to carry out the regimen, and if so, make appropriate referrals.

CHAPTER 1.12

MITRAL VALVE PROLAPSE

GENERAL INFORMATION

Mitral valve prolapse is a condition in which the leaflets/cusps of the mitral valve billow back into the left atrium during systole resulting in impaired closure of the mitral valve. The cause is not always clear, but the condition can result from connective tissue disorders (most commonly), rheumatic damage, or ischemic heart disease. Persons with mitral valve prolapse are generally asymptomatic, even though a few have thickened mitral leaflets that create a significant risk of morbidity and sudden death. Clinical manifestations when present include a midsystolic ejection murmur, a high-pitched late systolic murmur, and atypical chest pain usually related to fatigue (the most common symptom). It is the most common form of valve disease in the United States, affecting young women between the ages of 14–30 most often.

NURSING DIAGNOSIS 1

 ANXIETY

Related to:

Fear of heart disease

Fear of the unknown

Defining Characteristics:

Restlessness

Anxiety

Decreased attention span

Expressed fear

Numerous questions

Goal:

Anxiety is decreased or relieved.

Outcome Criteria:

✔ The patient verbalizes that anxiety has been relieved.

✔ The patient has no physiological symptoms of anxiety.

✔ The patient asks appropriate questions relevant to his or her health status.

NOC *Anxiety self-control*
Acceptance: Health status
Coping enhancement

INTERVENTIONS	RATIONALES
Assess for verbal and nonverbal signs of anxiety and fear.	Helps to detect the presence of anxiety and to allow for early intervention to prevent physiological alterations.
Monitor the intensity of anxiety/ fear by having patient rate on a numerical scale.	Allows for a more objective measure of anxiety and fear levels.
Encourage patient to verbalize fears and anxiety regarding diagnosis, needed interventions, and health status.	For most people, any diagnosis that is cardiac-related creates anxiety. Recognition of fear and anxiety is the first step to coping with issues and to avoidance of negative feelings.
Teach patient relaxation techniques (such as slow, purposeful breathing) and encourage their use.	Reduces anxiety and creates a feeling of comfort
Reassure the patient by explaining disease process, all procedures, treatment options, and required lifestyle changes.	Fear of the unknown contributes to anxiety; knowing what to expect helps the patient maintain a sense of control.
Stay with patient during acute episodes of shortness of breath or pain, or if fear and anxiety are evident.	Allows the nurse to offer comfort, care, and assurances to reduce anxiety and fear.
Administer anti-anxiety medications, as ordered.	Assists with decreasing the patient's anxiety level.

NIC *Anxiety reduction*
Calming technique
Presence

Evaluation

Assess the patient for the degree that fear or anxiety has been controlled. The patient should verbalize his or her feelings and indicate whether interventions have produced a comfortable state of anxiety and fear. Determine if the patient understands mitral valve prolapse and the impact that it may have on health status. During evaluation, be sure to inquire about the use of coping strategies and relaxation techniques. Determine whether the patient understands the disease process and prescribed treatment regimens.

Community/Home Care

The patient will need to develop coping strategies and relaxation techniques to utilize in the home setting. The nurse must adequately equip the patient with knowledge necessary to make them feel in control. An understanding of what to expect from physiological alterations will assist the patient to control the disease and prevent complications. In the home, the patient may be able to reduce anxiety more quickly through use of common everyday activities such short walks, reading, meditating, listening to the radio, and spending time with emotionally supportive family and friends.

Documentation

Using the numerical scale, document the degree of fear or anxiety the patient is experiencing. In addition, include any verbal, nonverbal, or physiological clues that could be indicators of anxiety or fear, such as restlessness, tachycardia, or diaphoresis. Interventions that the nurse implements to treat anxiety or fear should be documented along with the patient responses. Instruction on relaxation techniques, coping strategies, the disease process, and any preoperative preparation should be documented in the patient record.

NURSING DIAGNOSIS 2

 ACUTE PAIN

Related to:
Progressive worsening of regurgitation
Abnormal tension on papillary muscles
Fatigue

Defining Characteristics:
Chest pain with fatigue or stress
Complaints of left-sided or substernal chest pain

Goal:
Pain is relieved.

Outcome Criteria

✔ The patient will verbalize that pain is alleviated.
✔ The patient will report feeling relaxed and calm.
✔ The patient's pulse will be within patient's baseline (< 100).

NOC *Pain level*
Pain control
Medication response

INTERVENTIONS	RATIONALES
Assess patient pain for intensity (using a pain rating scale), location, and precipitating factors.	Identifying intensity, precipitating factors, and location will assist in accurate diagnosis and treatment, and assist the patient to prevent the pain. Using a pain rating scale will objectively quantify the intensity of pain.
Assess cardiac status: heart sounds, pulse, blood pressure. Inquire about palpitations.	Helps to establish a baseline and to detect changes that may indicate a change in cardiac output; palpitations sometimes occur due to dysrhythmias.
Assess patient for the presence of stress and for engagement in activities immediately prior to onset of pain.	Both stress and fatigue can cause the atypical chest pain of mitral valve prolapse and both need to be addressed.

(continues)

(continued)

INTERVENTIONS	RATIONALES
Administer analgesics as ordered.	Mild analgesics are usually given; nitrates are avoided.
Administer other cardiac-specific medications as ordered, including beta blockers or calcium channel blockers.	Helps to control palpitations and to reduce pain.
Teach the patient to avoid excessive use of caffeine products, including diet supplements.	Caffeine is a stimulant and can exacerbate symptoms, especially palpitations.
Teach and encourage the use of non-pharmacological measures to control pain, such as music therapy, relaxation techniques, and guided imagery.	The chest pain of mitral valve prolapse is often caused by emotional stress, and relaxation techniques can assist in reducing stress and enhance the effects of pharmacological measures.
Implement measures to avoid fatigue: pace activities, rest often, and gradually increase exercise participating in aerobic activities.	Chest pain is caused by fatigue, not exertion; pacing activities and increasing stamina can reduce fatigue as a precipitating factor.

NIC *Energy management*
Pain management

Evaluation

Determine to what degree the goals and outcome criteria have been achieved. The patient is able to identify what precipitated the pain and to what degree relief has been achieved. Evaluation should include a pain rating and the effective use of non-pharmacological measures to treat and prevent pain.

Community/Home Care

Patients with heart disease should always be cognizant of what activities or situations precipitate pain. The patient should be able to establish a plan for dealing with these once at home. Because cardiac pain generally creates some degree of anxiety, the use of relaxation techniques should prove beneficial for both the pain and the anxiety. It is important to teach the patient what to do when pain occurs and when to seek medical attention. Helping the patient to establish a realistic exercise program will assist in preventing pain by increasing tolerance and avoiding fatigue. Generally, patients with mitral valve prolapse require no specific treatment, but rather a

treatment of symptoms. Patients should be taught what symptoms might indicate mitral regurgitation and concomitant problems that would require interventions.

Documentation

Chart the descriptors of pain and include in the patient record any activities that may have precipitated the chest pain. The interventions implemented for relief are charted, including non-pharmacological measures. Document the vital signs and the patient response to interventions, including a re-assessment of pain level using a pain-rating tool. Any teaching done should also be documented.

NURSING DIAGNOSIS 3

 ## DEFICIENT KNOWLEDGE

Related to:

New diagnosis of heart disease
Misinformation

Defining Characteristics:

States lack of understanding of information
Requests information about disease
Discussion about disease contains incorrect or incomplete information

Goal:

The patient verbalizes an understanding of the disease process and the prescribed regimen.

Outcome Criteria

✔ The patient verbalizes a desire to learn the necessary information.

✔ The patient verbalizes understanding of the disease process and interventions required.

✔ The patient demonstrates knowledge of medications and changes in lifestyle—such as exercise, diet, avoidance of fatigue, and stress reduction—required to promote health.

✔ The patient verbalizes that he or she has resources to manage the regimen.

✔ The patient verbalizes a willingness to keep appointments and follow the prescribed regimen.

Knowledge: Disease process
Knowledge: Medications
Knowledge: Diet
Compliance behavior

INTERVENTIONS	RATIONALES
Assess the patient's current knowledge regarding mitral valve prolapse.	The patient may have some knowledge about mitral valve disease, and teaching should begin with what the patient already knows.
Assess patient for readiness and willingness to learn.	Various factors, including denial, can affect a patient's desire to learn. If the patient is not ready or willing to learn, he or she will be unlikely to incorporate necessary changes into his or her lifestyle.
Teach information that is simple first and only as much as the patient feels he or she can handle at a given session.	Patient will learn and retain knowledge better when information is segmented into smaller components, and simple information must be understood before the patient can understand more complex information.
Teach patient and family/ significant others: — Mitral valve prolapse disease process — Possible etiologies — Medications: beta blockers, calcium channel blockers (rationale for use, side effects, dosage, frequency, scheduling) — Check with health care provider before taking over-the-counter medications — Diet: avoid caffeine products as ordered — When to seek health care follow-up — Exercise methods and role of exercise in cardiac health — Stress reduction and relaxation techniques	Knowledge of the disease and treatment gives the patient a sense of control that will enhance the patient's compliance.
Offer printed materials and other audiovisual learning aides.	Printed and audiovisual learning aides enhance the learning process.
Consider the patient's religious and cultural practices when teaching.	Teaching that considers religious and cultural practices is a holistic approach that will enhance compliance.

Have the patient or family repeat the information and encourage them to ask questions.	Allows the nurse to hear in the patient's own words what was taught and makes it easier to know what information may need to be reinforced.
Assess the patient's financial status to establish that the patient has the resources required to be compliant.	Helps to ensure that the patient has the needed resources to be compliant, especially with expensive medications.

Learning readiness enhancement
Learning facilitation
Teaching: Prescribed medication
Teaching: Disease process
Teaching: Prescribed diet
Exercise promotion

Evaluation

Evaluate whether the outcomes have been achieved. The patient should verbalize an understanding of the medical regimen, including medications and lifestyle changes that are required to control symptoms. The nurse must determine whether the client is willing to be compliant and whether the patient has the resources to be compliant.

Community/Home Care

The patient with mitral valve prolapse is treated on an outpatient basis. Successful management is dependent upon the patient's willingness to follow the prescribed regimen, most importantly controlling symptoms such as fatigue, chest pain, and palpitations. Medications such as beta blockers and calcium channel blockers may cause annoying side effects, and patients may discontinue them without consulting their health care provider. Of particular concern may be side effects of fatigue and sexual alterations (impotence and decreased libido). It is crucial to teach relevant to side effects so that when these side effects occur the patient understands that it is acceptable to contact the health care provider to discuss a revision or change in the regimen. Included in the instruction is a word of caution about taking over-the-counter medications that may contain cardiac stimulants that can exacerbate cardiac symptoms such as ephedrine, diet pills, and pseudoephedrine. The patient needs to know the signs and symptoms of complications that may occur with mitral prolapse such as mitral regurgitation. It is also important that the patient has his or her blood pressure checked on a regular basis. The patient should keep a log that would document symptoms (such as chest pain), what may have precipitated them, what relieved them, and results of blood pressure checks.

Documentation

Document the content taught and the learner's understanding of the content. Include in the documentation the titles of any printed materials given and the methods used to evaluate learning. The areas that may require further teaching or reinforcement should also be documented. Always include whether the patient has verbalized a need for financial assistance to carry out the regimen, and if so make appropriate referrals. Document questions and concerns the patient may have so that subsequent health care providers can follow up.

NURSING DIAGNOSIS 4

 FATIGUE

Related to:

Cardiac disease

Defining Characteristics:

Verbalization of being tired

Verbalization of a lack of energy

Inability to carry out normal activities

Chest pain occurs when fatigued

Goal:

Fatigue will be relieved.

Outcome Criteria

✔ The patient is able to perform activities of daily living.

✔ The patient verbalizes that fatigue has improved or been eliminated.

✔ The patient will report absence of chest pain secondary to fatigue.

NOC *Activity tolerance*
Endurance
Energy conservation
Nutritional status: Energy

INTERVENTIONS	RATIONALES
Obtain subjective data regarding normal activities and limitations.	Helps to determine the effect fatigue has on normal functioning.
Monitor patient for signs of excessive physical and emotional fatigue.	Use as a guideline for adjusting activity.
Encourage periods of rest and activity.	Conserves oxygen and prevents undue fatigue.
Monitor response to activity (pulse, blood pressure, dyspnea).	Increased pulse and respirations, along with dyspnea, indicate an intolerance to activity.
Schedule activities so that excessive demands for oxygen and energy are avoided; for example, space planned activities away from meal times.	Digestion requires energy and oxygen; participation in activities close to meals will cause increased fatigue because of insufficient energy reserves.
Gradually increase activity as tolerated.	Use the results to indicate when activity may be increased or decreased.
Limit visitors during acute illness.	Socialization for long periods may cause fatigue.
Increase intake of high-energy foods such as meat (especially organ meats), poultry, dried beans and peas, whole grains, and foods high in vitamin C.	These foods enhance energy metabolism, increase oxygen-carrying capacity, and provide ready sources of energy.
Encourage patient to plan activities when he or she has the most energy, usually early in the day.	Helps to prevent fatigue, which may increase the risk for chest pain.

NIC *Energy management*

Evaluation

Obtain subjective information from the patient regarding the presence of fatigue. The patient should gradually report the ability to participate in activities of daily living and other normal activities with no fatigue. Determine if chest pain has occurred, and if so, conduct a complete evaluation of the pain experience including interventions that relieved the pain.

Community/Home Care

Patients with mitral valve prolapse should understand that even when at home, fatigue may persist. The patient must understand how to adjust his or her activity in response to feelings of fatigue, possibly even arranging for rest or nap periods in the afternoon. Attention to good nutrition should continue with intake of foods that are good sources of iron, vitamin C, and protein. Avoidance of fatigue at home will decrease the likelihood of chest pain. Health care workers should inquire about type of employment that the patient has to determine if fatigue may be a result of work-related activities. If so, the patient will need to be taught how to prevent work-related fatigue or how to manage it.

Documentation

Chart the specific complaint of fatigue to include what activities the patient has been performing. Document interventions implemented to address fatigue, being sure to document food intake. Assess and document the patient's sleep patterns to determine whether this is contributing to the fatigue. Document whether the patient has chest pain and any interventions implemented to relieve it.

CHAPTER 1.13

MITRAL VALVE STENOSIS/REGURGITATION

GENERAL INFORMATION

Rheumatic fever is the most common cause of both mitral regurgitation and mitral stenosis. The disease causes the valve leaflets to become thickened, calcified, rigid, and scarred. In mitral stenosis and regurgitation, the valve leaflets actually fuse at the commissures of the chordae tendineae, causing the valve leaflets to shorten and retract, interfering with normal valve closure. Stenosis is the actual thickening and stiffening of the valves causing a narrowing of the opening, and regurgitation is the leak that occurs due to the stenosis. Mitral regurgitation can also be caused by a myocardial infarction with a resulting distended left ventricle. A distended left ventricle causes physiologic displacement of the papillary muscles attached to the chordae tendineae that control closure of the mitral valve. If the papillary muscle ruptures due to ischemia, infarction, or trauma, mitral regurgitation will also occur. If mitral stenosis and/or regurgitation continues, the left atrium will have excess blood flow (retrograde) and left arterial pressures will increase. An increase in left atrial pressure will cause a retrograde increase in pressure on the pulmonary veins, causing a back flow of fluid into the lungs, which results in pulmonary edema. The left atrium also begins to hypertrophy due to the decreased amounts of blood it holds due to the regurgitation. Clinical manifestations will vary dependent upon the cause. In acute mitral regurgitation, the patient will exhibit symptoms of pulmonary edema including rapid respirations, crackles in lungs, thready peripheral pulses, onset of a systolic murmur, and in many instances signs of shock. Patients with chronic mitral regurgitation may be asymptomatic until the onset of the classic signs of left ventricular failure, which includes progressive dyspnea, fatigue, crackles, peripheral edema, and a third heart sound. Clinical manifestations of mitral valve stenosis include dyspnea with expectoration of bloody sputum, fatigue, a loud first heart sound as well as a loud snap sound, the presence of a diastolic murmur, and palpitations.

NURSING DIAGNOSIS 1

DECREASED CARDIAC OUTPUT

Related to:

Valve malfunction affecting cardiac output via preload and afterload

Regurgitation of blood into the left atrium

Decreased pump effectiveness of left ventricle

Defining Characteristics:

Loud, high-pitched systolic murmur, referred to as holosystolic murmur (regurgitation)

Tachycardia

Distended jugular veins with right ventricular failure

Loud S_1, opening snap, diastolic murmur (low-pitched) with stenosis

Palpated diastolic thrill (with stenosis)

Palpated forceful downward displacement of apical impulse (regurgitation)

Palpable thrill

Fatigue and weakness

Dyspnea on exertion

Tachycardia

Decreased SaO_2

Pulmonary edema

Lung crackles

Hemoptysis (stenosis)

Goal:

Adequate cardiac output is achieved.

Outcome Criteria

✔ Breath sounds are clear bilaterally.

✔ The patient's pulse rate is < 100.

✔ The patient reports no shortness of breath and oxygen saturation is > 90 percent.

✔ The patient verbalizes an understanding of the disease process and treatment options.

NOC *Cardiac pump effectiveness*
Cardiac disease: Self-management
Medication response

INTERVENTIONS	RATIONALES
Assess cardiac status for the following abnormalities: blood pressure (note decreases or changes in pulse pressure), pulse (tachycardia), respirations (increased rate), heart sounds (noting presence of S_3, S_4, loud S_1, murmurs, palpitations), presence of dysrhythmias on cardiac monitor (atrial fibrillation), palpable thrills, and skin temperature.	These are all symptoms of disease progression and indicators of the heart's inability to maintain adequate output and perfusion to vital organs.
Assess for crackles along with rate, rhythm, and quality of respirations, distended neck veins, peripheral edema, paroxysmal nocturnal dyspnea, and cyanosis.	Helps to detect early any symptoms of left- or right-sided heart failure.
Assess urine output for quantity.	As cardiac output decreases, perfusion to kidneys may decrease and be manifested as decreased output.
Monitor results of diagnostic and laboratory tests: — EKG: stenosis: right axis deviation, atrial fibrillation, left atrial enlargement, right ventricular hypertrophy; regurgitation: left atrial enlargement and atrial fibrillation — Echocardiography: restricted movement of mitral valve leaflets (stenosis); thickening of ventricle wall and thickened valve leaflets — Chest x-ray: for ventricular hypertrophy and pulmonary congestion	Results of these tests provide definitive diagnosis as well as clues to status of disease, damage to the myocardium, renal function, and response to treatments.
— Cardiac catherization: for definite diagnosis and severity of the disease — Cardiac enzymes: for indication of damage to the myocardial tissue — Electrolytes, BUN, serum creatinine: for increases that are indicative of renal dysfunction	
Monitor oxygen saturation and arterial blood gases.	Provides information regarding the heart's ability to perfuse distal tissues with oxygenated blood.
Give supplemental oxygen if signs of left ventricular failure are present.	In acute or severe mitral regurgitation, signs of left heart failure are present; supplemental oxygen makes oxygen available for gas exchange.
Encourage physical and mental rest.	Resting decreases myocardial oxygen demand, reducing the workload of the heart.
Administer diuretics as ordered to the patient with signs of failure.	Helps to reduce vascular sodium and reduce vascular fluid load.
Administer digitalis preparations as ordered for the patient with heart failure.	Digitalis has a positive inotrophic effect on the myocardium, which strengthens the force of contraction thus improving cardiac output.
Administer angiotensin-converting enzyme inhibitors as ordered.	Helps to reduce peripheral arterial resistance (afterload), pulmonary vascular resistance, and improve cardiac output; also reduces pulmonary congestion and peripheral edema.
Give anticoagulants as ordered if atrial fibrillation is present.	A common complication of atrial fibrillation is clot/thrombus formation caused by pooling of blood in poorly contracting or noncontracting atria, and prophylactic treatment is required to prevent emboli from reaching other organs.
Monitor for blood in stools, urine, emesis, and saliva, and monitor INR or PT.	Allows for early detection of signs of bleeding or hemorrhage secondary to anticoagulant therapy.
Assist with activities, particularly ambulation.	Patients with mitral valve disease often have respiratory symptoms predisposing them to activity intolerance.

(continues)

(continued)

INTERVENTIONS	RATIONALES
Restrict sodium in diet.	Helps to prevent or decrease fluid retention and decrease the workload of the heart.
Collaborate with surgeons to prepare the patient for surgery (balloon valvuloplasty, annuloplasty, or prosthetic valve replacement) and implement pre-op teaching for surgical intervention.	Depending on the patient, surgical intervention may be necessary. Valvulotomy is performed to surgically separate the thickened valve leaflets or the fused commissures; valve replacement surgery should be performed before left heart performance is compromised. For mitral valve stenosis, the treatment of choice is a mitral commissurotomy (surgically separate thickened valve leaflets or the fused commissures); for mitral regurgitation treatment is an open surgical valvuloplasty (to suture the torn leaflets, cordae tendineae); annuloplasty is performed to repair the ring that holds the valve leaflets or to repair chordae tendineae or papillary muscles; preoperative teaching reduces anxiety and enhances post-operative recovery.
Teach patient signs and symptoms of post-operative infection and emphasize the need to notify all health care providers of valvular disease.	Cardiac valve disease predisposes the patient to infections in general and particularly around the site of artificial valves; mitral stenosis patients may have frequent pulmonary infections. Prophylactic treatment with antibiotics is needed before dental work or surgery.
Teach the patient to avoid aspirin and any medications that contain aspirin.	These will potentiate the effect of anticoagulants and place the patient at high risk for hemorrhage.
Teach the patient about disease process, required activity restrictions, medical regimens, and surgical options.	Informing the patient about disease process and possible treatments increases the likelihood of compliance with prescribed regimen.
For the patient who has surgery, follow general cardiac surgery post-operative care guidelines (see Nursing Care Plan "Coronary Artery Bypass Graft/Valve Replacement").	Post-operative care for cardiac surgery requires special units with unit-specific protocols and intensive monitoring.

NIC   *Oxygen therapy*
Cardiac care: Acute
Hemodynamic regulation
Vital signs monitoring
Circulatory care

Evaluation

Determine whether the patient's cardiac output has improved and that there are no signs of heart failure. Evidence for a positive outcome includes clear breath sounds, absence of edema, urine output of at least 30 ml/hour, and pulse and blood pressure returned to patient's baseline. In addition, the patient should be able to tolerate activities without extreme fatigue. Determine whether the patient has understood teaching about disease and treatment options, including surgical interventions.

Community/Home Care

Patients with asymptomatic mitral stenosis and regurgitation are monitored closely for disease progression, making compliance with follow-up appointments extremely important. For patients with mitral stenosis and regurgitation, surgery may be indicated, but the patient is usually treated for a period of time at home prior to surgical intervention. For all patients, there is a need to implement strategies at home to prevent fatigue. This includes understanding how to balance activity and rest in order to conserve energy. A gradual increase in activities is required so as not to overtax the cardiac system. The patient needs to be able to monitor self for signs of heart failure, including weight gain, difficulty breathing, and edema. The patient with mitral stenosis is at high risk for thrombo emboli development on the leaflets and for atrial fibrillation, which causes emboli as well. For these patients, anticoagulants are a mainstay of therapy creating a need for in-home monitoring for bleeding (examination of all body fluids for blood and lab studies for INR or PT). The patient should be taught to avoid activities that are likely to cause bruising or bleeding and to use a soft padded toothbrush. It is crucial that the patient learns how to check his or her pulse and note irregularities. The patient, home health nurse, or other health care provider should monitor blood pressure regularly. If the patient has had surgery, attention should be given to wound care, prevention of infection at site of replacement valve or external wound, monitoring of cardiac status, and a gradual return to normal activities. Whether the patient has had valve replacement surgery or is being treated medically, the nurse should determine the availability of resources needed for positive patient outcomes.

Documentation

In the patient record, document the status of achievement of the stated outcome criteria. Document the patient's tolerance for activity, noting pulse before and after activity as well as the oxygen saturation level. Findings from a cardiac assessment should be included, such as the presence of any signs and symptoms of heart failure. Pulse and blood pressure should be noted as well as peripheral pulses. Any teaching that has been done regarding the disease process, pre-operative teaching, and patient's understanding of teaching should be documented in the patient record.

NURSING DIAGNOSIS 2

ACTIVITY INTOLERANCE

Related to:

Decreased cardiac output secondary to valvular disease

Defining Characteristics:

Tachycardia that persists > 3 minutes after activity ends

Shortness of breath

Tachypnea

Syncope

Rhythm changes with activity

Goal:

The patient will tolerate selected activities.

Outcome Criteria

✔ The patient will perform activities of daily living without shortness of breath.

✔ The patient will identify activities that cause fatigue and shortness of breath.

✔ The patient's pulse rate and respirations will return to baseline in 3 minutes or less following cessation of activity.

NOC *Activity tolerance*
Energy conservation
Endurance

INTERVENTIONS	RATIONALES
Ensure rest; create a rest schedule.	Decreases cardiac workload.
Assist with activities as needed.	Conserves energy and reduces myocardial oxygen demand; patient lacks enough oxygen reserves to perform activities independently.
Progress activities gradually from getting out of bed to taking short walks.	Allows the patient the opportunity to develop tolerance for activity over time.
Have oxygen available for use if patient becomes short of breath.	Initial activity may produce shortness of breath; having oxygen readily available enables the nurse to intervene quickly to restore respiratory status.
Pace activities and provide for rest periods before and after activity.	Helps to reduce workload of the heart by conserving energy and decreasing oxygen demands.
Inform patient to cease any activity that causes shortness of breath, chest pain, or dizziness.	These are indicators of intolerance to activity, and the level of activity should be evaluated.
Monitor response to activity (increased pulse, increased respiratory rate and dyspnea, lightheadedness, pallor, palpitations).	Increased pulse and respirations, along with dyspnea, indicate an intolerance to the activity; in addition, lightheadedness, pallor, and palpitations may indicate cardiac decompensation.
Rearrange the room (home or hospital) so that there is minimal movement required to gain access to the toilet, phone, chair, etc.	Provides easy access with a minimum of effort to decrease fatigue/exhaustion.
Collaborate with other disciplines, such as physical and respiratory therapy, as ordered to assist with activities in the hospital and to establish guidelines for at-home activities.	Respiratory therapy may need to provide portable oxygen when patient first starts activity, and physical therapy can assist with monitoring activity.
Teach patient and family needed information about diet, energy conservation, prescribed activity limitations, as well as reportable signs and symptoms indicative of cardiac decompensation.	Education will assist the patient to be compliant with the therapeutic regimen and prevent a crisis.

NIC   *Activity therapy*
        Energy management

Evaluation

Examine the degree to which the patient has achieved the outcome criteria as stated. The patient should be able to walk short distances to the bathroom without experiencing shortness of breath or tachycardia; if these are present, the patient should return to baseline within 3 minutes. The patient should verbalize his or her understanding of activity limitations and be able to identify those activities that cause symptoms. With time and gradual increase in activities, the patient should report better tolerance.

Community/Home Care

Patients with mitral disease frequently experience fatigue and exertional dyspnea at home and need to learn to adapt to this health status change. The home environment should be discussed with the patient to identify layout of the home (stairs, distance to bathroom and kitchen) and furniture placement to determine what changes may be necessary in order for the patient to maneuver with the least amount of energy expenditure. The patient should be taught how to progress activities at home as well as how to prioritize which activities should be done and which activities may require higher energy. An occupational therapist may be helpful in this endeavor by also presenting information on work/task simplification. The dietitian could be useful in assisting the patient and family in selecting foods that provide sources of energy. The patient can start an activity journal to record all activities along with the response (pulse rate and respiratory rate), including length of time of the activity. It is important that the patient refrain from a completely sedentary lifestyle.

Documentation

Document the patient's specific activity goals and progress towards the established outcome criteria. Include in the patient record specific patient behaviors in terms of response to activity. Always document the specific activities that the patient has attempted. If other disciplines are involved in the patient's care, such as physical therapy, document these visits.

NURSING DIAGNOSIS 3

 ANXIETY

Related to:
    Fear of disease, surgery, unknown outcome
    Activity limitations

Defining Characteristics:
    Restlessness
    Anxiety
    Decreased attention span
    Expressed fear
    Numerous questions

Goal:
    Anxiety is decreased or relieved.

Outcome Criteria

✔ The patient verbalizes that anxiety had been relieved.

✔ The patient has no physiological symptoms of anxiety.

✔ The patient states that he or she is relaxed.

✔ The patient asks appropriate questions relevant to his or her health status.

NOC   *Anxiety self-control*
        Acceptance: Health status
        Coping enhancement

INTERVENTIONS	RATIONALES
Assess for verbal and nonverbal signs of anxiety and fear.	Helps to detect the presence of anxiety and to provide for early intervention to prevent physiological alterations.
Monitor the intensity of anxiety/fear by having patient rate on a numerical scale.	Allows for a more objective measure of anxiety and fear levels.
Encourage patient to verbalize fears and anxiety regarding diagnosis, needed interventions, and health status.	Recognition of fear and anxiety is the first step to coping with issues and to avoidance of negative feelings.
Teach patient relaxation techniques, such as slow, purposeful breathing and guided imagery, and encourage their use.	Reduces anxiety and creates a feeling of comfort.

INTERVENTIONS	RATIONALES
Reassure the patient by explaining disease process, all procedures, treatment options, and required lifestyle changes.	Fear of the unknown contributes to anxiety; knowing what to expect helps the patient maintain a sense of control.
Stay with patient during acute episodes of shortness of breath, pain, or if fear and anxiety are evident.	Allows the nurse to offer comfort, care, and assurances to reduce anxiety and fear.
Administer anti-anxiety medications, as ordered.	Helps to assist with decreasing the patient's anxiety level.

NIC   *Anxiety reduction*
       Calming technique
       Presence

Evaluation

Assess the patient for the degree that fear and anxiety have been controlled. The patient should verbalize his or her feelings and indicate whether interventions have produced a comfortable state of anxiety and fear. Determine if the patient understands mitral stenosis and regurgitation and the impact they may have on health status. During evaluation, be sure to inquire about the use of coping strategies and relaxation techniques. Determine whether the patient understands the disease process and prescribed treatment regimens.

Community/Home Care

The patient will need to develop coping strategies and relaxation techniques to utilize in the home setting. The nurse must adequately equip the patient with knowledge necessary to make him or her feel in control. An understanding of what to expect from physiological alterations will assist the patient to control the disease and prevent complications. In the home, the patient may be able to reduce anxiety more quickly through use of common everyday activities such as taking a short walk, reading, meditating, and listening to the radio, and through the emotional support of family and friends. For the patient who is awaiting surgery, it is important to control anxiety before time of surgery through pre-operative teaching regarding post-operative expectations.

Documentation

Using the numerical scale, document the degree of fear or anxiety the patient is experiencing. In addition, include any verbal, nonverbal, or physiological clues that could be indicators of anxiety or fear, such as restlessness, tachycardia, or diaphoresis. Interventions that the nurse implements to treat anxiety or fear should be documented along with the patient responses. In the patient record, document instruction of relaxation techniques, coping strategies, disease process, and any pre-operative preparation.

CHAPTER 1.14

MYOCARDIAL INFARCTION

GENERAL INFORMATION

A myocardial infarction (MI) occurs when blood flow to a portion of the myocardium becomes occluded. This occlusion/blockage leads to localized ischemia and subsequent necrosis of the myocardial muscle. It is caused by the narrowing of one or more coronary arteries due to atherosclerotic plaques, a thrombus, or vascular spasm. The sequelae of events that follow are a result of a lack of sufficient oxygen and nutrients to the myocardium as a result of inadequate tissue perfusion. Myocardial infarction is usually manifested by a sudden onset of severe pain that may last from minutes to days. The pain is usually described as crushing, sharp, squeezing, or burning and is typically located substernally, radiating into the left arm or jaw that is unrelieved by rest. The pain associated with myocardial infarction can occur at rest, during activity, or during sleep. Other common symptoms include nausea and vomiting, diaphoresis, shortness of breath, and initially elevations of blood pressure and pulse. Myocardial infarction may also have a number of atypical presentations, including an absence of the classical pain. An atypical presentation is commonly noted in the elderly, in women, and in patients with chronic diseases such as diabetes mellitus. The primary goal of medical and nursing interventions is reperfusion of the myocardial muscle.

NURSING DIAGNOSIS 1

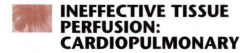

INEFFECTIVE TISSUE PERFUSION: CARDIOPULMONARY

Related to:

Obstructed flow of blood to myocardium

Myocardial ischemia when oxygen demand exceeds supply

Defining Characteristics:

Tachycardia

Chest pain

Dyspnea

Pain lasts more than 5 minutes, unrelieved by rest or nitroglycerin

Goal:

Adequate cardiac perfusion will be re-established.

Outcome Criteria

✔ The patient's blood pressure and heart rate return to baseline.

✔ The patient will verbalize that pain has been alleviated.

✔ The patient's EKG changes will improve and return to baseline.

✔ The patient will show signs of reperfusion (resolution of ST segment depression, abrupt cessation of chest pain, sudden onset of ventricular dysrhythmias).

NOC	*Circulation status*
	Tissue perfusion: Cardiac
	Vital signs
	Pain level
	Pain control
	Medication response

INTERVENTIONS	RATIONALES
Assess patient pain for onset, quality, intensity, location, and precipitating factors.	Identifying intensity, precipitating factors, and location will assist in accurate diagnosis.

INTERVENTIONS	RATIONALES
Assess cardiac and circulatory status: heart sounds, pulse, blood pressure, temperature, respirations, peripheral pulses, skin temperature, and skin color.	Establishes a baseline and helps to detect changes that may indicate a change in cardiac output or perfusion; vital signs should be monitored frequently, as often as every 15 minutes during the first few hours after admission. An S$_4$ may be heard and the pulse may be rapid and weak.
Assess respiratory status (rate, rhythm, crackles, shortness of breath, cyanosis), arterial blood gases, and oxygen saturation (pulse oximetry).	Helps to detect changes in the respiratory status that would indicate heart failure. Arterial blood gases would also provide information regarding metabolic state. If decreased tissue perfusion is widespread, anaerobic metabolism occurs with subsequent metabolic acidosis.
Monitor cardiac rhythms on continuous patient monitor and the results of a 12 lead EKG.	Reveals abnormal tracings that would indicate infarction or ischemia. In the presence of MI characteristic changes include ST segment elevation (STEMI), T wave inversion, and an abnormal Q wave. In some cases there is non-ST wave elevation (NSTEMI).
Prepare patient for insertion of any catheters for invasive monitoring (pulmonary artery catheter, intra-arterial line), and monitor readings as ordered or according to agency protocol.	The pulmonary artery catheter can evaluate left ventricular and overall cardiac function (cardiac output) through measurements of pressures in the right atrium, pulmonary artery, and left ventricle. The arterial line allows direct monitoring of systolic, diastolic, and mean arterial blood pressure.
Assess results of cardiac enzymes (total CPK, CK-MB, total LDH, LDH-1, LDH-2, troponin, myoglobin, C-reactive protein) ordered by physician.	These enzymes elevate in the presence of myocardial infarction at differing times and monitoring them assists in ruling out a myocardial infarction as the cause of the chest pain.
Anticipate dysrhythmias secondary to ischemia and infarction: premature ventricular contraction (PVC), ventricular tachycardia, ventricular fibrillation, AV block (especially with anterior wall infarct), bradydysrhythmias	Dysrhythmias are common, occurring in 80 percent of patients following myocardial infarction. Early detection is key to treatment and decreased mortality. The type of dysrhythmia depends upon
(especially with inferior wall infarction).	the area of the myocardium affected. Risk of ventricular fibrillation, the most common cause of sudden death, is greatest in the first 4 hours.
Monitor for change in mental status: restlessness, confusion, and agitation.	These are indicators of decreased cerebral tissue perfusion as a result of decreased cardiac output.
Establish intravenous line with large bore catheter.	Intravenous lines are required for administration of medications quickly and for better absorption. In some instances two lines are required for simultaneous administration of medications and because of incompatibility of medications.
Administer thrombolytic agents (streptokinase, tissue plasminogen activator) as ordered or according to agency protocol.	These agents dissolve the thrombus by targeting the fibrin component of the coronary thrombus and should be given within 6 hours of the coronary event. Contraindications for their use include recent stroke; known bleeding disorders; or recent abdominal, head, or spine surgery.
Evaluate for positive response (relief of chest pain, reperfusion dysrhythmias, ST segment returns to normal) and negative response (signs of bleeding: elevated pulse, decreased blood pressure, blood in body fluids) to thrombolytic administration.	Positive responses indicate a reperfusion of the myocardium, and negative signs indicate bleeding has occurred as a side effect of administration.
Administer morphine sulfate as ordered or according to agency protocol.	Decreases myocardial oxygen demand; reduces anxiety; reduces pain.
Administer amiodarone intravenously as ordered.	For prophylaxis and treatment of life-threatening ventricular dysrhythmias; decreases peripheral resistance and increases coronary blood flow.
Administer nitroglycerin as ordered.	Medications such as the vasodilator nitroglycerin enhance blood flow to the myocardium, reducing amount of blood returning to the heart and decreasing preload, which in turn decreases workload of the heart and the demand of the myocardium for oxygen.

(continues)

(continued)

INTERVENTIONS	RATIONALES
Administer cardio-selective beta blockers as ordered (usually within the first 24 hours).	To slow heart rate and decrease the force of cardiac contraction, thus prolonging the period of diastole and increasing myocardial perfusion while reducing the force of myocardial contraction; also decreases oxygen consumption by the myocardium.
Assess response to medications.	Determines effectiveness of medication and whether further interventions are required. Continued chest pain represents continued ischemia and damage to the myocardium.
Provide oxygen and monitor oxygen saturation via pulse oximetry, as ordered.	Oxygenation increases the amount of circulating oxygen in the blood, and therefore increases the amount of available oxygen to the myocardium, decreasing myocardial ischemia and pain.
Establish a quiet environment.	Reduces the energy demands on the patient.
Elevate head of bed.	Improves chest expansion and oxygenation.
Provide small meals or liquids as ordered and feed the patient.	Reduces cardiac workload required of digestion; feeding the patient conserves energy.
Assess urine output.	As cardiac output decreases, perfusion to kidneys may decrease resulting in impaired kidney function with resultant decreased urinary output.

NIC *Cardiac care: Acute*
  Respiratory monitoring
  Hemodynamic regulation
  Invasive hemodynamic monitoring
  Acid/base monitoring
  Pain management
  Oxygen therapy
  Vital signs monitoring

Evaluation

Evaluate the degree to which the outcome criteria has been met. The patient should report an absence of pain. Hemodynamic monitoring should reveal stable myocardium function; vital signs should return to baseline. The extent to which the myocardium has been reperfused should be evaluated by examining the cardiac monitor strips and EKG changes.

Community/Home Care

The patient who has had a myocardial infarction will require frequent follow-up once at home. Most patients experience some degree of anxiety regarding their prognosis and their limitations. Lifestyle changes are crucial to success of the therapeutic regimen and may prove to be difficult for the patient. The availability of support persons, such as family, friends, and support groups, to assist in the plan will enhance success and serve to allay some anxiety. When at home, many patients may be anxious about the possibility of pain and engage in extreme self-limiting of activities. While many patients may have concern for sexual activity and/or sexual functioning following a myocardial infarction, few may be willing to initiate discussion of the topic. The health care provider has a responsibility to discuss this issue and give the patient needed information regarding sexual performance as it relates to cardiac function. The patient should be referred to a home health agency for follow-up and to a cardiac rehabilitation program. It is important to teach the patient what to do if pain occurs and when to seek medical attention. Changes in lifestyle, such as exercise, stress reduction, and heart-healthy diets may be required to improve cardiac health. Referral to a dietitian may be required for diet instruction. As with any regimen, recommendations should consider the possible influence of any cultural or religious practices on the patient's willingness to comply. Availability of resources, such as finances and transportation, needs to be investigated prior to discharge.

Documentation

Document all baseline assessment findings (particularly cardiovascular and respiratory) and subsequent findings, including vital signs. Readings from hemodynamic monitoring should be charted according to agency requirements. Chart patient complaints of pain, interventions implemented for relief, and the patient's response. All interventions should be documented according to agency protocol to include the patient's response to the intervention. Particular attention should be given to the documentation of the patient's response to medical treatments, such as thrombolytic therapy. Any untoward findings, such as bleeding or decreased urinary output, should also be included in the patient record. Teaching should be documented with a clear indication of what was taught and the patient's understanding of the content.

NURSING DIAGNOSIS 2

 ## ACUTE PAIN

Related to:

Decreased myocardial oxygenation, ischemia

Defining Characteristics:

Complains of chest pain radiating to arm, jaw, or other atypical place

Facial grimace/moaning

Goal:

Pain is relieved.

Outcome Criteria

✔ The patient reports that pain has been relieved.

NOC *Pain level*

Pain control

Medication response

INTERVENTIONS	RATIONALES
Assess onset, characteristic, location, and intensity of pain.	Gives indications of severity of myocardial damage, and helps rule out other causes of pain.
Administer oxygen, as ordered, to maintain oxygenation saturation at > 92 percent.	Improves myocardial oxygenation and decreases myocardial ischemia, which causes pain.
Administer pain medications (usually IV: nitroglycerin or morphine sulfate) as ordered.	Reduces pain and anxiety; vasodilation and sedative effects improve myocardial oxygen consumption and reduce myocardial oxygen demand.
Maintain a calm, quiet environment.	Helps to relax patient and decrease anxiety.

Administer beta blockers as ordered.	Blocks stimulation of the sympathetic nervous system, which in turn slows heart rate and reduces systolic blood pressure, thus decreasing oxygen consumption.
Administer calcium channel blockers as ordered.	Calcium channel blockers lead to increased vasodilation, which leads to decreased myocardial oxygen consumption.
Assess patient response to medication.	Helps to determine if further interventions are required.
Place patient in a comfortable position, usually upright.	Decreases anxiety; upright position improves chest expansion and oxygenation.

NIC *Pain management*

Oxygen therapy

Evaluation

Assess the patient for resolution of chest pain. A pain-rating scale or the absence of nonverbal indicators can be used to evaluate the outcome. If the pain is not completely resolved, explore new methods for relief.

Community/Home Care

The patient may have some degree of anxiety when discharged about the possibility of experiencing chest pain and therefore may actually limit all activities. Discussion of activities that may cause the patient to have chest pain should be identified. The patient will need to know how to prevent chest pain and what to do if pain is not relieved. A modification of activities while the patient is going through cardiac rehabilitation will be required. Follow-up with the health care provider is important to monitor cardiac status and the progression of activities. Medications for chest pain, such as nitroglycerin tablets, will probably be prescribed, and the patient will need to understand when and how to take them, as well as the common side effects to be expected. The patient should be encouraged to participate in activities that increase cardiac function, ideally through a cardiac rehabilitation program.

Documentation

Chart a description of the pain in the patient's own words. Document all interventions, pharmacological and non-pharmacological, implemented for pain relief. Always document the patient response to the interventions and the degree to which pain relief was obtained (total relief or just a reduction). If nitroglycerin is given, document according to agency standards to include amount of time required for relief; if relief was not obtained and subsequent medications such as morphine were given, document this thoroughly in the record.

NURSING DIAGNOSIS 3

 ## ACTIVITY INTOLERANCE

Related to:

Increased oxygen demands when activity increases, causing myocardial ischemia

Weakness and fatigue

Defining Characteristics:

Chest pain with exertion

Goal:

The patient is able to tolerate activities.

Outcome Criteria

✔ The patient is able to walk 10 feet without shortness of breath.

✔ The patient is able to progress activities each day.

✔ The patient performs activities without pain.

NOC *Activity tolerance*

Energy conservation

INTERVENTIONS	RATIONALES
Obtain subjective data from the patient regarding normal activities prior to onset of the myocardial infarction.	Determines the effect the heart attack has had on the patient's ability to be active and allows for a better plan for future activity regimen.
Progress activity as ordered and in keeping with cardiac rehabilitation protocol; usually bedrest is maintained for the first 24 hours, followed by bedside commode and short periods out of bed in chair.	Slow progression of activities allows the myocardium to adapt; if increased physical activity causes pain, activity should be reduced until oxygenation is adequate and pain control has been achieved.
Encourage periods of rest and activity during the day; nursing staff should provide assistance as needed.	Conserves oxygen.
Gradually increase activity as tolerated and share guidelines for progression with patient.	Activities should be increased gradually, as tolerated, to avoid overtaxing cardiac system.
Teach the patient about the cardiac rehabilitation program required to improve patient's activity tolerance.	Knowledge of a specific program of activity will provide a guideline to follow and enhance compliance. Cardiac rehabilitation is an activity program that begins with admission to the hospital and continues through the outpatient recovery phase; it includes phases of activity with periodic medical evaluation, education, and modification of risk factors.
Monitor vital signs and oxygen saturation before and after activity.	Use the results to indicate when activity may be increased or decreased.
Teach patient about appropriate expectations for sexual activity and the use of nitroglycerin.	Patient may have concern about future sexual activity; nitroglycerin taken before sexual activity can decrease the chance of chest pain by increasing the supply of oxygen to the myocardium.
Teach patient how to organize activities once at home and what to do if pain occurs. If patient lives alone, explore the feasibility of in-home assistance for household chores until recovery is complete.	Gives patient a sense of control and helps decrease anxiety; performance of chores may not be tolerated for a period of time.

NIC *Cardiac precautions*

Energy management

Teaching: Prescribed activity/exercise

Evaluation

Evaluate whether the patient has achieved the stated desired outcomes. The patient verbalizes that he or she is able to carry out desired activities without chest pain. After engaging in activity, the patient's pulse, blood pressure, and respirations return to baseline values following rest. The patient should verbalize an understanding of the cardiac rehabilitation program and requirements for continued activity at home.

Community/Home Care

Ensure that the patient has all of his or her questions answered regarding activities allowed and increasing endurance. As an outpatient, the patient should actively participate in a cardiac rehabilitation program that can provide guidance with activities as well as medical supervision in the initial phase of recovery. Once at home, the patient should be aware of the increased demands on the cardiac system when climbing stairs. If bedrooms are upstairs, the patient may have to make other sleeping arrangements temporarily until activity tolerance has improved. It is important that the patient is at ease asking and getting answers to concerns about ability to engage in sexual activities. The proper protocol for nitroglycerin administration as needed for chest pain or anticipated exertion should be discussed. In rural areas, formal cardiac rehabilitation programs may not be an option, so the patient will need structured detailed instructions on activity programs. A health care provider should follow up to ensure that the patient is adapting to changes in health status.

Documentation

The nurse should chart the patient's tolerance for activity, including vital signs, oxygen saturation, and presence/absence of chest pain. Document types of activities the patient is able to perform and duration of the activity. If referrals have been made for cardiac rehabilitation programs, document this in the notes.

NURSING DIAGNOSIS 4

 ANXIETY

Related to:

Chest pain

Threat to self-image

Fear of dying

Deficient knowledge

Defining Characteristics:

Restlessness

Denial

Anger

Verbalizes anxiety

Goal:

Anxiety is relieved.

Outcome Criteria

✔ The patient verbalizes that anxiety has been reduced.

✔ The patient states that he or she is relaxed.

✔ The patient has no physiological signs of anxiety.

✔ The patient asks appropriate questions about disease.

NOC *Anxiety control*
         Acceptance: Health status

INTERVENTIONS	RATIONALES
Have patient rate anxiety on a numerical scale.	Allows for a more objective measure of anxiety level.
Provide oxygen, as ordered.	Helps patient to breathe easier so that he or she faces less physical stress (which can lead to anxiety).
Control pain, as appropriate and as ordered.	Reduction of pain will help to reduce anxiety level.
Reassure patient by explaining myocardial infarction, treatments, and tests.	Fear of the unknown contributes to higher levels of anxiety; knowing what to expect helps the patient maintain control of environment.
Encourage patient to verbalize concerns about health status.	Verbalizing concerns can help patient deal with issues and avoid negative feelings.
After an acute cardiac episode, educate patient/family concerning disease and treatment modalities.	An educated patient/family can be more proactive in helping the patient prevent/control pain and anxiety; gives patient a sense of control; during acute episodes the patient may not be able to learn effectively.
Stay with patient during episodes of pain and use a calm manner.	Allows the nurse to offer comfort, care, and assurances to reduce anxiety and fear.
After the acute cardiac episode is controlled, teach patient relaxation techniques (such as slow, purposeful breathing) and encourage their use.	During the acute phase the patient may not be ready to learn. Teaching reduces anxiety and creates a feeling of comfort.

NIC *Anxiety reduction*
      Calming technique
      Emotional support
      Presence

Evaluation

Assess the patient for the extent that they are free of anxiety. The patient should verbalize that anxiety is reduced and that he or she feels comfortable. Assess the patient for physiological signs of anxiety, such as increased pulse and sweating. During evaluation, be sure to inquire about the use of relaxation techniques. The patient will also need to report that he or she understands the disease process that has changed his or her health status.

Community/Home Care

The patient will need to know how to control anxiety in the home setting. It is crucial that health care providers equip the patient with knowledge to make the patient feel in control of his or her health. A patient who knows how to treat the chest pain and modify his or her lifestyle accordingly will have fewer incidences of anxiety and fear. By ensuring that the patient understands the health care regimen and knows what to do if acute symptoms develop, the health care provider may prevent unnecessary emergency room visits.

Documentation

Document the degree of anxiety experienced by the patient. Using some type of numerical rating scale similar to the pain scale will provide health care providers with a more objective measure of the degree of anxiety the patient is experiencing. Document any physiological or observable signs of anxiety, such as restlessness, tachycardia, or diaphoresis. Interventions implemented to treat these should be documented, along with subsequent assessments to determine their effectiveness.

NURSING DIAGNOSIS 5

INEFFECTIVE THERAPEUTIC REGIMEN MANAGEMENT

Related to:

Insufficient knowledge of myocardial infarction

New onset of disease

Complex nature of therapeutic regimen

Defining Characteristics:

Asks questions/has concerns

Asks no questions about health status

Denies having serious illness

Goal:

Patient verbalizes an understanding of required treatments and changes in lifestyle.

Outcome Criteria

✔ The patient verbalizes a desire to learn necessary information.

✔ The patient verbalizes a willingness to keep appointments and follow prescribed regimen.

✔ The patient demonstrates knowledge of myocardial infarction.

✔ The patient demonstrates knowledge of medications and changes in lifestyle such as diet, activity restrictions, and stress reduction required to promote health.

NOC *Knowledge: Disease process*
      Knowledge: Treatment regimen
      Compliance behavior

INTERVENTIONS	RATIONALES
Assess patient's current knowledge as well as his or her ability to learn and readiness to learn.	Teachings need to be tailored to the patient's ability and willingness to learn for maximum effectiveness.
Identify a family member or significant other who will also learn the content and assist the patient with compliance.	This person can reinforce the teaching and assist with implementation if the client becomes incapable of follow through.
Create a quiet environment conducive to learning.	Environmental noise and distractions can prevent the learner from focusing on what is being taught.
Teach the learners about the pathophysiology of myocardial infarction, including complications, in the initial teaching session.	Patient must understand what the disease is and how it affects the body before understanding the rationale for treatments.

INTERVENTIONS	RATIONALES
Be attuned to the patient's religious and cultural practices when teaching.	Culturally competent care that also considers religious practices is a holistic individualized approach that will enhance compliance.
Make appropriate referrals to a dietitian for instruction about the prescribed diet, including information about sodium, fat, and cholesterol restrictions, taking into consideration the patient's normal diet and any cultural/religious needs.	Understanding the rationale for these interventions will enhance compliance and considering cultural/religious preferences will increase the likelihood that the prescribed changes will be assimilated into the patient's routine.
Teach the learners about prescribed medications (nitroglycerin, beta blockers, aspirin, calcium channel blockers, digoxin) or others, as ordered, including information about action, side effects, and dosing schedule.	Knowledge of why the medication is needed and how it works will focus on the importance of the medication. Identification of side effects will minimize anxiety if these untoward effects should occur.
Teach the patient the activity regimen, particularly about the cardiac rehabilitation program. Include in the teaching required activity restrictions, how to progress exercise gradually while monitoring responses, and how to determine when to eliminate an activity. Inform the patient to stop any activity that produces chest pain or dizziness.	Incorporation of exercise into daily routine is needed to strengthen cardiac muscle.
Teach the patient which signs and symptoms to report to a health care provider: increased shortness of breath, chest pain unrelieved by nitroglycerin, swelling of feet and ankles, and severe activity intolerance.	Monitoring for signs and symptoms early can prevent a crisis that requires hospitalization.
Teach patient and family/significant others about relaxation techniques.	Practicing relaxation decreases anxiety and decreases oxygen consumption by myocardium.
Ask patient to repeat information and ask questions as needed.	This allows the nurse to hear in the patient's own words what was taught and makes it easier to know what information may need to be reinforced.
Establish that the patient has the resources required to be compliant.	If needed resources such as finances, transportation, and psychosocial support are not available, the patient cannot be compliant.
Refer to appropriate disciplines as needed (social worker, dietitian, home health nurse, physical therapist, etc.).	These disciplines can provide additional services to help the patient be compliant with prescribed regimen.
Give printed material of the information covered in teaching session to the patient.	The patient may be more comfortable at home knowing that there is printed material for future reference.

NIC *Teaching: Prescribed activity/exercise*
Teaching: Prescribed diet
Teaching: Disease process
Teaching: Prescribed medication
Learning readiness enhancement
Learning facilitation

Evaluation

Evaluate the degree to which the patient has achieved the expected outcomes. The patient verbalizes an understanding of the therapeutic regimen, including change in lifestyle behaviors that are required. When asked, the patient is able to repeat all information for the nurse and asks questions about the prescribed regimen (activity, diet, disease process). The patient can identify all medications by name and report the common side effects as well as the dosing schedule. The patient should be able to inform the nurse when health care assistance should be sought. The nurse must determine whether the patient is capable of being compliant, as well as whether the patient expresses a willingness to comply. Once this is established, it is crucial to determine that the patient has the necessary resources and information to manage his or her heart disease effectively.

Community/Home Care

For patients who have had a myocardial infarction, home care is crucial. Once at home, the patient may be anxious or unsure about the medical regimen. Successful management will depend on the patient's understanding of the information provided in teaching sessions and the internal motivation to implement health-promoting behaviors. Changes in lifestyle may be difficult at first, and reinforcement through follow-up home visits or telephone consultation may be required. Because of the complexity of the regimen with a variety of medications, activity requirements, and diet changes, the risk for non-compliance is high. The patient will need to establish a routine that includes activity and rest, medication scheduling, and meals. Special diets generally require more thought, planning, and preparation, so the person who prepares meals will need to plan for this additional time. The patient needs clear-cut instructions from a cardiac rehabilitation program for progression of activity, such as guidelines for a home walking program. As the patient resumes more of his or her normal activity following a myocardial infarction, he or she may discover that some activities cannot be resumed. Frequently, the patient has questions regarding resumption of sexual activities but feels uncomfortable initiating the topic, so the nurse or other health care provider following the patient should breach the subject. Cardiac support groups may provide social support and allay anxiety but may not be available in rural areas.

The health care provider must work with the patient to determine a realistic approach to rehabilitation and cardiac health that considers the patient's culture, socioeconomic resources, social support systems, and religion.

Documentation

Document the specific content taught and the titles of printed materials given to the patient or family. Chart the patient's understanding of the content and the methods used to evaluate learning. The nurse must clearly indicate areas that need to be reinforced. After the teaching session is complete, the nurse should determine if the patient indicates a willingness to comply with health care recommendations. If the teaching included a significant other, indicate this in the documentation. In addition, any referrals made should be documented in the patient record.

CHAPTER 1.15

PERICARDITIS: ACUTE

GENERAL INFORMATION

Pericarditis is an inflammation of the pericardial sac and the outer layer of the myocardium. Most often it is idiopathic, but it may occur as a result of an infection (usually viral), or it may be primary. Other causes include connective tissue disease (such as lupus erythematosus), uremia, malignancy, postmyocardial infection (Dressler's syndrome), or post-pericardiotomy/ectomy. Classic symptoms of acute pericarditis are chest pain with a pericardial friction rub and a low-grade fever. The disease most often affects men under the age of 50.

NURSING DIAGNOSIS 1

 ACUTE PAIN

Related to:

Pericardial inflammation

Defining Characteristics:

Complaint of sharp chest pain

Increased pain with respirations, coughing or activity

Goal:

Pain has been relieved.

Outcome Criteria

The patient will verbalize that pain has been relieved 30 minutes after interventions. The patient will verbalize an understanding of what causes pain.

NOC *Pain level*
Pain control
Comfort level

INTERVENTIONS	RATIONALES
Assess for location, intensity, quality, and precipitating factors.	Identifying these will assist in accurate diagnosis and treatment.
Have the patient rate pain intensity using a pain-rating scale.	Provides a more objective description of level of pain.
Assess heart sounds for abnormalities.	A pericardial friction rub is a characteristic sign of pericarditis, and in the presence of pericardial effusion heart sounds may sound distant or muffled.
Assess respiratory status.	Helps detect early signs of respiratory complications; in the presence of pericardial effusion, dyspnea and coughing may occur.
Monitor patient for signs of cardiac tamponade (paradoxical pulse, narrowed pulse pressure, dyspnea, tachycardia, distended neck veins, decreased blood pressure, diminished or absent pulses in carotid or femoral arteries during inspiration).	If pericardial effusion develops, the fluid in the pericardial sac may cause increased compression of the myocardium, which severely compromises cardiac output; monitoring for signs increases chance for early intervention to prevent a medical emergency.
Take vital signs, including temperature, every 4 hours.	Detects the presence of fever or signs of cardiac complications.
Monitor results of diagnostic and laboratory tests (CBC, ESR, cardiac enzymes, EKG, chest x-ray, CT scan).	Tests such as cardiac enzymes and EKG will help to rule out myocardial infarction; CBC will reveal an elevated WBC indicative of inflammation/ infection; ESR elevation will indicate acute inflammation; chest x-ray will reveal cardiac enlargement if the patient has pericardial effusion; CT scan will show more definitive films of the cardiac system and may be ordered if pericardial effusion is suspected.

(continues)

(continued)

INTERVENTIONS	RATIONALES
Administer analgesics (usually high doses of aspirin and NSAIDs) as ordered.	Reduces inflammatory response, reduces fever, and provides analgesia.
Assist in treating underlying causes (administer antibiotics if bacterial infectious process, give corticosteroids for patients with systemic causes, such as lupus or rheumatoid arthritis).	Treating the underlying cause will alleviate the pain.
Assist patient in assuming a sitting position, leaning forward; provide over-bed table to rest on; avoid recumbent positions.	Reduces pericardial pain by preventing the heart from making contact with thoracic wall/lung pleura.
Implement strategies to reduce anxiety (see nursing diagnosis "Anxiety").	Anxiety often intensifies the pain experience.
Assess effectiveness of interventions to relieve pain.	Determines whether interventions have been effective in relieving pain or whether new strategies need to be employed.

NIC *Pain management*
   Analgesic administration
   Anxiety reduction

Evaluation

The patient is able to report that the pain has been relieved or alleviated following interventions. The degree to which the patient is able to identify precipitating factors and assist in the management of the pain through anxiety reduction and relaxation techniques is assessed.

Community/Home Care

The patient will be at home where treatment with anti-inflammatory and analgesic medications will be continued to treat the pain. It is important that the patient at home understands clearly the role of these medications in the resolution of pericarditis. Instruct the patient to take medications with food or milk to prevent the gastrointestinal (GI) distress that often accompanies long-term therapy. At home the patient will need to monitor self for signs of GI bleeding, such as blood in stool or vomiting of blood. A home-health nurse or other health care worker should examine the patient's other medications to be sure that there are no interactions. Follow-up care should monitor the patient for development of chronic

constrictive pericarditis. The patient will need to know what type of manifestations would indicate cardiac complications that would require that they return to the physician.

Documentation

Document in the patient's own words the description of the pain and his or her rating of the level of pain. Chart the patient's response to all interventions. Include in the documentation assessments made relevant to the cardiac and respiratory systems. Specific assessments that are required include heart sounds and temperature. All teaching should be indicated in the patient record with an indication of the patient's level of understanding.

NURSING DIAGNOSIS 2

ANXIETY

Related to:
   Severe chest pain

Defining Characteristics:
   Restless
   Verbalizes anxiety

Goal:
   Anxiety is relieved.

Outcome Criteria

✔ The patient states that anxiety level has been reduced.

✔ The patient reports that he or she is relaxed.

NOC *Anxiety self-control*

INTERVENTIONS	RATIONALES
Have patient rate anxiety on a numerical scale.	Allows for a more objective measure of anxiety level.
Control pain, as appropriate and as ordered.	Reduction of pain will help to reduce anxiety level.
Reassure patient by explaining the process of the disease (acute pericarditis).	Fear of the unknown contributes to higher levels of anxiety; knowing what to expect helps the patient maintain a sense of control.

INTERVENTIONS	RATIONALES
Encourage the patient to verbalize concerns about health status.	Verbalizing concerns can help the patient deal with anxiety.
Educate the patient/family concerning pericarditis and treatment modalities.	An educated patient/family can be more proactive in controlling pain and anxiety; gives patient a sense of control.
Stay with the patient during episodes of pain and use a calm manner.	Allows nurse to offer comfort, care, and assurances to reduce anxiety and fear.
Teach patient relaxation techniques (such as slow, purposeful breathing) and encourage their use.	Reduces anxiety and creates a feeling of comfort.

NIC *Anxiety reduction*
Calming technique
Emotional support

Evaluation

Assess the patient for the extent that he or she is free of anxiety. The patient should verbalize that anxiety is reduced and that he or she feels comfortable. Assess the patient for physiological signs of anxiety, such as increased pulse and sweating. During evaluation, be sure to inquire about the use of relaxation techniques. The patient will also need to report that he or she understands the disease process that has changed his or her health status.

Community/Home Care

The patient will need to know how to control anxiety in the home setting. It is crucial that health care providers equip the patient with knowledge to make the patient feel in control of his or her health. A variety of anxiety-reducing strategies should be explained to the patient and their use encouraged at home. Simple methods such as reading, deep breathing, or guided imagery can be used at any time. A patient who understands his or her diagnosis (pericarditis), including prognosis and how to treat the pain, will have fewer incidences of anxiety and fear. Be sure that the patient understands the medication regimen, including rationale for use, actions, and side effects. Written instructions on dosing may prove to be beneficial for reference at a later time. By ensuring that the patient understands the health care regimen and knows what to do if symptoms of complications develop, the health care provider may prevent unnecessary emergency room visits.

Documentation

Document the degree of anxiety experienced by the patient. Using some type of numerical rating scale similar to the pain scale will provide health care providers with a more objective measure of the degree of anxiety the patient is experiencing. Document any physiological or observable signs of anxiety, such as restlessness, tachycardia, or diaphoresis. Interventions that have been implemented to treat these should be documented along with subsequent assessments to determine their effectiveness.

NURSING DIAGNOSIS 3

INEFFECTIVE BREATHING PATTERN

Related to:

Pain with respiratory movement

Pericardial inflammation

Defining Characteristics:

Shallow respirations

Guarded respirations

Goal:

Respirations will be effective for gas exchange.

Outcome Criteria

✔ Respiratory rate will be at patient's baseline (14–24).

✔ Respirations will be effective in maintaining oxygen saturation at > 90 percent.

✔ The patient will not experience shortness of breath.

NOC *Respiratory status: Ventilation*

INTERVENTIONS	RATIONALES
Assess respiratory system by noting respiratory rate, depth, chest expansion, rhythm, and breath sounds.	Establish a baseline for comparison for early detection of cardiopulmonary complications and to determine if the patient's breathing is shallow, which decreases ability to ventilate effectively for adequate gas exchange.

(continues)

(continued)

INTERVENTIONS	RATIONALES
Monitor oxygen saturation and arterial blood gases as ordered.	Provides information on effectiveness of respirations.
Encourage the use of splints or pillows if pain is present.	Splinting the chest when breathing allows for comfort by providing support.
Encourage deep breathing and coughing.	Increases chest expansion, air movement, and prevents atelectasis.
Control pain through use of prescribed analgesics.	Respiratory movement causes pain, especially with inspiration, and causes the patient to breathe shallowly in an effort to prevent pain.
Position patient in an upright position leaning forward.	Decreases pericarditis pain and provides for maximum chest expansion.

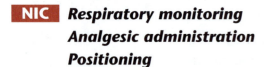

NIC *Respiratory monitoring*
Analgesic administration
Positioning

Evaluation

Evaluate the patient's respiratory status to determine if outcomes have been met. The patient's respirations should be within baseline or between 14–24 breaths per minute. Breath sounds should be clear with movement of air at bases, and there should be no shortness of breath. Pulse oximetry should reveal an oxygen saturation of > 90 percent.

Community/Home Care

At home, the patient should continue to practice deep breathing as long as pericarditis pain persists. It should be stressed that once at home the patient will need to maintain activity as prescribed to enhance respiratory functioning and prevent atelectasis. The patient needs to recognize signs and symptoms that may indicate respiratory complications from atelectasis (fever, congestion, shortness of breath) such as pneumonia. If respiratory status becomes compromised, the patient and family should contact a health care provider for follow-up care.

Documentation

Document respiratory assessment findings to include respiratory rate, depth, rhythm, and breath sounds. Describe exactly how the patient is breathing. Results of pulse oximetry should be documented as well. Chart planned deep-breathing exercises and positions that the patient assumes for comfort of respirations. Always include in the patient record the patient's specific response to therapeutic interventions.

CHAPTER 1.16

PULMONARY HYPERTENSION AND COR PULMONALE

GENERAL INFORMATION

Pulmonary hypertension is defined as the presence of increased pressure in the pulmonary artery that is continuous (systolic > 30 mm Hg and diastolic > 15 mm Hg). Pulmonary hypertension will occur because of resistance (from disease) or an obstruction in the lungs. Because the right side of the heart works harder to overcome the resistance in the lungs, the right ventricular wall thickens, causing the right ventricle to hypertrophy until it can no longer handle the work to overcome the resistance, which leads to right-sided heart failure. Primary pulmonary hypertension is a rare occurrence, with no known cause. Secondary pulmonary hypertension is more common and is caused by reduced size of the pulmonary vascular bed, which may be due to vasoconstriction or widespread vessel destruction or obstruction (Lemone and Burke, 2004). Clinical manifestations include those of the underlying respiratory disease, as well as dull, retrosternal chest pain, and syncope on exertion. Primary pulmonary hypertension is a progressive disorder that primarily affects women between the ages of 30–40 years and most often results in death within 4 years if not treated with bilateral lung transplantation (Lemone and Burke, 2004).

Cor pulmonale is defined as the dilation and hypertrophy of the right ventricle with subsequent right-sided heart failure. It occurs most often as a result of sustained pulmonary hypertension secondary to chronic obstructive pulmonary disease. Other conditions affecting the lungs that would cause pulmonary obstructions include reactive airway disease, bronchitis, bronchiectasis, and cystic fibrosis, as well as a pulmonary embolism. Certain restrictive lung diseases can also cause back pressure into the right ventricle and result in cor pulmonale: pneumonia, atelectasis, sarcoidosis, and interstitial fibrosis. Clinical manifestations are those of the underlying respiratory disease as well as those of right-sided heart failure, such as distended neck veins, peripheral edema, chronic productive cough, dyspnea, and wheezing.

NURSING DIAGNOSIS 1

IMPAIRED GAS EXCHANGE

Related to:

Alveolar wall damage

Stiffening of pulmonary vasculature

Increased pulmonary vascular resistance

Defining Characteristics:

Dyspnea on exertion

Fatigue

Wheezing

Chronic productive cough (cor pulmonale)

Retrosternal or substernal pain (cor pulmonale)

Exertional syncope

Goal:

Gas exchange is adequate.

Outcome Criteria

✔ Oxygen saturation is > 90 percent.

✔ The patient's respiratory rate is within baseline.

✔ The patient reports no dyspnea/shortness of breath.

NOC *Respiratory status: Ventilation*
Respiratory status: Gas exchange
Tissue perfusion: Pulmonary
Vital signs

INTERVENTIONS	RATIONALES
Assess respiratory status: skin color, breath sounds, respiratory rate, rhythm, quality, effort.	Establishes baseline information about respiratory function.
Assess oxygen saturation using pulse oximetry and arterial blood gases, as ordered.	Helps to determine status of oxygen to tissues and monitor for respiratory acidosis.
Monitor for altered mental status: restlessness, anxiety, and confusion.	These symptoms may indicate decreased oxygenation to cerebral tissues.
Provide supplemental oxygen as ordered.	Helps to maximize oxygen saturation and relieve shortness of breath.
Place in high Fowler's position.	This position allows for better chest expansion and subsequent air exchange.
Give bronchodilators as ordered (orally or inhaled via nebulizer, or handheld inhaler) and evaluate effectiveness.	Opens narrowed airways and improves gas exchange.
If thick secretions are present due to underlying lung disease, give mucolytics or expectorants.	Assists with mucous excretion, which will help to clear lungs of substances that cause obstruction and increased vascular resistance.
Have patient perform coughing and deep breathing.	Prevents stasis of secretions, open airways and improves gas exchange.
Allow a balance of rest and activity; encourage rest before and after activity assisting with activities of daily living.	Conserves oxygen reserves and prevents exacerbation of hypoxia.
Stay with patient during activities, especially during acute episodes of shortness of breath.	Allows nurse to monitor for exertional syncope and to prevent injury.
Teach patient about disease process, treatments required, and home care (see nursing diagnosis "Ineffective Management of Therapeutic Regimen").	Knowledge of disease and treatment required enhances compliance and allows patient to be in control.

NIC *Oxygen therapy*
Respiratory monitoring
Acid/base management:
   Respiratory acidosis
Positioning

Evaluation

Evaluate the status of outcome criteria. The patient should have indicators of good gas exchange, such as even, easy respirations and an oxygen saturation of at least 90 percent. Blood gas analyses should indicate an absence of respiratory acidosis and oxygen levels between 80 and 100 percent. The patient should report an absence of shortness of breath and respirations within baseline.

Community/Home Care

For patients with pulmonary hypertension or cor pulmonale, the progression of the disease depends on the chronicity of the underlying cause. The common lung diseases that cause these conditions almost always require some long-term use of home treatments. Usual activity patterns may need to be adjusted in the home until any shortness of breath is controlled. The patient will need to learn how to balance rest and activity based on his or her usual activity pattern, which may necessitate naps or obtaining assistance with household chores. Determining which activities are tolerable and which ones are not will require a period of trial and error. Patients who have continued shortness of breath and low oxygen saturation levels may need to consider home oxygen. If home oxygen is initiated, an assessment of the home environment for safety hazards such as open heating sources should be made. Availability of the financial resources to purchase oxygen and oxygen supplies is determined prior to discharge from the health care agency. The patient will need teaching regarding how to use oxygen and proper care of oxygen equipment. Teaching becomes crucial so that the patient and significant others can effectively demonstrate management of the disease. Referrals may need to be made to respiratory therapists, social workers, and a home health nurse for in-home follow-up.

Documentation

Included in the documentation should be a complete respiratory assessment. Chart all interventions and the patient's specific response. Results of oxygen saturation readings should be documented in addition to the patient's response to activity. Any teaching in preparation for discharge needs to be clearly documented with indications for further teaching that may be required. All referrals should be documented in the patient record as well.

NURSING DIAGNOSIS 2

FLUID VOLUME EXCESS

Related to:

Sustained increased pressure in pulmonary vasculature

Right ventricular hypertrophy

Pulmonary vasoconstriction

Defining Characteristics:

Jugular vein distention

Peripheral edema

Increased respirations

Increased blood pressure

Goal:

Fluid volume excess is decreased.

Outcome Criteria

✔ The patient will demonstrate weight loss.

✔ The patient's edema will be absent or decreased.

✔ The patient will have no distended neck veins.

NOC *Fluid balance*

Electrolyte and acid/base balance

Fluid overload severity

INTERVENTIONS	RATIONALES
Assess location and extent of edema particularly in extremities.	Helps to assess severity of the fluid excess.
Assess breath sounds for crackles.	Helps to detect early any signs of left heart failure; crackles are an indicator of fluid in the lungs and the patient should be monitored for worsening or improvement as an indicator of disease status and response to interventions.
Place patient in high Fowler's position.	Minimizes cardiac workload and decreases fluid return to the heart.
Administer diuretics, such as Lasix, as ordered.	Inhibits the reabsorption of sodium and chloride, thereby causing an increased fluid output by the kidneys.

Administer oxygen as ordered.	Improves oxygenation and peripheral perfusion.
Weigh patient daily at the same time, on the same scale, with an empty bladder, in the morning before breakfast.	The most accurate method of determining fluid volume loss is through daily weighing; 1 kilogram of weight loss = 1 liter of fluid lost. Morning weights are a better reflection of true weights since most people accumulate fluid as the day progresses.
Implement a diet low in sodium.	Sodium increases fluid retention; thus, decreasing the amount of dietary sodium intake will decrease the amount of retained fluid.
Implement fluid restrictions as ordered if respiratory symptoms or peripheral edema are pronounced.	Restricting the fluid intake can assist in decreasing circulating volume, thereby decreasing cardiac workload.
Obtain accurate intake and output.	Helps to monitor the balance between fluid consumed and urinary output; output also gives an indicator of renal perfusion.
Monitor electrolytes (especially potassium).	Diuretics cause an abnormal excretion of electrolytes.
Provide potassium supplements as ordered.	Replaces urinary potassium loss caused by diuretics.
Protect edematous skin in extremities and sacrum.	Fluid in tissue inhibits adequate circulation to the tissue, predisposing the patient to skin breakdown.
Monitor blood pressure and pulse.	Blood pressure and pulse may be elevated if the patient is experiencing the acute phase of heart failure due to pulmonary hypertension or cor pulmonale, but after therapy is implemented the patient may become hypotensive secondary to diuretic therapy.

NIC *Fluid management*

Electrolyte monitoring

Evaluation

Patient has weight loss, and urinary output is > intake. Edema is absent or decreasing, with no pitting edema. Skin in edematous dependent areas should be intact. Jugular vein distention has been alleviated.

Blood pressure returns to baseline and if left heart failure was present, breath sounds are clear. Any abnormal laboratory results return to normal levels. The patient should report the absence of shortness of breath.

Community/Home Care

Ensure that the patient at home understands the importance of monitoring fluid status. Weighing daily at home will allow the patient to notice subtle changes in fluid retention. Patients should be instructed to note clothing that becomes too tight in a short period of time, which is an indicator of fluid retention. Show the patient how to assess for development of edema. If fluid retention is detected, the patient should contact a health care provider. At home, the patient needs to limit the intake of salt and sodium rich foods. The patient should be taught how to read food labels for sodium content. Ask the patient to list the foods he or she normally has in his or her diet and use this information as a means to teach the patient about high-sodium foods. Diet instructions for home should consider the patient's normal diet, financial resources for purchase of food, and any cultural or religious preferences and restrictions. Have the patient keep a log of food and fluid intake as well as weight. Assist the patient to develop a schedule for taking prescribed diuretics that is mindful of his or her lifestyle and daily routines. Stress the need for follow-up care with a health care provider for monitoring of fluid status.

Documentation

Always document the extent to which the outcome criteria have been achieved. Record intake and output, blood pressure, pulse, weights, breath sounds, and the patient's understanding of the therapies for eliminating fluid excess.

NURSING DIAGNOSIS 3

ACTIVITY INTOLERANCE

Related to:

Impaired oxygen transport secondary to right sided heart failure because of altered pulmonary vasculature

Chronic hypoxemia

Defining Characteristics:

Dyspnea/shortness of breath with exercise

Tachypnea

Reports of fatigue

Exertional syncope

Goal:

The patient's activity level increases.

Outcome Criteria

✔ The patient will perform activities of daily living without shortness of breath.

✔ The patient will report improved ability to engage in activities such as ambulation without syncope or dyspnea.

NOC *Activity tolerance*
      Energy conservation
      Endurance

INTERVENTIONS	RATIONALES
Administer oxygen as ordered.	Improves oxygenation and thus allows an increased activity level.
Assist with activities as needed.	Conserves energy and reduces oxygen demand; the patient lacks enough oxygen reserves to perform activities independently; syncope is a common problem for secondary pulmonary hypertension and predisposes the patient to injury. Assisting with activities allows for monitoring or response to activity and enhances safety.
Progress activities gradually from getting out of bed to taking short walks.	Allows the patient an opportunity to develop a tolerance for activity over time.
Pace activities and provide rest periods before and after activity.	Reduces the demand for oxygen.
Monitor response to activity (pulse, respiratory rate, dyspnea, syncope).	Increased pulse and respirations, along with dyspnea, indicate an intolerance to the activity; syncope with exertion is a common complaint for patients with secondary pulmonary hypertension.

INTERVENTIONS	RATIONALES
Monitor electrolytes.	Treatment of the fluid excess of right-sided failure with diuretics often causes electrolyte imbalances that can cause muscle weakness and fatigue, which may in turn prevent a patient from participating in activity.
Inform patient to stop any activity that causes shortness of breath, chest pain, or dizziness.	These indicate intolerance to activity, and the level of activity being performed should be evaluated.
Collaborate with other disciplines, such as physical therapy and respiratory therapy, as ordered, to assist with ambulation.	Respiratory therapy may be needed to provide oxygen when the patient first starts an activity program, and physical therapy can assist with monitoring activity progression.

NIC *Activity therapy*
Energy management

Evaluation

The patient is able to tolerate the performance of self-care activities, and is able to walk short distances without fatigue or shortness of breath. The patient verbalizes an understanding of the need to progress activities gradually, restrict activity as needed, conserve energy, and monitor response to activity.

Community/Home Care

Patients with pulmonary hypertension and cor pulmonale may never return to their baseline level of activity performance. At home, the patient must understand how to continue progression of activities until the maximum level of functioning is achieved. Instructions should include specific activity goals, monitoring response to activity, and energy conservation. Home maintenance will require that the patient evaluate which of their usual activities or routines can be continued. The home environment is assessed for factors such as stairs and distance to the bathroom from patient's usual resting place to determine if adaptations to the environment are required.

Documentation

Document the specific activity goals prescribed for the patient. When the patient attempts an activity, document the exact activity and the patient's response to the activity. Specifically include the patient's pulse before and after activity, any complaints of shortness of breath, and any complaints of syncope.

NURSING DIAGNOSIS 4

 DECREASED CARDIAC OUTPUT

Related to:
Decreased ability of the right ventricle to pump blood into the pulmonary circulation
Accumulation of blood into venous circulation

Defining Characteristics:
Increased heart rate
Diminished peripheral pulses
Peripheral edema
Shortness of breath with activity
Neck vein distention
Chest pain

Goal:
Cardiac output will be maintained.

Outcome Criteria

✔ The patient achieves adequate cardiac output as evidenced by blood pressure and pulse within the patient's baseline.
✔ The patient will have a urinary output of > 30 ml/hour.
✔ The patient will have strong peripheral pulses.
✔ The patient will have absence of or reduced peripheral edema.

NOC *Cardiac pump effectiveness*
Circulation status
Respiratory status: Gas exchange

INTERVENTIONS	RATIONALES
Assess for abnormal heart and lung sounds, along with rate, rhythm, and depth of respirations.	Helps to detect the presence of left-sided failure which often occurs with right-sided failure. A third heart sound develops as the heart tries to fill a distended ventricle and the left ventricle becomes less compliant.

(continues)

(continued)

INTERVENTIONS	RATIONALES
Monitor results of laboratory and diagnostic tests (chest x-ray, electrocardiogram, blood urea nitrogen, electrolytes, creatinine).	Results of these tests provide clues to status of disease and response to treatments.
Monitor oxygen saturation and arterial blood gases.	Provides information regarding heart's ability to perfuse distal tissues with oxygenated blood.
Assess for hepatomegaly and abnormal liver enzymes as ordered.	Pulmonary hypertension and cor pulmonale resulting in right-sided failure cause liver engorgement that may alter hepatic functioning.
Assist patient in assuming a high Fowler's position.	Allows for better chest expansion, thereby improving pulmonary capacity.
Give oxygen as indicated by patient symptoms, oxygen saturation, and arterial blood gases.	Makes more oxygen available for gas exchange, assisting to alleviate signs of hypoxia and subsequent activity intolerance.
Administer diuretics, such as Lasix, as ordered.	Helps to reduce vascular sodium and right ventricular fluid load, decreasing peripheral edema. Diuretics prevent the reabsorption of sodium and chloride in the loop of Henle that causes water to be excreted along with the electrolytes.
Administer inotropic/cardiac glycoside agents (digitalis preparations) as ordered for signs of left-sided failure, and monitor for toxicity.	Digitalis has a positive inotropic effect on the myocardium that strengthens contractility, thus improving cardiac output.
Administer calcium channel blockers as ordered (such as Cardizem).	Reduces peripheral arterial resistance (afterload), pulmonary vascular resistance, and improves cardiac output, as well as exercise tolerance.
Administer vasodilators as ordered for patients with primary pulmonary hypertension.	Decreases right ventricular overload by dilating pulmonary blood vessels.
For patients with primary pulmonary hypertension unresponsive to other therapies, prepare for administration of Epoprostenol as prescribed according to agency protocol.	Decreases pulmonary vascular resistance through vasodilation.
Encourage periods of rest and assist with all activities.	Reduces cardiac workload and minimize myocardial oxygen consumption.

If retrosternal or sternal pain occurs, give analgesics as ordered.	Provides comfort and decreases oxygen demand.
Teach patient about disease, treatments, prognosis, and required home care.	Provides patient with needed information for management of disease and for compliance.

NIC   *Oxygen therapy*
Cardiac care: Acute
Hemodynamic regulation
Vital signs monitoring

Evaluation

The patient's cardiac output is improved. Examine the extent to which the stated outcome criteria have been achieved. The patient's peripheral edema has decreased or been alleviated and lungs are clear to auscultation. Blood pressure and pulse return to the patient's baseline and urinary output is at least 30 ml per hour on average. There is no jugular vein distention, and the patient reports no exertional dyspnea or syncope.

Community/Home Care

Patients with pulmonary hypertension and cor pulmonale will require follow-up at home because of the chronicity of the disease. For those with primary pulmonary hypertension, assistance with home management should be provided because of the short survival period in the absence of lung transplantation. If transplantation is to be undertaken, extensive teaching is required to be sure the patient is prepared for post-transplant care (see nursing care plan "Organ Transplantation"). If the medication epoprostenol is to be given at home, the patient and family will need in-home follow-up or a team of in-home providers to administer the drug and to ensure that the central lines are functional. There should be a gradual increase in activity with monitoring of response in terms of shortness of breath, increased respiratory rate, exertional syncope, and increased pulse. Patients, or their family members or significant others, need to assess the patient daily for edema, pulse rate, and chest discomfort, documenting these in a journal or notebook. In addition, weights should be recorded frequently and reported to the health care provider. It is important that the patient be supported and assisted with in-home activities while still maintaining as much independence as possible. Home care follow-up by a health care professional is required to ensure understanding and compliance with the medical regimen. This is particularly crucial for medications because most heart failure patients require a polypharmacy approach to treatment. Adherence to the regimen may be influenced by such things as work schedules, diets, religion, social support systems, and beliefs about health.

Documentation

Always document the status of achievement of outcome criteria with specific patient behaviors. Chart the blood pressure, pulse, breath sounds, assessments made relevant to edema, distended neck veins, output, and the patient's tolerance for activity. All interventions and teaching should be a part of the documentation. Include in the patient record his or her understanding of the disease process and response to the therapeutic interventions.

NURSING DIAGNOSIS 5

INEFFECTIVE THERAPEUTIC REGIMEN MANAGEMENT

Related to:

Complexity of therapeutic regimen

Insufficient knowledge

Lack of motivation

Defining Characteristics:

Verbalizes a desire to manage the prescribed regimen from the healthcare provider

Verbalizes difficulty with integrating one or more aspects of the prescribed treatment regimen

Shows no interest in learning the regimen

Goal:

The patient understands the therapeutic regimen as prescribed.

Outcome Criteria

✔ The patient demonstrates knowledge of the disease, signs, and symptoms, and verbalizes the need for follow-up health care.

✔ The patient verbalizes an understanding of medications prescribed, including their purpose/ action, side effects, and dosing schedule.

✔ The patient verbalizes an understanding of the need to incorporate activity into lifestyle as prescribed by the health care provider and verbalizes a willingness to follow activity as prescribed.

✔ The patient verbalizes an understanding of a low-sodium diet and is able to identify high-sodium foods from a list.

NOC *Knowledge: Disease process*
Knowledge: Diet
Knowledge: Medication
Knowledge: Energy conservation
Compliance behavior
Treatment behavior: Illness or injury

INTERVENTIONS	RATIONALES
Assess readiness of the patient to learn (motivation, cognitive level, physiological status).	The patient must be motivated to learn, have the capability to learn the content, and be free of distractions from learning, such as pain and shortness of breath.
Identify a family member or significant other who will also learn the content and assist the patient with compliance.	This person can reinforce the teaching and assist with implementation if the client becomes incapable of follow-through.
Create a quiet environment conducive to learning.	Environmental noise can prevent the learner from focusing on the content being taught.
Teach the learners about the pathophysiology of the disease, including complications, in the initial teaching session.	The patient must understand what the disease is and how it affects the body before understanding the rationale for treatments.
Teach the learners about the prescribed diet, including sodium restriction and possible potassium replacement if on diuretics, taking into consideration the patient's normal diet and any cultural/religious considerations.	Understanding the rationale for these interventions will enhance compliance, and considering cultural/religious preferences will increase the likelihood that the prescribed changes will be assimilated into the patient's routine.
Teach the learners about prescribed medications, including their action, side effects, and dosing schedule.	Knowledge of why the medication is needed and how it works will focus the importance of the medication. Identification

(continues)

(continued)

INTERVENTIONS	RATIONALES
	of side effects will minimize anxiety if these untoward effects should occur.
Teach learners about the required activity restrictions, including how to progress exercise gradually while monitoring responses and that some preferred activities may need to be eliminated. Instruct the learner to eliminate any activity that produces chest pain or dizziness.	Incorporation of exercise into daily routine is needed to strengthen cardiac muscle.
Teach the patient which signs and symptoms to report to a health care provider.	Monitoring for signs and symptoms early can prevent a crisis that requires hospitalization.
Evaluate the patient's understanding of all content covered by asking questions.	Helps to identify areas that require more teaching and to ensure that the patient has enough information to ensure compliance.
Give the patient written information.	Provides reference at a later time and for review.

NIC *Teaching: Prescribed activity/exercise*
Teaching: Prescribed diet
Teaching: Disease process
Teaching: Prescribed medication

Evaluation

The patient is able to repeat all information for the nurse and asks questions about the prescribed regimen (activity, diet, disease process). The patient can identify all medications by name and report the common side effects as well as the dosing schedule.

The patient should be able to inform the nurse when health care assistance should be sought.

Community/Home Care

For patients with pulmonary hypertension and cor pulmonale, home care is crucial to prevent crisis situations. In general, for patients with secondary pulmonary hypertension and cor pulmonale, the care required is similar to that for patients with COPD (see nursing care plan "COPD"). Follow-up care should focus on assessing the patient's ability to carry out the medical regimen and any financial or human resources that may be required. Vital signs and cardio-respiratory status need to be monitored in the home to detect early signs of left-sided failure. The patient should be encouraged to keep a log of vital signs, weight, and activity progression to share with health care providers. As the patient resumes more of his or her normal activities, he or she may discover that some activities cannot be resumed. In-home oxygen may be required at some point for the underlying causative disease, and if so the patient will need instructions on set-up, use, storage, and safety. If the patient smokes, he or she should be assisted to stop for two major reasons: nicotine causes vasoconstriction and worsens an already compromised cardiopulmonary system. The health care provider must work with the patient to determine a realistic activity regimen. For the patient with primary pulmonary hypertension, in-home administration of medications via a central line or port will necessitate in-home follow-up by a visiting nurse or team. In addition, for patients with primary pulmonary hypertension, the visiting nurse or other health care provider should be attuned to the need to address the patient's psychological state, especially anticipatory grieving and depression due to the short life expectancy. The severity of the disease and its poor prognosis may require that preparations be made for institutional care at some point.

CHAPTER 1.17

SHOCK: HYPOVOLEMIC

GENERAL INFORMATION

Hypovolemic shock occurs when there is an excessive loss of intravascular volume, whether through loss of blood, blood products, or other body fluids. Hypovolemic shock is the most commonly seen category of shock. The loss of volume could be due to actual loss of the fluid from the body or from shifting of fluid volume out of the circulating volume into extravascular spaces, such as that which occurs with sepsis, ascites, or burns. It can be caused by blood loss due to major trauma, massive crush injuries, gastrointestinal bleeding, a ruptured thoracic or aortic aneurysm, major burn injury, excessive diaphoresis, excessive vomiting, and excessive diarrhea. The decrease in circulating volume causes a decrease in venous return to the heart, decreased preload, and subsequently decreased cardiac output with impaired tissue perfusion. The body attempts to compensate for the loss and maintain cardiac output by selectively supplying blood to vital organs and shutting down perfusion to others. Manifestations of this compensation include tachycardia, increased rate and depth of respiration, and decreased urine output. This compensatory mechanism can only sustain tissue function temporarily, and if the process is not reversed, shock occurs. The degree of hypovolemic shock will depend upon the amount of blood/fluids lost, the rate of the loss, the age and physical condition of the patient, and the patient's compensatory mechanism response. Other clinical manifestations of hypovolemic shock include pale, cool, clammy skin; anxiety, confusion, and agitation; and decreased blood pressure.

Shock is divided into four classes by some:

—Class I: loss of up to 750 ml, up to 15 percent blood loss,

—Class II: loss of 750–1000 ml, 15 to 30 percent blood loss

—Class III: loss of 1500–2000, 30 to 40 percent blood loss

—Class IV: loss of 2000 ml or more, 40 percent or more blood loss (Phipps, Monahan, Sands, Marek, & Neighbors, 2003)

NURSING DIAGNOSIS 1

 DEFICIENT FLUID VOLUME

Related to:

Blood/fluid loss

Decreased circulating volume

Defining Characteristics:

Restlessness, agitation

Tachycardia

Hypotension

Delayed capillary refill (> 2 seconds)

Cool, clammy skin

Decreased urinary output

Goal:

Adequate fluid volume will be restored.

Outcome Criteria

✔ The patient's skin will be warm and dry; mucous membranes will be moist.

✔ The patient's blood pressure and pulse will be within pre-shock baseline.

✔ Urinary output will be ≥ 30 ml/hour.

NOC *Fluid balance*

INTERVENTIONS	RATIONALES
Establish IV access with large bore catheter (16 gauge or larger).	IV access is crucial to treatment; large gauge catheters allow for fluids to be given quickly and blood products will run best in large catheters.

(continues)

(continued)

INTERVENTIONS	RATIONALES
Administer IV fluid replacement as ordered: isotonic crystalloids such as 0.9 percent sodium chloride or lactated ringers—replace at a 3:1 ratio (3x as much fluid as the amount of fluid lost). For rapid volume expansion, human serum albumin may be given.	Fluid replacement is required to re-establish cardiac stability and circulating volume. Crystalloids are replaced at a 3:1 ratio with estimated blood loss because ⅔ of crystalloid solution diffuses out of vascular space into interstitial spaces.
If the patient is not improved (remains hypotensive) after rapid infusion of 2 liters of crystalloid fluid, prepare to administer blood. If hypovolemia is caused by blood loss, infusion of whole blood may be ordered.	Blood can be replaced at a 1:1 ratio because it remains in the intravascular volume; it is used to increase oxygen carrying capacity particularly if hemoglobin is < 12.
Warm all solutions administered for fluid replacement.	Rapid infusion of large amounts of cool or room temperature solutions can cause a drop in core body temperature.
If bleeding is present, control bleeding, as ordered or required.	External bleeding may be controlled with direct pressure, pulse-point pressure, or tourniquet. Internal bleeding may require surgical exploration.
Insert indwelling urinary catheter.	In shock states, the kidneys are hypoperfused as a compensatory mechanism and output decreases; as shock is corrected, urine output should increase. The indwelling catheter is used to accurately measure urinary output.
Monitor cardiac status: blood pressure, pulse (quality and rate), pulse pressure, and capillary refill.	Changes in blood pressure and pulse give information relevant to stage of shock. Initially, blood pressure may be normal to only slightly decreased due to compensatory mechanisms. In the compensatory and progressive stages, blood pressure decreases; pulse is rapid and thready. Capillary refill is an indicator of perfusion; in shock it is > 2 seconds.
Monitor skin temperature and color for baseline and during treatment for improvement.	Pale, cool, clammy skin indicates decreased perfusion. As treatment progresses, skin should be warm and return to normal color.
Monitor oxygen saturation using pulse oximetry. The ear or nose may need to be used.	Oxygen saturation indicates ability to perfuse tissues; in the presence of decreased cardiac

	output, perfusion to the fingers or toes may not be sufficient to obtain readings in these sites.
Monitor results of laboratory studies: hemoglobin and hematocrit, arterial blood gases, BUN, electrolytes.	Hematocrit fluctuates in response to fluid status; severe absolute loss from volume would produce a decrease in hematocrit with further drops during aggressive fluid resuscitation due to hemodilution; the hemoglobin may be decreased. If volume loss is due to third spacing, hematocrit may be high initially and decrease as fluid is restored to the intravascular space. Arterial blood gases are done to determine oxygen and carbon dioxide levels; shock often causes metabolic acidosis due to anaerobic metabolism as the respiratory and cardiac systems are unable to sustain adequate oxygenation to tissues. BUN and electrolytes would give indicators of renal function; BUN may be elevated initially, but decrease due to hemodilution of fluid replacement.
Treat the cause of the fluid loss as ordered. For diarrhea, give antidiarrheal medications; for vomiting, give anti-emetics; for ascites, give diuretics or albumin; for hemorrhaging, identify source and stop by applying pressure or surgical interventions and replace loss with blood or blood products.	Correction of underlying cause controls and corrects the fluid deficit.
If blood is administered, monitor for transfusion reaction (see nursing care plan "Blood Transfusion").	Transfusion reactions may occur due to allergenic response or immune response and need to be treated promptly.

NIC   *Fluid management*
Fluid monitoring
Fluid resuscitation
Hypovolemia management
Intravenous insertion
Intravenous therapy
Shock management: Volume
Emergency care

Evaluation

Assess the patient for return of normal fluid volume. The patient's blood pressure should return to baseline or be > 70 systolic. The pulse should be strong and regular and at the patient's baseline or only slightly increased. Skin should be warm and color should return to the patient's normal appearance. Renal function should not be impaired, with an hourly output on the average of 30 ml/hour. Following fluid replacement, the patient should also be assessed for fluid overload, which may occur in the elderly and those with chronic left ventricular disease.

Community/Home Care

Patients treated for shock secondary to deficient fluid volume have normal fluid status restored prior to discharge home. Patients experiencing the deficit secondary to vomiting or diarrhea should receive education regarding prevention of shock and the need to seek medical assistance in a timely manner. At home, the patient may not require any follow-up because this is an acute situation that for the most part has no long-term complications. Fatigue may be an issue that will need to be addressed at home, and can be handled simply by informing the patient to perform activities as tolerated until stamina/endurance is re-established. The health care provider may want the patient to return for a follow-up appointment to ensure that parameters such as hemoglobin, hematocrit, and renal function studies have returned to normal.

Documentation

In this emergency situation, document initial assessment findings and follow-up findings such as blood pressure, pulse, respirations, temperature, breath sounds, skin status, and mental status. If there is an obvious bleeding source document site, give an estimate of blood loss and measures implemented to stop the bleeding. Document all interventions, such as intravenous catheter insertion, fluids initiated (type, rate), indwelling catheter insertion with description of urine returned (amount, color). Be specific when charting patient responses to treatment so that other health care providers can clearly determine improvement or deterioration. If hemodynamic monitoring is initiated, document readings as required by agency/unit specific protocols.

NURSING DIAGNOSIS 2

 DECREASED CARDIAC OUTPUT

Related to:
>   Inadequate intravascular volume
>   Failure of compensatory mechanisms

Defining Characteristics:
>   Tachycardia
>   Decreased oxygen saturation
>   Skin cool to touch
>   Peripheral cyanosis
>   Diminished peripheral pulses
>   Delayed capillary refill > 2 seconds
>   Urinary output > 30 ml/hour
>   Narrowing pulse pressure

Goal:
>   Adequate cardiac output is restored.

Outcome Criteria

✔ The patient has pulse rate between 60–100.

✔ The patient's skin is warm and dry.

✔ Perfusion is restored as evidenced by absence of peripheral cyanosis and capillary refill is < 2 seconds.

✔ Urinary output is > 30 ml/hour average.

✔ The patient's blood pressure returns to the patient's baseline.

NOC *Circulatory status*
Tissue perfusion: Cardiac
Tissue perfusion: Peripheral
Tissue perfusion: Cerebral
Cardiac pump effectiveness
Vital signs

INTERVENTIONS	RATIONALES
Place patient with trunk flat, head no higher than 10 degrees, and legs elevated 20 degrees.	This position increases venous return to the heart from the periphery.

(continues)

(continued)

INTERVENTIONS	RATIONALES
Give oxygen as ordered.	Maintains PO$_2$ at > 90 percent; due to hyperfusion, tissues may be hypoxic; this increases amount of oxygen available for gas exchange.
Establish intravenous access and maintain fluid replacement as ordered (see nursing diagnosis "Deficient Fluid Volume").	Replacing intravascular volume is necessary to improve cardiac output.
Assess blood pressure and pulse every 15 minutes.	Changes in blood pressure and pulse give indicators to patient status. When a patient is in shock, a decreased blood pressure with narrowing pulse pressure may be noted; the pulse may be rapid, weak, and thready.
Assess neck veins.	Absence of visible neck veins when the patient is supine indicates decreased circulating volume.
Assess urinary output via an indwelling urinary catheter every hour.	Decreased urinary output (less than 30 ml/hour) indicates decreased perfusion to kidneys and progression of shock.
Assess skin temperature and color.	As shock progresses, the perfusion to skin and periphery is inadequate to maintain warmth or normal color.
Assess peripheral pulses.	As shock progresses, peripheral pulses become weak, diminished, or absent because the heart is unable to maintain perfusion to extremities.
Assess mental status: level of consciousness, confusion, agitation.	Changes in mental status indicate a decrease in cerebral tissue perfusion and indicates an inability of the body's compensatory mechanism to provide adequate oxygenation to cerebral tissue.
Assess respiratory status, noting adventitious breath sounds.	Decreased cardiac output leads to decreased perfusion to lungs causing crackles and dyspnea.
Assist with hemodynamic monitoring according to agency/unit protocol (pulmonary artery	Helps to more accurately assess progression of shock and to evaluate patient response to

pressure and central venous pressures and arterial pressures).

treatment; these measures can give information to evaluate left ventricular function (cardiac output) and fluid status.

Maintain bedrest.	Decreases the workload of the heart.

NIC *Invasive hemodynamic monitoring*
Cardiac care
Fluid management
Fluid monitoring
Shock Management: Volume
Vital signs monitoring

Evaluation

Note the degree to which outcome criteria have been achieved. The patient should demonstrate adequate cardiac output or improvement in abnormalities. Peripheral pulses should be present; skin should return to its normal color and when touched should be warm. If cardiac output is improved, perfusion to the kidneys should be adequate with the patient producing at least 30 ml of urine per hour on average. The pulse should be within the patient's baseline and should be strong and regular. The parameters from invasive hemodynamic monitoring should show improvement and a gradual return to normal. Arterial blood gases should return to normal or show compensation and oxygen saturation should be > 90 percent.

Community/Home Care

Patients who have experienced hypovolemic shock will need to know how to gradually increase activities when at home with a balance of rest and activity. The patient will need to monitor his or her response to activity noting any shortness of breath, increased respiratory rate, or increased pulse rate. If these occur, the patient should simply rest until the symptoms abate. Home care follow-up may be required for some patients, especially if they verbalize feelings of anxiety or lack of knowledge about the emergency situation that necessitated in-hospital care. If hypovolemic shock was caused by such things as severe diarrhea, vomiting, or dehydration, the patient will need to know how to prevent a reoccurrence. For most patients, once fluid status is re-established, cardiac output is restored and no further interventions are required in the home. However, a follow-up appointment is needed to be sure that the patient has returned to a normal level of functioning.

Documentation

Chart the results of all assessments made, particularly respiratory and cardiac system assessments, including respiratory effort, capillary refill, blood pressure, pulse, skin temperature, and urinary output. All interventions should be documented in a timely fashion with the patient's specific response to the intervention. Chart readings from hemodynamic monitoring according to agency/unit protocol. Always include the patient's psychological status: whether he or she appears anxious, restless, or fearful, and whether significant others are present. Document all vital signs in accordance with agency protocol.

NURSING DIAGNOSIS 3

ANXIETY

Related to:

Emergency health problem

Unknown health status

Defining Characteristics:

Tachycardia

Restlessness

Verbalization of anxiety, concern, fear

Goal:

Anxiety is relieved.

Outcome Criteria

✔ The patient reports feeling calm and relaxed.

✔ The patient verbalizes that anxiety has been reduced or alleviated.

✔ The patient asks appropriate questions regarding hypovolemic shock or any aspect of treatment.

NOC *Anxiety self-control*
      Symptom control

INTERVENTIONS	RATIONALES
Assess for verbal and nonverbal signs of anxiety and fear, including increased heart rate.	Helps to detect the presence of anxiety and for early intervention to prevent physiological alterations.
Monitor the intensity of anxiety/fear by having the patient rate on a numerical scale.	Allows for a more objective measure of anxiety and fear levels.
Encourage patient to verbalize fears and anxiety regarding health status (shock).	Admitting that one is fearful or anxious is required in order to implement strategies to cope with the current emergency situation.
Teach patient relaxation techniques (such as slow, purposeful breathing and guided imagery) and encourage their use.	Reduces anxiety and creates a feeling of comfort.
Reassure the patient by explaining procedures, treatments, and critical care environment.	Fear of the unknown contributes to anxiety; knowing what to expect helps the patient maintain a sense of control.
Stay with patient during critical times and during periods when fear and anxiety are evident.	Allows nurse to offer comfort, care, and assurances to reduce anxiety and fear.
Allow family/significant others to visit liberally, if possible, and keep them informed of patient's status. Encourage touching the patient.	The presence of significant others often has a calming effect on critically ill patients.

NIC *Anxiety reduction*
      Calming technique
      Presence

Evaluation

Assess the patient for the degree that fear/anxiety has been controlled. The patient should verbalize his or her feelings and indicate whether interventions have produced a comfortable state of anxiety and fear. Determine if the patient understands hypovolemic shock and interventions required for treatment by the health care provider and the patient. During evaluation, be sure to inquire about the use of coping strategies and relaxation techniques.

Community/Home Care

Coping strategies and relaxation techniques to utilize in the home setting will need to be developed by the patient. The nurse must adequately equip the patient with knowledge necessary to make him or her feel in control. An understanding of what to expect from a diagnosis of hypovolemic shock will assist the patient to feel in control. In the home, the patient may be able to reduce anxiety more quickly through use of common everyday activities, such as walking, reading, meditating, listening to music, and spending time with emotionally supportive family and friends.

Documentation

Using the numerical scale, document the degree of fear or anxiety the patient is experiencing. Also, include any verbal, nonverbal, or physiological clues that could be indicators of anxiety or fear, such as restlessness, tachycardia, or diaphoresis. Document interventions that the nurse implements to reduce or eliminate anxiety and fear, along with the patient responses. Document instruction of relaxation techniques and the disease process.

CHAPTER 1.18

SHOCK: CARDIOGENIC

GENERAL INFORMATION

Cardiogenic shock occurs when the heart fails to accomplish its task as a pump, resulting in a cardiac output that is unable to maintain perfusion. The etiological factors involved in cardiogenic shock are disease processes that cause ventricular ischemia (myocardial infarction, open heart surgery, cardiac arrest), structural problems (valvular disorders, septal rupture, papillary muscle rupture, ventricular aneurysm, cardiomyopathies, intracardiac tumors), and dysrhythmias (tachydysrhythmias, bradydysrhythmias). Myocardial infarction is the most common cause of cardiogenic shock (Lemone and Burke, 2004), but there are numerous other causative factors, including structural problems, cardiomyopathies, severe systemic hypertension, and sepsis. Despite the wide array of causes, the pathophysiological presentation is the same. Disruption of blood flow through the coronary arteries causes myocardial muscle ischemia. If ischemia is not corrected, myocardial tissue damage will occur, resulting in impaired tissue perfusion and a subsequent decrease in stroke volume; cardiac output decreases as left ventricular end-diastolic pressure rises, and shock ensues. Ironically, decreased tissue perfusion also occurs to myocardial muscle, causing further myocardial ischemia. To compensate for the shock state, heart rate increases, which further increases myocardial oxygen demand and worsens myocardial ischemia. The end result is widespread alterations in tissue perfusion, including cerebral and renal. Therapeutic interventions are directed towards improving cardiac output and increasing tissue perfusion while decreasing myocardial ischemia. Cardiogenic shock occurs in 5–10 percent of patients who experience myocardial infarctions. The mortality rate in cardiogenic shock is > 70 percent (Lemone and Burke, 2004).

NURSING DIAGNOSIS 1

 DECREASED CARDIAC OUTPUT

Related to:

Myocardial dysfunction secondary to myocardial ischemia

Defining Characteristics:

Tachycardia

Hypotension

Narrowing pulse pressure

Dyspnea

ECG changes (ischemia/MI)

Dysrhythmias

Increased cardiac isoenzymes

Increased pulmonary pressure

Weak, thready pulses

Tachypnea

Cyanosis

Decreased urine output

Decreased peripheral pulses

Mental status changes

Goal:

Cardiac output is increased.

Outcome Criteria

✔ Vital signs return to patient's baseline.

✔ Pulse is strong and regular.

✔ Urine output is 30 ml/hour or more.

✔ There is no cyanosis.

✔ Peripheral pulses are strong.

✔ The patient is alert, with baseline orientation, and is experiencing no agitation.

NOC *Cardiac pump effectiveness*
Tissue perfusion: Cardiac
Circulatory status

INTERVENTIONS	RATIONALES
Assess vital signs: note abnormalities of blood pressure < 90 and pulse greater than 100; note the quality of the beats and assess heart sounds for rate, rhythm, and quality.	Low blood pressure with a narrow pulse pressure, increased heart rate, and a weak and thready pulse indicates an inability to perfuse vital organs seen in the progressive stage of shock. Thorough assessment of heart sounds will allow early detection of dysrhythmias and other parameters that indicate cardiogenic shock. A diminished S_1 and S_2 may be auscultated due to decreased contractility.
Position patient with head of bed elevated 30 degrees and legs slightly elevated.	This position promotes venous return and improves cardiac output.
Assess peripheral pulses.	Absent or severely diminished peripheral pulses indicate impaired perfusion to distal cells.
Assess breath sounds along with rate, rhythm, and quality of respirations.	As shock progresses the patient may develop crackles because of interstitial pulmonary edema; respiratory rate increases to compensate for metabolic acidosis.
Assess mental status.	Helps to detect changes caused by decreased cerebral blood flow.
Monitor arterial blood gases.	Blood gases provide information on progression of shock; patients in cardiogenic shock experience respiratory alkalosis early in the syndrome and metabolic acidosis later as metabolism at the cellular level becomes anaerobic.
Monitor oxygen saturation continuously.	Provides information about respiratory status and perfusion to tissues.
Administer high flow oxygen to keep SaO_2 > 90 percent via non-rebreather mask, as ordered.	Maximizes oxygen saturation and reduce hypoxia and cyanosis.
Initiate two IV access lines with large bore needles and prepare for insertion of central line, as ordered.	For the emergency administration of medications and fluids.
Administer inotropic medications—dopamine, dobutamine, and low doses of epinephrine—as ordered.	Improves myocardial contractility and increase systolic pressure thereby improving cardiac output.
Administer vasodilating agents as ordered: nitroglycerin (Tridil) and sodium nitroprusside (Nipride).	Vasodilating agents are used in cardiogenic shock that is accompanied by increased systemic vascular resistance and excessive vasoconstriction to decrease afterload, cause vasodilation, and improve coronary artery circulation.
Assist with insertion of intra-aortic balloon pump (IABP) according to agency guidelines.	The IABP is a diastolic assist device that improves coronary artery perfusion and decreases systemic vascular resistance (SVR), which will improve cardiac output and tissue perfusion.
Obtain pulmonary artery wedge pressure (PAWP).	PAWP is a direct reflection of left ventricular pressure and can be used to assess cardiac function and guide fluid volume replacement.
Keep patient warm or at a normal body temperature.	Prevents an increase in metabolic rate that would increase metabolic demands for oxygen.
Insert indwelling urinary catheter as ordered and monitor intake and output.	Helps to monitor fluid balance as an indicator of renal perfusion.

NIC *Shock management: Cardiogenic*
Vital signs monitoring
Invasive hemodynamic monitoring
Hemodynamic regulation
Circulatory care
Cardiac care: Acute
Oxygen therapy

Evaluation

Evaluation is made by examining the extent to which the patient has achieved the stated outcomes. Cardiac output is increased, as demonstrated by blood pressure and pulse returning to patient's baseline. Pulse is strong and regular, and peripheral pulses are present. Renal output of > 30 cc/hour reflects adequate perfusion to kidneys. PAWP reflects adequate left ventricular function. Respiratory status has stabilized, as demonstrated by arterial blood gases that are normal, clear breath sounds, and regular rate. The patient should return to his or her baseline mental status.

Community/Home Care

Patients with decreased cardiac output due to cardiogenic shock are critically ill, and home recovery may be extensive. Referrals to cardiac rehabilitation programs or cardiac support groups may be made. The patient should be taught how to take his or her pulse and to monitor responses to activity such as shortness of breath and increased heart rate. The patient may require the services of a home health nurse who can reinforce teaching and monitor response to continued therapies such as medications, oxygen, and rest. Assessment should be made of factors in the patient's environment and usual routine that enhance or inhibit compliance. It is crucial that the patient and home care providers understand the prescribed medical regimen and verbalize a willingness to be compliant. Fatigue and loss of stamina/endurance are common reasons for the prolonged recovery and return to normal routines. If family members are not available, the patient may need the services of a home health aide or an assistant to do household chores such as cleaning or cooking. The nurse should make sure that the patient knows what to do if problems arise and the importance of follow-up appointments.

Documentation

The patient's response to all therapeutic interventions is charted in the patient record. Document the status of achievement of goals and outcome criteria. Include in the patient chart objective indicators such as pulse, blood pressure, readings from invasive monitoring devices, and specific responses to activity. Intake and output, vital signs, and medication administration are documented according to agency guidelines. Prior to discharge from the hospital, documentation should be made of education provided and the patient's understanding of the prescribed regimen. Referrals made to such entities as cardiac support groups, cardiac rehabilitation programs, and home health services should be noted.

NURSING DIAGNOSIS 2

 IMPAIRED GAS EXCHANGE

Related to:

Decreased cardiac output

Decreased availability of oxygenated blood for exchange of gases at the capillary membrane level

Defining Characteristics:

Hypoxia

Tachycardia

Tachypnea

Dyspnea

Decreased oxygen saturation

Cyanosis

Pale, cool, clammy skin

Goal:

Gas exchange will be adequate.

Outcome Criteria

✔ Arterial blood gases will be within normal ranges.
✔ Oxygen saturation will reach 90–100 percent.
✔ Skin color will be normal.
✔ Respirations will be unlabored.
✔ Vital signs will return to patient's baseline range.

NOC *Respiratory status: Gas exchange*

INTERVENTIONS	RATIONALES
Assess respiratory status to include breath sounds, respiratory rate, rhythm, and depth.	Increased pulmonary vascular pressures cause fluid to accumulate in the alveolar spaces, causing congestion, which in turn translates into crackles and increased rate and depth of respiration in an effort to improve gas exchange.
Position patient with head slightly elevated.	Improves chest expansion.
Administer high-flow supplemental oxygen by mask.	Maximizes oxygen saturation in the circulating blood volume.

(continues)

(continued)

INTERVENTIONS	RATIONALES
Monitor arterial blood gases and oxygen saturation as ordered.	In shock, the patient initially has respiratory alkalosis, but progresses to respiratory and metabolic (as cells function anaerobically) acidosis. Arterial blood gases will detect these changes and provide a means for monitoring the extent of hypoxemia and response to treatment.
Assess skin for cyanosis, pallor, and temperature, being sure to check mucous membranes for darker-skinned patients.	Due to peripheral vasoconstriction and decreased peripheral tissue perfusion, the skin becomes cool and cyanotic or pale. In darker-skinned patients, changes in color are more easily detected in mucous membranes.
Assist with institution of mechanical ventilation with positive-end expiratory pressure (PEEP), as ordered (see nursing care plan for the patient on mechanical ventilation).	Ensures delivery of a specified amount and percentage of oxygen at predetermined intervals.

NIC *Oxygen therapy*
     Respiratory monitoring
     Ventilation assistance

Evaluation

Examine specific patient responses to interventions that would indicate that the patient's oxygenation status is improved. Arterial blood gas and oxygen saturation level will be in normal ranges, indicating an absence of hypoxia and hypoxemia. Breath sounds will be clear, and respirations will be unlabored and return to patient's baseline rate. Cyanosis, if present, should be absent following institution of measures to correct decreased gas exchange.

Community/Home Care

Health care providers should determine if home oxygen is needed, and if so, appropriate referrals should be made. For most patients, this will not be the case, as oxygenation problems are corrected with resolution of the shock. However, the patient will need to understand the concept of oxygen supply and demand as it relates to activity. Methods to improve endurance should be taught to the patient prior to discharge home. The patient needs to gradually increase activities and monitor the response in terms of respirations and feelings of easy fatigue. Any activity that causes shortness of breath should be stopped and attempted later. Short periods of rest throughout the day may be needed in the early days following discharge to decrease oxygen demand. Follow-up is needed to ensure compliance with medical regimen and home health nurses may be needed for a period of time to monitor the patient's progress towards optimal functioning. Assessment of the patient's ability to follow all prescribed interventions should be made, taking into consideration religion, cultural practices, health beliefs, and availability of needed financial resources.

Documentation

Documentation includes extent to which outcomes are achieved. Chart the type of oxygen administration and the amount being delivered in the patient record. Document results of arterial blood gases and oxygen saturation according to agency guidelines. Results of a respiratory assessment should be made with documentation of breath sounds, respiratory rate, depth, and rhythm. Skin color, including that of mucous membranes, should be documented. Any verbalizations of activity intolerance—shortness of breath, fatigue—are documented.

NURSING DIAGNOSIS 3

 ANXIETY

Related to:
    Fear of dying
    Strange environment (critical care unit)
    Serious illness

Defining Characteristics:
    Expressions of fear
    Restlessness and anxiety
    Tachycardia

Goal:
    Anxiety is decreased or alleviated.

Outcome Criteria

✔ The patient reports being less anxious.

✔ The patient demonstrates no outward signs of anxiety such as restlessness or agitation.

NOC *Anxiety self-control*
         Anxiety level
         Comfort level
         Coping

INTERVENTIONS	RATIONALES
Assess level of anxiety (mild, moderate, severe); have patient rate on a scale of 1–10 with 10 being the greatest.	Provides a more objective and meaningful measure of anxiety.
Using a calm, reassuring manner, keep patient informed of all that is going on, including information about therapeutic interventions.	Communication of interventions being implemented in a straightforward manner may help to relieve anxiety by reducing the fear of the unknown and gives the patient a sense of well-being.
Stay with the patient if possible and allow family members to visit.	Provides emotional support and promotes a sense of comfort.
Encourage patient to verbalize fears and concerns.	Verbalization of fears contributes to dealing with concerns.
Control multiple sources of stimuli, which could cause sensory overload.	Over-stimulation can worsen anxiety.
Seek spiritual consult as needed or requested by the patient and or family.	Meeting the patient's spiritual needs helps the patient and family to deal with fears through use of spiritual or religious rituals.
Teach relaxation techniques, such as guided imagery and pursed lip breathing. Encourage their use along with distraction or music therapy.	These measures help to reduce anxiety by relaxing the patient.

NIC *Anxiety reduction*
         Coping enhancement
         Emotional support

Evaluation

Physiological signs of anxiety such as tachycardia will be absent. The patient will verbalize a decrease in anxiety and fear. Restlessness and agitation will be absent.

Community/Home Care

At home, the patient will need to practice relaxation techniques that can reduce anxiety. If the patient practices an organized religion, in-home visits by the religious/spiritual counselor should be planned. This provides an avenue for expression of concerns and fears. Nurses should assess which coping mechanisms work for the patient and encourage their use by the patient at home. Encourage the patient to identify quiet activities that help him or her to relax and ask the patient to practice them at scheduled times during the day. Suggested activities may include reading, music, computer games, meditation, and short walks. The relationship between anxiety and increasing oxygen demands by the myocardium should be explained so that the patient can understand the importance of controlling fears and anxiety. If questions should arise at home regarding the patient's health status or prescribed regimen, the patient should have a means of contact with a health care provider for answers.

Documentation

The degree to which the patient has decreased anxiety should be documented in the patient record. The degree of anxiety the patient is experiencing is recorded using a rating system that provides an objective way to relay to others the extent of the anxiety. Document whether the patient is able to verbalize a feeling of decreased anxiety and whether there are outward signs of anxiety. Blood pressure and pulse rates should be documented because anxiety often causes an increase in both vital signs. Record in the chart which strategies have been successful in decreasing or relieving anxiety.

CHAPTER 1.19

SHOCK: NEUROGENIC

GENERAL INFORMATION

Distributive shock is a generic term for a decrease in vascular resistance and extreme vasodilation that results in a maldistribution of vascular volume. There are three categories of distributive shock: septic shock, anaphylactic shock, and neurogenic shock. Neurogenic shock occurs due to a decrease in sympathetic tone that results in a free-flow of parasympathetic responses that cause vasodilation with pooling of blood in the venous and capillary systems. This reaction can occur as the result of deep general anesthesia, epidural anesthesia, heat exposure, CNS depressant by drugs, a spinal cord injury, or a brain stem injury at the medulla. In any event, patients who suffer from neurogenic shock have some loss of sympathetic nervous system tone that causes extensive vasodilation with massive pooling of blood in the venous and capillary systems. Because of decreased venous return, cardiac output decreases; the most common resultant clinical manifestations are decreased blood pressure and bradycardia, which is often described as bounding. Other changes include mental status changes, decreased urine output, and problems with temperature regulation (poikilothermia) and a risk for hypothermia. This type of shock is usually transient and responds well to fluid volume therapy.

NURSING DIAGNOSIS 1

 DECREASED CARDIAC OUTPUT

Related to:

Vasodilation

Pooling of blood in venous system

Defining Characteristics:

Severe hypotension

Bradycardia

Variations in body temperature (low or normal)

Mental status changes (restless, agitated, anxious)

Decreased urinary output

Decreased central venous pressure

Goal:

Patient's cardiac output is restored.

Outcome Criteria

✔ The patient has a pulse rate between 60–100.

✔ The patient is not agitated or restless; reports decreased anxiety.

✔ Urinary output is > 30 ml/hour average.

✔ Blood pressure returns to patient's baseline.

NOC *Circulatory status*
Tissue perfusion: Cardiac
Tissue perfusion: Peripheral
Tissue perfusion: Cerebral
Vital signs

INTERVENTIONS	RATIONALES
Place patient with trunk flat, head not higher than 10 degrees, and legs elevated 20 degrees.	This position increases venous return to the heart from the periphery.
Give oxygen as ordered.	Helps to maintain PO$_2$ at > 90 percent; due to hypoperfusion, tissues may be hypoxic and supplemental oxygen increases amount of oxygen available for gas exchange.
Complete a thorough cardiovascular assessment: cardiac rate, rhythm, and vital signs.	Helps to detect abnormalities and establish baseline for evaluation of response to interventions. In neurogenic

INTERVENTIONS	RATIONALES
	shock, assess for abnormalities of hypotension, normal or slow pulse, cool, clammy skin (in initial stages the extremities are pink and warm because of the increased blood in the venous circulation, but in the later stages the skin becomes cool and clammy). All of the above manifestations occur because of massive vasodilation, with subsequent changes in cardiac effectiveness.
Assess blood pressure and pulse every 15 minutes.	Changes in blood pressure and pulse give indicators to patient status. In shock, a decreased blood pressure with narrowing pulse pressure may be noted, the pulse may be rapid, weak, and thready; in neurogenic shock, the pulse may be bradycardic.
Assess temperature at least every 4 hours or more often as ordered and document.	Patients with neurogenic shock may experience poikilothermia (assuming the temperature of surrounding environment) and be unable to regulate temperature to normal levels. The massive vasodilation also contributes to insensible heat loss. Assessing temperature often will allow for early intervention.
Assess urinary output via an indwelling urinary catheter every hour.	Decreased urinary output (less than 30 ml/hour) indicates decreased perfusion to kidneys and progression of shock.
Assess skin temperature and color.	If shock progresses, the perfusion to skin and periphery is inadequate to maintain warmth or normal color; in the early stages, the extremities are warm and pink due to pooling of blood there, but as shock progresses, the extremities become cool and clammy due to lack of perfusion.
Assess peripheral pulses.	As shock progresses, peripheral pulses become weak, diminished, or absent, as the heart is unable to maintain perfusion to extremities.
Assess mental status for level of consciousness, confusion, or	Changes in mental status indicate a decrease in cerebral

INTERVENTIONS	RATIONALES
agitation, and assess for pertinent neurological history noting any abnormalities specific to neurogenic shock: cool, clammy skin above the level of any injury; priapism; history of recent spinal anesthesia; history of recent head/ neck trauma; neck pain, then loss of sensation.	tissue perfusion and an inability of the body's compensatory mechanism to provide adequate oxygenation to cerebral tissue; neurological injuries may produce clinical manifestations other than change in level of consciousness and could contribute to neurogenic shock.
Assess respiratory status, noting adventitious breath sounds.	Decreased cardiac output leads to decreased perfusion to lungs, causing crackles and dyspnea. Increased respiratory rate or a varying rate may be noted.
Assist with hemodynamic monitoring according to agency/ unit protocol (pulmonary artery pressure and central venous pressures and arterial pressures).	Helps to assess more accurately the progression of shock and to evaluate patient response to treatment; these measures can give information to evaluate left ventricular function (cardiac output) and fluid status.
Establish intravenous access and maintain fluid replacement as ordered (see nursing diagnosis "Deficient Fluid Volume").	Helps to compensate for relative volume depletion due to vasodilation, replacing intravascular volume as needed to improve cardiac output; most instances of neurogenic shock respond to fluid replacement.
Administer medications as ordered such as vasopressors or alpha-adrenergic agonists.	Vasoactive medications are given for their vasoconstrictive properties to increase venous return to the heart and to improve pumping ability of the myocardium. An increase in heart rate occurs leading to increased cardiac output and increased blood pressure. A vasopressor such as dopamine increases cardiac output and increases blood pressure and can increase heart rate. An alpha-adrenergic agonist such as phenylephrine causes an increased venous return and increases systolic and diastolic pressures.
Maintain bedrest.	Decreases the workload of the heart.
Assist in the treatment of the underlying cause of neurogenic shock (spinal cord injury, etc.) as ordered.	Neurogenic shock is usually transient and corrects with fluid therapy. The causative factor needs to be addressed in order to ensure physiological stability.

NIC *Invasive hemodynamic monitoring*
Cardiac care
Fluid management
Fluid monitoring
Shock management: Vasogenic
Vital signs monitoring

Evaluation

Note the degree to which outcome criteria have been achieved. The patient should demonstrate adequate cardiac output or improvement in abnormalities. Peripheral pulses should be present and skin should be warm and dry. If cardiac output is improved, perfusion to the kidneys should be adequate with the patient producing at least 30 ml of urine per hour on average. The pulse should be within the patient's baseline and should be strong and regular. The parameters from invasive hemodynamic monitoring should show improvement and a gradual return to normal. Arterial blood gases should return to normal or show compensation and oxygen saturation should be > 90 percent.

Community/Home Care

Patients who have experienced neurogenic shock will need to know how to gradually increase activities when at home with a balance of rest and activity. The patient will need to monitor his or her response to activity, noting any shortness of breath, increased respiratory rate, or increased pulse rate. Home care follow up may be required for some patients, especially if they verbalize feelings of anxiety or lack of knowledge about the emergency that necessitated in-hospital care. For patients with neurogenic shock, if the causative alteration has been treated or alleviated (anesthesia, central nervous system depression, medications, etc.), there may be no need for further post-hospital care. However, for patients who have had head or spinal injury, neurogenic shock may be resolved, but there may be lingering issues relevant to care (see specific nursing care plans relevant to head and spinal cord injury). For most patients, specific attention to decreased cardiac output caused by shock is not required once fluid status is re-established and cardiac output is restored. However, a follow-up appointment is needed to be sure

that the patient has returned to his or her normal level of functioning.

Documentation

Chart the results of all assessments made, particularly of the neurological and cardiac system. Chart intake and output hourly, or according to agency protocol, including presence of intravenous infusions. All interventions should be documented in a timely fashion, including the patient's specific response to the intervention. Chart readings from hemodynamic monitoring according to agency/unit protocol, paying particular attention to blood pressure and pulse. Temperatures should be taken at least every 4 hours and documented to detect early hypothermia. Always include the patient's psychological status—whether he or she appears anxious, restless, fearful, and whether significant others are present.

NURSING DIAGNOSIS 2

 DEFICIENT FLUID VOLUME

Related to:
    Vasodilation
    Capillary permeability
    Decreased venous return

Defining Characteristics:
    Tachycardia
    Hypotension
    Delayed capillary refill (> 2 seconds)
    Cool, clammy skin
    Decreased urinary output

Goal:
    Circulating volume will be restored from venous system.

Outcome Criteria

✔ The patient's skin will be warm and dry.
✔ The patient will have blood pressure and pulse within pre-shock baseline.
✔ Urinary output will be ≥ 30 ml/hour.

NOC *Fluid balance*

INTERVENTIONS	RATIONALES
Establish IV access with large bore catheter (16 gauge or larger), as ordered.	IV access is crucial to treatment; large gauge catheters allow for fluids to be given quickly, and blood products will run best in large catheters.
Administer IV fluid replacement, as ordered.	Crystalloids such as 0.9 percent sodium chloride or lactated ringers—replace at a 3:1 ratio (3x as much fluid as the amount of fluid lost) because ⅔ of crystalloid solution diffuses out of vascular space into interstitial spaces. For rapid volume expansion, may give human serum albumin.
Warm all solutions administered for fluid replacement.	Rapid infusion of large amounts of cool or room-temperature solutions can cause a drop in core body temperature.
Insert indwelling urinary catheter to accurately measure urinary output.	In shock states, the kidneys are hypoperfused as a compensatory mechanism and output decreases; as shock is corrected, urine output should increase.
Monitor cardiac status: blood pressure, pulse (quality and rate), pulse pressure, and capillary refill.	Changes in blood pressure and pulse give information relevant to stage of shock. The blood pressure in neurogenic shock is low and the pulse is bradycardic. In the compensatory and progressive stages of shock, the blood pressure may decrease further, and the pulse becomes rapid and thready. Capillary refill is an indicator of perfusion; in shock it is > 2 seconds.
Monitor skin temperature and color for baseline, and during treatment for improvement.	Pale, cool, clammy skin indicates decreased perfusion due to decreased circulating volume secondary to venous and capillary pooling. As treatment progresses, skin should be warm and return to normal color.
Monitor oxygen saturation using pulse oximetry.	Oxygen saturation indicates ability to perfuse tissues.
Monitor results of laboratory studies: hemoglobin and hematocrit, arterial blood gases, BUN, electrolytes.	Hematocrit fluctuates in response to fluid status; drops may be noted during aggressive fluid resuscitation due to hemodilution; the hemoglobin may be decreased. The

hematocrit may be high initially and decrease as fluid is restored to the intravascular space. Arterial blood gases are done to determine oxygen and carbon dioxide levels; shock often causes metabolic acidosis due to anaerobic metabolism as the respiratory and cardiac systems are unable to sustain adequate oxygenation to tissues. BUN and electrolytes would give indicators of renal function; BUN may be elevated initially, but decrease due to hemodilution of fluid replacement.

Treat the underlying cause of the shock as ordered (see nursing diagnosis "Decreased Cardiac Output").	Correction of underlying cause controls and corrects the fluid deficit.

NIC   ***Shock management: Vasogenic***
Emergency care
Fluid management
Intravenous insertion
Intravenous therapy

Evaluation

Assess the patient for indications that the vascular volume has been restored. The patient's blood pressure should return to baseline or be > 70 systolic. The pulse should be strong and regular and at the patient baseline or only slightly increased. Skin should be warm and color should return to the patient's normal appearance. Renal function should not be impaired, with an hourly output on the average of 30 ml/hour. Following fluid replacement, the patient should also be assessed for fluid overload, which may occur in the elderly and those with chronic left ventricular disease.

Community/Home Care

Patients treated for deficient fluid volume secondary to neurogenic shock have normal vascular fluid volume restored prior to discharge home. For the patient with neurogenic shock, stabilization of injuries or elimination of causative factors such as medications or anesthesia should correct the shock without residual effects. At home, the patient may not require any follow-up relevant to fluid status as this is an acute situation that for the most part has no long-term complications. Fatigue may be an issue at home and can be handled simply by informing the patient to perform activities as tolerated until stamina/endurance is re-established. The health care provider may want the patient to return for a follow-up appointment to ensure that parameters such as hemoglobin, hematocrit, and renal function studies have returned to normal.

Documentation

In this emergency situation, document initial assessment findings such as blood pressure, pulse, respirations, temperature, breath sounds, skin status, and mental status. In addition, document the findings from a thorough neurological assessment, with attention to what has caused the neurogenic shock. Chart intake and output according to agency policy, but for the patient experiencing shock, at least every hour. Document all interventions, including intravenous catheter insertion, fluids initiated (type, rate), and indwelling catheter insertion with description of urine returned (amount, color). Be specific when charting patient responses to treatment so that other health care providers can clearly determine improvement or deterioration. If hemodynamic monitoring is initiated, document readings as required by agency/unit's specific protocols.

NURSING DIAGNOSIS 3

 ## ANXIETY

Related to:

    Emergency health problem

    Unknown health status

Defining Characteristics:

    Tachycardia

    Restlessness

    Verbalization of anxiety, concern, fear

Goal:

    Anxiety is relieved.

Outcome Criteria

✔ The patient has no signs of anxiety (restlessness, agitation).

✔ The patient verbalizes that anxiety has been reduced or alleviated.

✔ The patient asks appropriate questions regarding neurogenic shock or any aspect of treatment.

NOC *Anxiety self-control*
           Symptom control

INTERVENTIONS	RATIONALES
Using a rating scale, have patient rate anxiety and assess for nonverbal signs of anxiety and fear, including increased heart rate, agitation, or restlessness.	Helps to detect the presence of anxiety and for early intervention to prevent physiological alterations.
Encourage patient to verbalize fears and anxiety regarding health status.	Recognition of fears and anxiety is the first step to understanding and coping.
Teach patient relaxation techniques (such as slow, purposeful breathing and guided imagery) and encourage their use.	Reduces anxiety and creates a feeling of comfort.
Explain what is happening, including procedures, treatments, and critical care or emergency room environment.	Reassures the patient; fear of the unknown contributes to anxiety; knowing what to expect helps the patient maintain a sense of control. For patients who have neurogenic shock secondary to spinal injuries, the anxiety may result from fear of paralysis.
Stay with patient during critical times and during periods when fear and anxiety are evident.	Allows the nurse to offer comfort, care, and assurances to reduce anxiety and fear.
Keep significant others/family informed of patient's status and allow them to stay with patient if possible.	The presence of significant others often has a calming effect on critically ill patients.

NIC *Anxiety reduction*
         Calming technique
         Presence

Evaluation

Assess the patient for the degree that fear/anxiety has been controlled. The patient should verbalize his or her feelings and indicate whether interventions have produced a comfortable psychological state, and whether anxiety and fear are improved. Assessment using an anxiety scale reveals that the level of anxiety has decreased. Determine whether the patient understands neurogenic shock and the interventions required for treatment by the health care provider and the patient. During evaluation, be sure to inquire about the use of coping strategies and relaxation techniques.

Community/Home Care

The patient will need to develop coping strategies and relaxation techniques to utilize in the home setting. The nurse must provide the patient knowledge necessary to make him or her feel in control. An understanding of what to expect from a diagnosis of neurogenic shock will assist the patient to feel in control. Adequate teaching needs to be done regarding emergency treatment that can be implemented prior to seeking health care. In the home, the patient may be able to reduce anxiety more quickly through use of common everyday activities, such as walking, reading, meditating, listening to music, and spending time with emotionally supportive family and friends. If neurogenic shock was caused by an injury such as head trauma or spinal cord injury, anxiety may persist as the patient copes with the possibility of long-term health problems. In this event, the health care provider must continue to monitor the patient for an extensive period of time to determine how he or she is managing anxiety.

Documentation

Using a numerical scale, document the degree of anxiety the patient is experiencing. In addition, include any verbal, nonverbal, or physiological clues that could be indicators of anxiety or fear, such as restlessness, tachycardia, or diaphoresis. Interventions that the nurse implements to treat anxiety or fear should be documented, along with the patient's responses. Document instruction of relaxation techniques and the disease process.

CHAPTER 1.20

SHOCK: SEPTIC

GENERAL INFORMATION

Septic shock occurs when sepsis (a severe form of infection) and or septicemia (an infection that has spread to the vascular system) is not detected early, or its treatment has not controlled or halted the infectious process. The causative organisms are many and range from viruses and bacteria to fungi; however, the most common agent is gram-negative organisms. The pathophysiology of septic shock is complex. Bacteria that have invaded the vascular system release endotoxins from their ruptured cell membranes into the circulation. A massive immune and inflammatory response occurs as the endotoxins damage the epithelial lining of small blood vessels, especially the lungs and kidneys. There is a disruption of normal coagulation and a release of vasoactive proteins. When septic shock occurs, there is profound vasodilation, severe hypotension, and severely diminished cellular perfusion, which, if uncorrected, will lead to death. Septic shock has distinct phases—early and late. Clinical manifestations in the early phase of septic shock include tachycardia, normal blood pressure or slightly hypotensive, elevated temperature, chills, warm, flushed skin, and tachypnea. During this period, the body attempts to compensate for the alterations by increasing cardiac output. As these mechanisms fail, clinical manifestations of the late phase of septic shock occur and include hypotension, cool and pale skin, decreased urine output, altered mental status, tachycardia, and tachypnea. The age groups at highest risk for sepsis are the very young (neonates) and the very old. Particular categories of patients at risk include those who are immunosuppressed; those who have chronic diseases such as liver failure, renal disease, or diabetes; those who have recently had an invasive surgical procedure; and those who have any type of indwelling catheter or drainage device (bladder, venous or arterial, renal).

NURSING DIAGNOSIS 1

 INFECTION*

Related to:

Invasion of host by virulent organism

Immunocompromise

Defining Characteristics:

Fever

Chills

Positive blood cultures, urine culture, sputum culture, wound culture

Hypotension

Tachycardia

Warm, flushed skin (early, warm phase)

Cool, clammy skin (late, cold phase)

Altered mental status (late phase)

Goal:

The patient's infection is resolved.

There are no further complications from infection.

Outcome Criteria

✔ The patient will be afebrile.

✔ The patient will have negative cultures by time of discharge.

✔ The patient's blood pressure and pulse will return to baseline.

NOC *Infection severity*

Knowledge: Infection control

INTERVENTIONS	RATIONALES
Monitor diagnostic studies: blood cultures, urine cultures, wound cultures or other cultures, CBC (complete blood count), chest x-ray.	Positive cultures provide evidence for cause of sepsis that precipitated the septic shock; most cases of septic shock are caused by gram-negative organisms; complete blood count will reveal elevated white blood cells; chest x-ray will rule out or confirm pulmonary infectious processes as a source of infection.
Monitor laboratory studies: serum lactate, BUN, creatinine, PT (prothrombin time) and APTT (activated partial thromboplastin time), arterial blood gases.	Serum lactate indicates impending metabolic acidosis as the body's metabolism becomes anaerobic; there is increased production of lactic acid; increases in BUN and creatinine provide clues about renal perfusion/function; abnormal PT and APTT occur due to the release of clotting factor XII in response to cellular damage. Blood gases may indicate metabolic acidosis.
Monitor temperature every 4 hours and assess for chills.	Helps to establish a baseline and monitor response to treatment; septic shock is characterized by a warm phase with elevated temperature, and a later phase known as the cold phase where temperature is low; chills often precede temperature elevations.
Institute measures to reduce temperature: administer antipyretics as ordered, apply cooling blanket, as ordered, or give a tepid sponge bath.	Helps to reduce temperature and decrease metabolic demands of the body.
Perform a complete cardio-respiratory assessment to include heart sounds, breath sounds, respiratory rate, use of accessory muscles for breathing, any shortness of breath, peripheral pulses, or capillary refill.	Allows for early detection of complications and response to treatment. As septic shock progresses, it will cause changes in total body perfusion as cardiac output decreases somewhat in part due to decreased circulating volume. Lungs try to compensate by ventilating faster (tachypnea).
Monitor results of oxygen saturation or arterial blood gases, as ordered.	When cardiac output decreases, oxygen supply to the body decreases, which causes

	decreased arterial oxygen levels and decreased oxygen saturation; these tests will allow the nurse to note any alterations in the respiratory system's ability to maintain oxygenation and gas exchange.
Assess neurological status, noting any abnormalities, such as decreasing level of consciousness, weakness, fatigue, or an inability to concentrate.	Patients experiencing septic shock may have decreases in mental status due to decreased oxygenation to cerebral tissues.
Assess patients thoroughly for infectious source: insertion sites of any drainage devices (urinary catheter, JP drains, hemovacs, other tubes), central lines, or other infusion devices for redness or other discoloration, drainage and swelling, and remove as required or ordered; assess any wounds for redness or other discoloration and purulent drainage; assess lungs for symptoms of pneumonia.	Foreign objects placed in body cavities are primary targets for invading organisms, as are wounds; stasis of secretions in the lungs also serves as a medium for bacteria growth especially in immobile, debilitated patients; infections cannot be successfully treated as long as these contaminated items remain in place.
If the patient has an infection that is transmissible to others, place the patient in isolation following agency isolation procedures.	Isolation precautions are needed to protect others from the spread of organisms.
Give oxygen as ordered and in accordance with arterial blood gases and oxygen saturation.	Septic shock causes impaired gas exchange and increases the work of breathing; oxygen will enhance oxygenation to tissues and decrease the work of breathing; supplemental oxygen is also needed to help decrease anaerobic metabolism.
Establish intravenous access with large bore needle and administer fluids as ordered; in most instances rapid infusion is required (see nursing diagnosis "Deficient Fluid Volume").	Intravenous fluids are required to replace decreased circulating volume and restore cardiac output.
Place patient in supine position with legs elevated to about 20 degrees, trunk flat, and head and shoulders higher than the chest.	Increases venous return to the heart, making more blood available for circulation and improving cardiac output.

(continues)

(continued)

INTERVENTIONS	RATIONALES
Institute strict intake and output.	Helps to monitor urinary output. In shock states, the kidneys are hypoperfused as a compensatory mechanism and output decreases; as shock is corrected urine output should increase.
If the patient is able to eat, give a diet high in calories and rich in iron, protein, and vitamin C.	Fatigue is common, and these measures will give the patient needed nutrients for energy and healing; iron-rich foods increase oxygen carrying capacity of the blood.
Administer antibiotics as ordered; broad-spectrum antibiotics should be given until culture results are obtained; monitor for side effects.	These medications will resolve the infection through bacteriocidal and bacteriostatic activities. Monitoring for side effects allows for dosage adjustment and prevention of complications.
In the hospital setting, implement strategies to prevent the spread of organisms: — Educate visitors regarding proper isolation procedures to be employed when visiting. — Be sure that isolation requirements are posted at doorway.	Organisms that cause sepsis can be virulent and easily transmissible; it is important to decrease the opportunity for transmission.

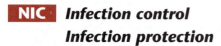 **NIC** *Infection control*
           Infection protection

Evaluation

Determine the extent to which the patient has achieved the expected outcomes. The patient should become afebrile, and there should be no signs or symptoms of infection. Cultures reveal an absence of active infection, and white blood cell count returns to normal. The patient should verbalize an understanding of the infectious process, treatment measures being implemented, and particularly those isolation precautions taken. Cardiac output will be restored, as will be demonstrated by blood pressure and pulse returning to patient's baseline.

Community/Home Care

The source of the infection should be resolved by time of discharge home. However, septic shock is a serious illness that leaves the patient feeling fatigued. At home, assistance may be needed for activities of daily living and household chores. The patient should be taught how to prevent infection and how to recognize the early signs of infection in order to reduce the risk of septic shock in the future. If the infection was caused by infection of medical treatment devices that the patient has to have at home, such as dialysis catheters, central lines, indwelling urinary catheters, and so forth, instructions for proper care should be reinforced to the family and patient. Given that a majority of patients who experience septic shock have other chronic illnesses or are debilitated, control or management of those diseases should be reinforced, particularly if they require invasive techniques such as catheters. Antibiotics may be continued after the patient is at home, and monitoring for side effects will be necessary. The nurse stresses to the patient the need to take the complete recommended course of medications. Continued attention to nutrition is required so that the patient returns to a normal state of energy. Effective teaching, including instruction about how to take a temperature, is crucial for the patient and family, and reinforcement is vital to ensure that the patient is managing the regimen as prescribed.

Documentation

Document the findings from a comprehensive assessment with special attention to the particular cause of the infection. Include patient-specific complaints such as fatigue, malaise or anorexia, chills, and vital signs. Always chart therapeutic interventions implemented and the patient's specific response to those interventions. Specific notes should be made relevant to initiation of intravenous fluids, measures to reduce fever, follow-up temperatures, and any specimens sent to the lab. Chart all medications according to agency protocols. All teaching and referrals are documented in the patient's record.

NURSING DIAGNOSIS 2

 DEFICIENT FLUID VOLUME

Related to:

    Increased capillary permeability

    Loss of fluid into interstitial space

    Peripheral vasodilation

Defining Characteristics:

> Decreased urine output
>
> Warm, dry skin
>
> Decreased blood pressure
>
> Tachycardia
>
> Elevated temperature

Goal:

> Fluid volume will be restored.

Outcome Criteria

✔ The patient's skin will be warm and dry, with no paleness.

✔ The patient's blood pressure and pulse will return to baseline.

✔ Urine output will be ≥ 30 ml/hour.

NOC   *Fluid balance*

INTERVENTIONS	RATIONALES
Assess fluid status by examining blood pressure, pulse, skin turgor, skin temperature, skin color, and urinary output.	Skin turgor will be poor for the patient with fluid deficit; cool skin that is pale or that has decreased color indicates poor perfusion and indicates shock progression. Decreased urinary output is seen in late septic shock. These conditions can give clues to the stage of shock, guide treatment, and monitor the patient response.
Assess cardiac status: blood pressure, pulse (quality and rate), pulse pressure, and capillary refill.	Changes in blood pressure and pulse give information relevant to stage of shock. Initially, blood pressure may be normal to only slightly decreased due to compensatory mechanisms. In the compensatory and progressive stages, blood pressure is decreased; pulse is rapid and thready. Capillary refill is an indicator of perfusion; in shock it is ≥ 2 seconds.
Assess oxygen saturation using pulse oximetry; it may be necessary to use the ear or nose.	Oxygen saturation indicates the ability to perfuse tissues; in the presence of decreased cardiac output, as is seen in late shock, perfusion to the fingers or toes may not be adequate enough to obtain readings, so it may be necessary to use the ear or nose.
Administer oxygen as ordered.	In shock, where there is decreased circulating fluid volume, oxygen transport to tissues is compromised, and supplemental oxygen is required to prevent or treat hypoxia.
Establish intravenous access with two large bore needles, preferably in large veins such as those in antecubital space, or assist with insertion with a central line and administer intravenous fluids rapidly as ordered, using caution in the elderly and in those with heart disease.	Restoring fluid to the intravascular space is necessary to improve cardiac output and restore perfusion. Fluid needs are dictated by patient parameters.
Insert indwelling urinary catheter and measure output hourly.	Helps to accurately assess urinary output; in shock states the kidneys are hypoperfused as a compensatory mechanism and output decreases; as shock is corrected, urine output should increase.
Monitor results of laboratory results: hematocrit, BUN, creatinine electrolytes.	Hematocrit fluctuates in response to fluid status; severe absolute loss from volume would produce a decrease in hematocrit with further drops during aggressive fluid resuscitation due to hemodilution; arterial blood gases are used to determine oxygen and carbon dioxide levels; shock often causes metabolic acidosis due to anaerobic metabolism as the respiratory and cardiac systems are unable to sustain adequate oxygenation to tissues. BUN and electrolytes are indicators of renal function. The BUN may be elevated initially but decrease due to hemodilution of fluid replacement.

NIC   *Fluid management*
       Fluid monitoring
       Hypovolemia management
       Intravenous insertion
       Shock management: Volume

Evaluation

Assess the patient for return of normal fluid volume. The patient's skin should be warm and dry, and should return to patient's baseline color. Blood pressure and pulse return to baseline or are only slightly outside the range. Renal function should stabilize, as demonstrated by urinary output increasing to 30 ml/hour. The patient should be assessed for fluid volume overload, which may occur in the elderly and those with chronic left ventricular disease.

Community/Home Care

Patients who have problems with fluid volume deficit have fluid status restored prior to discharge home. At home, the patient may not require any follow-up with regards to fluid status because this is an acute situation that for the most part has no long-term implications. The issue of fatigue may need to be addressed at home, but this could be handled by teaching the patient how to increase activities as tolerated until stamina is restored to baseline. The health care provider may want the patient to return for a follow-up appointment to ensure that parameters such as hemoglobin, hematocrit, and renal function studies have returned to baseline and fluid status have been maintained.

Documentation

Document findings from a comprehensive assessment with attention to blood pressure, pulse, and skin (color, temperature, turgor). Urine output should be charted according to agency policies, but at least every hour. Interventions implemented to correct fluid deficits (type and amount of fluid infused) are to be included in the patient chart with documentation of the patient's response to the intervention. Always document whether the patient met the proposed outcome criteria.

NURSING DIAGNOSIS 3

DECREASED CARDIAC OUTPUT

Related to:

    Late septic shock

    Inadequate intravascular volume

    Failure of compensatory mechanisms

Defining Characteristics:

    Tachycardia

    Decreased blood pressure

    Narrowing pulse pressure

    Decreased oxygen saturation

    Skin cool to touch

    Peripheral cyanosis/Oral cyanosis

    Diminished peripheral pulses

    Delayed capillary refill > 2 seconds

    Urinary output < 30 ml/hour.

Goal:

    Adequate cardiac output is restored.

Outcome Criteria

✔ The patient has pulse rate between 60–100.

✔ The patient's skin is warm and dry.

✔ Perfusion is restored as demonstrated by absence of peripheral cyanosis, and capillary refill is < 2 seconds.

✔ Urinary output is > 30 ml/hour average.

✔ The patient's blood pressure returns to baseline.

NOC   *Circulatory status*

    Tissue perfusion: Cardiac

    Tissue perfusion: Peripheral

    Tissue perfusion: Cerebral

    Cardiac pump effectiveness

    Vital signs

INTERVENTIONS	RATIONALES
Place patient with trunk flat, head not higher than 10 degrees, and legs elevated 20 degrees.	This position increases venous return to the heart from the periphery.
Give oxygen as ordered.	Helps to maintain PO$_2$ at > 90 percent; due to decreased perfusion tissues may be hypoxic; supplying oxygen increases the amount of oxygen available for gas exchange.
Assess cardiac status: take blood pressure and pulse every 15 minutes; monitor results of EKG.	Changes in blood pressure and pulse give indicators of patient status. In shock, decreased blood pressure with narrowing pulse pressure may be noted;

INTERVENTIONS	RATIONALES
	the pulse may be rapid, weak, and thready; the EKG would demonstrate effects on the cardiac system, such as dysrhythmias.
Assess neck veins.	Absence of visible neck veins when the patient is supine indicates decreased circulating volume.
Assess urinary output via an indwelling urinary catheter every hour.	Decreased urinary output ($<$ 30 ml/hour) indicates decreased perfusion to kidneys and progression of shock.
Assess skin temperature and color.	As shock progresses, the perfusion to skin and periphery is inadequate to maintain warmth or normal color.
Assess peripheral pulses.	As shock progresses, peripheral pulses become weak, diminished, or absent as the heart is unable to maintain perfusion to extremities.
Assess mental status, noting level of consciousness, confusion, or agitation.	Changes in mental status indicate a decrease in cerebral tissue perfusion and indicate an inability of the body's compensatory mechanism to provide adequate oxygenation to cerebral tissue.
Assess respiratory status, noting adventitious breath sounds.	Decreased cardiac output leads to decreased perfusion to lungs, causing crackles and dyspnea.
Assist with hemodynamic monitoring as ordered according to agency/unit protocol (pulmonary artery pressure and central venous pressures and arterial pressures).	Helps to more accurately assess progression of shock and to evaluate patient response to treatment; these measures can give information to evaluate left ventricular function (cardiac output) and fluid status.
Maintain fluid replacement as ordered (see nursing diagnosis "Deficient Fluid Volume").	Replacing intravascular volume is necessary to improve cardiac output.
Maintain bedrest.	Decreases the workload of the heart.
Treat the underlying cause of decreased cardiac output: septic shock/infection (see nursing diagnosis "Infection").	Removing the cause of shock and restoring depleted vascular volume should restore cardiac output.
Give inotropic medications (dopamine, dobutamide as	Dopamine increases systolic and pulse pressure and improves

ordered and monitor according to agency/unit protocols.

circulation to the renal vessels; dobutamide increases cardiac output and decreases total systemic vascular resistance, improves venous return.

NIC *Invasive hemodynamic monitoring*
Cardiac care
Fluid management
Fluid monitoring
Shock management: Volume
Vital signs monitoring

Evaluation

Note the degree to which outcome criteria have been achieved. The patient should demonstrate adequate cardiac output or improvement in abnormalities. Peripheral pulses should be present and skin should be warm to the touch. If cardiac output is improved, perfusion to the kidneys should be adequate, with the patient producing at least 30 ml of urine per hour on average. The pulse should be within the patient's baseline and should be strong and regular. The parameters from invasive hemodynamic monitoring should show improvement and a gradual return to normal. Arterial blood gases should return to normal or show compensation, and oxygen saturation should be $>$ 90 percent.

Community/Home Care

Cardiac output has been restored to normal at the time of discharge, but some effects may last for a short time. Patients who have experienced septic shock will need to know how to gradually increase activities when at home with a balance of rest and activity. The patient will need to monitor his or her response to activity, noting any chest pain, shortness of breath, increased respiratory rate, or increased pulse rate. Home care follow-up may be required for some patients, especially if they verbalize feelings of anxiety or lack of knowledge about the emergency situation that necessitated in-hospital care. If septic shock was caused by an infection acquired outside the hospital setting, the patient should be taught how to implement strategies to prevent infections, such as urinary tract infections, respiratory infections, and infections due to the presence of foreign devices in the body including drainage tubes, dialysis catheters, etc. Instruction of the patient and family should include how to cleanse or care for any tube, catheters, or drainage devices, with the patient or family member demonstrating the skills, and teaching the patient how to count his or her pulse and respirations. For most patients, once fluid status is reestablished, cardiac output is restored and no further interventions are required in the home. However, a follow-up appointment is necessary to be sure that the patient has returned to his or her normal level of functioning.

Documentation

Chart the results of all assessments made, particularly respiratory and cardiac. All interventions should be documented in a timely fashion with the patient's specific response to the intervention. Chart medications, vital signs, intake and output, and readings from hemodynamic monitoring according to agency/unit protocol. Always include the patient's psychological status: whether he or she appears anxious, restless, or fearful, and whether significant others are present.

NURSING DIAGNOSIS 4

 ## ANXIETY

Related to:

Emergency health problem

Unknown health status

Defining Characteristics:

Tachycardia

Restlessness

Verbalization of anxiety, concern, fear

Goal:

Anxiety is relieved.

Outcome Criteria

✔ The patient reports feeling calm and relaxed.

✔ The patient verbalizes that anxiety has been reduced or alleviated.

✔ The patient asks questions regarding health status, septic shock, or any aspect of treatment.

NOC   *Anxiety self-control*
       Symptom control

INTERVENTIONS	RATIONALES
Assess for verbal and nonverbal signs of anxiety and fear, including increased heart rate.	Helps to detect the presence of anxiety and allows for early intervention to prevent physiological alterations.
Monitor the intensity of anxiety/ fear by having patient rate on a numerical scale, if capable.	Allows for a more objective measure of anxiety and fear levels.
Encourage patient to verbalize fears and anxiety regarding health status (shock).	Recognition of fears and anxiety is the first step to coping.
Teach patient relaxation techniques (such as slow, purposeful breathing) and encourage their use.	Reduces anxiety and creates a feeling of comfort.
Reassure the patient by explaining procedures, treatments, and critical care environment.	Fear of the unknown contributes to anxiety; knowing what to expect helps the patient maintain a sense of control.
Stay with patient during critical times and during periods when fear and anxiety are evident.	Allows the nurse to offer comfort, care, and assurances to reduce anxiety and fear.
Keep significant others/family informed of patient's status and allow for visitation.	Family members may also be anxious, which may prevent them from being a source of emotional support for the patient; addressing their need for information makes them more able to provide support for the patient; the presence of significant others often has a calming effect on critically ill patients.

NIC   *Anxiety reduction*
       Calming technique
       Presence

Evaluation

Assess the patient for the degree that fear and anxiety has been controlled. The patient should verbalize his or her feelings and indicate whether interventions have produced a comfortable state of anxiety and fear. Determine whether the patient understands septic shock and interventions required for treatment by the health care provider and the patient. During evaluation, be sure to inquire about the use of coping strategies and relaxation techniques.

Community/Home Care

Being in the critical care environment is anxiety-provoking for most patients, and even when the sepsis has been successfully treated, the patient may still have a sense of despair. Even though the problems associated with septic shock are resolved at time of discharge, the patient may still be anxious about the overall experience, and may need to develop coping strategies and relaxation techniques to utilize in the home setting. The nurse must adequately prepare the patient with the knowledge necessary to make him or her feel in control. An understanding of what to expect from a diagnosis of septic shock will assist the patient to feel in control. In the home, the patient may be able to reduce anxiety more quickly through use of common everyday activities such walking, reading, meditating, listening to music, and spending time with emotionally supportive family and friends.

Documentation

Using a numerical scale, document the degree of fear or anxiety the patient is experiencing. In addition, include any verbal, nonverbal, or physiological clues that could be indicators of anxiety or fear, such as restlessness, tachycardia, or diaphoresis. Interventions that the nurse implements to treat anxiety or fear should be documented along with the patient's responses. Teaching regarding relaxation techniques and the disease process should be documented.

CHAPTER 1.21

SHOCK: ANAPHYLACTIC

GENERAL INFORMATION

Distributive shock is a generic term for a decrease in vascular resistance and extreme vasodilation that results in a maldistribution of vascular volume. There are three categories of distributive shock: anaphylactic shock, neurogenic shock, and septic shock. Anaphylactic shock occurs when there is an antigen/antibody response in a sensitized person when exposed to an allergen/antigen. Shock does not usually occur with the first exposure to an allergen, but rather on subsequent exposures after the body has developed specific immunoglobulin E against the offending substance or allergen. Following this, with each exposure large amounts of histamine are released in response, which causes vasodilation and increased capillary permeability leading to loss of fluid from the circulating volume. There is extensive vasodilation with massive pooling of blood in the venous and capillary systems. In addition, histamine also causes bronchial hyperactivity and constriction of smooth muscles, such as those in the lungs, which results in bronchospasm and laryngospasm producing characteristic symptoms of respiratory distress with wheezing and shortness of breath. Serotonin, which has vasoconstrictive properties, is also released, adding to the increased capillary permeability in the lungs. With this permeability, fluid is unable to remain in the vasculature of the lungs and instead leaks out into the alveoli, producing symptoms of pulmonary congestion. Anaphylaxis progresses quickly, with clinical manifestations often occurring within minutes of exposure to the offending substance, and if unchecked, death can occur within minutes. Common triggers include medications, exposure to latex, contrast media, certain foods, and environmental substances such as hay or insect bites/stings. In addition to the symptoms of respiratory distress, clinical manifestations of anaphylactic shock include profound decreased blood pressure; edema in lips, tongues, and eyelids; diaphoresis, weakness; sneezing; itching;

hives; mental status changes; and, as shock progresses, decreased urinary output. As a result of decreased venous return, cardiac output decreases, with resultant clinical manifestations of decreased blood pressure, mental status changes, slow pulse, and decreased urine output.

NURSING DIAGNOSIS 1

DECREASED CARDIAC OUTPUT

Related to:

Vasodilation

Pooling of blood in venous system

Decreased capillary permeability

Defining Characteristics:

Severe hypotension

Tachycardia

Feeling of uneasiness

Diaphoresis

Sneezing

Weakness

Mental status changes (restless, agitated, anxious)

Decreased urinary output

Goal:

The patient's cardiac output is improved.

Outcome Criteria

✔ The patient has a pulse rate between 60–100.

✔ The patient's blood pressure returns to patient's baseline.

✔ The patient has no wheezing or shortness of breath.

✔ Urinary output is > 30 ml/hour average.

✔ The patient has no signs of anxiety, such as agitation or restlessness, and reports decreased anxiety.

NOC   *Circulatory status*
Tissue perfusion: Cardiac
Tissue perfusion: Peripheral
Tissue perfusion: Cerebral
Vital signs

INTERVENTIONS	RATIONALES
Place patient with trunk flat, head not higher than 10 degrees, and legs elevated 20 degrees.	This position increases venous return to the heart from the periphery.
Give oxygen as ordered.	Assists in relieving respiratory distress; due to hypoperfusion, tissues may be hypoxic; oxygen is needed to increase the amount of oxygen available for gas exchange and to maintain PO_2 at > 90 percent.
Complete a thorough cardiovascular assessment: cardiac rate and rhythm, vital signs.	Detects abnormalities and establishes a baseline for evaluation of response to interventions. In anaphylactic shock, expect hypotension, tachycardia, dysrhythmias, and warm skin, all of which occur because of massive vasodilation with subsequent changes in cardiac effectiveness.
Assess blood pressure and pulse every 15 minutes.	Changes in blood pressure and pulse give indicators to patient status. In shock, decreased blood pressure with narrowing pulse pressure may be noted (an indication of progressive shock); the pulse may be rapid, weak, and thready.
Assist in identification of causative agent (food, insect bite, medications, other substances) and initiate interventions to treat the cause as ordered.	Identification of the causative agent will assist in correct treatment and prevention of future episodes.
Assess urinary output via an indwelling urinary catheter every hour.	Decreased urinary output (< 30 ml/hour) indicates decreased perfusion to kidneys and progression of shock.
Assess skin temperature and color.	As shock progresses, the perfusion to skin and periphery is inadequate to maintain warmth or normal color.
Assess peripheral pulses.	As shock progresses, peripheral pulses become weak, diminished, or absent, as the heart is unable to maintain perfusion to extremities.
Assess mental status: level of consciousness, confusion, agitation.	Changes in mental status indicate a decrease in cerebral tissue perfusion and an inability of the body's compensatory mechanism to provide adequate oxygenation to cerebral tissue.
Assess respiratory status, noting adventitious breath sounds: for patients experiencing anaphylaxis, assess for wheezing, stridor, and other signs of respiratory distress.	Decreased cardiac output leads to decreased perfusion to lungs, causing crackles and dyspnea; histamine causes a leak of fluid into alveoli, also causing pulmonary congestion, which manifests itself as crackles; histamine also causes smooth muscle constriction in the lungs, causing bronchospasms and laryngospasms, which manifests as wheezing and stridor.
Assist with hemodynamic monitoring according to agency/unit protocol (pulmonary artery pressure and central venous pressures and arterial pressures).	Helps to assess progression of shock more accurately and to evaluate patient response to treatment; these measures can give information to evaluate left ventricular function (cardiac output) and fluid status.
Establish intravenous access, and administer and maintain fluid replacement as ordered.	Compensates for relative volume depletion due to vasodilation; replacing intravascular volume is necessary to improve cardiac output.
Administer medications as ordered (epinephrine IV; Benadryl PO or IV; bronchodilators, metaproterenol/beta agonists, steroids). If symptoms of anaphylaxis do not stabilize or abate and shock progresses, administer vasoactive drugs (dopamine, dobutamine) as ordered.	In anaphylaxis, antihistamines decrease the amount of circulating histamines that caused vasodilation; epinephrine acts directly on alpha and beta receptors, strengthens myocardial contraction, and increases cardiac output. In addition, it inhibits histamine release, and as a result decreases respiratory symptoms, particularly bronchospasm. Vasoactive medications are given for their vasoconstrictive properties to increase venous

(continues)

(continued)

INTERVENTIONS	RATIONALES
	return to the heart and to improve pumping ability of the myocardium, which elevates blood pressure.
Maintain bedrest.	Decreases the workload of the heart.
Assess the patient for a quick reversal of symptoms of respiratory distress and decreased cardiac output in response to interventions. Note respiratory status, particularly breath sounds, effort, and rate; pulse; blood pressure; output; mental status, especially anxiety; and presence of any other symptoms of allergic reaction such as hives and itching.	Helps to evaluate the effectiveness of interventions and determine the need for further actions.

 NIC *Anaphylaxis management*

Invasive hemodynamic monitoring

Cardiac care

Fluid management

Fluid monitoring

Shock management: Vasogenic

Vital signs monitoring

Evaluation

Note the degree to which outcome criteria have been achieved. Respiratory status has stabilized with no wheezing or distress. The patient should demonstrate adequate cardiac output or improvement in abnormalities. Peripheral pulses should be present, and skin when touched should be warm. If cardiac output is improved, perfusion to the kidneys should be adequate, with the patient producing at least 30 ml of urine per hour on average. The pulse should be within the patient's baseline and should be strong and regular. The parameters from invasive hemodynamic monitoring should show improvement and a gradual return to normal. Arterial blood gases should return to normal or show compensation, and oxygen saturation should be > 90 percent.

Community/Home Care

Anaphylactic shock is a critical event when it occurs, but in most instances, once it has been treated the patient has no health care problems that require in-home care. The most critical part of home care involves educating the patient on how to prevent a reoccurrence by identifying the trigger that caused the reaction. Instruct the patient and significant other or family members about strategies required to prevent shock when exposed to offending triggers (see nursing diagnosis "Deficient Knowledge"). Wearing of a Medic-Alert bracelet is crucial so that others know about the allergy. For most patients, specific attention to decreased cardiac output caused by shock is not required once adequate fluid status is re-established and cardiac output is restored. However, a follow-up appointment is necessary to be sure that the patient has returned to his or her normal level of functioning and has followed through with obtaining the bracelet.

Documentation

Chart the results of all assessments made, particularly respiratory and cardiac. Chart intake and output hourly or according to agency protocol, including presence of intravenous infusions. Document all interventions in a timely fashion with the patient's specific response to the intervention. For patients who had anaphylactic shock, document an assessment of the skin for rashes and redness and for edema, especially of the lips, eyes, and tongue. Chart readings from hemodynamic monitoring according to agency/unit protocol. Always include the patient's psychological status: whether he or she appears anxious, restless, or fearful, and whether significant others are present.

NURSING DIAGNOSIS 2

INEFFECTIVE BREATHING PATTERN

Related to:

　　Bronchospasm

　　Laryngeal edema

　　Allergic reaction

　　Facial edema

Defining Characteristics:

　　Wheezing

　　Stridor

　　Decreased oxygen saturation

Dyspnea

Tachypnea

Abnormal blood gases (decreased pO_2 and increased $pCO_{2)}$

Restlessness and anxiety

Goal:

The patient's respiratory status returns to baseline.

Outcome Criteria

✔ Respiratory rate and effort will be at the patient's baseline.

✔ The patient will have no wheezing or stridor.

✔ The patient will have no cyanosis.

✔ Oxygen saturation will be > 90 percent.

✔ Arterial blood gases are normal or improved.

✔ The patient will demonstrate no signs of anxiety, such as restlessness or agitation.

NOC *Respiratory status: Airway patency*
Respiratory status: Ventilation
Allergic response: Systemic

INTERVENTIONS	RATIONALES
Assess respiratory status: breath sounds, respiratory rate, oxygen saturation; note abnormalities such as wheezing, stridor, dyspnea, presence of cyanosis, retractions, use of accessory muscles, flaring of nostrils, angioedema.	Abnormal breathing patterns may signal worsening of condition; stridor, retractions, and flaring of nostrils indicate a significant decline in respiratory status; angioedema of the facial area or mouth contributes to the inability to breathe by restricting intake of air. Assessments allow the nurse to monitor response to interventions.
Monitor patient for signs of occluded airway: cyanosis, cessation of wheezing, absence of breath sounds over lungs, holding throat, and continuous coughing.	If bronchospasm is severe, there may be no air movement, and therefore no wheezing; the patient may cough almost continuously in an attempt to open the airway.
Monitor arterial blood gases as ordered.	Initially ABG analysis will reveal respiratory alkalosis as the tachypnea blows off more carbon dioxide, but as the airway narrows, the lungs are unable to blow off carbon dioxide and acidosis is noted.
Assess for anxiety and reassure patient with presence.	The patient experiencing anaphylaxis is already anxious because of the allergic response; being unable to breathe causes more anxiety and fear; the patient needs a calming presence; anxiety increases the demand for oxygen.
Provide humidified oxygen, as ordered, to maintain oxygen saturation at > 90 percent.	Improves oxygenation to cells.
Establish intravenous access as ordered.	Ensures a route for rapid-acting medications.
Administer epinephrine as ordered.	Inhibits histamine release, reduces pulmonary congestion, and decreases laryngospasm as well as bronchospasm by its effect on both alpha and beta receptors.
Place the patient in high Fowler's position if possible and support with an over-bed table as needed.	Maximizes chest excursion and subsequent movement of air.
Assist respiratory therapist with administration of beta-adrenergic agonists (such as albuterol, metaproterenol) via nebulizer or metered dose inhaler as ordered and monitor for side effects.	Stimulates $beta_2$-adrenergic receptor sites in the pulmonary system to increase levels of cAMP, which relaxes smooth muscles causing bronchodilation and reducing bronchospasm; common side effects include tremors, tachycardia, and anxiety.
Administer corticosteroids (such as Solu-Medrol® IV, Prednisone PO, Flovent inhaled) or antihistamines (Benadryl®), as ordered, and monitor for side effects.	Corticosteroids suppress the inflammatory response and decrease mucosal edema; systemic side effects from short-term oral or IV administration include elevated blood-sugar levels and GI upset with oral medications; effects from inhaled corticosteroids include candidiasis, hoarseness, dry cough; antihistamines block the release of histamine, which causes bronchiole constriction; side effects include drowsiness and dry mouth.
Teach patient about prevention, medications, and home care (see nursing diagnosis "Deficient Knowledge").	Knowledge increases the chance that the patient can engage in health-promoting behaviors to prevent future allergic reactions.
If the patient's respiratory status does not improve, assist with implementation of mechanical	If stridor occurs, the patient will be unable to maintain effective respiratory efforts for oxygenation

(continues)

(continued)

INTERVENTIONS	RATIONALES
ventilation and transfer to a critical care environment.	and will need the assistance of intubation.
Inform family or significant others regarding patient's condition.	Emergencies such as anaphylaxis often cause anxiety and fear in family members and significant others. Holistic nursing care recognizes the importance of family and seeks to allay anxiety in the family members as well as in the patient.

NIC *Presence*
Respiratory monitoring
Oxygen therapy
Ventilation assistance

Evaluation

Assess the patient to determine the extent to which the outcome criteria have been met. Assessments of the respiratory system should reveal that acute respiratory symptoms of anaphylaxis, such as wheezing, have been resolved. The patient should be breathing effortlessly, and even though some mild wheezing may be noted, this should be improved. ABGs and oxygen saturation should indicate adequate oxygenation, and there should be no cyanosis.

Community/Home Care

The patient who has experienced respiratory distress due to anaphylaxis may not need any monitoring when discharged home. The patient and family will be able to implement strategies to manage future allergic reactions themselves with the use of EpiPens or Benadryl. Prior to discharge from the acute setting, the patient should attempt to identify known allergens in the home environment. Common precipitating factors are foods, insect or bee stings, medications, and cats. If possible, allergens should be minimized or alleviated altogether before the patient enters the home. The patient and family will need to know the signs of allergic reactions that indicate a possible progression to respiratory symptoms and what interventions could be implemented prior to seeking emergency care. The patient and family members will also need thorough information on medications (see nursing diagnosis "Deficient Knowledge"). All patients who have experienced anaphylactic shock should carry medical information on their person and wear a Medic-Alert bracelet to alert others.

Documentation

Note specifically the findings from a comprehensive respiratory assessment, changes in breath sounds in response to interventions, and the patient's emotional state. Include in the patient record all interventions carried out for the patient, and the patient's response. Document the introduction of new medication regimens and the patient's response or lack thereof. If the patient is able to participate in care, including self-care activities and coughing/deep breathing, document this in the chart. Vital signs and oxygen saturation should be documented according to agency protocol. Any teaching initiated should be charted with a clear indication of what was taught and to whom. Always include in the documentation the patient's progress towards achievement of the stated outcome criteria.

NURSING DIAGNOSIS 3

 IMPAIRED SKIN INTEGRITY

Related to:
    Allergic reaction

Defining Characteristics:
    Itching
    Edema of lips, eyelids
    Urticaria
    Redness/discoloration

Goal:
    The patient's skin will return to normal state.

Outcome Criteria

✔ The patient's skin will not be red or discolored.

✔ The patient will have no rashes or hives.

✔ Edema of lips, tongue, face, or eyelids will be alleviated.

NOC *Allergic response: Localized*
Tissue integrity: Skin mucous membranes

INTERVENTIONS	RATIONALES
Assess for urticaria/hives/rashes, pruritus; edema of lips, eyelids, and tongue; and redness. Inquire about ingestion of recent foods and drugs or exposure to other possible allergens, such as animals, hay, mold, etc.	For patients experiencing anaphylactic shock, exposure to an offending substance causes a hypersensitivity reaction that often produces skin changes such as redness, rash, and edema of the facial area.
Administer medications as ordered to relieve symptoms (such as Benadryl or epinephrine).	Benadryl or other antihistamines will block histamine release, decreasing symptoms; epinephrine will relieve sympathetic system responses and ultimately decrease swelling in the facial area as well as decrease amount of circulating histamine.
Apply ice pack to area of itching.	Decrease discomfort caused by pruritus.
Apply anti-itch lotions or ointments as ordered (such as Caladryl, hydrocortisone).	Increases comfort.
Encourage the patient to avoid scratching areas of rash or redness.	Scratching can lead to excoriation and further alterations in skin integrity.
Avoid putting substances containing alcohol or perfume or harsh deodorant soaps on affected areas.	The skin is sensitive, and harsh products and alcohol can further dry the area, making itching worse and contributing to excoriation.
If the patient has difficulty not scratching, especially during sleep, encourage him or her to wear soft gloves.	The discomfort from itching may be so severe that scratching is inevitable. During sleep, the patient is not aware that he or she is scratching. Having the patient wear soft gloves minimizes trauma to the skin.
Wear an eye patch at night if edema is present in area of eye.	If swelling of the eye is extensive and prevents complete closure of the eye, a patch will protect the eye from dryness or damage.
Assess skin, eyes, face, tongue, and other areas for improvement following interventions.	Helps to detect improvement, resolution, or a need for revision of therapeutic interventions.

 NIC *Skin surveillance*
Eye care
Allergy management

Evaluation

The patient's skin has returned to a normal state. The patient verbalizes no complaints of itching and areas of redness; hives or rash are resolved. In addition, edema of the eyes, face, or other areas has been eliminated. The patient experienced no further alterations in skin, and no areas of excoriation are noted.

Community/Home Care

The patient who has impaired skin integrity due to an allergic reaction may possibly go home with some symptoms still present. Continued care of skin at home may include applying substances for itching and monitoring for complete resolution of edema of eyes or other areas. The patient requires education regarding how to care for the skin, especially with respect to rashes, hives, and itching. Simple measures to employ at home include taking cool baths rather than hot ones, as hot water tends to make pruritus worse, and avoidance of everyday household products that can worsen symptoms, such as perfumed body lotions, soaps, and common household cleaning products. If the causative agent for the reaction is known, the patient should avoid it at all times, and if contact occurs, institute measures quickly to prevent problems. This may include taking a dose of Benadryl or possibly use of an EpiPen in accordance with discharge instructions from the physician. The patient should always have these items close at hand and be encouraged to carry them when traveling away from home. This is especially true for food allergies, because often the specific content of food (especially in the case of additives) is not always known, especially when the patient is eating at a restaurant or a friend's house.

Documentation

Document findings from the assessment of all skin, especially skin beneath clothing on back as well as the tongue, mucous membranes, and the eyes. Describe specifically what types of skin changes are seen, including their specific locations. Inspect for edema over the entire body but especially around the eyes and on the feet, hands, and tongue. Document all therapeutic interventions employed. After interventions, always document the patient's response and improvement, or changes required.

NURSING DIAGNOSIS 4

 ### ANXIETY

Related to:

Emergency health problem

Unknown health status

Defining Characteristics:

Tachycardia

Restlessness

Verbalization of anxiety, concern, fear

Goal:

Anxiety is relieved.

Outcome Criteria

✔ The patient is not agitated or restless.

✔ The patient verbalizes that anxiety has been reduced or alleviated.

✔ The patient asks questions regarding anaphylactic shock or any aspect of treatment.

NOC *Anxiety self-control*

Symptom control

INTERVENTIONS	RATIONALES
Assess for verbal and nonverbal signs of anxiety and fear; have patient rate anxiety using a rating scale.	Helps to detect the presence of anxiety and for early intervention to prevent physiological alterations; a rating scale provides a more objective measure of anxiety; increased pulse rate and diaphoresis are physiological indicators of anxiety.
Encourage patient to verbalize fears and anxiety regarding health status.	Recognition of fears and anxiety is the first step to understanding and coping.
Teach patient relaxation techniques (such as slow, purposeful breathing) and encourage their use.	Reduces anxiety and creates a feeling of comfort.
Explain the situation, including procedures, treatments, and critical care or emergency room environment.	Reassures the patient; fear of the unknown contributes to anxiety; knowing what to expect helps the patient maintain a sense of control. Patients who are having difficulty breathing or can feel their lips or other areas swelling
	due to allergic reactions most often feel in a state of panic and are fearful.
Stay with patient during critical times and during periods when fear and anxiety are evident.	Allows the nurse to offer comfort, care, and assurances to reduce anxiety and fear.
Keep significant others and family members informed of the patient's status and allow them to stay with the patient if possible.	The presence of significant others often has a calming effect on seriously ill patients.

NIC *Anxiety reduction*

Calming technique

Presence

Evaluation

Assess the patient for the degree that fear/anxiety has been controlled by use of a rating scale. The patient should verbalize his or her feelings and indicate whether interventions have produced a comfortable psychological state, and whether anxiety and fear have subsided. Determine whether if the patient understands anaphylactic shock and interventions required for treatment by the health care provider and the patient.

Community/Home Care

For the patient who has experienced anaphylactic shock, anxiety may persist for a while due to the fear that another exposure to the offending substance may produce the same consequences. In this situation, the patient will need to develop coping strategies and relaxation techniques to utilize in the home setting. The nurse must prepare the patient by providing the knowledge necessary to make him or her feel in control. An understanding of what to expect from a diagnosis of anaphylactic shock will assist the patient to feel less anxious and more relaxed. Adequate teaching is necessary regarding prevention and emergency treatment that can be implemented prior to seeking health care. In the home, the patient may be able to reduce anxiety more quickly through use of common everyday activities such as a walking, reading, meditating, and listening to music.

Documentation

Using a numerical scale, document the degree of fear or anxiety the patient is experiencing. In addition, include any verbal, nonverbal, or physiological clues that could be indicators of anxiety or fear such as restlessness, tachycardia, or diaphoresis. Interventions that the nurse implements to treat anxiety or fear should be documented, along with the patient's responses. Instruction of relaxation techniques and the disease process should be documented.

NURSING DIAGNOSIS 5

 ### DEFICIENT KNOWLEDGE

Related to:

Insufficient knowledge of anaphylaxis and its treatment

No previous history of the problem

Defining Characteristics:

Asks questions/has concerns

Has had no other health care visit for anaphylaxis

Asks no questions

Verbalizes a lack of knowledge

Goal:

The patient verbalizes an understanding of anaphylactic shock and its treatment.

Outcome Criteria

✔ The patient verbalizes a desire to learn necessary information.

✔ The patient verbalizes a willingness to keep appointments and follow the prescribed regimen.

✔ The patient demonstrates knowledge of anaphylaxis and how to prevent it.

✔ The patient demonstrates knowledge of medication (Benadryl) and correct use of the EpiPen.

NOC *Knowledge: Disease process*
Knowledge: Treatment regimen
Compliance behavior

INTERVENTIONS	RATIONALES
Assess readiness of patient to learn (motivation, cognitive level, physiological status).	The patient must be motivated to learn, have the capability to learn the content, and be free of distractions from learning, such as pain and shortness of breath.
Assess patient's current knowledge.	The teacher needs to ascertain what the patient already knows and build on this.
Teach the simplest information first.	Patients can understand simple concepts easily and then can build on those to understand more complex concepts.
Identify a family member or significant other who will also learn the content and assist the patient with compliance.	This person can reinforce the teaching and assist with implementation if the client becomes incapable of follow-through, especially in an emergency situation.
Create a quiet environment conducive to learning.	Environmental noise can prevent the learner from focusing on what is being taught.
Teach the learners about the pathophysiology of anaphylaxis, including complications.	The patient must understand what the disease is and how it affects the body before understanding the rationale for treatments.
Teach the learners about prescribed medications (see nursing diagnoses "Decreased Cardiac Output" and "Ineffective Breathing Pattern"), including action and side effects.	Knowledge of why the medication is necessary and how it works will help the patient to focus on the importance of the medication. Identification of side effects will minimize anxiety if these untoward effects should occur.
Teach the patient to take medications as ordered (generally): — Benadryl (or other antihistamines) with exposure to offending substance — Epinephrine when respiratory symptoms begin, or other symptoms are unrelieved by Benadryl	Taking antihistamines and epinephrine prior to onset of serious symptoms can prevent respiratory symptoms.
Teach the patient about the importance of tracking events/substances that trigger allergic reactions and how to minimize them.	The patient must understand triggering factors in order to control them and prevent future problems; for many patients, all allergies may not be known; keeping attuned to the environment to identify other allergens can assist the patient to avoid anaphylactic reactions.
Instruct patient and family member on when and how to use an EpiPen.	In the event of an emergency, when the patient is having extreme difficulty breathing and health care assistance is not available, the patient or family

(continues)

(continued)

INTERVENTIONS	RATIONALES
	can be instructed to administer a preloaded dosage of epinephrine using an EpiPen.
Teach the patient which signs and symptoms to report to a health care provider.	Monitoring for signs and symptoms early can prevent a crisis that requires hospitalization. It is important for patients with known serious allergies to know when to seek health care assistance to avoid complications.
Teach patient proper care of rashes, hives, and itching skin (see nursing diagnosis "Impaired Skin Integrity").	Proper skin care can prevent serious impairments to tissue integrity, such as open wounds.
Evaluate the patient's understanding of all content covered by asking questions; have patient and family member demonstrate use of EpiPen.	Identifies areas that require more teaching and ensures that the patient has enough information to comply; if the patient can demonstrate correct procedure for administering medications, he or she will feel more comfortable using them when needed, and anxiety should be decreased.
Give the patient written information.	Provides reference at a later time and allows for review.
Establish that the patient has the resources required to be compliant.	If needed resources such as finances, transportation, and psychosocial support are not available, the patient cannot be compliant.

NIC *Learning readiness enhancement*
Learning facilitation
Teaching: Psychomotor skill
Teaching: Disease process
Teaching: Prescribed medication

Evaluation

Evaluate the degree to which the patient has achieved the outcome criteria relevant to the teaching sessions. The patient is able to repeat all information for the nurse and asks questions about the prescribed recommendations. The patient should demonstrate the ability to administer medication in an emergency via the EpiPen. The patient should be able to inform the nurse when health care assistance should be sought for any allergic reaction.

Community/Home Care

The patient will need to be able to implement strategies to treat anaphylaxis should it occur again in the home setting. It is important that the patient know how to prevent future occurrences by constantly monitoring the environment for offending substances and informing others, particularly other health care providers. Adequate financial resources should be in place for purchase of the EpiPen and Benadryl. The patient may prefer to use liquid preparations of Benadryl as these tend to exert their action more quickly than tablets or capsules. It is important for the patient to have access to both of these medications when leaving home, in case of emergency. This is especially true when traveling via airplane, train, or bus where luggage is stored in separate compartments. Keeping the medication in a small travel bag kept with the patient at all times is preferable. If the patient cannot afford the medication, assistance with obtaining it should be made through social services prior to discharge from the acute care setting. Some follow-up may be required to ensure that the patient has returned to a normal level of functioning and that any respiratory or skin alterations have resolved. During the follow-up visits with health care providers, the patient should be questioned regarding his or her understanding of the content taught, especially use of the EpiPen, which may save his or her life.

Documentation

Document the specific content taught and the titles of printed materials given to the patient or family. Chart the patient's understanding of the content and the methods used to evaluate learning. Document the patient's successful demonstration of the proper use of the EpiPen. The nurse must clearly indicate areas that need to be reinforced. After the teaching session is complete, the nurse should note whether the patient indicates a willingness to comply with health care recommendations. If the teaching included a significant other, indicate this in the documentation. In addition, any referrals made should be documented in the patient's record.

UNIT 2
RESPIRATORY SYSTEM

CHAPTER 2.22

ASTHMA

GENERAL INFORMATION

Asthma (known as reactive airway disease) is a chronic inflammatory process that causes airway inflammation with bronchoconstriction and bronchospasm; mucosal edema; and mucus secretion, which contributes to airway obstruction. It is usually triggered by an allergic response to an inhalant, a food product, stress, or a response to extreme changes in ambient temperature. Typically, the patient has recurring episodes of wheezing (most often heard on expiration), breathlessness, coughing, and chest tightness. These manifestations produce hypoxia and extreme patient anxiety. The onset of symptoms may be abrupt at the time of exposure to the trigger or delayed up to 4–12 hours after exposure to the trigger, and either may resolve spontaneously or endure for hours or days. The clinical manifestations and the course of the attacks are variable and unpredictable. Immediate therapeutic intervention is aimed at reducing bronchospasm, loosening mucous plugs so that they can be expelled, and decreasing inflammation/edema of respiratory tissue. Status asthmaticus is asthma that continues and becomes worse despite treatment with standard asthma medications. Status asthmaticus is a life-threatening condition. Approximately 14 million Americans have asthma, and the incidence has increased 60 percent since the 1980s. It is estimated that there are 5000 deaths each year due to asthma, and asthma as a cause of hospitalization is highest among African Americans (Lewis, Heitkemper, and Dirksen, 2004).

NURSING DIAGNOSIS 1

INEFFECTIVE AIRWAY CLEARANCE

Related to:

Bronchospasm

Increased thick mucous secretions

Ineffective cough

Airway mucosal edema

Defining Characteristics:

Expiratory wheezes

Decreased oxygen saturation

Cyanosis

Dyspnea

Tachypnea

Abnormal blood gases (decreased pO_2 and increased pCO_2)

Restlessness and anxiety

Goal:

Patient's airway is patent.

Outcome Criteria

✔ The patient's breath sounds will be clear.

✔ The patient will expectorate mucous.

✔ The patient will have no cyanosis.

✔ Oxygen saturation will be > 90 percent.

✔ Arterial blood gases are normal or improved.

NOC **_Asthma control_**
Respiratory status: Airway patency
Respiratory status: Ventilation
Allergic response: Systemic

INTERVENTIONS	RATIONALES
Assess respiratory status: breath sounds, respiratory rate, oxygen saturation; note abnormalities such as dyspnea, presence of cyanosis, retractions, use of	Abnormal breathing patterns may signal worsening of condition; retractions and flaring of nostrils indicate a significant decline in respiratory

INTERVENTIONS	RATIONALES
accessory muscles, flaring of nostrils.	status; assessment establishes baseline and monitors response to interventions.
Monitor patient for signs of occluded airway: cyanosis, cessation of wheezing, absence of breath sounds over lungs, holding throat, and continuous coughing.	If bronchospasm is severe, there may be no air movement, and therefore no wheezing. Be very careful when auscultating the chest to pay particular attention to the sound of any air movement, as focusing on picking up wheezing may cause one to miss the fact that there is no air movement; patient may cough almost continuously in an attempt to open the airway.
Assess arterial blood gases as ordered.	ABGs provide data for treatment regarding the lungs' ability to oxygenate tissues; initially ABG analysis will reveal respiratory alkalosis as the tachypnea blows off more carbon dioxide, but as the airway narrows, the lungs are unable to blow off carbon dioxide and acidosis is noted.
Assess for anxiety and reassure patient with presence.	Being unable to breathe causes anxiety and fear; the patient needs a calming presence; anxiety increases the demand for oxygen.
Establish intravenous access.	Ensures a route for rapid-acting medications.
Place patient in high Fowler's position and support with overbed table as needed.	Maximizes chest excursion and subsequent movement of air.
Assist respiratory therapist with administration of beta-adrenergic agonists (such as albuterol, metaproterenol) via nebulizer or metered dose inhaler as ordered, and monitor for side effects.	Stimulates beta$_2$-adrenergic receptor sites in the pulmonary system to increase levels of cAMP, which relaxes smooth muscles causing bronchodilation reducing bronchospasm; common side effects include tremors, tachycardia, and anxiety.
Administer corticosteroids (such as Solu-Medrol IV, prednisone PO, Flovent inhaled) as ordered, and monitor for side effects.	Suppresses the inflammatory response, decreases mucosal edema; systemic side effects from oral or IV administration include cushingoid appearance (with long term use), acne, bruising, increased appetite,

INTERVENTIONS	RATIONALES
	muscle weakness, and, with oral intake, GI upset; effects from inhaled corticosteroids include candidiasis, hoarseness, and dry cough.
Encourage expectoration of secretions and assess the viscosity, amount, and color of secretions.	Thickened secretions of asthma are more likely to occlude the airway; making this observation would allow for implementation of measures to thin and loosen the secretions; the color of secretions allows for early detection of color changes due to infection.
Monitor for signs and symptoms of respiratory infection: fever, rales, increased mucous production, elevated white blood cell count, and chest x-ray reports.	The presence of infection can worsen asthma; monitoring for signs of infection allows for early treatment that can prevent complications.
Provide humidified oxygen, as ordered, to maintain oxygen saturation at > 90 percent.	Loosens secretions, making them easier to expectorate with coughing; improves oxygenation.
Administer methylxanthine derivatives as ordered, and monitor for side effects.	Causes bronchodilation by blocking phosphodiesterase, which increases cAMP, which in turn alters intracellular calcium ion movement, producing bronchodilation; side effects include dizziness, palpitations, tachycardia, nausea, and vomiting.
Assist patient with coughing and deep breathing.	Mobilizes secretions and prevents atelectasis.
Increase fluid intake.	Assists with liquefying secretions and enhancing ability to clear from airways.
Provide for periods of rest and activity, assisting with activities as needed.	Decreases demand for oxygen and likelihood of reoccurrence of acute episode.
Teach patient about disease, prevention of acute exacerbations, medications, home care (see nursing diagnosis "Deficient Knowledge").	Knowledge increases the chance that the patient can engage in health-promoting behaviors and take control of disease.
Monitor results of pulmonary function tests, such as peak expiratory flow rate (PEFR) and forced expiratory volume (FEV).	Gives information regarding extent of disease and effect on adequate respiration. PEFR is used to monitor response to treatment, and FEV reflects degree of airway patency.

NIC *Airway management*
Asthma management
Cough enhancement
Presence
Respiratory monitoring
Oxygen therapy
Ventilation assistance

Evaluation

Assess the client to determine the extent to which the outcome criteria have been met. Assessments of the respiratory system should reveal that acute symptoms of asthma or, more specifically, ineffective airway clearance have been resolved. The patient's airway should be clear; the patient should be able to cough with expectoration of secretions, and the patient should be breathing easy. Breath sounds should be present, and even though some mild wheezing may be noted on expiration, this should be improved. ABGs and oxygen saturation should indicate adequate oxygenation, and there should be no cyanosis. If criteria have not been met, determine whether expected outcomes were realistic or simply that more time for achievement is needed. In the latter case, note the degree of progress the patient is making towards meeting the outcomes.

Community/Home Care

The patient with a diagnosis of asthma will need monitoring for a period of time by a health care professional when discharged home. The patient and family members will be able to implement strategies to manage the disease themselves with the use of metered dose inhalers and in-home nebulizers. Prior to discharge form the acute setting, the patient should attempt to identify known triggers in the home environment. Common precipitating factors are dust, mold, smoke, smell of paint, open flames in fireplaces, and kerosene heaters. If possible, these should be minimized or alleviated all together before the patient enters the home. The patient and family members will need to know the signs of acute exacerbations and airway obstruction, what interventions could be implemented prior to seeking emergency care, and thorough information on medications (see nursing diagnosis "Deficient Knowledge"), and measures to prevent respiratory infection.

Documentation

Document a comprehensive respiratory assessment. Include in the patient record all interventions carried out for the patient, and the patient's response. Note specifically the findings from a thorough follow-up respiratory assessment, changes in breath sounds in response to interventions, and the patient's emotional state. Document the introduction of new medication regimens and the patient's response or lack thereof. If the patient is able to participate in care, including self-care activities and coughing/deep breathing, document this in the chart. Vital signs and oxygen saturation should be documented according to agency protocol. Any teaching initiated should be charted with a clear indication of what was taught and to whom. Always include in the documentation the patient's progress towards achievement of the stated outcome criteria.

NURSING DIAGNOSIS 2

 ACTIVITY INTOLERANCE

Related to:
Hypoxia
Decreased pO_2
Increased oxygen demands with activity

Defining Characteristics:
Gasp for breath during activities
Wheezing during activities
Inability to perform any physical activity

Goal:
The patient is able to tolerate activities.

Outcome Criteria

✔ The patient is able to perform activities of daily living without wheezing or shortness of breath.
✔ The patient states that he or she is comfortable with activity performance.

NOC *Activity tolerance*
Energy conservation
Endurance

INTERVENTIONS	RATIONALES
Obtain subjective data from the patient regarding normal activities prior to onset of acute episodes of asthma and current activity status.	Helps to determine the effect asthma has had on the patient's ability to be active and allows for a better plan for future activity regimen.
Have patient use oxygen immediately prior to activity in the acute setting.	Improves oxygenation and provides for oxygen reserves to be used with increased demand.
Monitor vital signs and oxygen saturation before and after activity.	Use the results to indicate when activity may be increased or decreased.
Assist with activities as needed.	Conserves energy and reduces oxygen demand; because of the restrictive disorder, the patient lacks enough oxygen reserves to perform activities independently.
Pace activities and encourage periods of rest and activity during the day.	Conserves oxygen.
Gradually increase activity as tolerated and share guidelines for progression with patient.	Activities should be increased gradually, as tolerated, which allows the lungs to adapt to increasing demands for oxygen.
Reduce level of activity as required in response to wheezing or shortness of breath.	If increased physical activity causes wheezing or shortness, activity should be reduced until oxygenation is adequate.
Discuss with the patient activities that would be appropriate at home and that would be within patient's activity tolerance.	Physical activity increases endurance and stamina.
Inform the patient to stop any activity that produces shortness of breath or wheezing.	These indicate an intolerance to activity, and the level of activity should be evaluated.

NIC *Activity therapy*
Energy management

Evaluation

Evaluate whether the patient has achieved the stated desired outcomes. The patient verbalizes that he or she is able to carry out desired activities without wheezing or shortness of breath. After engaging in activity and following rest, the patient's pulse, blood pressure, and respirations return to baseline values.

Community/Home Care

Ensure that the patient has all of his or her questions answered related to activities allowed and how to increase endurance. The patient with asthma may be hesitant to engage in usual activities for fear of wheezing. It is important that the patient know how to adjust activities and understands that activity has a role in adapting to the disease by increasing endurance and stamina. Even though the patient may not require the services of a visiting nurse, follow-up visits with a health care provider are necessary. During these visits, the patient should be questioned about activity performance and tolerance. Discussions related to the indiscriminant use of inhalers for minor shortness of breath and wheezing should be initiated, because often times discontinuance of the activity can relieve the symptoms.

Documentation

The nurse should chart the patient's tolerance for activity, including vital signs and presence/absence of wheezing or shortness of breath in response to activity. Document types of activities the patient is able to perform and duration of the activity. If oxygen is needed for activity performance, document the type and method of delivery and the rate of flow. Include in the patient's chart all interventions employed to address the problem and whether the patient has achieved the specific outcome criteria. If the criteria have not been met, document what progress has been made and any revisions to the plan of care.

NURSING DIAGNOSIS 3

 ANXIETY

Related to:

Wheezing

Inability to breathe effectively

Defining Characteristics:

Restlessness

Verbalization of anxiety

Diaphoresis

Verbalization of fear, not wanting to be left alone

Goal:

  Anxiety is relieved.

Outcome Criteria

✔ The patient verbalizes that anxiety has been reduced.

✔ The patient appears relaxed (no restlessness or agitation).

✔ The patient has no physiological symptoms of anxiety (tachycardia, diaphoresis).

✔ The patient asks appropriate questions about disease.

NOC *Anxiety control*
     Acceptance: Health status

INTERVENTIONS	RATIONALES
Have patient rate anxiety on a numerical scale.	Allows for a more objective measure of anxiety level.
Provide oxygen, as ordered.	Assists patient to breathe easier so that the patient faces less physical stress (physical stress can lead to anxiety).
Implement strategies to manage respiratory status (see nursing diagnosis "Ineffective Airway Clearance").	Correction of the alterations in respiratory status "unable to breathe" will help to reduce anxiety level.
Reassure patient by explaining the disease and treatments that are being implemented to correct breathing.	Inability to breathe contributes to anxiety because of the fear that interventions may not work quickly enough; knowing what to expect helps the patient maintain control of environment.
Encourage patient to verbalize concerns about health status.	Verbalizing concerns can help patient deal with issues and avoid negative feelings.
Stay with patient during episodes of shortness of breath and wheezing, and use a calm manner.	Allows the nurse to offer comfort, care, and assurances to reduce anxiety and fear.
Allow family to visit liberally if patient desires.	Family may provide emotional support that calms the patient and promotes a sense of comfort.
Teach patient relaxation techniques (such as slow, purposeful breathing) and encourage their use.	Reduces anxiety and creates a feeling of comfort.

NIC *Anxiety reduction*
     Calming technique
     Emotional support
     Presence

Evaluation

Assess the patient for the extent that he or she is free of anxiety. The patient should verbalize that anxiety is reduced and that he or she feels comfortable. Assess the patient for physiological signs of anxiety, such as increased pulse and sweating. During evaluation, be sure to inquire about the use of relaxation techniques. The patient will also need to report that he or she understands the disease process (asthma) that has changed his or her health status.

Community/Home Care

The patient will need to know how to control anxiety in the home setting. It is crucial that health care providers equip the patient with knowledge to make the patient feel in control of his or her health. A patient who knows how to treat the shortness of breath and wheezing of asthma and modify his or her lifestyle accordingly will have fewer incidences of anxiety and fear. The patient should be encouraged to keep a log of what makes him or her anxious and how anxiety is resolved. Keeping emergency medication easily accessible is recommended to decrease concern that the patient may not be able to get to it when necessary. By ensuring that the patient understands the health care regimen and knows what to do if acute symptoms develop, the health care provider may prevent unnecessary emergency room visits.

Documentation

Document the degree of anxiety experienced by the patient. Using some type of numerical rating scale similar to the pain scale will provide health care providers with a more objective measure of the degree of anxiety the patient is experiencing. Document any physiological or observable signs of anxiety, such as restlessness, tachycardia, or diaphoresis. Interventions implemented to treat these should be documented, along with subsequent assessments to determine their effectiveness.

NURSING DIAGNOSIS 4

 ## DEFICIENT KNOWLEDGE

Related to:

> Insufficient knowledge of asthma and its treatment
>
> No previous history of disease (asthma)

Defining Characteristics:

> Asks questions/has concerns
>
> Has had repeated hospital visits for asthma
>
> Has no questions
>
> Verbalizes a lack of knowledge/understanding

Goal:

> The patient verbalizes an understanding of asthma and its treatment.

Outcome Criteria

✔ The patient verbalizes a desire to learn necessary information.

✔ The patient verbalizes a willingness to keep appointments and follow prescribed regimen.

✔ The patient demonstrates knowledge of the disease (asthma).

✔ The patient demonstrates knowledge of prescribed medications.

✔ The patient demonstrates correct use of metered dose inhaler or in-home nebulizer and EpiPen.

NOC *Knowledge: Disease process*
Knowledge: Treatment regimen
Compliance behavior

INTERVENTIONS	RATIONALES
Assess readiness of patient to learn (motivation, cognitive level, physiological status).	The patient must be motivated to learn, have the capability to learn the content, and be free of distractions to learning, such as pain and shortness of breath.
Assess the patient's current knowledge.	The teacher needs to ascertain what the patient already knows and build on this.
Start with the simplest information first.	Patients can understand simple concepts easily and then build on those to understand more complex concepts.
Identify a family member or significant other who will also learn the content and assist the patient with compliance.	This person can reinforce the teaching and assist with implementation if the client becomes incapable of follow-through.
Create a quiet environment conducive to learning.	Environmental noise can prevent the learner from focusing on the content being taught.
Teach the learners about the pathophysiology of asthma in the initial teaching session, including complications.	The patient must understand what the disease is and how it affects the body before understanding the rationale for treatments.
Teach the learners about prescribed medications (see nursing diagnosis "Ineffective Airway Clearance"), including action, side effects, dosing schedule, correct use of inhalers, and proper technique for administering medications through a nebulizer.	Knowledge of why the medication is necessary and how it works will focus on the importance of the medication. Identification of side effects will minimize anxiety if these untoward effects should occur.
Teach the patient to take bronchodilators prior to other medications or inhalers.	Bronchodilators dilate/open narrowed airways and enhance absorption and effectiveness of other medications/inhalers.
Teach the patient about the importance of tracking events/substances that trigger attacks and how to minimize them. In general, teach the patient to avoid smoke, dust, and mold, and to keep away from heat sources such as kerosene heaters and wood burning fireplaces.	The patient must understand triggering factors in order to control them and prevent avoidable asthma attacks; the triggers listed here are common ones that could lead to an acute episode.
Teach the patient how to use a peak flow meter and how to interpret data.	Helps to assess symptom severity and can be used as a guide to adjust medications.
Instruct patient in relaxation techniques.	Informing the patient of relaxation techniques may help him or her reduce the severity of the attacks.
Instruct patient on when and how to use an EpiPen.	In the event of an emergency when the patient is having extreme difficulty breathing and health care assistance is not available, the patient can self-administer a preloaded dosage of epinephrine using an EpiPen.

(continues)

(continued)

INTERVENTIONS	RATIONALES
Teach the patient how to use an incentive spirometer and the rationale for its use.	Use and understanding of an incentive spirometer will help the patient to determine when to seek health care assistance earlier in the disease's acute phases.
Teach learners about activity, including how to progress exercise gradually while monitoring responses. Patients need to understand as well that some preferred activities may need to be eliminated. Inform the patient to eliminate any activity that produces wheezing, chest pain, or dizziness.	Incorporation of exercise into daily routine is necessary to regain stamina and maintain respiratory functioning.
Teach the patient which signs and symptoms to report to a health care provider.	Monitoring for signs and symptoms early can prevent a crisis that requires hospitalization. It is important for asthmatic patients to know when to seek health care assistance to avoid complications.
Evaluate the patient's understanding of all content covered by asking questions; have the patient demonstrate use of inhalers, nebulizers, and the EpiPen.	Helps to identify areas that require more teaching and to ensure that the patient has enough information to ensure compliance; if the patient can demonstrate correct procedure for administering medications through inhalers and nebulizers, he or she will feel more comfortable using them when needed and anxiety should be decreased.
Give the patient written information.	Provides for reference at a later time, and allows for review.
Establish that the patient has the resources required to be compliant.	If needed resources such as finances, transportation, and psychosocial support are not available, the patient cannot be compliant.

NIC *Learning readiness enhancement*
Learning facilitation
Teaching: Psychomotor skill
Teaching: Disease process
Teaching: Prescribed medication

Evaluation

Evaluate the degree to which the patient has achieved the outcome criteria relevant to the teaching sessions. The patient is able to repeat all information for the nurse and asks questions about the prescribed regimen. The patient can identify all medications by name and report the common side effects as well as the dosing schedule. Asthmatic patients should demonstrate the ability to give their own medications via metered dose inhaler, nebulizer, and EpiPen. The patient should be able to inform the nurse when health care assistance should be sought for acute exacerbations.

Community/Home Care

The patient will need to implement the medical regimen in the home setting. The success of treatment for asthma depends upon the degree to which the patient has received adequate teaching and has subsequently understood and internalized it. The patient with asthma will need to know how to prevent acute exacerbations by constantly monitoring the environment for triggers including emotional stress. Keeping a log of what he or she was doing prior to the onset of any acute episode will assist the patient to be proactive in disease management and is crucial to preventing crises. Adequate financial resources should be in place for purchase of medications and supplies prior to time of discharge. Investigation into this issue and appropriate assistance with this should be made through social services prior to discharge from the acute care setting. It may be helpful for the patient to have a notebook with all instructions in it for easy reference. This notebook should have a section or page for medication schedule, including spacing of oral meds, inhalers, and any nebulizer treatments, as well as a section on how to prevent and treat acute asthmatic attacks and how to prevent infections. Follow-up care should focus on assessing the patient's ability to perform nebulizer treatments and use of the spirometer to assess airway status. During follow-up visits with health care providers, the patient should be questioned about the information previously taught, with particular focus on how he or she uses inhalers, because in many instances patients overuse them, creating a risk for cardiac complications. Teaching can be reinforced at this time.

Documentation

Document the specific content taught and the titles of printed materials given to patient or family. Chart the patient's understanding of the content and the methods used to evaluate learning. The patient's successful demonstration of the proper use of nebulizers, metered dose inhalers, and the EpiPen should be documented. The nurse must clearly indicate areas that need to be reinforced. After the teaching session is complete, the nurse should note whether the patient indicates a willingness and the ability to comply with health care recommendations. If the teaching included a significant other or family members, indicate this in the documentation. In addition, document any referrals made in the patient record.

CHAPTER 2.23

CHRONIC OBSTRUCTIVE PULMONARY DISEASE

GENERAL INFORMATION

Chronic obstructive pulmonary disease (COPD) is a descriptive label applied to disorders of the respiratory system that obstruct flow of air through the pulmonary system. This limited airflow can occur because of destruction of alveoli function (emphysematous type) or chronic congestion due to thick mucous and mucosa edema (bronchitic type). One type may dominate, but for many patients seen in the acute care setting some aspects of both types are present. Ninety percent of patients with COPD have a significant history of cigarette smoking for many years. The patient with chronic obstructive pulmonary disease (COPD) will have the most difficulty exhaling. Therefore, pCO_2 levels in COPD patients will, as expected, be higher than normal. Emphysema usually occurs because of a long-term history of smoking or inhaled pollutants that produce inflammation and/or irritation and loss of elasticity of lung tissue. These pollutants could be chemicals, coal dust, or lint and dust from working in cotton mills. This causes the alveoli to rupture, forming larger air spaces known as blebs or bullae. Because of a decreased surface area for gas exchange to occur and an inelasticity of the bleb/bullae walls (causing air-trapping), the patient's demand for oxygenated blood cannot be met. For some patients, emphysema is caused by a genetic deficiency in alpha$_1$ anti-trypsin, which would prohibit proteolytic enzymes from destroying the lungs, but this accounts for only 1 percent of all cases. In emphysema, the patient may have a diagnosis for years without any significant demonstration of symptoms. Dyspnea is the first symptom, and is controlled by adjusting activities accordingly. However, as the disease progresses, the patient begins increasing the use of accessory muscles to breathe and hyperinflation occurs, which over time creates the characteristic barrel chest appearance. These patients have scant secretions. Chronic bronchitis is characterized by excessive mucous secretion, defined as a productive cough for 3 or more months over 2 consecutive years. The patient with bronchitis has chronic inflammation in the airways with excessive mucous production due to constant irritation. Normal ciliary movement is impaired due to the inflammation as well as the damage caused by irritants, thus placing the patient at high risk for infection. The presence of mucous in the airways not only causes obstruction of airflow, but also leads to bronchospasm, further limiting air movement. Early clinical manifestations include cough with production of large amounts of thick mucous and, later in the disease, signs of right-sided heart failure may be evident. As COPD progresses, the shortness of breath becomes so pronounced that the patient is unable to perform even simple activities of daily living. When end stage disease is noted, the patient is on oxygen and appears somewhat debilitated, because even eating requires use of oxygen reserves.

NURSING DIAGNOSES 1

INEFFECTIVE BREATHING PATTERN

Related to:

Destruction of alveoli

Obstruction of airflow

Bronchospasm

Tenacious secretions

Defining Characteristics:

Severe dyspnea

Sitting up, leaning forward, hands on knees

Use of accessory muscles of respiration

Abnormal blood gases

Abnormal inspiratory/expiratory ratio

Goal:

Patient's respirations are regular.

Outcome Criteria

✔ The patients respirations are easy and < 28.

✔ The patient reports a decrease in shortness of breath.

✔ The patient is able to cough up secretions.

✔ The patient's arterial blood gases return to baseline.

NOC *Respiratory status: Gentilation*
Respiratory status: Gas exchange
Vital signs

INTERVENTIONS	RATIONALES
Assess respiratory system by noting respiratory rate, depth, chest expansion, rhythm, breath sounds, arterial blood gases, pulse oximetry, and skin color, and note any of the following abnormalities: — Severe dyspnea that has progressively worsened — Cyanosis (nailbeds, lips) — Sitting up, with hands on knees, leaning forward — Use of accessory muscles of respiration — Prolonged expiratory phase — Clubbing of fingers — Barrel chest — Difficulty talking (due to shortness of breath) — Cough productive of thick secretions	Any of these abnormalities would indicate the status of the respiratory system and progression of disease; also establishes a baseline for future comparisons.
Assist patient in assuming a high Fowler's position or position of choice for easy respiration, such as leaning forward on overbed table.	Maximizes thoracic cavity space, decreases pressure from diaphragm and abdominal organs, and facilitates use of accessory muscles.
Provide humidified, low-flow (2 liters/min) oxygen, as ordered.	Provides some supplemental oxygen to improve oxygenation and to make secretions less viscous. However, caution should be taken when administering oxygen to COPD patients. In people without lung disease the stimulus to breathe comes from rising levels of pCO$_2$; however because these levels are always high in the COPD patient, the drive to breathe comes from a hypoxic drive (low pO$_2$). If oxygen is given at high rates, it may take away the drive to breathe, resulting in respiratory arrest.
Administer bronchodilators, such as methylxanthine derivatives (aminophylline IV, theophylline PO), as ordered, and monitor for side effects.	Causes bronchodilation and reduces bronchospasm, improving air flow; side effects include dizziness, palpitations, tachycardia, nausea, and vomiting. These are older medications; newer medications via metered dose inhalers may be more effective, but these older medications may still be used in some practices.
Administer corticosteroids (such as Solu-Medrol IV and prednisone PO, Flovent inhaled) as ordered, and monitor for side effects.	Suppresses the inflammatory response, decreases mucosal edema; systemic effects from oral or IV administration include cushingoid appearance, acne, bruising, increased appetite, muscle weakness, and with oral intake, GI upset; effects from inhaled corticosteroids include candidiasis, hoarseness, dry cough, and nose bleeds.
Administer or assist respiratory therapist with administration of beta-adrenergic agonists (such as albuterol and metaproterenol) via nebulizer or metered dose inhaler, as ordered, and monitor for side effects.	Stimulates beta$_2$-adrenergic receptor sites in the pulmonary system to increase levels of cAMP, which causes relaxation of smooth muscle, in turn causing bronchodilation reducing bronchospasm; common side effects include tremors, tachycardia, and anxiety.
Give anticholinergic agents (such as Atrovent) via inhaler.	These agents have bronchodilator properties with fewer side effects. A combination drug (Combivent), which contains Atrovent and albuterol is available.
Administer IV fluids and increase oral fluids (2000–3000 ml/day as tolerated), as ordered.	Helps to improve hydration state and decrease secretions.
Administer expectorants (bronchitis patients), as ordered.	Enhances expectoration of secretions of previously ineffective cough.

(continues)

(continued)

INTERVENTIONS	RATIONALES
Administer antibiotics if respiratory infection is present, or prophylactically, as ordered.	Helps to prevent or eradicate respiratory infection (i.e., pneumonia), to reduce secretions, and to end inflammation.
Provide chest physiotherapy, as ordered.	Mobilizes thick secretions and facilitates clearing of lung fields.
Assist with activities of daily living as required.	The patient with COPD may lack sufficient oxygen reserves to perform activities, especially during acute exacerbations; even eating may cause severe dyspnea.
Assess cardiac system for signs of right-sided heart failure and side effects of medications (tachycardia, decreased heart sounds, jugular vein distention, peripheral edema), and institute appropriate interventions to address (see "Heart Failure" care plan).	The increased work of breathing causes an increase in pressure in the pulmonary vasculature, which overworks the right ventricle. Tachycardia can be caused by medications and by the heart's attempt to compensate for decreased oxygen. Jugular vein distention and peripheral edema represents right-sided heart failure. Decreased heart sounds are noted due to distance between stethoscope and heart secondary to increased AP diameter.
Teach patient how to decrease shortness of breath by restructuring activities.	Knowing how to control shortness of breath will help patient cope and have optimal functioning; knowledge also decreases anxiety.
Teach pulmonary hygiene: prevention of infections, maintaining optimal health, flu and pneumonia vaccine (see nursing diagnosis "Ineffective Management of Therapeutic Regimen").	Protecting against infections can prevent acute exacerbations and subsequent hospitalizations.

NIC   *Respiratory monitoring*
Cough enhancement
Oxygen therapy
Positioning

Evaluation

The patient should show indications that breathing patterns have returned to baseline and are effective in meeting the body's need for oxygen. The rate should return to baseline, preferably between 12–24 breaths per minute, and be unlabored. For the patient who has thick secretions, the ability to expectorate these would be a positive outcome. The return of arterial blood gases to the patient's baseline or to within normal range should be expected.

Community/Home Care

In the home setting, the patient may continue to experience some shortness of breath dependent upon the severity of disease. Patients will need to know how to tailor their lives to adapt to the change in respiratory function (see nursing diagnosis "Deficient Knowledge"), with attention to how to manage acute episodes of shortness of breath. Performance of activities of daily living, household chores, and leisure activities may present challenges for the patient. The patient may need to incorporate rest periods into his or her daily routine to prevent increased oxygen demands and fatigue. When the patient has activities planned that include physical activity, such as showering/taking tub baths, shopping, going out for meals, or going on trips, he or she should spend some time resting first; if on home oxygen, administer oxygen prior to activity as needed. Utilizing new ways of breathing, such as pursed lip breathing and leaning forward over a table or with hands on knees, will provide the patient with methods to improve intake of air. The nurse should question the patient regarding his or her occupation, ability to return to work, and impact that the type of work may have on respiratory function. Follow-up care should focus on assessing for progression of the disease and changes that may be required to preserve as much lung function as possible. A health care provider should ensure that the patient understands all medications that are prescribed, including in home oxygen, metered dose inhalers, or nebulizers. It is important that the patient understand how to prevent upper respiratory infections particularly through the use of immunizations against influenza and pneumonia.

Documentation

Chart the results of a comprehensive assessment of the respiratory and cardiac systems. Note respiratory rate, chest expansion, use of any accessory muscles, breath sounds, and results of pulse oximetry. If the patient expectorates, document the amount, color, and consistency. When new treatments are initiated, such as the use of metered dose inhalers, nebulizers, or oral medications, chart this in the record according to agency guidelines and document any patient teaching completed. Document subjective data exactly as the patient states it. Include in the patient's chart all interventions employed to address ineffective breathing pattern and any patient response to the interventions that would indicate the problem has been resolved. If the patient's breathing has not improved, indicate how the plan has been revised.

NURSING DIAGNOSIS 2

 ## IMPAIRED GAS EXCHANGE

Related to:

Lower airway (alveolar) wall destruction preventing adequate exchange of gases of respiration

Airway obstruction (secretions) preventing adequate oxygenation

Ineffective breathing pattern

Defining Characteristics:

Severe dyspnea

Tachypnea

Sitting up, leaning forward

Use of accessory muscles of respiration

Agitation

Decreased oxygen saturation

Abnormal arterial blood gases (highly elevated pCO_2, decreased pO_2)

Goal:

Gas exchange is adequate.

Outcome Criteria

✔ The patient's arterial blood gases return to baseline or normal and oxygen saturation is > 90 percent.

✔ The patient's skin color improves.

✔ The patient's respiratory rate is within baseline.

✔ The patient reports no dyspnea/shortness of breath.

✔ The patient exhibits no agitation or restlessness.

NOC *Respiratory status: Ventilation*
Respiratory status: Gas exchange
Vital signs

INTERVENTIONS	RATIONALES
Assess respiratory status: skin color, breath sounds, respiratory rate, rhythm, quality, effort.	Establishes baseline information about respiratory function.
Assess oxygen saturation using pulse oximetry and arterial blood gases as ordered.	Helps to determine the status of oxygen to tissues and monitor for respiratory acidosis. Note that for many patients with COPD, some degree of respiratory acidosis is always present, but arterial blood gases will demonstrate compensation.
Provide supplemental low-flow oxygen as ordered.	Helps to maximize oxygen saturation and relieve shortness of breath; in people without lung disease, the stimulus to breathe comes from rising levels of pCO_2; however, because these levels are always high in the COPD patient, their stimulus to breathe comes from a hypoxic drive (low pO_2), and if oxygen is given at a high rate, it may take away the drive to breathe.
Place the patient in high Fowler's position or leaning over an overbed table, or leaning forward with hands on knees.	These positions allow for better chest expansion and subsequent air exchange.
Monitor for altered mental status: restlessness, anxiety, or confusion.	These symptoms may indicate decreased oxygenation to cerebral tissues.
Give medications as ordered (bronchodilators, corticosteroids, beta-adrenergic agonists) and evaluate effectiveness (see nursing diagnosis "Ineffective Breathing Pattern").	Opens narrowed airways; decreases inflammation and improves gas exchange.
If thick secretions are present, give mucolytics or expectorants, as ordered.	Assists with mucous excretion to clear lungs of substances that cause obstruction and increased vascular resistance.
Have patient perform coughing and deep breathing if able.	Prevents stasis of secretions, opens airways, and improves gas exchange.

(continues)

(continued)

INTERVENTIONS	RATIONALES
Encourage the use of pursed lip breathing and diaphragmatic breathing.	Minimizes air trapping; pursed lip breathing particularly assists the emphysema patient to keep airways open longer during expiration; diaphragmatic breathing uses the larger muscles of respiration, which helps to conserve energy.
Allow a balance of rest and activity; encourage rest before and after activity, assisting with activities of daily living.	Helps to conserve oxygen reserves and to prevent exacerbation of hypoxia. COPD patients tire easily and lack oxygen reserves; thus, when they become very tired, they may not be able to continue the work of breathing.
Monitor for weight loss, especially in the patient with emphysema.	Weight loss occurs due to the increased energy and oxygen required for eating, and also because of the feeling of satiety that occurs because the flattened diaphragm compresses abdominal organs.
During acute exacerbations, provide small meals that are easily digested or nutritional supplements, as ordered.	The patient may not have enough oxygen reserves to eat; large complex meals require oxygen for digestion, further depleting oxygen reserves in the already compromised patient; it is important that the patient have adequate nutrition to prevent weight loss and maintain optimal health status.

NIC *Oxygen therapy*
Respiratory monitoring
Acid base management:
*   Respiratory acidosis*
Positioning

Evaluation

Evaluate the status of the outcome criteria. The patient should have indicators of good gas exchange, such as even, easy respirations, good skin color, and an oxygen saturation of at least 90 percent. Blood gas analyses should indicate an absence of respiratory acidosis or show compensation and oxygen levels between 80–100 percent. The patient should report an absence of shortness of breath and a respiratory rate within baseline. Mental status should return to baseline levels and the patient should not be restless or agitated.

Community/Home Care

For most patients with COPD, gas exchange will always be a problem, as the disease is a progressive one. The patient will need to learn how to adapt to this change in health status while preserving optimal functioning. At home, the patient may notice activity intolerance in the form of shortness of breath when performing usual activities, such as mowing the lawn, doing laundry, taking walks, or other simple tasks, because of the inability of the diseased lungs to supply adequate oxygen during times of increased need. Teaching should be undertaken to assist the patient and family to cope with limitations and to make the necessary changes. The goal becomes one of maintaining an optimal state of health while keeping the patient as functional as possible. Simple suggestions, such as mowing only half the lawn, purchasing a riding mower (if financially possible), doing only half the household chores at a time, resting immediately before activity, and using new methods of breathing, can keep the patient active for a long period of time. Keeping a log of episodes of shortness of breath and activities that precipitate shortness of breath may be helpful in demonstrating where changes can be made. As the disease progresses, the need for in-home oxygen and nebulizer treatments must be investigated. It is crucial that the patient understand the rationale for use of all medications, when to contact a health care provider, and the need for immunizations against influenza and pneumonia (see nursing diagnosis "Deficient Knowledge").

Documentation

Included in the documentation should be a complete respiratory assessment with specific attention to breath sounds, skin color, effort of breathing, any complaints of shortness of breath, and the patient's level of comfort with his or her breathing. In addition, include the patient's response to activity. Chart all interventions, including any teaching done and the patient's specific response. Results of oxygen saturation readings and arterial blood gases should be documented as they represent the best measure of gas exchange. If the patient still has indicators of impaired gas exchange, these should be specifically noted along with any needed revisions to the plan of care that should be made.

NURSING DIAGNOSIS 3

 ## ACTIVITY INTOLERANCE

Related to:

Hypoxia

Decreased pO_2

Increased oxygen demands with activity

Defining Characteristics:

Shortness of breath/dyspnea

Patient reports "gasping for breath" during activities

Unable to perform any physical activity

Goal:

The patient is able to tolerate activities.

Outcome Criteria

✔ The patient is able to perform activities of daily living without shortness of breath.

✔ The patient states that he or she is comfortable with activity performance.

✔ The patient states that shortness of breath is improved following cessation of activity, and the patient's respiratory rate returns to baseline within 10 minutes.

NOC *Activity tolerance*
     Energy conservation
     Endurance

INTERVENTIONS	RATIONALES
Obtain subjective data from the patient regarding normal activities prior to onset of acute exacerbations of COPD and current activity status.	Helps to determine the effect COPD has had on the patient's ability to be active and allows for a better plan for a future activity regimen.
Reduce level of activity as required in response to shortness of breath.	If increased physical activity causes wheezing or shortness of breath, activity should be reduced until oxygenation is adequate.
Assist with activities as needed.	Helps to conserve energy and reduce oxygen demand; because of the obstructive disorder, the patient lacks enough oxygen reserves to perform activities independently.
Pace activities and encourage periods of rest and activity during the day.	Conserves oxygen.
Monitor vital signs and oxygen saturation before and after activity.	Use the results to indicate when activity may be increased or decreased.
Gradually increase activity as tolerated and share guidelines for progression with the patient.	Activities should be increased gradually, as tolerated, to avoid overtaxing the patient.
Discuss with the patient activities that would be appropriate once at home and that would be within patient's activity tolerance.	Physical activity increases endurance and stamina.
Have patient use oxygen immediately prior to activity in the acute setting and in the home as the disease progresses.	Improves oxygenation and provides for oxygen reserves to be used with increased demand.
Inform the patient to stop any activity that produces shortness of breath or wheezing.	These indicate an intolerance to activity, and the level of activity should be evaluated.
Encourage intake of foods that are high in iron and protein.	Iron has a role in oxygen transport and increases energy level; protein provides nutrients for energy and metabolism.
If shortness of breath is not relieved by rest, give prn oxygen or albuterol treatments, as ordered.	Causes bronchodilation, increases airflow, and relieves acute symptoms.

NIC *Activity therapy*
     Energy management

Evaluation

Evaluate whether the patient has achieved the stated desired outcomes. The patient verbalizes that he or she is able to carry out desired activities without wheezing or severe shortness of breath. After the patient engages in activity, his or her pulse, blood pressure, and respirations return to baseline values following rest. Pulse oximetry readings reveal an oxygen saturation of > 90 percent following rest.

Community/Home Care

Ensure that the patient has all of his or her questions answered related to activities allowed and increasing endurance. The patient with COPD may be hesitant to engage in any activities for fear of becoming short of breath. The patient should develop a daily routine that initially begins with short walks around the home and performance of activities of daily living. If the patient remains at home rather than going to work, he or she should not become completely sedentary, but should incorporate increasing amounts of activity into his or her day. It is important that the patient know how to adjust activities and understands that activity has a role in adapting to the disease by increasing endurance and stamina. The patient should keep an activity log with documentation of date, type of activity, duration of activity, and response to the activity (any shortness of breath or increased respiratory or heart rate). If untoward symptoms occur during activity, the patient should record what he or she did to relieve symptoms and how long it took to return to his or her baseline respiratory status. Even though the patient may not require the services of a visiting nurse, follow-up visits with a health care provider are needed. During these visits, the patient can share his or her activity log, which will provide valuable information to the health care provider regarding activity performance and tolerance. When mild shortness of breath or wheezing occurs the patient should be encouraged to cease activity and rest in order to relieve the symptoms, rather than using an inhaler.

Documentation

The nurse should chart the patient's tolerance for activity, including vital signs and presence/absence of wheezing or shortness of breath in response to activity. Include in the record any concerns the patient may have regarding the ability to perform activities of daily living or other activities once at home. Document types of activities the patient is able to perform and duration of the activity. Include in the patient's chart all interventions employed to address the problem and whether the patient has achieved the specific outcome criteria. If the criteria have not been met, document what progress has been made and any revisions to the plan of care.

NURSING DIAGNOSIS 4

 ### RISK FOR INFECTION

Related to:

Chronic respiratory disease process

Retention of thick secretions

Poor nutritional status

Decreased activity

Defining Characteristics (If Infection Occurs):

Chest congestion

Fatigue

Poor hydration status

Increased white blood cell count

Fever

Immobility

Goal:

The patient will not acquire a respiratory infection.

Outcome Criteria

✔ The patient will have no symptoms of respiratory infections such as fever, elevated white blood cell counts, or expectoration of mucopurulent sputum.

✔ The patient verbalizes an understanding of measures to prevent infection, such as adequate nutrition, activity, and immunizations.

NOC *Immunization behavior*
Nutritional status
Knowledge: Infection control

INTERVENTIONS	RATIONALES
Monitor for signs of infection: elevated white blood cell count, fever, coughing with expectoration of mucopurulent sputum.	Helps to detect the presence of infection early and initiate early interventions.
Increase fluid intake.	Moistens secretions so that they can be expectorated and not harbor bacteria.
Administer antibiotics, as ordered.	Antibiotics should be given prophylactically to prevent infection or to treat causative organisms found on sputum culture.
Increase level of activity per patient tolerance.	Helps to improve oxygenation and decrease secretion retention.
Encourage the intake of foods high in protein and vitamin C; discuss with the patient how to meet nutritional needs adequately.	Protein and vitamin C are required for immune system functioning and healing; the patient's general well-being and resistance to disease can be adversely affected by poor diet.

INTERVENTIONS	RATIONALES
Encourage the patient to take the influenza and pneumonia vaccines as appropriate and as ordered, and provide a list of locations where the vaccines can be obtained.	The patient with COPD is at high risk for acquiring upper respiratory infection because of secretions, absence of normal ciliary actions in upper airways, and compromised lung function; taking these vaccines can prevent infections that could cause acute exacerbations of the disease and severely compromise respiratory function requiring hospitalization.
Give medications as ordered (bronchodilators, beta adrenergic agonist, corticosteroids).	Helps maintain respiratory function in an optimal state.
Have patient rinse mouth following use of inhalers.	Helps to prevent development of oral fungal infections such as candidiasis.
During acute exacerbations, limit exposure to crowds and limit visitors, especially children.	Reduces exposure to microorganisms that can be transported via droplets and hand-to-hand contact.
Teach patient and family the signs and symptoms of infection and when to report them to the health care provider.	Allows for early initiation of treatment.

 NIC   *Infection control*

Infection protection

Immunization/vaccination management

Nutrition management

Evaluation

The patient has no symptoms of infection. Temperature remains normal and there is no elevation in white cell count. The patient reports that mucous is not purulent, and there is no shortness of breath other than what is normally present with activity.

Community/Home Care

The patient with COPD will always be at high risk for development of upper respiratory infections. It is important that the patient be able to verbalize the signs and symptoms of respiratory infections that should be reported to the health care provider. Upper respiratory infections can pose a serious threat to the patient's well-being, causing acute exacerbations that may require a lengthy hospitalization. Avoiding areas, such as crowded shopping centers, where infections are easily transmitted may be required, especially during winter months. For elderly patients, contact with grandchildren who have a common cold should also be avoided, as this may be enough to cause an acute exacerbation. Good handwashing should be practiced by the patient, especially following activities where there is likely to be significant handshaking, such as a religious service. Maintaining an optimal level of respiratory functioning by engaging in activity as tolerated as well as adequate intake of fluid and nutrition will assist in efforts to prevent infection. Of crucial importance is the patient's willingness to receive the influenza and pneumonia vaccines to prevent these two infections, which would further compromise respiratory function and in almost all instances require hospitalization for the COPD patient. The patient will usually have a variety of options for receiving these vaccines, such as special flu clinics, hospital clinics, health care providers' offices, local health departments, and senior centers.

NURSING DIAGNOSIS 5

INEFFECTIVE COPING

Related to:

Shortness of breath with activity

Need for limitations on normal functioning

Chronic nature of COPD

Progressive nature of COPD

Defining Characteristics:

Verbalizes that it is difficult to accept condition

Frequent hospitalizations for exacerbations

Verbalizes an inability to cope with activity limitations

Goal:

The patient will state an ability to cope with chronic illness.

Outcome Criteria

✔ The patient will identify one successful coping mechanism.

✔ The patient will verbalize satisfaction with management of illness and states feeling in control.

NOC   *Acceptance: Health status*
Adaptation to physical disability
Psychosocial adjustment:
   Life change
Coping

INTERVENTIONS	RATIONALES
Appraise the patient's understanding of the disease process.	Helps to ascertain that the patient has the correct information on which to make decisions.
Encourage the patient to verbalize fears, feelings, and anxiety about the disease (COPD); the needed interventions; and the change in functioning.	The first step in coping with a situation is to recognize and discuss feelings.
Be available to the patient to listen and use a calm, reassuring approach.	Often patients need to talk openly and freely about their feelings and concerns; taking time to listen provides a means of coping for the patient.
Explore with the patient how he or she normally copes with stressful situations and help him or her to identify new ways of coping.	Strategies that have worked before may be successful again, and new strategies can be explored to add to the patient's repertoire of coping methods.
Arrange for a spiritual consult, as appropriate.	Many people defer to their religion or spirituality for comfort during times of crisis or stress.
Teach the patient relaxation techniques (such as slow purposeful breathing, guided imagery) and encourage their use.	Reduces anxiety and creates a feeling of comfort.
Discuss openly with the patient the typical progression of the disease and interventions that will be required, such as long-term oxygen use, extreme limitation, in activities over time, medications, and eventual respiratory failure.	Knowing what to expect decreases the unknown and allows the patient to be prepared for the disease progression by establishing appropriate coping strategies before they are required in an emergency.
Stay with patient during any acute episode of shortness of breath.	Allows the nurse to offer comfort, care, and assurances in order to reduce anxiety that could add to the feeling of being unable to cope.
Encourage use of available support systems or organized support groups for patients with respiratory disorders.	Discussion with others can provide the patient with new information on established ways of coping with some of the problems that occur with respiratory disease.
For patients who have progressed to severely compromised lung function or with end-stage disease, discuss advance directives as appropriate or according to agency protocol.	Advance directives initiated by the patient before the disease is in its final stages can provide the health care provider with specifics about desired care and decreases anxiety and further stress for family members.
Support family members as they adjust to the change in health status of the patient and possible role performance changes.	Providing support to the family, talking with the family members, and encouraging verbalization of their concerns and questions will prepare them to better assist the patient to cope with chronic illness.

NIC   *Coping enhancement*
Emotional support
Support group

Evaluation

In order to establish that the outcome criteria have been met, the patient must willingly identify available coping strategies that can be used in adapting to this chronic disease. In addition, the patient should verbalize that he or she will be able to manage and control the disease. Indicators of effective coping might be that the patient asks questions regarding the progression of the disease and how to deal with the shortness of breath that accompanies it.

Community/Home Care

At home, the patient will need to focus on the positive and continue to explore and utilize a variety of coping strategies. Identification of limitations and how to deal with them will assist the patient to set realistic goals for activity and functioning. The presence of supportive family and friends during times of crisis or when the patient feels out of control can help the patient focus on the positive. Because the disease can endure for a long period of time (usual survival time from time of diagnosis is 10 years), the patient will need to adapt gradually to an increasing debilitation, with some periods being easier to adapt to than others. Due to this longevity, the family will need to discuss how long-term care will be provided if family members cannot care for the patient in the home. This issue frequently results in some degree of ineffective coping. During follow-up, the patient should be assessed for the presence of depression that may require interventions and for noncompliance with treatment recommendations. Ineffective coping may be compounded by issues of money and will increase the anxiety the patient may experience. COPD is a leading cause of disability and lost wages due to absence from work. The impact of this on the family's functioning and well-being should be monitored with social workers involved as needed. In addition, the availability of resources for medications and other treatments should be assessed by the health care provider, and appropriate referrals made. Discuss with the patient, the family, or significant other the changes that may have occurred in role performance due to the disease. If support groups are available in the patient's geographic area, this information should be provided to the patient and family and participation encouraged.

Documentation

Document that the patient has achieved the stated outcome criteria. An assessment of the patient's emotional state and verbalizations of concern (in the patient's specific verbatim words) regarding the disease should be documented. Place in the patient's record his or her stated ways of coping and what resources the patient has available to use. Document any teaching that has been implemented to help with coping strategies. Chart all interventions carried out to achieve the outcomes; however, if the patient is not coping effectively, document revisions made to the plan of care and any referrals made.

NURSING DIAGNOSIS 6

 ## DEFICIENT KNOWLEDGE

Related to:

Insufficient knowledge of COPD and its treatment

No previous history of disease

Defining Characteristics:

Asks questions/has concerns

Has had repeated hospital visits for exacerbations of COPD

Has no questions

Verbalizes a lack of knowledge/understanding

Goal:

Patient verbalizes an understanding of COPD and its treatment.

Outcome Criteria

✔ The patient verbalizes a desire to learn necessary information.

✔ The patient verbalizes a willingness to keep appointments and follow the prescribed regimen.

✔ The patient demonstrates knowledge of the disease (COPD).

✔ The patient demonstrates knowledge of prescribed medications.

✔ The patient demonstrates correct use of metered dose inhaler or in-home nebulizer and in-home oxygen.

NOC *Knowledge: Disease process*
Knowledge: Treatment regimen
Compliance behavior

INTERVENTIONS	RATIONALES
Assess readiness of patient to learn (motivation, cognitive level, physiological status).	The patient must be motivated to learn, have the capability to learn the content, and be free of distractions from learning, such as pain and shortness of breath.
Assess patient's current knowledge.	The teacher needs to ascertain what the patient already knows and build on this.
Start with the simplest information first.	Patients can understand simple concepts easily and then can build on those to understand more complex concepts.
Identify a family member or significant other who will also learn the content and assist the patient with compliance.	This person can reinforce the teaching and assist with implementation if the client becomes incapable of follow-through.

(continues)

(continued)

INTERVENTIONS	RATIONALES
Create a quiet environment conducive to learning.	Environmental noise can prevent the learner from focusing on what is being taught.
Teach the learners the pathophysiology of COPD in the initial teaching session, to include progression, effect on functioning/activity, and complications.	The patient must understand what the disease is and how it affects the body before understanding the rationale for treatments.
Teach the learners about prescribed medications (see nursing diagnosis "Ineffective Breathing Pattern") including action, side effects, dosing schedule, and correct use of inhalers (including use of a spacer) and nebulizers (adding medications, using equipment); teach the patient to rinse mouth after using inhalers.	Knowledge of why the medication is necessary and how it works will focus the importance of the medication. Use of spacers with inhalers improves medication delivery; nebulizers are frequently used to administer bronchodilators. Identification of side effects will minimize anxiety if these untoward effects should occur; rinsing the mouth will decrease drying of the mouth and prevent oral candidiasis.
Teach patient about the importance of tracking events/situations/substances that trigger an acute episode of shortness of breath (such as smell of paint, dust, kerosene heat, smoke) and how to minimize them.	The patient must understand factors that precipitate shortness of breath and acute exacerbations in order to control them and prevent avoidable hospitalizations.
Teach the patient how to use in-home oxygen as required, including: — Setting up a specific type of oxygen — Turning the system on and setting the appropriate rate — Determining whether the tank needs replacing — Cleansing or replacing supplies — Taking safety precautions: no smoking, no open flames near oxygen, post signs "oxygen in use" — General information on combustibility of oxygen	As the disease progresses, the patient will need oxygen to maintain optimal oxygen reserves and provide for performance of daily activities; knowledge of its operation empowers the patient. Safety precautions are required due to the combustibility of oxygen.
Instruct patient in relaxation techniques.	Informing patient of relaxation techniques may help reduce anxiety and shortness of breath.
Provide the patient with information regarding adequate	These foods provide energy. Excess carbohydrates should be

nutrient intake: high protein, high iron, vitamin C foods, need for nutritional supplements, small frequent meals.	avoided because the metabolism of carbohydrates produces carbon dioxide; eating frequent small meals decreases the amount of energy and oxygen required for digestion, thus avoiding shortness of breath and fatigue.
Teach the patient how to use and understand an incentive spirometer.	Use and understanding of an incentive spirometer will help the patient to determine when to seek health care assistance earlier in the acute phases of the disease.
Teach learners about activity, including how to progress exercise gradually while monitoring responses; make sure the patient understands that some preferred activities may need to be eliminated. Instruct the patient to eliminate any activity that produces wheezing, chest pain, dizziness, or severe shortness of breath.	Incorporation of exercise into daily routine is necessary to regain stamina and maintain respiratory functioning.
Teach the patient which signs and symptoms to report to a health care provider (i.e., respiratory infections).	Monitoring for signs and symptoms early can prevent a crisis that requires hospitalization. It is important for COPD patients to know when to seek health care assistance to avoid complications.
Teach the patient breathing techniques: — Diaphragmatic: Place one hand on chest and one on abdomen, inhale with mouth open while pushing with the abdominal muscle, keeping the hand on the chest. Exhale slowly. — Pursed lip breathing: Inhale through the nose with mouth closed, exhale slowly through pursed lips (pucker as if you were whistling).	Using the diaphragm and abdominal muscles will increase chest expansion; pursed lip breathing keeps airway open longer by maintaining positive pressure and prevents air trapping.
Evaluate the patient's understanding of all content covered by asking questions; have the patient return demonstrate use of inhalers, nebulizers, and oxygen equipment.	Identifies areas that require more teaching and ensures that the patient has enough information to comply; if the patient can demonstrate correct procedure for administering medications, he or she will feel more comfortable using them when needed, and anxiety should be decreased.

INTERVENTIONS	RATIONALES
Give the patient written information.	Provides for reference at a later time, and for review.
Establish that the patient has the resources required to be compliant.	If needed resources such as finances, transportation, and psychosocial support are not available, the patient cannot be compliant.

NIC *Learning readiness enhancement*
Learning facilitation
Teaching: Psychomotor skill
Teaching: Disease process
Teaching: Prescribed medication

Evaluation

Evaluate the degree to which the patient has achieved the outcome criteria relevant to the teaching sessions. The patient is able to repeat all information for the nurse and asks questions about the prescribed regimen. The patient can identify all medications by name and report the common side effects as well as the dosing schedule. COPD patients should demonstrate the ability to give their own medications via metered dose inhaler or nebulizer and be able to self-administer oxygen if prescribed. The patient should be able to inform the nurse when health care assistance should be sought for acute exacerbations or respiratory infections.

Community/Home Care

The patient will need to implement the medical regimen in the home setting. The success of treatment for COPD depends upon the degree to which the patient has received adequate teaching and has subsequently understood and internalized it. Patients with COPD will need to know how to prevent acute exacerbations by constantly monitoring the environment for situations that expose them to organisms that could cause an upper respiratory infection, including the common cold, or that may trigger shortness of breath, such as noxious odors. Keeping a log of activities prior to the onset of any acute episode of shortness of breath will help the patient to be proactive in disease management and is crucial to preventing crises. The patient may need continued evaluation to ensure that learning has occurred and been sustained. Follow-up care should focus on assessing the patient's ability to perform nebulizer treatments, use metered dose inhalers, and use oxygen equipment correctly. Adequate financial resources should be in place for purchase of medications and rental of respiratory therapy supplies. Assistance with this should be made through social services prior to discharge from the acute care setting. During follow-up visits with health care providers, the patient should be questioned about how he or she uses inhalers because in many instances patients overuse them, creating a risk for cardiac complications. The family will need to recognize that the life expectancy of the patient with COPD is lengthy and that long-term care may be a possibility in the end stage of the disease if an in-home care provider is not available. As with any teaching, the patient's culture, ethnicity, religion, and value system must be considered when making recommendations for a therapeutic regimen if compliance is to be achieved.

Documentation

Document the specific content taught and the titles of printed materials given to the patient or family. Chart the patient's understanding of the content and the methods used to evaluate learning. The patient's successful demonstration of the proper use of nebulizers, metered dose inhalers, and oxygen therapy should be documented. The nurse must clearly indicate areas that need to be reinforced. After the teaching session is complete, the nurse should note whether the patient indicates a willingness to comply with and an ability to comply with health care recommendations. If the teaching included a significant other, indicate this in the documentation. In addition, any referrals should be documented in the patient record.

CHAPTER 2.24

HEMOTHORAX AND PNEUMOTHORAX: SIMPLE AND TENSION

GENERAL INFORMATION

A hemothorax occurs secondary to a blunt chest trauma or a penetrating injury that causes blood to accumulate in the thoracic cavity. A simple hemothorax is a blood loss of < 1500 ml of blood, and a massive hemothorax is a blood loss of more than 1500 ml. A pneumothorax occurs when there is a breach in the pulmonary pleura and the pleural space is exposed to positive atmospheric pressure. When air enters the thoracic cavity, this loss of negative pressure and the very elastic lung tissue will collapse partially or totally. Any thoracic injury that allows accumulation of atmospheric air in pleural space results in a rise in intrathoracic pressure and a reduction in vital capacity. Pneumothoraces can be divided into three types: simple, traumatic, and tension pneumothorax. A simple pneumothorax is a condition in which air enters the thoracic cavity, through either a hole in the lung parenchyma, a hole in the bronchus or the trachea, or a hole in the chest wall. Patients can experience a simple pneumothorax as the result of a sudden rupture of a bleb or a cyst (which is also known as spontaneous pneumothorax) or because of trauma. Traumatic pneumothorax is a condition in which air escapes from a laceration in the lung itself and enters the pleural space or enters the pleural space through a wound in the chest wall. It can occur with almost any type of trauma including stab wounds, chest trauma, insertion of central lines, or thoracentesis. Traumatic pneumothorax is often accompanied by hemothorax. Open pneumothorax, a kind of traumatic pneumothorax, occurs when a wound in the chest wall is large enough to allow air to pass freely in and out of the thoracic cavity with each attempted respiration. A sucking sound is heard and structures of the mediastinum shift toward the uninjured side with each inspiration and in the opposite direction with expiration. Tension pneumothorax is a life-threatening pneumothorax that occurs when a hole in the airway structures or the chest wall permits air to enter the thoracic cavity during inspiration, but the air becomes trapped during exhalation. The pressure in the intrathoracic space will continue to increase until the lung collapses. With each breath, tension and positive pressure continues to increase within the affected pleural space. The lung on the opposite side will be compressed and the heart, great vessels, and trachea will shift to the opposite side of the chest (known as mediastinal shift). This will cause kinking of the superior and inferior vena cavae, diminishing venous return to the heart, decreasing diastolic filling, and subsequently a decrease in cardiac output. Death can be rapid if the condition is not corrected. Tension pneumothorax usually results from a penetrating injury to the chest, blunt trauma to the chest, or during use of a mechanical ventilator. Clinical manifestations of hemothorax or pneumothorax vary dependent upon the size of the pneumothorax/hemothorax and the cause, but include chest pain, respiratory distress (which may be minimal in simple pneumothorax), tachypnea, signs of air hunger, decreased movement of affected side, and absent breath sounds over the affected area. In tension pneumothorax, the patient displays air hunger, agitation, hypotension, tachycardia, tracheal deviation to the unaffected side, and agitation as hypoxemia increases.

NURSING DIAGNOSIS 1

INEFFECTIVE BREATHING PATTERN

Related to:

Severe chest pain

Partially/totally collapsed lung

Trauma to chest wall or lung

Defining Characteristics:

Shallow respirations

Tachypnea

Use of accessory muscles of respiration

Pale to cyanotic skin color

Decreased oxygen saturation

Abnormal arterial blood gases (ABGs), primarily decreased pO_2 (hypoxia) and increased pCO_2 (due to incomplete respiratory excursion)

Patient anxiety

Absent or diminished breath sounds over affected lung

Decreased movement of affected side

Pain with respiratory movement

Goal:

The patient's respirations are regular.

Outcome Criteria

✔ Breath sounds are present over affected area.

✔ Oxygen saturation is > 90 percent.

✔ Arterial blood gases are normal.

✔ Respiratory rate will be 12–24 per minute.

NOC *Respiratory status: Ventilation*
Respiratory status: Gas exchange

INTERVENTIONS	RATIONALES
Assess respiratory status by noting respiratory rate, depth, chest expansion, rhythm, breath sounds, or jugular vein distention; if tension pneumothorax is suspected, assess for mediastinal shift seen on x-ray and jugular vein distension, and feel/observe for tracheal deviation.	Establishes a baseline for comparison for early detection of complications or worsening condition.
Assist with insertion of chest tube into intrathoracic space as directed and connect to water seal drainage system.	Helps to relieve air, to re-establish negative pressure, and to re-expand the lung; in the case of hemothorax, helps to remove blood from pleural space.
If time permits, administer analgesic prior to insertion of chest tube.	Chest tube insertion can be uncomfortable, and in the case of hemothorax, a larger tube is required to remove blood, which causes more discomfort.
Administer oxygen, as ordered.	Improves oxygenation and decreases hypoxia.
Assist patient in assuming a semi- or high Fowler's position.	Helps to maximize intrathoracic space.
Monitor results of arterial blood gases and oxygen saturation.	Allows evaluation of respiratory adequacy and response to treatments.
Implement strategies to maintain chest tubes and drainage system: — Maintain a closed system and tape all connections (to prevent air leaks). — Maintain suction at pressure ordered (helps maintain negative pressure). — Check water seal and water level frequently (to ensure proper functioning). — Loop the tubing and secure to patient gown (prevents direct pressure on tube itself; prevents sensation of tube pulling out when moving). — Record any output from tube at least every shift or according to agency policy marking the level on the drainage chamber; this is especially important in hemothorax to allow for estimation of blood loss. — Keep dressing intact around entry site.	Proper functioning of the drainage system and chest tube is crucial to success of the intervention; securing the tube prevents inadvertent dislodging.
Encourage patient to cough and deep breathe every 2 hours following chest tube insertion and encourage ambulation, if allowed.	Maximizes ventilation and minimizes risk of atelectasis.
Monitor chest x-ray reports.	Allows assessment of improving or worsening of lung collapse and determines continued need for tube.
Assess patient for signs of infection: site-redness around dressing, fever, increased pain at insertion site; pulmonary-purulent sputum, cough, fever, pleuritic type chest pain.	A break in the skin provides a portal of injury for organisms, and limited movement due to the presence of tube in chest wall following injury places patient at high risk for pneumonia.

NIC *Respiratory monitoring*
Oxygen therapy
Tube care: Chest
Positioning

Evaluation

The patient should show indications that the lung has re-expanded and respiratory status is improving. Breath sounds should be noted over the affected lung. Respirations should be easy with equal chest expansion bilaterally and a rate of 12–24 per minute. Drainage from the chest tube should have decreased or stopped. Arterial blood gases and oxygen saturation results should provide evidence that breathing patterns are able to achieve adequate gas exchange.

Community/Home Care

At time of discharge, the pneumothorax/hemothorax has been resolved. Once at home the patient may continue to have some soreness in the site of the chest tube and require mild analgesics. A simple dressing may still be required at the site, and if so, the patient can change as directed. Because the possibility of infection at the chest tube insertion site remains, the patient should note drainage, redness, or any discoloration at the site and elevated fever immediately. If the pneumothorax was spontaneous, the patient should be able to identify the signs and symptoms of a pneumothorax, because the risk of reoccurrence is high, and understand the need to seek immediate health care if he or she should experience these symptoms. The patient will need to increase activities gradually, as tolerated.

Documentation

Document respiratory assessment findings, including breath sounds, respiratory rate, effort of breathing, chest expansion, and findings that would indicate hemothorax/pneumothorax. If there are chest wall wounds, document a thorough assessment of them as well. Include in the patient record the presence of the chest tube and equipment for drainage, amount of output from the tube every shift, and a description of the drainage. Always document all interventions carried out and the patient's response to them if any. If the patient verbalizes concerns regarding health status or treatments, include this in the documentation as well.

NURSING DIAGNOSIS 2

 DECREASED CARDIAC OUTPUT

Related to:

Tension pneumothorax causing mediastinal shift, kinking of great vessels

Decreased venous return secondary to tension pneumothorax

Decreased diastolic filling secondary to tension pneumothorax

Defining Characteristics:

Tachycardia

Hypotension

Muffled heart sounds

Decreased pulse quality

Peripheral cyanosis

Decreasing level of consciousness

Tracheal deviation

Agitation

Profuse diaphoresis

Goal:

Cardiac output will be maintained or restored.

Outcome Criteria

✔ The patient's pulse rate will be < 100 beats per minute.

✔ The patient's blood pressure will return to baseline.

✔ The patient's skin color improves with no cyanosis.

✔ The patient is alert with no signs of agitation.

NOC *Cardiac pump effectiveness*
Circulatory status
Respiratory status: Gas exchange
Vital signs

INTERVENTIONS	RATIONALES
Assist patient in assuming a semi-Fowler's position with legs elevated 20 degrees.	Semi-Fowler's position maximizes intrathoracic cavity space, and elevating the legs slightly increases venous return to the heart from the periphery.

INTERVENTIONS	RATIONALES
Give oxygen as ordered and as indicated by arterial blood gases and oxygen saturation.	Due to hypoperfusion tissues may be hypoxic; oxygen is given to maintain pO_2 at > 90 percent and to increase the amount of oxygen available for gas exchange.
Assess respiratory status noting absent breath sounds, tracheal deviation, increased effort of breathing, asymmetrical chest expansion and movement, increased rate.	Continued presence of these signs indicates unresolved tension pneumothorax, which, if untreated, could lead to shock and death due to cardiac tamponade.
Assist with insertion of chest tube as required and implement other strategies to address tension pneumothorax (see nursing diagnosis "Ineffective Breathing Pattern").	Once excess air is removed from the intrathoracic space, venous return to the heart will return to normal and cardiac output should return to normal; correction of the underlying cause of the decreased cardiac output (tension pneumothorax) will restore cardiac output.
Assess blood pressure and pulse every 15 minutes.	Changes in blood pressure and pulse give indicators to patient's status. In tension pneumothorax, a decreased blood pressure with narrowing pulse pressure may be noted; the pulse may be rapid, weak, and thready, indicating a serious cardiac output problem, which may lead to shock.
Assess urinary output via an indwelling urinary catheter every hour.	Decreased urinary output (< 30 ml/hour) indicates decreased perfusion to kidneys and a decrease in cardiac output.
Assess skin temperature and color.	As cardiac output deteriorates, the perfusion to skin and periphery is inadequate to maintain warmth or normal color.
Assess peripheral pulses.	Weak or diminished peripheral pulses indicate the heart is unable to maintain perfusion to extremities.
Assess mental status: level of consciousness, confusion, agitation.	Changes in mental status indicate a decrease in cerebral tissue perfusion and indicate an inability of the body's compensatory mechanism to provide adequate oxygenation to cerebral tissue.
Assist with hemodynamic monitoring according to agency/unit protocol (pulmonary artery pressure and central venous pressures and arterial pressures).	Helps to assess cardiac output more accurately and to evaluate patient's response to treatment; these measures can give information to evaluate left ventricular function (cardiac output) and fluid status.
Maintain intravenous access and give fluids, as ordered.	Access is necessary for emergency medications required to improve cardiac output.

NIC *Invasive hemodynamic monitoring*
Cardiac care: Acute
Vital signs monitoring
Respiratory monitoring
Tube care: Chest
Oxygen therapy

Evaluation

Note the degree to which outcome criteria have been achieved. The patient should demonstrate adequate cardiac output or improvement in abnormalities. Peripheral pulses should be present and skin, when touched, should be warm. If cardiac output is improved, perfusion to the kidneys should be adequate, with the patient producing at least 30 ml of urine per hour on average. The pulse should be within the patient's baseline and should be strong and regular. The parameters from invasive hemodynamic monitoring should show improvement and a gradual return to normal. Arterial blood gases should return to normal or show compensation, and oxygen saturation should be > 90 percent. All symptoms of tension pneumothorax should be improved or alleviated.

Community/Home Care

Patients who have experienced decreased cardiac output as a result of tension pneumothorax will need to know how to increase activities gradually when at home with a balance of rest and activity. The patient will need to monitor his or her response to activity, noting any shortness of breath, increased respiratory rate, or increased pulse rate. With the resolution of the tension pneumothorax, the cardiac output should resolve quickly, and the need for home care follow-up may not be required.

If the pneumothorax was spontaneous, the patient should be taught the signs and symptoms indicating a need for emergency care, as reoccurrences are common. For most patients, once respiratory function is re-established, cardiac output is restored, and no further interventions are required in the home. However, a follow-up appointment is needed to be sure that the patient has returned to his or her normal level of functioning.

Documentation

Chart the results of comprehensive assessments made, particularly the respiratory and cardiac systems, with attention to continuing symptoms of pneumothorax/hemothorax. The nurse should note the status of the chest tube system, including type and amount of drainage. All interventions should be documented in a timely fashion with the patient's specific response to the intervention. Chart readings from hemodynamic monitoring, pulse, and blood pressure according to agency/unit protocol. Always include the patient's psychological status: whether he or she appears anxious or restless, and whether significant others are present. Document any complaint made by the patient.

NURSING DIAGNOSIS 3

DEFICIENT KNOWLEDGE

Related to:

> New onset of condition
>
> Lack of information regarding pneumothorax/ hemothorax
>
> Fear and anxiety secondary to altered respiratory status

Defining Characteristics:

> Anxiety following insertion of chest tube
>
> Asks many or no questions

Goal:

> The patient verbalizes an understanding of the injury and the treatment required.

Outcome Criteria

✔ The patient verbalizes a willingness and desire to learn the necessary information.

✔ The patient verbalizes an understanding of the injury (pneumothorax, hemothorax) and interventions required.

✔ The patient understands the purpose of the chest tube and safety precautions needed.

✔ The patient will demonstrate how to get out of bed and ambulate with the chest tube system in place.

✔ The patient will be able to identify signs and symptoms of infection.

NOC *Knowledge: Disease process*
Knowledge: Health behavior
Treatment behavior: Illness or injury

INTERVENTIONS	RATIONALES
Assess readiness of client to learn (motivation, cognitive level, physiological status).	The patient must be motivated to learn, have the capability to learn the content, and be free of distractions from learning, such as pain and shortness of breath.
Assess what the patient already knows.	The patient may have some knowledge about disease/injury and its treatment, and teaching should begin with what the patient already knows.
Create a quiet environment conducive to learning.	Environmental noise can prevent the learner from focusing on what is being taught.
Teach the learners about the pathophysiology of pneumothorax and hemothorax, including complications.	The patient must understand what the disorder is and how it affects the body before understanding the rationale for treatments.
Teach the patient about the functioning of the chest tube and drainage system.	Understanding the rationale for these interventions will enhance patient's willingness to comply with regimen and decrease anxiety.
Demonstrate to the patient how to move in and out of bed with the chest tube; have the patient return the demonstration.	Many patients express apprehension about getting out of bed with a chest tube drainage system, not realizing that immobility can contribute to more complications such as pneumonia. Demonstration will allow patient to feel comfortable with activity.

INTERVENTIONS	RATIONALES
Teach the patient which signs and symptoms to report to a health care provider (reoccurrence of pneumothorax, infection).	Monitoring for signs and symptoms early can prevent a crisis that requires hospitalization.
Evaluate the patient's understanding of all content covered by asking questions.	Identifies areas that require more teaching and ensures that the patient has enough information to comply.
Give the patient written information.	Provides reference at a later time, and allows for review.

NIC **Teaching: Prescribed activity/exercise**

Teaching: Disease process

Teaching: Psychomotor skill

Teaching: Procedure/treatment

Evaluation

The patient is able to repeat all information for the nurse and asks questions about the pneumothorax/hemothorax and its treatment, specifically the chest tube. The patient is able to demonstrate to the nurse how to get out of bed with the chest tube and to identify measures to ensure proper functioning of the tube. The patient should be able to inform the nurse when health care assistance should be sought, specifically signs and symptoms of infection.

Community/Home Care

For patients who have experienced a pneumothorax/hemothorax, the problem should be resolved prior to discharge, and in-home follow-up care is rarely required. Follow-up care with a health care provider focuses on assurance that respiratory function has returned. As the patient resumes more of his or her normal activity, he or she may discover that some activities cause shortness of breath, but this should resolve with time. Considerations for the prevention of infection should be reinforced to the family and patient.

Documentation

Document all content taught and the patient's understanding. Include in the documentation an assessment of the chest tube insertion site, noting status of dressings and the chest tube drainage system. In addition, include the patient's ability to demonstrate the proper method of ambulation and mobility with the chest tube system. Any area that requires further teaching should be clearly indicated in the record. Chart any questions or concerns that the patient has verbalized. Always include the names of any printed literature given to the patient for reinforcement.

CHAPTER 2.25

LUNG CANCER

GENERAL INFORMATION

Lung cancer is the leading cause of cancer deaths in both men and women across all races. It is estimated that 85 percent of lung cancer cases can be traced to cigarette smoking. Inhaled substances such as asbestos also contribute to some cases, but the disease is 10 times more likely in cigarette smokers. Most lung cancers (90 percent) are bronchogenic, arising in the epithelium of the bronchi in the upper portion of the lungs. Cancers of the lung are divided into small cell lung cancer (25 percent of all cancers) and non-small cell lung cancer (75 percent). Further division of non-small cell lung cancers includes squamous cell, adenocarcinoma, and large cell undifferentiated. Small cell carcinomas grow more rapidly than the others, have a high rate of metastasis, and a poorer prognosis with a survival rate of 2 years or less when treated. Squamous cell carcinoma has a slower growth rate, with metastasis most often limited to the thoracic area, and the patient may demonstrate symptoms of obstruction of an airway or respiratory infections such as pneumonia. Adenocarcinomas are also slow growing, with a high probability of metastasis to the brain and are the predominant lung cancer in nonsmokers. Large cell cancers, which are larger tumors than adenocarcinomas, are slow growing, with the brain being a common site for metastasis. Even though the most common types of lung cancers grow slowly, for most people the disease is well advanced when diagnosed, with 55 percent of patients having metastasis at the time of diagnosis. Clinical manifestations vary by type and include chronic cough, hemoptysis, and, if airway obstruction is present, wheezing and shortness of breath may be seen. Dull aching chest pain may indicate tumor invasion into the mediastinum. With metastasis to the brain, the patient may demonstrate confusion, headache, and problems with balance and gait.

Later in the disease, the patient may experience bone pain, weight loss, and fatigue. The incidence of lung cancer increases as one ages, with a higher incidence in people between the ages of 50 and 70 years of age.

NURSING DIAGNOSIS 1

INEFFECTIVE BREATHING PATTERN

Related to:

Presence of tumor

Chest pain

Defining Characteristics:

Complaint of dull, aching pain or pleuritic chest pain

Tachypnea

Dyspnea

Decreased oxygen saturation

Abnormal ABGs (lowered pO_2)

Frequent cough

Goal:

The patient exhibits improved breathing pattern.

Outcome Criteria

✔ Respiratory rate will be at baseline (12–24 breaths per minute).

✔ The patient states that shortness of breath is relieved.

✔ Arterial blood gases and oxygen saturation will be within normal range.

NOC *Respiratory status: Ventilation*
Respiratory status: Gas exchange

INTERVENTIONS	RATIONALES
Assess respiratory status: breath sounds, use of accessory muscles, rate, depth, chest excursion, sputum for color and consistency, coughing.	Establishes a baseline and monitors for response to interventions; patients with lung cancer often have hemoptysis and frequent coughing.
Monitor arterial blood gases and oxygen saturation.	Results will provide accurate assessment of ability to ventilate effectively and allow for prompt attention to abnormalities that may signal problems.
Monitor results of diagnostic studies: chest x-rays, bronchoscopy, CT scan, and sputum from an early morning specimen for cytology.	A chest x-ray gives the first clue to disease; a CT scan is one of the most effective means of establishing a diagnosis and can also be used to identify metastasis to the bone and brain; bronchoscopy allows for direct visualization of the lungs and airway, permitting a biopsy, which is the best way to establish a definitive diagnosis of lung cancer; sputum for cytology allows one to obtain malignant cells for analysis.
Administer oxygen, as ordered.	Improves oxygenation and oxygen saturation.
Assist patient in assuming a semi-Fowler's position.	Maximizes pulmonary excursion; reduces pressure from diaphragm and abdominal organs.
Implement strategies to control and treat pain (see nursing diagnosis "Acute Pain").	Patients with pain often attempt to relieve pain by guarding the chest, preventing adequate chest expansion and subsequent depth of respirations.
Have patient cough and deep breathe every 2 hours.	Maximizes airway space and prevents atelectasis.
Teach controlled breathing.	Compensates for altered breathing patterns.
Educate and prepare the patient for diagnostic studies: bronchoscopy, CT scans, etc.; and treatment interventions for lung cancer: thoracotomy for segmental resection, lobectomy, wedge resection, pneumonectomy or radiation, and chemotherapy (see nursing diagnosis "Deficient Knowledge").	Diagnostic studies assist with accurate diagnosis, and ineffective breathing pattern will continue until medical interventions are employed to treat the tumor.
Support the patient in coping with a diagnosis of lung cancer.	Lung cancer generally has a poor prognosis and the patient may need support in coping

	with it (see nursing diagnosis "Anticipatory Grieving").
If surgery has been performed (with the exception of pneumonectomy), implement strategies to maintain chest tubes and drainage system: — Maintain a closed system and tape all connections (to prevent air leaks). — Maintain suction at pressure ordered (helps maintain negative pressure). — Check water seal and water level frequently (to ensure proper functioning). — Loop the tubing and secure to patient's gown (prevents direct pressure on tube itself; prevents sensation of tube pulling out when moving). — Record any output from tube at least every shift or according to agency policy, marking the level on the drainage. — Keep dressing intact around entry site.	Proper functioning of the drainage system and chest tube is crucial to success of the intervention; pinning the tube to the patient gown prevents inadvertent dislodging.
Encourage patient to cough and deep breathe every 2 hours following chest tube insertion and encourage ambulation if allowed.	Maximizes ventilation and minimizes risk of atelectasis.
Assess patient for signs of infection: chest tube insertion site: redness around dressing, fever, increased pain at insertion site; pulmonary: purulent sputum, cough, fever, pleuritic type chest pain.	Breaks in the skin provide a portal of entry for organisms, and limited movement due to the presence of tube in chest wall following surgery places patient at high risk for pneumonia.
Encourage cessation of smoking, particularly if cancer is caught early and possibility of long-term survival is good following surgery.	Smoking is the number one causative factor for lung cancer, and cessation is required for health maintenance.

NIC *Respiratory monitoring*
       Oxygen therapy
       Positioning

Evaluation

Evaluate the extent to which the patient has achieved the stated outcomes. The patient's respirations should be unlabored with equal chest expansion bilaterally. Respiratory rate should be within the patient's baseline normal (12–24 per minute), and the patient should report that respiratory effort is comfortable for them. Arterial blood gases and oxygen saturation results should indicate effectiveness of respirations by staying within normal limits.

Community/Home Care

The patient with lung cancer is still faced with the possibility of ineffective breathing pattern dependent upon the success of treatments utilized. For the patient who had successful removal of the diseased lung, ineffective breathing pattern may be completely resolved. For patients who are treated palliatively with radiation and chemotherapy, the problem will persist throughout their survival time. At time of discharge home, the patient should have discussed the possibilities for relief of respiratory symptoms through in-home use of relaxation techniques, controlled breathing, pain control, and at some point the use of oxygen at home (see nursing diagnosis "Deficient Knowledge"). The nurse visiting the home should reinforce teaching and determine the need for further assistance with self-care activities due to shortness of breath. In the home, it will be important for the patient to understand and be able to carry out the prescribed treatment regimen possibly, which may include chemotherapy and radiation therapy. The psychological toll on the patient with lung cancer is great given the poor prognosis at time of diagnosis for most patients. A visiting nurse or other health care provider should evaluate the patient once discharged to ensure that the patient is coping with the diagnosis of lung caner (see nursing diagnosis "Anticipatory Grieving with Risk for Ineffective Coping"). Because treatment will require returns to health care facilities for chemotherapy or radiation therapy, this is a prime opportunity for assessment. Prior to discharge home, the nurse, physician, or social worker should determine the availability of adequate resources for the patient to be compliant with prescribed treatments with appropriate referrals as required. For those patients who choose not to undergo treatments of any type, this decision should be supported. Spiritual consults may be useful at time of diagnosis but may also be beneficial to the patient at home as he or she grapples with an uncertain prognosis and a potentially challenging course of treatment.

Documentation

Document all initial and subsequent respiratory assessments according to agency protocols, specifically breath sounds, respiratory rate, chest excursions, and any dyspnea. The information recorded should also include oxygen saturation and arterial blood gases. When invasive diagnostic procedures such as bronchoscopy are performed, complete assessments or flow sheets according to agency/unit protocol, including the return of the patient's gag reflex. Document assessment of sputum expectorated, noting the presence of blood, and include documentations of any specimen collected for laboratory analysis. Chart all interventions implemented to treat any problem and the specific patient responses. If the patient has undergone surgery and has chest tubes, document chest tube output every shift or according to protocol. Assessments of the surgical site and chest tube site should also be documented. Include in the patient record any teaching implemented and the patient's understanding. Document any referrals made in the patient's chart as well.

NURSING DIAGNOSIS 2

ACUTE PAIN

Related to:

Presence of lung tumor causing pressure

Impairment of lung tissue

Defining Characteristics:

Complaint of dull, aching pain or pleuritic chest pain

Severe pain (later in the disease)

Goal:

Pain control is achieved.

Outcome Criteria

✔ The patient will verbalize that pain is reduced or relieved.

NOC *Pain level*

Pain control

Comfort level

Medication response

INTERVENTIONS	RATIONALES
Administer oxygen, as ordered.	Decreases tissue ischemia that contributes to pain.
Assess pain by having the patient rate pain for intensity using a pain rating scale.	Gives a more objective assessment of the pain intensity.
Administer analgesics, usually narcotic agents such as morphine, intravenously, by mouth, or through fentanyl patches as ordered, being sure that the patient has medications available for breakthrough pain. Give medications on a regular around-the-clock dosing schedule.	Provides pain relief and decreases anxiety; around-the-clock scheduled medication administration helps prevent breakthrough pain; pain increases the need for oxygen.
Teach appropriate relaxation techniques and other distraction techniques, such as guided imagery and music.	Enhances the effects of pharmacological interventions.
Assess effectiveness of interventions to relieve pain.	Determines effectiveness of interventions in relieving pain, or whether new strategies need to be employed. As the disease progresses, more potent and larger doses of analgesics may be required.
Refer to a pain specialist, if available, for assessment of pain medication needs and for education of family and patient.	A pain specialist will be able to collaborate with the physician, nurses, and the patient to develop a plan to control pain to the patient's satisfaction; educating the patient will dispel myths regarding cancer patients' addiction to narcotics that often discourage medication use and prohibit adequate pain control.
Establish a quiet environment.	Enhances effects of analgesics; decreases oxygen demands.
Elevate head of bed.	Improves chest expansion and oxygenation.

NIC *Pain management*
Analgesic administration
Anxiety reduction

Evaluation

The patient is able to report that the pain has been relieved or alleviated following interventions. Based on pain rating scales, the patient's pain has decreased. The degree to which the patient is able to

assist in the management of the pain through anxiety reduction and relaxation techniques is assessed.

Community/Home Care

Home care required for the management of pain will depend on the type of lung cancer, the stage of the cancer, and the type of treatment employed. For the patient being treated with chemotherapy and radiation, the problem will probably become more pronounced as the disease progresses, as these treatments only provide tumor shrinkage and slowing of growth. Initially, pain medications may be given by mouth to obtain satisfactory pain control. However, in the later stages, pain control may require the services of hospice or a home nurse when more invasive means of administering narcotics may be needed for control. In terminal phases, decisions will be made regarding the patient's ability to be pain-free and possibly sedated, versus the family's desire to have the patient alert. Ineffective in-home management of pain may cause undue emotional stress for the patient and family, necessitating hospitalization. Teaching the patient how to utilize non-pharmacological measures to enhance the effects of analgesics will be crucial to obtaining satisfactory outcomes. Assessing pain control is an important facet of follow-up care by the home health nurse, hospice, or other health care worker, and should include the patient's ability to purchase prescribed analgesics.

Documentation

Document in the patient's own words the description of the pain and his or her rating of the level of pain. Chart all interventions and the patient's response. Include in the documentation assessments made relevant to the respiratory system. All teaching should be indicated in the patient record with an indication of the patient's level of understanding. Document referrals to pain specialists.

NURSING DIAGNOSIS 3

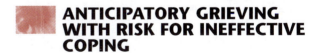

ANTICIPATORY GRIEVING WITH RISK FOR INEFFECTIVE COPING

Related to:

Diagnosis of lung cancer

Fear of dying

Poor prognosis

Defining Characteristics:

Anger

Expressions of fear

Restlessness and anxiety

Crying

Expresses distress at potential loss

Goal:

The patient demonstrates effective coping and grieving.

Outcome Criteria

✔ The patient identifies one coping mechanism to be used during anticipatory grieving.

✔ The patient verbalizes fears and concerns.

✔ The patient reports being less anxious about the diagnosis of lung cancer.

✔ The patient demonstrates no outward signs of anxiety, such as restlessness or agitation.

NOC *Grief resolution*

Anxiety control

Comfort level

Coping

INTERVENTIONS	RATIONALES
Assess level of anxiety (mild, moderate, severe); have patient rate on a scale of 1–10, with 10 being the greatest.	Gives the nurse a better perception of extent of the anxiety.
Keep patient informed of all that is going on, including information about diagnostic tests and therapeutic interventions.	Providing the patient with straightforward information on treatments and what to expect may help to relieve anxiety and enhance coping.
Use a calm, reassuring manner with the patient.	Gives the patient a sense of well-being.
Stay with patient as possible and allow family to visit liberally.	Provides emotional support and promotes a sense of comfort.
Encourage the patient to verbalize fears, concerns, and expressions of grief; listen to the patient attentively.	Verbalization of fears contributes to dealing with concerns; being attentive relays empathy to the patient.
Control multiple sources of stimuli, which could cause sensory overload.	Overstimulation can worsen anxiety.

Seek spiritual consult as needed or requested by the patient and or family.	Meeting the patient's spiritual needs helps him or her to deal with fears through use of spiritual or religious rituals.
Recognize the role of culture in the patient's method of grieving and the ability to verbalize fears and concerns.	Culture often dictates how a person grieves, and the nurse must recognize this in order to support the patient in a successful grief process.
Engage patient and family in open dialogue regarding options for treatments and care.	During the final stages of disease, the patient and family may not be able to care for the patient alone; discussion of care options early in the disease allows the patient to be more in control, giving him or her a sense of empowerment that may help the patient to cope with the disease.
Assess the patient to determine his or her feelings regarding the diagnosis of lung cancer and the prognosis, and support the patient as appropriate by answering questions and making referrals. Ask the patient how the nurse can assist in his or her grief work.	Assisting the family members to deal with the diagnosis and prognosis will enhance their ability to cope with serious illness and grieve appropriately.
Provide the patient and family with information regarding advance directives and support decisions made.	Allows the patient and family the opportunity to plan for the patient's wishes in the event that he or she becomes unable to make his or her own decisions.

NIC *Grief work facilitation*

Coping enhancement

Emotional support

Spiritual support

Evaluation

Evaluate the extent to which the outcome criteria have been achieved. The patient should be assessed for behaviors that would indicate adjustment to the diagnosis of lung cancer. The patient should verbalize his or her fears and concerns and be able to identify one way to cope with the diagnosis of cancer. The extent to which the patient displays appropriate coping behaviors should be noted. If the patient is unable to talk about the diagnosis and communicate concerns, the nurse should explore further new interventions to assist the patient.

Community/Home Care

Nurses should assess which coping mechanisms work best for the patient in anticipatory grieving and encourage their use by the patient at home, realizing that new strategies may need to be utilized as the disease progresses. Problems with grieving may continue for a long period of time, and follow-up by a health care provider can detect ineffective coping. Family should be taught what is appropriate anticipatory grieving and coping and what is not. Extreme isolation and depression should be noted and reported to a health care provider. For many patients and families, spiritual/religious rituals provide a means of coping with difficult stressful situations. In-home visits by the patient's religious or spiritual leader may be a source of great comfort for both the patient and the family. The patient's culture may dictate how he or she grieves and with whom he or she shares this process. It is crucial that the nurse and family support the patient as needed to foster a healthy psychological state, recognizing that anger and denial are common. As the disease progresses the patient may require new strategies for coping with the disease and the anticipated loss of life. The patient may benefit from quiet periods of meditation during the day. Support to long-term caregivers will be important, as they too need support during the grieving process. Hospice can play an important role in the home situation through provision of counselors, chaplains, and in-home care providers. If questions should arise at home regarding the patient's health status or prescribed regimen, the patient should have a means of contacting a health care provider for answers.

Documentation

The degree to which the patient has verbalized his or her feelings and has demonstrated decreased anxiety should be documented in the patient record. A rating system provides an objective way to relay to others the extent of the anxiety. Document whether the patient is able to discuss the diagnosis of lung cancer, as this is the beginning of the anticipatory grief process. Chart the patient's verbalizations as the patient states them and include in the record strategies utilized by the patient in the grief process. Document findings from an assessment of the patient's psychological state, including the presence of depression, anger, crying, or sadness. Document referrals to hospice or religious leaders.

NURSING DIAGNOSIS 4

 DEFICIENT KNOWLEDGE

Related to:

New disease

Complex treatment protocol

Misunderstanding of information

Defining Characteristics:

Many or no questions

Verbalizes a lack of knowledge/understanding

Goal:

The patient will understand lung cancer and its treatment.

Outcome Criteria

✔ The patient verbalizes a desire to learn necessary information.

✔ The patient verbalizes an understanding of diagnostic procedures (bronchoscopy, sputum analysis, CT scan).

✔ The patient verbalizes an understanding of lung cancer treatment options (surgery, radiation, chemotherapy), including untoward effects of treatment and possible complications of lung cancer, such as pan-neoplastic syndromes.

✔ The patient verbalizes an understanding of pain management.

✔ The patient verbalizes an understanding of oxygen therapy.

✔ The patient verbalizes an understanding of follow-up care required and expresses a willingness to comply.

NOC *Knowledge: Disease process*
Knowledge: Treatment regimen
Compliance behavior

INTERVENTIONS	RATIONALES
Assess the patient's current knowledge as well as his or her ability to learn and readiness to learn.	The teacher needs to ascertain what the patient already knows and build on this; if the patient is not capable of learning or is not ready to learn,

(continues)

(continued)

INTERVENTIONS	RATIONALES
	teaching will not be effective due to disinterest or inability to understand. The patient may not be ready to learn if in a state of denial or if extremely angry.
Start with the simplest information and move to complex information.	Patients can understand simple concepts easily and then can build on those to understand more complex concepts.
Instruct the patient regarding bronchoscopy: procedure, biopsy, withholding food and liquid for 8 hours before procedure and until gag reflex returns post-procedure, possibility of sore throat post-procedure.	Teaching before the test decreases anxiety and prepares the patient for what to expect.
Collaborate with the physician to teach patient and significant others: — Disease process of lung cancer, staging, and possible treatments — Pain medications (narcotics) used to treat cancer pain including dosage, frequency, side effects, scheduling, interactions with other medications; answer questions or concerns regarding dependence — Signs and symptoms that would indicate a need to seek health care (poor pain control, new onset of severe shortness of breath, sudden sharp chest pain)	Knowledge of disease, treatments required, and prevention of complications empowers the patient to take control and be compliant.
Instruct patient regarding radiation: — Method of action — Course/duration of treatment, usually 5 treatments each week for 6 weeks — Signs and symptoms of radiation pneumonitis (dyspnea on exertion, cough, or fever), esophagitis (sore throat and dysphagia), and pericarditis (new onset chest pain) — Skin changes to note include redness, sloughing, and tenderness	Radiation is used with almost all types of lung cancer even when surgery is employed and the patient needs to be informed. The radiated skin is sensitive and lotions, creams, ultraviolet rays, rubbing, etc., may cause burning and skin sloughing and interfere with radiation. The patient must know how to protect the skin from impairment; knowing what to expect in terms of radiation helps the patient to be more compliant and feel more in control.
— Skin care: do not apply soap, ointments, lotions, creams, or powder to area; refrain from using deodorant; do not rub, scrub, or scratch the area; do not try to wash off markings; avoid exposing the treated area to the sun during the treatment and for 1 year following treatments — Wear loose-fitting clothes; for women, bras may need to be avoided	
Teach patient and family about chemotherapy and its effects: — Method of action — Specific agents used for treatment — Alopecia: assist the patient to plan for hair loss by investigating the purchase of wigs (females) or having hair cut short and using hair for a specially made wig or for men shaving before alopecia occurs; find a resource that could teach women how to prepare fashionable head wraps — Nausea/vomiting: teach to use antiemetics before meals prophylactically; avoid foods with strong odors, and in the hospital setting have lids removed from trays outside the room (when lids are removed from food trays the smell is often overwhelming to the GI system and causes nausea); attempt frequent small meals, avoiding spicy foods — Care of access sites: prevention of infection by use of aseptic techniques and procedures according to agency protocol — Control of fatigue: balance of rest and activity; on chemotherapy days, a designated nap time should be scheduled — Prevention of infection: chemotherapy causes a depression of white blood cells, predisposing the patient to infection; avoid people with	Knowledge of what to expect helps the patient to prevent complications and to cope with untoward side effects and better equips them to take responsibility for managing the illness and engaging in self-care. Being proactive in addressing areas such as alopecia and nausea/vomiting reduces anxiety.

INTERVENTIONS	RATIONALES
infections, especially upper respiratory infections, and large crowds; practice good hand hygiene; know WBC counts	
Teach family and patient about oxygen therapy: set-up of equipment, care of equipment (when to replace tubing, mask or cannula cleaning), storage of equipment, safety requirements (no smoking or open flames), indicators for use of oxygen.	Oxygen at home is required for most lung cancer patients as the disease progresses. Including oxygen therapy in instruction information prepares the patient and family for the time when it is needed.
Provide patient and family with information on hospice and other community service agencies, such as the American Cancer Society.	These agencies can assist with durable medical equipment, in-home care providers, support, and other services.
Assess the patient's and family's understanding of all teaching by encouraging them to repeat information and ask questions as needed.	This allows the nurse to hear in the patient's own words what was taught and makes it easier to know what information may need to be reinforced.
Establish that the patient has the resources required to be compliant, such as transportation to chemotherapy treatments and radiation therapy.	If needed resources such as finances and transportation to follow-up appointments are not available, the patient cannot be compliant; the nurse will need to make necessary referrals. This may be a real problem for patients from remote and rural areas, especially if family support is not available.

NIC *Learning readiness enhancement*
Learning facilitation
Teaching: Disease process
Teaching: Prescribed medication

Evaluation

Evaluate the degree to which the patient has achieved the outcome criteria relevant to the teaching sessions. The patient should verbalize an understanding of content presented by repeating the information, particularly the disease process, treatments (radiation, chemotherapy, surgery), and medications, including oxygen therapy. The nurse must determine if the patient is capable of being compliant with the recommended regimen. If further teaching

is required at time of discharge, the appropriate referrals should be made to continue education.

Community/Home Care

The patient will need to implement the medical regimen in the home setting over an extended period of time. The success of this implementation will be dependent upon the degree to which the patient has received adequate teaching and has subsequently understood and internalized it. In most instances, the patient will need to return to an outpatient facility for chemotherapy or radiation therapy. At home, the patient will likely experience fatigue, hair loss, and nausea and vomiting as a result of treatments. A visiting nurse should assess the patient for these expected, untoward effects of treatment and determine that the effects are not severe. For the patient receiving chemotherapy, it is important to monitor the patient's weight if the patient is experiencing nausea and vomiting. Health care providers or dietitians can assist the patient to prepare a diet that is both nutritional and easy to digest with foods that are least likely to cause GI upset. Encourage the patient at home to take antiemetics prophylactically. The nurse or dietitian should be sure that any menu or diet developed considers cultural or religious preferences and financial resources of the patient. Radiation therapy patients will need to be monitored for ability to care for skin properly and prevent further tissue destruction. When oxygen therapy is needed the provider should ensure that the family and the patient know how to operate and care for the equipment. At home, the environment may need to be rearranged to accommodate durable medical equipment that may be needed later in the disease such as hospital beds, bedside commodes, and oxygen equipment. If homes are heated with open flame sources, such as kerosene heaters, fireplaces, or woodstoves, adjustments and careful placement of oxygen supply is warranted. Teachers should recognize that there may not be any alternatives due to financial costs of changing heating systems. In this instance, discussions with the patient and family must center on the best possible scenario for safety given the patient's home-heating situation. Pain control is a big part of home care and will require frequent follow-up to ensure patient satisfaction. Ensure that the patient or family member understands how to manage pain with both medications and non-pharmacological methods (see nursing diagnosis "Acute Pain").

Those healthcare workers providing follow-up care need to ensure that the family and patient understand that dependence should not be a concern for the cancer patient and that comfort is the ultimate goal. Because of the multifaceted approach to treatment of lung cancer and the numerous instructions that the patient and family need, it may prove helpful to set up a resource folder or notebook that contains printed literature regarding such things as medication schedules, use of oxygen, care of supplies, signs and symptoms to be reported, important telephone numbers, and other recommendations that must be carried out at home. This will make it easier for the patient to find what is needed. As the patient is seen on a regular basis for chemotherapy or radiation, health care providers can use these opportunites to determine whether further teaching or reinforcement is required.

Documentation

Document the specific content taught and the titles of any printed documents given to the patient. Include in the chart the patient's degree of understanding of the content and the methods used to evaluate learning. Any areas that need to be reinforced should be documented to ensure appropriate follow-up. If family members are present for the teaching sessions, document this in the chart, and always document any referrals made.

CHAPTER 2.26

MECHANICAL VENTILATION

GENERAL INFORMATION

Mechanical ventilation is performed when a patient is unable to sustain adequate ventilatory efforts, adequate tidal volume, and/or requires supplemental oxygen delivered under positive pressure for a variety of reasons. In the majority of cases, mechanical ventilation is a temporary measure that will end when the patient is able to maintain his or her own adequate ventilatory efforts. There are, however, those patients who will require long-term or permanent mechanical ventilation. The various modes of ventilatory assistance include assist control mode, controlled mandatory ventilation, and synchronized intermittent mandatory ventilation (SIMV). Assist control ventilation, the most commonly used mode, provides a preset tidal volume but is sensitive to the patient's own inspiratory efforts. Ventilators set in the synchronized intermittent mandatory ventilation mode have a preset ventilatory rate as well as tidal volume, but allow for the patient to breathe spontaneously between ventilator breaths at his or her own rate and tidal volume. This mode can be used for weaning by gradually decreasing the number of breaths to be made by the ventilator, allowing the patient to breathe spontaneously. The third mode of mechanical ventilation is controlled ventilation, which is the least used mode. In this mode, used for patients who are unable to initiate spontaneous breaths, the patient receives a set tidal volume at a set ventilatory rate. Any efforts by the patient to breathe on his or her own are blocked by the ventilator.

NURSING DIAGNOSIS 1

IMPAIRED SPONTANEOUS VENTILATION

Related to:

Neuromuscular disorders

Fatigue

Loss of respiratory drive (in midbrain)

Respiratory disease

Defining Characteristics:

Inability to use muscles of respiration (main and accessory)

Severely compromised respiratory rate and depth

Fatigue

Decreased oxygen saturation

Decreased pO_2 (< 60)

Diminished vital capacity/tidal volume

Respiratory arrest

Respiratory rate very low

Respirations very labored

Patient is using accessory muscles of respiration

Patient unable to sustain ventilatory efforts

Goal:

Mechanical ventilation provides adequate ventilatory rate, rhythm, and volume.

Outcome Criteria

✔ The patient returns to spontaneous ventilation.

✔ Arterial blood gas values demonstrate pO_2 between 90–100 percent.

✔ Oxygen saturation will be > 90 percent.

NOC *Mechanical ventilation response: Adult*

Respiratory status: Ventilation

Respiratory status: Gas exchange

INTERVENTIONS	RATIONALES
Assess vital signs.	Changes in vital signs may signal complications; tachycardia and tachypnea often result from hypoxemia and hypercapnia.
Assess respiratory status: lip color, bilateral chest expansion, respiratory rate, respiratory effort, rhythm; note the presence of bilateral equal breath sounds.	Lips are an excellent place to note cyanosis, which if present would indicate impaired gas exchange; lung sounds may reveal adventitious sounds such as crackles, rhonchi, or wheezing as well as diminished sounds over some areas dependent on the causative factors for impaired ventilation; bilateral equal breath sounds give evidence of proper placement of endotracheal tube.
Explain the intubation procedure and mechanical ventilation to the patient and family.	It is important for the patient to have knowledge of therapeutic interventions and to understand their purpose; information can decrease anxiety related to equipment, seriousness of respiratory status, and the inability to talk.
Assist physician or respiratory therapist with endotracheal intubation (ET) and ventilator set-up as required or ordered.	Placement of an endotracheal tube will provide a means through which adequate ventilations can be delivered to meet metabolic demands for oxygen.
Once the ET tube is in place, mark the level at which the tube touches the patient's teeth or nose.	Provides a reference point for checking minimal changes in tube placement. The tube can slip into the mainstem bronchus.
Ensure that the mechanical ventilator is set at the proper settings for the various modes to meet the patient's needs; check every hour or according to agency/unit protocol. Assess the settings routinely according to agency/unit protocol and re-evaluate patient needs: oxygen concentration (FIO_2), ventilatory rate, tidal volume, airway pressures (peak inspiratory pressure, continuous positive airway pressure), inspiratory/expiratory ratio, sigh volume and rate, humidity, and water and air temperature, PEEP (if ordered).	Each patient's needs will vary, and the patient's need for mechanical ventilation may be unique. Predetermine what the outcome goals will be and then assist with adjusting the ventilator, as ordered or according to agency protocol, to meet the patient's goals.
Be attentive to ventilator alarms and ensure that they are functional, including high-pressure and low-exhaled-volume/low-pressure alarms. Identify the cause of the alarm and correct as indicated or notify appropriate personnel.	High-pressure alarms sound when peak inspiratory pressure reaches a set level, which can be caused by a variety of factors, including increased secretions and displacement of the ET tube. Low-exhaled-volume alarms may occur if there is a leak in the ventilator that prevents a breath from occurring, which often happens if the patient is disconnected from the ventilator or is no longer breathing spontaneously (SIMV). Alarms require immediate attention from the nurse to preserve respiratory function.
Monitor for signs of respiratory infection, such as elevated white blood cell (WBC) count, increased sputum production, change in color of sputum, thick sputum, fever, crackles in lung.	Because the patient on mechanical ventilation is immobile, and generally in a compromised state, the risk for development of atelectasis predisposes the patient to respiratory infection.
Monitor arterial blood gases for changes.	Blood gases are the best measure of effectiveness of the mechanical ventilation; oxygen levels that are too low or too high signal a need for readjustment and can cause complications for the patient.
Empty condensation/water (from the humidifier) in the ventilator tubing into drainage collection receptacles.	Water in the tubing can be a breeding place for organisms and if allowed to remain in the tubing could possibly drain back into the humidifier.
Administer mouth care every two hours.	The mouth dries easily due to the lack of intake and because the mouth is constantly open.
Assess skin around ET tube or tracheostomy every 4 hours for redness or other color changes, tenderness, and warmth.	Helps to detect early any signs of breakdown or irritation.
Move the endotracheal tube to the opposite side of the mouth every 24 hours or according to unit/agency protocol.	The tube can cause trauma to the soft tissue of the mouth, and repositioning prevents breakdown/ulceration of the mouth.
Apply soft wrist restraints as needed.	Prevents pulling at tubes.
Turn patient every two hours.	Relieves pressure on skin and prevents skin breakdown.

INTERVENTIONS	RATIONALES
Administer muscle-paralyzing agents and/or sedatives as ordered.	Many patients who are intubated "fight" the ventilator, increasing the work of breathing and the demand for oxygen.
Suction orally or endotracheally as needed.	Maintains a patent airway and prevents resistance.
Monitor patient for decreased cardiac output: hypotension, fluid retention.	Hypotension is caused by increased intrathoracic pressure that is subsequent to use of the ventilator. The increased pressure on the chest wall impairs the return of blood to the heart. Fluid retention is caused by a homeostatic mechanism that causes the kidneys to preserve fluid in response to decreased blood flow through the renal system.
Assess the patient for signs and symptoms of barotraumas: tissue swelling in the neck, chest, and face; crepitus, unequal chest expansion with decreased breath sounds on one side; chest x-ray reveals pneumothorax; deteriorating blood gases. If detected, notify physician and assist as needed to correct.	Positive pressure and excess volume delivered cause overdistention and rupture of alveoli with subsequent release of air into the interstitial spaces in the pulmonary system. The result can be pneumothorax, signaled by unequal chest expansion as well as decreased breath sounds over affected lung and subcutaneous emphysema. If barotraumas go undetected and untreated, respiratory function is further compromised.

NIC *Artificial airway*
       Mechanical ventilation
       Respiratory monitoring
       Ventilation
       Oxygen therapy

Evaluation

Determine the degree to which the outcome criteria have been met. The patient's respiratory status should be stabilized with arterial blood gases within normal range. The patient's oxygen saturation is > 90 percent, and the patient is tolerating the mechanical ventilator. There is no evidence of complications from use of the ventilator, such as subcutaneous emphysema or pneumothorax.

Community/Home Care

The patient who has been on a mechanical ventilator may have continued problems with respiration once discharged, dependent upon the initiating cause of the respiratory difficulty. For some patients, weaning from the ventilator may not be possible so that care in an alternative setting such as a rehabilitation center or a long-term care center may be required. If this is the case, the family must be prepared to cope with this change in function and role performance. The primary care provider should give a realistic portrayal of the patient's prognosis or chance for weaning. The family may need assistance with coping and planning for placement through utilization of social workers or spiritual counselors. For the patient who is able to go home, respiratory function may still be compromised, and the patient will need to be monitored for ability to adequately meet oxygenation needs. Visits by a nurse will be beneficial for a short time following discharge to monitor respiratory status and ensure that the patient and family are able to identify signs of respiratory problems (shortness of breath, cyanosis, severe dypsnea, extensive use of accessory muscles for respiration). A gradual increase in activities, as tolerated, will assist the patient to increase stamina, but there remains a need to monitor response to activity. Because of the presence of foreign objects (endotracheal tube) in the upper respiratory system, the risk for infection is present after discharge and the patient should know the signs and symptoms to report to a health care provider. Follow-up care is critical to be sure that the patient's blood gases and oxygen saturation are normal.

Documentation

Chart the settings of the ventilator according to the agency/unit protocol. A comprehensive respiratory assessment is documented to include breath sounds, respiratory rate, chest expansion, description of any sputum, and patient's skin color. Note each time that the patient requires suctioning including amount, color, and consistency of sputum suctioned. Document the position of the endotracheal tube according to protocol, as well as all interventions employed to maintain the ventilator and assessments for complications. Chart the patient's response to all interventions and include any signs of fear or anxiety.

NURSING DIAGNOSIS 2

 ### INEFFECTIVE AIRWAY CLEARANCE

Related to:

Inability to sustain ventilatory efforts

Inability to protect airway (absence of gag reflex)

Presence of secretions

Presence of endotracheal tube

Defining Characteristics:

Restlessness and anxiety

Inability to cough

Presence of obstruction

Cyanosis

Diminished/absent breath sounds

Goal:

The patient's airway will remain patent.

Outcome Criteria

✔ The patient's airway is open and free from debris or secretions.

✔ The patient has clear, bilateral breath sounds.

✔ The patient's oxygen saturation is > 90 percent.

NOC *Respiratory status: Airway patency*
Respiratory status: Ventilation

INTERVENTIONS	RATIONALES
Assess breath sounds, oxygen saturation, and arterial blood gases.	Helps to establish baseline, response to interventions, and note drops in oxygen levels.
Assess the viscosity, amount, and color of secretions.	Thickened secretions are more likely to occlude the airway; noting this would allow for early implementation of measures to thin secretions; the color of secretions allows for early detection of color changes due to infection.
Suction as needed based on respiratory assessment, hyperoxygenating before and after suctioning. Findings that indicate a need for suctioning include crackles and frequent sounding of the high-pressure alarms on the ventilator.	Keeps the endotracheal tube (or other airway) free from obstruction and airway compromise; hyperoxygenating provides oxygen reserves and decreases hypoxia caused by suctioning.
Provide warm, humidified oxygen as ordered.	Helps to liquefy secretions and make them easier to mobilize and suction.
Ensure that "sigh" mechanism is functional on ventilator: rate and volume.	The sigh mechanism causes hyperexpansion of the lungs/alveoli and prevents atelectasis and fluid build-up in non-aerated areas.
Turn the patient frequently, at least every 2 hours.	Helps to mobilize secretions and avoid pooling of secretions.
Ensure adequate fluid intake intravenously or enterally.	Fluids will help keep secretions liquefied.

NIC *Airway management*
Airway suctioning
Respiratory monitoring
Oxygen therapy
Ventilation assistance

Evaluation

Assess the patient to determine the extent to which the outcome criteria have been met. The patient's airway should be clear, and the patient's blood gas analysis and oxygen saturation should reveal adequate oxygenation. Breath sounds should be clear, and there should be no cyanosis. If criteria have not been met, determine if expected outcomes were realistic or whether more time is needed for achievement. In this case, note the degree of progress the patient is making towards meeting the goals.

Community/Home Care

The patient who has been on a ventilator may only need short-term follow-up monitoring by a health care professional when discharged home. Airway clearance may not be an issue upon discharge, but because the patient who requires mechanical ventilation has been critically ill, some follow-up for the underlying cause is warranted. The patient and family will need to implement strategies to prevent increased production of secretions, such as maintaining fluid intake and increasing activity as tolerated to mobilize secretions. Teaching the patient how to cough and deep breathe can assist the patient to prevent respiratory infections by expanding the lungs and preventing stasis of secretions.

Documentation

Document the patient's breath sounds, color, and oxygen saturation. Include in the patient record all interventions carried out for the patient to address ineffective airway clearance, particularly suctioning, and the patient's response. Note specifically the amount, viscosity, and color of secretions obtained from suctioning. If the patient is able to participate in care, including initiating coughing, document this in the chart. Document vital signs according to agency protocol.

NURSING DIAGNOSIS 3

IMPAIRED VERBAL COMMUNICATION

Related to:

Endotracheal intubation

Defining Characteristics:

Is unable to speak

Goal:

The patient will be able to communicate needs.

Outcome Criteria

✔ The patient is able to communicate via a method that achieves this goal.

✔ The patient will use a communication board to express his or her needs.

✔ The patient will be able to express needs by use of writing or pointing to words.

NOC *Communication*

Communication: Expressive

INTERVENTIONS	RATIONALES
Assess the patient's ability to communicate; determine whether the patient can read and write.	Establishes that the patient is able to use alternative communication methods.
Provide the patient with alternatives to verbal communication: communication board, pencil and paper, Magic Slate, or chalkboard, if the patient is able to read and write. Provide picture cards if the patient cannot read or write.	This provides a method of communication until the patient is able to speak. When an endotracheal tube is in place, the patient will be unable to speak, as the tube prevents the passage of air over the vocal cords when the cuff is inflated properly.
If the patient is unable to use hands to write or point, teach the patient to signal using eye blinks, hand squeezing, nodding, or other means of nonverbal communication, etc.	Much information can be communicated using simple gestures to signal "yes" and "no" as well as other simple commands.
Take time to work with the patient in communication efforts, being patient and not rushing him or her.	Rushing the patient to communicate causes frustration and may make the patient stop trying.
Arrange for a speech therapy consultation.	Speech therapists can provide methods for the intubated, ventilated patient to communicate by evaluating the patient's specific capabilities.
Keep call light available and ensure that the patient has the ability to call for help if needed. Arrange for the occupational therapist to assist with development of nontraditional signaling methods if the patient is unable to move and cannot use call bell.	Always provide a means for the patient to be able to call for help whenever needed. Always respond promptly to a call for assistance.
Offer assurances to the patient and family that speech will be possible after the endotracheal tube is removed.	Inability to talk creates anxiety, and offering assurance and information to the family and patient can decrease this.

NIC *Communication enhancement: Speech deficit*

Anxiety reduction

Evaluation

Evaluate the progress the patient has made in ability to communicate. Establish what needs to be done to further enhance nonverbal communication with the patient. Evaluate whether the patient is able to communicate using a communication board, writing, or pointing. Determine whether the patient is frustrated or satisfied with attempts at communication.

Community/Home Care

Once the endotracheal tube has been removed, the patient's problem with verbal communication should be resolved. Many patients with endotracheal tubes feel embarrassed, causing them to refrain from efforts at communication, as well as frustrated at trying to make others understand them. At home, communication should not be an issue that needs follow-up. However, a related issue may be hoarseness from having the tube in place. The patient should utilize simple strategies such as gargling to resolve this.

Documentation

Document all communication strategies utilized with the patient. Include an evaluation of the patient's efforts to communicate and which strategies work best. Always include an assessment of the patient's emotional state and responses to all interventions. Chart any referrals made for assistance with communication and the outcomes of any suggested recommendations.

NURSING DIAGNOSIS 4

 ANXIETY

Related to:

Presence of endotracheal tube

Inability to talk

Defining Characteristics:

Fear that airway will become obstructed

Restlessness

Verbalization of anxiety

Goal:

The patient's anxiety level is reduced.

Outcome Criteria

✔ The patient reports being less anxious.

✔ The patient demonstrates no outward signs of anxiety, such as restlessness or agitation.

NOC *Anxiety control*
Comfort level

INTERVENTIONS	RATIONALES
Assess level of anxiety (mild, moderate, severe); have patient rate on a scale of 1–10, with 10 being the greatest.	Gives the nurse a better perception of extent of the anxiety.
Keep patient informed of all that is going on, including information about therapeutic interventions.	Communication in a calm and straightforward manner may help to relieve anxiety.
Ensure that the call bell/light button is readily accessible to the patient; respond to needs related to the endotracheal tube promptly: need for suctioning, coughing episodes.	Changes in respiratory status caused by mucous build-up and coughing can add to anxiety and fear. Knowing that help is readily accessible can help to reduce the patient's anxiety level and makes the patient feel confident that needs will be met and complications prevented; gives the patient a sense of control.
Use a calm, reassuring manner with the patient.	Gives the patient a sense of well-being.
Stay with patient as possible and allow family to visit.	Provides emotional support and promotes a sense of comfort.
If possible, encourage the patient to communicate fears and concerns about being on the ventilator.	Recognizing fears contributes to dealing with concerns and decreases anxiety.
Control multiple sources of stimuli that could cause sensory overload.	Overstimulation can worsen anxiety.
Give the patient and family information about the ventilator and endotracheal tube.	Knowledge decreases anxiety by giving the patient a sense of control.
Assist the patient with new strategies for communication.	The inability to communicate or the need to learn new communication techniques can cause frustrations that lead to anxiety.

NIC *Anxiety reduction*
Emotional support

Evaluation

Evaluate the extent to which the outcome criteria have been achieved. Physiological signs of anxiety, such as tachycardia and diaphoresis, will be absent. The patient will communicate a decrease in anxiety and fear. Restlessness and agitation will be absent. The patient reports that he or she is not frustrated with attempts at communication.

Community/Home Care

The patient may need no follow-up at home regarding anxiety. Once the ventilator is discontinued and the endotracheal tube is removed, the patient's anxiety may dissipate. Being in a critical care unit predisposes the patient to anxiety and fear regarding health status, and after discharge to home some concerns may still surface. Follow-up care with a health care provider should examine the patient's psychological well-being. If the patient remains anxious due to fear of alterations in respiratory status, the patient will need to practice relaxation techniques that can reduce anxiety. Nurses should assess which coping mechanisms work for the patient and encourage their use by the patient at home. The relationship between anxiety and increasing oxygen demands should be explained to the patient so that he or she can understand the importance of controlling fears and anxiety.

Documentation

The degree to which the patient has decreased anxiety should be documented in the patient record. A rating system provides an objective way to relay to others the extent of the anxiety. Document whether the patient is able to verbalize a feeling of decreased anxiety and whether there are outward signs of anxiety. Include in the documentation what specific events seem to contribute to anxiety episodes and what strategies are employed to relieve or reduce it. Blood pressure and pulse rates should be documented, as anxiety often causes an increase in both vital signs.

NURSING DIAGNOSIS 5

RISK FOR DYSFUNCTIONAL VENTILATORY WEANING RESPONSE

Related to:

Inability to wean patient from mechanical intubation

Prolonged ventilator dependence

Defining Characteristics:

Anxious and restless when mechanical ventilation is disconnected

Unable to sustain ventilatory efforts when mechanical ventilation is discontinued

Blood gases abnormal when mechanical ventilation is discontinued

Goal:

The patient is able to be weaned from the ventilator.

Outcome Criteria

✔ The patient is able to be weaned from the ventilator and his or her arterial blood gases are within normal limits.

✔ The patient is able to sustain spontaneous ventilatory efforts.

NOC *Mechanical ventilation weaning response: Adult*
Respiratory status: Ventilation

INTERVENTIONS	RATIONALES
Ensure that vital signs and breath sounds are within the patient's baseline normal limits prior to weaning.	If vitals signs are abnormal or breath sounds demonstrate diminished sound or adventitious sounds, the patient may be unable to sustain spontaneous ventilatory efforts. If the patient is febrile, his or her metabolic needs will increase, and oxygen adjustments will also increase.
Ensure that the patient has adequate strength (especially in muscles of respiration).	Weaning from a mechanical ventilator takes significant respiratory muscle strength and endurance.
Reassure the patient that coming off the ventilator will be successful and that, if there are difficulties, help will be close by to correct the problem.	The patient may be afraid to lose the security of mechanical ventilation.
Teach the patient the steps that will be used to wean him or her from the ventilator.	Anxiety will be reduced if the patient knows what will be happening.
Evaluate arterial blood gases (ABG) and recent chest x-ray to ascertain readiness for removal of mechanical ventilation.	The chest x-ray should demonstrate absence of congestion and reflect relatively clear lung fields. ABGs should be within normal limits with the patient on a fractional inspired oxygen percentage (FIO_2) of 40 percent or less.
In collaboration with the respiratory therapist and physician, adjust the ventilator settings than can "test" the patient's ability to sustain spontaneous respiration.	Setting the ventilator to test if the patient can "trigger" own ventilation efforts provides backup in the event spontaneous ventilations do not occur.
Assist with strategies of weaning as ordered or required: removing	The respiratory system must be reconditioned to breathe

(continues)

(continued)

INTERVENTIONS	RATIONALES
the ventilator for brief periods during which oxygen is administered, with these periods gradually increased until the patient is able to ventilate independently for a specified time; decreasing the number of mandatory ventilator-assisted breaths gradually. During weaning, monitor patient's ability to tolerate weaning by examining arterial blood gases, oxygen saturation, presence of dyspnea, and overall respiratory status.	independently. Assessments of the respiratory system must be made to ensure that the patient can tolerate weaning.
Plan other nursing care activities around weaning activities, arranging weaning activities at a time when the patient is well rested.	The patient needs to be well rested to avoid fatigue and increased oxygen demands on a compromised respiratory system.
Assure the patient that it may take several trials to reach successful weaning.	Knowing that weaning may take time and is not always successful at first will decrease anxiety and alert the patient as to what can be expected.

NIC *Mechanical ventilation*
Mechanical ventilatory weaning

Evaluation

Evaluate whether the patient has been able to tolerate removal from the ventilator. A respiratory assessment that includes oxygen saturation, efforts at respiration, breath sounds, and any dyspnea should be noted.

Community/Home Care

This problem should no longer be an issue for the patient once at home. Once the patient has been weaned from the ventilator, it is necessary for him or her to remain in the hospital setting where his or her respiratory status will be monitored. At home, the patient will continue to recuperate from a critical illness and will require a gradual return to functioning. The patient is taught how to progress activities and monitor respiratory status, noting any dyspnea. For the patient who cannot be weaned from the ventilator, transfer to a rehabilitation center or other long-term care facility will be necessary.

If the family undertakes care of the patient with a ventilator at home, intensive education should be undertaken to include operation of the ventilator, suctioning, respiratory assessment, troubleshooting, and care of equipment, etc. In-home visits from a visiting nurse will be required to reinforce the teaching and to provide encouragement and support. The visiting care provider should assess caregivers for caregiver role strain and provide information on support groups.

Documentation

Chart all interventions implemented in efforts to wean the patient from the ventilator. Document the results of a respiratory assessment before and after attempts at weaning. Include arterial blood gases, oxygen saturation results, and whether the patient is able to sustain ventilatory efforts independently. If weaning is not successful, document the specific patient responses to the efforts.

NURSING DIAGNOSIS 6

 RISK FOR INFECTION

Related to:

Endotracheal intubation

Less-than-adequate pulmonary function

Possible damaged pulmonary tissue

Defining Characteristics (If Infection Occurs):

Foul-smelling, thick pulmonary secretions

Decreased lung sounds; pulmonary congestion/consolidation

Changes in vital signs

Tachycardia

Fever

Goal:

The patient will not acquire a respiratory infection.

Outcome Criteria

✔ The patient will be afebrile.

✔ WBC count will be normal.

✔ Sputum will be clear and thin.

NOC *Nutritional status*
Infection severity

INTERVENTIONS	RATIONALES
Monitor for signs of infection: elevated WBC, fever (take temperature every 4 hours), coughing with expectoration of mucopurulent sputum (note an increase in amount and viscosity).	Helps to detect early the presence of infection and initiate early interventions.
Monitor chest x-ray reports for consolidation, congestion, or atelectasis.	These findings indicate the possible presence of infection; atelectasis predisposes the patient to pneumonia.
Increase fluid intake intravenously or enterally.	Moistens secretions so that they can be expectorated and will not harbor bacteria.
Administer antibiotics, as ordered.	Antibiotics should be given to prevent infections or to treat causative organisms found on sputum culture.
Provide enterally substances high in protein and vitamin C.	Protein and vitamin C are required for immune system functioning and healing, the patient's general well-being and resistance to disease can be adversely affected by poor diet.
Use sterile aseptic technique when suctioning the patient.	Prevents introduction of organisms into the respiratory system.
Limit visitors and post signs warning visitors with upper respiratory infections or colds not to visit.	Reduces exposure to microorganisms that can be transported via droplets and hand-to-hand contact.
Practice good hand hygiene when working with the patient.	Many organisms are transported via hands of health care workers and readily cause infection in compromised hosts.

NIC *Infection control*
Infection protection
Nutrition management

Evaluation

The patient has no symptoms of infection. Temperature remains normal and there is no elevation in white cell count. The patient's secretions are of usual viscosity and a normal color (not purulent). Ordered chest x-rays reveal no evidence of pneumonia.

Community/Home Care

The patient who has been on a ventilator will be at high risk for development of upper respiratory infections for a period of time following extubation. It is important that the patient or family be able to verbalize the signs and symptoms of respiratory infections that should be reported to the health care provider. Because patients are in a compromised state following a critical illness, upper respiratory infections can pose a serious threat to the patient's well-being, and should be prevented. The patient should avoid areas such as crowded shopping centers, where infections are easily transmitted. Good hand washing should be practiced by the patient, especially following activities where there is likely to be significant handshaking, such as after a religious service. Maintaining an optimal level of respiratory functioning by engaging in activity as tolerated, adequate intake of fluid, and adequate nutrition will assist in efforts to prevent infection. If the patient is being discharged on a ventilator, the risk for infection persists, especially if the patient has a chronic disorder such as Guillain-Barre syndrome, amyotrophic lateral sclerosis, or quadriplegia, and the care providers will need to be vigilant in their efforts to prevent infection.

Documentation

Chart the results of a thorough respiratory assessment to include breath sounds and a description of any secretions obtained from suctioning. Include in chart notations the patient's temperature and pulse rate every 4 hours. All interventions employed to prevent or treat infection are charted, and if any signs and symptoms are detected, these are noted with attention to revisions to the plan of care to address them.

CHAPTER 2.27

MODIFIED/RADICAL NECK SURGERY/LARYNGECTOMY

GENERAL INFORMATION

Radical neck surgery and laryngectomies are usually done to remove a cancerous/malignant tumor of the head or neck and metastasis to lymph nodes of the neck, muscles, nerves, and other tissues. Both neck dissection and laryngectomy may be done in modified or radical procedures. In radical neck dissections, the soft tissue from the lower part of the mandible down to the clavicle is removed along with the cervical lymph nodes, the sternocleidomastoid muscle, internal jugular vein, eleventh cranial nerve, the submaxillary salivary gland, and in some cases part of the thyroid and parathyroid glands. The patient who undergoes a radical neck dissection is left with extensive disfigurement, and skin grafts with flaps are required. Because the eleventh cranial nerve is responsible for the shoulder, the patient is left with shoulder drop. A modified neck dissection will spare the jugular vein, the sternocleidomastoid muscle, and the eleventh cranial nerve. In a laryngectomy, the larynx may be partially or totally removed. For the patient with a tumor that occurs in only a portion of the larynx, a partial laryngectomy can be performed, which spares the vocal cords and preserves the voice; however, the voice is usually hoarse. A total laryngectomy is performed when the cancer extends beyond the vocal cords, and in this instance the entire larynx along with the epiglottis, the hyoid bone, one or more tracheal rings, and thyroid cartilage are all removed. Following a total laryngectomy, there is no voice capability and a permanent tracheostomy is required. After complete removal of the larynx, there are a variety of methods to establish speech for the patient, including use of a voice prosthesis, esophageal speech, or an electronic artificial larynx.

NURSING DIAGNOSIS 1

INEFFECTIVE AIRWAY CLEARANCE

Related to:

Mucous plugs

Edema

Hemorrhage

Absence of cough

Presence of laryngectomy/tracheostomy tube

Defining Characteristics:

Tachypnea

Decreased breath sounds

Edema in surgical site

Thick mucous

Decreased oxygen saturation

Abnormal blood gases with decreased oxygen

Goal:

The patient's airway is patent.

Outcome Criteria

✔ Breath sounds will be clear.

✔ The patient will have no cyanosis.

✔ Oxygen saturation will be > 90 percent.

✔ Arterial blood gases (ABGs) will be within normal limits.

NOC *Respiratory status: Airway patency*
Respiratory status: Ventilation

INTERVENTIONS	RATIONALES
Assess respiratory status: breath sounds, respiratory rate, oxygen saturation, and arterial blood gases (ABGs).	Establishes a baseline and monitor response to interventions.
Monitor patient for signs of occluded airway: cyanosis, whistling sound from tracheostomy or laryngectomy tube, holding throat, absent or diminished breath sounds.	The airway may obstruct without the patient being able to notify health care worker.
Assess the viscosity and color of secretions; note any bleeding.	Thickened secretions are more likely to occlude the tracheostomy; recognizing this would allow for implementation of measures to thin secretions; the color of secretions allows for early detection of color changes due to infection and hemorrhage.
Provide humidified oxygen, as ordered.	The humidification function of the upper airway does not function with a tracheostomy, so humidified oxygen is given to help liquefy secretions and ensure adequate oxygenation.
Suction the tracheostomy or stoma as ordered and prn, providing oxygen before and after suctioning.	Removes secretions and prevents airway obstruction; oxygen prevents hypoxia.
Administer mucolytic agents as ordered.	Liquefies secretions to facilitate removal.
Administer bronchodilator agents, as ordered.	Dilates bronchioles, which facilitates movement of secretions.
Maintain sterile technique when with tracheostomy site or tracheostomy tube.	Prevents introduction of infectious organisms into the respiratory system.
Avoid movement of tracheostomy tube unnecessarily.	Movement causes irritation to trachea and discomfort for the patient.
Assist patient with coughing and deep breathing every 2 hours.	Mobilizes secretions and prevents atelectasis.
Clean around tracheostomy/laryngectomy site and replace inner cannula with a new disposable one every shift. If older model reusable metal tracheostomy/laryngectomy tube is used, remove inner cannula, cleanse according to agency procedure, and replace.	Clears airway debris that has adhered to the side of the tube and minimizes the risk for infection.

Monitor for signs and symptoms of respiratory infection: fever, rales, increased mucous production, elevated white blood cell count, chest x-ray reports.	Initiates treatment early and prevents complications.

NIC　*Airway management*
Airway suctioning
Cough enhancement
Respiratory monitoring
Oxygen therapy
Ventilation assistance

Evaluation

Assess the client to determine the extent to which the outcome criteria have been met. The patient's airway should be clear, and the patient should be able to cough with expectoration of secretions. Breath sounds should be clear and there should be no cyanosis. Oxygen saturation should be > 90 percent, and blood gases should be within normal range. If criteria have not been met, determine whether the expected outcomes were realistic or whether more time is needed for achievement. In the latter case, note the degree of progress the patient is making towards meeting the goals.

Community/Home Care

The patient with a tracheostomy or laryngectomy tube may need long-term monitoring by a health care professional when discharged home. In some instances, the patient and family will be able to care for the tracheostomy themselves; in some cases care will always be provided by a visiting nurse. The patient and family must know how to handle emergencies that could arise. Specifically, the patient and family will need to know the signs of airway obstruction and how to relieve it in the home until medical personnel can reach them. Performance of tracheostomy care (see nursing diagnosis "Deficient Knowledge"), suctioning, and measures to prevent respiratory infection are important aspects of in-home care that the patient and family need to understand. The patient should avoid becoming sedentary but make conscious efforts to move around the home or engage in some type of physical activity to prevent statis of secretions. In addition, fluids should be taken liberally to help thin secretions. It is crucial that the patient have all needed supplies for tracheostomy care, so there needs to be an assessment of the patient's financial resources. Health care providers visiting the home should give attention to the patient's psychological state, as disfigurement from the laryngectomy and/or neck dissection along with the tracheostomy is a visible change in anatomy that can disturb body image. Question the patient about his or her social life and general sense of well-being to ascertain if the patient may be socially isolating him or herself (see nursing diagnosis "Disturbed Body Image").

Documentation

Document a comprehensive respiratory assessment. Include in the patient record all interventions carried out for the patient and the patient's response. Note specifically secretions, suctioning, tracheostomy or laryngectomy tube care, and drainage from surgical sites. If the patient is able to participate in care, including initiating coughing, document this in the chart. Document vital signs according to agency protocol. Chart any teaching initiated with a clear indication of what was taught and to whom.

NURSING DIAGNOSIS 2

IMPAIRED SKIN INTEGRITY

Related to:

Surgical procedures of neck dissection and laryngectomy

Presence of drainage tubes

Reconstructive surgery for radical neck dissection using skin flaps

Defining Characteristics:

Presence of surgical incisions

Fever

Elevated white blood count

Redness, swelling, drainage around stoma

Foul smell from tracheostomy tube

Elevated wound skin flap

Goal:

Incision heals without complications.

Infection is prevented or eliminated.

Outcome Criteria

✔ The patient's surgical site has no redness or other discoloration, purulent drainage, or heat.

✔ The surgical sites are well approximated.

✔ The patient remains afebrile.

✔ White blood cell count remains within normal limits.

✔ The surgical site heals and remains intact.

NOC *Wound healing: Primary intention*

INTERVENTIONS	RATIONALES
Monitor surgical sites and all flaps every hour; look for healthy color.	Ensures adequate blood flow to the surgical site and reconstruction site; skin that is darkened, blue, or pale indicates decreased blood supply and should be reported immediately.
Monitor surgical site and drainage tube insertion sites for signs and symptoms of infection: redness, swelling, purulent drainage.	Early identification of infection can expedite treatment and prevent irreparable damage to site.
Maintain patency of drainage devices and assess drainage from Hemovac® drains or other drainage tubes for amount, color, and consistency.	The drainage device helps maintain position of skin flaps; if not draining properly, the drainage may build up under the flap and damage the graft by impeding arterial blood supply to the graft and venous drainage from the site; drainage may be bloody initially, but should become serosanguineous.
Take temperature every 4 hours.	Detects signs of infection.
Provide careful oral and stoma hygiene as ordered.	Decreases the number of bacteria and other organisms.
Change dressings as ordered and clean area using sterile technique, cleansing site of drainage devices last.	Maintenance of a clean incisional site decreases the number of organisms and reduces chance of infection.
Administer antipyretics (acetaminophen [Tylenol]), as ordered.	Reduces fever.
Administer antibiotics, as ordered: IV (intravenously) or PO (by mouth).	Reduces the number of infective organisms and eliminates or prevents infection.
Administer corticosteroids, as ordered.	Reduces local inflammation.

INTERVENTIONS	RATIONALES
Restrict visitors with colds, etc.	Reduces the likelihood of patient exposure to infective agents.
Support head when moving patient.	Reduces strain and trauma to operative site.
Encourage adequate nutritional intake orally, parenterally, or enterally with intake of protein, vitamin C, and iron.	Adequate nutrient intake, especially of vitamin C, protein, and iron, is required for healing and tissue repair.

NIC *Incision site care*

Infection control

Nutrition management

Wound care

Wound care: Closed drainage

Evaluation

Evaluate the degree to which the outcome criteria have been met. The surgical site should be intact healing by primary intention with incision well approximated. Redness, swelling, purulent drainage, and heat should be absent from the site. Drainage from the drainage devices should be serosanguineous and should be decreasing in amount. The patient should be afebrile, and white blood cell counts should return to normal.

Community/Home Care

The status of the surgical site may remain a problem after the patient has been discharged home. If the patient has had reconstructive surgery, the site will need to be examined by a health care provider to ensure that blood flow to the area is sustained. Whether the patient has a tracheostomy, laryngectomy tube, or stoma, he or she will need to be taught how to care for it as prescribed by the health care provider, with attention to how to properly cover when showering/bathing. In addition, good handwashing before touching the site should be stressed. The patient may also feel more comfortable covering the tracheostomy, stoma, or laryngectomy tube with some type of covering for cosmetic reasons and to prevent entry of organisms that may cause respiratory infection. The patient will need to understand the importance of good nutrition in complete wound healing. Eating may be difficult, but attention to adequate amounts of vitamins and minerals is crucial (see nursing diagnosis "Imbalanced Nutrition").

The importance of completing any ordered medications such as antibiotics once at home should be stressed. The risk for infection remains, and the family will need to know what symptoms may signal the onset of infection. If any evidence of infection is found, the patient should be instructed to contact the health care provider. Visits from a nurse will be beneficial to ensure that proper wound care is being performed and to monitor healing of both the surgical and skin flap sites.

Documentation

Document assessment findings of the surgical sites to include color, approximation, drainage, etc., being sure to note any sign of infection. Also include in the chart dressing changes and type of dressing applied. Chart the status of drainage devices or tubes indicating the color, amount, and consistency of drainage. Document vital signs according to agency protocol, as ordered for postoperative patients.

NURSING DIAGNOSIS 3

IMBALANCED NUTRITION: LESS THAN BODY REQUIREMENTS

Related to:

Tracheostomy tube

Laryngectomy tube

Dysphagia

Odynophagia

Inability to eat

Defining Characteristics:

Difficulty swallowing

Loss of appetite

Loss of weight

Refuses to eat

Eats little of food served

Goal:

Adequate dietary/fluid intake is ensured.

Outcome Criteria

✔ The patient does not lose weight.

✔ The patient consumes 50 percent of food served.

✔ The patient tolerates enteral feedings without nausea, vomiting, or diarrhea.

NOC *Swallowing status: Oral phase*
Nutritional status: Food and
*   fluid intake*
Nutritional status: Nutrient intake
Oral hygiene
Sensory function: Taste and smell

INTERVENTIONS	RATIONALES
Assess laboratory results: albumin, electrolytes, glucose, protein (total), and iron.	These are indicators of nutritional status.
Assess the patient's ability to eat/drink and whether he or she has difficulty chewing or swallowing.	Identifies specific problems the patient may be experiencing and allows intervention accordingly.
Weigh patient and monitor weight daily.	Establishes a baseline for comparison and as patient progresses allows for early intervention for nutritional deficits.
Monitor intake and output.	Assures adequate hydration needed for wound healing and liquefaction of secretions.
Consider dietitian consult to ascertain the patient's ability to take in enough food to meet caloric demand and to determine the patient's likes, dislikes, and preferences within the prescribed diet and with consideration to cultural or religious preferences.	For patients who have had a total laryngectomy, the sense of taste and smell have been disrupted; the patient will be more likely to consume foods that he or she likes and that are a part of his or her normal diet.
Provide for tube feedings if necessary and as ordered and monitor for side effects (nausea, vomiting, and diarrhea).	Because of the difficulty in chewing and swallowing following surgery on the head and neck, enteral feedings may be necessary to maintain the calories, nutrients, and vitamins required for healing.
Encourage the patient to adopt a pureed or soft diet (foods that are soft and slippery, such as custards and ice cream), consumed in small, frequent meals.	Food may be more tolerable in small portions; there is less risk of aspiration, and the food is easier to chew and to digest (patients who have had total laryngectomy cannot aspirate because there is no connection between the trachea and the esophagus).
Stay with the patient the first time food or liquids are taken orally.	Allows nurse to assess the ability to eat or drink and to intervene if aspiration occurs.
Allow adequate time for meals.	The patient may take longer to eat due to structural changes in the neck and/or mouth.
Provide privacy during meals.	The patient may be embarrassed because swallowing is not precise and food may spill out of mouth.
Keep suction apparatus connected at bedside.	Allows for emergency intervention in case the patient is unable to chew and swallow effectively.
Consult with speech therapist or appropriate discipline to assist patient with assessment of swallowing ability.	All patients undergoing neck surgery have some dysphagia or odynophagia, and many must learn to swallow again.

NIC *Nutritional monitoring*
Nutritional management
Swallowing therapy

Evaluation

The patient's nutritional state is stable and the patient has a satisfactory method for nutrient intake. Assess the patient's weight and determine that the patient is not losing weight. The patient should be ingesting at least 50 percent of food served and, if on enteral feedings, should be tolerating them without nausea, vomiting, or diarrhea. Laboratory results should reveal a normal level of albumin as well as total protein and electrolytes. Prior to discharge, the patient should be able to eat and drink without pain or difficulty.

Community/Home Care

Difficulties with eating and drinking may continue at home for the patient who has had a laryngectomy or neck dissection. The patient will need to continue efforts to ingest enough food and nutrients to meet metabolic demands of healing. A home nurse needs to monitor the patient's nutritional status on a regular basis to detect excessive weight loss and to note reports of decreased intake due to pain, anxiety, fear of choking, etc. The family can assist the patient by preparing foods that are easy to chew and swallow, that the patient likes, and that have nutritional value. The patient needs encouragement to eat and even at home may prefer privacy for meals because of drooling, special chewing and swallowing, and the extended time it takes for meals. Small, frequent meals and appropriate snacks that are easily chewed and swallowed are means of increasing intake. Have the patient keep an intake diary along with weights to share with the health care provider. If enteral feedings are to be administered in the home, the family and/or patient will need to learn all aspects of this skill or the services of a nurse will be required. In some instances, the patient may receive enteral feedings via a pump at night while asleep. This may be the recommendation for patients who cannot tolerate bolus feedings or for those who can consume some food during the day but not enough to meet nutritional needs. Consultation with a social worker may be warranted to arrange for acquisition of supplies particularly if the pump is to be used. Return to the preoperative nutritional state may take considerable time. If problems with nutrition and weight loss occur, the patient needs to contact a health care provider for more aggressive measures.

Documentation

Chart the patient's weight daily. Include in the chart assessments made during the patient's efforts to eat for the first time. Document any difficulty that the patient experiences during meals, particularly pain, difficulty swallowing, or difficulty chewing and any interventions implemented to address them. Record intake and output according to agency protocol, being sure to document the percentage of food consumed. If the patient verbalizes concerns, include this in the chart. Document the placement of enteral feeding tubes as well as the patient's tolerance to feedings. Always document any referrals made to other disciplines, such as the nutritionist and the social worker.

NURSING DIAGNOSIS 4

IMPAIRED VERBAL COMMUNICATION

Related to:

> Absence of larynx and vocal cords
>
> Presence of tracheostomy or laryngectomy tube
>
> Neck dissection

Defining Characteristics:

> Unable to talk

Goal:

> The patient is able to communicate.

Outcome Criteria

✔ The patient will use a communication board to express his or her needs.

✔ The patient will be able to express needs by writing or pointing to words.

✔ The patient will use esophageal speech, an electrolarynx, or tracheoesophageal prosthesis (voice prosthesis) for communication.

NOC *Communication*
Communication: Expressive

INTERVENTIONS	RATIONALES
Assess patient's ability to communicate; determine if patient can read and write.	Establishes that the patient is able to use alternative communications methods.
Provide patient with an alternative to verbal communication: communication board, pencil and paper, Magic Slate, or chalkboard if the patient is able to read and write; picture cards if the patient cannot read or write.	This provides a method of communication until the patient is able to speak. When a tracheostomy tube is in place, the patient will be unable to speak because air will not pass the vocal cords to produce the vibrations necessary to produce sounds.
If the patient is unable to use hands to write or point, teach the patient to signal using eye blinks, hand squeezing, nodding, or other means of nonverbal communication.	Much information can be communicated using simple gestures to signal "yes" and "no" as well as other simple commands.
Arrange for a speech therapist consult.	Speech therapists can assist the patient with communication methods, including adjunct devices to facilitate communication.
Teach patient how to cover tracheostomy when surgical healing allows.	Covering the tracheostomy opening permits air to flow over the larynx allowing for speech.
Consult with the physician regarding the use of a special tracheostomy tube that allows speech, such as a Communitrach.	These tracheostomy tubes have a one-way valve that closes with exhalation allowing for speech.
Take time to work with patient in communication efforts, being	Rushing the patient to communicate causes frustration

(continues)

(continued)

INTERVENTIONS	RATIONALES
patient and not rushing him or her.	and may make the patient stop trying to communicate.
Utilize a speech therapist for assistance in establishing the best speech methodology and to educate the patient and family about the following options: — Tracheoesophageal prosthesis: a tracheoesophageal puncture (TEP) creates a fistula between tracheal wall and anterior esophagus; the prosthesis, which has a one-way shunt valve, is fitted into the fistula, and sound can be created by covering the tracheostomy stoma. — Electrolarynx: a battery-operated device that is held to the neck and that creates vibrations that are then transmitted to the mouth; another one delivers a tone into the mouth via a plastic tube inserted into the corner of the mouth using the lips, tongue, and mouth muscles to form the words. — Esophageal speech: uses swallowed air to form words.	These methods allow effective communication by the patient, and the speech therapist is best qualified to assist the patient. The physician makes the decision for the TEP.
Provide privacy and emotional support for the patient who is learning new speech strategies.	All of the above methods of speech require motivation and practice for effective use; encouragement and support enhance that motivation and decrease anxiety. Privacy may be required in the early stage of learning as the patient becomes more comfortable with new speech.
Provide the family with resources for further information: the American Cancer Society, the American Speech and Hearing Association, and the International Association of Laryngectomies.	These organizations/agencies provide literature and information about other resources to assist the patient and family in coping with the issues surrounding having a laryngectomy and impaired speech.

NIC *Communication enhancement:*
Speech deficit
Learning Facilitation
Anxiety reduction

Evaluation

Evaluate the progress the patient has made in his or her ability to communicate. Establish what needs to be done to further enhance nonverbal communication with the patient. Evaluate whether the patient is able to communicate using a communication board, writing, or pointing. Assess the effectiveness of communication using electrolarynx, esophageal speech, or the voice prosthesis. Determine if the patient is frustrated or satisfied with attempts at communication.

Community/Home Care

For the patient who has had a laryngectomy, the inability to communicate verbally may prove to be the biggest challenge when discharged home. Many patients feel embarrassed, particularly in public; they also experience frustration at trying to make others understand, and may refrain from efforts at communication. The patient can practice new communication strategies with family members or in private. The patient must be encouraged to continue with new communication strategies, and this is where social support systems can be most beneficial. As family and friends display acceptance, encouragement, and patience, the patient will become more comfortable with communication knowing that others understand. If this does not happen, the patient may socially isolate him or herself, which could lead to emotional stress. Other patients or support group members may be helpful in assisting the patient with communication and may provide tips and pointers acquired through trial and error. Follow-up care should give attention to not only the physiological realm of care but to this very critical aspect of the patient's well-being.

Documentation

Document all communication strategies utilized with the patient. Include an evaluation of the patient's efforts to communicate and of the strategies to determine which work best. Always include an assessment of the patient's emotional state and responses to all interventions. Chart any referrals made for speech and the outcomes of their recommendations. When speech devices or techniques are employed to enhance communication, document the patient's ability and willingness to use them.

NURSING DIAGNOSIS 5

 ANXIETY

Related to:

Presence of tracheostomy/laryngectomy tube and new way to breathe

Inability to talk

Defining Characteristics:

Expresses fear that he or she will be unable to communicate

Anxiety

Restlessness

Verbalization of anxiety

Goal:

The patient's anxiety level is reduced.

Outcome Criteria

✔ The patient reports being less anxious.

✔ The patient demonstrates no outward signs of anxiety, such as restlessness or agitation.

NOC *Anxiety control*
      Comfort level

INTERVENTIONS	RATIONALES
Assess level of anxiety (mild, moderate, severe); have patient rate on a scale of 1–10, with 10 being the greatest.	Gives the nurse a better perception of extent of the anxiety.
Assess the patient to determine if he or she appears sad, crying, depressed, withdrawn, angry, concerned that people will make fun of him or her, worried that family will reject him or her, or embarrassed about disfigurement. Determine whether the family members appear tentative, concerned over their reaction to the patient's appearance, or supportive, and whether they express feelings about the patient's appearance.	Early detection of grieving, anxiety, and depression can afford the patient early treatment and avoid severe depression and isolation. The family's reaction to the patient's disfigurement will affect how the patient accepts the physical change. Noting negative family reactions can afford the nurse the opportunity to assist the family to accept the changes that have occurred, which will help to achieve more positive outcomes for the patient.
Keep the patient informed of all that is going on, including information about therapeutic interventions.	Communication of information about therapeutic interventions in a calm and straightforward manner may help to relieve anxiety.
Ensure that the call bell/light button is readily accessible to the patient; respond to needs related to the tracheostomy promptly, such as the need for suctioning and coughing episodes.	Changes in respiratory status caused by mucous build-up and coughing can add to anxiety and fear. Knowing that help is readily accessible can help to reduce the patient's anxiety level and makes the patient feel confident that needs will be met and complications prevented.
Use a calm, reassuring manner with the patient.	Gives the patient a sense of well-being.
Stay with patient as possible and allow family to visit.	Provides emotional support and promotes a sense of comfort.
Encourage the patient to communicate fears and concerns about the tracheostomy/laryngectomy tube and the inability to talk.	Recognizing fears contributes to dealing with concerns.
Control multiple sources of stimuli, which could cause sensory overload.	Overstimulation can worsen anxiety.
Teach patient and family about the tracheostomy and the use of new communication techniques.	Knowledge decreases anxiety by giving the patient a sense of control.
Assist the patient with new strategies for communication and allow him or her to be a part of the decision regarding what type communication strategy to use.	The inability to communicate or the need to learn new communication techniques can cause frustrations that lead to anxiety.
Explore possible relaxation techniques and coping strategies, and teach as appropriate.	Use of relaxation techniques and coping strategies, especially those that have worked in the past, reduces anxiety and fear and enhances positive outcomes.

NIC *Anxiety reduction*
      Emotional support

Evaluation

Evaluate the extent to which the outcome criteria have been achieved. Physiological signs of anxiety, such as tachycardia, will be absent. The patient will verbalize a decrease in anxiety and fear. Restlessness and agitation will be alleviated. The patient reports that he or she is not frustrated with attempts at communication and that he or she has employed relaxation techniques.

Community/Home Care

The patient will need to have follow-up at home possibly regarding tracheostomy care, laryngectomy tube care, skin care, and communication. Oftentimes the patient is anxious because of a perceived lack of knowledge regarding the tracheosotmy/laryngectomy tube or stoma and also about the reaction of others to his or her changed appearance. If the patient remains anxious due to fear of alterations in respiratory status and the presence of an alteration in outward appearance, the patient will need to practice relaxation techniques that can reduce anxiety. Nurses should assess which coping mechanisms work for the patient and encourage their use by the patient at home. The relationship between anxiety and increasing oxygen demands should be explained to the patient, so that he or she can understand the importance of controlling fears and anxiety. Anxiety may be reduced for the patient and family by encouraging participation in support groups. The patient should feel comfortable with knowledge of how to handle emergencies should they arise.

Documentation

The degree to which the patient has decreased anxiety should be documented in the patient record. A rating system provides an objective way to relay to others the extent of the anxiety. Document whether the patient is able to verbalize a feeling of decreased anxiety and whether there are outward signs of anxiety. Include in the documentation what specific events seem to contribute to anxiety episodes and what strategies are employed to relieve or reduce it. Blood pressure and pulse rates should be documented as anxiety often causes an increase in both vital signs.

NURSING DIAGNOSIS 6

 DISTURBED BODY IMAGE

Related to:

  Physical disfigurement post-surgery

  Loss of voice

Defining Characteristics:

  Withdrawal

  Social isolation

  Depression

  Negative statements about physical appearance

  Attempts to cover stoma, tracheostomy/laryngectomy tube when visitors are present

Goal:

  The patient accepts the change in physical appearance and continues social activities and interpersonal relationships.

Outcome Criteria

✔ The patient states a willingness to look at and touch surgical site.

✔ The patient learns and participates in care of tracheostomy/laryngectomy tube.

✔ The patient verbalizes a satisfaction with body appearance.

NOC *Body image*

INTERVENTIONS	RATIONALES
Provide assurance that feelings are very normal post-operatively.	Stops the patient from thinking that his/her feelings are abnormal.
Allow the patient privacy when bathing, dressing, or at dressing changes.	Allows the patient time to adjust to appearance without concern for how others react.
Encourage patient to communicate feelings about changes in physical appearance.	Talking about the changes may sometimes be the beginning of acceptance.
Teach the patient methods to cover the tracheostomy, laryngectomy, or stoma in a tasteful, unobtrusive way with scarves or other clothing; recommend clothes that may cover the neck disfigurement, such as items with standup collars or turtlenecks.	Minimizes visibility of the site to others, which may make the patient more comfortable.
Teach the patient and family how to care for the laryngectomy tube, stoma, or tracheostomy.	If the patient is comfortable with self-care, that comfort level may translate into acceptance for the change in appearance and incorporation of body appearance change into a positive self-image.

INTERVENTIONS	RATIONALES
Teach the patient to do shoulder strengthening exercises three times a day.	Shoulder drop is one additional change in physical appearance that may occur; these exercises can improve shoulder drooping that occurs with radical neck dissection.
Monitor patient's feelings about self, interpersonal relationships with family members and friends, withdrawal, social isolation, fear, anxiety, embarrassment by appearance, fear appearance will frighten loved ones, desire to be alone.	Detects early alterations in social functioning; prevents unhealthy behaviors and allows early intervention through referral to counseling.
Encourage patient to participate in at least one outside/public activity each week once health status permits.	Prevents patient from isolating self from others.
Identify the effects of the patient's culture or religion on perception of body image.	A patient's culture and religion often help define his or her reactions to changes in body image and self-worth.
Identify community support groups, if available, such as laryngectomy club or lost cord club.	Discussions with other patients with a similar situation allows the patient an opportunity to share thoughts with and hear thoughts from those who understand what the patient is going through; provides the patient with support and the courage to move forward in terms of acceptance of the change.
Assist the patient in identifying coping devices/diversionary activities.	Provides diversionary activities so that not all thoughts are on disfigurement.
Arrange for psychosocial counseling.	Provides psychological assistance to the patient and psychosocial evaluation.
Allow the patient/family to grieve the loss of normal functioning; allow the patient/family time and privacy to do this.	It is appropriate to grieve for the loss of function of body parts that are vital to everyday life; supporting the family and patient will enhance healthy adaptation.

NIC   *Body image enhancement*
Emotional support

Support group
Socialization enhancement

Evaluation

The patient is able and willing to learn about the care of the tracheostomy, laryngectomy tube, or stoma site, and begin to participate in self-care. Time is required for the patient to assimilate the change in body appearance completely into his or her self-perception. It is crucial that the nurse evaluate to what degree the patient is beginning to do this. Look for behaviors such as touching the site, looking at the disfigurement in the mirror, or asking appropriate questions. Communication of feelings and concerns relevant to the change in appearance should be taken as a positive sign that progress towards meeting outcome criteria is being made.

Community/Home Care

At home, continued monitoring of the patient's perception of body image is needed. The nurse who visits will need to be alert to subtle hints that may indicate that the patient has not completely adapted to the change in body appearance. Ascertain that the patient is willing to care for the site appropriately in the home. The patient should look at the site and self in a mirror each day, which may assist the patient to assimilate the change into his or her body image and become accustomed to the change in appearance.

Open discussions regarding the change in appearance and interventions to prevent social isolation and withdrawal should continue with patient and family. Community support groups should be explored, as they provide a forum for expression of feelings with others who may have similar experiences. Encourage the family and the patient to attend social activities initially with close friends or other relatives with whom the patient feels most comfortable.

Documentation

Chart any specific behaviors or verbalizations that may indicate an altered body image. Include all interventions that have been employed to address this issue and the patient's response. Note when and if the patient begins to ask questions and participate in care. All referrals should be documented in the patient record.

NURSING DIAGNOSIS 7

 DEFICIENT KNOWLEDGE

Related to:

Care of tracheostomy, laryngectomy tube, and stoma

Radical neck surgery

New communication methods

Defining Characteristics:

Many or no questions

Verbalizes a lack of knowledge/understanding

Unable to perform new procedures for care

Goal:

The patient or significant other will know how to perform tracheostomy, stoma, or laryngectomy tube care.

The patient will be able to communicate.

Outcome Criteria

✔ The patient indicates a desire to learn necessary information.

✔ The patient knows the purpose of the tracheostomy or laryngectomy tube.

✔ The patient and or family demonstrates proper care of laryngectomy tube, tracheostomy, or stoma.

✔ The patient expresses an understanding of the care required at home.

✔ The patient demonstrates an understanding of new communication techniques.

✔ The patient verbalizes an understanding of follow-up care required and expresses a willingness to comply.

NOC *Knowledge: Treatment procedures*
Knowledge: Infection control
Knowledge: Treatment regimen
Knowledge: Health resources

INTERVENTIONS	RATIONALES
Assess the patient's current knowledge and his or her ability to learn and readiness to learn.	The teacher needs to ascertain what the patient already knows and build on this; if the patient is not capable of learning or is not ready to learn, teaching will not be effective due to disinterest or inability to understand.
Start with the simplest information and move to complex information.	Patients can understand simple concepts easily and then can build on those to understand more complex concepts.
Teach patient and significant others: — Purpose of tracheostomy and laryngectomy tube — Tracheostomy and laryngectomy tube care: cleansing, replacing, and suctioning (demonstrate this to family and patient) — Prevention of infection by covering openings with stoma guard or other covering to prevent particles from entering respiratory system — Importance of avoiding swimming or immersion in any water — Need to cover stoma or tubes when coughing — Surgical incision skin care: keep clean and dry; inspect for drainage and redness — Shoulder strengthening exercises to prevent or stabilize shoulder drop — Interventions for emergencies — Signs and symptoms of complications that would indicate a need to seek health care — Proper storage of supplies	Knowledge of how to carry out tracheostomy care, care of laryngectomy tube, incisional care, and prevention of complications empowers the patient to take control and be compliant.
Provide rationales for performing each step in all skills taught.	Rationales for the steps increase understanding.
Allow adequate time for task mastery and have the patient or significant other demonstrate performance of tracheostomy care and suctioning as often as required for him or her to become comfortable with procedure, performing the skills one step at a time.	The person performing the care should feel comfortable performing the procedure before discharge to home, and the nurse needs to know that the patient can correctly perform this activity prior to discharge.
Teach patient and family measures to prevent infection: good handwashing, especially when working with tracheostomy or laryngectomy tube, stomas, or surgical site; avoidance of	The patient's first line of defense against organisms into the respiratory system is lost and vigilance is required to prevent respiratory infection.

INTERVENTIONS	RATIONALES
crowds, especially during flu season; adequate fluid intake; taking of flu and pneumonia vaccines; adequate balanced nutrition.	
Teach the patient and family when the patient should be suctioned and how to suction.	Most patients with a tracheostomy or laryngectomy tube occasionally have increased mucous secretions that require suctioning; knowledge empowers the patient and can decrease anxiety.
Teach the patient the importance of adequate nutrition, especially with patients experiencing difficulty swallowing.	At home, without monitoring by the nursing staff, the patient may experience alterations in nutrition or lose interest in food. Stressing the importance of nutrition to the family and the patient will increase the possibility that the patient will be compliant with requirements.
Teach administration of enteral feedings if ordered and have the patient and the family demonstrate the skill.	Because of the severity of the dissection, some patients may not be able to ingest enough food to meet the body's requirements and will go home with instructions to take food by mouth and supplements via tube feeding.
Assess the patient and family's understanding of all teaching by encouraging them to repeat information, demonstrate all skills, and ask questions as needed.	This allows the nurse to hear in the patient's own words what was taught and makes it easier to know what information may need to be reinforced.
Give the patient or family printed material that outlines the procedures and all information presented.	Printed materials can serve as a backup when the patient is at home and needs review or reinforcement.
Refer patient to home health nursing for follow-up and reinforcement of teaching once the patient is at home.	Once at home, the patient and family may have questions about the care of surgical site, laryngectomy tube, tracheostomy care, or suctioning that require reinforcement; the nurse also needs to be sure that procedures are being performed correctly.
Establish that the patient has all care supplies required to be compliant.	If needed resources such as supplies, finances, and transportation to follow-up appointments are not available, the patient cannot be compliant; the nurse will need to make necessary referrals.

NIC *Learning readiness enhancement*
Learning facilitation
Teaching: Psychomotor skill

Evaluation

Evaluate the degree to which the patient has achieved the outcome criteria relevant to the teaching sessions. The patient should verbalize an understanding of content presented by repeating the information. It is crucial that the patient or family demonstrate correct performance of all psychomotor skills, such as tracheostomy care, suctioning, care of a laryngectomy tube, care of incisions, and correct utilization of new communication techniques. The nurse must determine if the patient is capable of being compliant with the recommended regimen. If further teaching is required at time of discharge, the appropriate referrals should be made to continue education.

Community/Home Care

The patient will need to implement the medical regimen in the home setting over an extended period. The success of this implementation will be dependent upon the degree to which the patient has received adequate teaching and has subsequently understood and internalized it, and the patient's level of motivation to participate in self-care. Crucial to successful in-home care are the patient's and family's abilities to perform tracheostomy care, laryngectomy tube care, wound care, and activities relevant to nutrition, especially if the patient is to receive enteral feedings. Discuss with the patient and family correct storage and care of all supplies. A hard plastic storage box that closes tightly can be used. The boxes can be labeled according to skills, such as "Feeding Supplies," "Tracheostomy Care," or "Skin Care," etc. A home nurse should follow up with the family and patient to ensure that all procedures are carried out comfortably in the home; the nurse may actually want to plan to be present the first time a procedure is done. The nurse should also assess the patient's ability to communicate effectively using new techniques demonstrated by the speech therapist. Depression and withdrawal are common in patients who have had laryngectomies and neck dissections, and may not be noted until the patient is at home. These conditions may manifest themselves in the patient's refusal to learn self-care activities. Adequate teaching may make the family and/or patient comfortable with what is required and will give them some sense of control that may assist them to move from a state of grief and denial to one of self-sufficiency and hope.

Documentation

Document the specific content taught and the titles of any printed materials given to the patient. Include in the chart the patient's degree of understanding of the content and the methods used to teach and evaluate learning. Document the patient's ability to perform the psychomotor skills required for incisional care, stoma care, tracheostomy care, or laryngectomy tube care. Any areas that need to be reinforced should be documented to ensure appropriate follow-up. If family members are present for the teaching sessions, document this in the chart, and always document any referrals made. Include information regarding the patient's and family's feelings, concerns, and fears about performing care in the home.

CHAPTER 2.28

NEAR-DROWNING

GENERAL INFORMATION

Near-drowning occurs when a patient survives, at least initially, a prolonged period under water (or other fluid). It occurs when the patient cannot remain afloat because he or she cannot swim, is exhausted, is traumatized, panics, or has an acute medical emergency, such as a myocardial infarction or seizure. Near-drownings can be divided into three categories and two types. The three categories are dry drowning, wet drowning, and secondary drowning. The two types of near-drowning are sea water/saltwater and freshwater. Dry drowning occurs when laryngeal-tracheal spasm occurs, preventing water from entering the trachea. When this occurs, however, oxygen is also prevented from entering the trachea and lungs, resulting in cerebral anoxia, cerebral edema, and coma or death. It is difficult to identify dry drowning as, once the victim becomes unconscious, laryngeal-tracheal spasm will stop and water will enter the trachea and lungs. Wet drowning, the most commonly seen type of near-drowning, occurs when, during frantic respiratory efforts, water enters the trachea and lungs and prevents oxygen from crossing the alveolar-capillary cellular membrane. Secondary drowning occurs when, after the initial insult and resuscitation, pulmonary edema, or aspiration pneumonia occurs. Seawater contains salt and is a hypertonic solution. Because of seawater's osmotic pull, when seawater aspiration occurs fluid will be pulled into the lungs causing pulmonary edema. Because fluid is pulled from blood, hemoconcentration and hypovolemia will also occur. Freshwater is a hypotonic solution and is also usually not clean; for example, pool, lake, or pond water are forms of freshwater that contain chlorine, algae, and other debris. Initially, because of the hypotonicity of the water, fluid will readily cross the alveolar-capillary cellular membrane where it is readily absorbed, causing hypovolemia. Because the water is not clean, surfactant breakdown occurs, causing the alveolar walls to break down and the fluid to enter the lungs once again, resulting in pulmonary edema. Clinical manifestations include decreased level of consciousness, cyanosis, apnea, rapid respirations, tachycardia, pink frothy sputum (sign of pulmonary edema), hypotension, and hypothermia.

NURSING DIAGNOSIS 1

 IMPAIRED GAS EXCHANGE

Related to:

Tracheobronchial spasms

Aspiration of fluid

Breakdown of surfactant, which leads to increased arteriole-capillary membrane permeability

Pulmonary edema

Defining Characteristics:

Tachypnea

Rales, rhonchi, or wheezes

Pink, frothy sputum

Cyanosis

Goal:

The patient will have adequate gas exchange.

Outcome Criteria

✔ Spontaneous respirations return.

✔ Arterial blood gases will improve and return to normal.

✔ Respiratory rate returns to normal (12–24/minute).

✔ Pulmonary adventitious sounds decrease or are absent.

✔ Cyanosis or pallor is relieved.

NOC *Respiratory status: Ventilation*
Respiratory status: Gas exchange
Vital signs

INTERVENTIONS	RATIONALES
Assess airway and clear as needed.	Prevents aspiration and allows better oxygenation.
Perform respiratory assessment: lung sounds, respiratory rate, depth, and rhythm.	Establishes a baseline and allows monitoring of response to treatment; in near-drowning, crackles may be heard due to fluid in lungs, and bronchospasms cause wheezing.
Monitor results of oxygen saturation and arterial blood gases (ABGs).	Helps to evaluate respiratory status, specifically hypoxemia/oxygenation to tissues; use as a guide to determine the need for mechanical ventilation; also helps to assess metabolic states: acidosis can occur as the tissues engage in anaerobic metabolism, with subsequent acid end-products of metabolism.
Assess for signs and symptoms of hypoxemia, such as altered mental status: restlessness, decreased level of consciousness, increased respiratory rate, cyanosis.	Changes in mental status indicate decreased cerebral oxygenation, and increased respiratory rate indicates the body's attempt to compensate; cyanosis indicates lack of oxygen to tissues.
Administer high-flow oxygen, as ordered, to maintain oxygen saturation at > 90 percent.	Maximizes oxygenation and decreases hypoxia.
Monitor diagnostic study results: chest x-ray.	Chest x-ray will show the presence of infiltrates.
Assess for signs of worsening respiratory function (pulmonary edema and acute respiratory distress), such as excessive fluid in lungs on auscultation, pink frothy sputum, labored rapid respirations, stridor, nasal flaring, and use of accessory muscles for breathing.	These indicate a lack of response to first-line interventions and the need for mechanical ventilation.
Anticipate the need for ventilatory assistance, as ordered.	Helps to improve breathing and ventilation. A bag-valve-mask device and/or intubation and a mechanical ventilator are possible methods.
Suction secretions only as needed.	Helps to maintain clear airway and provide maximum oxygenation; however, suctioning can cause an increase in intracranial pressure.
Give packed red blood cells, as ordered.	Increases oxygen-carrying capacity of the blood.
Administer antibiotics, as ordered.	Reduces effects of pulmonary contamination, especially with freshwater.
Give bronchodilators, as ordered.	Helps to treat bronchospasms.

NIC *Oxygen therapy*
Respiratory monitoring
Airway management

Evaluation

Examine the degree to which the outcome criteria have been achieved. The patient should have arterial blood gases (ABGs) that are returning to normal and oxygen saturation readings > 90 percent. The patient's lungs should be clear to auscultation and no signs or symptoms of pulmonary edema or hypoxemia should be present. The respiratory rate should be at the patient's baseline (12–24). All assessments and diagnostic studies should indicate an improvement in respiratory status.

Community/Home Care

For patients who have experienced a near-drowning, information on primary prevention should be discussed. The patient, once recovered, should be given instructions on signs and symptoms that would indicate complications, such as the development of pneumonia or respiratory distress once at home. If the patient is not being hospitalized except for observation, he or she should know that some effects may not be apparent until 24–48 hours after the event, and may include neurological deficits. Teaching should include the specific signs and symptoms that would indicate a need for seeking health care. For the more acutely ill patient who experienced more serious effects from the near-drowning, the neurological damage may be permanent, and once at home the patient may require assistance from a personal care assistant and a visiting nurse. Assisting the family to make decisions regarding long-term care if home care is not feasible should be coordinated with a multidisciplinary team. The family may also need assistance with coping strategies due to the sudden change in health status of the patient.

Documentation

Document the findings from a comprehensive respiratory assessment with particular attention to indicators of the status of the patient's ability to maintain adequate gas exchange. Chart all interventions implemented and the patient's specific response. Include in the documentation whether the patient has met the outcome criteria with specific behaviors such as respiratory rate, oxygen saturation, and effort of breathing. If the patient is not improving, document the specific problems that continue and how the plan of care has been revised. Chart the results of specific monitoring activities, such as continuous oxygen saturation or blood pressures, according to agency protocol.

NURSING DIAGNOSIS 2

 ## FLUID VOLUME EXCESS

Related to:

Fluid aspiration

Fluid shift into the alveoli (saltwater)

Pulmonary edema

Absorption of water into circulating volume (freshwater)

Defining Characteristics:

Pulmonary rales, rhonchi

Pink, frothy sputum

Tachycardia

Increased hematocrit, decreased hemoglobin (due to shift of fluid from vascular space to pleural tissue)

Increased pulmonary artery wedge pressure, central venous pressure

Congestion on chest x-ray

Tachypnea

Electrolyte imbalance

Goal:

Fluid volume excess is decreased.

Outcome Criteria

✔ The patient's breath sounds will be clear.

✔ The patient will have no distended neck veins.

✔ Sputum will no longer be frothy.

✔ The patient will have a respiratory rate at baseline (12–24).

NOC *Fluid balance*
Electrolyte and acid/base balance
Fluid overload severity

INTERVENTIONS	RATIONALES
Assess fluid status: breath sounds, presence of jugular vein distention, urine output, color of urine, sputum color, and consistency.	Helps to assess severity of fluid excess: rales indicate pulmonary congestion, frothy sputum represents pulmonary edema, jugular vein distention indicates vascular overload, concentrated urine indicates loss of circulating volume as is seen when fluid shifts from vascular space to pleural tissue.
Assess vital signs, especially blood pressure and respiratory rate.	Freshwater aspiration causes hypovolemia and subsequent elevated blood pressures; saltwater aspiration causes hypervolemia and subsequent decreases in blood pressures; fluid in the lungs can cause increased work of breathing and an increased rate as the lungs attempt to maintain gas exchange.
Monitor serum electrolytes and osmolality.	In saltwater aspiration, serum sodium and chloride may be high; osmolality is increased; in freshwater, aspiration electrolytes and osmolality may be reduced.
Monitor hematocrit.	Elevated hematocrit will be seen in hypovolemia, as is seen in saltwater near drowning, and will be decreased in hypervolemia seen with freshwater near-drowning.
Establish intravenous access.	Provides a method of delivering medications and fluids if needed.

(continues)

(continued)

INTERVENTIONS	RATIONALES
Give intravenous fluids and electrolytes as ordered.	Corrects fluid volume shift and electrolyte imbalances.
Administer oxygen, as ordered.	Improves oxygenation and pulmonary function.
Assist with the placement of hemodynamic monitoring lines and monitor central venous pressure and pulmonary wedge pressure according to agency protocol.	These measures give accurate information on fluid status and effects on cardiac output.
Administer diuretics, as ordered (possibly Lasix).	Inhibits the reabsorption of sodium and chloride, thereby causing an increased fluid output by the kidneys, decreasing excess fluid in lungs.
If the patient is able to take fluids or food by mouth, give low sodium substances.	Sodium increases fluid retention.
Assure accurate intake and careful monitoring of output, especially if the patient has pulmonary edema.	Helps to monitor fluid balance between fluid consumed or administered and urinary output.

NIC *Fluid management*
      Electrolyte monitoring

Evaluation

The patient should have achieved the stated outcome criteria. Evaluate fluid status by assessing for breath sounds that are clear or improving. If sputum is present, it should be of normal color and consistency. Serum electrolytes and osmolality return to normal or show improvement. Dyspnea secondary to fluid congestion in lungs should be relieved with a respiratory rate between 12–24. Blood pressure should return to baseline.

Community/Home Care

When the patient is at home following a near-drowning, fluid status has usually been satisfactorily resolved, and in the absence of underlying disease additional problems may not occur. However, some effects of near-drowning may occur up to 48 hours later in the patient who never lost consciousness and was only kept for observation for 24 hours. The patient should be educated about signs and symptoms of fluid overload, such as increasing shortness of breath, a congested cough, production of pink frothy sputum, and an increased respiratory rate. Follow-up with a health care provider should be sought if these occur.

Documentation

Document all assessment findings, particularly those that indicate fluid status: breath sounds, jugular vein distention, or changes in blood pressure. Chart interventions initiated and the patient's response to them that would indicate achievement of outcome criteria. Include in the chart vital signs and readings from other monitoring according to agency policy. If the patient's fluid status has not improved, document the specific patient assessments noted and how the plan is revised. Intake and output should be recorded. Any teaching done with patient and family should be documented.

NURSING DIAGNOSIS 3

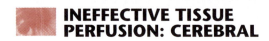 **INEFFECTIVE TISSUE PERFUSION: CEREBRAL**

Related to:
    Decreased cardiac output
    Hypoxemia
    Increased intracranial pressure
    Cerebral edema

Defining Characteristics:
    Decreased level of consciousness
    Agitation, restlessness
    Diminished cranial nerve reaction
    Dilated, sluggish, or nonresponsive pupil(s)

Goal:
    The patient's cerebral tissue perfusion improves.

Outcome Criteria

✔ Level of consciousness improves (the patient is alert).

✔ The patient's score on the Glasgow Coma Scale improves.

✔ The patient is not agitated or restless.

NOC *Cognition*
      Neurological status: Cerebral
      Neurological status: Consciousness

INTERVENTIONS	RATIONALES
Assess neurological status every hour according to agency guidelines or through use of the Glasgow Coma Scale.	Establishes a baseline and allows monitoring of response to therapy.
Monitor for increased intracranial pressure (ICP) via nursing assessments (change in LOC, vital signs, pupillary changes) or an intracranial pressure monitor.	A change in level of consciousness is an early indication of increasing ICP; increased systolic blood pressure and pulse pressure and bradycardia are late indications. Increased ICP may indicate cerebral edema and cerebral hypoxia.
Administer high-flow oxygen, as ordered.	Maintains adequate oxygenation.
Administer osmotic diuretics, as ordered (mannitol).	Relieves cerebral edema and decreases intracranial pressure.
Elevate head of bed 30 degrees and keep head in neutral position.	Decreases intracranial pressure and promotes drainage of cerebral fluid.
Administer sedatives cautiously, as ordered.	Reduces anxiety, retching, and Valsalva, all of which increase intracranial pressure but may mask signs and symptoms of neurological problems.
Assist as ordered or allowed with barbiturate coma.	Decreases cerebral metabolic needs and ICP, and prevents neurological damage.
Anticipate administration of anticonvulsants.	Prevents seizures. Seizures cause tremendous increases in intracranial pressure.
Administer corticosteroids as ordered.	Reduces cerebral edema and intracranial pressure.

NIC *Cerebral perfusion promotion*
      Neurologic monitoring

Evaluation

An evaluation of the patient in relation to cerebral tissue perfusion examines the accomplishment of the outcome criteria. The patient should demonstrate an amelioration of neurological status, as demonstrated by improved level of consciousness. The Glasgow Coma Scale score should demonstrate an improvement and vital signs should return to normal. Intracranial pressure should be decreasing or return to normal.

Community/Home Care

Alterations in cerebral tissue perfusion should be resolved prior to discharge to home. If alterations continue that may indicate permanent changes in cerebral function, the patient may need extended care in another facility after the acute episode is resolved. Referrals to appropriate disciplines, such as social work for placement, are appropriate, and a holistic approach to assisting the family to cope with a significant change in health status of the patient is required. For the patient who goes home, in-home care is individualistic according to the deficits present. The family will need assistance in identifying what the home care needs or services may be and developing a plan of action in conjunction with nursing or other disciplines.

Documentation

Chart a thorough neurological assessment of the patient, including signs and symptoms of increased ICP, readings from the ICP monitor (if used), and the results of the Glasgow Coma Scale. Document interventions and the patient's specific response to them. If emergency interventions are required for occurrences such as onset of seizures or deterioration in neurological status, document precisely a description of the occurrence and the nursing interventions employed. Be specific about the patient's achievement of the stated outcome criteria in the patient's chart.

NURSING DIAGNOSIS 4

 DECREASED CARDIAC OUTPUT

Related to:
   Fluid shift into lungs, which leads to decreased circulating volume
   Hypoxemia
   Dysrhythmias secondary to hypothermia

Defining Characteristics:
   Tachycardia
   Hypothermia

Cool, clammy cyanotic skin

Hypotension

Weak, thready pulse

Decreased peripheral pulses

Goal:

The patient exhibits improved cardiac output.

Outcome Criteria

✔ The pulse rate is < 100 but > 60.

✔ Blood pressure is at patient's baseline.

✔ No dysrhythmias are noted.

✔ Skin color returns to baseline.

✔ Urine output will be > 30 ml/hour.

NOC *Cardiac pump effectiveness*
Circulation status
Respiratory status: Gas exchange
Tissue perfusion: Cerebral
Tissue perfusion: Peripheral
Vital signs
Medication response

INTERVENTIONS	RATIONALES
Monitor for tachycardia, dysrhythmias, abnormal heart sounds (murmur, S_3, S_4), and blood pressure.	Assessment of cardiac status gives early clues to cardiac status and response to interventions and establishes the patient's baseline.
Assess for signs of heart failure (cyanosis, jugular venous distention, dependent edema, cool and pale extremities, diminished peripheral pulses, capillary refill > 2 seconds, dyspnea on exertion).	Helps to detect severity of cardiac alterations and progression; as the ventricles lose ability to pump, pulmonary congestion and peripheral blood flow becomes worse.
Monitor temperature frequently.	Allows for baseline readings and for monitoring of response to interventions to correct hypothermia.
Assess for changes in mental status (confusion, restlessness, agitation).	These indicate decreased cerebral tissue perfusion.
Assess arterial blood gas (ABG) results and oxygen saturation level.	These are measures of the ability of the heart to perfuse tissues with oxygenated blood.
Administer supplemental oxygen, as ordered, based on results of ABGs and oxygen saturation.	Maximizes amount of oxygen available for gas exchange, assists to alleviate signs of hypoxia, and decreases workload of myocardium.
Monitor results of any ordered diagnostic tests such as EKG, echocardiogram, and chest x-ray.	These tests reveal definitive diagnosis and aid in monitoring response to interventions (EKG will show any dysrhythmias, echocardiogram will show chamber size and thickness as well as systolic and diastolic function, chest x-ray will show any pulmonary congestion).
Monitor urine output.	Decreased urine output < 30 ml/hour may indicate decreased tissue perfusion to the kidneys.
Assess skin for color and temperature.	Establishes a baseline and helps to monitor response to therapy; pale, cool skin indicates decreased perfusion.
Initiate measures to rewarm patient, such as warmed intravenous fluids, warm humidified oxygen, placing a covering on head, and rewarming blankets (see nursing care plan "Hypothermia").	To correct an underlying cause of altered cardiac function, core body temperature may be significantly reduced following immersion in cold water; covering the head prevents heat loss from the body. Be cautious with peripheral rewarming, which can cause vasodilation and further loss of volume from circulation, adding to the decreased cardiac output.
Administer inotropic agents—cardiac glycosides (digoxin)—as ordered.	Inotropic agents increase the force of myocardial contractility, resulting in increased cardiac output.
Treat metabolic and respiratory acidosis with sodium bicarbonate, as ordered.	Decreases respiratory effort required to correct acidosis naturally and to decrease the oxygen demand on the myocardium.
Assist with monitoring of cardiac output by examining CVP, pulmonary capillary wedge pressure, etc., as ordered.	These invasive measurements give a more accurate measurement of cardiac output.
Monitor serum electrolytes, BUN, Digoxin levels, liver enzymes, as ordered.	These tests may be abnormal because of the near-drowning or as an effect of medication regimens.

NIC   *Cardiac care acute*
        Oxygen thearpy
        Vital signs monitoring
        Medication management

Evaluation

The patient has no signs of decreased cardiac output. Breath sounds are clear and urinary output has been maintained at or above 30 ml/hour. The patient's pulse and blood pressure have returned to baseline/normal. Dysrhythmias have been resolved, and the patient's core temperature has returned to normal. Assessment reveals that the patient has been able to reestablish adequate perfusion also evidenced through warm, dry skin that is normal in color for the patient.

Community/Home Care

The patient who has decreased cardiac output secondary to near-drowning should have this corrected prior to discharge. At home, the patient may initially need to make adaptations in lifestyle to accommodate temporary changes in health status that may impact work, social activities, and self-care ability. Because of the fatigue that often follows critical illnesses, strategies for energy conservation should be discussed with the patient who experienced decreased cardiac output. If symptoms of decreased cardiac output persist following discharge, the patient will need referral for follow-up care and may require an in-home nurse to monitor pulse and blood pressure.

Documentation

Chart the status of achievement of outcomes with specific patient behaviors. Include pulse, blood pressure, oxygenation saturation, heart sounds, and breath sounds. Document all indicators of cardiac output and tissue perfusion. Include in the chart the interventions employed and the patient's response to the interventions. Rhythm strips from cardiac monitoring should be included in the chart to indicate resolution of any dysrhythmias. Be sure to include results of frequent temperature monitoring and information from invasive hemodynamic monitoring.

CHAPTER 2.29

PNEUMONIA

GENERAL INFORMATION

Pneumonia is a disease process involving inflammation of lung tissue. Pulmonary inflammation caused by bacteria, viruses, fungus, or parasites is classified as infectious pneumonia. Infectious pneumonia typically results when microorganisms enter the normally sterile lungs from the nasopharynx and produce inflammation of the lung parenchymam. Because of the inflammation, the alveoli fill with fluid or mucous, and gas exchange cannot take place at a the alveolar-capillary-cellular membrane level. Microorganisms can also enter the lungs from the bloodstream in septicemia, from infected lymph, or from infected pleural fluid. Pulmonary inflammation caused by aspiration of gastric contents, inhalation of toxic gases, or radiation therapy is classified as noninfectious pneumonia. Noninfectious pneumonia commonly evolves into infectious pneumonia as bacteria colonize the inflamed pulmonary tissue. People are more susceptible to pneumonia when they are debilitated, have a long history of smoking, have primary cardiovascular or pulmonary conditions, are diabetics, are immunosuppressed, aspirate gastric contents, have a foreign body in the airway, or experience rapid changes in environmental temperatures. Pneumonia is classified as hospital-acquired (HAP) or community-acquired (CAP). Streptococcus pneumoniae, a gram-positive organism, is the most common form of CAP. Gram-negative bacteria account for approximately 80 percent of HAP cases, with *Pseudomonas aeruginosa* being the most common causative agent. Clinical manifestations have a rapid onset and vary to some extent depending upon the type of pneumonia, but generally include fever, shaking chills, cough with production of rust-colored or purulent sputum, pleuritic chest pain, rales/crackles on auscultation, and diminished breath sounds. Pneumonia is the sixth leading cause of death in the United States, accounting for approximately 90,000 deaths (Lewis, Heitkemper, and Dirksen, 2004). This care plan addresses the patient who is experiencing a microbial pneumonia (bacterial, viral, or fungal).

NURSING DIAGNOSIS 1

IMPAIRED GAS EXCHANGE

Related to:

Pneumonia/inflamed lung tissue

Presence of fluid and mucous in lungs

Invasion of host by infecting organisms

Consolidation of mucous/fluid in specific lung lobes preventing transfer of gases across the alveolar-capillary-cellular membrane

Defining Characteristics:

Fever

Diminished breath sounds

Severe dyspnea

Tachypnea

Crackles/wheezes

Difficulty in raising secretions

Decreased oxygen saturation

Abnormal blood gases

Goal:

Infection will be resolved, and the patient will have adequate gas exchange.

Outcome Criteria

✔ The patient will have clear breath sounds.

✔ The patient will be afebrile.

✔ The patient will have no purulent sputum.

✔ The patient will not experience dyspnea.
✔ Respiratory rate will be < 28.
✔ Oxygen saturation will be > 94 percent.
✔ Arterial blood gases (ABGs) will return to baseline.

NOC *Respiratory status: Airway patency*
Respiratory status: Ventilation
Respiratory status: Gas exchange
Infection severity

INTERVENTIONS	RATIONALES
Perform a complete respiratory assessment: respiratory rate, rhythm, chest expansion, ease of breathing, use of accessory muscles, pursed lip breathing, breath sounds, mucous expectoration (thick secretions, purulent, blood tinged, foul smelling), perioral cyanosis, tachypnea, dyspnea, pulse oximetry; and monitor laboratory and diagnostic tests such as sputum cultures, complete blood cell count, arterial blood gases (ABGs), and chest x-rays.	Because of airway inflammation and mucus accumulation, pneumonia can cause fluid in the lungs and increase the work of breathing, resulting in impaired gas exchange. These assessments provide data to use for planning interventions and assessing progress. Sputum cultures identify the causative organisms; arterial blood gases (ABGs) demonstrate decreased oxygen concentration and in the absence of chronic lung disease, respiratory alkalosis is present; CBC shows elevated white blood cells; chest x-ray will confirm the presence of fluid in lungs or areas of consolidation.
Obtain subjective data from patient or significant other, including history of recurrent respiratory infection, history of chronic respiratory disease, and history of smoking.	Knowledge of the patient's respiratory health status contributes to information that can assist in determining other factors that may have contributed to the pneumonia or influence its treatment.
Assist patient to semi-Fowler's or Fowler's position.	Sitting upright allows the diaphragm to descend, resulting in easier breathing.
Administer oxygen as ordered or as indicated by arterial blood gases (ABGs).	Pneumonia causes increased mucous production and fluid retention in lungs, which decrease adequate gas exchange; supplemental oxygen provides additional oxygen for tissue oxygenation.
Administer antibiotics, as ordered, and monitor for side effects. Initially, broad spectrum antibiotics are ordered until results of sputum cultures are available. Common antibiotics include *Streptococcus pneumoniae:* azithromycin, penicillin G, doxycycline, clarithromycin; *Staphylococcus aureus:* nafcillin, vancomycin; *Pseudomonas aeruginosa:* Cipro, Levaquin.	Helps to stop the proliferation of microorganisms; the most common side effects include GI upset (nausea, vomiting, diarrhea) and allergic reaction (urticaria, rash).
Take temperature every 4 hours or as ordered.	Infectious processes cause an increase in temperature.
Administer antipyretics (Tylenol) as ordered.	Helps to reduce temperature.
Provide comfort measures: change linens and clothing as needed.	Following temperature spikes and chills, linens and clothing may become saturated due to perspiration.
Encourage adequate fluid intake to 2000 cc per day.	Helps to thin and liquefy secretions.
Administer mucolytics, as ordered.	Decreases mucus viscosity.
Administer bronchodilators, as ordered.	Dilates airways, enhancing the ability to exchange gases and to facilitate mucus mobilization.
Provide chest physiotherapy: postural drainage, chest percussion, and vibration, or assist respiratory therapist as required.	Loosens mucus plugs thus increasing area available for gas exchange.
Encourage coughing and deep breathing with mucus expectoration.	Coughing and deep breathing cause alveoli to open and loosen mucous to help clear the airways.
Assess mucus amount, color, and consistency.	Helps to detect improving status of pneumonia; amount should be decreasing and viscosity should be thinning following interventions; green, brown, or purulent mucus indicate continued presence of pneumonia.

NIC *Respiratory monitoring*
Airway management
Temperature regulation
Vital signs monitoring
Chest physiotherapy
Fever treatment

Evaluation

Evaluate the extent to which the outcome criteria have been met. The patient has bilaterally equal, clear breath sounds. Oxygen saturation is > 90 percent and arterial blood gases (ABGs) indicate adequate gas exchange. Mucous expectoration decreases and color returns to normal. The patient is experiencing no shortness of breath, and respiratory rate returns to the patient's baseline.

Community/Home Care

For the patient with pneumonia, care continues in the home following discharge from the hospital. At home, interventions are focused on continuing improvement in respiratory status and complete alleviation of infection. If expectoration of mucous is persistent, the patient should create a wastebasket at home with a paper or plastic bag liner (grocery bags can be used) specifically for disposal of soiled tissues to limit spread of organisms to other members in the household. Even at home, the patient should practice good hand hygiene, washing the hands frequently while applying friction. The patient needs to continue with intake of fluids to keep secretions thin and easily expectorated. Placing water bottles close to the patient will increase the likelihood that the patient will drink freely and achieve the goal of at least 2000 ml per day. Water is the best liquid, but if the patient desires, liquids such as ginger ale, apple juice, and lemonade may also be used. Nutrition consisting of foods rich in vitamin C, iron, and protein is needed for healing and recovery, but especially for energy. Even though the patient may feel well, normal household activities may produce shortness of breath and fatigue. The patient will need to schedule periods of rest throughout the day (see nursing diagnosis "Activity Intolerance"). It should be stressed to the patient that antibiotics should be taken until gone to ensure that the infection is satisfactorily eradicated. Although the patient may welcome visitors, caution should be taken as visitors who mean well could be a new source of infection. Precautions with visitors include avoiding anyone who is coughing, avoiding people with young children—especially those in day care, and refraining from shaking hands. Although home visits may not be required if the patient has support persons at home, follow-up is needed to assess the patient's respiratory status.

Documentation

Chart the findings from a thorough respiratory assessment, including breath sounds, pulse oximetry, mucous amount, color and consistency, respiratory rate and rhythm, use of accessory muscles, and any complaints offered by the patient. Include in the chart all interventions employed to treat the respiratory problems and note the patient's response to interventions. Document the patient's temperature, and if elevated, chart medications given to treat the fever and a follow-up temperature. Chart any changes to the plan of care in response to new data, such as pulse oximetry or blood gas results. Even though respiratory therapists (RT) chart their interventions, the nurse should include in the patient record the visit by the therapist and any observations noted following therapies carried out by RT, such as increased mucous production or coughing.

NURSING DIAGNOSIS 2

ACTIVITY INTOLERANCE

Related to:
  Actual respiratory infection
  Hypoxia
  Decreased pO_2
  Increased oxygen demands with activity

Defining Characteristics:
  Shortness of breath during activities
  Inability to perform physical activity
  Complaints of fatigue

Goal:
  The patient is able to tolerate activities.

Outcome Criteria

✔ The patient is able to perform activities of daily living without shortness of breath.

✔ The patient states that he or she is comfortable with activity performance.

✔ The patient states that shortness of breath is improved following cessation of activity, and the patient's respiratory rate returns to baseline within 5 minutes.

NOC *Activity tolerance*
Energy conservation
Endurance

INTERVENTIONS	RATIONALES
Obtain subjective data from patient regarding normal activities prior to onset of pneumonia; monitor for labored breathing, fatigue, and exhaustion.	Helps to determine the effect pneumonia is having on the patient's ability to be active.
Reduce level of activity as required in response to shortness of breath.	If increased physical activity causes wheezing or shortness of breath, activity should be reduced until oxygenation is adequate.
Assist with activities as needed.	Conserves energy and reduces oxygen demand; patients with pneumonia lack enough oxygen reserves to perform activities independently.
Pace activities and encourage periods of rest and activity during the day.	Conserves oxygen.
Monitor vital signs and oxygen saturation before and after activity.	Use the results to indicate when activity may be increased or decreased.
Gradually increase activity as tolerated and share guidelines for progression with patient.	Activities should be increased gradually, as tolerated, to avoid overtaxing the patient.
Discuss with the patient activities that would be appropriate once at home that would be within patient's activity tolerance.	Physical activity increases endurance and stamina; following pulmonary infection, return to normal activity level may take time.
Have the patient use oxygen immediately prior to activity in the acute setting.	Improves oxygenation and provides for oxygen reserves to be used with increased demand.
Inform the patient to stop any activity that produces shortness of breath or wheezing.	These indicate an intolerance to activity, and the level of activity should be evaluated.
Encourage intake of foods high in iron and that are good sources of energy (protein).	Iron has a role in oxygen transport and increases energy level.

NIC *Activity therapy*
Energy management

Evaluation

Evaluate whether the patient has achieved the stated desired outcomes. The patient verbalizes that he or she is able to carry out desired activities without wheezing or severe shortness of breath. After engaging in activity, the patient's pulse, blood pressure, and respirations return to baseline values following rest. Pulse oximetry readings reveal an oxygen saturation of > 90 percent following rest.

Community/Home Care

Ensure that patient has all of his or her questions answered related to activities allowed and how to increase endurance. The patient who has had pneumonia and experienced shortness of breath may be hesitant to engage in any activities for fear of becoming short of breath. It is important that the patient know how to adjust activities and understand that activity has a role in increasing endurance and stamina. Even though the patient may not require the services of a visiting nurse, follow-up visits with a health care provider are needed. During these visits, the patient should be questioned regarding activity performance and tolerance. It is anticipated that in the absence of chronic lung disease, activity intolerance will be a short-term problem that completely resolves with time.

Documentation

The nurse should chart the patient's tolerance for activity to include vital signs and presence/absence of wheezing or shortness of breath in response to activity. Oxygen saturation following activity should be assessed and documented. Document types of activities the patient is able to perform and duration of the activity. Include in the patient's chart all interventions employed to address the problem and whether the patient has achieved the specific outcome criteria. If the criteria have not been met, document what progress has been made and any revisions made to the plan of care.

NURSING DIAGNOSIS 3

 ACUTE PAIN

Related to:

Inflammation of lung tissue

Pulmonary infection

Episodes of coughing

Defining Characteristics:

Complaint of pleuritic chest pain (especially on inspiration)

Tachypnea

Goal:

Pain control is achieved.

Outcome Criteria

✔ The patient will verbalize that pain is relieved.

NOC *Pain level*

Pain control

Comfort level

Medication response

INTERVENTIONS	RATIONALES
Assess pain status to determine precipitating factors, location, and intensity.	Helps to determine the cause of pain and to determine treatment required.
Have patient rate pain intensity using a pain rating scale.	Gives a more objective assessment of the pain intensity.
Administer mild analgesics, as ordered.	Provides pain relief; pain increases the need for oxygen.
Refrain from giving cough suppressants unless at bedtime.	Even though some pain may be caused by frequent coughing, cough suppressants are given sparingly because they eliminate the ability to mobilize and expectorate secretions; they may be given at bedtime to promote rest.
Establish a quiet environment.	Enhances the effects of analgesics; decreases oxygen demands.
Elevate head of bed.	Improves chest expansion and oxygenation.
Use non-pharmacological measures to reduce pain, such as relaxation techniques, distraction techniques such as guided imagery, and splinting chest when coughing.	Enhances effects of pharmacological interventions.
Assess effectiveness of interventions to relieve pain.	Helps to determine whether interventions have been effective in relieving pain or whether new strategies need be to employed.

NIC *Pain management*

Analgesic administration

Evaluation

The patient is able to report that the pain has been relieved or alleviated following interventions. The degree to which the patient is able to assist in the management of the pain through non-pharmacological measures such as relaxation techniques is assessed.

Community/Home Care

Once the pneumonia has been resolved and coughing decreases, the pain should be alleviated. If the patient has had severe coughing episodes, the chest area may be sore at time of discharge, but again this should subside in a short period of time. Home care required for this problem should be minimal and would consist of mild analgesic medications and rest as needed. It is important that the patient at home understand clearly the importance of reporting any severe pleuritic pain to a health care provider, as this may signal a new problem.

Documentation

Document in the patient's own words the description of the pain and their rating of the level of pain using a pain assessment tool. Chart all interventions employed for the relief of pain and the patient's response. If pain persists, document this in the chart along with indications of revisions to the planned interventions. Include in the documentation assessments made relevant to the respiratory system.

NURSING DIAGNOSIS 4

 DEFICIENT KNOWLEDGE

Related to:

Lack of information about pneumonia and treatment

Defining Characteristics:

  Ask no questions

  No prior experience with pneumonia

  Ask many questions

  Is noncompliant

Goal:

  The patient and family members will verbalize understanding of the disease and treatment.

Outcome Criteria

✔ The patient will verbalize a willingness to comply with the treatment regimen.

✔ The patient will verbalize an understanding of antibiotic therapy.

✔ The patient will verbalize an understanding of the need for increased fluid intake.

✔ The patient will indicate a willingness to obtain pneumonia vaccine.

NOC *Knowledge: Disease process*
      Knowledge: Health behavior
      Treatment behavior: Illness
          or injury

INTERVENTIONS	RATIONALES
Assess the readiness of the patient to learn (motivation, cognitive level physiological status).	The patient must be motivated to learn, have the capability to learn the content, and be free of distractions from learning, such as pain, shortness of breath, and emotional distress.
Assess what the patient already knows.	The patient may have some knowledge about pneumonia, and teaching should begin with what the patient already knows.
Create an environment conducive to learning.	Environmental noise can prevent the learner from focusing on the content being taught.
Teach incrementally from simple to complex.	The patient and family members will learn and retain knowledge better when information is presented in small segments.
Teach the learners: — Pathophysiology of pneumonia — Importance of maintaining adequate fluid intake	When the patient and family members understand the disease process and treatment, improved disease

(2000–3000 cc per day) to liquefy secretions — Need to take all of prescribed antibiotics — How to protect oneself from infection from others (avoid crowds and children with colds, refrain from shaking hands, limit visitors) — Role of nutrition in recovery — Proper disposal of used tissues — Follow-up care	control occurs, complications decrease, and hospital stay and repeat hospitalizations are reduced.
Assess compliance with prescribed treatment regimen.	With knowledge and understanding, compliance should increase.
Evaluate the patient's understanding of the content covered by asking questions.	Identifies areas that require more teaching and ensures that the patient has enough information to ensure compliance.
Give the patient written information.	Provides reference at a later time.

NIC *Teaching: Disease process*
      Discharge planning
      Teaching: Individual

Evaluation

The patient is able to repeat all information for the nurse and asks questions about pneumonia and possible outcomes. The patient verbalizes a willingness to comply with treatment regimen during hospitalization or at home, especially antibiotic therapy and fluid intake. The patient and family members are able to identify reportable signs and symptoms that would result in early intervention.

Community/Home Care

For the patient with uncomplicated pneumonia, the hospital stay is short, which dictates that knowledge deficits are addressed early. A majority of patients who have had pneumonia will not require further education or follow-up in the home. The most critical aspect of in-home care is continuing antibiotic therapy until all medication has been consumed. Once at home and feeling better, the patient may be inclined to stop taking antibiotics. A schedule can be developed in collaboration with the patient listing the remaining doses so that the patient can simply cross them out when taken. This documentation can be brought back to the health care provider at time of follow-up. The patient may need reinforcement from family members or significant others regarding avoidance of crowds, limitation of visitors, and hand hygiene, as well as the feasibility of obtaining a pneumonia vaccine. Prior to discharge, health care workers can determine that the patient understands the role of nutrition and fluid intake in the continued recovery from pneumonia. The effectiveness of teaching in this area will be determined when the patient returns for follow-up appointments to assess respiratory status.

Documentation

Document all content taught and the patient's verbalization of understanding. Attend to documentation of any specific concerns that the patient or family members express. Include in the documentation the patient's willingness to comply with all recommendations made regarding fluid intake, nutrition, hand hygiene, pneumonia vaccine, and antibiotic therapy. Clearly indicate in the record any area that requires further teaching. Always include the names of printed literature given to the patient.

CHAPTER 2.30

PULMONARY EMBOLUS

GENERAL INFORMATION

Pulmonary embolus (PE) results when a thrombus becomes dislodged from the vascular system, most commonly from the lower extremities following deep vein thrombosis (DVT), and then floats into the pulmonary vasculature until it becomes wedged in a branch of the pulmonary artery, creating a partial or total obstruction and pulmonary infarction. Pulmonary embolus can also originate when fat, amniotic fluid, or air enters the vascular system. The most common sites for thrombus formation are the right side of the heart, the lower extremities, and the pelvis. The obstruction of blood circulation that occurs with pulmonary emboli affects both perfusion and ventilation. Clinical manifestations depend on the extent to which blood flow is obstructed in the pulmonary circulation and the size of the embolus. The most common manifestations include dyspnea and pleuritic chest pain. Other symptoms include tachypnea, crackles on auscultation, anxiety, restlessness, skin color changes, and tachycardia. Pulmonary embolus may often be confused with other diagnoses that produce similar signs and symptoms, such as pneumothorax, myocardial contusion, and myocardial infarction. Of the deaths from pulmonary embolus, 50 percent occur within the first 2 hours.

NURSING DIAGNOSIS 1

IMPAIRED GAS EXCHANGE

Related to:

Pulmonary artery obstruction, which leads to decreased lung perfusion

Pulmonary physiologic shunting because of surfactant loss, causing alveolar collapse

Defining Characteristics:

Dyspnea

Pleuritic chest pain

Decreased oxygen saturation

Abnormal arterial blood gases (ABGs)

Skin color cyanotic

Tachypnea

Tachycardia

Rales (crackles)

Anxiety

Restlessness

Feeling of impending doom

Cough with occasional hemoptysis

Goal:

Gas exchange will improve.

Outcome Criteria

✔ Oxygen saturation is > 90 percent.

✔ Arterial blood gases (ABGs) are normal.

✔ Respirations are unlabored.

✔ Pleuritic chest pain is absent or reduced.

✔ V/Q scan returns to normal.

NOC *Respiratory status: Gas exchange*

INTERVENTIONS	RATIONALES
Assess respiratory status, including respiratory rate, rhythm, depth, and breath sounds; continue to monitor frequently throughout treatment.	The blockage of pulmonary blood flow can cause increased pulmonary vascular pressure with fluid accumulation in the lungs. This in turn translates into crackles and increased rate and depth of respiration in an effort to improve gas exchange.

(continues)

(continued)

INTERVENTIONS	RATIONALES
Monitor arterial blood gases (ABGs) and oxygen saturation, as ordered.	In pulmonary embolus, both ventilation and perfusion are affected, causing a decrease in oxygen saturation. Respiratory alkalosis may be present due to tachypnea and hyperventilation but can progress to acidosis as ventilation becomes seriously compromised; blood gases and oxygen saturation readings provides a means for monitoring the extent of hypoxemia and response to treatment.
Assess skin for cyanosis, pallor, and temperature, being sure to check mucous membranes of darker-skinned patients.	Due to decreased peripheral tissue oxygenation/perfusion, the skin becomes cool and cyanotic or pale. Changes in color can be detected more easily in mucous membranes in darker-skinned patients.
Monitor lung scans and chest x-rays.	Perfusion lung scans inject a radioactive flagged substance into the bloodstream and in the area of occlusion the isotope is undetected, suggesting a lack of perfusion; chest x-ray shows infiltrates.
Monitor D-dimer tests.	D-dimer is a fragment of fibrin that occurs with lysis of a clot; elevations indicate the presence of a thrombus.
Institute bedrest and position patient in a semi- or high Fowler's position.	Maximizes lung excursion and increases thoracic space. Decreases pressure of diaphragm and abdominal organs. Bedrest during acute episodes prevents further movement of emboli and minimizes oxygen demand.
Administer oxygen, as ordered.	Maximizes oxygen saturation in the circulating blood volume, decreases hypoxemia.
Administer anticoagulants (Heparin) as ordered: regular infractionated Heparin intravenously using an infusion device, maintaining a continuous infusion without interruption and Coumadin by mouth after initial treatment phase with Heparin (approximately 5 days).	Heparin deactivates clotting factors IX, X, XI, and XII to prevent further clot formation. Coumadin diminishes the formation of prothrombin by the liver. It also disrupts formation of extrinsic clotting factors VII, IX, and X. Coumadin is initiated prior to discharge,

	and the patient receives both Heparin and Coumadin for several days because of the time required to achieve sufficient therapeutic blood levels of the Coumadin.
Monitor the patient's bleeding studies (APTT for Heparin, PT or INR for Coumadin) for levels that are lower or higher than the agency therapeutic range; if noted, adjust anticoagulant dose per agency protocol or as ordered to achieve therapeutic blood levels.	Levels that are lower than the therapeutic range prolong treatment and predispose the patient to complications; levels that are higher than therapeutic predispose the patient to hemorrhage.
Anticipate administration of thrombolytic agents (streptokinase, urokinase, tissue plasminogen activator), as ordered.	Thrombolytics may be given to dissolve larger clots in the very early stage and act by activating the conversion of plasminogen to plasmin, the enzyme that degrades fibrin; fibrinogen; and other proteins into soluble fragments.
Monitor for bleeding secondary to anticoagulant or fibrinolytic therapy, examining all body fluids for blood (urine, feces, saliva, emesis).	Patients on anticoagulants often experience abnormal bleeding from body orifices that require adjustments in dosing; monitoring of coagulation studies and early detection can prevent massive hemorrhage.
Have patient brush teeth with a soft bristle brush, and apply pressure to any puncture site.	Even minor skin trauma can cause abnormal bleeding.
Assess the patient for response to treatment by re-evaluating the signs and symptoms of pulmonary embolism.	Improvement in initial symptoms such as pleuritic chest pain, tachypnea, dyspnea, and decreased oxygen saturation indicate beginning resolution of the clot.

NIC *Embolus care: Pulmonary*
Oxygen therapy
Respiratory monitoring
Ventilation assistance

Evaluation

Evaluate the degree to which the interventions have alleviated the patient's symptoms. Examine specific patient responses to interventions that would indicate that the patient's oxygenation status has improved. The patient should be free of pleuritic chest pain, respirations should be unlabored at the patient's baseline rate, and breath sounds should be clear. Continue to evaluate the patient's overall respiratory status, looking for indications that adequate oxygenation and gas exchange are occurring. Arterial blood gases (ABGs) and oxygen saturation should be normal, indicating the absence of hypoxia and hypoxemia. The patient should report that he or she feels better and is not anxious.

Community/Home Care

The patient needs to practice health promotion behaviors that include preventing the development of subsequent thrombi in the extremities. At home, the patient needs to continue with ambulation and avoidance of positions that cause stasis or pooling of blood. It will be important for the nurse to question the patient regarding availability of resources to purchase long-term oral anticoagulants. The patient will need to monitor self for abnormal bleeding and report this to the health care provider immediately. Follow-up home health care will include blood draws for anticoagulation studies or establishment of appointments at outpatient laboratories. Because of the possibility of reoccurrence in the future, the patient should be aware of the signs and symptoms of deep vein thrombosis (DVT) as well as those of pulmonary emboli. The patient will need methodical, well-planned teaching relevant to disease prevention and medications, especially side effects of the anticoagulants (see nursing diagnosis "Deficient Knowledge").

Documentation

Document a thorough assessment of respiratory status, noting the continued presence of or absence of signs and symptoms of pulmonary embolism. It is crucial to document precise indicators such as dyspnea, hemoptysis, oxygen saturation, and any pleuritic chest pain. Chart all interventions implemented and the patient's response. If anticoagulant protocols are revised in response to bleeding studies, be sure to include this in the documentation, and if possible, the data that supports the need for change. Be sure to include any patient complaints precisely as the patient states them.

NURSING DIAGNOSIS 2

INEFFECTIVE BREATHING PATTERN

Related to:

Pleuritic chest pain

Hypoxia

Extreme apprehension

Defining Characteristics:

Complaint of pleuritic chest pain

Tachypnea

Dyspnea

Decreased oxygen saturation

Abnormal arterial blood gases (ABGs) (lowered pO_2)

Skin pale/cyanotic, cool, clammy

Use of accessory muscles of respiration

Goal:

The patient exhibits an improved breathing pattern.

Outcome Criteria

✔ Respiratory rate will be at baseline (12–24 breaths per minute).

✔ The patient states that shortness of breath is relieved.

✔ The patient does not use accessory muscles for breathing.

NOC *Respiratory status: Ventilation*

Respiratory status: Gas exchange

INTERVENTIONS	RATIONALES
Assess respiratory status: breath sounds, use of accessory muscles, respiratory rate and depth, and chest excursion.	Establishes a baseline and monitors for response to interventions.
Administer oxygen, as ordered.	Improves oxygenation and oxygen saturation.
Assist patient in assuming a semi-Fowler's position.	Maximizes pulmonary excursion; reduces pressure from diaphragm and abdominal organs.

(continues)

(continued)

INTERVENTIONS	RATIONALES
Administer analgesics, as ordered.	Patients with pain often guard chest, preventing adequate chest expansion and subsequent depth of respirations; relieves pain and decreases anxiety.
Have patient cough and deep breathe.	Maximizes airway space and prevents atelectasis.
Consider intubation and mechanical ventilation if blood gases and oxygen saturation continue to deteriorate.	Improves oxygenation, blood gases, and oxygen saturation.
Teach controlled breathing.	Compensates for altered breathing patterns.
Implement measures to improve gas exchange (see nursing diagnosis "Impaired Gas Exchange").	Improving gas exchange is required to alleviate patient symptoms.

NIC *Airway management*
Respiratory monitoring
Oxygen therapy
Acid/base monitoring
Positioning

Evaluation

Evaluate the extent to which the patient has achieved the stated outcomes. The patient's respirations should be unlabored with equal chest expansion bilaterally. Respiratory rate should be within normal (12–24 per minute), and the patient should report that his or her respiratory effort is comfortable.

Community/Home Care

By the time of discharge home, the patient should have relief of all symptoms that suggested a pulmonary embolism. In the home, it will be important for the patient to understand and be able to carry out the prescribed medical regimen, including anticoagulant therapy and safety precautions. These include avoiding injury and recognizing the signs and symptoms of deep venous thrombus, pulmonary embolus, and hemorrhage (see nursing diagnoses "Impaired Gas Exchange" and "Deficient Knowledge").

Documentation

Document all initial and subsequent respiratory assessments according to agency protocols. Chart all interventions implemented to treat the problem and the specific patient responses. If the patient complains of difficulty breathing, document this along with the nursing interventions initiated, and the patient's response. Include in the patient record any teaching implemented and the patient's understanding. If follow-up is required, document this in the patient's chart as well.

NURSING DIAGNOSIS 3

 ## ACUTE PAIN

Related to:
> Pulmonary artery obstruction
> Lung tissue ischemia

Defining Characteristics:
> Complaint of severe pleuritic chest pain (especially on inspiration)
> Tachypnea
> Tachycardia
> Anxiety

Goal:
> Pain control is achieved.

Outcome Criteria

✔ The patient will verbalize that pain is relieved.
✔ The patient will verbalize a decrease in anxiety.

NOC *Pain level*
Pain control
Comfort level
Medication response

INTERVENTIONS	RATIONALES
Administer oxygen, as ordered.	Decreases tissue ischemia.
Have patient rate pain for intensity using a pain rating scale.	Gives a more objective assessment of the pain intensity.

INTERVENTIONS	RATIONALES
Administer analgesics, as ordered.	Pain increases the need for oxygen and increases anxiety, and therefore needs to be relieved.
Administer anticoagulants/ thrombolytics, as ordered.	Eliminates the emboli and clears the pulmonary artery, decreasing tissue ischemia, which is the cause of the pain.
Establish a quiet environment.	Enhances effects of analgesics, decreasing oxygen demands.
Elevate head of bed.	Improves chest expansion and oxygenation.
Assess effectiveness of interventions to relieve pain.	Helps to determine whether interventions have been effective in relieving pain or whether new strategies need to be employed.
Teach appropriate relaxation techniques and other distraction techniques, such as guided imagery.	Enhances effects of pharmacological interventions.

NIC *Pain management*
Analgesic administration
Anxiety reduction

Evaluation

The patient is able to report that the pain has been relieved or alleviated following interventions. The degree to which the patient is able to assist in the management of the pain through anxiety reduction and relaxation techniques is assessed.

Community/Home Care

Once the pulmonary embolus has been resolved, the pain should be alleviated. Home care required for this problem should be minimal and would consist of mild analgesic medications as needed. It is important that the patient at home understand clearly the importance of reporting any severe pleuritic pain to a health care provider, as this may signal further pulmonary emboli. At home, the patient will need to monitor self for signs of bleeding, such as blood in stool or vomiting of blood, which may occur secondary to anticoagulant therapy. A home health nurse or other health care worker should assess the patient's other medications to be sure that there are no interactions between anticoagulants and analgesics. Caution the patient against use of over-the-counter analgesics without consultation with a health care provider.

Documentation

Document in the patient's own words the description of the pain and his or her rating of the level of pain. Chart all methods used to alleviate or reduce the pain and the patient's response. Include in the documentation assessments made relevant to the cardiac and respiratory systems. All teaching should be indicated in the patient record with an indication of the patient's level of understanding.

NURSING DIAGNOSIS 4

 ANXIETY

Related to:
> Fear of dying
> Strange environment (critical care unit)
> Serious illness

Defining Characteristics:
> Expressions of fear
> Restlessness and anxiety
> Tachycardia

Goal:
> Anxiety is decreased or alleviated.

Outcome Criteria

✔ The patient reports being less anxious.
✔ The patient demonstrates no outward signs of anxiety, such as restlessness or agitation.

NOC *Anxiety control*
Comfort level
Coping

INTERVENTIONS	RATIONALES
Assess level of anxiety (mild, moderate, severe); have patient rate on a scale of 1–10 with 10 being the greatest.	Gives the nurse a better perception of extent of the anxiety.

(continues)

(continued)

INTERVENTIONS	RATIONALES
Keep patient informed of all that is going on, including information about therapeutic interventions.	When the patient is aware of what is being done, why, and what to expect, he or she will be less anxious.
Use a calm, reassuring manner with the patient.	Gives the patient a sense of well-being.
Stay with the patient as much as possible, especially during acute episodes of shortness of breath or pain, and allow family to visit.	Provides emotional support and promotes a sense of comfort.
Encourage the patient to verbalize fears and concerns.	Verbalization of fears contributes to dealing with concerns.
Control multiple sources of stimuli, which could cause sensory overload.	Overstimulation can worsen anxiety.
Seek spiritual consult as needed or requested by the patient and or family.	Meeting the patient's spiritual needs helps him or her to deal with fears through spiritual or religious rituals.

NIC *Anxiety reduction*
     Coping enhancement
     Emotional support

Evaluation

Evaluate the extent to which the outcome criteria have been achieved. Physiological signs of anxiety such as tachycardia will be absent. The patient will verbalize a decrease in anxiety and fear. Restlessness and agitation will be absent.

Community/Home Care

If the patient remains anxious due to fear of a reoccurrence of the pulmonary embolus while at home, he or she will need to practice relaxation techniques that can reduce anxiety. The relationship between anxiety and increasing oxygen demands should be explained to the patient, so that he or she can understand the importance of controlling fears and anxiety. Nurses should assess which coping mechanisms work for the patient and encourage their use by the patient at home. Simple activities, such as reading, listening to quiet music, meditating, or taking a short walk, may help the patient relax. Be sure

that the patient receives information on how to contact the health care provider. Knowing that there is a means to get answers to questions when or if they arise at home also may decrease the patient's anxiety.

Documentation

Document the degree to which the patient has decreased anxiety in the patient record. A rating system provides an objective way to relay to others the extent of the anxiety. Document whether the patient is able to verbalize a feeling of decreased anxiety and whether there are outward signs of anxiety. Blood pressure and pulse rates should be documented, as anxiety often causes an increase in both vital signs.

NURSING DIAGNOSIS 4

 DEFICIENT KNOWLEDGE

Related to:

   Acute illness

   Treatment protocol

   Misunderstanding of information

Defining Characteristics:

   Many or no questions

   Verbalizes a lack of knowledge/understanding

Goal:

   The patient will understand pulmonary embolism and the steps necessary to prevent complications.

Outcome Criteria

✔ The patient verbalizes a desire to learn necessary information.

✔ The patient verbalizes an understanding of pulmonary embolism: causes, prevention, complications.

✔ The patient expresses an understanding of the treatment regimen for pulmonary embolism, including activity restrictions, anticoagulant medications, and untoward effects of treatment.

✔ The patient verbalizes an understanding of follow-up care required and expresses a willingness to comply.

NOC *Knowledge: Disease process*
Knowledge: Treatment regimen
Compliance behavior

INTERVENTIONS	RATIONALES
Assess the patient's current knowledge as well as his or her ability to learn and readiness to learn.	The teacher needs to ascertain what the patient already knows and build on this; if the patient is not capable of learning or is not ready to learn, teaching will not be effective due to disinterest or inability to understand.
Start with the simplest information and move to complex information.	Patients can understand simple concepts easily and then can build on those to understand more complex concepts.
Teach the patient and family members: — Disease process of pulmonary embolism — Primary prevention: the most common risk factor for developing pulmonary embolism (deep vein thrombosis) and its causes (sitting for prolonged periods, crossing legs, dehydration, obesity, immobility, smoking, etc.) — Medications (anticoagulants) used to treat pulmonary embolism including rationale for use, dosage, frequency, side effects, scheduling, interactions with other medications — Avoiding use of over-the-counter medications, such as aspirin or aspirin containing products (these potentiates the effects of the anticoagulants due to antiplatelet aggregation property) — Importance of wearing a Medic Alert bracelet and carrying a wallet card stating that the patient is receiving anticoagulants — Signs and symptoms of complications that would indicate a need to seek health care (abnormal bleeding, new	Knowledge of disease, treatments required, monitoring needed, and prevention of complications empowers the patient to take control and be compliant.
onset of shortness of breath, sudden sharp chest pain, restlessness) — Need to monitor all body fluids for blood (urine, saliva, feces, sputum) — Need for follow-up care: blood draws for coagulation studies — Avoiding straight razor for shaving (men or women), as even a mild nick can bleed profusely — Need to apply constant pressure to any bleeding site	
Instruct patient on the correct use of anti-embolic or compression stockings if ordered. Have patient return demonstrate application of these devices.	Anti-embolic stockings are difficult to apply, and the nurse needs to know that the patient can correctly perform this activity prior to discharge. These stockings prevent venous stasis.
Teach the patient and family members about activity and position requirements, including bedrest and avoidance of crossing legs.	Even though some physicians allow limited ambulation in patients with pulmonary embolism, bedrest is usually required in the early stages until all symptoms subside. Bedrest prevents further movement of the emboli. Crossing of legs causes constriction of blood flow in extremities, which can cause a DVT and put the patient at further risk for additional pulmonary emboli.
Assess the patient's and the family members' understanding of all teaching by encouraging them to repeat information and ask questions as needed.	This allows the nurse to hear in the patient's own words what was taught and makes it easier to know what information may need to be reinforced.
Establish that the patient has the resources required to be compliant.	If needed resources such as finances and transportation to follow-up appointments are not available, the patient cannot be compliant; the nurse will need to make necessary referrals.

NIC *Learning readiness enhancement*
Learning facilitation
Teaching: Disease process
Teaching: Prescribed medication

Evaluation

Evaluate the degree to which the patient has achieved the outcome criteria relevant to the teaching sessions. The patient should verbalize an understanding of content presented by repeating the information, particularly the disease process and medications. The nurse must determine if the patient is capable of being compliant with the recommended regimen. If further teaching is required at time of discharge, the appropriate referrals should be made to continue education.

Community/Home Care

Education of the patient is required in order for the patient to implement the medical regimen in the home setting. The ability to implement the recommendations will be dependent upon the degree to which the patient has received adequate teaching from the nurse or other health care provider and has subsequently understood it. The patient will need to follow a routine that includes administration of anticoagulants and self-assessment of bleeding. Precautions to be taken in the home include using of soft toothbrushes, using electric razors for shaving, and avoiding of trauma that could produce bleeding. Even though the patient may not want to engage in observation of his or her bowel movements or urine, it should be stressed that this should be done to detect bleeding from the urinary system and GI tract that may occur if bleeding times increase beyond the therapeutic range. If coagulation studies are to be done by the home nurse or at an outpatient center, the patient should be clear about appointment time and whether to take the anticoagulant medication on that day. It is crucial that the patient understand that the medication regimen will continue past the time that symptoms dissipate and the importance of continuing the therapy until discontinued by the health care provider. The interaction of other medications with anticoagulants should be discussed, especially commonly used over-the-counter products such as aspirin. The nurse and patient should discuss risk factor for pulmonary embolism and DVT development and ascertain if any risk factors continue to exist for the patient and the feasibility of their elimination. Question the patient about occupation, usual positions when sitting, and activity.

Documentation

Document the specific content taught and the titles of any printed documents given to the patient. Include in the chart the patient's degree of understanding of the content, particularly medications and the methods used to evaluate learning. Document specifically the patient's ability to perform the psychomotor skill of applying anti-embolism stockings, as well as any areas that need to be reinforced, to ensure appropriate follow-up. If family members are present for the teaching sessions document this in the chart, and always document any referrals made.

CHAPTER 2.31

RESPIRATORY ACIDOSIS

GENERAL INFORMATION

Respiratory acidosis is a disorder of acid/base balance characterized by an increase in carbonic acid in the form of partial pressure of carbon dioxide in the arterial blood (pCO_2) > 45 mm Hg, causing the arterial blood pH to decrease below 7.35. The bicarbonate buffering system is activated when respiratory acidosis occurs, resulting in increased bicarbonate production and reabsorption by the kidneys. Renal buffering can be effective in normalizing the pH if enough time has passed for bicarbonate levels to increase in the blood and if the magnitude of the respiratory acidosis is not too severe. Acute respiratory acidosis, such as occurs with status asthmaticus, respiratory arrest, or post-anesthesia respiratory depression, is typically uncompensated and therefore physiologically dangerous because of the low pH levels that develop and may result in death if not corrected. Chronic respiratory acidosis, such as occurs with chronic obstructive pulmonary disease (COPD)—emphysema and chronic bronchitis—is typically well compensated by elevated bicarbonate levels in the blood and therefore better tolerated. Patients with chronic respiratory acidosis, such as COPD, often develop acute respiratory problems such as pneumonia that result in worsening of their baseline respiratory acidosis. Because the renal system's compensatory mechanism of increased bicarbonate buffering is slow to develop, the formerly compensated respiratory acidosis becomes partially compensated, posing serious physiologic dysfunction. Clinical manifestations of respiratory acidosis can include dyspnea, tachypnea, dizziness, headache, mental status changes, and in severe cases, cyanosis.

NURSING DIAGNOSIS 1

 IMPAIRED GAS EXCHANGE

Related to:

Hypoventilation from effects of drugs (narcotics, anesthesia, alcohol intoxication, drug overdose)

Air trapping from obstructive pulmonary disease

Fatigue from prolonged respiratory distress

Airway obstruction from thick mucous, bronchospasm, or aspiration

Pulmonary infection

Defining Characteristics:

Arterial blood gas (ABG): pH is decreased to < 7.35 and pCO_2 is elevated to > 45 mm Hg

Hypoxemia

Dypsnea

Tachypnea

Goal:

Acid/base balance will be restored.

Outcome Criteria

✔ The pH level will return to normal range.

✔ Carbon dioxide levels will be within normal limits.

✔ Oxygen saturation will be between > 93 percent (chronic CO_2 retainers O_2 sat: 88–92 percent)

✔ Respiratory rate will be < 28.

✔ The patient will breathe without dyspnea or excessive accessory muscle use.

NOC *Respiratory status: Ventilation*
Respiratory status: Gas exchange

INTERVENTIONS	RATIONALES
Assess respiratory system, including rate, depth, effort, rhythm, use of accessory muscles,	Helps to determine a baseline in order to evaluate response to treatment; decreasing

(continues)

(continued)

INTERVENTIONS	RATIONALES
breath sounds, presence of cough, skin color, and mental status.	respiratory rate along with deterioration in other assessment parameters may signal respiratory failure.
Monitor arterial blood gases (ABGs).	Helps to determine acid/base status; in respiratory acidosis, the pH will be lower than normal and the carbon dioxide level will be higher than normal.
Assess oxygen saturation.	Helps to detect hypoxemia.
Assist patient to semi-Fowler's or Fowler's position.	Sitting upright allows diaphragm to descend, resulting in easier breathing and improved gas exchange.
Administer oxygen, as ordered, to maintain oxygen saturation > 93 percent (chronic CO_2 retainers O_2 sat: 88–92 percent).	Promotes tissue oxygenation.
Assess ease of breathing, use of accessory muscles, pursed lip breathing, complaints of dyspnea, and cyanosis.	Impaired gas exchange can cause increased work of breathing and fatigue.
Encourage patients with a history of chronic obstructive or restrictive pulmonary disease (asthma, COPD: emphysema, chronic bronchitis) to lean forward and rest elbows on bedside table.	This position can help alleviate air trapping and improve gas exchange.
Encourage patients with history of chronic obstructive pulmonary disease (COPD) to practice pursed-lip breathing.	Pursed-lip breathing can help alleviate air trapping and improve gas exchange.
Administer naloxone (Narcan) as ordered if narcotic/opiate overdose is suspected.	Naloxone is a narcotic antagonist that is useful in reversing respiratory depression associated with opiates.
Administer bronchodilators, as ordered.	Dilates airways and facilitates gas exchange.
Monitor for signs of pulmonary infection and collaborate with physician, if present, regarding antibiotic administration.	Green, brown, or purulent mucous along with fever, crackles, and impaired gas exchange can indicate pneumonia.
Prepare for mechanical ventilation.	Patients who do not respond to conservative management of impaired gas exchange may require mechanical ventilation.

NIC *Acid/base monitoring*
Acid/base management
Respiratory monitoring
Airway management

Evaluation

Evaluate the status of outcome criteria. The patient should have indicators of good gas exchange, such as even, unlabored respirations, and an oxygen saturation of at least 90 percent. Blood gas analyses should indicate an absence of respiratory acidosis by a return of pH and carbon dioxide to normal levels, or compensation has occurred and oxygen levels are between 80–100 percent. Respiratory rate should return to the patient's baseline.

Community/Home Care

For most patients, respiratory acidosis is corrected quickly by treating the cause and is not a problem in the home environment unless the patient has a chronic respiratory condition such as COPD. Teaching the patient how to control his or her breathing so that he or she can revert to a steady rhythmic type of respiration is crucial so that the person can blow off excessive carbon dioxide. Cough and deep breathing exercises should be taught to the patient, and he or she should be encouraged to perform these throughout the day when at home, especially if the patient has conditions predisposing him or her to reoccurrence of respiratory acidosis. This method of breathing opens airways more, assisting in the elimination of carbon dioxide and preventing atelectasis, which can cause pneumonia. Community and in-home care is centered on preventing or controlling those respiratory problems that place the patient at risk for respiratory acidosis. Patients and family members should know the signs of respiratory acidosis and respiratory infection, because infection frequently causes acidosis as respirations become inadequate for gas exchange due to the presence of secretions in the airways. The patient should avoid crowds in the home and community and other persons with colds, practice good hand washing, and receive appropriate immunizations for flu and pneumonia. If symptoms of infection or acidosis occur, the patient should return to the health care provider.

Documentation

Included in the documentation should be a complete respiratory assessment with specific attention to a description of how the patient is breathing and whether the patient feels comfortable with his or her breathing. Chart all interventions employed to address respiratory status and hypoventilation and the patient's specific response. Results of oxygen saturation readings and arterial blood gases (ABGs) should be documented as they represent the best measure of gas exchange. If the patient still has indicators of impaired gas exchange, such as uncompensated respiratory acidosis (decreased pH and increased carbon dioxide), these should be specifically noted along with needed revisions to the plan of care.

NURSING DIAGNOSIS 2

INEFFECTIVE AIRWAY CLEARANCE

Related to:

> Pulmonary infection
> Decreased level of consciousness

Defining Characteristics:

> Thick mucous
> Difficulty expectorating mucous
> Diminished breath sounds
> Dyspnea
> Adventitious breath sounds
> Coughing
> Tachypnea

Goal:

> The patient's airway is patent.

Outcome Criteria

✔ The patient will maintain clear airways with bilaterally equal and clear breath sounds.

✔ The patient will have no cyanosis.

✔ Oxygen saturation will be > 93 percent (for chronic retainers of carbon dioxide, 88–92 percent).

✔ The patient's pCO_2 will be within normal (35–45 mm Hg), or at patient's baseline for patients with COPD.

NOC *Respiratory status: Airway patency*

INTERVENTIONS	RATIONALES
Perform a respiratory assessment frequently: breath sounds, respiratory rate, depth and effort, skin color.	Establishes a baseline and guides treatment.
Administer bronchodilators, as ordered.	Dilates airways and facilitates mucous mobilization.
Provide chest physiotherapy: postural drainage, chest percussion, and vibration.	Loosens mucous plugs.
Encourage coughing and mucus expectoration.	Clears the airways.
Encourage intake of 2000–3000 ml of fluid daily.	Fluid helps to thin secretions.
Administer mucolytics, as ordered.	Decreases mucous viscosity.
Suction airways if patient is unable to expectorate mucous.	Clears the airways.
Encourage patient to reposition self every 2 hours or ambulate.	Activity prevents stasis of secretions and helps clear the airway.
If the patient is expectorating, assess mucus amount, color, and consistency.	Green, brown, or purulent mucus can indicate pneumonia.
Administer antibiotics, as ordered.	Treats or prevents infection.

NIC *Respiratory monitoring*
Airway management
Airway suctioning

Evaluation

Evaluate the extent to which the patient has met the outcome criteria. The patient is able to cough and to expectorate mucus, and mucous is not green, brown, or purulent. There are no signs of cyanosis. The patient has bilaterally equal and clear breath sounds. The patient is afebrile and is not dyspneic. Arterial blood gases and oxygen saturation results are within normal range, or at least at the patient's baseline.

Community/Home Care

The patient who has respiratory acidosis secondary to ineffective airway clearance due to an acute problem will probably not need assistance at home. If the airway clearance problem has been caused by excessive mucous production due to a chronic problem, such as chronic bronchitis, attention in the home will need to address implementation of strategies to prevent mucous accumulation. The patient will need to establish a plan for intake of fluids to thin secretions, using thin liquids such as apple juice or cranberry juice and avoiding substances such as milk or milkshakes or juices with pulp. An effective, inexpensive way to help open airways is to have the patient stand in the shower or sit in the bathroom with the hot water running and inhale the steam/mist, or the patient can purchase a humidifier for use. Practicing coughing and deep breathing should also be incorporated into the patient's daily schedule. Expectoration of mucous is encouraged and the patient should be informed of the importance of observing the mucous for color and consistency while also noting if there seems to be an increase in amount. The patient can keep a log of how he or she is treating the airway patency problem, keeping track of medications, turn/cough/deep breathe activities, presence of mucous with color noted, and daily fluid intake. This can be helpful when the patient returns to the health care provider. The patient should know to return for follow-up care if symptoms persist or worsen, as demonstrated by increasing shortness of breath, difficulty expectorating mucous, thicker mucous, and odor or color changes.

Documentation

Document a comprehensive respiratory assessment, including breath sounds, respiratory rate and effort, production of mucous, skin color, and any complaints of shortness of breath. The results of arterial blood gases (ABGs) and oxygen saturations are charted according to agency protocol. All interventions carried out to relieve ineffective airway clearance are included in the record. Note the patient's efforts at coughing and deep breathing. Always include in the documentation the patient's progress towards achievement of the stated outcome criteria.

CHAPTER 2.32

RESPIRATORY ALKALOSIS

GENERAL INFORMATION

Respiratory alkalosis is an acute process involving a decrease in carbonic acid measured as the partial pressure of carbon dioxide in the arterial blood (pCO_2) of < 35 mm Hg, causing the arterial blood pH to increase above 7.45. It is most often caused by hyperventilation, usually secondary to anxiety. If respiratory alkalosis persists over an extended period, the kidneys' bicarbonate buffering system starts to compensate by eliminating bicarbonate and decreasing bicarbonate production. Renal buffering can be effective in normalizing the pH if enough time has passed for bicarbonate levels to decrease in the blood, and if the magnitude of the respiratory alkalosis is not too severe and the underlying problem is corrected in a timely fashion. The longer the duration of the respiratory alkalosis, the more likely total compensation of the pH by the kidneys is to occur. Acute respiratory alkalosis, such as occurs with hysteria, anxiety attacks, pain, acute asthma exacerbation, or pulmonary embolism, is typically uncompensated. Other causes of respiratory alkalosis include salicylate poisoning, congestive heart failure, or central nervous system problems such as tumors, infections (septicemia), stroke or head trauma, and mechanical ventilation. In alkalotic states, there are increased rates of binding of extracellular calcium with albumin, decreasing the serum concentration levels of calcium and rendering the neuromuscular system more excitable and the patient prone to development of symptoms of hypocalcemia if the alkalosis is uncorrected. Clinical manifestations of respiratory alkalosis are dizziness, lightheadedness, confusion, tachycardia, nausea/vomiting, numbness and tingling in extremities, and tremors. The aim for treatment is to identify and treat the underlying cause so that carbonic acid levels in the blood increase, resulting in the pH decreasing below 7.45.

NURSING DIAGNOSIS 1

IMPAIRED GAS EXCHANGE

Related to:

Loss of respiratory acid

Ineffective breathing pattern: increased respiratory rate and/or depth

Defining Characteristics:

pH > 7.45

pCO_2 is < normal (< 35 in most labs)

Hypoxemia

Tachypnea

Use of accessory muscles

Goal:

The patient's acid/base balance will be restored.

Outcome Criteria

✔ Arterial blood gas pH will be within normal limits.

✔ Carbon dioxide level will be within normal limits (35–45).

✔ Oxygen saturation will be > 93 percent (chronic CO_2 retainers O_2 sat: 88–92 percent).

✔ Respiratory rate will be at the patient's baseline.

✔ The patient will breathe comfortably, without dyspnea or excessive accessory muscle use.

NOC *Respiratory status: Ventilation*
Respiratory status: Gas exchange
Vital signs

INTERVENTIONS	RATIONALES
Assess respiratory rate, depth, ease of breathing, use of accessory muscles, complaints of anxiety, numbness or tingling of extremities and face.	Helps to detect clinical manifestations associated with hyperventilation and consequent respiratory alkalosis; numbness and tingling are a result of decreased calcium levels.
Assess arterial blood gases (ABGs) noting increased pH and decreased carbon dioxide levels.	Helps to determine acid/base status and validate severity of the problem.
Assess oxygen saturation.	Allows confirmation of hypoxemia.
Administer oxygen, as ordered, to maintain O_2 saturation >93 percent.	Promotes tissue oxygenation (chronic CO_2 retainers O_2 sat: 88–92 percent).
Coach the patient in ways to slow respiratory rate.	Rapid respirations cause loss of carbon dioxide, resulting in respiratory alkalosis.
Encourage the patient to talk to you.	Talking will cause a decrease in respiratory rate and can be a distraction from his or her breathing.
Encourage patient to breathe into cupped hands or a paper bag.	This will cause the patient to rebreathe carbon dioxide and decrease respiratory alkalosis.
Treat underlying cause.	Removes the trigger for increased breathing.
Stay with patient and offer reassurance.	Decreases anxiety, which is a contributing factor for hyperventilation.
Administer anti-anxiety medication, as ordered.	Decreases anxiety, which is a cause of or contributing factor for hyperventilation.
Monitor neurological system: level of consciousness; motor/sensory function; anxiety; agitation; confusion; hyperreflexia; tetany; seizures; headache; vertigo; dizziness; tinnitis; and paresthesias of the face, hands, or feet.	These are indicators of neurological impairment that may be caused by decreased serum calcium levels or the acid/base imbalance itself and require treatment.
Assist with identification of causes other than anxiety: salicylate poisoning, brain tumors, pain, asthma exacerbation, stroke, and septicemia.	Even though anxiety and hyperventilation are the most common causes of respiratory alkalosis, other disorders should not be overlooked.

Teach the patient how to prevent a recurrence of hyperventilation or acute anxiety through use of controlled breathing and relaxation techniques.	Controlled breathing slows the respiratory rate, preventing the abnormal loss of carbon dioxide. Relaxation techniques help control breathing and subsequently decrease anxiety.

NIC   *Oxygen therapy*
Respiratory monitoring
Acid/base monitoring
Acid/base management:
*   Respiratory alkalosis*

Evaluation

Evaluate the status of outcome criteria. The patient should have indicators of good gas exchange, such as even, easy respirations, and an oxygen saturation of at least 90 percent. Blood gas analyses should indicate an absence of respiratory alkalosis by a return of pH and carbon dioxide to normal levels or show compensation and oxygen levels between 80–100 percent. The patient should exhibit an absence of hyperventilation and respirations within baseline. There should be no neurological changes that would indicate the presence of decreased calcium levels (tetany).

Community/Home Care

For most patients, respiratory alkalosis is corrected quickly by treating the cause and is not a problem in the home environment. If the patient is prone to anxiety attacks or panic attacks, he or she is likely to have future episodes of respiratory alkalosis. It is crucial to teach the patient how to control his or her breathing in order to revert to a slow rhythmic type of respiration so that too much carbon dioxide is not exhaled upon expiration. The patient can do this by taking a deep breath in and counting to 10 slowly as he or she exhales. Not only will this slow the rate, but it also helps the patient to relax, which may decrease anxiety. Showing the patient how to breathe into a paper bag and explaining how it works will provide the patient with one other mechanism to control hyperventilation in the home. Keeping a log of episodes of hyperventilation and what activities precipitated them may be helpful in demonstrating where changes can be made.

Documentation

Include in the documentation a complete respiratory assessment with specific attention to describing how the patient is breathing and whether the patient feels comfortable with his or her breathing. Chart all interventions employed to address anxiety and hyperventilation and the patient's specific response. Results of oxygen saturation readings and arterial blood gases (ABGs) should be documented as they represent the best measure of gas exchange. If the patient still has indicators of impaired gas exchange, such as uncompensated respiratory alkalosis (increased pH and decreased carbon dioxide), note these specifically along with revisions to the plan of care.

NURSING DIAGNOSIS 2

 ANXIETY

Related to:

Stress

Situational/maturational crises, conflict

Pain

Hypoxemia

Defining Characteristics:

Expressed anxiety

Restlessness, jitters, shaking, twitching

Tachypnea

Tachycardia

Pupillary dilation

Hypertension

Diaphoresis

Goal:

Anxiety is relieved.

Outcome Criteria

✔ The patient verbalizes that anxiety has been reduced.

✔ The patient's respirations are easy and < 28.

✔ The patient reports feeling relaxed.

✔ The patient has no physiological signs of anxiety (tachycardia, diaphoresis, papillary dilation).

NOC *Anxiety control*

INTERVENTIONS	RATIONALES
Have patient rate anxiety on a numerical scale.	Allows for a more objective measure of anxiety level.
Provide oxygen, as ordered.	This assists patient to breathe easier.
Implement strategies to manage hyperventilation: — Have patient breathe into a paper bag — Have patient perform relaxed purposeful breathing by taking deep breath in and then releasing/expiring to the count of 10	Correction of the rapid respirations will help to reduce anxiety level.
Encourage patient to verbalize concerns about anxiety or panic attacks.	Verbalizing concerns can help patient deal with issues and avoid negative feelings.
Stay with patient during acute episodes of anxiety and use a calm manner.	Allows the nurse to offer comfort, care, and assurances to reduce anxiety and fear.
Administer anti-anxiety agents as ordered.	Pharmacological interventions may be needed to reduce symptoms of anxiety.
Teach the patient relaxation techniques, such as deep breathing and guided imagery, and encourage their use as well as attempting meditation and quiet music.	Reduces anxiety and creates a feeling of comfort.

NIC *Anxiety reduction*
Calming technique
Emotional support
Presence

Evaluation

Assess the patient for the extent that he or she is free of anxiety. The patient should verbalize that anxiety is reduced and that he or she feels comfortable. Assess the patient for physiological signs of anxiety, such as increased pulse and sweating. During evaluation, be sure to inquire about the use of relaxation techniques. The patient should report that he or she understands how to control anxiety attacks and stop hyperventilation.

Community/Home Care

The patient will need to know how to control anxiety in the home setting. It is crucial that health care providers provide the patient with knowledge to make the patient feel in control of his or her emotional and psychological health. A patient who knows how to treat anxiety will have fewer incidences of anxiety attacks and fear. The patient should be sure to have paper bags available and know how to control breathing. By ensuring that the patient understands how to treat anxiety and subsequent hyperventilation at home, the health care provider may prevent unnecessary emergency room visits.

Documentation

Document the degree of anxiety experienced by the patient. Using some type of numerical rating scale similar to the pain scale will provide health care providers with a more objective measure of the degree of anxiety the patient is experiencing. Document any physiological or observable signs of anxiety, such as restlessness, tachycardia, or diaphoresis. Interventions implemented to treat anxiety should be documented along with subsequent assessments to determine their effectiveness. Chart the patient's understanding of teaching related to controlling anxiety.

CHAPTER 2.33

TRACHEOSTOMY

GENERAL INFORMATION

A tracheostomy/tracheotomy is a surgical incision made into the trachea to create an airway (temporary or permanent) when there is an obstruction above the trachea or the patient is experiencing respiratory failure and needs the benefit of reduced airway resistance. The procedure is generally elective and is often used to maintain prolonged mechanical ventilation. The tracheostomy opening is kept patent with a disposable tracheostomy tube, a specially designed tube for this procedure. A tracheostomy is also performed when there is need for a more permanent airway than endotracheal intubation can provide.

NURSING DIAGNOSIS 1

 IMPAIRED GAS EXCHANGE

Related to:

Airway obstruction

Presence of tracheostomy

Thick secretions

Ineffective cough

Defining Characteristics:

Decreased oxygen saturation

Cyanosis

Tachycardia

Restlessness and agitation

Goal:

The patient's airway is patent, and adequate gas exchange is restored.

Outcome Criteria

✔ Breath sounds will be clear.

✔ The patient will have no cyanosis.

✔ Arterial blood gases (ABGs) will return to normal.

✔ Oxygen saturation will be > 90 percent.

NOC *Respiratory status: Airway patency*
Respiratory status: Ventilation

INTERVENTIONS	RATIONALES
Assess respiratory status: breath sounds, respiratory rate, oxygen saturation.	Helps to establish a baseline and monitor response to interventions.
Monitor patient for signs of occluded airway: cyanosis, whistling sound from tracheostomy, holding throat.	Airway may obstruct without the patient being able to notify a health care worker.
Provide humidified oxygen, as ordered.	The humidification function of the upper airway does not function with a tracheostomy; using humidified oxygen liquefies secretions and ensures adequate oxygenation.
Assess the viscosity and color of secretions.	Thickened secretions are more likely to occlude the tracheostomy; noting this would allow for implementation of measures to thin secretions; the color of secretions allows for early detection of color changes due to infection.
Suction the tracheostomy as ordered and prn, providing oxygen prior to suctioning and post-suctioning to prevent hypoxia.	Removes secretions and prevents airway obstruction.
Maintain sterile technique when working with tracheostomy site or tracheostomy tube.	Prevents the introduction of infectious organisms into the respiratory system.
Avoid unnecessary movement of tracheostomy tube.	Movement causes irritation to the trachea and discomfort for the patient.

(continues)

(continued)

INTERVENTIONS	RATIONALES
Assist patient with coughing and deep breathing.	Mobilizes secretions and prevents atelectasis.
Clean around tracheostomy site and replace inner cannula with a new disposable one every shift. If old-fashioned reusable metal tracheostomy tube is used, remove inner cannula, cleanse according to agency procedure, and replace.	Clears airway debris that has adhered to the side of the tube and minimizes the risk of infection.
Monitor for signs and symptoms of respiratory infection: fever, rales, increased mucous production, elevated white blood cell count, and chest x-ray reports.	Helps to initiate treatment early and prevent complications.

NIC *Airway management*
Airway suctioning
Cough enhancement
Respiratory monitoring
Oxygen therapy
Ventilation assistance

Evaluation

Assess the patient to determine the extent to which gas exchange has been restored and the outcome criteria have been met. The patient's airway should be clear, and the patient should be able to cough with expectoration of secretions. Breath sounds should be clear, and there should be no cyanosis. Results of oxygen saturation readings and arterial blood gases (ABGs) should be within normal range or improved. If criteria have not been met, determine whether expected outcomes were realistic or whether more time is necessary for achievement. In the latter case, note the degree of progress the patient is making towards meeting the outcomes.

Community/Home Care

The patient with a tracheostomy may need long-term monitoring by a health care professional if discharged to the home. In some instances, the patient and family will be able to care for the tracheostomy themselves; in some cases care will always be provided by a visiting nurse. The patient and family will need to know the signs of airway obstruction and how to relieve it, tracheostomy care including suctioning (see nursing diagnosis "Deficient Knowledge"), and measures to prevent respiratory infection. It is crucial that the patient have all needed supplies for tracheostomy care, so there needs to be an assessment of the patient's financial resources. Supplies for tracheostomy care can be kept in a container, such as a heavy plastic storage box with a snap-on lid bought from any retail store that sells household supplies. The patient and family must be aware of how to handle emergencies that could arise, such as mucous plugs. Health care providers visiting the home should give attention to the patient's psychological state, as the tracheostomy is a visible change in anatomy and body image may be disturbed. Question the patient about his or her social life and general sense of well-being to ascertain if the patient may be socially isolating him or herself (see nursing diagnosis "Disturbed Body Image").

Documentation

Document a comprehensive respiratory assessment. Include in the patient record all interventions carried out for the patient and the patient's response. Note specifically secretions, suctioning, and tracheostomy care. If the patient is able to participate in care, including initiating coughing, document this in the chart. Vital signs should be documented according to agency protocol. Any teaching initiated should be charted with a clear indication of what was taught and to whom.

NURSING DIAGNOSIS 2

IMPAIRED VERBAL COMMUNICATION

Related to:
Presence of tracheostomy tube

Defining Characteristics:
Inability to talk

Goal:
The patient is able to communicate.

Outcome Criteria

✔ The patient will use a communication board to express one need.

✔ The patient will be able to express needs by writing or pointing to words.

NOC *Communication*
Communication expressive

INTERVENTIONS	RATIONALES
Assess the patient's ability to communicate; determine whether the patient can read and write.	Establishes that the patient is able to use alternative communications methods.
Provide the patient with alternative to verbal communication, such as a communication board, pencil and paper, Magic Slate, or a chalkboard, if the patient is able to read and write. Provide picture cards if the patient cannot read or write.	This provides a method of communication until the patient is able to speak. When a tracheostomy tube is in place, the patient will be unable to speak because air will not pass the vocal cords to produce the vibrations necessary to produce sounds
If the patient is unable to use hands to write or point, teach the patient to signal using eye blinks, hand squeezing, nodding, or other means of nonverbal communication.	Much information can be communicated using simple gestures to signal "yes" and "no" as well as other simple commands
Arrange for a speech therapist consult.	Speech therapists can assist the patient with communication methods, including adjunct devices to facilitate communication.
Teach the patient how to cover tracheostomy when respiratory status allows.	Covering the tracheostomy opening permits air to flow over the larynx, allowing for speech.
Consult with physician regarding the use of a special tracheostomy tube that allows speech, such as a Communitrach.	These tracheostomy tubes have a one-way valve that closes with exhalation, allowing for speech.
Take time to work with the patient in communication efforts, without rushing him or her.	Rushing the patient to communicate causes frustration and may make the patient stop trying to communicate.

NIC *Communication enhancement:*
Speech deficit
Anxiety reduction

Evaluation

Evaluate the progress the patient has made in ability to communicate. Determine whether the patient is able to express needs. Establish what needs to be done to further enhance nonverbal communication with the patient. Evaluate whether the patient is able to communicate using a communication board, writing, or pointing. Determine whether the patient is frustrated or satisfied with attempts at communication and whether the use of the new Communitrach would be beneficial.

Community/Home Care

For the patient with a tracheostomy, the inability to communicate verbally may prove to be the biggest challenge when he or she is discharged home. Many patients feel embarrassed and may refrain from efforts at communication due to this as well as to frustration at trying to make others understand him or her. Have the patient practice verbal communication skills in a private place several times a day. The patient must be encouraged to continue with new communication strategies, and this is where social support systems can be most beneficial. As family and friends display acceptance, encouragement, and patience the patient will become more comfortable; through communication, the patient knows that others understand. If this does not happen, the patient may socially isolate him or herself, which could lead to emotional stress. Follow-up care should give attention to not only the physiological realm of care but to this very critical aspect of the patient's well-being.

Documentation

Document all communication strategies utilized with the patient. Include an evaluation of the patient's efforts to communicate and of which strategies work best. Always include an assessment of the patient's emotional state and responses to all interventions. Chart any referrals made for speech and the outcomes of any recommendations.

NURSING DIAGNOSIS 3

ANXIETY

Related to:

Presence of tracheostomy and new way to breathe

Defining Characteristics:

    Fear that airway will become obstructed

    Restlessness

    Verbalization of anxiety

Goal:

    The patient's anxiety level is reduced.

Outcome Criteria

✔ The patient reports being less anxious.

✔ The patient demonstrates no outward signs of anxiety, such as restlessness or agitation.

NOC *Anxiety control*
      Comfort level

INTERVENTIONS	RATIONALES
Assess level of anxiety (mild, moderate, severe); have the patient rate on a scale of 1–10 with 10 being the greatest.	Gives the nurse a better perception of extent of the anxiety.
Keep the patient informed of all that is going on, including information about therapeutic interventions.	Communication of what is happening in a calm and straightforward manner may help to relieve anxiety.
Ensure that the call bell/light button is readily accessible to the patient; respond to needs related to the tracheostomy promptly, such as the need for suctioning or coughing episodes.	Changes in respiratory status caused by mucous build-up and coughing can add to anxiety and fear. Knowing that help is readily accessible can help to reduce the patient's anxiety level, and makes the patient feel confident that needs will be met and complications prevented.
Use a calm, reassuring manner with the patient.	Gives the patient a sense of well-being.
Stay with patient as possible and allow the family to visit.	Provides emotional support and promotes a sense of comfort.
Encourage the patient to communicate fears and concerns about the tracheostomy.	Recognizing fears contributes to dealing with concerns.
Control multiple sources of stimuli, which could cause sensory overload.	Overstimulation can worsen anxiety.
Teach the patient and family about tracheostomy.	Knowledge decreases anxiety by giving the patient a sense of control.
Assist the patient with new strategies for communication.	The inability to communicate or the need to learn new communication techniques can cause frustrations that lead to anxiety.
Explore possible relaxation techniques and coping strategies, and teach these as appropriate.	Use of relaxation techniques and coping strategies that have worked in the past reduces anxiety and fear and enhances positive outcomes.

NIC *Anxiety reduction*
      Emotional support

Evaluation

Evaluate the extent to which the outcome criteria have been achieved. Physiological signs of anxiety, such as tachycardia, will be absent. The patient will verbalize a decrease in anxiety and fear, and restlessness and agitation will be absent. The patient reports that he or she is not frustrated with attempts at communication and that he or she has employed relaxation techniques.

Community/Home Care

The patient will need to be followed at home regarding tracheostomy care. Often the patient is anxious because of a perceived lack of knowledge regarding the tracheostomy or others perceptions of his or her changed appearance. If the patient remains anxious due to fear of alterations in respiratory status and the presence of an alteration in outward appearance, he or she will need to practice relaxation techniques that can reduce anxiety. Assuring that the patient knows how to respond to respiratory problems that may arise and understands how to care for the tracheostomy can also reduce the possibility of anxiety. Nurses should assess which anxiety-reducing strategies work for the patient and encourage their use by the patient at home. The relationship between anxiety and increasing oxygen demands should be explained to the patient, so that he or she can understand the importance of controlling fears and anxiety. The patient should feel comfortable with knowledge of how to handle emergencies should they arise.

Documentation

Document the degree to which the patient has decreased anxiety in the patient record. A rating system provides an objective way to relay to others the extent of the anxiety. Document whether the patient is able to verbalize a feeling of decreased anxiety and whether there are outward signs of anxiety. Include in the documentation what specific events seem to contribute to anxiety episodes and what strategies are employed to relieve or reduce it. Blood pressure and pulse rates should be documented as anxiety often causes an increase in both vital signs.

NURSING DIAGNOSIS 4

DEFICIENT KNOWLEDGE

Related to:

Care of tracheostomy and suctioning

Defining Characteristics:

Many or no questions

Verbalizes a lack of knowledge/understanding about the tracheostomy

Unable to perform new procedures for care

Goal:

The patient, a family member, or a significant other will know how to perform tracheostomy care.

Outcome Criteria

✔ The patient indicates a desire to learn necessary information.

✔ The patient knows the purpose of the tracheostomy.

✔ The patient and or family demonstrates proper tracheostomy care and suctioning techniques.

✔ The patient expresses an understanding of the care required for the tracheostomy.

✔ The patient verbalizes an understanding of follow-up care required and expresses a willingness to comply.

NOC *Knowledge: Treatment procedures*
Knowledge: Infection control
Knowledge: Treatment regimen
Knowledge: Health resources

INTERVENTIONS	RATIONALES
Assess the patient's current knowledge as well as his or her ability to learn and readiness to learn.	The teacher needs to ascertain what the patient already knows and build on this; if the patient is not capable of learning or is not ready to learn, teaching will not be effective due to the patient's disinterest or inability to understand.
Start with the simplest information and move to complex information.	Patients can understand simple concepts easily and then can build on those to understand concepts that are more complex.
Teach patient and significant others: — The purpose of tracheostomy — Tracheostomy care: cleansing, replacing, and suctioning (demonstrate this to family and patient) — Indications for suctioning — Oxygen therapy (how to administer, care for supplies, safety precautions) — Prevention of infection by covering opening with stoma guard or other covering to prevent particles from entering respiratory system — Importance of covering opening when coughing — Interventions for emergencies — Signs and symptoms of complications that would indicate a need to seek health care — Storage and care of supplies	Knowledge of how to carry out tracheostomy care and prevention of complications empowers the patient to take control and be compliant.
Provide rationales for performing each step in all skills taught.	Rationales for the steps increase understanding.
Allow adequate time for task mastery and have the patient or significant other return demonstrate performance of tracheostomy care and suctioning as often as required to become comfortable with procedure, performing the skills one step at a time.	The person performing the care should feel comfortable performing the procedure before discharge home, and the nurse needs to know that the patient can correctly perform this activity prior to discharge.
Teach patient and family measures to prevent infection: good hand washing, especially when working with tracheostomy;	The patient's first line of defense against organisms into the respiratory system has been lost, and vigilance

(continues)

(continued)

INTERVENTIONS	RATIONALES
avoidance of crowds, especially during flu season; adequate fluid intake; taking of flu and pneumonia vaccines, and adequate balanced nutrition.	is required to prevent respiratory infection.
Teach the patient oxygen therapy, as most patients with a tracheostomy have in-home oxygen to be used as needed; include delivery methods, safety requirements (no smoking or open flames), indicators for use of oxygen, care of equipment (when to replace tubing, mask, or cannula; cleaning).	Knowledge empowers the patient and can decrease anxiety; there is a need to have information relevant to oxygen so that the patient and family are already equipped to implement oxygen therapy if it is needed.
Assess the patient and family members' understanding of all teaching by encouraging them to repeat information, demonstrate all skills, and ask questions as needed.	This allows the nurse to hear in the patient's own words what was taught, allows for observation of skill performance to ensure the procedure is correct, and makes it easier to know what information may need to be reinforced.
Give the patient or family printed material that outlines the procedure and all information presented.	Printed materials can serve as a backup when the patient is at home and needs review or reinforcement.
Refer patient to home health nursing for follow-up and reinforcement of teaching once the patient is at home.	Once at home, the patient and family may have questions about the tracheostomy care or suctioning; the nurse also needs to be sure that procedures are being performed correctly.
Establish that the patient has the tracheostomy care supplies required to be compliant.	If needed resources such as finances and transportation to follow-up appointments are not available, the patient cannot be compliant; the nurse will need to make necessary referrals.

NIC *Learning readiness enhancement*
Learning facilitation
Teaching: Psychomotor skill

Evaluation

Evaluate the degree to which the patient has achieved the outcome criteria relevant to the teaching sessions. The patient should verbalize an understanding of the content presented by repeating the information. It is crucial that the patient or family demonstrate correct performance of tracheostomy care, suctioning, and application of oxygen. The nurse must determine whether the patient is capable of being compliant with the recommended regimen in terms of obtaining supplies, performing skills, and having necessary human and financial resources for assistance, as well as transportation for appointments. If further teaching is required at time of discharge, the appropriate referrals should be made to continue education.

Community/Home Care

The patient will need to implement the medical regimen in the home setting over an extended period. The success of this implementation will be dependent upon the degree to which the patient has received adequate teaching and has subsequently understood and internalized it. Home environments must be assessed for safety hazards (open flame heat sources and proper storage space) relevant to oxygen therapy. Even though the patient may not be on oxygen continuously at home, oxygen is required because of the risk for hypoxia secondary to suctioning or in case of respiratory complications. Crucial to successful in-home care is the patient and family's ability to perform tracheostomy care and suctioning. A home nurse should follow up with the family and patient to ensure that the procedure is carried out comfortably in the home and may actually want to plan to be present the first time the procedure is done. The nurse visiting the home should assess the environment, determine that equipment is stored properly, and provide recommendations as needed. Tracheostomy care supplies can be easily stored in a hard plastic storage box with a lid (purchased in any retail store) and labeled accordingly. Colorful covers for oxygen tanks not being used or suction apparatus can be made from fabric remnants of bright bed sheets.

Documentation

Document the specific content taught and the titles of any printed materials given to the patient. Include in the chart the patient's degree of understanding of the content and the methods used to teach and evaluate learning. Document the patient's ability to perform the psychomotor skill of tracheostomy care and suctioning. In addition, document any areas that need to be reinforced, to ensure appropriate follow-up. If family members are present for the teaching sessions, document this in the chart, and always document any referrals made.

 DISTURBED BODY IMAGE

Related to:

Presence of tracheostomy

Defining Characteristics:

Attempts to cover tracheostomy when visitors are present

Self-isolation

Negative statements about physical appearance

Goal:

The patient accepts the tracheostomy and continues social activities and interpersonal relationships.

Outcome Criteria

✔ The patient states willingness to look at and touch the tracheostomy site.

✔ The patient learns and participates in care of tracheostomy.

✔ The patient verbalizes satisfaction with body appearance.

NOC *Body image*

INTERVENTIONS	RATIONALES
Encourage the patient to communicate feelings about tracheostomy.	Talking about the tracheostomy may sometimes be the beginning of acceptance.
Teach the patient methods to cover the tracheostomy in a tasteful, unobtrusive way with scarves or other clothing.	Minimizing the visibility of the tracheostomy to others may make the patient feel better.
Teach patient and family how to care for the tracheostomy.	If the patient is comfortable caring for the tracheostomy, that comfort level may translate into acceptance for the tracheostomy and incorporation of body appearance change into a positive self-image.
Monitor the patient's feelings about self, interpersonal relationships with family members and friends, withdrawal, social isolation, fear, anxiety, embarrassment by appearance, fear that appearance will frighten loved ones, desire to be alone.	Helps to detect early alterations in social functioning and prevent unhealthy behaviors.
Encourage the patient to participate in at least one outside/public activity each week once health status permits.	Prevents the patient from isolating self from others.
Identify the effects of the patient's culture or religion on body image.	A patient's culture and religion often help define his or her reactions to changes in body image and self-worth.
Identify community support groups, if available.	Discussions with other patients with a similar situation who will be able to share thoughts with the patient will be beneficial and help the patient to deal with the change; in addition, the patient will be able to hear thoughts from those who understand what the patient is going through; this provides the patient with support and the courage to move forward in terms of acceptance of the change.

NIC *Body image enhancement*
Emotional support
Support group
Socialization enhancement

Evaluation

The patient is able and willing to learn about the care of the tracheostomy and begin to participate in self-care. Time is required for the patient to assimilate the change in body appearance into his or her self-perception completely. It is crucial that the nurse evaluate to what degree the patient is beginning to do this. Look for behaviors such as touching the site, looking at the tracheostomy in the mirror, or asking questions about its care. Communication of feelings and concerns relevant to the tracheostomy should be taken as a positive sign that progress towards meeting outcome criteria is being made.

Community/Home Care

At home, continued monitoring of the patient's body image is needed. The nurse who visits will need to be astute to subtle hints that may indicate that the patient has not completely adapted to the change in body appearance. Open discussions regarding this change and interventions to prevent social isolation and withdrawal should continue with the patient and family. Community support groups should be explored and encouraged, as they offer the patient and family a means to discuss their concerns openly with others who have had similar experiences. Association with others in the support group also allows the patient to socialize without concern that others may be staring at him or her, as other group members will have had experience with loved ones with the same type of alteration or be patients themselves. Small goals for the patient should be set. A starting place may be going to a public place once a week, perhaps an area where the patient is comfortable such as a religious or civic organization, or a park. If at any time the health care provider detects that the patient is becoming depressed or is totally socially withdrawn, other approaches to helping the patient adjust to disturbed body image should be implemented.

Documentation

Chart any specific behaviors or verbalizations that may indicate an altered body image. Include all interventions that have been employed to address this issue and the patient's response. Note when and if the patient begins to ask questions or expresses an interest in the care for the tracheostomy. Document all referrals in the patient record.

CHAPTER 2.34

TUBERCULOSIS (TB)

GENERAL INFORMATION

Tuberculosis (TB) is generally a primary respiratory disease caused by the bacterial agent mycobacterium TB. TB is a contagious disease whose primary means of transmission is through inhalation of TB-infected droplets, spreading from one human to another. Usually transmission is through coughing or sneezing; however, the organism can be spread when the infected person speaks or sings. The organism is slow growing. Even though TB is a respiratory disease, it can affect any organ. Secondary sites for TB are kidneys and genitourinary tract; cerebral meninges; and the bones and joints. With initial infection and in the early stages, there may be no symptoms; the disease may be identified on routine skin testing or chest x-ray. Common clinical manifestations of active disease when present are nonspecific and include fatigue, malaise, anorexia, weight loss, low-grade fevers, night sweats, and cough. The cough causes the person to seek medical advice, as it is frequent with the production of mucopurulent sputum and often blood-tinged sputum.

TB is a public health concern that showed a significant increase in incidence in the late 1980s and 1990s. Part of this increase has been attributed to the presence of TB in AIDS/HIV patients. Groups that are at higher risk of development of the disease are the immunosuppressed, the homeless, substance abusers, and those in correctional facilities. In the United States, immigrants have TB rates 8 times higher than that of people born in the United States. Case rates for blacks, Hispanics, and Native Americans are 7–8 times that of whites, while Asians and Pacific Islanders in the United States have a 20 times higher rate (Lemone and Burke, 2004). Those living in impoverished conditions, especially in urban areas, are also at higher risk. Adding to the problem of resurgence of cases is the emergence of multi-drug–resistant strains of mycobacterium TB.

NURSING DIAGNOSIS 1

 INFECTION (ACTUAL)*

Related to:

 Invasion of mycobacterium TB

Defining Characteristics:

 Positive tuberculin skin test

 Chest x-ray demonstrates active disease

 Culture positive for mycobacterium TB

 Low-grade fever

 Night sweats

 Cough with expectoration

 Fatigue

Goal:

 Infection will be resolved.

Outcome Criteria

✔ The patient will have three negative cultures following treatment.

✔ The patient will be afebrile.

✔ The patient will have no further symptoms, such as night sweats, cough, and fatigue.

✔ The patient will verbalize an understanding of isolation precautions required.

NOC *Infection severity*

 Community risk control:
   Communicable disease

 Knowledge: Infection control

INTERVENTIONS	RATIONALES
Monitor diagnostic studies: PPD (purified protein derivative) skin test for TB (also called Mantoux),	PPD is the initial screening for TB but is not diagnostic for active disease, only exposure to *(continues)*

(continued)

INTERVENTIONS	RATIONALES
pulmonary function studies, sputum culture/smear, bronchial washings culture/smear, chest x-ray, CBC (complete blood count).	the organism. A positive reading is represented by erythema and induration of > 10 mm after 48 hours; for immunocompromised patients such as HIV/AIDS patients an induration of > 5 mm is considered positive because of a delayed type hypersensitivity response, and in some cases no reaction to the PPD (anurgic) occurs at all. Sputum culture that is positive for mycobacterium TB provides a positive diagnosis; however, the organism is slow-growing, and it may take up to 4 weeks to be detected in the sputum specimen. Sputum smear for acid-fast bacilli is a quicker way to identify the tubercle bacillus; bronchial washings for culture and smears are obtained via bronchoscopy if the patient is unable to produce a sputum specimen; chest x-ray will demonstrate active disease. Complete blood count (CBC) will reveal elevated white blood cells.
Perform a complete respiratory assessment to include temperature every 4 hours, breath sounds, respiratory rate, presence of cough and expectoration (note color, amount, consistency, presence of blood); take a history from the patient noting recent travel to foreign countries or contact with relatives with TB.	Helps to detect symptoms of disease and their resolution, and to monitor the patient's response to treatment; the history may give clues as to where the patient may have contacted the disease.
Monitor results of oxygen saturation or arterial blood gases (ABGs), if ordered.	Reveals any alterations in the respiratory system's ability to maintain oxygenation and gas exchange.
If the patient is hospitalized, place him or her in respiratory isolation and follow agency isolation procedures, wearing a mask when entering the room and a gown and gloves if soiling is expected.	A special well-ventilated negative pressure room with scheduled air exchange is required, and use of isolation protocols is necessary to protect others.

Administer anti-TB medications as ordered, including isoniazid (INH), rifampin, ethambutol, pyrazinamide (PZA), and streptomycin, usually in a regimen of three different medications, and monitor for side effects:

— Isoniazid (INH) is a part of all treatment plans; monitor for peripheral neuropathy (tingling, numbness burning in hands or feet) and hepatotoxicity (anorexia, nausea, malaise, yellow skin, elevated liver enzymes, which should be done monthly during treatment for those at risk such as the elderly and alcoholics)

— Rifampin is a broad-spectrum antibiotic used with INH; monitor for signs of hepatotoxicity/hepatitis (elevation of liver enzymes, yellow skin, anorexia, nausea, malaise), which is the most common side effect of concern; rifampin frequently colors the urine red-orange, and patients should be aware of this to prevent alarm

— Pyrazinamide (PZA) is the third agent in the most common regimen (INH, rifampin, and PZA); monitor for hepatotoxicity as noted above; monitor for hyperuricemia, skin rash, and GI distress

— Ethambutol is only bacteriostatic, so is always used with other agents; monitor for optic neuritis resulting in blurred vision and disturbance of color discrimination; may recommend baseline testing of vision before therapy

— Streptomycin: monitor for injury to eighth cranial nerve, resulting in hearing loss and disturbance in balance, making elderly clients particularly prone to falls; monitor renal function studies (BUN, creatinine)

Anti-TB regimens always contain two or more drugs to decrease the risk for development of drug-resistant organisms. These medications will resolve the infection through bacteriocidal and bacteriostatic activities and protect the health of the larger community by stopping transmission. Monitoring for side effects allows for dosage adjustment and prevention of complications.

INTERVENTIONS	RATIONALES
Give oxygen as ordered and in accordance with arterial blood gases (ABGs) and oxygen saturation.	Respiratory infections cause impaired gas exchange and increase the work of breathing; oxygen will enhance oxygenation to tissues and decrease the work of breathing.
Place the patient in semi- or high-Fowler's position.	Increases chest excursion and ability to breathe adequately.
Have the patient cough and deep breathe.	Maximizes airway space and enhances expectoration of mucous.
In the hospital setting, implement strategies to prevent the spread of organisms: — Teach patient correct handling of secretions, and to cover mouth and nose when coughing or sneezing. — Keep tissues at bedside; tape plastic bag to bedrail for disposal or place wastebasket directly beside bed. — Teach and encourage use of frequent proper handwashing after handling secretions. — If patient leaves room, have him or her wear a mask. — Educate visitors regarding proper isolation procedures to be employed when visiting. — Be sure that isolation requirements are posted at the doorway. — Keep the door closed at all times.	Proper disposal of infectious items and minimizing droplet contact from person to person is standard to the prevention of the spread of organisms and is crucial to protect the public health.
Increase fluids if not contraindicated.	Helps to thin secretions.
Give a diet high in calories and rich in iron, protein, and vitamin C.	Fatigue is common, and these measures will give the patient needed nutrients for energy and healing. Iron-rich foods increase oxygen-carrying capacity of the blood.
Collaborate with other disciplines to protect community by assisting with identification of contacts and education of family for screening and prophylactic treatment.	Identifying contacts and providing prophylactic treatment of people who screen positive is crucial to halting the spread of disease and protection of lung function.
Conduct extensive teaching to the patient and family prior to discharge from hospital, or if in	Noncompliance is a serious threat with the regimen because of its length, and teaching is

the community setting, on repeated visits to an outpatient facility (see diagnosis "Ineffective Management of Therapeutic Regimen/Deficient Knowledge").

Make necessary referrals to the community health department or provide follow-up and assistance with carrying out the medication regimen.

crucial to teach the patient and others the importance of compliance with medication regimen exactly as prescribed.

TB is a public health concern, and follow-up with a public health entity is required.

NIC *Infection control*
Health screening
Communicable disease management
Infection protection
Medication management
Respiratory monitoring

Evaluation

Determine the extent to which the patient has achieved the expected outcomes. The patient should become afebrile, and the cough should diminish with little or no expectoration. Other symptoms, such as night sweats, also abate. Fatigue should improve, as should the patient's appetite. The patient should verbalize an understanding of the treatment measures being implemented and particularly those isolation precautions taken.

Community/Home Care

All patients with a diagnosis of TB will require some degree of follow-up and management by a public health program for prevention and management of communicable disease in keeping with the Centers for Disease Control guidelines. The patient, when discharged home, needs to be assessed for the ability to self-manage the disease and may require in-home visitation for further assessment and teaching reinforcement. The nurse should establish that the patient is taking all medications as prescribed by the physician and knows the importance of staying on the regimen for its duration. Follow-up sputum specimens will be needed to ascertain the effectiveness of treatment, and the patient needs to be clear on how and when these are to be done. There is no need for airborne precautions at home if family members have already been exposed to the disease. If the patient needs to go outside the home before cultures are negative, he or she should wear a mask and always avoid crowds. Cultures usually are negative within three months, and after three negative culture the patient is no longer considered infectious and can return to work or school. With special populations, such as the homeless or those at high risk for noncompliance, some area health departments have programs that require patients to come in to be observed taking the medications. Throughout the regimen, the patient should be monitored for side effects of the medications and referred appropriately for medical assistance. Effective teaching is crucial for the patient and family, and reinforcement is vital to ensure that the patient is managing the regimen as prescribed (see nursing diagnosis "Deficient Knowledge").

Documentation

Document the findings from a comprehensive respiratory assessment, with special attention to the presence or absence of cough and a description of the sputum. Include patient-specific complaints, such as fatigue, malaise, or anorexia. Always chart therapeutic interventions implemented and the patient's specific response to those interventions. Record results of PPD skin testing according to agency protocol. Document all teaching and referrals in the patient's record.

NURSING DIAGNOSIS 2

DEFICIENT KNOWLEDGE/INEFFECTIVE MANAGEMENT OF THERAPEUTIC REGIMEN

Related to:

New diagnosis of TB

Insufficient knowledge of TB

Noncompliance with therapeutic regimen due to lack of understanding

Complexity of prescribed regimen

Defining Characteristics:

Asks many questions

No prior history with TB

Asks no questions about health status

Verbalizes a lack of knowledge/understanding

Goal:

The patient verbalizes an understanding of required treatment regimen.

Outcome Criteria

✔ The patient verbalizes a desire to learn necessary information.

✔ The patient verbalizes a willingness to keep appointments and follow the prescribed regimen.

✔ The patient demonstrates knowledge of TB and how to prevent transmission.

✔ The patient demonstrates knowledge of medications to include name, dosage, scheduling, and side effects.

NOC   *Knowledge: Disease process*
        Knowledge: Treatment regimen
        Compliance behavior

INTERVENTIONS	RATIONALES
Assess the patient's current knowledge, as well as his or her ability to learn, readiness to learn, and risk for noncompliance.	Teachings need to be tailored to the patient's ability and willingness to learn for maximum effectiveness; assessment of the patient for likelihood of noncompliance will allow the nurse to intervene early.
Identify a family member or significant other who will also learn the content and assist the patient with compliance.	This person can reinforce the teaching and assist with implementation if the client becomes incapable of follow-through.
Create a quiet environment conducive to learning.	Environmental noise and distractions can prevent the learner from focusing on the content being taught.
Teach the learners the following information about TB: — Disease process of TB — Prevention of transmission to others (cover mouth when sneezing or coughing, proper disposal of tissues, good handwashing, avoidance of crowds) — In-home care required — Medications: (isoniazid,	Knowledge empowers the patients to take control and be compliant; stressing adherence to the regimen as prescribed will prevent relapse/reoccurrence of TB; often noncompliance becomes a problem because of the length of time of the regimen and a lack of understanding of the importance of completing the medications; identification

INTERVENTIONS	RATIONALES
rifampin, pyrazinamide, ethambutol, streptomycin) or others, as ordered, including action, side effects (see nursing diagnosis "Actual Infection"), dosing schedule, anticipated duration of therapy, and importance of adhering to the regimen for the duration as prescribed — Importance of good nutrition — Signs and symptoms of complications to be reported — Importance of complying with follow-up appointments for sputum cultures, chest x-rays, etc.	of side effects will minimize anxiety if these untoward effects should occur.
Be attuned to the patient's religious and cultural practices when teaching.	Culturally competent care that also considers religious practices is a holistic individualized approach that will enhance the likelihood that the prescribed changes will be assimilated into the patient's routine.
Teach the patient which signs and symptoms to report to a health care provider.	Monitoring for signs and symptoms early can prevent a crisis that requires hospitalization.
Ask the patient to repeat information and ask questions as needed.	This allows the nurse to hear in the patient's own words what was taught and makes it easier to know which information may need to be reinforced.
Establish that the patient has the resources required to be compliant.	If needed resources such as finances, transportation, and psychosocial support are not available, the patient cannot be compliant.
Refer to appropriate disciplines as needed or required for communicable diseases (social worker, public health agency, etc.).	These disciplines can provide additional services to help the patient be compliant with the prescribed regimen.
Give printed material to patient of information covered in the teaching session.	The patient may be more comfortable at home knowing that there is printed material for future reference.

NIC *Teaching: Disease process*
Teaching: Prescribed medication

Learning readiness enhancement
Learning facilitation

Evaluation

Evaluate the degree to which the patient has achieved the expected outcomes. The patient verbalizes an understanding of the content taught regarding the therapeutic regimen, particularly prescribed medications, is able to repeat all information for the nurse, and asks questions about the information. The patient should be able to identify all medications by name and report the common side effects as well as the dosing schedule and the length of time to take the medications. The patient should be able to inform the nurse about signs and symptoms that would necessitate contact with a health care provider. The nurse must determine that the patient is capable of being compliant, and it should also be ascertained whether the patient expresses a willingness to comply with the somewhat lengthy regimen. Once this is established, it is crucial to determine that the patient has the necessary resources and information to manage his TB at home.

Community/Home Care

For patients with TB, community and home care is crucial. Because of the complexity of the regimen with a variety of medications and the longevity of the therapy, the risk for noncompliance is high. Once at home, the patient may be unsure about ability to comply with the medical regimen. Successful management will depend on the patient's understanding of the information provided in teaching sessions and the internal motivation to implement health-promoting behaviors. The patient will need to implement strategies to prevent the transmission of the tubercle organism, including a basic strategy of covering mouth and nose when coughing or sneezing. Proper disposal of tissues in the home is important, and the client should use plastic bags to contain the tissues. Until sputum cultures are negative, the patient should not go to work or school and should wear a mask if out in public. Follow-up by a community health nurse is required once the patient is at home to check on medication administration and check for signs and symptoms of medication side effects. A large poster that outlines the schedule for medications can be made and posted in a prominent place. If it is determined that the patient is noncompliant, measures should be implemented to protect the public, such as identifying another person to administer the medications to the patient or having the patient travel to a clinic to be observed taking the medications.

Instructions regarding nutrition become most important once the patient is at home in order to help resolve fatigue and stamina. It will be important for health care providers to determine if the patient has incorporated these teachings into their routine by taking a dietary history that specifically asks about the preparation of nutritious meals that include foods high in vitamin C and protein. The patient's nutritional status and energy levels at subsequent appointments should be assessed to ensure that the patient is returning to his or her normal level of functioning as the disease improves.

Documentation

Document the specific content taught and the titles of printed materials given to patient or family. Chart the patient's and family member's understanding of the content, particularly the medication regimen and the methods used to evaluate learning. The nurse must clearly indicate areas that need to be reinforced. After the teaching session is complete, the nurse should assess whether the patient indicates a willingness to comply with health care recommendations. If the teaching included a family member or significant other, indicate this in the documentation. In addition, any referrals made should be documented in the patient record.

NURSING DIAGNOSIS 3

FATIGUE

Related to:

Infectious process (TB)

Fever

Decreased nutrition due to anorexia

Defining Characteristics:

Verbalization of being tired

States a lack of energy

Inability to carry out normal activities

Goal:

Fatigue will be relieved.

Outcome Criteria

✔ The patient is able to perform activities of daily living.

✔ The patient verbalizes that fatigue has improved or been eliminated.

NOC *Activity tolerance*
   Endurance
   Energy conservation
   Nutritional status: Energy

INTERVENTIONS	RATIONALES
Obtain subjective data regarding normal activities and limitations.	Determines the effect fatigue has on normal functioning.
Monitor the patient for signs of excessive physical and emotional fatigue.	Use as a guideline for adjusting activity.
Encourage periods of rest and activity.	Conserves oxygen and prevents undue fatigue.
Schedule activities so that excessive demands for oxygen and energy are avoided; for example, space planned activities away from meal times.	Digestion requires energy and oxygen; participation in activities close to meals will cause increased fatigue because of insufficient energy reserves.
Gradually increase activity as tolerated.	Use the results to indicate when activity may be increased or decreased.
Limit visitors during acute illness.	Socialization for long periods may cause fatigue.
Increase intake of high-energy foods such as meat (especially organ meats), poultry, dried beans and peas, whole grains, and foods high in Vitamin C.	These foods enhance energy metabolism, increase oxygen-carrying capacity, and provide ready sources of energy needed in hypermetabolic states such as infection and fever.
Encourage the patient to plan activities for time when he or she has the most energy, usually early in the day.	Prevents fatigue.

NIC *Energy management*

Evaluation

Obtain subjective information from the patient regarding the presence of fatigue. The patient should gradually report the ability to participate in activities of daily living and other normal activities with no fatigue.

Community/Home Care

Patients with TB should understand that even when at home, fatigue may persist until the infectious process is resolved. The patient must understand how to adjust activity in response to feelings of fatigue, possibly even arranging for rest or nap periods in the afternoon. Attention to good nutrition should continue with intake of foods that are good sources of iron, vitamin C, and protein. With the assistance of the nurse or a dietitian, develop a sample menu for the patient. Those giving nutritional recommendations can also make a list of foods that are acceptable for improving energy (such as those rich in iron) and make copies for the person who prepares the meals. The sample menu and list of foods should only be developed after consultation with the patient to consider cultural or religious restrictions, the patient's likes and dislikes, and his or her usual dietary routine. If fatigue persists for extended periods, the patient may need to seek health care to investigate the possibility of other causes of the fatigue.

Documentation

Chart the specific complaint of fatigue to include what activities the patient has been performing. Document interventions implemented to address fatigue, especially food intake. An assessment of the patient's sleep patterns and any strategies implemented to enhance sleep should also be documented.

CHAPTER 2.35

UPPER AIRWAY OBSTRUCTION

GENERAL INFORMATION

The upper airway can become obstructed for a variety of reasons, including tumors, blood emesis, tongue, fractured larynx, respiratory secretions and very commonly, aspiration of a foreign body. Maintenance of a patent airway is paramount in sustaining oxygenation to the body and maintaining life. Most patients automatically attempt to clear an occluded airway by coughing, provided that the cough mechanism is intact neurologically. Some groups of patients who are at high risk for airway obstruction include post-operative patients; patients with neurological impairments that have affected the gag/cough reflex, such as those resulting from cerebrovascular accidents or spinal cord injuries; those who are sedated; and the mentally challenged, who may be prone to placing foreign objects in their mouths. Interventions to re-establish the airway include Heimlich maneuver, cricothyrotomy, or tracheostomy.

NURSING DIAGNOSIS 1

INEFFECTIVE AIRWAY CLEARANCE

Related to:

Airway obstruction, mechanical or physiologic, causing hypoxia

Defining Characteristics:

Absent respirations

Cyanosis

Tachycardia

Nasal flaring

Wheezing

Stridor

Dyspnea

Holding throat and attempting to communicate

Goal:

The patient's airway is patent.

Outcome Criteria

✔ The patient's breath sounds will be present.

✔ The patient will have no cyanosis.

✔ The patient will be alert.

✔ The patient will have normal respirations without stridor, wheezing, nasal flaring, or dyspnea.

NOC *Respiratory status: Airway patency*
Respiratory status: Ventilation

INTERVENTIONS	RATIONALES
Assess respiratory status: breath sounds, respiratory rate, oxygen saturation, dyspnea, presence of cyanosis, retractions, use of accessory muscles, flaring of nostrils.	Absence of breath sounds may be noted; abnormal breathing patterns may signal worsening of condition; retractions, stridor, and flaring of nostrils indicate a significant decline in respiratory status and airway patency; establishes baseline and monitors response to interventions.
Monitor patient for signs of occluded airway: cyanosis, cessation of wheezing, a high-pitched sound or stridor when inhaling, inability to speak, absence of breath sounds over lungs, holding throat, or continuous coughing.	Occlusion of the airway results in no air movement, and therefore no breath sounds. Holding the throat and being unable to speak are classic signs of choking, and the patient may cough almost continuously in an attempt to open the airway.
Clear airway through suctioning or the Heimlich maneuver; if the patient becomes unconscious, perform the Heimlich maneuver and a finger sweep to remove	Blood and emesis can be removed via suctioning; the Heimlich maneuver forces air from the thoracic cavity to dislodge obstructions caused

INTERVENTIONS	RATIONALES
the object; or, if the object is visible, remove with ring forceps or suction.	by a foreign body, and physical removal of visible objects will clear the airway.
If surgical intervention is required for a cricothyrotomy or tracheostomy, prepare the patient according to agency protocol and assist as ordered.	Cricothyrotomy provides a temporary airway in an emergency situation, and tracheostomy provides a more permanent airway.
Assess mental status during periods when airway is obstructed and immediately following.	Lack of oxygen for even short periods can affect cerebral oxygenation, resulting in changes in mental status and level of consciousness.
Monitor arterial blood gases (ABGs) and oxygen saturation, as ordered.	ABG analysis will reveal respiratory acidosis, as the lungs are unable to expel carbon dioxide, and oxygen levels will be low, as the lungs are unable to take in oxygen and exchange gases.
Assess for anxiety and reassure the patient with presence.	Being unable to breathe causes anxiety and fear; the patient needs a calming presence; anxiety increases the demand for oxygen.
Provide humidified oxygen, as ordered, to maintain oxygen saturation at >90 percent.	Restores oxygenation to tissues.
Establish intravenous access.	Ensures a route for rapid-acting medications.
Place the patient in a high Fowler's position.	Maximizes chest excursion and subsequent movement of air.
Perform frequent respiratory assessments following reestablishment of airway: oxygen saturations, respiratory rate, rhythm, depth, color, and breath sounds.	Detects improvements in oxygenation status.
Monitor the patient for signs of aspiration into lungs: abnormal breath sounds, fever, and increased secretions.	Frequently when foreign objects (especially food) are in the airway, some particles may be aspirated into lungs and may cause aspiration pneumonia; monitoring the patient allows detection of early symptoms that may require further treatment.

NIC *Airway management*
Cough enhancement
Presence

Respiratory monitoring
Oxygen therapy
Ventilation assistance

Evaluation

Assess the client to determine the extent to which the outcome criteria have been met. Assessments of the respiratory system should reveal that acute symptoms of airway obstruction have been resolved. The patient's airway should be clear; the patient should be able to speak and should be breathing easy. Breath sounds should be present, and even though some mild wheezing may be noted as the respiratory system attempts to reestablish adequate respirations, this should be improved. Arterial blood gases (ABGs) and oxygen saturation should indicate adequate oxygenation, and there should be no cyanosis. The patient should be alert and back at a normal level of consciousness.

Community/Home Care

Little home care is required for the patient who has experienced airway obstruction, except as it applies to other disease processes that may have been present. If the patient has a tracheostomy as a result of upper airway obstruction, some assistance may be needed (see nursing care plan "Tracheostomy"). The patient and family should be aware of causes of obstruction and how to prevent a reoccurrence. Elderly patients, especially those with dentures, should be encouraged to chew food well before swallowing. Once at home, the patient who is mentally challenged should be closely monitored for the presence of objects that can be easily placed into the mouth. The patient and family will need to know the signs of airway obstruction and what interventions could be implemented prior to seeking emergency care. Family members may want to learn the Heimlich maneuver.

Documentation

Document a comprehensive respiratory assessment, including respiratory status during obstruction and the patient's status once problem has been resolved. Of particular note should be breath sounds, color, oxygenation status, respiratory rate, depth, and any nonverbal signs from the patient that he or she is having difficulty breathing. Include in the patient record interventions carried out to relieve the obstruction and the patient's response. If surgical interventions were required, document preparations carried out in preparation for surgery and postoperative nursing care provided. Note specifically changes in breath sounds in response to interventions and the patient's emotional state. Document vital signs according to agency protocol. Always include in the documentation the patient's progress towards achievement of the stated outcome criteria.

NURSING DIAGNOSIS 2

 ### IMPAIRED GAS EXCHANGE

Related to:

Hypoxia resulting from airway obstruction

Defining Characteristics:

Cyanosis

Decreased oxygen saturation

ABGs demonstrate hypoxia

Decreased level of consciousness

Goal:

Gas exchange is adequate.

Outcome Criteria

✔ The patient's arterial blood gases return to normal and oxygen saturation is > 90 percent.

✔ The patient's skin color improves.

✔ The patient's respiratory rate is within baseline.

✔ The patient reports no dyspnea/shortness of breath.

✔ The patient's level of consciousness improves.

NOC   *Respiratory status: Ventilation*
Respiratory status: Gas exchange
Vital signs

INTERVENTIONS	RATIONALES
Assess respiratory status: skin color, breath sounds, respiratory rate, rhythm, quality, and effort.	Establishes baseline information about respiratory function.
Assess oxygen saturation using pulse oximetry and arterial blood gases (ABGs), as ordered.	Helps to determine the status of oxygen to tissues and to monitor for respiratory acidosis.
Monitor for altered mental status: restlessness, anxiety, and confusion.	These symptoms may indicate decreased oxygenation to cerebral tissues.
Provide supplemental oxygen as ordered.	Maximizes oxygen saturation, overcomes oxygen deficit that occurred with obstruction, and relieves shortness of breath.
Place in high Fowler's position.	This position allows for better chest expansion and subsequent air exchange.
Give bronchodilators if ordered (orally or inhaled via nebulizer or handheld inhaler) and evaluate effectiveness.	Opens narrowed airways and improves gas exchange; airways that have become obstructed may have bronchospasms following establishment of a patent airway.
If thick secretions are present due to underlying lung disease, give mucolytics or expectorants.	Assists with mucous excretion to clear lungs of substances that cause obstruction and increased vascular resistance.
Have patient perform coughing and deep breathing if able.	Prevents stasis of secretions, opens airways, and improves gas exchange.
Allow a balance of rest and activity; encourage rest before and after activity, assisting with activities of daily living.	Conserves oxygen reserves and prevents exacerbation of hypoxia.

NIC   *Oxygen therapy*
Respiratory monitoring
Acid base management:
     Respiratory acidosis
Positioning

Evaluation

Evaluate the status of outcome criteria. The patient should have indicators of good gas exchange, such as even, easy respirations, good skin color, and an oxygen saturation of at least 90 percent. Blood gas analyses should indicate an absence of respiratory acidosis and oxygen levels between 80–100 percent. The patient should report an absence of shortness of breath and respirations within baseline. Mental status should return to baseline levels and the patient should not be restless or agitated.

Community/Home Care

For most patients, once the airway obstruction has been relieved, gas exchange is also corrected.

The patient may notice some fatigue when at home due to loss of oxygen reserves, but this also should resolve. Resting for short periods during the day can help with fatigue until the patient's usual energy level returns. Good nutrition rich in iron can assist the patient with energy. These simple measures at home should be all that is required. If any indicators of impaired gas exchange persist, such as intolerance to activities, the patient should know to contact his or her health care provider.

Documentation

Included in the documentation should be a complete respiratory assessment. Chart all interventions and the patient's specific response. Document the results of oxygen saturation readings and arterial blood gases (ABGs), as they represent the best measure of gas exchange. If the patient still has indicators of impaired gas exchange, these should be specifically noted along with any revisions to the plan of care made.

UNIT 3
NEUROLOGICAL SYSTEM

CHAPTER 3.36

ALZHEIMER'S DISEASE

Alzheimer's disease is an irreversible central nervous system disorder classified as a form of dementia and characterized by progressive deterioration of intellectual functioning. The etiology of Alzheimer's disease is unknown, but current theories include the loss of neurotransmitter stimulation by choline acetyltransferase, viral infections, and genetic defects. Pathophysiologically, the disease is characterized by neuritic plaques and neurofibrillary tangles (fibers that are twisted inside neurons). The degenerative changes that take place result in a decreased number of functioning neurons leading to the clinical manifestations seen in the disease. Alzheimer's disease is typically categorized into three stages. Stage I is demonstrated in the earliest sign of disease: short-term memory loss that is initially mild and is usually attributed to "becoming forgetful." There is decreased attention span, some mild personality changes, and often the patient forgets the names of objects. During this phase, it is easy to mask the deficits from others. Stage II shows more obvious impaired cognition with more pronounced personality changes, with the patient demonstrating agitation, sometimes violent behavior, serious memory deficits, confusion, inability to write as usual, or to recognize objects by touch. In addition, the patient begins to wander, which poses a serious safety problem. As this stage progresses, the patient's ability to make decisions and use judgment become more impaired, along with the presence of poor social skills and motor skills, leading to a limited ability to perform activities of daily living. It is during this stage that family members must make decisions regarding driving and allowing the patient to cook or be alone. Stage III of the disease is characterized by a total inability to care for self, with communication and motor skills totally lacking and the patient becoming bedridden and totally incontinent. In addition, a large number of patients experience difficulties eating. It is during this stage that the family usually makes decisions regarding alternative living arrangements. Dementia of the Alzheimer's type (DAT) represents approximately two-thirds of all types of dementia (Lemone and Burke, 2004). DAT has a usual onset between age 50 and 60, and the disease is estimated to affect over 4 million Americans. There are no diagnostic tests to confirm the disease, but other causes for the symptoms such as electrolyte imbalances, vitamin deficiencies, thyroid disease, parathyroid disease, hypoglycemia, and excessive use of drugs and alcohol are ruled out.

NURSING DIAGNOSIS 1

 ### DISTURBED THOUGHT PROCESSES (EARLY STAGE)

Related to:

Effects of disease

Decreased number of functioning neurons

Defining Characteristics:

Inability to make decisions

Confusion

Getting lost

Inability to continue conversations

Impaired judgment

Goal:

The patient will be oriented to reality to the extent possible.

Outcome Criteria

✔ The patient will state his or her name.

✔ The patient will state where he or she is.

✔ The patient will participate in daily activities.

✔ The patient will recall one meaningful experience from his or her past.

NOC *Cognition*
Cognitive orientation
Memory
Information processing
Decision-making

INTERVENTIONS	RATIONALES
Assess patient's level of cognitive impairment/deficit monitoring for reality perceptions, expression ability, memory, recognition, impaired judgment, impaired memory (does not recognize family members), decreased concentration, increased inappropriate activity (e.g., undressing, climbing out of bed), verbal aggressiveness, physical aggressiveness, confusion.	Establishes a baseline of the patient's functioning for planning care and monitoring for stabilization or improvement. In the early stage, cognitive impairment may be slowed with medical intervention.
Provide a low-stimulation environment.	Numerous stimuli coming into the patient increase confusion because of the amount of cognition required for processing.
Call patient by name and tell him or her where he or she is.	Orients the patient to reality and attempts to preserve function; reality orientation is only appropriate in early disease.
Place familiar objects in the patient's rooms (pictures, favorite chairs, or pillows, etc.) and label pictures with names.	Familiar objects help orient the patient to reality; demented patients can often remember familiar objects, and these also help decrease agitation.
Have patient wear glasses or hearing aids at all times if possible.	These will assist the patient to identify sensory input correctly.
Play the radio or television at certain periods of the day when the time and date are likely to be told or shown (i.e. during the news).	Hearing the time and date will serve as reality orientation for the patient.
Talk to the patient and ask him or her to tell stories about his or her past.	The patient's long-term memory may still be intact, and talking about things remembered provides comfort.
Assist the patient in decision-making regarding basic needs, but allow the	With a limited need for detailed cognitive function, the patient will feel more
patient to perform as much self-care as possible.	in control and not agitated; allowing him or her to participate in care promotes independence that may help maintain some degree of cognitive function and maintains optimal function.
Give one instruction at a time and repeat instructions as needed.	The patient cannot process more than one command at a time; repetitions assist the patient in retaining information.
Speak slowly, calmly, and with short phrases, and adjust communication style to the patient's needs.	Speaking slowly allows the patient time to think and process; too many phrases in one statement may be too much for the patient to process.
Maintain routines in care if possible, whether at home or in other settings.	Routines enhance the likelihood that the patient will remember what to expect and promotes a feeling of security; decreases agitation.
Administer cholinesterase inhibitor medications, such as Aricept® (donepezil hydrochloride) and Exelon® (rivastigmine), as ordered, and monitor for side effects.	In the early stages of Alzheimer's, these medications are given to raise the acetylcholine level in the cerebral cortex to improve cognitive function. However, the benefits are short-term only. Common side effects include headache, nausea/vomiting, and diarrhea, but these usually subside in about 1 week.

NIC *Reality orientation*
Dementia management

Evaluation

Determine whether the stated outcome criteria have been met. In the early stage of the disease, the patient should be able to state his or her name and where he or she is. Participation in daily activities to their maximum capability should be allowed. The patient communicates about meaningful life experiences from long-term memory. Inability to meet outcome criteria indicates progression from the early stage of the disease and the need to revise the plan of care.

Community/Home Care

Care of the patient with Alzheimer's disease at home will prove to be challenging as cognitive functioning continues to deteriorate, leaving the family with the dilemma of how to cope. Early in the disease process, the family or significant other can implement all of the above interventions to attempt to preserve as much cognitive function as possible and slow the memory loss. Making each day routine and creating a familiar environment may help the patient with memory loss. Orienting the patient to reality calmly and firmly sometimes helps in early disease. Place a large colorful calendar in a prominent place so the patient can see the year and date. Plan periods when the patient can have a one-on-one conversation with a special person (family member or friend). If the patient is still able, encourage reading or word puzzles. Even simple tasks such as choosing clothes can make the patient's thought processes worse. In some instances, home videos of earlier times will increase a patient's ability to continue to recognize family members and also provide comfort to the person. The greatest threat to well-being is when the confusion and memory loss create issues of safety. Common occurrences are forgetting to turn stoves off or leaving food cooking on the stove and forgetting how to get back home when driving (see nursing diagnosis "Risk for Injury"). The family and significant others will need to remain astute observers in order to detect deteriorating cognitive function and implement strategies that will allow the patient to remain as independent as possible. It is important that the family make determinations regarding the patient's ability to manage his or her own affairs (business, financial, and health care decisions) early in the disease before a crisis occurs. Family members will need to be assisted in their efforts to cope with the changing personality and functional levels of their loved one as they make tough decisions regarding care options as the patient's mental and physical status deteriorate. Even though medications help the memory loss and cognitive function, its benefits tend to disappear after several years.

Documentation

Document the findings from a complete neurological/ psychological assessment. Be sure to specify what the patient can and cannot do, and the extent of cognitive impairments. If the patient is in the hospital setting, document any medications given and the presence of any side effects. Always include in your documentation any teaching done with family or significant others. Document all

interventions added to the plan of care for the patient, whether in the hospital or as part of a home health caseload.

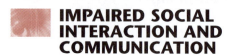

NURSING DIAGNOSIS 2

IMPAIRED SOCIAL INTERACTION AND COMMUNICATION

Related to:

　　Reduced cognitive abilities

　　Loss of memory

　　Judgment deficits

　　Disorientation

Defining Characteristics:

　　Inappropriate use of language

　　Inappropriate social behaviors

　　Social isolation

　　Inability to recognize family members and friends

Goal:

　　The patient engages in social interactions that are appropriate for his or her cognitive level and behavioral response.

Outcome Criteria

✔ The patient will have one social activity per week.

✔ The patient will have a reasonable and appropriate conversation with one person.

INTERVENTIONS	RATIONALES
Encourage frequent but brief visits by family and friends other than the caregiver.	These types of visits provide minimally stimulating, short periods where the patient may interact. Frequency may help with memory in early stages.
Encourage frequent periods of social interaction by caregivers (hospital or home).	The patient will get used to these short interactions and may be able to modify behaviors, as expectations are minimal.
Discuss things that were of interest to the patient.	Talking about things that were pleasant and enjoyable to the patient may help to stimulate recall; be aware that the disease may prevent the patient from responding.

INTERVENTIONS	RATIONALES
Provide opportunities for social interactions appropriate for the patient's level of functioning, such as taking a walk with one other person, having a visit from a clergy, looking at old photographs, watching an old movie with scenes that may be familiar, or going for a ride.	Simple interactions that do not threaten the patient can decrease confusion and thus agitation; this will help to keep the patient's frustration level low. On the other hand, if the patient is bored, confusion may also increase and cognitive function decrease more.
Set limits.	When the patient's behavior becomes unacceptable, clear limits must be set. The patient should be corrected or removed from the situation.
When communicating with the patient, talk directly to him or her; use simple sentences, ask one question at a time, do not rush the patient, and above all do not argue with the patient.	Simple communication techniques are required to prevent agitation and frustration by the patient. Simple, unrushed communication will enhance the likelihood that the patient will respond favorably. Arguing with the patient increases agitation and anxiety, and may lead to emotional or violent outbursts.
Plan for rest periods in home or hospital.	Fatigue tends to increase confusion and agitation, precluding the patient from appropriate social interactions/communications.
During meals, enhance appropriate social interactions by removing distractions and making the table simple in appearance. Serve the patient one or two foods at a time.	Having numerous items on the table around the patient allows his or her thoughts to wander away from the task at hand, which is eating. Likewise, having to decide between what to eat may produce anxiety, as the patient cognitively cannot make such a choice. Frustration may occur, which could further affect ability to remain socially active, even with family members.
Investigate the possibility of attendance at senior centers or Alzheimer's day care centers.	These sites are designed to work with people who may need encouragement to interact, and staff members have usually received some training in communicating with people with acute confusion. This is a method of keeping the patient in a structured social environment and provides respite for caregivers.

NIC *Behavior management*
Calming technique
Dementia management
Limit setting
Socialization enhancement

Evaluation

Determine if the outcome criteria have been met. The patient should be able to participate in social activities or interactions, as conditions allow, with at least one person. The patient is able to communicate with caregivers or other family members without agitation.

Community/Home Care

It is important for caregivers and family members to continue to engage the patient in social interactions for as long as possible. Activities at home that allow for interaction with others must be simple and relaxed, as stressful interactions or situations may create anxiety, frustration, and agitation. Suggested activities include quiet walks with one person, short visits with familiar people, or participation in small group activities such as those at senior centers or Alzheimer's day care centers. Communication with the patient with DAT may become challenging as the disease progresses, making social activities impossible or extremely difficult. Many DAT patients experience prosopagnosia (an inability to recognize self or other familiar people), which makes social interactions even more difficult. Caregivers should place pictures of familiar people who are likely to visit in the home and label the pictures with names in bold bright letters. Periodically reminiscing with the patient about these people by calling their names may also encourage the patient to talk more. All family members should be taught appropriate socialization strategies and communication techniques, as outlined in the interventions above.

Documentation

Include in the patient record the patient's ability to interact with others, especially the appropriateness of conversation. Document all strategies employed to enhance social interactions and communications, as well as information shared with family members on how to communicate or enhance interactions. In addition, document in the record any referrals made to social workers or community resources, such as adult day care centers.

NURSING DIAGNOSIS 3

 ### RISK FOR INJURY

Related to:

Impaired cognitive function

Confusion

Poor judgment

Decreased motor skills

Defining Characteristics:

Leaves cooking stove on

Leaves food on stove

Falls

Locks self out of house

Unable to state home address

Drives carelessly

Wanders away from home

Cannot care for self

Goal:

The patient will be safe.

Outcome Criteria

✔ The patient will not sustain injury from the stove.

✔ The patient will not be involved in an automobile accident.

✔ The patient will not become lost.

✔ A safe, healthy home or institutional environment is provided.

✔ The family is able to access the resources available in the community.

NOC *Safe home environment*

Risk detection

Risk control

INTERVENTIONS	RATIONALES
Assess home environment for unsafe conditions, and remove or minimize any hazards.	Removal of hazardous objects may prevent the patient from harming him or herself.
When it is determined that the patient cannot safely cook, remove knobs from stove or	As the disease progresses, forgetfulness worsens; patients who try to cook increase the
place safety caps or covers over them.	risk for injury; implementing simple safety measures prevents injuries.
As cognitive function deteriorates, stop patient from driving by taking keys to automobiles.	Patients will attempt to drive, not realizing their own cognitive impairment, and become disoriented in familiar territory, creating frustrations that lead to inability to manipulate the highway; in many instances, patients become lost. At this point, the patient becomes a threat to others' safety; taking keys protects the patient and the public.
Remove dangerous cleansing substances from kitchen cabinets or put safety caps on all such items.	Liquids in colorful containers in the kitchen may be mistaken for juices.
Put safety caps on all medications and keep away from the patient.	Due to cognitive impairment with short-term memory loss, the patient may not be able to determine whether he or she has had his or her medications and may take an overdose.
Have the patient wear an identification bracelet at all times with his or her name and the number of a contact person.	If the patient wanders off or becomes lost while driving, others can identify them and notify caregivers.
Involve the patient in activities, such as walks or housework.	These activities decrease restlessness and boredom.
When the patient is found wandering, calmly redirect him or her to another desirable place.	Redirecting the patient towards a different place can distract the patient from his or her original destination and return the patient back to a safe environment. The patient has very little short-term memory and therefore may not recall where he or she was were headed.
If the patient smokes, remove cigarettes and matches or lighters.	Ensures safety of patient and others.
Remove any guns or other weapons and lock in a safe place.	The patient may not recognize these items as dangerous and cannot recall their proper use, predisposing the patient and others to injury.
Caregivers should keep a spare key with them or keep one somewhere outside.	It is likely that in the early stages of the disease the patient may go outside the home and inadvertently lock the door, or

INTERVENTIONS	RATIONALES
	the patient may lock the door while inside leaving the caregiver locked outside. The patient may be unable to follow commands to unlock the door; having a spare key available can prevent frustrations.
Provide constant supervision as the disease progresses.	As the disease progresses, the patient may experience apraxia (inability to use objects correctly) and agnosia (loss of sensory comprehension), which increase the risk for unintentional self-inflicted injury.
Provide meals for the patient that can be warmed in the microwave and allow the patient to assist with warming as abilities allow.	Meals that are prepared in advance by the caregiver that do not require much preparation will facilitate meal preparation and decrease frustration by the patient. Other options include agencies such as Meals on Wheels.
Determine whether assistance is required.	A home health aide or other similar service may be utilized so that the patient is assured adequate personal care each day.
If possible, place large bright pieces of tape on floors by doorways/exits or place purchased appliqué stop signs on doors.	The patient will be attracted to these, causing them to become distracted from their original plan of attempting to exit the home. The caregiver can then redirect the patient.
When the patient is hospitalized, he or she should be placed close to the nurse's station and away from stairwells or other exits.	Being close to the nurse's station allows for better supervision, and removal from close proximity to exits prevents easy escape.

NIC *Environmental management: Safety*

Risk identification

Surveillance: Safety

Evaluation

Outcome criteria have been achieved. The patient is protected in the home or institutional setting. Throughout the disease, the patient does not sustain injury or injure others. There are no instances of fires, automobile accidents, being lost, or wandering.

Community/Home Care

Safety at home is a major issue for both family and patient. For a period of time, the patient may be safe in his or her own home where the surroundings are familiar, but as the patient's thought processes continue to deteriorate, the ability to make good decisions and judgments also decreases, making familiar environments dangerous. The biggest safety issues involve cooking and driving. Taking car keys from a loved one is usually an emotionally charged event, as in most instances the patient does not agree to the action. This signals a major change in the patient's ability to function independently, but the action is required to ensure the safety of the patient and others. The loss of cooking capabilities may serve as a source of frustration, especially for women, but must cease due to the high risk for setting the home on fire. The local fire department may offer suggestions for how to disable the stove knobs, or appliance stores can offer assistance on how to remove knobs. Simple measures such as placing a key outside or keeping one with a neighbor can prevent frustration if the nurse or caregiver needs to enter the house but the patient refuses entry or cannot understand how to unlock the door. The patient should wear an identification bracelet with his or her name and contact information inscribed on it. The family should check frequently to be sure that the bracelet remains on, as the patient's confusion may cause him or her to remove it from time to time. Bracelets that look like a regular piece of jewelry are less likely to be removed by the patient. Many in-home alarm systems have mechanisms that announce which door is being opened without the actual burglar alarm sounding. This would be an ideal mechanism to activate in the home as it would alert the caregiver to doors opening and allow them to check to see if it were the patient exiting. As family members attempt to safety-proof the home, they may experience psychological stress as they realize that their loved one is losing the ability to care for him or herself. It is at this time that the family or caregiver may require the assistance of support groups specifically for Alzheimer's caregivers or home health agencies (see nursing diagnosis "Caregiver Role Strain"). At home, the caregiver and family members will need to examine the interventions listed above and tailor them to meet the needs of the patient, with a major focus on ensuring patient safety. The family may also find other helpful hints on safety from the Alzheimer's Association, the Alzheimer's Disease and

Related Disorders Association, or the Alzheimer's Disease Education and Referral Center.

Documentation

Chart in the patient record teaching done with the family regarding measures to take to ensure safety of the patient. Document all interventions employed to protect the patient and the patient's emotional response. Any concerns and fears that the family expresses should be charted. Referrals to community agencies are included in the patient record.

NURSING DIAGNOSIS 4

SELF-CARE DEFICIT: BATHING/HYGIENE, TOILETING, FEEDING, DRESSING/GROOMING

Related to:

Impaired cognitive function

Poor motor skills

Confusion

Progression of disease

Defining Characteristics:

Unable to dress self appropriately

Incontinent of urine and feces

Requires assistance with eating

Unable to bathe self

Goal:

The patient's basic needs of hygiene, dressing/grooming, feeding, and toileting will be met.

Outcome Criteria

✔ The patient will not choke or aspirate on foods.

✔ The patient will consume enough food to avoid weight loss.

✔ The patient will be clean and have no body odors.

✔ The patient will remain dry.

✔ The patient will have regular bowel movements and be cleansed.

✔ The patient will have no skin breakdown due to urine or fecal incontinence.

INTERVENTIONS	RATIONALES
Assess the patient's ability to perform activities of daily living.	Determine what type and how much assistance the patient may require.
Encourage the patient to do as much as possible.	Participating in care, even in limited ways, helps to maintain function and provides stimulation for the patient. This fosters some sense of independence.
When assisting the patient, divide the tasks to be done into simple steps and give instructions simply and one at a time.	The patient can follow through on simple step-by-step instructions but cannot process detailed instructions; simple instructions also decrease the chance of frustration or agitation when the patient cannot follow through.
Bathing: Offer the patient a bath regularly and make this as routine as possible, recognizing that the patient may not accept a daily bath. Gather supplies for the patient and proceed to instruct the patient if the patient is unable to follow through with bathing independently. Caregivers may need to be as simplistic as telling the patient to "wet the cloth, put soap on the cloth, now rub cloth on your arm," and so forth. Do not argue with the patient about taking a bath; leave supplies in plain view, which may stimulate the patient to want to use them. Provide a bath to the patient in late disease.	Elderly patients do not necessarily need daily total baths; arguing with the patient only increases agitation and may make the patient more uncooperative. When the patient sees the items needed for the bath, he or she may decide to use them. However, in the later stages the caregiver will need to bathe the patient.
Dressing/Grooming: Use clothes that are easy for the patient to put on. Place an entire outfit together on a hanger, including items such as underwear, socks/hose, shirt, and pants. Place items needed for personal care such as toothbrushes, toothpaste, combs, and hairbrushes within the patient's view to stimulate the patient to use them.	As motor skills deteriorate, the ability to dress becomes more difficult, especially the use of zippers, buttons, and ties. Gathering an entire outfit limits the decision-making required of the patient. In later stages, the patient will require total assistance for dressing.
Toileting: Take the patient to the bathroom at scheduled intervals (every 2 hours) for urination. For bowel movements, take the patient to the bathroom following breakfast. When the patient	Scheduled trips to the bathroom may increase the likelihood that the patient will use the bathroom and prevent incontinent episodes. Thirty minutes to 1 hour following breakfast is the natural

INTERVENTIONS	RATIONALES
becomes incontinent, check him or her frequently, and keep the patient clean and dry.	time for increased peristalsis, which improves likelihood that bowel evacuation will occur. In stage two, the patient becomes incontinent because of loss of cognitive function, and in stage 3 the patient is totally dependent for all needs and is usually bedridden, requiring incontinent pads and frequent checking and cleaning to prevent skin breakdown.
Limit fluids after 6 p.m. in the evening.	Limiting fluids in the evening will decrease the patient's nighttime incontinent episodes.
Feeding: Create a pleasant environment for meals. Allow the patient to feed self for as long as possible. Offer finger foods or foods easy to manipulate with a fork or spoon, but do not place more than a couple of food items on the plate at a time. As the ability to use utensils decreases, provide finger foods, such as sandwiches and chunks of vegetables. As the disease progresses, caregivers may need to tell the patient to chew and swallow with each bite. Do not force-feed the patient. If the patient resists eating, leave the food within sight so that the patient can see it and consume it later.	These efforts decrease the frustration that can come with being unable to feed oneself appropriately. In some instances, the patient does not have adequate cognitive functioning to remember to get the next bite of food or to chew it and swallow it. In late disease, the patient will require feeding by a caregiver and may eventually progress to the stage of not being able to chew and swallow.
Turn bedridden patients turn every 2 hours.	Relieves pressure on areas at high risk for skin breakdown (see nursing care plan "Pressure Ulcers").

NIC *Self-care assistance: Toileting*

Self-care assistance: Dressing/grooming

Self-care assistance: Feeding

Self-care assistance: Bathing/grooming

Evaluation

All outcome criteria have been achieved or reasons for non-achievement are noted. The patient is bathed and kept clean, dry, and odor-free. The patient eats appropriately and is able to participate in mealtime activities. Incontinent episodes are minimized by taking the patient to the bathroom at scheduled intervals or as requested. No skin breakdown occurs. The patient has his or her self-care needs met with minimal incidences of agitation.

Community/Home Care

Adjusting to the patient's decreasing ability to take care of his or her most basic needs often creates a great challenge for in-home caregivers. As the patient's mental status deteriorates, he or she may refuse to bathe or change clothes for several days, not realizing why it is necessary to do so. Attempts to force the patient to comply are usually futile, only creating agitation and frustration for both patient and caregiver. Efforts to increase compliance will need to be creative. In some instances, just leaving cues for the patient that may peak his or her curiosity will work, such as leaving a brightly colored towel and washcloth within the patient's view along with other personal care items. Purchase clothing that pulls on easily, avoiding small buttons that require significant dexterity. The patient may not be able to make multiple decisions regarding selection of clothes, such as picking out a blouse to go with pants. Place clothing items together to make an entire ensemble so that the patient's decision-making is simple. Protect the clothing during mealtimes, as getting the patient to change when soiled may prove to be difficult. If possible, involve the patient in the preparation of meals on a limited basis. It is important that the patient have enough time to eat, and that independence is maintained as long as possible. Caregivers should prepare foods for the patient that are nutritious but also easy for the patient to eat. For instance, instead of serving a chicken breast, which the patient may get frustrated trying to eat, offer chicken fingers or legs that the patient can easily eat without having to use fork or knife. Due to the short-term memory loss, patients frequently report that they have not eaten even though meals have been consumed; in this case offer the patient simple snacks that are low in calories or fats, such as fresh vegetables or fruits, or toast and juice. During the early stages of Alzheimer's the patient may remain able to respond to signals for the need to toilet him or herself. However, as time progresses, the patient simply cannot respond and may be unable even to locate the bathroom. Caregivers should take note of the patient's usual pattern of voiding and having bowel movements and establish a scheduled toileting plan that mimics the patient's normal routine. Taking the patient to the bathroom every 2 hours for urination may assist in keeping the patient dry, and encouraging him or her to sit on the toilet for a period of time following breakfast will assist in bowel evacuation. If the patient has an easy view of the bathroom, he or she may be prompted to use it, and some caregivers have suggested placing a picture of a bathroom or commode on the door of the bathroom for this purpose. Having a portable toilet in plain view for the patient is another way of prompting use of the bathroom. All of these efforts will require patience and a time commitment by the caregiver. As cognitive function continues to deteriorate, other behaviors that may occur include fecal smearing by the patient or using inappropriate sources for elimination such as the trashcan, as the patient may perceive this as the appropriate place for the activity. For many families, the decision to institutionalize the patient occurs when the patient becomes incontinent, especially of bowel. As the disease takes its toll, the patient becomes totally dependent for all activities of daily living and may even stop communicating in any way. The family needs to plan for the care requirements when this stage is reached. When addressing the self-care needs of the patient, the nurse and family must consider the agencies that are available to provide some in-home assistance for personal care and seek out referrals.

Documentation

Whether the patient is in the home or in an institution, a health care provider should document the level of functioning for the patient in all areas of self-care. Document incontinent episodes and record intake and output as required. In addition, include in the record the ability or willingness of the patient to eat and how much the patient eats. Chart any interventions employed to enhance self-care efforts and whether they have been successful.

NURSING DIAGNOSIS 5

CAREGIVER ROLE STRAIN

Related to:

    Change of pattern in daily activities for caregiver

    Caregiver is unfamiliar with the type of care that must be provided

    Caregiver must also work outside the home

    Caregiver gets no breaks

    Community resources unknown, unavailable, or not affordable

Defining Characteristics:

    Caregiver expresses frustration, anger, and sadness

    Caregiver states that he or she does not know how to care for loved one

    Caregiver not satisfied with community resources

    Caregiver unable to provide level of care required

Goal:

    The caregiver reports satisfaction with caregiving role.

    The caregiver is able to recognize when he or she can no longer handle the complete or partial care of the patient.

Outcome Criteria

✔ The caregiver reports that he or she is not experiencing stress.

✔ The caregiver identifies at least one source of support.

✔ The caregiver verbalizes the ability to handle the responsibilities of caring for the patient and coordinating care of the patient.

NOC   *Caregiver emotional health*
               Caregiver lifestyle disruption
               Caregiver stressors
               Caregiver well-being

INTERVENTIONS	RATIONALES
Teach the caregiver about the disease and the disease process.	Understanding the disease assists the caregiver in understanding why the patient is behaving the way he or she is and what to expect in the future.
Assist the caregiver in planning for care of the patient.	The caregiver will need assistance in planning for the care of the patient, including access to home health care and other community services. The

INTERVENTIONS	RATIONALES
	caregiver can plan for scheduled breaks away from the patient.
Encourage the caregiver to express feelings about his or her role as a caregiver, allowing time for venting frustrations, anxieties, and fears.	The first step towards coping with a change in life is to identify positive and negative feelings about the situation.
Teach the caregiver how to care for the patient properly, including communication techniques and techniques to provide basic needs of toileting, feeding, bathing, and dressing (see nursing diagnoses "Disturbed Thought Processes" and "Self-Care Deficits")	Having the knowledge to care for the patient decreases anxiety.
Encourage the caregiver to identify and utilize relaxation and stress reduction techniques, such as music therapy, quiet walks, meditation, exercise, etc.	The caregiver must utilize these strategies to prevent stress and anxiety that may negatively influence his or her ability to be an effective care provider.
Encourage the primary caregiver to identify one other family member, friend, or significant other who can provide short periods of relief.	The caregiver may need short periods of relief in order to run errands or regroup his or her thought processes, especially on demanding days.
Encourage the use of outside services, such as Meals on Wheels or home health aides, in the home.	These services can relieve some of the hardship of providing care to the Alzheimer's disease patient and allow the patient to remain in the home.
Refer the caregiver to local chapters of the Alzheimer's Association or Alzheimer's Disease and Related Disorders Association to identify location and meeting dates/times for support groups.	These organizations offer educational materials and sponsor support groups. Participation in support groups allows the caregiver to talk to others and garner support from others that are experiencing the same challenges. Caregivers may also benefit from sharing experiences and strategies for handling particular situations.
Provide referral for social services consult to investigate the feasibility of respite care or participation of the patient in day care programs specifically for Alzheimer's disease patients.	The caregiver may need to find respite care for extended periods of time to allow for caregiver rest or for a daily program so that the caregiver can work or rest. Social services can assist the caregiver in identifying appropriate community resources, support groups, and services for financial aid and patient placement when it becomes necessary.
Support the family in decision-making regarding institutionalization of the patient, if required.	Many family members experience conflicts when faced with the decision to place the patient in an alternative living arrangement such as a nursing home but also recognize that they can no longer provide 24-hour nursing care. They need to be supported in their decisions.

NIC *Caregiver support*
Respite care
Home maintenance assistance
Support group

Evaluation

Decide if the outcome criteria have been met. The caregiver should be able to verbalize both positive and negative feelings about being a caregiver. Ideally, the caregiver reports an ability to provide care without undue stress. The caregiver identifies sources of support, including relaxation and coping strategies as well as the willingness to use respite care when needed.

Community/Home Care

The caregiver will discover that as the disease progresses the ability to remain positive about the role of caregiver may prove more challenging. It should be stressed to the caregiver to seek out assistance prior to becoming burned out or so stressed that their physical and mental health suffer. Encouraging the caregivers to take time to care for themselves is crucial. Simple stress-reducing activities such as making time for walking or reading can enhance the sense of calm that is required to cope with the Alzheimer's disease patient. Visits by religious or spiritual leaders may also be a source of stress reduction for the caregiver. Support groups can provide emotional support, as well as give specific information about what to expect based on the real life experiences of others. Depression may become apparent in caregivers if respite periods from care giving are not taken on some level (a few hours, a few days, or one day). Home health aides can relieve some of the responsibilities of providing direct patient care. Even though many caregivers may feel guilty for involving outsiders in care, the primary caregiver should be supported in his or her decisions. A referral to social services may be required to investigate placements in nursing homes or other facilities.

Documentation

Document an assessment of the caregiver's current psychological state, including his or her specific verbalizations of concern. Chart teaching done regarding stress and relaxation techniques. All referrals made are included in the record, particularly referrals to agencies that provide respite care, long-term care, and or day care centers.

CHAPTER 3.37

BELL'S PALSY

GENERAL INFORMATION

Bell's palsy is the sudden onset of paralysis of the facial nerve (cranial nerve VII), which results in the patient's inability to move the muscles for facial expression. The condition usually occurs unilaterally, and may be transient or permanent. The patient experiences complete paralysis on the affected side of the face; the patient cannot wrinkle his or her forehead, close the eyelid, or smile. The paralysis onset occurs within 2 to 5 days of an initial episode of facial pain or pain behind the ear. The patient's inability to close the eyelid leaves the eye exposed and vulnerable. Other clinical manifestations include numbness and stiffness of the affected side of the face, unilateral loss of taste, constant tearing, mask-like appearance to face, and facial drooping of one side. Generally, there is no change in the patient's condition for approximately two weeks. After that, the patient may begin to recover from the paralysis, exhibiting voluntary movement of the affected facial muscles in 3 to 4 weeks. However, there is no way to predict a patient's prognosis. Approximately 80 percent of all patients recover in a short period of time—a few weeks to a few months; however, some patients may not begin to recover until 6 months, and maximum recovery may take a year. Unfortunately, not all patients will experience complete recovery.

Several theories have been suggested about the cause of Bell's palsy, including trauma or compression of the nerve and infection with some link to the herpes simplex virus. The disorder strikes men and women equally. Though individuals may be affected at any age, they are most likely to be between 20 and 60 years old. There are no diagnostic or laboratory tests specific to the disease to aid in confirming a diagnosis.

NURSING DIAGNOSIS 1

 DEFICIENT KNOWLEDGE

Related to:

Need for information regarding Bell's palsy and its prognosis

No previous history of disease

Defining Characteristics:

Asks questions/has concerns

Has no questions

Verbalizes a lack of knowledge

Is anxious

Goal:

The patient verbalizes an understanding of Bell's palsy and its treatment.

Outcome Criteria

✔ The patient verbalizes a desire to learn necessary information.

✔ The patient demonstrates knowledge of disease (Bell's palsy).

✔ The patient demonstrates knowledge of prescribed medications.

✔ The patient verbalizes an understanding of the prognosis.

✔ The patient verbalizes a willingness to keep appointments and follow the prescribed regimen.

NOC *Knowledge: Disease process*
Knowledge: Treatment regimen
Compliance behavior

INTERVENTIONS	RATIONALES
Assess readiness of the patient to learn (motivation, cognitive level, physiological status).	The patient must be motivated to learn, have the capability to learn the content, and be free of distractions from learning, such as pain.
Assess the patient's current knowledge.	The nurse needs to ascertain what the patient already knows and build on this.
Start with the simplest information first.	Patients can understand simple concepts easily and then can build on those to understand concepts that are more complex.
Identify a family member or significant other who will also learn the content and assist the patient with compliance.	This person can reinforce the teaching and assist with implementation if the client becomes incapable of follow-through.
Create a quiet environment conducive to learning.	Environmental noise can prevent the patient or family from focusing on the content being taught.
Provide information about the pathophysiology and clinical manifestations of Bell's palsy in the initial teaching session, including — Sudden onset of paralysis of the facial nerve with exact cause unknown — Clinical manifestations: asymmetrical facial appearance, unilateral facial droop, inability to close eye on affected side, inability to grimace or smile, inability to wrinkle forehead, inability to whistle, drooling, inability to keep food and fluid in mouth, difficulty chewing, facial pain on affected side and behind ear, loss of nasolabial folds	The patient must understand what the disease is and how it affects the body before understanding the rationale for treatments.
Teach the patient and family about prescribed medications (corticosteroids), including action, side effects, dosing schedule, tapering of dose at end of therapy.	Corticosteroids decrease inflammation of the nerve and decrease pain; the patient must understand the side effects of water retention and GI upset. If the patient does not understand the need for tapering, he or she may alter the schedule and inadvertently take the wrong dose. Knowledge of why the medication is necessary and how it works will focus the importance of the medication.

	Identification of side effects will minimize anxiety if these untoward effects should occur.
Teach patient how to communicate effectively and implement strategies to enhance communication: — Encourage patient to speak slowly. — Use a writing pad, chalk board, Magic Slate, computer. — Inform the patient that normal speech usually returns. — Collaborate with physician to arrange for a speech therapy consult.	Speaking slowly may help others more easily understand the patient's speech. With alternate communication methods, the patient can communicate when his or her words cannot be understood. If the patient knows that his or her speech problem is self-limiting, the frustration levels will decrease. A speech therapist can work with the patient to develop short-term communication methods and can ensure that maximum function is maintained until the paralysis resolves.
Teach patient proper protection of eye on affected side: — Wear dark glasses when outside or for cosmetic purposes (eye doesn't close). — Wear a patch or shield at night or tape eye closed to prevent drying of cornea. — Even though there may be excessive tearing, the cornea can still dry due to constant exposure; use artificial tears to keep cornea moist.	The eye needs to be protected to prevent corneal abrasion. The patient may want to use dark eyeglasses or sunglasses to shield the eyes' appearance from others, as the eye may remain open and the eyelids are everted.
Collaborate with the physical therapist to teach the patient facial massage.	Facial massage exercises help the patient regain tone.
Teach the patient which signs and symptoms to report to a health care provider.	Monitoring for worsening pain or paralysis, or inability to take adequate food, should be reported to rule out other neurological deficits and prevent a crisis that requires hospitalization.
Evaluate the patient's understanding of all content covered by asking questions.	Identifies areas that require more teaching and ensures that the patient has enough information to ensure compliance; if the patient can demonstrate correct procedure for administering medications, he or she will feel more comfortable using them when needed, and anxiety should be decreased.
Give the patient written information.	Provides reference at a later time, and for review.

INTERVENTIONS	RATIONALES
Establish that the patient has the resources required to be compliant.	If needed resources such as finances, transportation and psychosocial support are not available, the patient cannot be compliant.

NIC *Learning readiness enhancement*
Learning facilitation
Teaching: Disease process
Teaching: Prescribed medication

Evaluation

Evaluate the degree to which the patient has achieved the outcome criteria relevant to the teaching sessions. The patient is able to repeat all information for the nurse, verbalizing an understanding of the pathophysiology of the disease, and asks questions about the prescribed regimen. The patient can identify all medications by name and report the common side effects as well as the dosing schedule. Patients with Bell's palsy should verbalize an understanding of the dosing schedule for corticosteroids and the concept of tapering. Following the teaching session the patient should be able to relate to the nurse which signs and symptoms to report to a health care provider.

Community/Home Care

The patient with Bell's palsy is treated almost exclusively in the home environment with corticosteroids and mild analgesics. Thus, it is crucial that the patient receive adequate teaching related to the disease and its prognosis in order to decrease anxiety. This anxiety is usually attributed to the patient's concern about whether his or her face will return to a normal appearance and function and whether his or her speech impairment will resolve. The nurse, physical therapist, or other health care workers will need to ensure that the patient is able to perform massage to the face to assist in maintaining muscle strength and function. At home, the patient and family will need to adapt food to consistencies that are easy for the patient to chew and swallow. This may mean offering soft foods and frequent small meals, as chewing with limited movement of the face makes eating a normal meal a tiring process (see nursing diagnosis "Imbalanced Nutrition: Less Than Body Requirements"). Initially, communica-

tion may be an issue for the patient due to the paralysis of the facial muscle. The patient will need to use alternative methods of communication until some facial movement returns. Informing the patient about alternative means of communication and assuring him or her that speech is likely to return to normal as function returns will decrease anxiety, frustration, and alterations to self-esteem. During follow-up visits with healthcare providers, the patient should be questioned on use of medications, perceived improvement of facial paralysis, and ability to eat adequate amounts of food.

Documentation

Document the specific content taught and the titles of printed materials given to patient or family. Chart the patient's understanding of the content and the methods used to evaluate learning. The patient's successful demonstration of facial massage and verbalized understanding of disease process and medications should be documented. The nurse must clearly indicate areas that need to be reinforced. After the teaching session is complete, the nurse should note whether the patient indicates a willingness to comply with health care recommendations. If the teaching included a significant other or family member, indicate this in the documentation. In addition, document any referrals made in the patient record.

NURSING DIAGNOSIS 2

 ACUTE PAIN

Related to:
    Inflammation of seventh cranial nerve

Defining Characteristics:
    Complaint of pain
    Facial grimacing on unaffected side
    Limited movement of face

Goal:
    The patient's pain is resolved.

Outcome Criteria

✔ The patient states pain has decreased 1 hour after intervention.

✔ The patient verbalizes methods to reduce pain.

NOC *Pain: Disruptive effects*
Pain level
Pain control

INTERVENTIONS	RATIONALES
Obtain a pain history and assess for onset, location, precipitating factors, relieving factors, and effect on function.	In Bell's palsy the patient history is used for accurate diagnosis. The patient reports a rapid onset (3 to 5 days) of facial or ear pain that helps validate the diagnosis. Knowing how pain affects function will provide information needed for treatment and to assist patient with home care needs.
Assess the patient's pain using a pain rating scale	Provides a more objective assessment.
Administer mild analgesics, as ordered.	Decreases pain.
Administer corticosteroids (prednisone) and any antivirals/antibiotics as ordered.	Decreases inflammation, nerve compression, and/or infection, thereby decreasing subsequent pain.
Collaborate with the physician to arrange for physical therapy consultation as allowed and assist with facial massage.	Physical therapists can provide the patient with facial massage exercises that may decrease the the pain response and help the patient regain tone. Massage also maintains circulation to the face.
Apply moist heat to affected side of face.	Aids muscle relaxation, decreases pain, and provides vasodilation and comfort.
Assess effectiveness of all interventions implemented for pain, particularly medications.	Helps to determine whether revisions in the plan of care are are required.
Protect the face from cold.	Cold may cause increased pain due to hyperesthesia in some patients.
Teach patient to close eyelids manually throughout waking hours and to instill artificial tears into eyes for patients who are unable to close eyes.	Extremely dry eyes can become painful; eyes must be protected from likelihood of corneal abrasion resulting from inability to close eyelid. Artificial tears can help maintain moisture in the eye.
Teach the patient how to patch or shield the eye during sleep.	Protects from injury that could cause pain.

NIC *Heat/cold application*
Analgesic administration
Pain management

Evaluation

Assess the degree to which the patient expresses satisfaction with pain control. Determine the effectiveness of the individual interventions in order to decide which ones work best or least for the patient. If pain persists, the nurse should determine whether there are other causes of the pain and should also investigate additional measures to relieve pain.

Community/Home Care

The patient with Bell's palsy is treated almost exclusively as an outpatient. The pain that occurs with Bell's palsy is generally manageable with mild analgesics, and in the home environment pain is not usually a top priority. At home, the patient should continue to massage the facial muscles and use heat as needed to enhance the effects of medications. Strategies in the home to address pain are explained to the patient, especially the correct dosing of the corticosteroids that must be tapered, usually after 7–10 days. Make the patient a dosing schedule using a calendar, writing the number of tablets for a particular day on that day's date. This can then be displayed in a prominent place. Side effects of analgesics and steroids should be thoroughly explained to the patient with an explanation of what to do if they should occur. Follow-up care with a health care provider is crucial in order to monitor disease progression and resolution and to determine whether further evaluation and additional treatment are required.

Documentation

Document the results of the pain assessment, along with all interventions implemented to address the pain. It is important that the record reflect as much description about the pain as possible: location, intensity, precipitating factors, and general descriptor of the type of pain. Chart the achievement of outcome criteria with specific patient behaviors that validate achievement. Include in the patient record the patient's verbalization of satisfaction with pain control.

NURSING DIAGNOSIS 3

 IMBALANCED NUTRITION: LESS THAN BODY REQUIREMENTS

Related to:

Inability to chew due to paralysis of facial muscle

Decreased sense of taste

Patient has difficulty eating

Patient has difficulty keeping fluids from dribbling out of mouth

Defining Characteristics:

Difficulty swallowing

Weight loss

States he or she cannot eat

Goal:

Nutritional status is maintained.

Outcome Criteria

✔ The patient is able to ingest a normal diet.

✔ The patient does not lose weight.

✔ The patient reports no difficulty swallowing.

NOC *Swallowing status*

Swallowing status:
Esophageal phase

Nutritional status:
Food and fluid intake

Weight: Body mass

INTERVENTIONS	RATIONALES
Collaborate with the physician to obtain consultation for swallowing studies to assess patient's ability to swallow a variety of food types.	Helps to determine the extent of difficulty in swallowing and to make decisions regarding type of diet required; swallowing is difficult due to paralysis of one side of the face.
Assess patient's ability to open mouth wide enough to consume adequate foods and chew.	The face, especially the mouth, is unilaterally paralyzed.
Consult with a dietitian as ordered or as necessary.	A dietitian can make recommendations for adequate nutrient intake to prevent weight loss and regarding food consistency and nutritional value.
Weigh patient on first contact with health care system and monitor weight at follow-up visits.	It is important to establish a baseline weight and monitor weight over the progression of the disease to determine if the patient is able to take in enough food.
Provide a variety of flavorful foods.	The patient with Bell's palsy has a loss of taste on the anterior portion of the tongue, and a variety of flavorful foods may entice the patient to eat.
Offer a soft diet with 5–6 small meals per day.	Soft foods are easier to chew. Because of the effort that goes into chewing when the face is paralyzed, the patient may become frustrated or fatigued and stop eating before enough nutrients have been consumed.
Encourage the patient to place foods on the unaffected side of mouth and chew on unaffected side.	The affected side of the face is paralyzed and may sag, making it difficult to keep food or liquids in that side of the mouth.
Encourage the patient to perform oral care after each meal.	Small amounts of food may become trapped in the jaw or around teeth because of the paralysis and could lead to bad breath, cavities, or candida infections. In addition, if the mouth is fresh, flavors of food will be enhanced.
Teach the patient all strategies/interventions to maintain or improve nutritional status and encourage their use at home.	The patient needs to implement strategies to promote swallowing, digestion, and maintenance of nutrition to prevent complications.

Evaluation

The patient reports that he or she is able to swallow without difficulty. Weight remains stable and patient states satisfaction with diet. The patient eats a normal diet. In addition, the patient should verbalize an understanding of all required interventions and rationales for implementation.

Community/Home Care

At home, the patient should continue to implement strategies to maintain nutritional status. Even though a nurse or other health care provider may not be required for home visits, the patient's nutritional status will need to be monitored through some mechanism. Because of the difficulty with eating, drooling, and chewing, it will be easy for the patient to become frustrated and lose interest in eating leading to a gradual loss of weight, which over time can become pronounced. The patient should have printed information available that gives nutritional content of food that he or she can consume easily. The dietitian or nurse should be sure through teaching that the patient is able to select foods that have nutritional value and not just substances that are easy to consume. Liquid nutritional supplements may be beneficial to the patient to consume between meals or as snacks, as they contain multiple nutrients. Because of the unilateral paralysis, it may be difficult to keep food and liquid in the mouth (drooling), and the patient may choose to isolate him or herself from others when eating due to embarrassment. The family should offer emotional support and encouragement for the patient to increase the likelihood that he or she will continue to try to eat. As the paralysis disappears, the patient should gradually resume the ability to consume a normal diet. The meal preparer should develop menus that incorporate softer foods that are easily chewed by the patient but that are also palatable to all members of the family. Follow-up visits with a health care provider should include an assessment of the patient's ability to chew and swallow along with a measurement of the patient's weight at each visit. A 24-hour recall of food intake with a calorie count can serve to identify the need for further intervention by a dietitian.

Documentation

Chart the patient's weight and the findings from an assessment of the patient's ability to chew and swallow. Document any complaints of facial pain when eating. Include in the patient record the percentage of food consumed and if less than adequate, assess the patient for possible reasons. Chart all interventions implemented to maintain adequate nutrition, the patient's response, and all teaching, including verbalization of understanding or the need for reinforcement. Document any referrals made.

NURSING DIAGNOSIS 4

DISTURBED BODY IMAGE

Related to:
Paralysis of face
Drooling
Masklike appearance to face
Inability to close eyelid
Lower eyelid everted
Sagging of mouth

Defining Characteristics:
Withdrawal
Social isolation
Depression
Negative statements about physical appearance
Attempts to cover face in the presence of others

Goal:
The patient accepts the change in physical appearance and continues social activities and interpersonal relationships.

Outcome Criteria

✔ The patient states willingness to look at and touch face.
✔ The patient does not verbalize negative feelings toward self.
✔ The patient verbalizes an understanding that paralysis is likely to resolve.

NOC *Body image*

INTERVENTIONS	RATIONALES
Encourage the patient to get feelings out in the open and assure the patient that his or her feelings are normal.	The patient should understand that his or her emotions are real and should be expected.
Encourage patient to communicate feelings about changes in physical appearance.	Talking about the changes may sometimes be the beginning of acceptance.
Teach patient methods to care for face to regain function and maintain muscle tone (see nursing diagnoses "Acute Pain" and "Deficient Knowledge").	Massaging the face can help the paralysis resolve and maintain muscle tone of face.
Monitor the patient's feelings about self, interpersonal relationships with family members and friends, withdrawal, social isolation, fear, anxiety, embarrassment by appearance, fear that appearance will be displeasing to loved ones, and desire to be alone.	Helps to detect early alterations in social functioning, prevent unhealthy behaviors, and intervene early through referral to counseling.
Encourage the patient to participate in at least one outside/public activity each week.	Prevents the patient from isolating self from others; because of difficulties with

INTERVENTIONS	RATIONALES
	communication, the patient may refrain from social interaction.
Identify the effects of the patient's culture or religion on body image.	A patient's culture and religion often help define his or her reactions to changes in body image and self-worth.
Assure the patient that a stroke has not occurred and that the changes are temporary in most cases.	The changes in the face are similar to those seen in patients with strokes, and the patient is fearful that the changes are permanent. Educating the patient on the prognosis may assist him or her to adapt to the changes and protect his or her body image.

NIC *Body image enhancement*
Emotional support
Support group
Socialization enhancement

Evaluation

The patient is willing and able to learn about the strategies to improve functioning and manage his or her own activities to the extent possible. Determine whether the patient is able to verbalize feelings regarding the facial paralysis and the impact it will have on role performance. Time is required for the patient to assimilate the change in body appearance into his or her self-perception completely. It is crucial that the nurse evaluate the degree to which the patient is beginning to do this. Communication of feelings and concerns relevant to the change in appearance should be taken as a positive sign that progress towards meeting the outcome criteria is being made.

Community/Home Care

At home, continued monitoring of the patient's perception of body image is needed. The health care provider who interacts with the patient during follow-up will need to be astute to subtle hints that may indicate that the patient has not completely adapted to the change in body appearance. For the patient with Bell's palsy, the change in facial appearance will be obvious to others as the face is paralyzed and takes on a masklike appearance, making speech sound different and conversation difficult, as well as noticeably impairing eating. The patient may be fearful or anxious about eating in public as well as talking to people outside of his or her family. However, it is important that family or significant others encourage continued participation in outside activities and avoidance of self-imposed isolation. Have the patient practice speech with one person until he or she is comfortable with communication. Open discussions regarding the changes and their accompanying frustrations are crucial to the patient's ability to maintain a positive body image. Religious or civic organizations of which the patient is a member may be a good place to start social interaction, as the patient may be comfortable with the people there and be more willing to attempt interactions.

Documentation

Chart any specific behaviors or verbalizations that may indicate an altered body image. Document a precise description of the physical change in appearance that is causing the disturbed body image. Include all interventions that have been employed to address this issue and the patient's response. Note when and if the patient begins to verbalize feelings regarding the change in facial appearance.

CHAPTER 3.38

CLOSED HEAD INJURY

GENERAL INFORMATION

Closed head injury is diagnosed when there is blunt force trauma to the head without an open skull fracture and the dura mater remains intact. Closed head injuries range from simple concussions, to focal injuries such as subdural or epidural bleeding, to diffuse axonal injury (DAI). A major concern for all patients with closed head injury is the risk for developing increased intracranial pressure from cerebral edema development, bleeding into brain tissue, and obstructive hydrocephalus. Acute care of the head injury patient includes frequent monitoring of neurologic status to detect signs of increased intracranial pressure and supportive care to minimize intracranial pressure. The patient's clinical manifestation will depend on the type of injury and the part of the brain affected but may include change in level of consciousness, headache, changes in pupil reactions, vomiting, visual disturbance, impaired memory, and amnesia of events immediately before and after the injury. Complications of head injury include hematomas and central nervous system infections that may develop due to the traumatic injury or monitoring devices, and long-term effects such as alterations in usual cognitive, behavioral, and motor function. Head injury patients often require extensive rehabilitation following the acute phase of illness. The leading causes of closed head injury are motor vehicle and bicycle accidents. Consequently, head injury prevention efforts focus on teaching about seat and lap belts, child safety seats, and bicycle and motorcycle helmets. Other causes of traumatic brain injury are varied, but include falls, sports injuries, and gunshot wounds. Traumatic brain injury is a leading cause of death and disability in the United States, with approximately 50,000 deaths each year. Males are more likely to sustain a head injury than females.

NURSING DIAGNOSIS 1

 INEFFECTIVE TISSUE PERFUSION: CEREBRAL

Related to:

Increased intracranial pressure (ICP)

Cerebral edema

Decreased cerebral perfusion pressure (CPP)

Ineffective breathing pattern

Defining Characteristics:

Altered level of consciousness

Restlessness

Goal:

Cerebral tissue perfusion will be restored.

Outcome Criteria

✔ The patient will not develop increased intracranial pressure.

✔ The patient will not develop seizures.

✔ The patient will be alert and oriented to person, place, and time.

✔ Vital signs will return to patient's baseline.

NOC *Neurological status*
Tissue perfusion: Cerebral

INTERVENTIONS	RATIONALES
Complete a thorough neurological assessment including specific assessments for signs of increased intracranial pressure: altered level of consciousness, pupillary changes, motor or sensory alterations, seizures, orientation, motor function, and	Head trauma may result in increased volume of any of the three components of the intracranial volume (brain tissue, blood, cerebrospinal fluid), which causes an increased pressure in the nonexpendable brain vault. Assessment findings

INTERVENTIONS	RATIONALES
speech. Use the Glasgow Coma Scale.	will give data to validate the presence or absence of increased intracranial pressure. Hematomas (most often acute subdural) are common following brain trauma, and symptoms also mimic those of increased intracranial pressure. Decreased level of consciousness is the earliest and one of the most sensitive signs of increased ICP.
Assess for cerebrospinal drainage from ears (otorrhea) or nose (rhinorrhea); if basilar skull fracture is suspected assess for blood behind tympanic membrane (hemotympanum) or ecchymosis over the mastoid process (Battle's sign) and periorbital ecchymosis (raccoon eyes).	Head trauma injuries may cause leakage of cerebrospinal fluid if the dura is disrupted, and skull fractures lead to abnormal bleeding.
Report any abnormalities to the physician.	Changes in cerebral tissue perfusion or signs of increased intracranial pressure must be reported quickly to prevent further assault on cerebral function. Invasive procedures may need to be implemented to relieve pressure.
Assist with placement of invasive monitoring devices to monitor for increased intracranial pressure (ICP) and cerebral perfusion pressure (CPP) and monitor according to agency protocol. Notify physician of elevations and treat as ordered.	Early detection and treatment of ICP is warranted to prevent further problems that may compromise CPP; inadequate CPP can result in brain tissue death. Normal ICP should be < 15 mm Hg, and readings above 20 are considered elevated; CPP should be above 70 mm Hg to ensure adequate perfusion. (CPP = MAP − ICP)
Monitor vital signs, especially blood pressure and pulse.	A rising systolic blood pressure, a slowing heart rate, and widened pulse pressure (Cushing's response) are classic indicators of increased ICP. Fever without an identifiable infection is a late sign of increased ICP that further increases ICP due to increased metabolic demands of the brain.
Assess for elevated temperature and administer antipyretics, as ordered.	Elevated temperature can increase the risk of cerebral edema and increased intracranial pressure by increasing cerebral metabolism.
Position the patient in semi-Fowler's position with head in midline alignment.	Facilitates venous drainage, which should decrease the intracranial pressure and improve cerebral perfusion. Reposition the patient only after validation that no neck or spinal injury has occurred.
Monitor oxygen and carbon dioxide levels through arterial blood gases (ABGs) and pulse oximetry.	Increased levels of carbon dioxide and decreased levels of oxygen may place the patient at further risk for complications. Interventions, such as causing the patient to hyperventilate and expel more carbon dioxide, may be required.
Prepare the patient for mechanical ventilation and hyperventilation.	Hyperventilation will decrease the pCO_2, which is a potent cerebral vasodilator.
Administer oxygen, as ordered.	Facilitates oxygenation of tissues.
Limit nursing care activities, allowing for periods of rest, and monitor for signs of ICP during all activities.	Turning and bathing increase intracranial pressure.
Administer osmotic diuretics, such as mannitol, as ordered.	Improves cerebral perfusion by decreasing cerebral edema.
Administer steroids, such as Decadron® or Solu-Medrol, as ordered.	Reduces edema caused by inflammation.
Support the blood pressure with vasoactive drugs to maintain the CPP as ordered.	Hypotension may endanger the cerebral perfusion.
Maintain a quiet, restful, dimly lit environment.	Decreases stress and stimulation of cerebral metabolism.
Restrict fluids to 1000–2000 ml/day.	Fluid volume influences the intracranial pressure; minimizing fluid volume can improve cerebral perfusion.
Monitor for seizures and implement safety measures to prevent injury; administer anticonvulsants, as ordered, if seizures occur.	Seizures increase cerebral metabolism and thus increase the intracranial pressure, which in turn decreases cerebral perfusion (see nursing care plan "Seizures" for nursing measures).
If the patient is alert, implement measures to avoid straining (Valsalva maneuver) when having a bowel movement or coughing.	These activities increase intra-abdominal and intrathoracic pressures that in turn increase ICP by interfering with venous drainage from the brain.

NIC *Neurologic monitoring*
Cerebral perfusion promotion
Intracranial pressure monitoring
Seizure precautions
Fluid management

Evaluation

The patient's condition stabilizes and no signs of increased intracranial pressure are present (blood pressure, pulse, and temperature are at the patient's baseline). Cerebral perfusion pressure is maintained, and the patient does not develop seizures. The patient is alert and oriented to person, place, and time.

Community/Home Care

Ineffective cerebral tissue perfusion resolves in a brief period and is not usually a problem once the patient has been discharged. However, it is a good idea to teach the family the signs and symptoms of increased intracranial pressure. The patient who has sustained a closed head injury may have a prolonged recovery period either at home or in a rehabilitation facility. While many patients recover completely from head injury, others will be left with residual, and sometimes serious, cognitive and musculoskeletal deficits. Patients often are unable to return to their usual level of cognitive functioning, especially with tasks that require concentration and memory. Many patients may attempt to return to work but find it impossible to function effectively. The family will need to discuss the prognosis of the patient with health care providers so that they can make realistic plans for care after the acute phase. For the patient expected to make a complete recovery, such a recovery will involve an extended period at home resting and participation in rehabilitation that includes occupational and physical therapy. Problems that may persist at home include bowel and bladder control, mobility, and fatigue. With continued work, these may resolve, and the patient can resume previous activities. The family will need to encourage independence to the extent possible, recognizing that some assistance may be necessary at times. A visiting nurse is recommended to assess neurological function and evaluate the degree to which the patient is returning to a normal level of function. The family will need to be educated on what to do in case seizures occur to facilitate patient safety (see nursing care plan "Seizures"). Chronic subdural

hematomas can develop over weeks or months and occur most often in the elderly. The family or caregiver needs to be taught the symptoms of subdural hematoma (confusion, sleepiness) so that prompt medical attention can be obtained if they occur. Because the most common causes of head injuries are motor vehicle accidents or bicycle accidents, the nurse can take the opportunity to teach the patient and family about healthy behaviors to prevent head injury, such as wearing helmets when cycling and seat belts when riding in automobiles. Some patients with a head injury have a total self-care deficit, and at-home care will need to be coordinated well by a case manager or social worker. At this time, the social worker will need to investigate whether the patient has the financial resources required to be compliant with the recommended regimen. If the patient is left with motor deficits, family members need to be taught correct patient handling techniques for use at home, including transferring from bed to chair and vice versa, and repositioning in bed. The family should demonstrate these skills prior to taking the patient home. If the patient has sustained a serious head injury without recovery of ability to eat, the family at home must learn how to feed the patient using a tube, either gastrostomy or nasogastric. Family members need to understand that the patient with deficits may have emotional outbursts due to frustrations over the deficits. Family members of patients with head injuries that do not require hospitalization may be anxious. Instructions for taking the patient home usually include waking the patient every 2 hours through the first 24 hours, monitoring the patient for nausea and vomiting, excessive sleepiness, dizziness, headaches that worsen especially when moving, and any seizure activity. They should realize how critical it is to notify the physician if any of these occur or call 911 and return the patient to the emergency department.

Documentation

Chart the results of a thorough neurological examination, including specific assessments for increased intracranial pressure, as well as readings from any invasive monitoring. Glasgow Coma Scale evaluations are documented according to the unit policy, usually a checklist. Describe in the record a description of the patient's behavioral response. Document all vital signs and medications according to agency procedures. Include in the record all interventions implemented to address altered cerebral tissue perfusion and whether the patient has met the stated outcome criteria. In addition, document any referrals made for follow-up care.

NURSING DIAGNOSIS 2

 ### INEFFECTIVE AIRWAY CLEARANCE

Related to:

Neurological impairment

Decreased level of consciousness

Defining Characteristics:

Dyspnea

Tachypnea

Inability to breathe without assistance

Arterial blood gases (ABGs) demonstrate hypercapnia and hypoxia

Goal:

The patient's airway remains patent.

Outcome Criteria

✔ Oxygen saturation is > 90 percent.

✔ Arterial blood gases (ABGs) are within normal level.

✔ Respirations are unlabored and < 24.

✔ The patient's breathing is maintained (through intubation/tracheostomy and mechanical ventilation, if necessary).

NOC *Respiratory status: Ventilation*

Respiratory status: Gas exchange

Vital signs

Mechanical ventilation respiratory: Adult

INTERVENTIONS	RATIONALES
Assess respiratory status by noting respiratory rate, depth, chest expansion, rhythm, breath sounds, pulse oximetry, and skin color (examine lip color and color of mucous membranes for dark-skinned patients).	Many patients with head injury are unconscious and have difficulty keeping airway open and maintaining adequate ventilation. Frequent assessments are needed to gather information on the status of the respiratory system, to establish a baseline for future comparisons, and to assist in determining when and if mechanical ventilation is required. Decreased breath sounds indicate atelectasis; decreased oxygen saturation and abnormal blood gases all indicate ineffective breathing pattern that affects gas exchange.
Place patient in a semi-Fowler's position with head elevated 30 degrees and in a neutral position.	Maximizes thoracic cavity space, decreases pressure from diaphragm and abdominal organs, facilitates use of accessory muscles, and prevents aspiration of stomach contents that may be refluxed; the head needs to be elevated to increase venous drainage from the brain.
Monitor arterial blood gases (ABGs) and oxygen saturation via pulse oximetry.	Arterial blood gases (ABGs) are the most accurate method for determining oxygenation status; pulse oximetry is a quick, easy assessment of oxygen saturation but cannot provide accurate information related to carbon dioxide levels or general gas exchange.
Give supplemental oxygen, as ordered.	The head injury patient may lack respirations effective enough to provide adequate oxygen; supplemental administration increases the amount of oxygen available to tissues.
Keep suction apparatus available and suction secretions only if absolutely necessary. If suctioning is needed, hyperventilate and hyperoxygenate before suctioning, as needed.	The patient will be unable to cough to remove secretions. If left alone, the secretions will accumulate and cause airway obstruction. However, suctioning also causes increased intracranial pressure and is used only if necessary to clear secretions. Hyperventilation reduces risk for development of hypoxemia.
Assist with placement of the patient on mechanical ventilation with endotracheal intubation/tracheostomy, as ordered or according to agency protocol (see nursing care plan "Mechanical Ventilation").	The unconscious patient may not be able to breathe on his or her own. Intubation will become necessary when pCO_2 increases, pO_2 decreases, and vital capacity drops, demonstrating severe hypoventilation.

(continues)

(continued)

INTERVENTIONS	RATIONALES
Turn patient every 2 hours.	The unconscious patient cannot reposition self, leading to accumulation of secretions that could cause pneumonia and subsequent obstructions to airway.
Provide chest physiotherapy, as ordered.	Mobilizes secretions that tend to accumulate when the patient is immobile and facilitates that all lung fields are clear.
Monitor for signs and symptoms of respiratory infection: elevated temperature, diaphoresis, thick secretions, and elevated white blood cell counts.	Respiratory infections are easily acquired due to immobility and decreased movement of respiratory muscles.

NIC   *Respiratory monitoring*
Artificial airway
Mechanical ventilation
Ventilation
Positioning

Evaluation

The patient's airway remains patent, and assessments show evidence that breathing patterns are effective in meeting the body's need for oxygen. Secretions do not obstruct airway, and upper airways are clear. The rate should preferably be between 12–24 breaths per minute and unlabored. Arterial blood gases (ABGs) should indicate an absence of hypercapnia or hypoxia; normal range should be expected.

Community/Home Care

For most patients who have sustained a serious head injury, care may be provided in alternative settings, such as extended care, nursing homes, or rehabilitation centers. If the brain-injured patient is cared for at home but does not require a ventilator, the family will need to monitor the patient's respiratory status—particularly the airway—closely. The family will need to be taught how to clear the airway, either through suctioning or chest physiotherapy, and how to monitor respiratory rate and depth as well as chest movement changes that would indicate ineffective patterns of respiration or airway obstruction. It is important to stress to the caregiver that the patient continues to be at risk for development of respiratory infection due to immobility. In-home caregivers should be taught

symptoms of respiratory infection, including elevated temperature, diaphoresis, increased expectoration of sputum and abnormal colors to sputum, as well as how to suction the patient orally. It is important that the family understand how to prevent upper respiratory infections, particularly through immunizations against influenza and pneumonia but also through aggressive repositioning and good hand hygiene. Care of any suction apparatus is also included in teaching, and should be undertaken according to guidelines specific for the type of supplies used. Oral suction devices should be kept in the plastic wrapper when not in use or should be wrapped in clean gauze. These should be discarded according to the manufacturer's guidelines, and if reused, should be washed well, rinsed thoroughly, and stored in a clean covering. If family members note signs of infection, they are to report to a health care provider immediately.

Documentation

Chart the results of a comprehensive assessment of the respiratory system. Note specific signs of airway obstruction, respiratory rate, chest expansion, use of any accessory muscles, breath sounds, skin color, and results of pulse oximetry. If the patient expectorates, or when the patient is suctioned, document the amount, color, and consistency. Chart the specific patient assessment findings that provided indicators for the need for suctioning and patient's response to suctioning. Document any family teaching completed. Include in the patient's chart all interventions employed to address ineffective airway clearance and the patient's response to the interventions that would indicate the problem has been resolved. If the patient is placed on mechanical ventilation, document this according to agency protocol along with the assessment findings that provided evidence for its need.

NURSING DIAGNOSIS 3

EXCESS FLUID VOLUME

Related Factors:

High risk for syndrome of inappropriate antidiuretic hormone secretion (SIADH)

Cerebral edema

Defining Characteristics:

Fluid retention

Decreased urine output

Concentrated urine

Edema

Hyponatremia

Goal:

The patient will have a normal fluid balance.

Outcome Criteria

✔ The patient will have no signs or symptoms of increased intracranial pressure and cerebral edema.

✔ The patient will have a normal serum sodium, osmolality, and specific gravity.

NOC *Fluid balance*
       Electrolyte acid/base balance

INTERVENTIONS	RATIONALES
Assess for signs and symptoms of SIADH: headache, changes in level of consciousness, muscle twitches, decreased urine output.	SIADH is a common complication of head injury, and symptoms are related to hyponatremia and water excess.
Assess for signs of excess fluid volume: signs of increased intracranial pressure, abnormal breath sounds, hand veins that do not flatten within 3–5 seconds when hand is raised above the level of the heart.	Excess fluid volume worsens cerebral edema and increased intracranial pressure.
Assess for neurological changes caused by decreasing levels of sodium: headache, apprehension, lethargy, hyperreflexia, muscle twitching.	Osmotic gradient changes occur across the blood-brain barrier and increase the water content of brain tissue that can cause these symptoms; sodium levels decrease with hemodilution of fluid retention that occurs with SIADH.
Monitor laboratory results: serum sodium, osmolality, and specific gravity of urine.	In states of fluid volume excess, the sodium and osmolality will be decreased due to hemodilution; cerebral tissue is sensitive to decreases in sodium.
Monitor intake and output accurately; weigh patient if not contraindicated.	Decreased output is a symptom of SIADH, and weight is a better measure of fluid gain; intake and output can detect imbalances.
Restrict fluid intake as ordered usually 1000–2000 ml/day.	Decreases total body water and risk of cerebral edema and increased intracranial pressure.
Administer diuretics, as ordered.	Decreases total body water and risk of cerebral edema and increased intracranial pressure.

NIC *Fluid monitoring*
       Fluid management

Evaluation

The patient has restricted fluid intake (1000–2000 ml/day). No signs or symptoms of cerebral edema and increased intracranial pressure have occurred. Urine output returns to normal at approximately 30 ml per hour. Serum sodium and osmolality will be normal.

Community/Home Care

Fluid volume excess is generally an acute care problem that has resolved by time of discharge. However, if the patient is discharged to the home, caregivers will need to monitor for cerebral edema by noting signs of increased intracranial pressure, such as vomiting, headache, restlessness, changes in pupil response, etc. Other more easily recognized signs of fluid excess related to SIADH are decreased output and weight gain. The caregiver, if unable to weigh the patient by standing him or her up, must be taught how to look for other signs of weight gain, such as clothing that becomes too tight quickly and edema that appears in legs, ankles, and around eyes. The caregiver should also measure urine to be sure that output is adequate and retention is not a problem. For the patient who is incontinent, the nurse can teach the caregiver how to measure output by weighing incontinent pads or briefs prior to disposal. If any signs of fluid volume excess or increased intracranial pressure are noted, notify the physician immediately.

Documentation

Chart the results of an assessment of fluid status on each shift to include intake and output according to agency protocol. If edema is present, chart the specific locations, also noting whether the patient has any other complaints. Chart compliance with fluid restrictions. Document findings from a neurological assessment along with any symptoms of increased intracranial pressure or fluid excess.

NURSING DIAGNOSIS 4

 ## IMPAIRED PHYSICAL MOBILITY

Related to:

Cerebral edema

Increased intracranial pressure

Altered level of consciousness

Cognitive impairment

Neuromuscular impairment

Decreased muscle strength or control

Defining Characteristics:

Limited ability to perform gross or fine motor skills

Uncoordinated or jerky movements

Difficulty turning and changing positions

Goal:

The patient will have no complications of immobility.

Outcome Criteria

✔ The patient will take the initiative on movement and position changes at least every 2 hours.

✔ The patient will not develop contractures.

✔ The patient will participate in physical therapy activities as tolerated.

NOC   *Mobility*

INTERVENTIONS	RATIONALES
Assess the patient's cognitive ability to initiate mobility and position changes.	Helps to determine need for assistance.
Assess the patient's physical ability to initiate mobility and position changes.	Helps to determine need for assistance.
Assist patient as needed to change positions at least every 2 hours.	Prevents complications of immobility.
Consult physical therapy, as ordered.	Physical therapists are expert practitioners for patients with impaired mobility.
Progress activity as tolerated from bed to chair, to ambulation if possible, or as ordered and directed by physician and physical therapy.	Assists patient in returning to highest level of function.
Perform range of motion exercises every 4 hours.	Maintains positions of function; range of motion helps with muscle strength and prevention of contractures.
Utilize assistive/supportive devices (as needed).	Some patients will benefit from assistive/supportive devices to maximize their mobility.
Encourage the patient to take initiative.	Helps the patient to progress toward independence with mobility routine.

NIC   *Positioning*
Exercise therapy: Ambulation
Exercise therapy: Joint mobility
Exercise therapy: Muscle control

Evaluation

The patient moves and changes position at least every 2 hours. The care provider encourages the patient to move and the patient takes the initiative on movement and position changes at least every 2 hours. Range of motion is performed every 4 hours and no contractures have developed. The patient participates in all prescribed activity with the assistance of physical therapy.

Community/Home Care

Head-injured patients may return home following the acute phase and receive physical therapy at home, or they may be discharged to rehabilitation centers or other extended care facilities for rehabilitation. The family should receive thorough information regarding the prognosis of recovery from head injury and its impact on mobility. In the acute phase following the injury, it is crucial that caregivers encourage the patient to participate in physical therapy or other activities to the fullest extent possible. Exercises using trapeze bars for shifting weight and repositioning are helpful and should be encouraged by caregivers. The physical therapist has a role in providing teaching to family and patients on the use of assistive devices for ambulation such as wheelchairs, walkers, or canes. The patient may become disillusioned as he or she realizes that the physical limitations are permanent, but he or she should be encouraged and given factual information about the rehabilitation prognosis. Assess the patient's feelings concerning limitations in mobility, any social isolation, and future disability, as well as feelings of depression. Concerns and needs may center on role performance at home: mowing the lawn, household chores such as laundry and cleaning, or self-care needs such as bathing and dressing. An assessment of the home is required in order to make suggestions for changes in the environment that promote independence and safety. Depending upon the severity of the limitations, some issues to be addressed include ability to move about the home, especially getting to the bathroom, getting in or out of the shower or tub, exiting the house if there are steps, and the ability and willingness to be mobile in the home. If the patient is wheelchair-bound following a head injury, a ramp may be required for entry and exit of the home. If the patient is unable to afford such a ramp, community resources such as churches or construction companies should be contacted to see if they could offer assistance. The social worker can be a vital piece of this puzzle. It is crucial that the patient understand the strategies required to maintain optional functioning of affected extremities (see interventions). In-home visits by a physical therapist for a period of time will be important to the patient's health maintenance so that appropriate instructions on exercises and on the use of assistive devices can be completed. Encourage the patient and significant other to utilize community resources, such as support groups.

Documentation

Document a thorough assessment of the patient's functional mobility, including muscle strength, ability to move independently, and use of assistive devices. If the patient is able to ambulate/move, detail the extent of his or her capabilities and participation. Chart any complications of immobility noted in accordance with agency protocol. Chart the implementation of interventions to address immobility, including instruction of the family, and whether these interventions have been effective.

CHAPTER 3.39

GUILLAIN-BARRE SYNDROME

GENERAL INFORMATION

Guillain-Barre syndrome (GB) is an acute degenerative disorder characterized by widespread inflammation of the ascending and descending nerves in the peripheral nervous system as the nerve roots and peripheral nerves are demyelinized. The etiology of Guillain-Barre has been associated with both cell and humoral-mediated autoimmune mechanisms several days to 3 weeks after a mild upper respiratory or gastrointestinal infection (viral or bacterial). A large number of cases of Guillain-Barre can be linked to infections with *Campylobacter jejuni*. The demyelinization of the nerves causes a loss of neurotransmission to the peripheral nerves, resulting in acute onset of ascending flaccid motor paralysis with eventual involvement of the respiratory system. Specific clinical manifestations vary from mild to severe, but generally include symmetrical muscle weakness beginning in the lower extremities and progressing upwards to include the diaphragm, numbness, severe pain that worsens at night, paresthesia, lack of reflexes, and inability to chew or swallow (facial nerve effects). Involvement of the diaphragm results an in inability to maintain respiratory function that necessitates mechanical ventilation. When the autonomic nervous system is affected, the patient demonstrates fluctuations in the blood pressure (hypotension, hypertension, frequent orthostatic hypotension), abnormal vagal responses (bradycardia, heart block, and asystole), and syndrome of inappropriate antidiuretic hormone secretion. Of those affected, 80 percent experience full recovery, another 6 percent will succumb to the disease, and the remainder will have some residual or debilitating disability resulting from the disease. The recovery period and rehabilitation period for those who recover extends from several months to years. It affects men and women of all ages.

NURSING DIAGNOSIS 1

IMPAIRED PHYSICAL MOBILITY

Related to:

Paresthesias

Paralysis of peripheral nerves and nerve roots causing muscle paralysis

Loss of sensation

Defining Characteristics:

Inability to ambulate or move independently

Inability to carry out activities of daily living

Decreased range of motion

Goal:

Adequate range of motion and positions of function are maintained/accomplished.

Outcome Criteria

✔ The patient's lower extremities will be able to move through range of motion.

✔ Contractures and foot drop are avoided.

✔ Complications of immobility do not occur (pneumonia, skin breakdown).

NOC *Mobility*

INTERVENTIONS	RATIONALES
Assess patient for range of motion and weakness as well as ability to reposition self or ambulate.	Helps to determine the current functional ability and to plan for appropriate interventions.
Obtain a history from the patient about mobility limitations and effect on ability to remain functional.	Helps to determine what adaptations in lifestyle need to be made and to determine the severity of mobility limitations.

INTERVENTIONS	RATIONALES
Encourage the patient to remain ambulatory for as long as the condition allows.	Limits the period of time that the patient is immobile; prevents complications of immobility and preserves function.
When or if the patient becomes immobile, have him or her get out of bed in a chair daily.	Prevents complications of prolonged bedrest, such as pneumonia, deep vein thrombosis (DVT), skin breakdown.
Collaborate with physician to arrange for physical therapy consultation for methods/ therapies to improve or preserve function, and for rehabilitation following the acute phase.	The physical therapist can implement a plan for improvement of weakness and for preservation of muscle tone. Eighty percent of patients with GB have a full recovery, and activity during the phase when symptoms are more pronounced can prevent the patient from losing muscle tone and becoming contracted, which would prevent adequate activity once the disease has resolved. Because of muscle weakness and loss of tone, the patient may have to relearn how to walk.
Reposition the patient every 2 hours. Provide trochanter rolls, pillow supports, and range of motion.	Maintains positions of function and comfort. Range of motion and proper positioning help to prevent contractures and other complications of immobility such as pneumonia, skin breakdown, DVT.
Assess patient skin for redness or skin breakdown every 2 hours when repositioning.	Pressure from immobility compresses blood vessels in high-risk areas, depriving them of nutrients and oxygenation, leading to skin death.
Teach the patient and family turning, lifting/moving techniques, correct body alignment, use of assistive devices, and how to perform range of motion.	Helps to maintain function as long as possible and prevent contractures. Even though a physical therapist may come into the home to work with the patient, family members may also be required to move and position the patient. During the recovery period when muscles are weak due to lack of use, the patient will need assistive devices.

Assist with plasmapheresis, as indicated by agency protocol.	Plasmapheresis is beneficial during the early phase of the disease (2 weeks) to remove antibodies from the blood, and is thought to expedite recovery.
Administer intravenous immunoglobin, as ordered.	Modifies severity of the disease and is thought to expedite recovery.
Administer medications as ordered, such as corticosteroids (prednisone).	Decreases autoimmune inflammation of the nerves in the peripheral nervous system.
Assess the patient for signs of DVT (heat and pain in calf, redness or other discoloration in calf).	Allows nurse to initiate treatment with anticoagulants. DVT is a complication of immobility.

NIC *Exercise therapy*
Joint mobility
Positioning

Evaluation

The patient maintains full range of motion of all extremities with no contractures. The patient participates in mobility activities and exercises to the extent possible. Skin breakdown and pneumonia do not occur as a result of being on bedrest. Following the acute phase, the patient is able to participate in physical therapy for reconditioning and strength.

Community/Home Care

Guillain-Barre syndrome is treated at home unless artificial ventilation is required or an in-home care provider is not available. The family should receive thorough information regarding the disease and its impact on mobility. In the acute phase of the disease, it is crucial that caregivers encourage the patient to remain mobile as long as possible. As the weakness progresses to paralysis, the attention in the home turns to preserving muscle tone, preventing contractures, and promoting as much self-care as possible. Range of motion exercises must be aggressive and frequent to prevent complications. Turning and repositioning are required to prevent skin breakdown and pneumonia. It would be easy for caregivers or family members to omit exercises if the patient does not want to participate, but everyone must understand the importance of this therapy. Because 80 percent of patients recover from the disorder, maintenance of muscle tone and prevention of contractures is necessary for future efforts at rehabilitation. Muscle tone and strength return during the recovery phase in descending order so that the patient may begin working on upper-body strength before paralysis of legs has resolved. Exercises using trapeze bars for shifting weight and repositioning are helpful and should be encouraged by caregivers. The physical therapist has a role in providing teaching to the patient and family members on the use of assistive devices for ambulation once paralysis resolves. The patient may become disillusioned during the phase of paralysis but should be encouraged and given factual information about the disease's progression and prognosis. Providing care for a totally dependent patient can prove to be challenging to family members, necessitating a change in routines. It is important that family members are supported in their care giving. Providing them with a visiting nurse who can assess how the patient is progressing and troubleshoot with the family can assist in reducing anxiety that may be present. The family will need to be equipped with a mental fortitude that withstands days of exhaustion, both physical and mental, as well as the ability to step away from the situation and ask for assistance in the care-giving role, especially given that the time required for recovery can range from several months to upwards of 2 years. If the patient makes no progress towards regaining mobility of his or her extremities, the caregivers may be faced with making decisions regarding alternative living arrangements, possibly in long-term care facilities.

Documentation

Chart the findings from an assessment of motor function and muscle strength. If the patient is able to ambulate or move, detail the extent of his or her capabilities and participation. Document all interventions implemented to address the issue of immobility, as well as instruction to the caregiver relevant to addressing immobility. Chart any complications of immobility noted in accordance with agency protocol.

NURSING DIAGNOSIS 2

IMPAIRED SPONTANEOUS VENTILATION

Related to:

Paralysis of diaphragm and chest wall muscles

Defining Characteristics:

Increasing fatigue

Increasing dyspnea, tachypnea

Inability to breathe without assistance

Decreased tidal volume and vital capacity

Arterial blood gases demonstrate hypercapnia and hypoxia

Goal:

The patient has adequate oxygenation.

Outcome Criteria

✔ Oxygen saturation is > 90 percent.

✔ Arterial blood gases (ABGs) are within normal level.

✔ Respirations are unlabored.

✔ Respiratory function returns and is unassisted.

✔ The patient's breathing is maintained (through intubation/tracheostomy and mechanical ventilation if necessary).

NOC   *Respiratory status: Ventilation*
          Respiratory status: Gas exchange
          Vital signs
          Mechanical ventilation response: Adult

INTERVENTIONS	RATIONALES
Assess respiratory system by noting respiratory rate, depth, chest expansion, rhythm, breath sounds, pulse oximetry, and skin color (examine lip color and color of mucous membranes for dark-skinned patients).	Provides information on the status of the respiratory system and progression of disease; also establishes a baseline for future comparisons; assists in determining when and if mechanical ventilation is required.
Assist the patient in assuming a high Fowler's position or position for easy respiration.	Maximizes thoracic cavity space, decreases pressure from diaphragm and abdominal organs, and facilitates the use of accessory muscles.
Monitor arterial blood gases (ABGs).	Arterial blood gases (ABGs) are the most accurate method for determining oxygenation status.

INTERVENTIONS	RATIONALES
Suction secretions.	The patient will be unable to cough to remove secretions. If left alone, the secretions will accumulate and cause airway obstruction and subsequent impairments in gas exchange.
Consider intubation/ tracheostomy and mechanical ventilation.	As Guillain-Barre syndrome ascends, the phrenic and intercostal nerves will become paralyzed, and the patient will not be able to breathe on his or her own. Intubation will become necessary when pCO_2 increases, and vital capacity drops, demonstrating severe hypoventilation.
Assist with placement on mechanical ventilation as ordered or according to agency protocol (see nursing care plan "Mechanical Ventilation").	The patient with Guillain-Barre syndrome often requires mechanical ventilation to maintain respirations as the diaphragm becomes paralyzed.
Turn the patient every 2 hours.	Prevents atelectasis in bases.
Provide chest physiotherapy, as ordered.	Mobilizes secretions that tend to accumulate when the patient is immobile and facilitates clear lung fields.
Monitor for signs and symptoms of respiratory infection: elevated temperature, diaphoresis, thick secretions, coughing.	Respiratory infections are easily acquired due to immobility and decreased movement of respiratory muscles.
Teach pulmonary hygiene: prevention of infections, maintaining optimal health, taking flu and pneumonia vaccines.	Protecting against infections can prevent acute respiratory illness and subsequent hospitalizations.
Provide mouth care every 2 hours.	Cleansing the mouth helps decrease the risk of pneumonia; patients on ventilators have easy entry ports for organisms via endotracheal tubes.

NIC *Respiratory monitoring*
Artificial airway
Mechanical ventilation
Ventilation
Positioning

Evaluation

The patient has adequate ventilation and can eventually be weaned off the ventilator. The patient should show indications that breathing patterns have returned to baseline and are effective in meeting the body's need for oxygen. The rate should return to baseline, preferably between 12–24 breaths per minute, and be unlabored. Respiratory function returns and is unassisted. The return of arterial blood gases (ABGs) to the patient's baseline or to within normal range should be expected.

Community/Home Care

If the patient is cared for at home without a ventilator, the family will need to monitor the patient's respiratory status closely. The caregiver should be taught how to monitor respiratory rate and depth, as well as chest movement changes that would indicate paralysis of the diaphragm. If such changes are noted, the patient will need to seek health care quickly. For the patient who has been on a ventilator in an extended-care facility, function of respiratory muscles generally returns over 2–3 weeks, and the patient is weaned. Once at home, the patient may experience some anxiety about the possibility of being unable to breathe again. It is important to stress to the caregiver that the patient continues to be at risk for development of respiratory infection due to the previous compromised respiratory status. It is anticipated that the patient will need to regain stamina and endurance and may experience some shortness of breath dependent upon the severity of disease. In-home caregivers should be taught symptoms of respiratory infection, including elevated temperature, diaphoresis, increased expectoration of sputum, and abnormal colors to sputum. Because full recovery takes months to upwards of 2 years, it is important that the patient understand how to prevent upper respiratory infections, particularly through the use of immunizations against influenza and pneumonia. If the patient is eating food orally, monitor for aspiration: coughing while eating and expectorating mucous that contains food particles. The patient with Guillain-Barre is at high risk for aspiration because of the paralysis of respiratory muscles and loss of gag reflex. Monitoring for this allows the family to intervene early to prevent respiratory complications, such as aspiration pneumonia. Follow-up care is necessary to monitor for resolution of the disease with a return to normal respiratory function.

Documentation

Chart the results of a comprehensive assessment of the respiratory system. Note respiratory rate, chest expansion, use of accessory muscles, breath sounds, and results of pulse oximetry. If the patient expectorates, document the amount, color, and consistency. Document any patient or family teaching completed. Include in the patient's chart all interventions employed to address ineffective breathing pattern, and the patient's response to the interventions that would indicate the problem has been resolved. If the patient is placed on mechanical ventilation, document this according to agency protocol along with the assessment findings that provided evidence for its need. Document settings and readings from the ventilator as required by agency guidelines.

NURSING DIAGNOSIS 3

 ACUTE PAIN

Related to:

>   Demyelination of peripheral nerves
>   Inflammation

Defining Characteristics:

>   Nocturnal pain
>   Severe pain
>   Paresthesia
>   Numbness

Goal:

>   Pain decreases and mobility is improved.

Outcome Criteria

✔ The patient states that pain has decreased 1 hour after intervention.
✔ The patient verbalizes methods to reduce pain.
✔ The patient is able to sleep without nocturnal pain disruptions.

NOC *Pain: Disruptive effects*
       Pain level
       Pain control

INTERVENTIONS	RATIONALES
Assess the patient's pain using a pain rating scale.	Provides a more objective assessment.
Assess or take history regarding time of onset, location, precipitating factors, relieving factors, and effect on function.	These will assist in accurate diagnosis and treatment; knowing how pain affects function will provide information needed to assist patient with home care needs. The patient's pain is worse at night, so measures to ensure adequate pain control are necessary to prevent alterations in sleep pattern.
Apply moist heat or cold.	Aids muscle relaxation and decreases pain; moist heat is able to penetrate deeper; if pain intensifies during acute phase or inflammation, cold can be used for analgesia properties as well.
Administer analgesic medications as ordered and monitor for effectiveness and side effects.	In the early phase of the disease, pain may only be relieved with opiate medications such as morphine. Large doses of medication may be required for pain relief in muscles.
Give all medications on a regular dosing schedule rather than prn.	Provides better relief and prevents the pain from becoming severe.
Give corticosteroids as ordered and monitor for side effects, which include elevations of blood sugar levels, water retention, and hypertension.	Corticosteroids relieve inflammation of peripheral nerves, which is the source of the paresthesias and pain.
Teach relaxation techniques such as music therapy, massage, distraction, and meditation.	These techniques enhance the effect of analgesics and may decrease reliance on medications for complete relief.

NIC *Simple relaxation therapy*
       Heat/cold application
       Analgesic administration
       Pain management

Evaluation

Assess the degree to which the patient reports pain has been relieved by interventions. The nurse should investigate additional measures to relieve persistent pain. Determine whether the patient is able to verbalize how to reduce pain.

Community/Home Care

The patient with Guillain-Barre syndrome is typically treated as an outpatient unless there is a need for mechanical ventilation. A major problem to be addressed is the management of muscular pain. A therapeutic regimen that allows for tolerable pain may require an extended period of trial and error with a variety of pharmacological and non-pharmacological measures. If able, the patient needs to learn how to implement relaxation techniques that enhance the therapeutic effects of medications. Family members may be required to learn how to use non-pharmacological measures to assist the patient, such as back rubs before bedtime and playing soothing music. Administration of medications is crucial, especially if the patient is to take opiates such as morphine in the home. Caregivers need to be taught side effects of the medications and how to monitor respiratory status to detect respiratory depression. Scheduling of the medication is important to achieve the best outcome; giving medications at bedtime has a dual purpose: enhancement of sleep and relief of pain. The patient will need to understand the side effects of all medications, many of which are significant, such as GI bleeding (corticosteroids) and respiratory depression (opiates). If measures are not effective in relieving the pain, a health care provider should be contacted for discussion of new pain relief measures.

Documentation

Include in the patient record the patient's verbalized perception of pain and satisfaction with pain control. Document all interventions utilized to treat pain. If the patient is at home for treatment, be sure that office visits document the specific therapeutic interventions prescribed for pain and whether they are effective.

NURSING DIAGNOSIS 4

 INEFFECTIVE PROTECTION

Related to:

Loss of neurotransmission to peripheral nerves
Motor paralysis

Lack of reflexes
Severely diminished deep tendon reflexes
Symmetrical paralysis that usually begins in the lower extremities and gradually ascends to chest and arms (including muscles of respiration) and then gradually (usually) resolves

Defining Characteristics:

Paresthesia
Numbness
Orthostatic hypotension
Dizziness

Goal:

The patient will sustain no injury.

Outcome Criteria

✔ The patient will not fall.
✔ The patient will not injure him or herself (cuts, burns, skin tears, etc.).
✔ The patient will have no signs or symptoms of infections (urinary, respiratory, central access sites, skin areas).
✔ The patient will verbalize an understanding of the necessary precautions needed to prevent infection and prevent injury.

NOC *Immune status*
Knowledge: Infection control
Risk control

INTERVENTIONS	RATIONALES
Assess patient for signs of injury such as bruising or skin tears.	Helps to detect injuries that occurred that the patient is unaware of. The patient with Guillain-Barre syndrome experiences decreased reflexes as well as paresthesia and numbness, which decreases the ability to feel the pain that may come with injury, especially in the lower extremities.
Assess skin color.	Skin color changes may be indicative of increased pressure on an area; skin may become pale due to impaired perfusion.

(continues)

(continued)

INTERVENTIONS	RATIONALES
Monitor for signs of respiratory infection: elevated white blood cells, purulent mucous, frequent expectoration, elevated temperature, coughing, decreased oxygen saturation, shortness of breath.	The patient with Guillain-Barre is at risk for respiratory infection due to immobility and ineffective breathing pattern (see nursing diagnosis "Impaired Spontaneous Ventilation").
Assess the patient for urinary retention (distended abdomen, decreased output) and signs of urinary infections (urine that is cloudy, malodorous, dark in color, elevated temperature, burning on urination).	Urinary retention may occur due to the lack of sensation to void. This retention predisposes the patient to infection due to stagnant urine.
Assist the patient with careful ambulation and/or range of motion exercises.	Due to dizziness, weakness, orthostatic hypotension, and numbness, the patient is at higher risk for falls; providing assistance decreases that risk. The patient with Guillain-Barre has muscle weakness of the lower extremities, making ambulation difficult; some patients have symmetrical paralysis that prevents walking at all. Both groups are unable to reposition themselves independently. Continuing exercises prevents muscle atrophy.
Practice good handwashing.	Handwashing is one of the best ways to stop the transmission of infection.
Restrict visitors who are sick and have the patient avoid crowds.	Visitors can transmit infection via colds, coughs, and handshakes; being in crowds increases the risk of acquiring respiratory infections from droplet infection.
Teach the patient and family members all safety precautions required related to falls and infection.	The patient needs to be informed in order to practice health promotion and disease prevention behaviors.

NIC *Risk identification*
Self-care assistance
Surveillance

Evaluation

Evaluate whether outcome criteria have been met. The patient should be free of injury such as falls, traumatic injury to skin, or undetected wounds. Respiratory infections have been prevented. The patient, if able, ambulates or repositions him or herself without injury, with the assistance of others. Both the patient and the family are able to verbalize safety precautions required.

Community/Home Care

The patient with Guillain-Barre syndrome will be at risk for ineffective protection until recovery occurs, or if symptoms are permanent, the risk will continue. The patient, family members, or other caregivers need to continue to practice safety-enhancing behaviors for physical injury and infections. The patient must be vigilant in preventing complications such as falls, impairments to skin integrity, and muscle atrophy due to paresthesia, numbness, and weakness. The patient should implement strategies to protect him or herself from injury, such as avoiding bumping into objects that may cause bruising or disruption of skin or rearranging furniture or removing rugs to make walking areas clear. Caregivers should examine the patient's extremities daily to look for signs of injury. Because the patient has weakness or paralysis in the lower extremities and is prone to experience orthostatic hypotension, the threat of injury is greater with movement and/or ambulation. This is especially true in the earlier phases of the disease when the patient is still coping with the fact of progressive weakness and ultimate paralysis, not always accepting the limitations imposed by the disease (see nursing diagnosis "Impaired Physical Mobility"). The second aspect of protection for the patient is preventing infections, especially respiratory, due to the involvement of the respiratory muscles/diaphragm. The patient with Guillain-Barre syndrome may want to avoid large crowds or other activities that may increase the risk for infection. The family can assist by being sure to turn the patient to prevent stasis of secretions and monitor for signs of respiratory infection such as coughing, runny nose, expectoration of purulent mucous, and elevated temperature. Practicing good handwashing techniques can minimize risk of infection. If possible, patients with young children or grandchildren should avoid them when they are sick with colds or the flu. At the first sign of infection, the patient should return to a health care provider for further assistance.

Documentation

Document the findings from a thorough assessment of the patient, especially the presence of bruises or skin impairments. If the patient falls while in a health care facility, follow agency protocol for documentation and assess the patient carefully for injury. In addition, document the patient's activity level and any negative responses to activity (increased blood pressure, fatigue, dizzy). If the patient has any signs of infection, even minor, document this in the patient record with a description of what interventions were carried out in response to the findings.

CHAPTER 3.40

HERNIATED NUCLEUS PULPOSA (HNP/RUPTURED DISK/SLIPPED DISK)

GENERAL INFORMATION

Herniated disk can occur due to repeated stress or trauma to the spine, poor body mechanics, or invertebral degeneration and can be partial or complete. The part of the disk known as the annulus is a ring of tissue that gives size and shape to the disk and holds the nucleus pulposus in place (Black and Hawks, 2005). When the disk herniates, the annulus becomes torn, allowing for the protrusion of the pulposa with narrowing of the intervertebra and an inability to absorb the shock of movement, etc. In addition, there is compression of nerve roots. The most common location for herniation is lumbosacral disks between lumbar vertebrae 4 and 5, and between lumbar vertebrae 5 and sacral vertebrae 1. Herniation of the disks in the cervical spine usually occurs between cervical vertebrae 5 and 6, and between cervical vertebrae 6 and 7. Risk factors for the development of herniated disks and lower back pain are heavy lifting, obesity, poor posture, and falls. Clinical manifestations include acute sudden, severe pain, and then later, chronic or recurrent lower back pain. Other complaints include muscle spasms, hyperesthesia (tingling, numbness), and worsening of pain by coughing, sneezing, bending and lifting, prolonged sitting, and lifting the leg straight. Herniated disks occur more often in men than women, and in people ages 30–50 years. Lower back pain is the leading cause of disability and absence from work for people under 45 years of age, making it a major costly health care problem in the United States.

NURSING DIAGNOSIS 1

ACUTE AND CHRONIC PAIN

Related to:

Herniated disc leading to nerve compression

Defining Characteristics:

Sharp back pain

Muscle spasms

Recurrent pain in lower back

Paresthesia

Inability to walk upright

Leaning to one side

Goal:

The patient's pain is manageable/tolerable.

Outcome Criteria

✔ The patient reports that pain has gradually decreased.

✔ The patient rates pain as < 5 on a pain rating scale.

✔ The patient verbalizes methods to reduce or prevent pain.

✔ The patient identifies aggravating factors.

NOC *Pain: Disruptive effects*
Pain level
Pain control

INTERVENTIONS	RATIONALES
Obtain a pain history and assess the patient for complaints of pain, increased pain with motion; increased pain with straight leg lifting (Lasègue's sign); severe sharp pain over area of herniation; pain that radiates into buttocks, legs, back; pain provoked by any sudden movement; patient's statements that his or her "back gave out."	These are all specific manifestations of herniated disks caused by compression of nerve roots and lack of ability of the nucleus pulposa to absorb the shock of movement.
Have the patient rate pain on a pain rating scale.	Helps to obtain a more objective measure of the pain.

INTERVENTIONS	RATIONALES
Administer analgesics, as ordered, on a regular schedule.	Analgesics will help for general pain relief; giving the medications on a regular schedule maintains serum levels and prevents pain from becoming severe.
Administer muscle relaxants (such as Valium®, Flexeril®, Robaxin®, carisoprodol), as ordered.	These medications relieve muscle spasms; as muscle spasm decreases, pain will also decrease.
Administer nonsteroidal anti-inflammatory agents (NSAIDs), as ordered.	NSAIDs decrease swelling and therefore decrease pressure on nerve roots, lessening pain and discomfort. Common side effects include GI upset and bleeding; monitor body fluids for blood and patient for nausea.
Administer COX-2 inhibitors as ordered; assess for effectiveness and monitor for side effects.	Used for its analgesic properties, these inhibit prostaglandin synthesis by inhibiting COX-2; they are also anti-inflammatory agents.
Assist with injection of corticosteroid agents into the area of herniation.	Combined with an anesthetic and injected into the affected area, corticosteroids decrease pain.
Encourage the patient to lose weight if he or she is overweight.	Obesity places more stress on the lumbar sacral area, increasing the pain.
Apply moist heat packs.	Aids muscle relaxation and decreases pain; moist heat is able to penetrate deeper.
Place a firm mattress or a board on the bed.	Provides support for the back.
Teach the patient how to manage chronic pain with a combination of pharmacological and non-pharmacological measures, such as relaxation techniques, guided imagery, and music therapy, and encourage their use.	Patients with chronic pain need to learn coping strategies that will assist them in handling persistent pain.
Arrange for a physical therapy consult.	The physical therapist is best equipped to develop a plan to decrease muscle spasms and relax muscles. A physical therapist will plan a rehabilitation regime that usually will include mild exercise, stretching, and other therapeutic interventions, such as ultrasound hydrotherapy, heat treatments, and hot and cold packs.
Prepare patient for TENS (Transcutaneous Electrical Nerve Stimulation) Unit, as ordered.	This therapy provides electrical stimuli that interrupt the transmission of pain signals.
Assess the effectiveness of all interventions with each health care visit.	The plan for pain management should be reviewed to determine if it has been effective and to allow for revisions if it has not been effective.
Teach the patient how to prevent irritation of herniated disk and nerve root by avoiding sudden turning, twisting, lifting, and positioning when sitting or lying that prevents pressure on herniated disk.	Identifying aggravating factors and eliminating them will assist in pain management.
If non-pharmacological measures are unsuccessful, anticipate surgical intervention and prepare the patient through pre-operative teaching.	Medical management is the first line of treatment; for patients who do not respond, surgery may be undertaken to relieve symptoms.

NIC *Simple relaxation therapy*
Heat/cold application
Analgesic administration
Pain management

Evaluation

Assess the degree to which the patient reports that pain decreases through interventions. The patient must report satisfaction with pain control. For pain that worsens, the nurse should investigate additional measures to relieve pain. Determine whether the patient is able to verbalize aggravating factors and how to reduce pain using a combination of pharmacological and non-pharmacological measures.

Community/Home Care

The patient with herniated disk is typically treated as an outpatient, with in-home care focused on management of pain. A therapeutic regimen that allows for tolerable pain may require an extended period of trial and error with a variety of pharmacological and non-pharmacological measures. If able, the patient needs to learn how to implement relaxation techniques that enhance medications. The patient needs to understand that at times when the pain intensifies, bedrest may be required. A physical therapist will need to consult with the patient to provide suggestions on correct positioning when sitting or lying, appropriate exercises, and the proper use of assistive devices such as pillows. Other suggestions for the patient include avoiding standing in one position for an extended period; exercise for short periods (15 minutes) twice a day; sleeping on a firm mattress; losing weight if overweight; refraining from positions where the lower back is strained, such as leaning forward; and avoidance of sitting for long periods of time. Activities such as swimming or walking should be encouraged. For women, high heeled shoes should be avoided as they tend to create an abnormal balance and place more strain on the lower back. The physical therapist should also teach the patient proper body mechanics for performing normal, routine tasks at work or home. The patient is encouraged to perform stretching exercises as ordered. For some patients, wearing corsets or commercial support devices (support belts) provides added support for the back and prevents pain or further injury. Health care providers should follow up to determine whether the pain prevents the patient from working or performing activities of daily living. If so, a change in regimen should be undertaken with the goal of making the patient as functional as possible. The patient will need to understand the side effects of all medications as many of them, such as GI bleeding and water retention, are significant. In addition, a side effect often overlooked with some NSAIDs is the decreased effectiveness of some antihypertensive medications when taken concurrently with NSAIDs, particularly ACE inhibitors and beta blockers such as atenolol. If the patient is prescribed narcotics for pain relief such as the opiates, teach him or her to increase fiber and fluid in the diet to offset the side effect of constipation. Because lower back pain can be disabling, the patient should be assessed for psychosocial problems, such as depression, anxiety, and ineffective coping. Counseling may be required to assist the patient to cope with what could be a chronic condition requiring changes in lifestyle, especially in the ability to earn income.

Documentation

Given that the patient is at home for treatment, it is important to be sure that office visits document the specific therapeutic interventions prescribed for pain and those utilized by the patient. Include in the patient record the patient's verbalized perception of pain control. In addition, keep records of the patient's report of how the pain has affected everyday

functioning, especially his or her ability to work, if appropriate. Physical therapists should document the patient's activity prescriptions clearly.

NURSING DIAGNOSIS 2

 IMPAIRED PHYSICAL MOBILITY

Related to:

Pain

Muscle spasm

Defining Characteristics:

Inability to stand up straight

Listing to one side

Reluctance to perform any type of physical activity

Limited range of motion, moves slowly

Goal:

The patient has improved physical mobility.

Outcome Criteria

✔ The patient is able to ambulate without pain in the lower back.

✔ The patient is able to perform activities of daily living.

✔ The patient reports that back pain is tolerable.

NOC *Mobility*
Knowledge: Body mechanics
Body mechanics performance
Body positioning: Self-initiated

INTERVENTIONS	RATIONALES
Monitor results of diagnostic tests: x-rays, computed tomography (CT) scan, MRI (magnetic resonance imaging), EMG (electromyography), myelogram, diskography.	X-rays can show structural abnormalities, CT scan helps identify location of herniation, MRI may reveal a narrowing of the spinal canal with extension of the disk material into it, myleography shows narrowing of the disk space and impingement of a spinal nerve root as well as the exact level of herniation, and results of a diskography will demonstrate changes in the disk.

INTERVENTIONS	RATIONALES
Obtain a history and assess the patient for: ability to walk with erect posture; ability to get up and down from chairs and perform activities of daily living; activity level when pain first occurred and following onset of pain; inability to stand upright; difficulty walking; severe pain when lifting something heavy, twisting torso, or during or after prolonged sitting; understanding of causative activities; decreased sensation; decreased deep tendon reflexes; decreased muscle strength; decreased muscle tone; limb weakness; paresthesia in limb(s); pain over area of herniation.	These are indicators of level of functioning and will provide information relevant to the extent of problems. This thorough history provides data for developing an individualized plan of care.
Obtain history from the patient about occupation, nature of work, trauma, sports in the past or present, and obesity past or present.	Helps to determine whether adaptations in lifestyle will need to be made and to decide whether lifestyle is a contributing factor.
Arrange for physical therapy consultation for methods/therapies to improve mobility (moist heat, ultrasound, hydrotherapy, gentle exercise, stretches, massage, ambulatory assistive devices).	Improves physical mobility by relaxing the back, relieving pain, and improving range of motion.
Implement strategies to alleviate pain (see nursing diagnosis "Acute and Chronic Pain").	Alleviating the pain will allow for better mobility.
Encourage regular exercises, such as walking on level surfaces, stretching, swimming, or water exercises specifically designed for patients with lower back pain.	Exercise helps maintain and restore function; maintains muscle tone and mobility; enhances pain control measures.
Encourage the patient to use assistive devices as prescribed (support belts, pillows when in bed, etc.).	Helps relieve stress on back when moving.
Teach the patient good posture, correct body mechanics, and body alignment: — Avoid twisting. — When in bed lie supine with small pillow under knees. — Use a side-lying position on unaffected side with pillow between knees. — Use a support belt when lifting. — Push objects rather than pulling. — When lifting, keep back straight and avoid bending at the waist; use large muscles. — Use a footstool when sitting to lessen back strain. — When sitting at work, change positions often.	Protects the back and reduces stress on vertebra.
Teach patient how to cope with chronic pain through use of medications and non-pharmacological measures (see nursing diagnosis "Acute and Chronic Pain").	Many patients become dependent and focus on what they cannot do rather than taking control of the disease. Patients must learn how to cope with pain on a daily basis and maintain optimum function.
Teach patient about herniated disk and its effect on mobility.	Knowledge about the disease and how it affects the body will give the patient a sense of control and allows for a better understanding of the role of prescribed therapeutic interventions.
Make referrals to support groups.	Support groups can offer emotional support as well as helpful tips on how to live with chronic pain.

Evaluation

Determine the degree to which the patient is achieving the established outcomes. The patient should report to the health care provider that he or she is able to perform routine household chores and activities of daily living. Assess the extent to which the patient is able to ambulate without pain as well as the effectiveness of interventions to enhance mobility.

Community/Home Care

Herniated disks are treated almost exclusively in the home environment. Initially, the patient may require some in-home assistance or adaptations in environment or lifestyles due to pain that prevents him or her from performing normal routines. As the pain becomes tolerable, the patient may start to resume activities, but the health care provider will need to monitor the effect that chronic pain and limited mobility has on effective functioning. Concerns and needs may center on performance of household chores such as laundry and cleaning, but more importantly, on the ability to work. Some occupations such as mill/factory work will not permit time off during the day for physical therapy or water exercises. The same may be true for people who work 12-hour shifts, and the outpatient centers may be closed at times that the worker is available. Creative strategies for incorporating structured physical therapy into these types of lifestyles are required. Referrals to physical therapy for a period of time will be important to the patient's health maintenance so that appropriate exercises, positioning, use of pillows for body alignment, and instructions on proper body mechanics can be completed. Stress to the patient the crucial role of exercise in the prescribed therapy and encourage him or her to make it a daily routine. Proper body mechanics, positioning, and movement can prevent further trauma to the disks of the vertebral column. In the home environment, it may be difficult to adhere completely to the prescribed regimen for movement. Usual home activities that one never considered damaging are now prohibited, such as bending down to pick up an item on the floor or picking up a small child or infant. It may be helpful to the patient to have the physical therapist, or nurse, make a list of seemingly routine tasks and activities that can aggravate the pain and thus limit mobility and functioning. In some areas, there may be special classes or support groups for persons with back problems, such as Back School.

Documentation

Document a thorough assessment of the patient's functional mobility. Include in the patient record all interventions recommended to the patient to address the problem of mobility. Document participation in physical therapy or other activities, such as water aerobics. A report of the patient's perception of the ability to be mobile should be included. Clearly document the effectiveness of all interventions for all members of the health care team. Record all teaching. This documentation will most likely be in a record in a physician's office or a home health agency and should be completed according to the agency protocol.

NURSING DIAGNOSIS 3

DEFICIENT KNOWLEDGE

Related to:

     Possible surgical intervention: laminectomy

Defining Characteristics:

     No prior knowledge of procedure

     Asks many questions

Goal:

     The patient verbalizes an understanding of surgical intervention.

Outcome Criteria

✔ The patient states the purpose of a laminectomy.

✔ The patient states how the procedure is performed.

✔ The patient states the pre-operative and post-operative care required when undergoing a laminectomy.

✔ The patient expresses an understanding of the care required at home.

✔ The patient verbalizes an understanding of follow-up care required and expresses a willingness to comply.

NOC   *Knowledge: Treatment regimen*
          Knowledge: Disease process

INTERVENTIONS	RATIONALES
Assess the patient's current knowledge as well as his or her ability and readiness to learn.	The nurse needs to ascertain what the patient already knows and build on this; if the patient is not capable of learning or is not ready to learn, teaching will not be effective due to disinterest or inability to understand.
Start with the simplest information and move to complex information.	Patients can understand simple concepts easily and then can build on those to understand more complex concepts.
Explain laminectomy to the patient: — Most common procedure for herniated disk — Anatomy and physiology of the vertebral column, and pathophysiology of herniated disk — Removal of a part of the vertebral lamina and nucleosus pulposa — Usual length of hospital stay is 2–3 days	Understanding the procedure will enhance post-operative outcomes.

INTERVENTIONS	RATIONALES
Teach the patient how to logroll and to refrain from using the bedrails for position changes.	Post-operatively, the patient will be turned by the nurse using logrolling techniques, and the patient needs to understand that this is required to maintain the spinal column in proper body alignment. Pulling on the side rails puts stress on the operative site.
Teach the patient how to use the incentive spirometer and how to cough and deep breathe.	These techniques will be required to prevent respiratory complications, such as atelectasis.
Inform the patient that post-operatively he or she will need to remain flat for a period of time, including for meals.	If the patient understands the need for this, anxiety will diminish and the patient will be more compliant.
Inform the patient that limited movement and ambulation will be allowed the first post-operative day.	Even though activity is prescribed by the physician, most patients are allowed out of bed the first post-op day. If patients are informed of this pre-operatively, they will not be surprised but can mentally prepare themselves for the challenge.
Teach patient to use pain control measures before pain becomes severe and to seek pain relief prior to the first time out of bed.	Pain that becomes severe is more difficult to relieve; if pain is managed, the patient is more likely to comply with activity recommendations.
Assess the patient's and family's understanding of all teaching by encouraging them to repeat information and ask questions as needed.	This allows the nurse to hear in the patient's own words what was taught and makes it easier to know what information may need to be reinforced.
Give the patient or family printed material that outlines the information taught.	Printed materials can serve as a backup when the patient is at home and needs review.

NIC　*Learning readiness enhancement*
　　　Learning facilitation

Evaluation

Evaluate the degree to which the patient has achieved the outcome criteria relevant to the teaching sessions. The patient should verbalize an understanding of the laminectomy procedure and pre-operative and post-operative care required. The nurse must determine whether the patient is capable of being compliant with the recommended regimen. If further teaching is required at time of discharge, the appropriate referrals should be made to continue education.

Community/Home Care

At home, the patient may not require the services of any health care personnel other than the physical therapist for reinforcement of activity requirements. Once at home, the patient must implement activity prescriptions, such as ambulation. The patient is not allowed to sit or stand for long periods, but should ambulate on a regular basis as recovery progresses. Stairs are avoided following laminectomy for several weeks because of the stress on the spinal column, making in-home adjustments necessary. If bedrooms are on second-floor levels, the patient will need to make other sleeping arrangements. In addition, if a patient lives in an apartment on an upper floor without elevators, a transport service with a stretcher will be needed to carry the patient upstairs. When out of bed at home, the patient should sit in a straight back chair. The patient will need to wear some type of thoracolumbar support device, a brace, or other support device for the back. Such devices may alter the way clothes look, and the patient may be hesitant to wear them in public, but the necessity of wearing such a dveice should be stressed. The recovery time following laminectomy varies, and it may take 6–12 months before the patient is able to return to normal functioning. Patients should understand that laminectomies do not always totally alleviate the pain. A health care provider needs to investigate the impact this may have on patients who are still employed, in terms of being able to meet financial obligations of health care and the home. Appropriate referrals for assistance should be made as deemed appropriate.

Documentation

Chart whether the stated outcome criteria have been achieved. Document the specific content taught and the titles of any printed materials given to the patient. Include in the chart the patient's degree of understanding of the content and the methods used to teach and evaluate learning. Document the patient's stated understanding of pain management and activity restrictions and recommendations. Chart the patients' ability to demonstrate use of the incentive spirometer and how to logroll. Any areas that need to be reinforced should be documented to ensure appropriate follow-up. If family members are present for the teaching sessions, document this in the chart, and always document referrals made for in-home assistance. Include information regarding the patient's and family's feelings or concerns about care at home.

CHAPTER 3.41

LOU GEHRIG'S DISEASE (AMYOTROPHIC LATERAL SCLEROSIS)

GENERAL INFORMATION

Lou Gehrig's disease or amyotrophic lateral sclerosis (ALS) is a degenerative disorder of the neurological system that results from a gradual degeneration and demyelination of motor neurons in the brain stem, cerebral cortex, and spinal cord. As the disease progresses, the affected neurons become unable to produce or transport necessary impulses to muscles. The eventual result is flaccid quadriplegia; however, there are no sensory or cognitive impairments. The earliest symptoms are weakness of hands and arms with fatigue. Other clinical manifestations include muscle atrophy of legs, dysarthria, dysphagia, atrophy of tongue and facial muscles, loss of fine motor skills, and increased deep tendon reflexes. Respiratory complications develop late in the disease and include dyspnea and ineffective airway clearance. ALS occurs most often in persons 40–60 years old with most cases seen in people in their early 50s and most often in men. A majority of patients diagnosed with ALS die within 2–5 years of diagnosis from respiratory failure or respiratory infection.

NURSING DIAGNOSIS 1

 IMPAIRED PHYSICAL MOBILITY

Related to:

    Degeneration of motor neurons

    Lack of impulses to extremities

Defining Characteristics:

    Weakness in hands, arms, and shoulders

    Fasciculations

    Increased deep tendon reflexes

    Muscle atrophy and paresis

    Progressive fatigue

    Loss of fine motor skills

    Weakness/paresis of trunk and legs (late in disease)

Goal:

    The patient is able to remain physically mobile, either through the use of assistive devices or with the help of a caregiver or family member.

    Adequate range of motion and positions of function are maintained/accomplished.

Outcome Criteria

✔ The patient's arms and hands will be able to move through range of motion.

✔ The patient's lower extremities will be able to move through range of motion.

✔ Complications of immobility do not occur (pneumonia, skin breakdown, contractures).

✔ The patient will be out of bed three times a day.

✔ The patient will be mobile with a wheelchair.

NOC *Ambulation: Wheelchair Mobility*

INTERVENTIONS	RATIONALES
Assess for alterations in motor function and note abnormalities such as weak extremities and decreased muscle mass and strength.	A baseline of function needs to be established; these are clinical manifestations of the disease.
Assess the patient for range of motion and weakness as well as ability to reposition self or ambulate.	Helps to determine the current functional ability and to plan for appropriate interventions.

INTERVENTIONS	RATIONALES
Obtain a history from the patient about mobility limitations and effect on ability to remain functional, especially with usual activities such as personal care.	Helps to determine what adaptations in lifestyle need to be made and the severity of mobility limitations.
Encourage the patient to remain ambulatory for as long as condition allows.	To limit the period of time that the patient is immobile, to prevent complications of immobility, and to preserve function.
When paresis extends to lower extremities and the patient becomes immobile, move the patient out of bed into a chair daily.	Prevents complications of prolonged bedrest such as pneumonia, DVT, and skin breakdown.
Arrange for physical therapy consultation for methods/ therapies to improve or preserve function for as long as possible.	The physical therapist can implement a plan for improvement of weakness and for preservation of muscle and prevention of contractures.
Reposition the patient every 2 hours or as requested. Provide trochanter rolls, pillow supports, and range of motion.	Maintains positions of function and comfort. The patient does not lose sensation and can detect discomfort from pressure/immobility; he or she may request repositioning. Range of motion and proper positioning help to prevent contractures.
Assess patient skin for redness or skin breakdown every 2 hours when repositioning.	Pressure from immobility compresses blood vessels in high-risk areas, depriving them of nutrients and oxygenation leading to skin death.
Teach patient and family turning, lifting/moving techniques, correct body alignment, use of assistive devices, and how to perform range of motion.	Maintains function as long as possible and prevents contractures. Even though a physical therapist may come into the home to work with the patient, family members may also be required to move and position the patient.
Administer medications, such as riluzole (Rilutek®), as ordered, and monitor for side effects.	Riluzole is a glutamate antagonist that protects the neurons against glutamic acid.
Encourage range of motion exercises at least three times a day.	Prevents contractures.
Assess for fatigue and encourage frequent rest periods throughout the day.	Rest and relaxation provide an opportunity to replenish the body's energy. Activity should be undertaken following a period of rest or early in the morning. Fatigue may exacerbate symptoms.
Note results of diagnostic test: EMG.	EMG is the only diagnostic test that provides evidence for the diagnosis.
Teach patient and family: — Disease process — Effect on functional ability — Prognosis: effect on communication, mobility, and eating, complete quadriplegia and death — Complications	The patient and family need to understand what to expect from the disease so preparations can be made before the situation reaches a crisis.

NIC *Exercise therapy*
Joint mobility
Positioning

Evaluation

The patient maintains full range of motion of all extremities with no contractures. The patient participates in mobility activities and exercises to the extent possible by using wheelchairs or other assistive devices. Skin breakdown and pneumonia do not result from bedrest. The patient does not fall while ambulating and is able to participate in self-care to the extent possible.

Community/Home Care

ALS is treated at home for most patients until they become totally dependent in activities of daily living, and the family or other caregiver can no longer manage them. The family should receive thorough information regarding the disease and its impact on mobility. Early in the disease, it is crucial that caregivers encourage the patient to remain mobile and participate in ambulation and exercise as long as possible. As the weakness/paresis in the upper extremities progresses through the hands, then shoulders and upper arms, the patient becomes unable to perform simple activities such as eating or dressing. At this point, the patient must rely on others for assistance, including exercising the affected extremities in an attempt to preserve some muscle tone, preventing contractures, and promoting as much self-care as possible. Other interventions, such as range of motion and the use of special braces and splints, should be initiated by the caregiver to prevent contractures that can develop quickly (within 1 week). Range of motion exercises must be aggressive and frequent, at least every 2 hours to prevent complications. Turning and repositioning are required to prevent skin breakdown and pneumonia, especially as the patient becomes more immobile. The physical therapist has a role in providing instruction to family and patients on the use of assistive devices such as walkers and wheelchairs for ambulation once independent ambulation is no longer possible due to extreme weakness and paralysis. Fatigue is a serious problem, making the patient's efforts at activity problematic. The patient should be encouraged to participate in activity following rest periods each day. As the patient's paralysis progresses to the point of the patient having no motor function, feelings of frustration, powerlessness, and even depression become more pronounced. Providing care for a totally dependent patient can prove to be challenging to family members, necessitating changes in routines. It is important that the family members are supported in their care giving in order to prevent caregiver role strain and the possibility of negative behaviors directed at the patient. Providing a visiting nurse who can assess how the patient is progressing and troubleshoot with the family can reduce anxiety. The family will need to be equipped with coping strategies that are successful in stressful times of physical and mental exhaustion. Caregivers will need to understand that it is okay to ask for and accept assistance in the care-giving role. Social services can assist with acquisition of durable medical supplies such as wheelchairs, hospital beds, and bedside commodes for use in the home. In addition, the social worker or case manager may be able to explain available financial resources for assistance. For ALS patients, there is no expectation that mobility will return, leading some caregivers to make decisions in favor of alternative living arrangements, possibly in long-term care facilities.

Documentation

Chart the findings from an assessment of motor function and muscle strength and provide an accurate description of the patient's motor activity. If the patient is able to ambulate or move, detail the extent of his or her capabilities and participation. Include in the documentation the use of special devices or assistive devices for ambulation. Document all interventions implemented to

address the issue of immobility, as well as instruction provided to the caregiver relevant to addressing immobility. If any complications of immobility are noted, these are charted in accordance with agency protocol.

NURSING DIAGNOSIS 2

 INEFFECTIVE AIRWAY CLEARANCE

Related to:

Weakness of respiratory muscles

Dysphagia

Atrophy of the tongue that makes aspiration likely

Defining Characteristics:

Coughing when eating

Shortness of breath

Crackles in lungs

Inability to expectorate sputum

Goal:

The patient's airway will remain clear.

Outcome Criteria

✔ The patient will have no shortness of breath.

✔ The patient will have clear breath sounds.

✔ The patient will state that breathing is easy.

✔ Respiratory rate will be < 28 per minute.

✔ Oxygen saturation will be > 90 percent.

NOC *Respiratory status: Airway patency*
Respiratory status: Ventilation

INTERVENTIONS	RATIONALES
Assess respiratory status: breath sounds (note adventitious sounds), respiratory rate, oxygen saturation, dyspnea, presence of cyanosis, use of accessory muscles, flaring of nostrils.	Abnormal breath sounds may be noted; abnormal breathing patterns may signal worsening of condition; flaring of nostrils indicate a significant decline in respiratory status and airway patency; establishes a baseline and allows monitoring of response to interventions.

INTERVENTIONS	RATIONALES
Monitor patient for signs of occluded airway: cyanosis, a high-pitched sound when inhaling, inability to speak, absence of breath sounds over lungs, holding throat, continuous coughing.	Occlusion of the airway results in no air movement, and therefore no breath sounds. Holding the throat and being unable to speak are classic signs of choking, and the patient may cough almost continuously in an attempt to open the airway.
Clear airway through suctioning or Heimlich maneuver; if the patient becomes unconscious perform Heimlich maneuver and finger sweep to remove object; or, if the object is visible, remove with ring forceps or suction.	Thick secretions or emesis can be removed via suctioning; the Heimlich maneuver forces air from the thoracic cavity to dislodge obstructions caused by a foreign body and physical removal of visible objects clears the airway.
Assess mental status during period when airway is obstructed and immediately following.	Lack of oxygen for even short periods can affect cerebral oxygenation, resulting in changes in mental status and level of consciousness.
If in the hospital setting, monitor arterial blood gases (ABGs) and oxygen saturation, as ordered.	ABG analysis will reveal respiratory acidosis, as the lungs are unable to expel carbon dioxide; oxygen levels will be low, as the lungs are unable to take in oxygen and exchange gases.
Assess for anxiety and reassure patient with presence.	The patient's inability to breathe causes anxiety and fear, which in turn increases the demand for oxygen; the patient needs a calming presence.
Provide oxygen if available in the home, as ordered.	Restores oxygenation to tissues.
Place patient in high Fowler's position.	Maximizes chest excursion and subsequent movement of air.
Monitor patient for signs of aspiration into lungs: abnormal breath sounds, fever, increased secretions.	Helps to detect early symptoms that may require further treatment in a hospital setting. Frequently, when foreign objects (especially food) are in the airway, some particles may be aspirated into lungs and may cause aspiration pneumonia.
When the patient eats, put him or her in high Fowler's position and feed him or her with the head flexed forward slightly.	This allows for better swallowing and propulsion of food through the esophagus with airway closed.
Feed slowly, giving small amounts; if the patient coughs during feeding, stop feeding immediately.	Prevents aspiration.
Always have suction equipment at bedside and teach the family how to use it.	Provides a means for removing food and secretions that may cause choking or aspiration because the patient can not expectorate them.
Encourage the family to turn the patient every 2 hours when he or she is confined to bed.	This promotes mobilization of secretions that can occlude airway.
Encourage intake of at least 2000 ml of fluids each day.	Fluids thin secretions and decrease the likelihood of stasis in the lungs.

NIC *Airway management*
Cough enhancement
Presence
Respiratory monitoring
Oxygen therapy
Ventilation assistance

Evaluation

Assess the patient to determine the extent to which the outcome criteria have been met. Assessments of the respiratory system should reveal that acute symptoms of airway obstruction have been resolved. The patient's airway should be clear; the patient should be able to speak and should be breathing easy. Breath sounds should be present and even, though some mild wheezing may be noted as the respiratory system attempts to reestablish adequate respirations; this should be improved. The patient should be alert and back at a normal level of consciousness.

Community/Home Care

The patient with ALS is maintained at home, where airway obstruction will continue to be a problem due to the loss of respiratory muscle function. The patient and family should be aware of causes of obstruction and how to prevent a reoccurrence. The ALS patient should be encouraged to chew food slowly and well before swallowing. A consult with a nutritionist or the speech pathologist may be helpful to the family to determine types of foods that can be chewed and swallowed easily. It is important that the patient eat sitting up; the family can use a comfortable chair with a tray, leaving the patient up for at least 1 hour following meals. Family members who are caring for the patient should learn how to suction the patient orally, and to the extent possible, the patient should also learn self-suctioning. Health care providers should make appropriate referrals to obtain the necessary equipment for use in the home ensuring that teaching with the opportunity for demonstration and questioning is available when the equipment is delivered. Follow-up care by an in-home nurse may be needed to be certain that the family understands how to work equipment, recognizing that suctioning may produce physiological discomfort for the patient and psychological discomfort for the caregiver. Teaching should also include how to assess the respiratory status of the patient, particularly signs of respiratory distress and aspiration. The patient and family will need to know the signs of airway obstruction and what interventions may be implemented prior to seeking emergency care.

Documentation

Health care providers should document a comprehensive respiratory assessment, including the family members' or caregivers' observations during any acute episodes of obstruction, and the patient's status once the problem has been resolved. Of particular note should be breath sounds, color, respiratory rate, depth, and any nonverbal signs by the patient that he or she is having difficulty breathing. Include in the patient record interventions carried out to relieve the obstruction and the patient's response. Note specifically changes in breath sounds in response to interventions and the patient's emotional state. Always include in the documentation the patient's progress towards achievement of the stated outcome criteria.

NURSING DIAGNOSIS 3

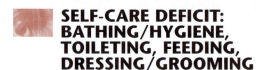

SELF-CARE DEFICIT: BATHING/HYGIENE, TOILETING, FEEDING, DRESSING/GROOMING

Related to:

Weakness and paresis of upper extremities (early)

Weakness and paresis of lower extremities (late)

Progression of disease

Defining Characteristics:

Unable to dress self appropriately

Continent of bladder and bowel but unable to get to bathroom independently

Requires assistance with eating

Unable to bathe self

Dysphagia

Goal:

The patient's basic needs of hygiene, dressing/grooming, feeding, and toileting will be met.

Outcome Criteria

✔ The patient will be clean and have no body odors.

✔ The patient will eat 75 percent of meals and not aspirate.

✔ The patient will remain continent of bowel and bladder.

✔ The patient will have no skin breakdown.

INTERVENTIONS	RATIONALES
Assess the patient's ability to perform activities of daily living.	Determines what type and how much assistance the patient may require.
Encourage the patient to do as much as possible.	Participating in care even in limited ways helps to maintain function, provides stimulation for the patient, and fosters some sense of independence.
Encourage the patient to participate in activity/schedule planning.	This will help the patient retain a sense of control and autonomy and meet his or her daily living needs.
Bathing: Offer the patient assistance with the bath as needed, but encourage the patient to do as much as physically possible; gather supplies for the patient.	The patient may be able to bathe self independently early in the disease, but the ability to perform bathing will decrease as weakness, fatigue, and paralysis of extremities worsens. It is important for the patient's self-esteem to allow him or her to remain as independent as possible. Eventually the patient may become totally dependent, requiring bathing by a caregiver.

INTERVENTIONS	RATIONALES
Dressing/grooming: Assess the patient's ability to dress and groom self. Use clothes that are easy for the patient to put on. Place items needed for personal care such as toothbrushes, toothpaste, combs, and hairbrushes within easy reach for the patient.	As motor skills deteriorate, the ability to gather supplies and dress becomes more difficult; the use of zippers, buttons, and ties becomes especially difficult, as fine motor skills are lost.
Toileting: Assist the patient as needed for toileting: help the patient to the bathroom as needed; once the patient has become dependent, take him or her to the bathroom at scheduled intervals (every 2 hours) for urination; for bowel movements, take the patient to the bathroom following breakfast.	Patients with ALS generally do not become incontinent, but scheduled trips to the bathroom may increase the likelihood that the patient will use the bathroom. Thirty minutes to 1 hour following breakfast is the natural time for increased peristalsis, which improves likelihood that bowel evacuation will occur. If the patient becomes totally dependent for all needs and is bedridden, incontinent pads and frequent checking and cleaning to prevent skin breakdown is required.
Assess patient for skin breakdown and turn every 2 hours.	Once the patient becomes immobile, the risk for breakdown increases due to pressure on areas prone to breakdown.
Increase fluids to 2000 ml/day but limit fluids after 6 p.m.	Increasing fluids helps prevent urinary stasis and risk for urinary tract infection; limiting the fluids in the evening will reduce the patient's nighttime incontinent episodes.
Feeding: Create a pleasant environment for meals. Assess the patient's ability to eat and what assistance may be needed. Allow the patient to feed him or herself for as long as possible, encouraging him or her to take small bites and chew carefully. Position the patient in upright position with head flexed forward. As the disease progresses, it is important to have a suction apparatus available in case the patient aspirates or chokes.	The patient with ALS has dysphagia due to atrophy of the tongue and facial muscles. Aspiration is a potential problem to anticipate; having a suction apparatus available is necessary in case airway patency becomes threatened. In some instances, the patient does not have adequate motor control to feed him or herself the entire meal.

Provide for sufficient rest periods between activities. Schedule significant activities early in the day.

With ALS, fatigue is always a problem and worsens as the day progresses; patients with ALS can become quite fatigued very easily. Rest is important to maximize activity periods.

NIC *Self-care assistance: Toileting*

Self-care assistance: Dressing/grooming

Self-care assistance: Feeding

Hair care

Self-care assistance: Bathing/grooming

Evaluation

All outcome criteria have been achieved, or reasons for non-achievement are noted. The patient is bathed and kept clean, dry, and odor-free. The patient eats at least 75 percent of the meals served without aspiration and is able to participate in mealtime activities. The patient remains continent by requesting assistance with toileting or by caregivers taking the patient to the bathroom at scheduled intervals. The patient has his or her self-care needs met.

Community/Home Care

Adjusting to the patient's decreasing ability to take care of his or her most basic needs often creates a great challenge for in-home caregivers. Involvement of upper extremities—hands and arms—occurs early in the disease, making it difficult for the patient to remain independent for skills such as bathing, dressing, or feeding self. Purchase clothing that pulls on easily, avoiding small buttons that require significant dexterity, as fine motor skills are lost. Changes in the function of the tongue and atrophy of facial muscles makes eating difficult and places the patient at significant risk for aspiration. It is important that the patient have enough time to eat and eat slowly, but independence should be maintained as long as possible. A critical intervention for in-home caregivers is learning how to operate a suction machine correctly and how to perform the Heimlich maneuver in case the patient aspirates. The patient may also learn how to suction the oral cavity. The family will need to pay attention to the amount the patient consumes to ensure that intake of food and fluids is adequate. Because of the frustrations of eating, the patient may eat less, and weight loss may occur. If so, supplemental intake of nutritious snacks or drinks should be incorporated into the patient's diet. The patient should be out of bed, sitting upright for meals if possible and remain upright for 1 hour after meals. In addition, when swallowing becomes difficult and the risk for aspiration is real, the patient should flex head forward when attempting to swallow. The patient with ALS does not lose the ability to respond to signals for the need to void or defecate, so incontinence does not occur. When the patient becomes totally dependent in terms of mobility, the caregiver can implement a scheduled toileting program to keep the patient dry. Caregivers should take note of the patient's usual pattern of voiding and having bowel movements, and establish a scheduled toileting plan that mimics the patient's normal routine. Thirty to sixty minutes following breakfast is the ideal time to sit the patient on the toilet for bowel evacuation. All of these efforts will require patience of and a time commitment by the caregiver. For many families, the decision to institutionalize the patient may occur when the patient becomes totally dependent for all care. When addressing the self-care needs of the patient, the family must consider the available resources that may provide some in-home assistance for personal care and seek out referrals.

Documentation

Whether the patient is in the home or in an institution, a health care provider should document the level of functioning for the patient in all areas of self-care. Document the patient's ability to toilet self, or assistance required, and record intake and output as required. In addition, include in the record the ability or willingness of the patient to eat and how much he or she eats. Chart any interventions employed to enhance self-care efforts.

NURSING DIAGNOSIS 4

IMPAIRED VERBAL COMMUNICATION

Related to:

Brain stem involvement

Atrophy of facial muscles

Atrophy of the tongue

Defining Characteristics:

Dysarthria

Goal:

The patient will be able to communicate needs and desires.

Outcome Criteria

✔ The patient will continue to talk for as long as possible, using simple words.

✔ The patient will use a communication board to express one need.

✔ The patient will be able to express needs by using pictures, writing, or pointing to words.

NOC *Communication*
Communication expressive

INTERVENTIONS	RATIONALES
Assess the patient's ability to communicate; determine whether the patient can read and write.	Establishes that the patient is able to use alternative communication methods.
If the patient is able to read and write, provide the patient with alternative to verbal communication: communication board, pencil and paper, Magic Slate, or chalkboard. Provide picture cards if the patient cannot read or write.	This provides an alternative method of communication. For the patient with ALS, the use of the hands may be impaired to the extent that he or she is unable to write.
If the patient is unable to use his or her hands to write or point, teach him or her to signal using eye blinks, nodding, or other means of nonverbal communication.	Much information can be communicated using simple gestures to signal "yes" and "no" as well as other simple commands.
Arrange for a speech therapist consult and utilize the speech therapist for assistance in establishing the best communication strategies and to educate the patient and family.	Speech therapists are best qualified to assist the patient with alternative communication methods, including adjunct devices.
Teach the patient how to speak slowly.	Even though the patient's speech may be understood by some, such as caregivers or family, others may not be able to understand, as the speech is altered from normal. Speaking slowly allows for better formation of words and allows others to listen more attentively.

INTERVENTIONS	RATIONALES
Take time to work with the patient in communication efforts; be patient and do not rush him or her.	Rushing the patient to communicate causes frustration and may make the patient stop trying to communicate.
Provide encouragement and emotional support for the patient who is learning new communication strategies.	Encouragement and support enhance patient motivation and decrease anxiety. Privacy may be required in the early stage of learning as the patient becomes more comfortable with new communication methods. The patient may feel comfortable with family but not with other people.

NIC   *Communication enhancement:*
   Speech deficit

   Learning facilitation

   Anxiety reduction

Evaluation

Evaluate the progress the patient has made in the ability to communicate. Establish what needs to be done to further enhance nonverbal communication with the patient. Evaluate whether the patient is able to communicate using a communication board, pictures, writing, nodding, blinking, or pointing. Determine whether the patient is frustrated or satisfied with attempts at communication.

Community/Home Care

For the patient who has ALS, the inability to communicate verbally may prove to be a challenging and frustrating aspect of the disease. As the tongue and facial muscles atrophy, the ability to formulate words for speech that can be understood deteriorates. Patients may feel embarrassed, particularly in public or around non-family members, and may refrain from efforts to communicate due to this as well as frustration at trying to make others understand. The patient must be encouraged to continue with new communication strategies, and this is where social support systems can be most beneficial. All caregivers should talk to the patient and have him or her respond verbally with words other than "yes" or "no" as long as the patient is capable of speech. As family and friends display acceptance,

encouragement, and patience, the patient will become more comfortable with communication knowing that others understand. If this does not happen, the patient may socially isolate him or herself, which could lead to emotional distress. Follow-up care should give attention to not only the physiological realm of care but to this very critical aspect of the patient's well-being.

Documentation

Document all communication strategies utilized with the patient. Include an evaluation of the patient's efforts to communicate and which strategies work best. Always include an assessment of the patient's emotional state and responses to all interventions. Chart any referrals made for speech and the outcomes of recommendations. When communication devices or techniques are employed to enhance communication, document the patient's ability and willingness to use them.

NURSING DIAGNOSIS 5

 INEFFECTIVE COPING: INDIVIDUAL AND FAMILY

Related to:

   Chronic progressive disease

   Life expectancy of 2–6 years

Defining Characteristics:

   Anger

   Expressions of fear

   Restlessness and anxiety

   Crying

   Expresses distress at potential loss of life

Goal:

   Coping is enhanced and anxiety decreased.

Outcome Criteria

✔ The patient identifies one coping mechanism to be used.

✔ The family verbalizes an understanding of the disease process.

✔ The caregiver identifies one coping mechanism to be used.

✔ The patient verbalizes fears and concerns.

✔ The patient and family report being less anxious.

✔ The patient demonstrates no outward signs of anxiety, such as restlessness or agitation.

NOC *Anxiety control*
Comfort level
Coping
Grief resolution

INTERVENTIONS	RATIONALES
Assess level of anxiety (mild, moderate, severe); have the patient rate on a scale of 1–10, with 10 being the greatest.	Gives the nurse an objective measure of extent of the anxiety.
Assess the patient and family to determine their feelings regarding the diagnosis of Lou Gehrig's disease and the patient's prognosis, and support them as appropriate by answering questions and making referrals.	Assisting the patient and family to deal with the diagnosis and prognosis will enhance their ability to cope with serious illness.
Keep the patient and family informed of all that is going on, including information about possible disease progression and interventions required at home.	Knowledge about the disease and what is required prepares the patient and family for the patient's future needs. Honesty concerning prognosis is the start to having the patient cope; communication in a straightforward manner may help to reduce anxiety.
Use a calm, reassuring manner with the patient.	Gives the patient a sense of well-being.
Encourage the patient and family to verbalize expressions of fear and concern about the possible loss of function; listen attentively.	Verbalization of fears contributes to dealing with concerns; being attentive relays empathy to the patient.
Have the patient and family identify at least one coping mechanism that has worked before and investigate new coping strategies.	Coping mechanisms that have worked in the past may help with current needs, but additional ones may be required because of the chronic, life-threatening nature of ALS.
Seek spiritual consult as needed or requested by the patient and/or family.	Meeting the patient's spiritual needs helps him or her to deal with fears through use of spiritual or religious rituals.
Recognize the role of culture in the patient's method of	Culture often dictates how a person grieves, copes, and

coping with life stressors, especially illness and the verbalization of fears and concerns, especially related to communication and mobility.

handles stressful situations; the nurse must recognize this in order to support the patient in a successful grief process.

Engage the patient and family in open dialogue regarding options for treatments and care.	During the final stages of the disease, the patient and family may not be able to care for the patient alone; discussion of care options early in the disease allows the patient to be more in control and gives him or her a sense of empowerment that may assist with coping with the disease.
Provide the patient and family with information regarding advance directives and support decisions that are made.	Allows the patient and family the opportunity to plan for the patient's wishes in the event that he or she becomes unable to make his or her own decisions.
Encourage the family or caregiver to seek assistance with care-giving activities and to attend support groups, if available.	The patient eventually becomes completely dependent, and the caregiver may need assistance to decrease stress and strain. Support groups can provide emotional support.

NIC *Coping enhancement*
Emotional support
Spiritual support
Grief-work facilitation

Evaluation

Evaluate the extent to which the outcome criteria have been achieved. The patient should be assessed for behaviors that would indicate adjustment to the diagnosis of ALS. The patient and family should verbalize their fears and concerns and be able to identify at least one coping strategy that they believe will be successful in dealing with ALS. Note the extent to which the patient displays appropriate coping behaviors. If the patient is unable to talk about the diagnosis and communicate concerns, the nurse should explore further new interventions to assist the patient.

Community/Home Care

Nurses visiting the home should assess which coping mechanisms work for the patient and family and encourage their use at home. Because the life expectancy for ALS is 2–6 years, the patient and family may experience symptoms of grieving. Family members should be encouraged to express any grief in their own way and acceptable coping strategies should be discussed. Extreme self-isolation and depression should be noted and reported to a health care provider. For many patients and families, spiritual/religious rituals provide a means of coping with difficult stressful situations. The patient's culture may dictate how he or she copes and grieves and with whom he or she shares this process. It is crucial that the nurse and family support the patient as needed to foster a healthy psychological state, recognizing that anger and emotional outburst are common. When this occurs, allow the patient to vent his or her feelings. The quiet presence of the caregiver at home may also help. As the disease progresses, the patient may require new strategies for coping with the disease and the anticipated loss of life. The patient as well as the caregiver may benefit from quiet periods of meditation during the day. Playing soothing music that the patient likes may also decrease anxiety. Support to long-term caregivers will be important, as they too need to be supported in a grief process. Visiting nurses from community agencies can play an important role in the home situation through provision of counselors, chaplains, and in-home care providers. If questions should arise at home regarding the patient's health status or prescribed regimen, the patient should have a means of contact with a health care provider for answers.

Documentation

Document coping strategies that the patient and family have identified as successful in the past. Include any suggestions given for new coping strategies. The degree to which the patient is able to verbalize feelings regarding having ALS and has decreased anxiety should be documented in the patient record. Chart the patient's verbalizations as the patient states them and include in the record coping mechanisms utilized by the patient. Record the level of anxiety present using a rating scale that provides an objective way to relay to others the extent of any anxiety. Document findings from an assessment of the patient's psychological state and whether there is depression, anger, crying, sadness, etc. Document any referrals to any agencies for assistance or to religious leaders.

CHAPTER 3.42

MENINGITIS

GENERAL INFORMATION

Meningitis is a disease involving inflammation of the meninges, the protective layers covering the brain and spinal column. Meningitis most commonly occurs secondary to infection by microorganisms but can also be related to chemical or mechanical irritation. Patients with head trauma, especially with a basilar skull fracture, are at high risk for meningitis development because of disruption of the protective blood-brain barrier. Bacterial meningitis is the most common form of meningitis. Bacteria that cause meningitis commonly inhabit the upper respiratory tract as part of the normal flora or proliferate during upper respiratory infections. It is unclear how bacteria enter the central nervous system, but the infecting bacteria cross the blood-brain barrier and cause inflammation of the meningeal layers. Increased intracranial pressure may develop from the meningeal edema and blockage of cerebrospinal fluid reabsorption. Cerebrospinal cultures are positive for bacteria growth in bacterial meningitis. Treatment of bacterial meningitis includes supportive care to minimize the intracranial pressure and antibacterial medications. Viral meningitis is also called "aseptic meningitis" because culture results are negative. Viral antigen assays may detect and identify the infecting viruses. Typically, viral meningitis is less severe than bacterial meningitis and tends to be self-limiting. Treatment involves supportive care to minimize the intracranial pressure and administration of antiviral medication when indicated. Fungal meningitis occurs in immunosuppressed patients and is considered an opportunistic infection. Prophylactic treatment with antifungal medications is commonly prescribed to prevent the development of fungal meningitis. When fungal meningitis develops, cerebrospinal cultures are positive for fungal growth. Treatment includes supportive care to minimize the intracranial pressure and administration of antifungal medications. Clinical manifestations of bacterial meningitis include fever and chills, nausea/vomiting, nuchal rigidity (neck stiffness), a headache (possibly severe), photophobia, changes in mentation that could range from restlessness or agitation to confusion, positive Brudzinski's sign (flexion of the neck that causes the hip and knee to flex), positive Kernig's sign (inability to extend the knee while the hip is flexed at a 90 degree angle), and in meningococcal meningitis a petechial rash. Both Brudzinski's sign and Kernig's sign indicate meningeal irritation. In viral meningitis, the same clinical manifestations are present but are much milder. All types of meningitis can affect people of any age and are most often seen in children. However, meningococcal meningitis has a higher incidence in children and young adults. For this reason, it is not uncommon to see meningococcal meningitis on college campuses and among military recruits where young adults have close contact and close living quarters.

NURSING DIAGNOSIS 1

 ### ACTUAL INFECTION*

Related to:

Direct invasion of organisms into the nervous system after head trauma or invasive procedures

Transport of organisms to the CNS via the blood from other sites of infection

Intrathecal medication administration

Immunodeficiency

Defining Characteristics:

Positive CSF culture and gram stain

Meningeal signs

Photophobia

Fever

Headaches

Stiff neck (nuchal rigidity)

Positive Brudzinski's sign

Positive Kernig's sign

Nausea and vomiting

Goal:

The meningeal infection will resolve.

Outcome Criteria

✔ The patient will have negative CSF culture and gram stain.

✔ The patient will not have signs and symptoms of meningitis.

✔ The patient will be afebrile.

NOC *Infection status*
       Infection severity

INTERVENTIONS	RATIONALES
Assess continued risk for meningitis.	Identifying the presence of risk factors can help with diagnosis; patients who live in college dormitories, military recruits, patients with head trauma, basilar skull fracture, ventricular shunts, and immunosuppression have increased risk for meningitis.
Monitor patient's neurological status including level of consciousness and changes in orientation, seizures, restlessness, increased intracranial pressure (increased blood pressure, decreased pulse, widening pulse pressure, vomiting), and worsening symptoms.	Irritation to the cerebral tissues can cause a varied neurological response including seizures, cerebral edema, and increased intracranial pressure (usually seen in bacterial infections).
Assess for stiff neck, headache, nausea/vomiting, Brudzinski's sign, Kernig's sign, petechial rash, (meningococcal meningitis) photophobia, and fever.	These are classic symptoms of meningitis.
Take temperature every 4 hours and administer antipyretics (usually Tylenol), as ordered.	Fever is caused by pyrogens from microorganisms; the fever is usually high and may remain elevated throughout treatment; fever also increases cerebral edema and increases the risk of seizures.
Provide alternative methods of temperature regulation, including dressing lightly, maintaining cool environmental temperature, tepid bath, or using cooling blanket.	These techniques can aid in reducing fever and maintaining normothermia.
Prepare to assist with lumbar puncture to collect CSF specimen in patients with increased risk and signs or symptoms of meningitis.	Facilitates microorganism detection, identification, and antibiotic sensitivity.
Monitor results of diagnostic tests: CSF for appearance, cell count, protein, glucose, culture, and bacteria; complete blood count; x-rays of sinuses and mastoids.	If it is bacterial meningitis, the fluid will be cloudy with increased white blood cells, increased protein, and decreased glucose, and the causative organism; in viral meningitis, the fluid will be clear with increased white blood cells, increased or slightly elevated protein, and normal glucose; complete blood count will be elevated; x-rays of sinuses and mastoids are done to try and find a causative source.
Administer antibiotics, as ordered.	Treats the infection and prevents the transmission of meningitis to others.
Keep the room dark and place a cool cloth over the eyes.	Darkened rooms enhance comfort for those patients with photophobia; the cool cloth relieves discomfort. A darkened room also decreases stimuli.
Administer medications for nausea and vomiting.	Vomiting is prevented or controlled as it can cause increased ICP, and to provide comfort for the patient.
Administer medications and employ non-pharmacological measures for headache.	Provides comfort; Tylenol may treat headache if not severe; cool packs to the head may also help.
Place the patient in isolation until CSF culture results are known.	Meningococcal infection (*Neisseria meningitides* organism) requires isolation to protect others from this contagious form of the disorder.

NIC *Neurological monitoring*
       Infection protection
       Infection control

Evaluation

Following interventions, the patient's neurological status should improve. The patient has negative CSF culture and gram stain. The patient does not demonstrate any meningeal signs or photophobia. Temperature has returned to normal and the patient offers no complaints.

Community/Home Care

Patients with bacterial meningitis are acutely ill and, following hospitalization, require convalescence at home. Instruction by a health care provider is crucial to ensure that the patient will understand and comply with the medical regimen. The patient with bacterial meningitis will need to take antibiotics for a period ranging between 7 and 21 days, depending on the causative organism. Once the patient begins to feel better, it is easy for him or her to believe that the antibiotics are not needed, and he or she may stop taking them. The nurse must stress to the patient the importance of completing the scheduled therapy for its duration until all antibiotics are consumed. The patient needs to understand that it may take several weeks before he or she returns to a normal level of activity and energy. Because of the possibility of fatigue, the patient will need to eat a nutritious diet consisting of high protein and high calorie foods. Family members or significant others can prepare food in small amounts and offer frequent small servings. Even after acute treatment, the patient may continue to have some neck soreness as a result of the nuchal rigidity. The patient may find comfort from warm compresses applied to the neck for scheduled periods during the day. Family and friends may have some concern and anxiety about whether the patient is able to transmit the disease to others. Assurance should be given to all that the patient has been on antibiotics and the period for transmission is past. Encourage the patient to return for all follow-up appointments and if any neurological symptoms persist to call a health care provider immediately.

Documentation

Document the findings from a complete neurological assessment, including the presence of symptoms of meningitis and any specific patient complaints. Chart medication administration and temperature in the appropriate places in the patient record according to agency guidelines. Include in the record all interventions implemented to treat the meningitis and the patient's response. If the patient experiences photophobia, chart this and the interventions carried out to relieve it. Document any verbalizations the patient makes verbatim.

NURSING DIAGNOSIS 2

 ACUTE PAIN

Related to:
    Meningeal inflammation

Defining Characteristics:
    Patient complaint of headache
    Grimacing, moaning
    Photophobia
    Guarding of neck

Goal:
    Pain and discomfort will be relieved.

Outcome Criteria

✔ The patient will state that headache has been relieved.
✔ The patient verbalizes that nuchal rigidity is improved.
✔ Photophobia has been relieved.

NOC *Pain: Disruptive effects*
        Pain level
        Pain control

INTERVENTIONS	RATIONALES
Assess the patient's pain using a pain rating scale.	Provides a more objective assessment.
Assess or take history regarding time of onset, location, precipitating factors, relieving factors and effect on function, complaint of headache, neck pain or stiffness.	These will assist in accurate diagnosis and treatment; knowing how pain affects function will provide information needed to assist patient with home care needs.
Apply moist heat to neck.	Aids muscle relaxation and decreases pain; moist heat is able to penetrate deeper; if pain intensifies, cold can be used for analgesic properties as well.

INTERVENTIONS	RATIONALES
Administer analgesic medications as ordered and monitor for effectiveness and side effects.	Headaches that accompany meningitis may be relieved with mild analgesics.
Give all medications on a regular dosing schedule rather than prn.	Provides better relief and prevents the pain from getting severe.
Position in semi-Fowler's position with head in midline position.	Facilitates venous drainage from head to minimize cerebral edema that contributes to the pain.
Keep lights off or on low settings in patient's room with curtains closed.	Photophobia commonly occurs secondary to meningeal inflammation, and dim lighting makes environment more comfortable.
Do not medicate to the point that neurological assessment and level of consciousness assessment are obscured.	Narcotic analgesics are often contraindicated because they depress the level of consciousness and make neurological assessment difficult.
Teach relaxation techniques, such as music therapy, massage, distraction, and meditation.	These techniques enhance the effect of analgesics and may decrease reliance on medications for complete relief.

NIC *Simple relaxation therapy*
Heat/cold application
Analgesic administration
Pain management

Evaluation

Assess the degree to which the patient reports that headache and neck pain has been relieved by interventions. For persistent pain, the nurse should investigate additional measures to relieve pain. Determine whether the patient is able to verbalize how to reduce pain.

Community/Home Care

The pain associated with meningitis typically has been relieved by the time the patient is at home. Some degree of neck soreness may persist for a period and require mild analgesics. The patient needs to learn how to implement relaxation techniques that enhance the therapeutic effects of medications. Using moist heat as well as analgesics may relieve the soreness in the neck and should be attempted.

The patient may need to experiment with positioning for comfort when sleeping. The patient may need to take medication before bedtime to achieve the two-fold outcome of enhancement of sleep and relief of pain. If no measures are effective in relieving the pain, a health care provider should be contacted for discussion of new pain relief measures.

Documentation

Document all measures implemented for pain relief. Include in the patient record the patient's verbalized perception of pain and satisfaction with pain control. For the patient who has persistent neck pain or headache, the health care provider should make note of this and include how the plan for pain control was revised. Once the patient is at home for treatment, be sure that office visits document the specific therapeutic interventions prescribed for pain.

NURSING DIAGNOSIS 3

 DEFICIENT KNOWLEDGE

Related to:

Lack of information about meningitis and treatment

Defining Characteristics:

No prior experience with meningitis

Asks no questions

Asks many questions

Goal:

The patient and family will verbalize understanding of meningitis.

Outcome Criteria

✔ The patient/family will verbalize understanding of the disease.

✔ The patient will state the names of medications used to treat meningitis and verbalize an understanding of the need to complete the regimen.

NOC *Compliance behavior*
Knowledge: Disease process
Knowledge: Treatment regimen
Knowledge: Medications

INTERVENTIONS	RATIONALES
Assess the patient's and family's knowledge base, willingness to learn, and readiness to learn.	Teaching must be tailored to the patient's or family members' ability, and the learners must be ready to learn in order to gain from education.
Teach incrementally: simple to complex.	The patient and family members will learn and retain knowledge better when information is presented in small segments, starting with the simple concepts first. The learners can then build on those to understand more complex information.
Teach the patient the following information: — Disease process of meningitis and treatment required — Medication: names, purpose, side effects, scheduling, and duration of treatment — Need for rest at home after hospitalization for bacterial meningitis — Prevention of infection	When the patient and family understand the disease process and treatment, improved disease control occurs, complications decrease, and, if the patient is hospitalized, the hospital length of stay may be reduced.
Provide written material of all information.	This serves as a reference in case the patient forgets what is taught.
Assess the patient's and/or family's understanding of all information taught by asking them to repeat the information.	This allows the nurse to hear in the patient's or family members' own words what was taught and makes it easier to know what information may need to be reinforced.

NIC *Teaching: Disease process*
Learning readiness enhancement
Learning facilitation
Teaching: Prescribed medication

Evaluation

Following the teaching session, the patient states a willingness to be compliant with all recommendations. The patient and family members can state what meningitis is, how it is contracted, and how it is treated. In addition, the patient and family members state the name of prescribed medications, side effects, dosages, and schedule.

Community/Home Care

The disease of meningitis is usually treated successfully, and the patient does not require services of any in-home health care providers. Management at home focuses on the patient taking the prescribed medications (antibiotics) for the duration of the prescribed time. It is difficult for many young people to understand the need for medications if they feel well; however, family support persons must monitor this and ensure that all antibiotics are consumed as ordered. Because the fever may persist throughout the course of treatment, antipyretics—usually Tylenol—may need to be taken at home. It may be beneficial to record the temperature along with medication taken so that this can be reported to a health care provider during follow-up visits. Tylenol is also useful for treatment of discomfort associated with meningitis, including neck soreness and headache. Some adolescents and young adults may have difficulty swallowing pills or gelcaps, and the patient or family members may want to use liquid preparations, but ability to measure doses accurately should be ascertained. For those persons who have meningococcal meningitis, fatigue may be a problem at home, and rest periods should be encouraged until recovery is complete. Quiet activities such as reading, computer games, or board games may provide diversional activities until energy levels return. If the patient has experienced seizures as a result of meningitis and has been prescribed anticonvulsants, the nurse should be sure that the family understands precautions to be taken in case of a seizure to protect the patient from injury, as well as understands the dosing and side effects of medications for seizure (see nursing care plan "Seizures"). The family should be able to verbalize the predisposing conditions for contracting meningitis.

Documentation

Chart teaching sessions in the patient record specifying the exact content taught, titles of printed materials given, and learners who were a part of the session. Document the patient's verbalization of understanding and whether he or she is willing to comply with the medication regimen. Include in the chart any referrals made, as well as where and when the patient is to receive follow-up care.

CHAPTER 3.43

MULTIPLE SCLEROSIS (MS)

GENERAL INFORMATION

Multiple sclerosis (MS) is a progressive degenerative disease of the central nervous system that affects both the brain and spinal cord. In most patients, it results in loss of motor functions and/or sensory functions in varying degrees. The cause of MS is not clearly known, but research points to a genetic component as well as a link to viral infections with a subsequent abnormal immune response. Characteristic pathophysiological findings include chronic inflammation, demyelination, and scarring in the CNS. Because of the demyelination of nerve fibers, transmission of impulses is altered, and in some cases, impulse transmission ceases altogether. Some patients may experience periods of exacerbations and remission, whereas others experience a chronic gradual deterioration in nervous system function. There are four categories of MS: the most common type is relapsing-remitting, which has periods of exacerbations with full recovery or partial recovery with some residual deficits; primary progressive type has a steady worsening of disease from the onset with occasional minor recovery; secondary progressive begins as with relapsing-remitting, but the disease steadily becomes worse between exacerbations; progressive relapsing is a rare form that continues to progress from the onset but also has exacerbations with or without full recovery (Lemone and Burke, 2004). Clinical manifestations depend on the area of the central nervous system affected and vary among patients, but commonly identified manifestations include fatigue (experienced by almost all patients), motor deficits (weakness, paralysis, and/or spasticity), intentional tremors (tremors that occur with intentional movement), altered visual acuity, paresthesias, and spastic bladders. Because of its debilitating effects on both the motor and sensory systems, patients often experience severe emotional distress and personality changes. These patients are often seen in the acute care setting when the disease exacerbates or when complications of the disease occur.

NURSING DIAGNOSIS 1

 IMPAIRED PHYSICAL MOBILITY

Related to:

Loss of motor activity

Loss of sensory perception

Muscle spasms

Intention tremors

Defining Characteristics:

Limb weakness

Dragging of foot and foot drop

Falls

Bruises on extremities

Ataxia leading to inability to ambulate

Goal:

The patient is able to remain physically mobile, either through the use of assistive devices or with the help of a caregiver or family member.

Adequate range of motion and positions of function are maintained/accomplished.

Outcome Criteria

✔ The patient's lower extremities will be able to move through range of motion.

✔ Contractures and foot drop are avoided.

✔ Complications of immobility do not occur (pneumonia, skin breakdown).

✔ The patient will be out of bed three times a day.

✔ The patient will be mobile with walker or wheelchair.

NOC *Ambulation: Wheelchair Mobility*

INTERVENTIONS	RATIONALES
Assess for alterations in motor function and note abnormalities such as weak extremities, decreased muscle tone, muscle spasms, intentional tremors, decreased fine motor abilities, and dragging of foot when walking.	A baseline of function needs to be established; these are clinical manifestations of the disease.
Assess patient for range of motion and ability to reposition self or ambulate.	Helps to determine the current functional ability and to plan for appropriate interventions.
Obtain a history from the patient about mobility limitations and effect on ability to remain functional, especially with usual activities such as personal care.	Helps to determine what adaptations in lifestyle need to be made and the severity of mobility limitations.
Encourage the patient to remain ambulatory for as long as condition allows.	Limits the period of time that the patient is immobile, prevents complications from immobility, and preserves function.
Get the patient out of bed into a chair three times daily when or if the patient becomes immobile.	Prevents complications from prolonged bedrest, such as pneumonia, DVT, and skin breakdown.
Arrange for physical therapy consultation for methods/ therapies to improve or preserve function for as long as possible.	The physical therapist can implement a plan for improvement of weakness and for preservation of muscle and prevention of contractures.
Reposition the patient every 2 hours. Provide trochanter rolls, pillow supports, range of motion.	Maintains positions of function and comfort. Range of motion and proper positioning help to prevent contractures.
Assess the patient's skin for redness or skin breakdown every 2 hours when repositioning.	Pressure from immobility compresses blood vessels in high-risk areas, depriving them of nutrients and oxygenation and leading to skin death.
Teach patient and family turning, lifting/moving techniques, correct body alignment, use of assistive devices, and how to perform range of motion.	Maintains function as long as possible and prevents contractures. Even though a physical therapist may come into the home to work with the patient, family members may also be required to move and position the patient.
Administer medications, such as corticosteroids (adrenocorticotrophic hormones	Treats exacerbations and achieves a remission; decreases inflammatory response
and prednisone) as ordered, and monitor for side effects.	and suppresses the immune system.
Administer immunosuppressive agents such as Imuran® and Cytoxan®, as ordered, and monitor for side effects.	Used to achieve immunosuppression and thus relieve exacerbations.
Administer muscle relaxants, such as baclofen, dantrolene, and Valium, as ordered, and monitor for side effects.	Relieves muscle spasms.
Administer immunomodulators, such as beta interferon (Betaseron®) and glatiramer acetate (Copaxone®), as ordered, and monitor for side effects.	Helps to treat exacerbations.
Encourage range of motion exercises at least three times a day.	Prevents contractures.
Use a foot board on beds.	Prevents foot drop.
Assess for fatigue and encourage frequent rest periods throughout the day.	Rest and relaxation provide an opportunity to replenish the body's energy. Activity should be undertaken following a period of rest or early in the morning. Fatigue may exacerbate symptoms.
Note results of diagnostic tests: computed tomography (CT) scan, MRI (magnetic resonance imaging), spinal tap/lumbar puncture, EEG (electroencephalogram), and evoked responses.	These provide evidence for the diagnosis and rule out other causes of symptoms.

NIC   *Exercise therapy*
        Joint mobility
        Positioning

Evaluation

The patient maintains full range of motion of all extremities with no contractures or foot drop. The patient participates in mobility activities and exercises to the extent possible using wheelchairs or other assistive devices. Skin breakdown and pneumonia do not occur because of being immobile. The patient does not fall while ambulating and is able to participate in self-care to the extent possible.

Community/Home Care

Multiple sclerosis is treated at home for many patients unless they become completely dependent in activities of daily living. The family should receive thorough information regarding the disease and its impact on mobility. Early in the disease, it is crucial that caregivers encourage the patient to remain mobile, participate in ambulation, and exercise as long as possible. As the weakness in the lower extremities progresses to spastic paralysis, the attention in the home turns to preserving muscle tone, preventing contractures, and promoting as much self-care as possible. Stretching exercises and the use of special braces and splints can serve to prevent contractures. Range of motion exercises must be aggressive and frequent to prevent complications. Turning and repositioning are required to prevent skin breakdown and pneumonia, especially as the patient becomes immobile. Fatigue is a serious problem, making the patient's efforts at activity problematic. Encouraging participation in activity should occur following rest periods each day. As the patient attempts to remain independent, intentional tremors of the upper extremities may create feelings of frustration as spills and dropping items become commonplace. An occupational therapist or physical therapist may be helpful in adapting frequently used items for use by the MS patient, especially utensils used at mealtime. The physical therapist has a role in providing instruction to the family and patients on the use of assistive devices such as walkers and wheelchairs for ambulation once independent ambulation is no longer possible due to spasticity. Providing care for a completely dependent patient can prove to be challenging to family members as it necessitates a change in routines, and it is important that the family members are supported in their care-giving. Providing them with a visiting nurse who can assess how the patient is progressing and troubleshoot with the family can assist in reducing anxiety that may be present. The family will need to be equipped with coping strategies that allow them to withstand days of physical and mental exhaustion, as well as the ability to step away from the situation and ask for assistance in the care-giving role. For MS patients, there is no expectation that mobility will return, causing some caregivers to make decisions in favor of alternative living arrangements, possibly in long-term care facilities.

Documentation

Chart the findings from an assessment of motor function and muscle strength, noting spasticity or intentional tremors. If the patient is able to ambulate or move, detail the extent of his or her capabilities and participation. Include in the documentation the use of special or assistive devices for ambulation. Document all interventions implemented to address the issue of immobility. Document instruction to the caregiver relevant to addressing immobility. If any complications of immobility are noted, document these in accordance with agency protocol.

NURSING DIAGNOSIS 2

SELF-CARE DEFICIT: BATHING/HYGIENE, TOILETING, FEEDING, DRESSING/GROOMING

Related to:

Spasticity

Intentional tremors

Progression of disease

Defining Characteristics:

Unable to dress self appropriately

Incontinent of bladder and bowel

Requires assistance with eating

Unable to bathe self

Goal:

The patient's basic needs of hygiene, dressing/grooming, feeding, and toileting will be met.

Outcome Criteria

✔ The patient will be clean and have no body odors.
✔ The patient will remain dry.
✔ The patient will be assisted in toileting for bowel movements and be cleansed.
✔ The patient will have no skin breakdown due to bowel or bladder incontinence.

INTERVENTIONS	RATIONALES
Assess the patient's ability to perform activities of daily living.	Determines what type of and how much assistance the patient may require.
Encourage the patient to do as much as possible.	Participating in care even in limited ways helps to maintain function and provides stimulation for the patient, fosters some sense of

(continues)

(continued)

INTERVENTIONS	RATIONALES
	independence, and maintains self-esteem.
Encourage the patient to participate in activity/schedule planning.	This will help the patient retain a sense of control and autonomy and meet his or her daily living needs.
Bathing: Offer the patient assistance with the bath as needed, but encourage patient to do as much as physically possible; gather supplies for the patient.	The patient may be able to bathe self independently early in the disease, but the ability to perform bathing may decrease as tremors and spasticity of extremities occur. It is important for the patient's self-esteem to allow him or her to remain as independent as possible for as long as possible. Eventually the patient may become completely dependent and require bathing by a caregiver.
Dressing/grooming: Assess the patient's ability to dress and groom self. Use clothes that are easy for the patient to put on. Place items needed for personal care, such as toothbrushes, toothpaste, combs, and hairbrushes, within easy reach for the patient.	As motor skills deteriorate, the ability to gather supplies and dress becomes more difficult, especially the use of zippers, buttons, and ties.
Toileting: Assess the patient for retention, incontinence, and urgency. Assist the patient to the bathroom as needed; once the patient is dependent, take him or her to the bathroom at scheduled intervals (every 2 hours) for urination; for bowel movements take the patient to the bathroom following breakfast. When the patient becomes incontinent, check frequently and keep him or her clean and dry. Assess the need for catheterization (intermittent or indwelling).	Scheduled trips to the bathroom may increase the likelihood that the patient will use the bathroom and prevent incontinent episodes. Thirty minutes to 1 hour following breakfast is the natural time for increased peristalsis, which improves likelihood that bowel evacuation will occur. If the patient becomes completely dependent for all needs and is bedridden, incontinent pads and frequent checking and cleaning to prevent skin breakdown will be required.
Cleanse the patient after any incontinent episode; apply protective ointment.	Prevents skin breakdown caused by urine.
Assess the patient for skin breakdown and turn every 2 hours.	Once the patient becomes immobile, the risk for breakdown increases due to pressure on areas prone to breakdown.

Increase fluids to 2000 ml/day but limit fluids after 6 p.m.	Increasing fluids helps prevent urinary stasis and risk for urinary tract infection; limiting the fluids in the evening decreases the number of nighttime incontinent episodes.
Feeding: Create a pleasant environment for meals. Assess the patient's ability to eat and what assistance may be needed. Allow the patient to feed self for as long as possible. If intentional tremors and spasticity worsen, encourage special eating utensils such as plate guards, and offer finger foods or foods easy to manipulate with a fork or spoon.	These efforts increase self-esteem and independence, and decrease the frustration that can come with being unable to feed him or herself appropriately. In some instances, the patient does not have adequate motor control to feed him or herself the entire meal.
Provide for sufficient rest periods between activities and schedule significant activities early in the day.	With MS, fatigue progresses as the hours of the day pass, and patients can become quite fatigued very easily. Rest is important to maximize activity periods.

NIC   *Self-care assistance: Toileting*

Self-care assistance: Dressing/ grooming

Self-care assistance: Feeding

Self-care assistance: Bathing/ grooming

Evaluation

All outcome criteria have been achieved, or reasons for non-achievement are noted. The patient is bathed and kept clean, dry, and odor-free. The patient eats appropriately and is able to participate in mealtime activities. Incontinent episodes are minimized by taking the patient to the bathroom at scheduled intervals or as requested. The patient has his or her self-care needs met.

Community/Home Care

Adjusting to the patient's decreasing ability to take care of his or her most basic needs often creates a great challenge for in-home caregivers. As the patient's physical abilities deteriorate, he or she is unable to bathe or change clothes independently. Purchase clothing that pulls on easily, avoiding small buttons that require significant dexterity. If possible, involve the patient in the preparation of meals on a limited basis. It is important that the patient have enough time to eat and that independence is maintained as long as possible. Caregivers should prepare foods for the patient that are nutritious but also easy for the patient to eat. For instance, instead of serving a chicken breast, which the patient may get frustrated trying to eat, offer chicken fingers or legs that the patient can easily eat without having to use fork or knife. The family will need to pay attention to the amount the patient consumes to ensure that intake is adequate. Because of the frustrations of eating, the patient may eat less and weight loss may occur. If so, supplemental intake of nutritious snacks or drinks should be incorporated into the patient's diet. Encouraging the patient to use a water bottle with an attached straw for drinks will allow for better intake of fluids as spills are prevented; the patient may be able to handle the water bottle without dropping it, and it appears very normal. An occupational therapist can adapt eating utensils to meet the needs of the patient for eating, such as forks with special handles or plates with guards to prevent food from spilling. During the early stages of MS, the patient may remain able to respond to signals for the need to toilet him or herself. However, as time progresses, the patient often develops bladder spasticity or simply cannot remain continent. It is at this point that the caregiver should implement a scheduled toileting program to keep the patient dry. Caregivers should take note of the patient's usual pattern of voiding and having bowel movements and establish a scheduled toileting plan that mimics the patient's normal routine. Taking the patient to the bathroom every 2 hours for urination may assist in keeping the patient dry, and encouraging him or her to sit on the toilet following breakfast will assist in bowel evacuation. All of these efforts will require patience and a time commitment by the caregiver. For many families, the decision to institutionalize the patient occurs when the patient becomes incontinent, especially of bowel incontinence. When addressing the self-care needs of the patient, the family must consider the available resources that may provide some in-home assistance for personal care and seek out referrals.

Documentation

Whether the patient is in the home or in an institution, a health care provider should document the level of functioning for the patient in all areas of self-care. Document incontinent episodes and record intake and output as required. In addition, include in the record the ability or willingness of the patient to eat and how much he or she eats. Chart any interventions employed to enhance self-care efforts, such as the use of special devices for eating. Document all teaching, including the content taught and the learners.

NURSING DIAGNOSIS 3

DISTURBED SENSORY PERCEPTION: VISUAL

Related to:

Optic nerve involvement

Cranial nerve (III–XII) involvement

Defining Characteristics:

Visual blurring

Impaired color perception

Decreased central visual acuity

Diminished vision

Decreased pupil reaction to light

Nystagmus

Diplopia

Eye pain

Goal:

The patient is able to compensate for impaired vision.

Outcome Criteria

✔ The patient states that blurring has improved.

✔ The patient states that eye pain is resolved.

✔ The patient has no injury due to decreased vision.

NOC *Sensory function: Vision*

 Vision compensation behavior

INTERVENTIONS	RATIONALES
Assess for alterations in vision: decreased vision, change in color perception, nystagmus, diplopia, eye pain, blurring, and decreased pupillary reaction.	Establishes a baseline of visual functioning to serve as a basis for assistance to the patient.

(continues)

(continued)

INTERVENTIONS	RATIONALES
Apply eye patches, if ordered, for diplopia.	Restricting movement of eyes and alternating eyes that are patched will relieve diplopia.
Assess for signs of pain in eye, such as keeping eyelids tightly closed, facial grimace, headache, and pain in globe of eye, and treat as ordered with mild analgesia.	Pain in the eye occurs due to involvement of optic nerve.
Encourage the patient to close eyes for periods of time throughout the day.	Rests the eyes and prevents eye fatigue.
Orient the person to the environment, especially if hospitalized.	Disturbances in vision are present, and the person needs to know where objects are to prevent injury.
Use books with large print; locate and use household items, such as clocks and remote controls, that have large numbers or letters.	Enhances the environment to compensate for diminished vision.
Assist the patient with meals, especially for those patients who experience decreased central visual acuity, by helping with menu selection and preparation of foods on the plate or tray; assure the patient that it is okay to get assistance.	The patient may not eat if he or she cannot readily find food.
Place frequently used objects within easy reach.	Prevents the patient from needing to search for what he or she needs, and enhances safety.
Inform the patient of colors of clothes and other items.	Decreases the patient's feeling of helplessness when selecting clothes and ensures that the patient has correct colored items.
Encourage eye examinations on a regular basis.	Helps to monitor progress or deterioration of eyesight and allows for early intervention.

NIC *Eye care*

Communication enhancement: Visual deficit

Environmental management

Evaluation

Assess the degree to which outcomes have been achieved. The patient reports an ability to compensate for decreased vision. There is an absence of diplopia and eye pain. The patient reports that there are no new variations in visual ability and is able to participate in activities of daily living.

Community/Home Care

For most patients with visual impairments due to MS, treatment is done on an outpatient basis through physicians' offices. The patient should be encouraged to seek health care to ensure early detection and treatment of any further visual problems. The nurse or health care provider should question the patient about how vision impacts performance of usual tasks. In some instances, impaired vision accompanied by muscle weakness and tremors make even the simplest tasks difficult. In the early stages of the disease, this is more trying, as the goal is to maintain functioning as long as possible. Evaluations should be made to determine what assistance the patient may need in the home environment to compensate for altered visual ability. Keeping the patient safe and functional are the goals of interventions to address visual impairments. Be sure that the patient's home environment remains the same so that the patient knows where all items are to prevent injury. Family members need to assist the patient with meals and ambulation as dictated by the patient. For the patient who is mobile, keep pathways clear of clutter and hazards, such as throw rugs. Brightly colored objects should be used when possible, as these may be easier for the patient to see. If the patient enjoys reading, locate libraries that have books in large print, or get books on tape. Household items used by the patient, such as telephones, clocks, and remote control devices, can be purchased with big numbers or letters. Signs and symptoms that necessitate immediate attention should be made clear to the patient and/or family members.

Documentation

Chart all assessments related to the status of the patient's vision. Document all interventions implemented, including patches, as well as the patient's response to interventions and understanding of all procedures. Document any instruction with a clear indication of the patient's understanding of information. All referrals are included in the patient record.

NURSING DIAGNOSIS 4

CAREGIVER ROLE STRAIN

Related to:

Change of pattern in daily activities for caregiver

Caregiver unfamiliar with the type of care that must be provided

Caregiver must also work outside the home

Caregiver gets no break

Community resources unknown, unavailable, or not affordable

Defining Characteristics:

Caregiver expresses frustration, anger, sadness

Caregiver states that he or she does not know how to care for loved one

Caregiver not satisfied with community resources

Caregiver unable to provide level of care required

Goal:

Caregiver reports satisfaction with care-giving role.

Caregiver is able to recognize when he or she can no longer handle the complete or partial care of the patient.

Outcome Criteria

✔ The caregiver reports that he or she is not experiencing stress or is able to cope with stress.

✔ The caregiver identifies at least one source of support.

✔ The caregiver verbalizes his or her ability to handle the responsibilities of caring for the patient and coordinating care of the patient.

NOC *Caregiver emotional health*
Caregiver lifestyle disruption
Caregiver stressors
Caregiver well-being

INTERVENTIONS	RATIONALES
Teach caregiver about MS.	Understanding the disease assists the caregiver in understanding why the patient is behaving the way he or she is and what to expect in the future.
Assist the caregiver to plan for care of the patient.	The caregiver will need assistance in planning for the care of the patient, including access to home health care and other community services. The caregiver can plan for scheduled breaks away from the patient.
Encourage the caregiver to express feelings about his or her role, allowing time for venting frustrations, anxieties, and fears.	The first step towards coping with a change in life is to identify positive and negative feelings about the situation.
Teach the caregiver how to properly care for the patient, including communication techniques and techniques to provide basic needs of toileting, feeding, bathing, and dressing (see nursing diagnosis "Self-Care Deficits").	Having the knowledge to care for the patient decreases anxiety.
Encourage the caregiver to identify and utilize relaxation and stress reduction techniques, such as music therapy, quiet walks, meditation, exercise, etc.	The caregiver must utilize these strategies to prevent stress and anxiety that may negatively influence his or her ability to be an effective care provider.
Encourage the primary caregiver to identify one other family member, friend, or significant other who can provide short periods of relief.	The caregiver may need short periods of relief in order to run errands or regroup his or her thought processes, especially on demanding days.
Encourage the use of outside services such as Meals on Wheels or home health aides in the home.	These services can relieve some of the hardship of providing care to a completely dependent patient and allow the patient to remain in the home.
Refer the caregiver to local chapters of the Multiple Sclerosis Society to identify location and meeting dates/times for support groups.	These organizations offer educational materials and sponsor support groups. Participation in support groups allows the caregiver to talk to and gather support from others who are experiencing the same challenges and share experiences and strategies for handling particular situations.
Provide referral for social services consult to investigate the feasibility of respite care especially once the patient becomes dependent.	The caregiver may need to find respite care for extended periods of time to allow for caregiver rest or for a daily program so that the caregiver can work or rest. Social services can assist the caregiver in identifying appropriate community

(continues)

(continued)

INTERVENTIONS	RATIONALES
	resources, support groups, and service for financial aid and patient placement, if it becomes necessary. The caregiver needs to be supported in his or her decisions.
Support the family in decision-making regarding institutionalization of the patient if required.	Many family members experience conflicts when faced with the decision to place the patient in an alternative living arrangement, such as a nursing home, but also recognize that they can no longer provide 24-hour nursing care.

NIC *Caregiver support*
Respite care
Home maintenance assistance
Support group

Evaluation

Decide whether the outcome criteria have been met. The caregiver should be able to verbalize positive and negative feelings about being a caregiver. Ideally, the caregiver reports an ability to provide care without undue stress. The caregiver identifies sources of support, including relaxation and coping strategies, as well as a willingness to use respite care when needed.

Community/Home Care

The caregiver will discover that as the disease progresses, the ability to remain positive about the role of caregiver may prove more challenging. It should be stressed to the caregiver that he or she should seek out assistance prior to becoming burned out or so stressed that his or her physical and mental health are suffering. It is crucial to encourage the caregiver to take time to care for him or herself. Simple stress-reducing activities, such as walking or reading can enhance the sense of calm required to cope with a completely dependent patient. If participation in an organized religion or civic group has been part of the caregiver's weekly routine, he or she should investigate the possibility of having other family members or friends stay with the patient in order to attend an occasional service or meeting. Support groups can provide moral support, as well as give specific information on what to expect based on real life experiences from other caregivers. Depression may become apparent in caregivers if respite periods from care giving are not taken on some level (a few hours, a few days, or one day). Home health aides can relieve some of the responsibilities of providing direct patient care and should be explored. Even though many caregivers may feel guilty for involving outsiders in care, the primary caregiver should be supported in his or her decisions. Referrals to social services may be required to explore placement in a nursing home or other facility.

Documentation

Document an assessment of the caregiver's current psychological state, including his or her specific verbalizations of concern. Chart teaching done regarding stress and relaxation techniques. Include all referrals made in the record, specifically referrals to agencies that provide respite care and long-term care, and/or day care centers.

CHAPTER 3.44

MYASTHENIA GRAVIS

GENERAL INFORMATION

Myasthenia gravis (MG) is a chronic neuromuscular disease thought to be caused by an autoimmune response that destroys some acetylcholine receptors while decreasing effectiveness of others. The result is significant muscle weakness and fatigue with the patient experiencing exacerbations and remissions. It is believed that the thymus gland is responsible for an autoantigen that stimulates the autoimmune response of myasthenia gravis; however, the exact nature of this relationship is unclear. In a large percentage of the patients with myasthenia gravis there are thymus hyperplasia or thymus gland tumors. Clinical manifestations depend on the muscles involved and severity of the disease, but general manifestations may include the most common ocular manifestations of diplopia and ptosis, dysarthria, dysphagia, fatigue, progressive muscle weakness that improves with rest and increases with activity, increasing weakness with sustained muscle contraction, change in facial muscles resulting in a smile looking like a snarl, and an inability to hold the head upright. The patient is also at risk for myasthenic crisis (exacerbation of muscle weakness due to under-medication or infection) or cholinergic crisis (due to over-medication). Both place the patient at risk for severe respiratory compromise due to increased weakness of the respiratory muscles. Myasthenia gravis occurs most often between the ages of 20 and 30 years of age and is seen more frequently in women when onset is before 40 years of age.

NURSING DIAGNOSIS 1

INEFFECTIVE BREATHING PATTERN

Related to:

Respiratory muscle weakness

Decrease in movement of diaphragm

Defining Characteristics:

Dyspnea

Ineffective cough

Evidence of poor gas exchange

Difficulty swallowing

Goal:

The patient's respiratory patterns will maintain adequate oxygenation.

Outcome Criteria

✔ The patient will verbalize that dyspnea has been relieved or has improved.

✔ Respiratory rate will be < 28.

✔ Oxygen saturation will be > 90 percent (hospital patients).

✔ Arterial blood gases (ABGs) will be within normal ranges (hospital patients).

✔ The patient is able to cough up secretions.

NOC *Respiratory status: Ventilation*
Respiratory status: Gas exchange
Vital signs

INTERVENTIONS	RATIONALES
Assess respiratory system by noting respiratory rate, depth, chest expansion, rhythm, breath sounds, skin color, and if hospitalized, arterial blood gases (ABGs) and pulse oximetry, and note abnormalities such as dyspnea that has worsened, cyanosis (of nailbeds and lips), use of accessory muscles of respiration, and difficulty talking (due to shortness of breath).	Any of these abnormalities would indicate status of respiratory system and progression of disease; also establishes a baseline for future comparisons.

(continues)

(continued)

INTERVENTIONS	RATIONALES
Assist the patient in assuming a high Fowler's position or position for easy respiration.	Maximizes thoracic cavity space, decreases pressure from diaphragm and abdominal organs, and facilitates use of accessory muscles.
Provide humidified, low-flow (2 liters/min) oxygen, as ordered.	Provides some supplemental oxygen to improve oxygenation and humidification; makes secretions less viscous.
Administer anticholinesterases such as Mestinon® or Prostigmin® 30 minutes to 1 hour before meals and monitor for side effects.	Facilitates impulse transmission by enhancing the effects of acetylcholine at receptor sites; side effects include nausea, vomiting, diarrhea, excess salivation, sweating, and bronchoconstriction.
Administer glucocorticoids (such as prednisone), as ordered, and monitor for side effects.	For immunosuppression that will decrease muscle weakness; systemic effects from oral administration include cushingoid appearance, acne, bruising, increased appetite, and GI upset.
Monitor for myasthenic crisis (tachycardia, tachypnea, cyanosis, absence of cough and swallow reflex, and respiratory distress).	Under-medication, anesthesia, surgery, or infection may cause myasthenic crisis; respiratory distress may become serious enough to warrant ventilatory support.
Monitor for cholinergic crisis (abdominal cramps, diarrhea, increased pulmonary secretions, and hypotension).	Over-medication is the usual cause of cholinergic crisis and noting symptoms early prevents major life-threatening effects.
Balance rest with activity through out the day.	Muscle weakness worsens as the day progresses.
Administer antibiotics if respiratory infection is present or suspected, as ordered.	Helps to eradicate respiratory infection; infections are a frequent cause of myasthenic crisis.
Provide chest physiotherapy, as ordered.	Mobilizes secretions from lung fields.
Assist with activities of daily living, as required.	The patient with myasthenia gravis, especially in the early phases before medication is effective or during exacerbation, experiences significant weakness and some fatigue. This makes it difficult to perform normal activities, especially during acute exacerbations, when even eating may cause dyspnea.

Teach the patient how to decrease shortness of breath by restructuring activities.	Knowing how to control shortness of breath will help patient cope and have optimal functioning and decreases anxiety.
Teach pulmonary hygiene: prevention of infections, maintaining optimal health, flu and pneumonia vaccine (see nursing diagnosis "Ineffective Management of Therapeutic Regimen").	Protecting against infections can prevent acute exacerbations and subsequent hospitalizations.

NIC *Respiratory monitoring*
Cough enhancement
Oxygen therapy
Positioning

Evaluation

The patient should show indications that breathing patterns have returned to baseline and are effective in meeting the body's need for oxygen. The rate should return to baseline, preferably between 12–24 breaths per minute, and be unlabored. The return of arterial blood gases (ABGs) to the patient's baseline or to within normal range should be expected.

Community/Home Care

In the home setting, the patient with MG should remain cognizant of respiratory status. Although many patients may never experience respiratory symptoms with their MG, the potential threat to respiratory function is serious. It is important that the patient understand how to prevent upper respiratory infections, particularly through avoidance of crowds, avoidance of people with colds, good hand hygiene, and the use of immunizations against influenza and pneumonia. It is important that the family and patient understand the importance of taking the medication as prescribed on time, as either over-medication or under-medication can cause respiratory distress that may warrant ventilatory support. Respiratory muscles are often weakened, especially during times of stress and at the end of tiring days. At home, the patient will need to have rest periods during the day to prevent increased weakness of respiratory muscles. If shortness of breath begins to occur with simple activities that have previously been tolerated, the patient should contact a health care provider for advice. The patient should perform tasks or activities that require more energy and oxygen in the early part of the day prior to the onset of fatigue. A health care provider should ensure that the patient understands all medications prescribed.

Documentation

Chart the results of a comprehensive history and assessment of the respiratory system. Note respiratory rate, chest expansion, use of accessory muscles, breath sounds, and results of pulse oximetry. Document any patient teaching completed. Document subjective data exactly as the patient states it especially any complaints of fatigue. Include in the patient's chart all interventions employed to address ineffective breathing pattern, and the patient's response to the interventions that would indicate the problem has been resolved. If the patient's breathing is no better, indicate how the plan will be revised.

NURSING DIAGNOSIS 2

IMBALANCED NUTRITION: LESS THAN BODY REQUIREMENTS

Related to:

Weakness of facial muscle

Weakness of mastication muscles

Fatigue when eating

Inability to hold head erect when eating

Defining Characteristics:

Decreased amount of food consumed

Complains of fatigue before meal is complete

Weight loss

Dysphagia

Goal:

The patient will maintain adequate nutrition.

Outcome Criteria

✔ The patient will eat 50 percent of meals served.

✔ The patient will not lose weight.

✔ The patient will not aspirate when eating.

NOC *Nutritional status: Food and fluid intake*
Nutritional status: Nutrient intake
Oral hygiene
Sensory function: Taste and smell

INTERVENTIONS	RATIONALES
Assess laboratory results: albumin, electrolytes, glucose, protein (total), and iron.	These give indications of nutritional status.
Assess the patient's ability to eat/drink, including difficulty chewing and swallowing, and monitor for nausea, vomiting, abdominal cramping, or diarrhea, which are side effects of medications used to treat MG.	Helps to identify specific problems the patient is experiencing and allows the nurse to intervene accordingly.
Weigh patient on first contact with health care system and monitor weight regularly.	Establishes a baseline for comparison and as patient progresses allows for early intervention for nutritional deficits.
Monitor intake and output.	Assures adequate hydration.
Consider dietitian consult to ascertain the patient's ability to take in enough food to meet caloric demand and to determine the patient's likes, dislikes, and preferences within the prescribed diet, giving consideration to cultural or religious preferences.	For patients who have myasthenia gravis, fatigue of the muscles needed for chewing causes early cessation of eating; offering the patient foods that he or she likes will at least increase the likelihood that he or she will consume some of the meal.
Have the patient sitting upright for all meals, with head tilted slightly towards chest, and remain up for 30–60 minutes following the meal.	This position prevents aspiration by allowing gravity to assist movement of food without reflux.
Encourage the patient to consume small frequent meals and nutritious snacks with soft foods on the menu.	Frequent small meals decrease the likelihood of fatigue; food may be more tolerable in small portions; soft food is easier to chew and to digest; nutritious snacks are a way to increase nutrients.
Encourage the patient to avoid trying to talk with food in his or her mouth and to try to focus on chewing and swallowing.	Talking and eating at the same time increases the risk of aspiration.

(continues)

(continued)

INTERVENTIONS	RATIONALES
Allow adequate time for meals.	The patient may take longer to eat due to weakness of muscles, difficulty chewing and swallowing, and fatigue of muscles of mastication.
Consult with a speech therapist or appropriate discipline to assist patient with assessment of swallowing ability.	These disciplines can evaluate swallowing ability and provide recommendations to the patient for strengthening muscles.
If the patient has evidence of aspiration, auscultate breath sounds for crackles or rhonchi.	Detects abnormal substances in lungs and allows for early intervention.

NIC *Nutritional monitoring*
Nutritional management
Swallowing therapy

Evaluation

The patient's nutritional state is stable and the patient has a satisfactory method for nutrient intake. Assess the patient's weight and determine that the patient is not losing weight. The patient should be ingesting at least 50 percent of food served without undue fatigue. Laboratory results should reveal a normal albumin level as well as total protein and electrolytes.

Community/Home Care

Difficulties with eating and drinking are common problems for the patient with MG in the home setting. The patient will need to implement strategies to enhance the ingestion of enough food and nutrients to meet metabolic demands. Most interventions will center on actions to prevent fatigue of the muscles needed for chewing. The patient should evaluate his or her normal diet and determine which foods are easy to chew. Nutritious items such as custards, ice cream, mashed potatoes, yogurt, or very soft vegetables are encouraged, as some of these slide down with very little effort. The patient should avoid or limit hard foods that require extensive chewing, such as fried pork chops or steak. Even in the home setting, the patient will need to eat sitting up and remain up for 30–60 minutes after meals to prevent aspiration and reflux. When the patient is eating, family members should not talk to the patient because the patient cannot simultaneously participate in conversation and chew effectively. A home nurse or other health care provider needs to monitor the patient's nutritional status on a regular basis to detect excessive weight loss and to note reports of decreased intake due to fatigue, anxiety, fear of choking, etc. Instructing the patient and family on how to keep a food diary and calorie count will be helpful in helping the health care provider examine nutritional intake and needs. The family can assist the patient by preparing foods that are easy to chew and swallow that the patient likes but that also have nutritional value. The patient needs encouragement to eat even when he or she may feel tired, and even at home he or she may prefer privacy for meals because of the extended time it takes to eat. The patient should be taught to take the anticholinesterase medications 30 minutes before meals to enhance ability to chew and swallow. If problems with nutrition and weight loss persist, the patient needs to contact a health care provider.

Documentation

In the hospital setting, chart the patient's weight daily, or in the home weigh the patient weekly. Document any difficulty that the patient experiences during meals, particularly early fatigue and aspiration, and any interventions implemented to address them. Record intake and output according to agency protocol, being sure to document the percentage of food consumed. Document all interventions implemented to address imbalanced nutrition in the patient record. If the patient verbalizes concerns, include this in the chart. Always document teaching done with the patient and any referrals made to other disciplines, such as dietitians and speech therapists.

NURSING DIAGNOSIS 3

 DEFICIENT KNOWLEDGE

Related to:

New onset of myasthenia gravis

Lack of information about the disease and its treatment

Defining Characteristics:

Asks no questions

Has many questions/concerns

Is anxious

Goal:

> The patient and family understand myasthenia gravis and its treatments.

Outcome Criteria

✔ The patient verbalizes an understanding of the disease process of myasthenia gravis.

✔ The patient expresses an understanding of the prescribed treatment regimen.

✔ The patient is able to identify medications prescribed including actions, side effects, and expected therapeutic responses.

✔ The patient verbalizes an understanding of the symptomatology that would indicate a need to seek health care.

NOC *Knowledge: Disease process*
Knowledge: Treatment regimen
Knowledge: Medication

INTERVENTIONS	RATIONALES
Assess the patient's current knowledge, ability to learn, and readiness to learn.	Any instruction should build on what the patient already knows; teachings need to be tailored to the patient's ability and willingness to learn for maximum effectiveness.
Teach incrementally: simple to complex.	The patient will learn and retain knowledge better when information is presented in small segments starting with simple concepts.
Instruct the patient and family about the disease: — Definition of myasthenia gravis — Medications ordered to control the disease, including side effects of glucocorticoids and anticholinesterases (see nursing diagnosis "Ineffective Breathing Pattern"). — Effect of disease on nutritional status and ability to eat (see nursing diagnosis "Imbalanced Nutrition: Less than Body Requirements") — When to seek emergency health care attention	Knowledge of disease and of treatment options improves patient outcomes and provides the patient and family with realistic expectations. When the patient and family understand the patient's disease process and medication regime, aspects of the disease process that can be controlled occur and complications of the disease decrease and/or repeat hospitalizations are reduced.
— Importance of activity restrictions and energy conservation	
Teach signs and symptoms of myasthenic crisis and cholinergic crisis: — Myasthenic crisis: elevated heart rate, elevated respiratory rate, restlessness, difficulty swallowing, increased diaphoresis — Cholinergic crisis: abdominal cramps; nausea/vomiting; increased difficulty chewing, swallowing, and speaking; severe muscle weakness	These are life-threatening emergencies that require immediate treatment to prevent respiratory failure.
Teach the patient about treatment options other than medications: — Thymectomy: removal of thymus gland; inform patient to expect chest tubes and incision on chest wall, need for turning/coughing/deep breathing excercises and incentive spirometry — Plasmapheresis: a process of plasma exchange to remove antibodies that contribute to symptoms of the disease, such as muscle weakness and fatigue; 3–5 treatments over 5–7 days.	The patient needs to understand the possible treatments available to control the disease.
Ask the patient and family to repeat the information and ask questions.	This allows the nurse to hear in the patient's own words what he or she understood.
Offer printed materials and other audiovisual aids.	Printed and audiovisual aids enhance learning.
Provide family members with literature about the disease and inform them of opportunities for increased learning.	When a patient's family members understand the disease process, they will be better able to assist the patient.
Establish that the patient has the resources required to be compliant when discharged.	If needed resources, such as finances for medication, transportation, and psychosocial support are not available, the patient cannot be compliant.

NIC *Learning readiness enhancement*
Learning facilitation
Teaching: Prescribed medication
Teaching: Disease process

Evaluation

Evaluate the degree to which the patient has achieved the expected outcomes. The patient and family verbalize an understanding of myasthenia gravis, planned treatment options, emergencies, and medications, and state that their questions have been answered. The patient and family indicate a willingness and ability to comply with interventions. The nurse should determine whether the patient has the necessary resources to be compliant with follow-up care.

Community/Home Care

Compliance with the prescribed regimen can only occur if the nurse takes the responsibility to educate the patient about all aspects of the plan. The patient will need to understand thoroughly the disease process and the role of medications in the treatment. The patient will need to balance work, activity, and rest, and may be required to make major adaptations in lifestyle if muscle weakness is not completely resolved. Emotional stress, excessive fatigue, and infections can exacerbate the condition and should be avoided to the extent possible. The patient will need to use relaxation techniques regularly and incorporate rest into his or her day, whether at work or at home. Teaching should incorporate any religious, cultural, or socioeconomic factors that may affect compliance. The outcome of successful teaching is that the patient and family will be able to monitor the patient's health status, including taking the pulse and identification of signs and symptoms that would indicate a need to see a health care provider, elevated pulse, increasing difficulty with chewing and swallowing, abdominal cramping, signs of respiratory problems, etc. Investigations should be made to determine whether the patient has the necessary resources to carry out the prescribed instructions.

Documentation

Document the specific content taught and the titles of any printed materials given to the family or patient. After the teaching session, document the degree to which the patient and/or family verbalize understanding and a willingness to comply. The nurse should indicate any areas that will require further instruction and note any referrals made.

CHAPTER 3.45

PARKINSON'S DISEASE

GENERAL INFORMATION

Parkinson's disease is a progressive degenerative disease that affects the neurons of the basal ganglia of the brain, resulting in an imbalance between dopamine and acetylcholine in the basal ganglia. Dopamine is a neurotransmitter responsible for the inhibitory effects of motor movements and acetylcholine is the neurotransmitter responsible for the excitatory effects. In Parkinson's disease, there is a decrease in the number of dopamine neurotransmitters so that acetylcholine is not inhibited. The most common characteristic manifestations of this pathophysiological process are unintentional tremors that occur at rest and are absent during sleep, a shuffling propulsive gait that is slow to initiate and difficult to stop, rigidity, akinesia/bradykinesia, and a forward tilt to the posture especially when walking. A classic symptom often noted is a "pill rolling" tremor where the thumb rolled across the palm, specifically along the second and third digits of the hand. Other manifestations include a masklike appearance to the face with a wide, open staring appearance, orthostatic hypotension, severe constipation, difficulties chewing and swallowing, and uncontrolled drooling. The disease is seen most often in people over 50 years of age and more often in men.

NURSING DIAGNOSIS 1

IMPAIRED PHYSICAL MOBILITY

Related to:

Imbalance of dopamine and acetylcholine

Degeneration of neurotransmitters

Defining Characteristics:

Shuffling gait

Difficulty stopping movement

Stooped posture

Loss of dexterity

Unintentional tremors

Rigidity

Goal:

The patient is able to maintain mobility.

Adequate range of motion and positions of function are maintained/accomplished.

Outcome Criteria

✔ The patient ambulates without injury.

✔ The patient will be out of bed three times a day.

✔ The patient will be mobile with a walker or wheelchair.

NOC *Neurological status:*
   Central motor control
   Ambulation
   Mobility

INTERVENTIONS	RATIONALES
Assess for alterations in motor function and note abnormalities characteristic of Parkinson's disease, such as unintentional tremors, shuffling gait with short hesitant steps, stooped posture, inability to stop quickly, decreased fine motor abilities, "pill rolling" movement of fingers, and rigidity of muscles with a masklike appearance to face.	A baseline of function needs to be established; these are clinical manifestations of the disease; assessment of motor function is needed regularly to evaluate progression of disease and response to treatment.
Obtain a history from the patient about mobility limitations and effect on ability to remain functional, especially with usual activities such as personal care.	Helps to determine what adaptations in lifestyle are necessary and to determine the severity of mobility limitations.

(continues)

(continued)

INTERVENTIONS	RATIONALES
Give dopamine replacement medications as ordered, (such as levodopa or levodopa-carbidopa/Sinemet®) and monitor for side effects.	Levodopa preparations are the mainstay of therapy, and most patients receive this class of medication; reduces Parkinson's symptoms by improving the synthesis/uptake of dopamine, restoring the balance of dopamine and acetylcholine in the brain. Side effects can be troubling, and the family needs to know about them; common side effects include nausea, vomiting, postural hypotension, psychosis, dyskinesias (abnormal movements such as head bobbling, tics), and hypertensive crisis when used with MAO inhibitors.
Avoid vitamins that contain pyridoxine (vitamin B_6) and limit foods rich in vitamin B_6 when patient is receiving levodopa.	Pyridoxine causes a decrease in the amount of levodopa that reaches the central nervous system.
Give dopamine agonist medications as ordered, such as pramipexole (Mirapex®), bromocriptine (Parlodel®), or pergolide (Permax®), and monitor for side effects.	Activates dopamine receptors in the brain. Side effects include hallucinations, confusion, agitation, dyskinesia, daytime sleepiness, constipation, and nausea. Sleep attacks—profound overwhelming sleepiness that occurs with rapid onset—may occur.
Administer COMT (catecholamine-O-methyl transferase inhibitors), such as entacapone, as ordered and monitor for side effects.	These medications prevent the breakdown of levodopa by COMT in the periphery, which diminishes the symptoms of Parkinson's disease. Side effects include vomiting, diarrhea or constipation, yellow-orange tinting to the urine; when combined with levodopa, side effects of dyskinesias, orthostatic hypotension, sleep disturbances, and hallucination may occur.
Administer MAO-B (monamine oxidase type B) inhibitors as ordered such as selegiline and monitor for side effects.	Selegiline has a neuroprotective effect and selectively inhibits the enzyme (monamine oxidase type B) that inactivates dopamine in the brain and is thought to slow the progression of the disease. It is a second- or third-line drug and is used with levodopa. The most common side effect specific to the drug

INTERVENTIONS	RATIONALES
	when used alone is insomnia; however, used in combination with levodopa the adverse effects of levodopa are intensified.
Administer dopamine releaser medication, such as amantadine, as ordered, and monitor for side effects.	Amantadine causes dopamine to be released from functioning dopaminergic terminals in the brain. Side effects are generally mild and include lightheadedness, dizziness, anxiety, nervousness, difficulty concentrating, and insomnia.
Administer anticholinergic agents, such as Artane® and Cogentin®, as ordered and monitor for side effects.	These agents block muscarinic receptors and restore the balance between dopamine and acetylcholine, reducing tremors and rigidity, but have no effect on bradykinesia. Common side effects include sedation, constipation, and dry mouth. This group of medications is used cautiously in the elderly because they may cause confusion and hallucinations.
Encourage the patient to remain ambulatory for as long as condition allows.	Limits the period of time that the patient is immobile; helps to prevent complications of immobility and to preserve function.
Provide assistance with ambulation activities and use assistive devices such as walkers and gait belts, as required. When the patient is using a fast, trot-like, shuffling gait, encourage him or her to stop after a short distance.	The patient is at risk for falls due to shuffling gait and posture. Assistance is needed to ensure safety. In addition, the patient often freezes in place while walking and may be unable to continue ambulation. When the patient is going at a trot pace with a stooped posture, he or she is more likely to fall; stopping will allow a slowing of ambulation, which can prevent falls.
Have the patient use a wide base of support when walking.	Gives more support and prevents falls.
Keep pathways clear of items that can be obstacles to ambulation, such as small area rugs, small pieces of furniture, and extension cords.	Blocked pathways can cause a hazard for the patient trying to maneuver about the home.
When or if the patient becomes immobile, help him or her get out of bed into a chair 2–3 times per day.	Helps to prevent complications of prolonged bedrest, such as pneumonia, DVT, and skin breakdown.

INTERVENTIONS	RATIONALES
Arrange for physical therapy consultation with the family for methods/therapies to preserve mobility for as long as possible.	The physical therapist can implement a plan for preservation of muscle and prevention of contractures.
Reposition the patient every 2 hours. Provide trochanter rolls, pillow supports, and range of motion at least three times a day.	Maintains positions of function and comfort. Range of motion and proper positioning help to prevent contractures.
Assess patient's skin for redness or skin breakdown every 2 hours when repositioning.	Pressure from immobility compresses blood vessels in high-risk areas, depriving them of nutrients and oxygenation, and leading to skin death.
Teach the patient and family turning, lifting/moving techniques, correct body alignment, use of assistive devices, and how to perform range of motion.	Helps to maintain function as long as possible and to prevent contractures. Even though a physical therapist may come into the home to work with the patient, family members may also be required to move and position the patient.
Provide assistance for self-care needs (feeding, toileting, bathing, dressing) as required while fostering independence.	Because of unintentional tremors and rigidity, the patient will require some assistance with activities of daily living (ADLs); independence should be maintained for as long as possible, and the patient should be allowed to function at his or her optimal level as the disease progresses.
Teach the patient and family about medication therapy (action, dosing, scheduling, side effects).	Medications are a main part of the treatment for Parkinson's disease, and the family needs adequate knowledge to implement the regimen in the home setting.

NIC *Exercise therapy*
Joint mobility
Positioning

Evaluation

The patient maintains full range of motion of all extremities with no contractures. The patient participates in mobility activities and ambulates or exercises to the extent possible by using assistive devices or people. The patient does not fall while ambulating and is able to participate in self-care to the extent possible.

Community/Home Care

Patients with Parkinson's disease are treated at home with the aim of keeping the patient as independent as possible for as long as possible. Medication therapy is started early in the disease to slow progression, and in many cases the patient is on more than one medication. Understanding the schedule for the medications and their side effects is important for the caregiver. The family should receive thorough information regarding the disease and its impact on mobility. Early in the disease, it is crucial that caregivers encourage the patient to remain mobile and participate in ambulation and exercise as long as possible. However, because of the characteristic trot-like shuffling gait, postural changes making the patient lean forward when walking, rigidity, and freezing in place that eventually occur in the disease, the family should understand that the patient will eventually require assistance with ambulation. When the patient becomes frozen (akinesia), the family members will need to help the patient initiate movement by having him or her rock back and forth or by touching his or her foot slightly with theirs. There may be a tendency to refrain from ambulating, making range of motion exercises more crucial in efforts to preserve function and prevent complications. Keeping the environment "ambulation friendly" by removing objects such as throw rugs, small tables, or decorative items from pathways needs to be implemented by the family. A physical therapist should teach the family techniques to use to assist the patient at home with mobility activities. Special grab rails in showers and high toilet seats should be installed. Using a wide base of support when walking helps balance, and clasping hands behind the back can improve or maintain posture. Family members or significant others should encourage the patient to change positions frequently to avoid freezing in one place. Stretching exercises and massage can loosen stiff muscles and should be done three times a day. The patient should not sit in easy chairs that are deep and soft because the movement required to lift out of the chair is often impossible. Firm chairs with hard armrests will be easier for the patient to get out of. Tremors may make eating and drinking from a cup difficult, and utensils may need to be adapted to prevent spilling. If tremors are sustained for long periods, the patient can hold items, such as a ball, in the hands when at rest to offer some degree of relief. Unintentional tremors may create feelings of frustration as spills and dropping items become commonplace. Providing the family with a visiting nurse who can troubleshoot with the family and assess how the patient is progressing can assist in reducing anxiety that may be present. There is no cure for Parkinson's disease, and medications tend to lose their effectiveness over time, causing some caregivers to make decisions about alternative living arrangements, possibly in long-term care facilities.

Documentation

Chart the findings from an assessment of motor function and muscle strength, noting any of the defining characteristics of Parkinson's disease, especially common findings such as rigidity, unintentional tremors, and shuffling gait. If the patient is able to ambulate or move, detail the extent of his or her capabilities and participation. Include in the documentation the use of special devices or assistive devices for ambulation, and chart medications according to agency guidelines. Document all other interventions implemented to address the issue of immobility, as well as instruction to the caregiver relevant to addressing immobility and medication administration. Any complications of immobility noted are charted in accordance with agency protocol.

NURSING DIAGNOSIS 2

 ## IMBALANCED NUTRITION: LESS THAN BODY REQUIREMENTS

Related to:

Akinesia

Difficulty chewing or inability to chew effectively

Difficulty swallowing

Defining Characteristics:

Has difficulty keeping food and fluids from dribbling out of mouth

Experiences weight loss

States he cannot eat, refuses food

Goal:

Nutritional status is maintained.

Outcome Criteria

✔ The patient is able to ingest a normal diet.

✔ The patient does not lose weight.

✔ The patient reports no difficulty swallowing.

NOC *Swallowing status*
Swallowing status:
Esophageal phase
Nutritional status:
Food and fluid intake
Weight: Body mass

INTERVENTIONS	RATIONALES
Assess the patient's ability to chew and swallow; use a variety of food types.	Helps to determine the extent of difficulty in swallowing and to make decisions regarding type of diet required; swallowing is difficult due to the rigidity/slow movement of muscles required for chewing and swallowing.
Assess the patient's ability to open his or her mouth wide enough to consume adequate food and to chew.	Patients frequently have difficulty opening the mouth and muscles required for chewing and swallowing become ineffective due to akinesia.
Consult with a dietician as ordered or as necessary.	The dietician can provide recommendations for adequate nutrient intake to prevent weight loss.
Weigh patient on first contact with health care system and monitor weight at follow-up visits.	It is important to establish a baseline weight and monitor weight over the progression of the disease to determine whether the patient is able to consume enough food.
Provide a variety of flavorful foods.	The patient is more likely to consume foods that are pleasant to the taste.
Offer a soft diet of 5–6 small meals, including thick or frozen liquids such as ice cream, cold liquid nutritional supplements (Ensure, Boost), milkshakes, or frozen juice.	Soft foods are easier to chew; because of the effort that goes into chewing, the patient may become frustrated or fatigued and stop eating before enough nutrients have been consumed; cold, thick liquid substances are easier to swallow.
Encourage the patient to place foods into the back of mouth.	Helps to prevent food and liquid from drooling out of oral cavity.
Provide extended periods of time for meals.	If the patient is rushed, he or she may become frustrated and anxious and lose interest in eating.
Teach the patient and family all strategies/interventions to maintain or improve nutritional	The patient needs to implement strategies to promote swallowing, digestion, and

INTERVENTIONS	RATIONALES
status, and encourage their use at home.	maintenance of nutrition.
Monitor laboratory results such as electrolytes, hemoglobin, albumin, and glucose.	These tests will provide clues to nutritional status.

NIC *Nutrition monitoring*
Nutrition management

Evaluation

The patient is able to consume foods and reports that he or she is able to swallow without difficulty. Weight loss does not occur, and the patient states satisfaction with diet. In addition, the patient and family should verbalize an understanding of all required interventions and rationales for implementation.

Community/Home Care

At home, the patient should continue to implement strategies to maintain nutritional status. Even though a nurse or other health care provider may not be required for home visits, the patient's nutritional status will need to be monitored through some mechanism. Because of the difficulty with chewing and swallowing it will be easy for the patient to become frustrated and lose interest in eating, leading to a gradual loss of weight, which over time can become pronounced. The patient should have printed information available that gives nutritional content of food that can be chewed and swallowed easily and is among the patient's preferred foods. The dietician or nurse should be sure through teaching that the patient is able to select foods that have nutritional value and not just substances that are easy to consume. Liquid nutritional supplements may be beneficial to consume between meals or as snacks, as they contain multiple nutrients. Because of the uncontrolled drooling, it may be difficult to keep food and liquid in the mouth, and the patient may choose to isolate him or herself from others when eating due to embarrassment. The family should offer emotional support and encouragement for the patient to increase the likelihood that he or she will continue to try to eat. The meal preparer should develop menus that incorporate more soft foods that are easily chewed by the patient but are also palatable to all members of the family.

Follow-up visits with a health care provider should include an assessment of the patient's ability to chew and swallow, along with obtaining a weight at each visit. A 24-hour recall of food intake with a calorie count can serve to identify the need for further intervention by a dietician. As the disease progresses, and the rigidity and akinesia make eating extremely difficult, the family will be faced with decision-making regarding artificial nutrition.

Documentation

Chart the patient's weight and the findings from an assessment of the patient's ability to chew and swallow. Include in the patient record the percentage of food consumed, and if less than adequate, assess the patient for possible reasons. Chart all interventions implemented, the patient's response, and all teaching, including verbalization of understanding or the need for reinforcement. If referrals are made, document these in the record.

NURSING DIAGNOSIS 3

 IMPAIRED VERBAL COMMUNICATION

Related to:
Motor dysfunction
Akinesia

Defining Characteristics:
Dysarthria
Monotone voice
Slow speech
Soft, muffled speech
Difficulty starting speech

Goal:
The patient will be able to communicate needs and desires.

Outcome Criteria

✔ The patient will continue to talk for as long as possible, using simple words.

✔ The patient will use a communication board to express one need.

✔ The patient will be able to express needs by writing or pointing to words or pictures.

NOC *Communication*
Communication expressive

INTERVENTIONS	RATIONALES
Assess patient's ability to communicate verbally and determine whether the patient can read and write.	Establishes a baseline and helps to determine whether the patient will be able to use alternative communication methods.
If the patient is able to read and write, provide patient with alternatives to verbal communication: communication board, pencil and paper, Magic Slate or chalkboard. Provide picture or word cards if the patient cannot read or write.	This provides an alternative method of communication. The use of the hands may be impaired due to tremors and rigidity to the extent that the patient is unable to write.
Arrange for a speech therapist consult, as ordered.	Speech therapists can assist the patient with communication methods, including adjunct devices to facilitate communication.
Teach the patient how to speak slowly.	Even though the patient's speech may be understood by some, such as caregivers and family, others may not be able to understand the patient, as the speech is altered from normal. Speaking slowly allows for better formation of words and allows others to listen more attentively.
Take time to work with the patient in communication efforts; do not rush the patient.	Rushing the patient to communicate causes frustration and may make the patient stop trying to communicate.
Have the patient speak slowly, purposefully, and loudly.	When the patient thinks consciously of speaking, the ability to form words may be easier; the voice of the Parkinson's patient is low and muffled, and speaking loudly makes it easier to hear him or her.
Teach the patient how to exercise facial muscles required for speech by singing, if possible.	The facial movement that occurs with singing helps to maintain tone in the muscles of the face and jaw that are required for speech.
Utilize speech therapist for assistance in establishing the best communication strategies and to educate the patient and family.	The speech therapist is best qualified to establish alternative methods for effective communication by the patient.

NIC *Communication enhancement:*
Speech deficit
Learning facilitation
Anxiety reduction

Evaluation

The patient continues to talk with those around them. Evaluate the progress the patient has made in ability to communicate. Establish what needs to be done to further enhance nonverbal communication with the patient. Evaluate whether the patient is able to communicate by using a communication board, writing, or pointing. Determine whether the patient is frustrated or satisfied with attempts at communication.

Community/Home Care

For the patient who has Parkinson's disease, the changes in verbal communication may prove to be a challenging and frustrating aspect of the disease. The patient's voice is low, and due to changes in innervation of the muscles that control the mouth, speaking may become difficult and slow. Patients may feel embarrassed, particularly in public or around outsiders, and may refrain from efforts at communication due to this as well as to frustration at trying to make others understand. The patient must be encouraged to continue with new communication strategies, and this is where social support systems can be most beneficial. The family should be taught how to help the patient with communication. As family and friends display acceptance, encouragement, and patience, the patient may become more comfortable with communication, knowing that others understand. A speech therapist may be of assistance in teaching the patient simple oral exercises that can enhance the ability to speak. If this does not happen, the patient may socially isolate him or herself, which could lead to emotional stress. Follow-up care should give attention to not only the physiological realm of care but to this very critical aspect of the patient's well-being.

Documentation

Document all communication strategies utilized with the patient. Include an evaluation of the patient's efforts to communicate and which strategies work best. Always include an assessment of the patient's emotional state and responses to all interventions. Chart any referrals made for speech and the outcomes of the recommendations. When communication devices or techniques are employed to enhance communication, document the patient's ability and willingness to use them.

NURSING DIAGNOSIS 4

 ### INEFFECTIVE COPING: INDIVIDUAL AND FAMILY

Related to:

Chronic, progressive disease

Need for care assistance

Loss of function

Defining Characteristics:

Angry

Expressions of fear

Restlessness and anxiety

Crying

Expressions of distress at loss of function

Goal:

Coping is enhanced, and anxiety is decreased or alleviated.

The patient and family members demonstrate new effective coping strategies.

Outcome Criteria

✔ The patient identifies one coping mechanism to be used.

✔ The family verbalizes an understanding of disease process.

✔ The caregiver identifies one coping mechanism to be used.

✔ The patient verbalizes fears and concerns.

✔ The patient reports being less anxious.

✔ The patient demonstrates no outward signs of anxiety, such as restlessness or agitation.

NOC *Adaptation to physical disability*

Anxiety control

Family coping

Coping

INTERVENTIONS	RATIONALES
Monitor for the presence of anxiety (mild, moderate, severe) by having patient rate on a scale of 1–10, with 10 being the greatest.	Gives the nurse an objective measure of the anxiety.
Assess the patient and family to determine his or her feelings regarding the diagnosis of Parkinson's disease and the patient's physical disability resulting from the disease, and support them as appropriate by answering questions and making referrals.	Assisting the patient and family to deal with the diagnosis and ensuing loss of function will enhance their ability to cope with serious illness.
Keep the patient and family informed of all that is going on, including information about possible disease progression and interventions required at home.	Knowledge about the disease and what is required prepares the family and patient for future needs. Honesty concerning the loss of function due to Parkinson's disease helps the patient begin to cope; communication in a straightforward manner may help to relieve any anxiety.
Use a calm, reassuring manner with the patient.	Gives the patient a sense of well-being.
Encourage the patient and family to verbalize fears, concerns, and expressions of possible loss of function. Listen attentively.	Verbalization of fears contributes to dealing with concerns; being attentive relays empathy to the patient.
Have the patient and family identify at least one coping mechanism that has worked before and investigate new coping strategies.	Coping mechanisms that have worked in the past may help with current needs, but additional ones may be required because of the chronic, debilitating nature of Parkinson's disease.
Seek spiritual consult as needed or requested by the patient and or family.	Meeting the spiritual needs of the patient helps the patient to deal with fears through use of spiritual or religious rituals.
Recognize the role of culture in the patient's and family's method of coping with life stressors, especially illness and the verbalization of fears and concerns related to communication and mobility.	Culture often dictates how a person grieves, copes, and adapts to illness/decreasing health; the health care provider must recognize this in order to support the patient and family.
Provide the patient and family with information regarding advance directives and support decisions that are made.	Allows the patient and family the opportunity to plan to fulfill the patient's wishes in the event he or she becomes unable to make his or her own decisions.

(continues)

(continued)

INTERVENTIONS	RATIONALES
Encourage the family or caregiver to seek assistance with care-giving activities and to attend support groups if available. Agencies such as the American Parkinson's Disease Association, the Parkinson's Disease Foundation, and the National Parkinson Foundation may be of assistance.	The patient eventually becomes completely dependent, and the caregiver may need assistance to decrease stress and strain. Support groups can provide emotional support.

NIC *Coping enhancement*
Emotional support
Spiritual support

Evaluation

Evaluate the extent to which the outcome criteria have been achieved. The patient should be assessed for behaviors that would indicate adjustment to the diagnosis of Parkinson's disease. The patient and family should verbalize their fears and concerns and be able to identify at least one coping strategy that they believe will be successful in dealing with the loss of function that occurs with Parkinson's disease. The extent to which the patient displays appropriate coping behaviors should be noted. If the patient is unable to talk about the diagnosis and communicate concerns, the nurse should explore further interventions to assist the patient.

Community/Home Care

Care providers should assess which coping mechanisms work for the patient and family and encourage their use at home. Parkinson's disease causes notable changes in the patient's functional ability, especially in areas of ambulation, speech, and eating. Families must work diligently to encourage the patient to remain as active as possible to maintain function for as long as possible. The patient may become self-conscious and depressed, often grieving this loss of function. The patient and family should be informed that it is acceptable to be anxious, angry, and fearful as he or she attempts to cope, and that these feelings are normal. However, extreme self-isolation and depression should be noted and reported to a health care provider. For many patients and families, spiritual/religious rituals provide a means of coping with difficult stressful situations. The patient's and family's culture may dictate how they cope and with whom they share this process. It is crucial that the nurse and family support the patient as needed to foster a healthy psychological state, recognizing that anger and emotional outburst are common. The patient as well as the caregiver may benefit from quiet periods of meditation during the day. Support to long-term home caregivers will be important, as they too need to be supported in their adjustment to a new role as caregiver for the patient once capacity for self-care diminishes. If questions should arise at home regarding the patient's health status or prescribed regimen, the patient should have a means of contact with a health care provider for answers.

Documentation

Document coping strategies that the patient and family have identified as successful in the past. Include any suggestions given for new coping strategies. Document the degree to which the patient is able to verbalize feelings regarding having Parkinson's disease and has decreased anxiety. Chart the patient's verbalizations as the patient states them, and include in the record coping mechanisms utilized by the patient. Record the level of anxiety present using a rating scale that provides an objective way to relay to others the extent of any anxiety. Document findings from an assessment of the patient's psychological state and whether there is depression, anger, crying, sadness, self-isolation, etc. Document any referrals to any agencies for assistance or to religious/spiritual leaders.

NURSING DIAGNOSIS 5

DISTURBED BODY IMAGE

Related to:

Drooling

Masklike appearance to face

Shuffling gait

Stooped posture

Defining Characteristics:

Withdrawal

Social isolation

Depression

Negative statements about physical appearance

Goal:

The patient accepts the change in physical appearance and continues social activities and interpersonal relationships.

Outcome Criteria

✔ The patient does not verbalize negative feelings toward self.

✔ The patient verbalizes an adaptation to or acceptance of body appearance.

✔ The patient verbalizes an understanding regarding physical changes due to Parkinson's disease.

NOC *Body image*

INTERVENTIONS	RATIONALES
Encourage the patient to vent his or her feelings and assure the patient that his or her feelings are normal.	The patient should understand that his or her emotions are real and should be expected.
Encourage the patient to communicate feelings about changes in physical appearance and functional status.	Talking about the changes may sometimes be the beginning of acceptance.
Monitor the patient's feelings about self, interpersonal relationships with family members and friends, withdrawal, social isolation, fear, anxiety, embarrassment by appearance, fear that appearance will be displeasing to loved ones, and desire to be alone.	Helps to detect early alterations in social functioning, prevent unhealthy behaviors, and intervene early through referral to counseling.
Encourage the patient to participate in at least one outside/public activity each week.	Prevents patient from isolating him or herself from others; because of difficulties with ambulation and speech, the patient may refrain from social interaction.
Identify the effects of the patient's culture or religion on his or her perception of body image.	A patient's culture and religion often help define his or her reactions to changes in body image and his or her sense of self-worth.

NIC *Body image enhancement*
Emotional support
Support Group
Socialization enhancement

Evaluation

The patient is able and willing to learn about the strategies to maintain functioning and manage his or her own activities to the extent possible. Determine whether the patient is able to verbalize feelings regarding the change in facial appearance, drooling, and gait, and the impact these changes may have on role performance. Time is required for the patient to assimilate the change in body appearance completely into his or her self-perception. It is crucial that the health care provider and family members evaluate the degree to which the patient is beginning to do this. Communication of feelings and concerns relevant to the change in appearance should be taken as a positive sign that progress is being made towards meeting the outcome criteria.

Community/Home Care

At home, continued monitoring of the patient's perception of body image is needed. The health care provider who interacts with the patient during follow-up will need to be alert to subtle hints that may indicate that the patient has not completely adapted to the change in body appearance and physical function. The change in facial appearance, speech, and gait will be obvious to others, as will drooling. Have the patient keep handkerchiefs with them to wipe saliva from drooling. Family members must encourage the patient to continue communication efforts in order to maintain speech. The patient may be fearful or anxious about eating in public as well as talking to outsiders. However, it is important that family members or significant others encourage continued participation in outside activities and avoidance of self-imposed isolation. Open discussions regarding the changes and their accompanying frustrations are crucial to the patient's ability to maintain a positive body image or at least an acceptance of the changes in his or her body. If the patient is an active member of a religious or civic group, that may be a good place to start social interaction, as the patient may have some sense of comfort with the people there and be more willing to attempt interactions.

Documentation

Chart any specific behaviors or verbalizations that may indicate an altered body image. Document a precise description of the physical changes in appearance that is causing the disturbed body image, such as drooling or alterations in gait, speech, and facial appearance. Include all interventions that have been employed to address this issue and the patient's response. Note when and if the patient begins to verbalize feelings regarding the change in facial appearance and body function.

CHAPTER 3.46

SEIZURES

GENERAL INFORMATION

A seizure is a period of abnormal electrical activity in the brain resulting in alterations in consciousness, motor and sensory function, and autonomic nervous system control. Seizure classification includes generalized seizures when both cerebral hemispheres are involved and partial seizures when only a portion of the cerebrum is involved. Tonic-clonic (formerly grand mal) and absence attacks (formerly petit mal) are examples of generalized seizures. All generalized seizures result in altered levels of consciousness. Tonic-clonic seizures present themselves as repetitive muscle contraction and relaxation. Airway compromise, apnea, incontinence of urine and stool, and increased metabolism with subsequent hypoglycemia are common sequelae of tonic-clonic seizures. Risk of injury is high during tonic-clonic seizures due to uncontrolled motor activity. Absence seizures, in which the patient stares blankly while intentional motor activity ceases, typically last 5–10 seconds or longer. Automatisms such as lip smacking or eyelid fluttering may occur during absence seizures. Partial or focal seizures may be simple if consciousness is not altered or complex if consciousness is altered. Twitching, lip smacking, eye blinking, or other repetitive movements may occur with partial seizures. Partial seizures may spread from one portion of the cerebrum to another, with consequent sequential spreading of motor and sensory manifestations from one part of the body to another. This is termed a Jacksonian seizure or Jacksonian march. Epilepsy is a term assigned to chronic seizure disorders. Persons with epilepsy are managed pharmacologically with anticonvulsant medications with the goal of a "seizure-free status." The leading cause of recurrent seizures in a person with epilepsy is sub-therapeutic serum anticonvulsant levels. Physiological alterations as well as noncompliance with medication regimen are possible causes for these decreased serum levels. Status epilepticus is a life-threatening condition in which seizure activity is continuous and can result in airway compromise, apnea, acidosis, hypoglycemia, and death. Administration of intravenous benzodiazepines, airway and ventilation management, and safety precautions are included in the care of a patient with status epilepticus.

NURSING DIAGNOSIS 1

RISK FOR INJURY

Related to:

Altered levels of consciousness

Tonic-clonic movements

Environment

History of seizures

Defining Characteristics:

None

Goal:

The patient will not be injured during a seizure.

Outcome Criteria

✔ The patient will state ways to enhance safety and will verbalize known auras.

✔ The patient will have no traumatic injury to tongue from biting.

✔ The patient's skin will be free from traumatic injuries.

✔ The patient will not sustain a fall injury (head injury, fractures, etc.).

NOC *Fall-prevention behavior*
Physical injury severity
Risk control
Seizure control
Risk detection

INTERVENTIONS	RATIONALES
Assess environment for safety hazards.	Detecting unsafe environmental factors facilitates arranging a safe environment.
Arrange environment for safety.	Decreases injury risk.
Pad side rails of bed with blankets.	Decreases risk of head or extremity trauma during seizure.
Maintain bed in low position with side rails elevated when patient is in bed.	Elevated rails decrease fall risk and bed in low position decreases fall distance should the patient fall out of bed.
Place nurse call system in easy reach.	Facilitates communication from patient to nurse when patient needs assistance.
Interview the patient and family regarding past seizures: characteristics of seizures, aura, date of last seizure, interventions required during/after last seizure, medication regimen, and compliance with medication regimen.	Aids in care planning to decrease injury risk.
Instruct the patient to notify the nurse immediately if he or she experiences an aura or change in the way he or she is feeling.	Some persons will experience an aura or change in the way they feel prior to a seizure, which would alert the nurse to be present to protect patient from injury.
Do not leave bedside when a seizure occurs.	Patients need to be monitored during a seizure.
Notify physician immediately when a seizure occurs.	Seizures can be life-threatening and medical intervention is required.
Assist the patient to a side-lying position.	Facilitates airway and breathing maintenance during the seizure.
Continuously monitor airway and breathing.	Airway obstruction by mucous, emesis, or the tongue may occur during seizures. Patients may also develop bradypnea or apnea.
Prepare to administer anticonvulsant medications as ordered (benzodiazepines such as Valium are commonly prescribed).	Stops the seizure in progress.
Monitor for respiratory insufficiency or apnea: oxygen saturation, respiratory rate, effort, and breath sounds.	Respiratory suppression is a common side effect of anticonvulsants administered during a seizure.
Administer oxygen and/or bag/ mask ventilation as needed.	Supports ventilation and gas exchange.
Following a seizure, start maintenance anticonvulsants (such as Dilantin® or Tegretol®), as ordered.	Prevents future seizures.

NIC *Surveillance*
Positioning
Seizure precautions
Seizure management

Evaluation

Determine that the outcome criteria have been met. The patient should be protected from injury if a seizure occurs. The patient should be able to report any auras to the nurse. No injury has occurred.

Community/Home Care

The patient will need to take medications at home to prevent seizures in the future. A thorough history of current medications is crucial because some medications (such as Reglan® and Wellbutrin®) lower the patient's threshold for seizures. It is important that the patient understand the medication dosing, schedule, and side effects. Dependent upon the medication prescribed, the patient may be able to take all medication in one dose rather than in divided doses, which should enhance compliance. Monitoring of serum levels of the medication is required, especially during initiation of therapy and following any changes in dose. The patient needs to understand the need for compliance with this follow-up, as under-medication may result in seizure activity and over-medication can cause serious side effects. If the patient is started on Dilantin, education should be given on the signs and symptoms of an infrequent but serious side effect of Johnson-Stevens syndrome that necessitates immediate medical attention. All other health care providers, such as the dentist, should be informed of the patient's use of Dilantin. If seizures do occur, the patient and family should understand what measures need to be taken for emergency care and how to protect the patient from injury. In some states, there are restrictions on persons diagnosed with seizures obtaining a driver's license, and the social worker or nurse should attempt to obtain this information for the patient. In some instances, specially trained dogs can be used to alert the patient of impending seizures. These animals are not widely used, but may prove beneficial for patients who have recurrent seizures not well controlled by medications. Location of the animal and the cost of such therapy may prohibit its widespread use. A Medic-Alert bracelet should be worn at all times to alert others to the medical condition.

Documentation

If seizures occur, document a description of the seizure, duration, and patient status following the seizure, including mental status (whether the patient is alert or lethargic) and vital signs. Chart results of a gross assessment for injuries. If the patient verbalizes feelings that may be signs of an impending seizure or reports having had an aura, chart this as well. Chart any medications administered according to agency protocol.

NURSING DIAGNOSIS 2

INEFFECTIVE THERAPEUTIC REGIMEN MANAGEMENT

Related to:

Complexity of therapeutic regimen

Lack of thorough understanding of need for compliance

Knowledge deficit related to seizures

Defining Characteristics:

Verbalizes concern regarding regimen

Noncompliance with medication regimen

Misunderstanding of therapeutic regimen

Goal:

The patient will be compliant with recommended medical regimen.

Outcome Criteria

✔ The patient will state a willingness to comply with the medical regimen, including follow-up care.

✔ The patient will state the names of medications used to treat his or her seizures.

✔ The patient will verbalize an understanding of the mechanism of action and side effects of medications.

✔ The patient will verbalize feelings regarding the diagnosis of seizures and the need to take medications to prevent them.

NOC *Compliance behavior*
Knowledge: Treatment regimen
Knowledge: Disease process
Knowledge: Medication

INTERVENTIONS	RATIONALES
Assess the patient's ability and readiness to learn.	The patient has to be ready and able to learn, or the teaching will not be successful.
Assess the patient's current knowledge and understanding of the therapeutic regimen.	Helps to determine what the patient already knows and understands about the therapeutic regimen and build on this.
Start with the simplest information first.	Patients can understand simple concepts easily and can then build on those to understand information that is more complex.
Review each medication, its purpose, dosage, schedule for administration, side effects, toxic effects, and interactions with other medications.	Compliance improves when patients understand medications and why they need them. Some anticonvulsants can be taken once a day and others will need to be taken two or three times a day.
Assist the patient and family with the creation of a medication log in which they record medication administration and also track medication side effects, adverse reactions, and serum levels of the medications. If seizures occur, document this in the medication log.	A log provides the patient and family with a way to remember all therapeutic interventions, especially medications, and recording serum levels of medications provides a written summary for review, especially in case of an emergency.
Provide written materials about each medication the patient is taking.	Provides resources for review, as patients often forget a large percentage of what they are taught.
Inform the patient of the need for scheduled, periodic blood draws to monitor serum levels of anticonvulsant medications and of parameters that would require a visit to a health care provider.	Sub-therapeutic levels are the most common reason for seizures in persons with a history of seizures. Likewise, elevated levels can predispose the patient to toxic effects. Serum levels will need to be drawn to ensure that the medication is therapeutic, and the patient needs to understand the rationale in order to be compliant.

INTERVENTIONS	RATIONALES
Assess the patient and family's understanding of all teaching by encouraging them to repeat information and ask questions as needed.	This allows the nurse to hear in the patient's own words what was taught and makes it easier to know what information should be reinforced.
Determine whether the patient has the financial resources for medications and follow-up care; make appropriate referrals to a social worker for assistance.	Medications are the mainstay of treatment for seizures and are required. If the patient does not have financial resources for medications or follow-up care, he or she cannot be compliant with the regimen. Social workers will be aware of sources of assistance.

NIC *Teaching: Disease process*
Learning-readiness enhancement
Learning facilitation
Teaching: Prescribed medication

Evaluation

The patient is able to verbalize an understanding of all aspects of medication therapy required for control of seizures. The patient reports that he or she understands the pathophysiology of seizures and states a willingness to comply with requirements of the medical regimen, including returning for laboratory tests to determine serum levels of medication. The patient is effectively managing the therapeutic regimen and verbalizes feelings about the diagnosis. The patient does not have a seizure.

Community/Home Care

The patient with seizures will not need the services of any health care providers in the home. Management of the regimen at home centers on taking medication as scheduled. With written instructions and labeling on the medication bottle, the patient should be able to follow the medication regimen as prescribed. Health care providers should stress to the patient the importance of returning to the designated laboratory to have blood drawn for serum levels of anticonvulsants. Keeping a medication log will be helpful to keep track of medication doses and any side effects. For patients who work outside the home, investigate the possibility of taking medications as one dose so the person does not have to remember to take medication while at work. This is especially true for patients who work in occupations

where the time to take a break or lunch may be random or sporadic making a set schedule difficult. If seizures occur, the patient should seek health care assistance to determine whether the medication dosage needs to be adjusted. Family members or significant others need to be taught what to do in case of a seizure to protect the patient from injury.

Documentation

Chart teaching sessions in the patient record, specifying the exact content taught, titles of printed materials given, and learners who were part of the session. Document the patient's report of understanding and whether he or she is willing to comply with the therapeutic regimen. Include in the chart where the patient needs to go for follow-up care and laboratory testing.

NURSING DIAGNOSIS 3

INEFFECTIVE AIRWAY CLEARANCE

Related to:

Altered level of consciousness during seizure

Positioning during seizure where airway is obstructed by tongue falling backwards

Vomiting during seizure

Mucous in airway

Defining Characteristics:

Snoring

Cyanosis

Hypoxemia

Thick mucus

Diminished breath sounds

Adventitious breath sounds: crackles, wheezes

Tachypnea/bradypnea

Goal:

The patient will maintain a clear airway.

Outcome Criteria

✔ The patient will have a patent airway.

✔ Breath sounds will be clear and equal bilaterally.

✔ The patient will not develop hypoxemia or cyanosis.

✔ Oxygen saturation will be > 94 percent.

NOC *Respiratory status: Airway patency*

INTERVENTIONS	RATIONALES
Evaluate breathing, skin color, and oxygen saturation during and after seizure.	Patients may experience ineffective airway clearance during and after seizures related to altered consciousness; ineffective airway clearance is manifested by snoring, noisy respirations, cyanosis, hypoxemia, and frothy mucous or emesis in mouth.
Place in side-lying position.	This position facilitates airway maintenance by allowing the tongue to fall to the side of the mouth and mucous or emesis to drain from the mouth.
Assess breath sounds and oxygen saturation.	Helps to evaluate the need for clearing the airway.
Keep suction setup at bedside and suction upper airway as needed.	Suction may be required to clear the upper airways of mucus or emesis (typically nasopharyngeal suctioning because the teeth generally are clenched shut during a seizure).
Administer oxygen as ordered for patients who are cyanotic or hypoxemic.	Ineffective airway clearance may result in hypoxemia; oxygen is needed to support gas exchange.
Do not force anything, including padded tongue blades or oral airways, into the mouth during a seizure.	These traditional interventions may occlude the airway and are no longer recommended.
Following the seizure, assess the patient's respiratory status.	Ensures that the patient's respiratory status has returned to baseline and that no further interventions are required.

NIC *Respiratory monitoring*
Airway management
Airway suctioning
Seizure precautions
Seizure management

Evaluation

If a seizure occurs, the patient's airway is kept patent. Breath sounds are clear and respirations are equal bilaterally. Oxygen saturation is 94 percent or above. The patient is not hypoxemic or cyanotic.

Community/Home Care

At home, the patient and family must understand what to do to maintain airway patency in the event of a seizure. Family members or significant others need to be taught how to perform emergency techniques to prevent airway occlusion with assurance that learning has occurred. Teaching should include how to place the patient in a side position to ensure that the tongue does not occlude the airway. It should be stressed to the family that no object should be placed in the mouth during a seizure because of the possibility of injuring the mouth and or further occluding the airway. If a seizure occurs in the home, measures should be undertaken to assess the patient's respiratory status following the seizure by noting any difficulty breathing, shortness of breath ("difficulty catching my breath"), or statements like "feels like something went down into my lungs." If any breathing difficutlies are noted, the patient should go to a nearby health care facility emergency room or urgent care facility, or call emergency personnel.

Documentation

Chart the results of a respiratory assessment conducted during and after the seizure. Note respiratory rate, chest expansion, and breath sounds. If the patient's airway was compromised during the seizure, document nursing interventions employed to address the problem, such as positioning on the side or suctioning. Include in the chart oxygen saturation results.

CHAPTER 3.47

SPINAL CORD INJURY (SCI)

GENERAL INFORMATION

The spinal cord is the nerve center of the body. It transmits impulses to and from the brain and the body to elicit movement and the sensation of pain. The spinal cord is well protected by the meningeal layer (the pia, the arachnoid, and the dura), cerebrospinal fluid, the bony vertebrae, and the paravertebral muscles. The anterior (front half) of the spinal cord contains motor (movement) tracts and the posterior (rear half) contains the sensory (pain, cold, etc.) tracts. Spinal cord injuries (SCIs) occur when the vertebral column is hyperextended, hyperflexed, distracted, compressed, bent laterally beyond normal limits, or over-rotated, and when axial loading occurs (large force to top of head). The vertebrae are fractured, dislocated, or subluxed. If the injury is located high in the cervical spine, the possibility of respiration impairment exists and will result in death if therapeutic interventions are not immediate. Types of spinal cord injuries are classified as cord concussion, cord contusion, cord laceration, and cord transection. Concussions usually produce transient deficits; contusions may result in temporary or permanent deficits; cord lacerations results in permanent deficits; and transections result in permanent disabilities below the level of the transection. The levels of spinal cord injury and resulting disability are

C1–C3: Quadriplegia; loss of all respiratory and muscle functions

C4–C5: Quadriplegia; loss of most muscle function, reduced pulmonary ability

C6–C7: Quadriplegia; may have some arm/hand sparing, some independence

C7–C8: Quadriplegia; usually has some arm/hand/digit sparing

T1–L1: Paraplegia; able to use arms/hands/digits, usually able to use muscles of respiration, patient is more independent

L1–sacrals: May have loss of bowels and bladder, varying motor and sensory loss at and below level of injury

The most common cause of spinal cord injuries is motor vehicle crashes, followed by diving incidents, and contact sports incidents. Approximately 12,000 people sustain spinal cord injuries each year, with 6000 of them sustaining paraplegia or quadriplegia. Of all spinal cord injuries that occur, the highest incidence is among 16 to 30 year olds. It is also interesting to note that 80 percent of the injuries occur in males, probably as the result of high-risk behaviors.

NURSING DIAGNOSIS 1

 INEFFECTIVE BREATHING PATTERN

Related to:

Spinal cord injury at C1–C5

Defining Characteristics:

Lack of respirations

Inability to use muscles of respiration

Diaphragmatic dystonia

Intercostal muscle dysfunction

Abdominal muscle dysfunction

Goal:

The patient's respiratory status will be maintained.

Outcome Criteria

✔ Oxygen saturations will be > 96 percent.

✔ Arterial blood gases (ABGs) will return to normal range.

✔ The patient's respiratory rate will remain < 28 but > 12.

NOC *Respiratory status: Ventilation*
Respiratory status: Gas exchange
Vital signs
Mechanical ventilation
   respiratory: Adult

INTERVENTIONS	RATIONALES
Assess respiratory system every hour initially during acute phase and every 4 hours once the patient is stable by noting respiratory rate, depth, chest expansion, rhythm, lung sounds, pulse oximetry, ability to cough, and skin color (examine lip color and color of mucous membranes for dark-skinned patients).	Provides information on the status of the respiratory system and extent of injury; also establishes a baseline for future comparisons. Assists in determining when and if mechanical ventilation is required. Patients with spinal cord injury at levels of C1–C5 experience serious loss of ability to maintain respiratory function due to effects on the phrenic nerve, which controls the diaphragm; such injuries require mechanical ventilation (complete to partial loss). Injuries at the level of T1–T7 affect innervation of the intercostal muscles, which may alter accessory muscles involved in respiratory function and decrease the patient's ability to cough effectively.
Monitor arterial blood gases (ABGs).	Monitoring arterial blood gases (ABGs) is the most accurate method for determining oxygenation status; edema of the spinal cord may impair adequate function of the phrenic nerve, making respirations ineffective in maintaining adequate gas exchange.
Assist with intubation/ tracheostomy and mechanical ventilation, as required.	The phrenic and intercostal nerves may be paralyzed as a result of the spinal cord injury, and the patient will not be able to breathe on his or her own, making mechanical ventilation necessary; patients with injuries above C4 are ventilator-dependent. Endotracheal intubation is done to gain and maintain access to the lower airway and to protect the lungs from aspiration. Mechanical

	ventilation is employed to assure adequate respirations by maintaining a constant rate and volume.
Assess the patient for other injuries in the area of the head and neck or chest.	Most spinal cord injuries are a result of automobile accidents, and other injuries that affect the respiratory system could be present, such as trauma to the chest.
Administer supplemental oxygen, as ordered and required based on arterial blood gas (ABG) analysis.	Supplemental oxygen is needed for adequate tissue oxygenation.
If the patient does not require mechanical ventilation, encourage coughing and deep breathing exercises or the use of an incentive spirometer every hour.	Expands alveoli of the lungs and assists with better gas exchange.
Ensure an open airway and have suction readily available; when suctioning, monitor the patient for vasovagal response.	The airway must be open and clear in order for oxygen to reach the lungs; patients with SCI are at higher risk for vasovagal response of severe bradycardia, which can be life-threatening.
Following the acute phase of injury, monitor for signs and symptoms of respiratory infection: elevated temperature, increased white blood cells, diaphoresis, or thick secretions.	Respiratory infections are easily acquired due to immobility and decreased movement of respiratory muscles.
If the patient is going home with a ventilator, teach appropriate caregivers how to care for the ventilator and how to assess respiratory status (see nursing care plan "Mechanical Ventilation").	Patients with SCI above C4 are ventilator-dependent and will be cared for in an extended care facility or at home with family, necessitating intense education with attention to anxiety control.

NIC *Respiratory monitoring*
Cough enhancement
Artificial airway
Mechanical ventilation
Ventilation

Evaluation

The patient should show indications that breathing patterns are effective in meeting the body's need for oxygen. The rate should return to baseline, preferably between 12–24 breaths per minute, and be unlabored. Respiratory function is maintained unassisted for injuries below C5 and on mechanical ventilation for injuries above C4. The return of arterial blood gases (ABGs) to the patient's baseline or to within normal range should be expected.

Community/Home Care

If the patient is cared for at home without a ventilator, the family will need to closely monitor the patient's respiratory status. The caregiver should be taught how to monitor respiratory rate and depth, as well as chest movement changes that would indicate paralysis of the diaphragm. If noted the patient will need to seek health care quickly. For the patient who has been on a ventilator in an extended care facility, function of respiratory muscles generally returns over 2–3 weeks, and the patient is weaned. Once at home, the patient may experience some anxiety about the possibility of being unable to breathe again. It is anticipated that the patient will need to regain stamina and endurance and may experience some shortness of breath dependent upon the severity of the SCI and its effect on mobility. For those patients with injuries above C4 that require permanent mechanical ventilation, the family will need extensive teaching regarding maintenance of the ventilator. A visiting nurse is crucial for the family who will be caring for a ventilator-dependent patient in the home. During the early period of home care, the nurse can work with family members as they gradually acquire competency in care and become more comfortable with the patient's requirements. Anxiety is a natural response to this new responsibility, and the nurse can also assist the family to cope with the change in life. Adjustments to the environment to accommodate the ventilator equipment may be needed. Smaller beds may be required to make room for ventilators and oxygen supplies, as well as wheelchairs or other medical equipment and supplies. Spouses may need to adjust to new sleeping arrangements and positioning for sleep. It is important to stress to the caregiver that the patient continues to be at risk for development of respiratory infection due to the previous compromised respiratory status. In-home caregivers should be taught symptoms of respiratory infection, including elevated temperature, diaphoresis, increased expectoration of sputum, and abnormal colors of sputum. It is important that the patient understand how to prevent upper respiratory infections, particularly through the use of immunizations against influenza and pneumonia. Follow-up care is necessary to monitor for stabilization of respiratory function.

Documentation

Chart the results of a comprehensive assessment of the respiratory system. Note respiratory rate, chest expansion, use of accessory muscles, breath sounds, and results of pulse oximetry. If the patient expectorates, document the amount, color, and consistency. Chart each time the patient is suctioned, with a description of the results. If the patient is on a ventilator, document settings and other assessments according to the unit protocol. Document any family or patient teaching completed. Include in the patient's chart all interventions employed to address ineffective breathing pattern and the patient's response to the interventions. Chart any referrals made for in-home care.

NURSING DIAGNOSIS 2

 ## DECREASED CARDIAC OUTPUT

Related to:

   Neurogenic or spinal shock

   Vasodilation

   Pooling of blood in venous system

   Decreased capillary permeability

Defining Characteristics:

   Severe hypotension

   Bradycardia (neurogenic)

   Mental status changes (restless, agitated, anxious)

   Decreased urinary output

   Decreased central venous pressure

Goal:

   The patient's cardiac output is restored.

Outcome Criteria

✔ The patient has a pulse rate between 60–100.

✔ The patient is not agitated or restless; reports decreased anxiety.

✔ Urinary output is > 30 ml/hour average.

✔ The patient's systolic blood pressure is > 90, and blood pressure returns to patient's baseline.

NOC *Circulatory status*
Tissue perfusion: Cardiac
Tissue perfusion: Peripheral
Tissue perfusion: Cerebral
Vital signs

INTERVENTIONS	RATIONALES
Assess for signs of neurogenic shock: bradycardia, decreased blood pressure, mental status changes, hypothermia, decreased urinary output, and cool, clammy skin.	Reveals abnormalities and establishes a baseline for evaluation of response to interventions. All of the above manifestations occur because of massive vasodilation with subsequent changes in cardiac effectiveness.
Give oxygen, as ordered.	Helps to maintain pO_2 at > 90 percent. Due to hypoperfusion tissues may be hypoxic; giving oxygen increases the amount available for gas exchange.
Assess blood pressure and pulse every 15 minutes.	Changes in blood pressure and pulse give indicators to patient status. In shock, a decreased blood pressure with narrowing pulse pressure may be noted; in neurogenic shock, the pulse may be bradycardic.
Assess temperature at least every 4 hours and document.	Patients with neurogenic shock may experience poikilothermia (assuming the temperature of surrounding environment) and be unable to regulate temperature to normal levels. The massive vasodilation also contributes to insensible heat loss. Assessing temperature often will allow for early intervention.
Assess urinary output via an indwelling urinary catheter every hour.	Decreased urinary output (< 30 ml/hour) indicates decreased perfusion to kidneys and progression of shock.
Assess skin temperature and color.	If shock progresses, the perfusion to skin and periphery is inadequate to maintain warmth or normal color; in the early stages, the extremities are warm and pink due to pooling of blood there, but as shock progresses, the extremities become cool and clammy due to lack of perfusion.
Assess peripheral pulses.	As shock progresses, peripheral pulses become weak, diminished, or absent as the heart is unable to maintain perfusion to extremities.
Assess mental status for presence of altered level of consciousness, confusion, or agitation, and assess for pertinent neurological history, noting any abnormalities specific to neurogenic shock such as cool, clammy skin above the level of any injury; priapism; and neck pain followed by loss of sensation.	Changes in mental status indicate a decrease in cerebral tissue perfusion and an inability of the body's compensatory mechanism to provide adequate oxygenation to cerebral tissue; neurological injuries may produce clinical manifestations other than change in level of consciousness and could contribute to neurogenic shock.
Assess respiratory status, noting adventitious breath sounds; for patients experiencing neurogenic shock, assess for tachypnea and in some cases varying changes in respiratory rate.	Decreased cardiac output leads to decreased perfusion to lungs, causing crackles and dyspnea.
Assist with hemodynamic monitoring according to agency/unit protocol (pulmonary artery pressure, central venous pressures, and arterial pressures).	Helps to more accurately assess progression of shock and to evaluate patient response to treatment; these measures can give information to evaluate left ventricular function (cardiac output) and fluid status.
Establish intravenous access and administer fluids, as ordered.	Patients need an access site for administration of emergency medications, and fluids are needed to reestablish cardiac output.
Administer medications as ordered; for neurogenic shock, administer medications, including vasopressors (such as dopamine) and alpha-adrenergic agonists (such as phenylephrine).	Vasoactive medications are given for their vasoconstrictive properties to increase venous return to the heart and to improve pumping ability of the myocardium. An increase in heart rate occurs leading to increased cardiac output and increased blood pressure. Dopamine increases cardiac output and blood pressure, and can also increase heart rate. Phenylephrine causes an increased venous return and increases systolic and diastolic pressures.
Maintain bedrest.	Decrease the workload of the heart.

NIC *Invasive hemodynamic monitoring*
Cardiac care
Fluid management
Fluid monitoring
Shock management: Vasogenic
Vital signs monitoring

Evaluation

Note the degree to which outcome criteria have been achieved. The patient should demonstrate adequate cardiac output or improvement in abnormalities. Peripheral pulses should be present and skin should be warm to the touch. If cardiac output is improved, perfusion to the kidneys should be adequate, with the patient producing at least 30 ml of urine per hour on average. The pulse should be within the patient's baseline and should be strong and regular. The parameters from invasive hemodynamic monitoring should show improvement and a gradual return to normal. Arterial blood gases (ABGs) should return to normal or show compensation and oxygen saturation should be > 90 percent.

Community/Home Care

Patients who have experienced neurogenic shock and are mobile will need to know how to gradually increase activities when at home with a balance of rest and activity. The patient will need to monitor his or her response to activity, noting any shortness of breath, increased respiratory rate, and increased pulse rate, as neurogenic shock can occur over an extended period. Patients who are not mobile will need to be monitored for continued or new symptoms of cardiovascular and neurological deficits that could signal a problem. Home care follow-up may be required for some patients, especially if they verbalize feelings of anxiety or lack of knowledge about their health status. In patients with neurogenic shock, if the causative alteration has been treated or alleviated (central nervous system depression, medications, etc.), there may be no need for further post-hospital care. However, in patients who have had head or spinal injury, neurogenic shock may be resolved, but lingering issues relevant to care may continue (see nursing diagnoses "Impaired Physical Mobility" and "Ineffective Breathing Pattern"; see also nursing care plan "Head Injury"). For most patients, specific

attention to decreased cardiac output caused by shock is not required once cardiac output is restored. However, a follow-up appointment is needed to be sure that the patient has returned to his or her normal level of functioning.

Documentation

Chart the results of all assessments made, particularly of the neurological and cardiac systems. Chart intake and output hourly or according to agency protocol, including presence of intravenous infusions. Document all interventions in a timely fashion with the patient's specific response to the intervention. Chart readings from hemodynamic monitoring according to agency/unit protocol, paying particular attention to blood pressure and pulse. Temperatures should be taken at least every 4 hours and documented to detect early hypothermia. Always include the patient's psychological status—whether he or she appears anxious, restless, or fearful—and whether significant others are present.

NURSING DIAGNOSIS 3

 IMPAIRED PHYSICAL MOBILITY

Related to:
    Spinal cord injury
    Loss of innervation to muscles

Defining Characteristics:
    Inability to move
    Paraplegia
    Quadriplegia

Goal:
    The patient will achieve maximum level of physical mobility.

Outcome Criteria

✔ The patient will participate in prescribed physical therapy.

✔ The patient will not sustain injury.

✔ The patient will be out of bed after spinal injury/neurological status is stabilized.

NOC *Mobility*

INTERVENTIONS	RATIONALES
Perform a complete neuromuscular assessment, including muscle tone, spasticity, movement, loss of reflexes, pain response, tactile response, and range of motion, and note extent of extremity paralysis.	Helps to determine the current functional ability and to plan for appropriate interventions. Spinal shock may occur, resulting in a loss of reflex below the level of injury when there is total cord dissection.
Assist with immobilization of the patient as required or ordered using halos or other traction devices.	All spinal injuries require immobilization to prevent movement of the spine. Cervical spine injuries create the danger of an extremely unstable spinal column, and injuries in this area require immediate immobilization that may last for extended periods.
Monitor results of diagnostic tests: computed tomography (CT) scans, MRI, x-rays (spine series, chest x-ray).	Helps to determine the extent of injury and ensure proper treatment.
Collaborate with the physician to arrange for physical therapy consultation for methods/ therapies to improve or preserve function, and/or rehabilitation following the acute phase.	The physical therapist can implement a plan for achieving maximum function and for preservation of muscle tone. Therapy is required to prevent loss of muscle strength/tone, to help control spasticity, and to prevent contractures. The physical therapist will evaluate the patient's potential for rehabilitation and start therapy within prescribed limitations to ensure that the patient can achieve a maximum level of mobility. Physical therapy usually starts as soon as the patient's neurological status stabilizes.
Once stable, turn the patient every 2 hours using logrolling techniques.	Prevents pressure on areas prone to breakdown.
If the patient is unable to engage in ambulatory activity with physical therapy, assist the patient in getting out of bed and into a chair daily and perform range of motion exercises every 4 hours once neurological injury is stable. Provide trochanter rolls, pillow supports, and/or splints for hands.	Prevents complications of prolonged bedrest such as pneumonia, DVT, skin breakdown, muscle loss, and contractures. Maximizing function and strength of uninvolved limbs is essential to possible independence. If range of motion is performed on affected limbs, some function and strength may return. Splints, braces, and proper

	positioning help to prevent contractures.
For patients with paraplegia, encourage participation in prescribed physical therapy activities to prepare for rehabilitation; teach transfer techniques and the use of a wheelchair, with attention to strengthening upper body.	All patients with spinal cord injury will need rehabilitation in a special center; this is especially true for those with paraplegia who have potential for self-care, including making transfers, driving, self-catheterization, etc. Preventing loss of muscle tone and mass is crucial to enhance success.
Teach the family turning, lifting/moving techniques, correct body alignment, use of assistive devices, and performing range of motion.	Maintains function as long as possible and prevents contractures. Even though a physical therapist may come into the home to work with the patient, family members may also be required to move and position the patient.
Refer patient to a social worker for discharge planning to a rehabilitation center where the patient can receive physical and occupational therapy.	All patients with spinal cord injuries require specialized rehabilitation to achieve maximum functional potential.

NIC *Exercise therapy*
Joint mobility
Positioning

Evaluation

The patient maintains full range of motion of all extremities with no contractures. The patient participates in mobility activities and exercises as prescribed by a physical therapist to the extent possible. Skin breakdown and pneumonia do not occur because of limited mobility. Following the acute phase of spinal cord injury, the patient is able to participate in physical therapy for teaching on transfer techniques, reconditioning, and strength.

Community/Home Care

Following the acute phase and a stay at a rehabilitation center or other extended care facility, the patient with a spinal cord injury may return home. The family will need thorough information regarding the changes in normal functions caused by the injury. In the acute phase of the injury, it is crucial that caregivers encourage the patient to participate in physical therapy or other activities to the fullest extent possible. For patients with injuries above C4, physical therapy and rehabilitation potential is limited and may focus only on preventing loss of muscle mass and prevention of contractures, as the patient has little potential for mobility. Exercises using trapeze bars for shifting weight and repositioning are helpful and should be encouraged by caregivers. The physical therapist provides education to the family and patients on the use of assistive devices, such as wheelchairs, walkers, or canes, for ambulation. The patient may become disillusioned as he or she realizes that the physical limitations are permanent, but he or she should be encouraged and given factual information about the rehabilitation prognosis. Assessments should be made of the patient's feelings concerning limitations in mobility, social isolation, and future disability as well as feelings of depression. Concerns and needs may focus on role performance at home and activities including mowing the lawn, household chores such as laundry and cleaning, or self-care needs such as bathing and dressing. An assessment of the home is required in order to make suggestions for changes in the environment that promote independence and safety. Issues to be addressed include ability to move about the home, especially getting to the bathroom, getting in or out of the shower or tub, exiting the house if there are steps, and the ability and willingness to be mobile in the home. If the patient is wheelchair-bound following a spinal cord injury, a ramp is required for entry and exit of the home. If the patient is unable to afford such a ramp, community groups such as religious organizations or construction companies should be contacted to see if they could offer assistance. The social worker can be a vital piece of this puzzle. It is crucial that the patient understand the strategies required to maintain optimal functioning of affected extremities (see "Interventions/Rationales"). In-home visits by a physical therapist for a period of time will be important to the patient's health maintenance and for completion of appropriate exercises and instructions on the use of assistive devices. Encourage the patient and family members or significant others to use community resources, such as support groups specifically for caregivers and patients with spinal cord injury. These groups can be invaluable in assisting the patient and family to cope.

Documentation

Document a thorough assessment of the patient's functional mobility, including muscle strength, presence of paralysis, and use of assistive devices. If the patient is able to ambulate or move, detail the extent of his or her capabilities and participation. Include in the patient record all interventions recommended to the patient to address the problem of mobility. Include a report of the patient's perception of the ability to be mobile. Clearly document the effectiveness of all interventions and instruction to the caregiver relevant to addressing immobility. If any complications of immobility are noted, chart these in accordance with agency protocol.

NURSING DIAGNOSIS 4

RISK FOR IMPAIRED SKIN INTEGRITY

Related to:

Immobility

Loss of sensation to pressure points

Defining Characteristics:

None

Goal:

The patient's skin will remain intact.

Outcome Criteria

✔ The skin will have no redness or other discoloration.

✔ No skin breakdown will occur.

NOC *Tissue integrity: Skin and mucous membranes*

Immobility consequences: Physiological

Risk control

Risk detection

INTERVENTIONS	RATIONALES
Complete a thorough skin assessment every shift noting areas of redness, pallor, edema, and any denuded or open areas, with particular attention to sacrum/coccyx, heels, ears, hips, and inner aspects of knees, ankles, and elbows.	A thorough assessment establishes a baseline; areas subject to pressure are at higher risk for breakdown, and these include most bony prominences.
Use the Braden risk assessment scale.	This is an objective method of assessing the patient's risk for skin breakdown and includes parameters such as sensory perception, moisture, activity, mobility, nutrition, friction, and shear. Information from this assessment adds to the general assessment and allows for planning to resolve causative factors.
Turn the patient every 2 hours using turn sheets and acceptable patient handling techniques (logrolling may be required), avoiding friction and shearing force.	Patients with spinal cord injuries are unable to sense the pressure on prone areas and immobility prevents self-repositioning; pressure causes vasculature to be compressed and unable to provide nutrients to the high-risk areas; friction and shearing damage the skin and underlying vasculature.
Post a turning schedule at the patient's bedside.	Ensures that all health care workers are aware of the need for turning; the schedule prevents the patient from being repositioned in a particular position too often.
Apply heel and elbow protectors bilaterally.	Prevents excoriation to bony areas.
Place thin pillows between knees.	Prevents bony areas of knees from rubbing against one another and causing skin breakdown.
Keep patient clean and dry by washing well (avoiding friction) with warm water after each incontinent episode of urine or stool; change sheets if patient is diaphoretic; apply protective ointment after cleansing.	Enzymes and chemicals found in urine and feces can irritate tissues, as can the moisture from urine. Hot water should be avoided as it causes dryness of the skin. Friction causes trauma to sensitive at risk skin. Cleansing is required after each episode to clean the irritants away from skin.

Institute use of special mattresses—air, water, or other—as ordered.	Special mattresses are intended to relieve pressure to high-risk areas, especially the sacrum and coccyx.
Avoid massaging bony prominences.	Pressure from massage increases the risk for ulcer formation due to excessive friction on areas already at risk.
Provide topical moisturizing agents, as ordered.	Skin that is dry and flaky is more likely to experience breakdown.
Assess the patient's hydration and nutritional status.	An adequate diet and hydration are necessary for healthy skin.
Teach family or other caregiver techniques for preventing skin breakdown.	If family members are planning to care for the spinal cord injury patient at home, they will need to know how to prevent skin breakdown that will continue to be a problem.

NIC *Pressure ulcer prevention*
Skin surveillance
Skin care: Topical treatments
Positioning

Evaluation

Determine that the patient has met the out-come criteria. The patient's risk for breakdown will be minimized. The patient's skin will remain intact with no areas of redness/discoloration or excoriation.

Community/Home Care

Most spinal cord injury patients go to rehabilitation centers or other extended care facilities for post-acute care. However, many of these patients go home after the maximal rehabilitation benefit has been achieved. For a number of patients, pressure ulcers are a common occurrence and in some instances necessitate hospitalization for skin grafting and serious infections. Prevention of skin breakdown can prevent serious complications. In the home, great detail should be given to teaching the family strategies to prevent skin breakdown. Because of alterations in sensory perception, nutrition status, elimination patterns, and hydration, the patient remains at high risk for breakdown. The family will need to implement strategies identified in the interventions section with emphasis placed on turning, positioning, and maintaining cleanliness of the skin. When dependent patients return home, the family often does not have a realistic perception of what total patient care involves. The nurse needs to enlist the family members to participate in the care while the patient is still hospitalized or in a rehabilitation center so that they may perform tasks while resources are available to answer questions and provide assistance. The most critical aspects of care in the home will be turning the patient religiously to relieve pressure on high-risk areas. A schedule that outlines which position the patient should be in at specific times will be helpful, particularly if there will be multiple caregivers. It is also crucial that the family learn how to use bed pillows or possibly a small rolled throw to support the patient in the side-lying position and smaller, semi-flat pillows between the knees to prevent rubbing of the bony inner aspects against each other. The family can also use a pillow or a smooth texture blanket to place beneath the feet to keep heels off the bed. The second area of emphasis in the home is handling incontinence. All too often, when patients experience urinary incontinence, caregivers remove soiled incontinence pads and replace with a clean one but never cleanse the skin. The harsh components of urine can continue to irritate the skin, contributing to breakdown. Family caregivers must be diligent in cleansing the skin well after each episode of incontinence (urine and stool) with mild soap and warm water. Commercially prepared wet wipes can be used, but can be rather expensive. There are many commercial barrier products on the market as well, but these are also expensive to use for totally incontinent patients. Good inexpensive substitutes that act as barriers, especially to urine, include petroleum jelly and zinc oxide paste (commonly used on babies). Even though the patient has on incontinent briefs, he or she should still be checked at least every 2 hours for wetness, and caregivers can check for wetness or stool at the same time they reposition the patient. In addition, the family will need to learn the initial signs of skin breakdown, such as redness/discoloration, pallor, warmth, or any open areas. Nutrition plays a vital role in preventing skin breakdown, and the family will need to encourage the patient to maintain adequate nutrients needed for tissue maintenance. If the family detects any change in the skin, a health care provider must be notified, and a visit from a nurse may be warranted.

Documentation

Chart the results of a thorough assessment of the patient's skin including the results of the Braden Skin Risk Assessment Scale. If any signs of impaired skin integrity are noted, chart them along with the interventions implemented to address the problem. Document all actions employed to prevent skin impairment, including teaching to caregivers. Most agencies have protocols established that nurses should follow when skin breakdown is detected, thus if any area of breakdown is detected, document according to protocol.

NURSING DIAGNOSIS 5

 ## DISTURBED BODY IMAGE

Related to:

Paralysis

Loss of function

Spasticity

Bowel and bladder incontinence

Defining Characteristics:

Withdrawal

Social isolation

Depression

Negative statements about physical appearance

Verbalizations regarding loss of function

Goal:

The patient accepts and adapts to the change in physical appearance and function, and interacts with others.

Outcome Criteria

✔ The patient states willingness to look at legs.

✔ The patient does not verbalize negative feelings toward self.

✔ The patient verbalizes an understanding of the extent of the injury.

✔ The patient verbalizes feelings of self-worth.

✔ The patient verbalizes an understanding that the paralysis may be permanent and will require rehabilitation.

NOC   *Body image*
Adaptation to physical disability
Psychosocial adjustment:
Life change
Self-esteem
Coping

INTERVENTIONS	RATIONALES
Encourage the patient to get his or her feelings out in the open and assure the patient that his or her feelings are normal.	The patient should understand that his or her emotions are real and should be expected.
Encourage the patient to communicate feelings about changes in physical appearance and function as well as the significance or meaning of the changes.	Talking about the changes may sometimes be the beginning of acceptance.
Inform the patient of interventions required to treat spinal cord injury (see nursing diagnosis "Impaired Physical Mobility").	Knowing the prognosis and what is required may assist the patient to start coping with the consequences of the injury.
Monitor the patient's feelings about him or herself, interpersonal relationships with family members and friends, withdrawal, social isolation, fear, anxiety, embarrassment by appearance, fear that appearance will be displeasing to loved ones, and desire to be alone.	Helps to detect early alterations in social functioning, prevent unhealthy behaviors, and intervene early through referral to counseling.
Help the patient to identify coping mechanisms and support persons.	Lifestyle changes and rehabilitation will be extensive and possibly frustrating; the patient will need ways to cope with the challenges and people to be supportive.
Assist the patient in identifying realistic goals and acceptance of dependency on others.	Realizing limitations and having realistic goals can prevent frustrations that decrease self-esteem.
Encourage the patient to participate in at least one visitation with a friend or family member and leave the hospital room.	Prevents patient from isolating him or herself from others.
Determine whether the patient's culture or religion has an impact	A patient's culture and religion often help define his or her

on his or her perception of body image and self-esteem.	reactions to changes in body image and self-worth; religion can also be a source of strength and an effective coping mechanism.
Monitor for changes in self-esteem: improvement or worsening.	Helps to determine whether the patient is moving in a positive direction in terms of accepting the condition or whether intense counseling is required. Recognize that denial and anger are common.
Arrange for a consult with a counselor, as required.	Spinal cord injuries with permanent paralysis cause a sudden major change in functional ability and emotional state; such a change is most often difficult to adjust to and the patient may need counseling beyond that which a nurse can provide.

NIC   *Self-esteem enhancement*
Body image enhancement
Emotional support
Support group
Socialization enhancement

Evaluation

The patient is able and willing to learn about the strategies to improve functioning and manage activities to the extent possible. Determine whether the patient is able to verbalize feelings regarding the paralysis and the impact it will have on role performance. Time is required for the patient to completely assimilate the change in body appearance and function into his or her self-perception. It is crucial that the nurse evaluate to what degree the patient is beginning to do this. Communication of feelings and concerns relevant to the changes should be taken as a positive sign that progress towards meeting the outcome criteria is being made.

Community/Home Care

At home, continued monitoring of the patient's body image and self-esteem is needed. The health care provider who interacts with the patient during follow-up will need to be alert to subtle hints that may indicate that the patient has not completely adapted to the change in body function. For the patient who has sustained a spinal cord injury, the change in function will be obvious to others, as the patient is required to use alternative means of mobility. The patient may be angry, fearful, or anxious about the impact the injury will have on the ability to function in all aspects of life, such as self-care, work, sexuality, etc. It is important that family or significant others encourage and support efforts at body image and self-esteem enhancement and avoidance of self-imposed isolation. Open discussions regarding the changes and their accompanying frustrations are crucial to the patient's ability to maintain a positive self-esteem and body image. Encourage the patient to look at him or herself in mirrors while sitting in wheelchair so that he or she can view his or her entire body. If the patient is an active member of civic or religious organizations, these may be good places to start social interaction, as the patient may have some sense of comfort with the people there and be more willing to attempt interactions. Counseling may be needed for a period of time to help the patient adjust to the changes and be an active participant in rehabilitation activities.

Documentation

Chart any specific behaviors or verbalizations that may indicate a low self-esteem and altered body image. Document a precise description of the physical change in appearance that is causing the disturbed body image. Include all interventions that have been employed to address this issue and the patient's response. Note when and if the patient begins to verbalize feelings regarding the change in function. Document any referrals made to spiritual or professional counselors.

NURSING DIAGNOSIS 6

AUTONOMIC DYSREFLEXIA

Related to:

Spinal cord injury above T6

Profound sympathetic nervous system response to obnoxious stimuli

Fecal impaction

Distended bladder

Urinary tract infections

Defining Characteristics:

Uncontrollable paroxysmal hypertension (systolic > 140, diastolic > 90)

Diaphoresis

Bradycardia

Headache described as pounding

Flushed skin on face

Goal:

Symptoms of autonomic dysreflexia will be eliminated.

Outcome Criteria

✔ Blood pressure will return to patient's baseline with a systolic < 140 and diastolic < 90.

✔ Heart rate will be > 60 beats per minute.

✔ The patient will offer no complaints of headache.

✔ The patient will have no bladder distention.

✔ The patient will not experience a fecal impaction.

NOC *Neurological status: Autonomic*
Urinary elimination
Bowel elimination
Vital signs

INTERVENTIONS	RATIONALES
Assess patient for risk factors for development of autonomic dysreflexia: bladder distention (80 percent of cases), constipation/impaction, restraining clothes, skin breakdown.	Helps to identify the specific causes and determine actions to prevent occurrence.
Assess for signs and symptoms of autonomic dysreflexia: profound elevations in blood pressure, slow pulse, diaphoresis, facial flushing, pounding headache, nausea.	These are signs of dysreflexia, and the patient needs to be monitored for these closely.
Assess for bladder distention every 2 hours.	Bladder distention is a leading cause of dysreflexia.
Prevent or relieve bladder distention by catheterizing the patient at specified intervals; if the patient has an indwelling catheter, ensure patency by checking that tubing is not kinked.	Bladder distention is the most common cause of autonomic dysreflexia; if patients have orders for catheterization, be sure that catheterization is performed prior to the patient leaving the floor for any tests or rehabilitative activities.

(continues)

(continued)

INTERVENTIONS	RATIONALES
Monitor bowel function for early treatment of constipation and prevention of impaction.	Constipation and impaction contribute to dysreflexia.
Place the patient on a bowel therapy program to include administration of fiber, laxatives, and liquids, and document bowel activity every shift.	These interventions can prevent constipation and fecal impaction.
If dysreflexia occurs take blood pressure every 2–3 minutes.	Reveals changes in blood pressure and improvement in the patient. The blood pressure may be high enough to precipitate a CVA.
Establish intravenous access.	Provides a route for emergency medications.
If blood pressure is sustained at extremely high levels, administer potent antihypertensives as ordered, such as Hyperstat®, Procardia®, or Apresoline®.	Emergency intervention is required to prevent complications, such as CVA.
Teach family members or other caregivers how to prevent autonomic dysreflexia.	If the patient is to go home, the family needs to know how to prevent its occurrence.

NIC   *Dysreflexia management*
          Vital signs monitoring
          Urinary catheterization:
             Intermittent
          Bowel management
          Urinary elimination management

Evaluation

Determine whether the patient has achieved the stated outcomes. The patient has no symptoms of autonomic dysreflexia, such as elevated blood pressure or pounding headache. Bladder distention will be relieved through natural processes or catheterization. The patient achieves a routine for bowel evacuation to prevent constipation or impaction.

Community/Home Care

Caregivers for the spinal cord injury patient at home will need to understand autonomic dysreflexia and how to prevent it. Careful attention to bladder emptying and bowel elimination is required to prevent this disorder, which can continue to be a threat for many months after the rehabilitative phase. Family members need to learn how to catheterize the patient to empty the bladder or to check for bladder distention regularly. Institution of a bowel plan to ensure regular bowel evacuation should be undertaken following appropriate education on symptoms of impaction, types of food needed in the diet, appropriate laxatives and suppositories, administration techniques, and best times for administration. The family should keep records of bowel elimination and urinary output to be sure that impaction and retention do not go undetected. If the patient complains of any of the symptoms of autonomic dysreflexia, the caregivers should know how to identify the causes and institute measures to alleviate them or to report to the nearest emergency care facility.

Documentation

Document an assessment of bladder and bowel function. Also include in the patient record all interventions implemented to prevent and treat autonomic dysreflexia. If the patient is catheterized, document the results on the intake and output record. Document bowel movements when they occur to include approximation of amount and consistency. Vital signs should be documented according to agency protocol. All medications administered, including laxatives, suppositories, or anti-hypertensives, are charted on the medication administration record.

CHAPTER 3.48

STROKE: CEREBROVASCULAR ACCIDENT (CVA)

GENERAL INFORMATION

A cerebrovascular accident (CVA) is caused by a sudden acute occlusion or rupture of a cerebral vessel that impairs cerebral blood flow. Ischemic strokes account for 85 percent of all strokes, with 61 percent of those being thrombotic (atherosclerotic) and 24 percent being embolic in nature. Hemorrhagic strokes account for the remaining 15 percent. Thrombotic strokes are caused by a thrombus formation in arteries supplying the brain or the cerebral artery itself as a result of atherosclerosis, hypertension, cerebral atrophy (from aging), smoking, use of birth control pills, diabetes, high cholesterol levels, valvular heart disease, and increased coagulability of blood, among other things. Atherosclerosis is the most frequent cause of thrombotic stroke so any impairment that contributes to atherosclerosis is implicated. Thrombotic strokes occur most often in people over 50 years of age during sleep or resting times. Embolic strokes may be caused by an embolus originating outside the brain that travels to the cerebral vessels and becomes lodged in one of the smaller, narrow vessels or at a site of bifurcation. Embolic strokes generally occur in younger populations during activity. Common risk factors for this type of stroke are atrial fibrillation, myocardial infarction, valvular prosthesis or surgery where stasis of blood caused the blood to clot. Hemorrhagic stroke (cerebral hemorrhage) usually results from chronic or acute hypertension (most common cause), ruptured aneurysms, arteriovenous malformations, brain tumors, and bleeding disorders. Hemorrhagic strokes have a rapid onset with loss of consciousness in over half of those affected, and complaints of a headache are common. Clinical manifestations of strokes will depend upon the type of stroke, the location, and the extent of the occlusion or hemorrhage. General manifestations are numerous and include hemiplegia, hemiparesis, paralysis, or paresis of face, slurred speech, aphasia, numbness of affected side, dysphagia, diplopia, homonymous hemianopia, agnosia, and apraxia. The term "brain attack" has been in use recently to stress the need for immediate intervention (just as in "heart attack") for maximum functionality and minimum residual effects.

NURSING DIAGNOSIS 1

 INEFFECTIVE TISSUE PERFUSION: CEREBRAL

Related to:

Vascular occlusion or hemorrhage

Defining Characteristics:

Decreased level of consciousness

Contralateral hemiparesis

Aphasia (expressive and/or receptive)

Sensory loss

Dysphagia

Dysarthria/slurred speech

Facial droop

Neglect syndrome

Homonymous hemianopsia

Spatial perceptual deficits

Hyporeflexia that progresses to hyperreflexia

Severe headache

Apraxia (loss of ability to carry out a learned activity or to use objects correctly when there is no paralysis)

Agnosia (inability to recognize a familiar object by use of senses)

Unilateral fixed/dilated pupils

Goal:

Cerebral tissue perfusion will be restored.

Outcome Criteria

✔ The patient exhibits an increased level of consciousness.

✔ The patient is able to express needs.

✔ The patient achieves maximum physical function.

✔ The patient's blood pressure will be within baseline.

NOC *Neurological status*
    Tissue perfusion: Cerebral

INTERVENTIONS	RATIONALES
Perform a complete neurological check/assessment as ordered using the Glasgow Coma Scale. In addition, assess for headaches and gag reflex; ascertain time of onset of symptoms.	Helps to detect abnormal findings and establish a baseline of impairments, which assists in planning care. The Glasgow Coma Scale is a widely used objective scale for assessment of neurological patients in the areas of consciousness (best verbal response), best motor response (muscle strength and movement), and pupillary reaction. In many agencies, blood pressure is added as a component. The time of onset of symptoms will be important in determining if thrombolytics can be used.
Take vital signs.	The vital signs give information relevant to patient status. Blood pressure may be elevated, respirations may be rapid, and pulse may be rapid. Depending upon the area involved, hypothalamus function may be affected, resulting in the inability to regulate temperature adequately with subsequent hyperthermia.
Perform a respiratory assessment, including arterial blood gases (ABGs) and pulse oximetry.	Determines airway patency and adequacy of oxygenation; adequate amounts of circulating oxygen are needed to maintain adequate cerebral oxygenation.
Note results of common diagnostic tests: computed tomography (CT) scan, MRI (magnetic resonance imaging), PET (positron emission tomography), digital subtraction angiography, doppler ultrasonography, EKG, APTT.	CT scan is the most common tool used to diagnose a stroke, typically done on admission to the health care system, and serial scans are done for several days after symptoms to detect progression or improvement of the stroke. MRI can give information on the extent of brain injury. PET provides information about tissue metabolism, brain structure, and damage from the stroke. Angiography/digital subtraction angiography is used to visualize the cerebral blood vessels as well as the carotid and vertebral arteries. Doppler ultrasonography obtains information on patency of carotid arteries using duplex scanning. EKG provides information on cardiac function. APTT is necessary to determine a baseline of clotting ability in case anticoagulants or thrombolytics are needed.
Assist patient in assuming a semi-Fowler's position with head midline.	Maintains airway, improves airway clearance, maximizes venous return from head and arterial flow to head; assists in decreasing intracranial pressure.
Administer oxygen, as ordered.	Maximizes cerebral oxygenation and reduces vasodilation (due to increased CO_2).
Establish intravenous access.	Intravenous access is required for administration of medications.
Assist with administration of thrombolytics—tissue plasminogen activator (tPA)—as ordered, and monitor for hemorrhage (deterioration in mental status, restlessness, dropping pulse and blood pressure, blood in body fluids).	The drug of choice is tPA, but this must be initiated within 3 hours of onset of symptoms. It acts by binding to the fibrin of the clot, causing enzymes to digest the fibrin and fibrinogen and resulting in lysis of the clot. Strict adherence to protocol is required, and it must be ascertained that the patient does not have a hemorrhagic stroke. CT scans need to be done quickly to confirm diagnosis in order to facilitate the timely administration of thrombolytics.
Administer aspirin or platelet inhibitors (Plavix®, Ticlid®,	These medications are used in strokes caused by emboli or

INTERVENTIONS	RATIONALES
Persantine®) that prevent platelet aggregation, as ordered.	thrombi to prevent platelets from adhering to the wall of the vessel at the site of the emboli or thrombi. This prevents further clot formation.
Administer anticoagulants (Coumadin, Heparin), as ordered.	In patients with thrombi or emboli, prevents further clot formation by interfering with clotting factors.
Administer antihypertensive agents, as ordered, for markedly elevated blood pressure.	Decreases blood pressure. Elevated blood pressure is common in patients with stroke, and for those patients with hemorrhagic stroke, it tends to be more severe, requiring treatment. Moderate increases are not treated. Decreasing the blood pressure too much may decrease cerebral blood flow/perfusion.
Administer steroids (such as Decadron), as ordered.	Decreases cerebral edema caused by inflammation.
Administer diuretic (such as mannitol), as ordered.	As an osmotic diuretic, mannitol decreases intracranial pressure and cerebral edema, increasing tissue perfusion.
Administer calcium channel blockers (such as nimodipine), as ordered.	Reduces spasms in cerebral arteries, thus increasing tissue perfusion.
Monitor for seizure activity.	The cerebral tissue may be more excitable, and increased ICP may cause seizures, further decreasing tissue perfusion.
Administer Dilantin, as ordered.	Controls seizure activity caused by increased intracranial pressure.
Decreases stimuli in the environment and group activities when providing care.	Excess movement/activity, excitability, and stress increase intracranial pressure, which can worsen symptoms.
If elevated temperature occurs, give antipyretics, use cooling blankets, or initiate other activities as ordered.	Lowers temperature and decreases metabolic demands and oxygen requirements of the body.

NIC *Cerebral perfusion promotion*
Intracranial pressure monitoring
Neurologic monitoring
Seizure precautions

Evaluation

There is evidence that cerebral tissue perfusion is being restored. The findings from use of the Glasgow Coma Scale have not deteriorated. The patient's level of consciousness has stabilized with blood pressure back to baseline. No complications are noted, and the patient is able to express needs. Motor activity has not worsened, and the patient is participating in rehabilitation. Arterial blood gases indicate adequate oxygen for perfusion to cerebral tissues.

Community/Home Care

For the patient who has had a stroke, care following hospitalization is focused on returning the patient to an optimal level of functioning. This recovery period may be extensive, but even though the patient seems to be stabilized or improving, cerebral tissue perfusion may continue to be a problem, as patients may have a reoccurrence. The family needs to know the signs and symptoms of decreased tissue perfusion that need to be reported, such as change in mental status, speech changes, and further impairment of motor activity (see nursing diagnosis "Impaired Physical Mobility"). The patient will need to continue to take prescribed medications that increase cerebral blood flow that may include an anti-platelet medication such as aspirin or Plavix, or a traditional blood thinner such as Coumadin. Even though most people do not want to examine their bodily eliminations, the patient on blood thinners or anti-platelet medications should examine urine and feces for blood; and if blood is noted, the patient should call the health care provider. A nurse following the patient at home should conduct a thorough neurological assessment to establish a baseline of function. Talking with the patient and any significant others can help the nurse to identify subtle changes that may be taking place, such as minute changes in strength or slight alterations in speech that might otherwise go undetected. The nurse and other members of the health care team should discuss the patient's specific needs so that appropriate resources can be obtained and appropriate referrals made. If there are residual deficits that impact ability to function independently, the team and patient/family must decide what alterations in the environment are necessary. The patient who has had a stroke may need to go to an extended care facility following the acute phase for rehabilitation or for permanent placement.

Documentation

Always note whether the patient has achieved the outcome criteria. Chart the findings from a complete neurological assessment, including parameters on the Glasgow Coma Scale. Document vital signs and pulse oximetry as required. All interventions carried out for the patient are included in the patient record. Medications are documented in accordance with agency protocol. Chart the patient's responses to therapeutic interventions, such as improvement in mental status, muscle strength, speech, and movement.

NURSING DIAGNOSIS 2

 ## IMPAIRED PHYSICAL MOBILITY

Related to:

Hemiparesis

Muscle weakness

Disuse

Unilateral neglect

Loss of proprioceptive skills

Defining Characteristics:

Inability to move extremities on one side

Loss of muscle strength on one side

Anosognosia (inability to recognize physical deficit)

Goal:

The patient will achieve maximum level of physical mobility.

Outcome Criteria

✔ The patient will not develop contractures.

✔ The patient will participate in prescribed physical therapy.

✔ The patient will not sustain injury.

NOC *Mobility*

INTERVENTIONS	RATIONALES
Assess patient for range of motion and extremity weakness, particularly on affected side as well as ability to reposition self or ambulate.	Determines the current functional ability and allows planning for appropriate interventions.
Obtain a history from the patient or family about mobility limitations and effect on ability to remain functional.	Determines what adaptations in lifestyle need to be made and the severity of mobility limitations.
Arrange for physical therapy consultation for methods/ therapies to improve or preserve function, and for rehabilitation following the acute phase.	The physical therapist can implement a plan for improvement of weakness and for preservation of muscle tone. Therapy is required to prevent loss of muscle strength/tone and to prevent contractures that can happen quickly. The physical therapist will evaluate the patient's potential for rehabilitation and start therapy within prescribed limitations to ensure that the patient can achieve a maximum level of mobility. Physical therapy usually starts as soon as the patient is stabilized, which may be as early as 48 hours after the onset of symptoms.
If the patient is unable to engage in ambulatory activity with physical therapy, help the patient to get out of bed and into a chair, as ordered.	Prevents complications of prolonged bedrest such as pneumonia, DVT, and skin breakdown.
Reposition the patient every 2 hours and perform range of motion every 4 hours. Provide trochanter rolls, pillow supports, and or splints for hands. Be sure the patient is not lying on arm of the affected side.	Maintains positions of function and comfort. Range of motion helps with muscle strength. Splints and proper positioning help to prevent contractures. Due to unilateral neglect and sensory alterations, the patient will not sense pressure from lying on the arm.
Assist patient with all transfer activities.	The patient may be weak from being in bed; with hemiparesis the risk for falls increases as the patient is not always aware of limitations or may deny limitations. The presence of sensory problems with spatial relationships and unilateral neglect also increases the risk for injury.
When the patient ambulates with walker or cane, instruct him or her to turn his or her head towards the affected side to examine the surrounding environment and avoid injury from bumping into objects.	The patient's visual field is decreased, creating a need to scan the environment by turning the head.

INTERVENTIONS	RATIONALES
Assess the patient's skin for redness/discoloration or skin breakdown every 2 hours when repositioning.	Pressure from immobility compresses blood vessels in high-risk areas, depriving them of nutrients and oxygenation and leading to skin death.
Teach the patient and family turning techniques, lifting/moving techniques, correct body alignment, use of assistive devices, and performing range of motion exercises.	Maintains function as long as possible and prevents contractures. Even though a physical therapist may come into the home to work with the patient, family members may also be required to move and position the patient. During the early period following a stroke the patient may need assistive devices.
Reinforce physical therapy teaching regarding use of wheelchairs and walkers, and proper transfer techniques.	The nurse is readily available to the patient for extended periods and can encourage the patient to practice new skills.

NIC *Exercise therapy*
     Joint mobility
     Positioning

Evaluation

The patient maintains full range of motion of all extremities with no contractures. The patient participates in mobility activities and exercises as prescribed by physical therapy to the extent possible. Following the acute phase of stroke, the patient is able to participate in physical therapy for teaching on use of assistive devices, transfer techniques, reconditioning, and strength building. Skin breakdown and pneumonia do not occur because of limited mobility. No injuries occur because of limited mobility or the patient's inability to recognize his or her physical deficits.

Community/Home Care

Stroke patients may return home following the acute phase and receive physical therapy at home, or they may be discharged to rehabilitation centers or other extended care facilities for rehabilitation. The family should receive thorough information regarding the disease and its impact on mobility. In the acute phase of the disease, it is crucial that caregivers encourage the patient to participate in physical therapy or other activities to the fullest extent possible. Exercises using trapeze bars for shifting weight and repositioning are helpful and should be encouraged by caregivers. The physical therapist has a role in providing teaching to family and patients on use of assistive devices for ambulation such as wheelchairs, walkers, or canes. Patients who wish to remain independent may pose a safety risk for caregivers as they deny the full extent of their limitations and attempt to ambulate, move, and transfer without assistance. The patient may become disillusioned as he or she realizes that the physical limitations are permanent but should be encouraged and given factual information about the rehabilitation prognosis. Assessments should be made of the patient's feelings concerning limitations in mobility, any social isolation, and concerns about future disability. Concerns and needs may center around role performance at home, mowing the lawn, household chores such as laundry and cleaning, or with self-care needs such as bathing and dressing. An assessment of the home is required in order to make suggestions for changes in the environment that promote independence and safety. Two-story homes with all bedrooms on the second floor pose a challenge for the patient with mobility limited to a walker or wheelchair, as climbing stairs is not possible. A rearrangement of rooms will be required to create a first-floor sleeping space. Unfortunately, it may be necessary to remove furniture to make room for easy wheelchair passage in certain areas. Other issues to be addressed include the ability to move about the home, especially getting to the bathroom, getting in or out of the shower or tub, or exiting the house if there are steps, as well as the ability and willingness to be mobile in the home. If the patient is wheelchair-bound following a stroke, a ramp may be required for entry and exit of the home. If the patient is unable to afford such a ramp, community resources such as religious and civic organizations or construction companies should be contacted to see if they are able to offer assistance. It is crucial that the patient understand the strategies required to maintain optimal functioning of affected extremities (see interventions). In-home visits by a physical therapist for a period of time will be important to the patient's health maintenance so that appropriate exercises and instructions on the use of assistive devices can be completed. Encourage the patient and family members to utilize community resources such as Stroke Clubs International and stroke support groups.

Documentation

Document a thorough assessment of the patient's functional mobility, including muscle strength, presence of paresis, and use of assistive devices. If the patient is able to ambulate or move, detail the extent of their capabilities and participation. Include in the patient record all interventions that have been recommended to the patient to address the problem of mobility. A report of the patient's perception of the ability to be mobile should be included. The effectiveness of all interventions should be clearly documented for all members of the health care team. Document instruction to the caregiver relevant to addressing immobility. If any complications of immobility are noted, chart these in accordance with agency protocol.

NURSING DIAGNOSIS 3

 SELF-CARE DEFICIT: BATHING/HYGIENE, TOILETING, FEEDING, DRESSING/GROOMING

Related to:

> Hemiparesis and weakness
>
> Facial drooping
>
> Impaired swallowing reflex due to impaired cranial nerve

Defining Characteristics:

> Unable to dress self appropriately
>
> Continent of urine and bowel but unable to get to bathroom independently
>
> Requires assistance with eating
>
> Unable to bathe self
>
> Dysphagia

Goal:

> The patient's basic needs of hygiene, dressing/grooming, feeding, and toileting will be met.

Outcome Criteria

✔ The patient will be clean and have no body odors.

✔ The patient will eat 75 percent of meals and not aspirate.

✔ The patient will remain continent of bowel and bladder.

✔ The patient will have no skin breakdown.

INTERVENTIONS	RATIONALES
Assess the patient's ability to perform activities of daily living.	Helps to determine what type and how much assistance the patient may require.
Encourage the patient to do as much as possible.	Participating in care, even in limited ways, helps to maintain function and provides stimulation for the patient; fosters some sense of independence and self-esteem.
Encourage patient to participate in activity/schedule planning.	This will help the patient retain a sense of control and autonomy, increase self-esteem, and meet his or her daily living needs.
Bathing: Offer the patient assistance with bathing as needed, but encourage the patient to do as much as physically possible; gather supplies for the patient.	The patient may be unable to bathe independently, and more than likely will need some assistance due to weakness, fatigue, or paralysis of extremities. It is important for the patient's self-esteem to allow him or her to remain as independent as possible.
Dressing/grooming: Assess the patient's ability to dress and groom him or herself; use clothes that are easy for the patient to put on. Place items needed for personal care, such as toothbrushes, toothpaste, combs, and hairbrushes, within easy reach and within the patient's visual field. Use Velcro fasteners for clothes if possible; slip-on shoes and pull-on pants or skirts will be helpful for those with hemiparesis. Assist the patient to place affected extremities into clothing first.	The ability to gather supplies and dress oneself (especially the use zippers, buttons, and ties) may be difficult due to hemiparesis or paralysis and generalized weakness.
Toileting: Assist the patient as needed for toileting; answer call bells promptly and assist the patient to the bathroom as needed. If the patient is dependent, take him or her to the bathroom at scheduled intervals (every 2 hours) for urination; for bowel movements, take the patient to the bathroom following breakfast. Use bedside	Patients who have experienced a stroke do not always become incontinent. If they do, scheduled trips to the bathroom may increase the likelihood that they will use the bathroom. Thirty minutes to 1 hour following breakfast is the natural time for increased peristalsis, which improves likelihood that bowel evacuation will occur.

INTERVENTIONS	RATIONALES
commodes as needed for patients with limited mobility or no mobility.	If the patient becomes completely dependent for all needs and is bedridden, incontinent pads and frequent checking and cleaning to prevent skin breakdown are required.
Assess the patient for skin breakdown and turn every two hours.	The risk for breakdown increases due to pressure on areas prone to breakdown and the presence of urine and feces on the skin if the patient is incontinent.
Increase fluids to 2000 ml/day, but limit fluids after 6 p.m.	Increasing fluids helps prevent urinary stasis and risk for urinary tract infection; limiting the fluids in the evening will decrease the patient's need for nighttime bathroom visits or incontinent episodes.
Arrange for a speech therapy consult to determine the patient's swallowing ability.	The speech therapist can conduct swallowing studies at bedside and determine whether the patient has an adequate gag reflex for intake of food orally. The speech therapist can develop a plan to address any swallowing issues.
Provide mouth care before meals.	Makes mouth fresh, enhances taste, and stimulates the flow of saliva to enhance mastication.
Feeding: Create a pleasant environment for meals. Assess the patient's ability to eat and what assistance he or she may need. Allow the patient to feed him or herself if possible and encourage him or her to take small bites and chew carefully. Place the patient in an upright position with head flexed forward and place food within his or her visual field. If hemiplegia and facial drooping are present, place food in the unaffected side of the mouth. Have suction apparatus available. Leave the patient up for 1 hour after meals. For patients with homonymous hemianopia, place food on the right side of the plate or direct the patient to turn his or her head to the left during eating.	The patient with a stroke may have dysphagia, and aspiration is a potential problem to anticipate. Having suction apparatus available is necessary in case airway patency becomes threatened. In some instances, the patient does not have adequate motor control to feed him or herself the entire meal. Due to visual sensory deficits (homonymous hemianopia), the patient cannot see the left side of the plate and will ignore food placed there.
Avoid thin liquids, and if recommended by a speech therapist, add thickening to liquids.	Thickened liquids are easier to swallow; however, do not thicken liquids to the point that they are no longer liquid, as some patients may not like the consistency.
Use special utensils such as food guards on plates, and nonslip bowls and cups. Consultation with occupational therapy may be required.	These items foster independence by allowing the patient to feed him or herself and minimize spills.
Encourage the patient to chew slowly and carefully after taking small bites.	Decreases the risk of choking and aspirating.
Monitor the patient's progress towards resuming some of self-care activities.	Helps to determine what resources will be needed at time of discharge.

NIC *Self-care assistance: Toileting*

Self-care assistance: Dressing/grooming

Self-care assistance: Feeding

Hair care

Self-care assistance: Bathing/grooming

Evaluation

All outcome criteria have been achieved or reasons for non-achievement are noted. The patient is bathed and kept clean, dry, and odor-free. The patient eats appropriately and is able to participate in mealtime activities. The patient remains continent by requesting assistance with toileting, or the health care worker takes the patient to the bathroom at scheduled intervals. The patient has self-care needs met and is making progress towards reaching maximum level of function.

Community/Home Care

The stroke patient's needs will vary depending on the type of deficits present at time of discharge. If the patient has hemiparesis, he or she will require assistance with most activities of daily living. A home health aide may be needed for bathing and dressing, especially in the early phase of rehabilitation. Dressing can be mastered by using clothes with easy fasteners, such as Velcro or large buttons, and pull-on garments. The patient or caregiver should be instructed to put the affected arm through sleeves first and affected legs through pants first. It is important that the patient assist as much as possible by pulling garments on with unaffected arm and hand. Eating may prove a challenge because the patient may have paresis of the dominant hand as well as a swallowing deficit. In the home, the patient should be out of bed for meals if possible, sitting upright and remaining upright for 1 hour after meals. Special utensils for feeding should be obtained prior to discharge from the hospital, and the patient should be encouraged to use them. Some patients may refrain from using special utensils or food guards due to embarrassment, but should be encouraged to use them. Other family members should be cautioned against staring at the patient who is trying to eat with the special devices. Some practice will be required, especially if the patient has not spent time in a rehabilitation center. It is important that the patient have enough time to eat and eat slowly, but also that independence is maintained as long as possible. If mobility is limited to paralysis on one side, a bedside commode may be useful. However, if the patient uses a walker or cane, ambulating to the bathroom during waking hours should be encouraged to foster independence, self-esteem, and the positive benefits of exercise. Pathways that the patient will use frequently should be clear of clutter or furniture that impedes ambulation. Prior to discharge home, the patient will need to practice transfer techniques (if within functional ability) alone and with a family member. Because beds and chairs in the home are significantly different from those in institutions, it may be helpful for a physical therapist or nurse to visit the home to evaluate the patient's ability to transfer using his or her own furniture. Adjusting to the patient's inability to take care of the most basic needs often creates a great challenge for family caregivers. All of these efforts will require the caregiver's patience and a time commitment. For many families, the decision to institutionalize the patient may occur if the patient is completely dependent for all care. When addressing the self-care needs of the patient, the family must consider resources available for in-home assistance for personal care and seek out appropriate referrals through the social worker or health care provider.

Documentation

Whether the patient is in the home or in an institution, a health care provider should document the level of functioning for the patient in all areas of self-care. Document his or her ability to toilet self or assistance required, and record intake and output as required. Also include in the record the ability of the patient to eat, percentage of food consumed, and whether any special utensils are employed. It is important to document the patient's mobility status. Even though physical therapy provides assistance with activity plans, the nurse should document the patient's ability to carry out the plan at other times, including transfer and any ambulation. If the patient demonstrates or verbalizes frustrations, document this as accurately as possible in the record. Chart any interventions employed to enhance self-care efforts and referrals made.

NURSING DIAGNOSIS 4

 IMPAIRED VERBAL COMMUNICATION

Related to:

Cerebral anoxia due to occlusion or hemorrhage

Loss of muscle tone in face, mouth, tongue

Involvement of dominant hemisphere (left hemisphere for most people)

Defining Characteristics:

Expressive aphasia

Receptive aphasia

Global aphasia

Dysarthria

Goal:

The patient will be able to communicate at maximum level of functional ability.

Outcome Criteria

✔ The patient will attempt to talk.

✔ The patient will use a communication board to express one need.

✔ The patient will be able to express needs by use of writing or pointing to words or pictures.

✔ The family expresses an understanding of the communication deficits and interventions required.

NOC *Communication*

Communication expressive

INTERVENTIONS	RATIONALES
Assess patient's ability to communicate; determine whether the patient can read and write.	Establishes that the patient is able to use alternative communications methods.
If the patient is able to read and write, provide the patient with alternatives to verbal communication: communication board, pencil and paper, Magic Slate or chalkboard. Provide picture cards if the patient cannot read or write.	This provides an alternative method of communication. For the patient who has had a stroke, the use of the hand needed for writing may be impaired to the extent that he or she is unable to write.
Collaborate with the physician to arrange for a speech therapist consult and utilize the speech therapist for assistance in establishing the best communication strategies and to educate the patient and family.	The speech therapist is best qualified to establish alternative methods for effective communication by the patient.
Teach the patient how to speak slowly.	Caregivers and family may understand the speech; however, others may not be able to understand the patient because the speech may be altered from normal. In addition, some patients often speak in low tones, almost whispers. Speaking slowly allows for better formation of words and allows others to listen more attentively.
Take time to work with the patient in communication efforts; do not rush the patient.	Rushing the patient to communicate causes frustration and may make the patient stop trying to communicate.
Face the patient when talking, and speak slowly; use questions that require short responses.	Enhances understanding and allows for simple answers that the patient can formulate.
Give instructions in short, simple phrases one thought at a time.	Enhances the patient's ability to comprehend.
Play recordings of favorite songs and encourage the patient to sing along.	Patients can often sing familiar tunes, even when they cannot speak clearly; singing helps strengthen the voice.
Provide encouragement and emotional support for the patient who is learning new communication strategies; understand that frustrations and anger may occur.	Encouragement and support enhance patient motivation and reduce anxiety. Privacy may be required in the early stage of learning as the patient becomes more comfortable with new communication methods.

	The patient may feel comfortable with family but not with other people.
Teach family appropriate communication techniques to be used with the patient.	The family members, especially those who will be caregivers, need to learn these in order to communicate effectively with the patient; when family members can communicate, they may in turn decrease the anxiety in the patient.

NIC *Communication enhancement: Speech deficit*
Learning facilitation
Anxiety reduction

Evaluation

Evaluate patient's progress in his or her ability to communicate. Establish what needs to be done to further enhance nonverbal communication with the patient. Evaluate whether the patient is able to communicate by using a communication board, writing, or pointing. The patient should be able to communicate needs to care providers. Determine whether the patient is frustrated or satisfied with attempts at communication.

Community/Home Care

For the patient who has had a stroke resulting in communication disorders, the inability to communicate verbally may prove to be a challenging and frustrating aspect of the disease. Patients may feel embarrassed, particularly in public or around outsiders, and may refrain from efforts at communication due to this as well as frustration at trying to make others understand them. An annoying occurrence for family may be the tendency of the patient to curse—even if he or she rarely or never cursed before—as a result of frustration or inability to communicate basic needs. The family needs to know that this is a common occurrence and should not become angered with the patient or draw undue attention to it. There may be times when the family will need to serve as a liaison for communication between the patient and others when they cannot understand the patient. The patient must be encouraged to continue all efforts at communication and should practice expressing self. Keep any items needed for communication close to the patient. Small canvas tote bags can be used for this purpose and can easily hang on the wheelchair, bed, or walker; these can also be taken outside the home with the patient. Use of new communication strategies should be continued, and this is where social support systems can be most beneficial. As family and friends display acceptance, encouragement, and patience, the patient will become more comfortable with communication knowing that others understand. If this does not happen, the patient may socially isolate him or herself, which could lead to emotional stress. Frustrations and emotional displays such as crying may occur, and at this time, the patient needs patience and support. The patient will need to continue to practice at home when rested and in a peaceful environment. Follow-up care should give attention to not only the physiological realm of care but to this very critical aspect of the patient's well-being.

Documentation

Document all communication strategies utilized with the patient. Include an evaluation of the patient's efforts to communicate, and which strategies work best. Always include an assessment of the patient's emotional state and responses to all interventions. Chart any referrals made for speech and the outcomes of recommendations. When communication devices or techniques are employed to enhance communication, document the patient's ability and willingness to use them.

NURSING DIAGNOSIS 5

DISTURBED SENSORY PERCEPTION: VISUAL, TACTILE

Related to:

Changes in nerve pathways

Inability to interpret, to integrate, or respond to stimuli

Defining Characteristics:

Hemianopia

Patient denies paralysis

Does not attempt to reposition extremity

Does not look at affected side

Inability to perceive pain or pressure

Unaware of where affected extremities are and their relationship to the environment

Goal:

The patient will not sustain injury.

Outcome Criteria

✔ The patient will touch the affected side.

✔ The patient will verbalize an ability to see objects in visual field.

✔ The patient will not fall.

✔ The patient will verbalize an understanding of the deficits.

NOC *Sensory function: Cutaneous*
Sensory function: Vision
Vision compensation behavior
Sensory function: Proprioception
Body positioning: Self-initiated

INTERVENTIONS	RATIONALES
Assess the patient's tactile sensory status with attention to response to pain (using a pinprick), touch (using a cotton ball or feather), or temperature (using a hot or cold object).	Determines the extent of the deficit; establishes a baseline for planning interventions and for providing safety.
Assess the patient's visual status by asking him or her to verbalize complaints such as double vision; note if patient leaves food on half of the plate or never looks toward side.	Double vision is common following a stroke; because of hemianopia, the patient may only see half of the food on his or her plate and ignores (unilateral neglect) or is unaware of the deficits on the affected side.
Assess the deficits in proprioception skills and assess for apraxia (inability to carry out learned voluntary acts) and agnosia (inability to recognize familiar objects).	Helps to determine the degree of compromise in the ability to move safely; deficits in proprioception skills prevent the patient from recognizing where body parts are in relation to the environment, creating a safety issue; apraxia and agnosia will prevent the patient from carrying out basic activities of daily living.
Approach the patient from the unaffected side in the early phase of stroke.	Visual disturbances can prevent the patient from seeing you if approached from affected side; note that the most common visual impairment is the loss of vision in a portion of the visual field for each eye.

INTERVENTIONS	RATIONALES
Teach the patient to scan the environment by turning the head from side to side.	The patient is unable to see towards the unaffected side; scanning allows visualization and enhances safety and helps to avoid bumping into objects if the patient is ambulatory.
Put needed objects within visual field.	Allows the patient to see objects.
If double vision is present, patch one eye every 4 hours while awake.	Patching one eye corrects double vision in the other eye.
Position the patient so that the eye with intact vision is towards the door.	Assures that the patient can see caregivers or visitors entering.
Encourage the patient to look at and touch the affected side as well as to check positioning.	Because of the loss of sensation and unilateral neglect, the patient may not recognize the affected side.
Encourage the patient to wash the affected side and massage while bathing.	This helps to reintegrate the body part into the patient's body image.
If unilateral neglect still persists after the stroke stabilizes, place some needed objects on affected side; place the involved arm where the patient can see it; and at times approach patient on affected side.	Encourages the patient to look at the affected side and get into the habit of turning the head to scan the environment; this helps the patient to compensate for loss of function of affected side.
Show the patient common objects that he or she may need to use and ask him or her to name them; have the patient to participate in as many aspects of care as possible.	The patient who has apraxia or agnosia will need to relearn names of common items and steps in activities required for existence. The family needs to be involved in this process, and an occupational therapist usually provides the needed assistance.
Inspect the affected side every shift for injury/trauma or edema.	Because the patient may not be able to sense pain or injury to the affected side, he or she cannot notify nurse of injury.
Elevate the affected arm on a pillow above the heart when the patient is in bed, and use a sling when he or she is ambulating.	Decreases the risk for edema; a sling can prevent the arm from dangling loosely.
Teach the family how to incorporate interventions for altered sensory perception into routines.	The caregiver will need to know how to protect the patient from injury due to altered sensory perception.

NIC *Positioning*
Unilateral neglect management
*Environmental management:
   Safety*
Fall prevention
Surveillance: Safety
Peripheral sensation management

Evaluation

Determine the degree to which the patient has met the outcome criteria. The patient should recognize the affected side and its deficit as demonstrated by touching it or repositioning it. The patient compensates for visual deficits by scanning the environment and turning the head. No falls, injuries, or trauma to affected side occurs.

Community/Home Care

Educating the patient and family regarding sensory deficits and unilateral neglect is vital. The interventions suggested for implementation in the hospital or rehabilitation center will also need to be accomplished in the home setting. Once at home, adaptations in the environment are made to promote safety. If the patient is ambulatory but has weakness on one side, be sure that the patient has a clear path for ambulation to prevent injury that he or she may not perceive due to loss of sensation. The family members or other caregiver should check positioning of the affected arm periodically to ensure that the patient is not lying on it or that it is not tangling loosely or possibly caught in a wheelchair spoke. If possible, also continue to remind the patient to check positioning of the affected arm. If the patient has unilateral neglect, the family members or other caregiver must continue to call the patient's attention to the affected side. This can be accomplished by placing frequently used items on the affected side, encouraging the patient to touch the affected extremities, and having the patient bathe that side. This forces the patient to turn in that direction and continue the process of compensation. Investigate the possibility of purchasing a full-length mirror to place in the patient's bedroom and have him or her look at him or herself in it daily. This allows the patient to view the entire body and recognize the affected side. Bath water should be tested for temperature with the unaffected arm or foot, and heating pads used on the affected side should be at a medium-low setting, as the patient may not sense if it becomes too hot. Teach the caregiver and patient to inspect the affected side for signs of trauma daily. The patient may need constant cues from caregivers to complete tasks due to apraxia and agnosia. Bedroom furniture or favorite chairs may need to be repositioned so that the patient can have his or her intact visual field facing the doorway or entry. Any deterioration in the patient's sensory status should be reported to a health care provider.

Documentation

Chart the results of a thorough assessment of the patient's sensory status, making particular notes of deficits such as decreased sensory perception (tactile, visual). If unilateral neglect is noted, document the specific patient behaviors that are evidence of its presence. Document interventions initiated to address the deficits and the patient's response relevant to stated outcome criteria. Include in the record instruction to the family and patient.

NURSING DIAGNOSIS 6

DEFICIENT KNOWLEDGE

Related to:

No previous history of stroke/new onset stroke

Lack of information about the disease and its treatment, prevention, and prognosis

The patient and/or family members have difficulty coping with situation

Defining Characteristics:

Asks no questions

Have many questions/concerns

Shows no interest in learning about disease

Presence of expressive and/or receptive aphasia

Extensive therapeutic regimen is required

Goal:

The patient and/or family members are knowledgeable about the disease and the prescribed regimen and have a post-discharge plan in place.

Outcome Criteria

✔ The patient and family members verbalize a desire to learn necessary information.

✔ The patient and family members demonstrate knowledge of stroke (pathophysiology, prognosis).

✔ The patient and family members verbalize an understanding of required treatments.

✔ The patient and family members demonstrate knowledge of medications and changes in lifestyle, such as diet, activity restrictions and stress reduction required to promote health.

✔ The patient and family members verbalize a willingness to keep appointments for physical therapy and to follow the prescribed regimen.

NOC　*Knowledge: Disease process*
　　　Knowledge: Treatment regimen
　　　Compliance behavior

INTERVENTIONS	RATIONALES
Identify a family member or significant other who will also learn the content and assist the patient with compliance.	This person can reinforce the teaching and assist with implementation if the patient becomes incapable of follow-through.
Assess the patient and family's current knowledge as well as their ability and readiness to learn; be prepared to use and respond to alternative methods of communication depending on the severity of the stroke and its effect on the patient.	Teachings need to be tailored to the ability and willingness of the learner to learn for maximum effectiveness; many stroke patients experience aphasia, which makes learning more difficult.
Create a quiet environment conducive to learning.	Environmental noise and distractions can prevent the learner from focusing on what is being taught.
Be attuned to the patient's religious and cultural practices when teaching.	Culturally competent care that also considers religious practices is a holistic individualized approach that will enhance compliance.
Teach the learners about the pathophysiology of stroke in the initial teaching session, including — Effects on functioning in areas of sensory perception, mobility, eating, communication — Rehabilitation plans — Possible complications	The patient must understand what the disease is and how it affects the body before understanding the rationale for treatments.

INTERVENTIONS	RATIONALES
Taking into consideration the patient's normal diet and any cultural/religious needs, make appropriate referrals to a dietician for teaching about the prescribed diet, including sodium, fat, and cholesterol restriction; texture restrictions; and use of thickeners for liquids.	Reduction of these substances in the diet reduces the risk for stroke and heart attack. Thickeners and restriction of thin liquids are required if the patient has dysphagia. Understanding the rationale for these interventions will enhance compliance and considering cultural/religious preferences will increase the likelihood that the prescribed changes will be assimilated into the patient's routine.
Teach the learners about prescribed medications such as those to prevent platelet aggregation (aspirin, Plavix, Ticlid, Persantine), antihypertensives, or others, as ordered, including action, side effects, and dosing schedule.	Knowledge of why the medication is needed and how it works will help the patient to focus on the importance of the medication. Identification of side effects will minimize anxiety if these untoward effects should occur.
Teach learners about the physical therapy regimen, including mobility limitations, transfer techniques, repositioning, range of motion, in-bed exercises, and use of assistive devices, as ordered, or reinforce teaching of physical therapist. If the patient is ambulatory at time of discharge, include information about how to progress exercise gradually while monitoring responses, understanding that some preferred activities may need to be eliminated. Instruct the patient to stop any activity that produces dizziness or chest pain.	A major component of the prescribed regimen is physical therapy to assist the patient to return to a maximum level of functioning. Incorporation of exercise into daily routine is needed to promote cardiac health as well as to strengthen extremities weakened by the stroke.
Teach the patient how to bathe and dress in the presence of paresis or paralysis on one side: bathe affected side and dress affected side first. Use easy pull-on clothes with large fasteners.	Makes dressing easier for the patient to control; if unaffected side is dressed first, the garments are harder to pull on the affected side because of limited "give."
Teach the family and patient strategies to be used during mealtime: — Take small bites and chew carefully.	These techniques can improve chewing, swallowing, and thus intake, while preventing aspiration.

— Sit upright for all meals with head flexed forward. — Place food within visual field if vision is impaired. — Place food on unaffected side if facial paresis is a problem. — Avoid thin liquids if swallowing is impaired.	
Teach the patient and family how to compensate for decreased sensory perception (see nursing diagnosis "Disturbed Sensory Perception: Visual, Tactile").	Decreased sensation and vision predispose the patient to injury due to an inability to perceive threats to physiological integrity; patient and caregivers need to know how to compensate to prevent injury.
Teach the patient which signs and symptoms to report to a health care provider, such as severe headache, new onset of weakness/paralysis, new onset aphasia, new onset of tingling or numbness, and new onset of altered visual acuity.	These are symptoms of stroke and may indicate a new stroke; monitoring for signs and symptoms early can prevent a crisis/emergency situation.
Ask the patient or other learners to repeat information and ask questions as needed.	This allows the nurse to hear in the patient's own words what was taught and makes it easier to know what information may need to be reinforced.
Establish that the patient has the resources required to be compliant.	If needed resources such as medical equipment (special utensils, walkers, wheelchairs, etc.), finances, transportation, and psychosocial support are not available, the patient cannot be compliant.
Give the patient printed material containing the information covered in the teaching session.	The patient may be more comfortable at home knowing that there is printed material for future reference.
Inform the patient and family about community groups available for support, such as stroke clubs and the National Stroke Association.	These organizations can provide educational information, and stroke clubs provide emotional support to caregivers and patients.

NIC *Teaching: Prescribed activity/exercise*
Teaching: Prescribed diet
Teaching: Disease process

Teaching: Prescribed medication
Learning readiness enhancement
Learning facilitation

Evaluation

Evaluate the degree to which the patient has achieved the expected outcomes. The patient or family member understands what a stroke is and how it has affected the patient. The patient or family verbalizes an understanding of the therapeutic regimen including change in lifestyle behaviors such as activity and diet. The patient or caregiver is able to repeat all information for the nurse and asks questions about the prescribed regimen, especially activity and medications. The patient or family can identify all medications by name and report the common side effects as well as the dosing schedule. The patient can identify for the nurse instances when he or she should seek health care assistance. At the end of educational sessions, the nurse must determine that the patient is capable of being compliant, and it should also be ascertained whether the patient expresses a willingness to comply. Once this is established, it is crucial to determine that the patient has the necessary resources and information to manage effectively.

Community/Home Care

For patients who have had a stroke and are not being discharged to a rehabilitation center, home care is crucial. Once at home, the patient may be anxious or unsure about his or her ability to manage the prescribed medical regimen. Successful management will depend on the patient's understanding of the information provided in teaching sessions and the internal motivation to implement health-promoting behaviors. Changes in lifestyle may be difficult at first, and reinforcement through follow-up home visits or telephone consultation may be required. Because of the complexity of the regimen with a variety of medications, physical therapy requirements, and changes in self-care ability, the risk for noncompliance is high. The patient will need to establish a daily routine that includes physical therapy either at home or in an outpatient center. In addition, the patient needs to implement other measures to regain or maintain function of extremities, such as range of motion and transfer techniques. It is anticipated that teaching and reinforcements will continue to be necessary as the patient and family strive to be compliant with all prescribed parts of the home regimen. The assistance of a dietician in the home for at least one visit to assist with questions regarding food and liquid consistency and preparation of more nutritional meals may be helpful. This person can work with the meal preparer to identify those food items on hand that are appropriate or not. Working through this in the comfort of one's own kitchen with commonly used food items may make retention of the information better. Stroke clubs or other support groups may provide social support and allay anxiety, but may not be available in some rural areas; the services of local religious or civic organizations may be a good substitute if the patient or family are members of such groups. During hospitalization, education must be thorough and culminate in the health care provider, the patient, and the family establishing a realistic approach to rehabilitation and attainment of optimal health that considers the patient's culture, socioeconomic resources, social support systems, and religion.

Documentation

Document the specific content taught and the titles of printed materials given to patient or family. Chart the patient's and family members' understanding of the content and the methods used to evaluate learning. The nurse must clearly indicate areas that need to be reinforced. After the teaching session is complete, the nurse should assess to determine whether the patient indicates a willingness to comply with health care recommendations. If the teaching included a significant other or family member, indicate this in the documentation. In addition, document any referrals made in the patient record.

CHAPTER 3.49

TRIGEMINAL NEURALGIA (TIC DOULOUREUX)

GENERAL INFORMATION

Trigeminal neuralgia (also called tic douloureux) is a chronic neurological disorder of the trigeminal nerve (cranial nerve V). It is characterized by a sudden, severe, electric shock-like or stabbing pain typically felt on one side of the jaw or cheek along the track of the nerve. The pain usually begins close to one side of the mouth and progresses upwards towards the ear and eye on the same side. The attacks of pain, which generally last several seconds to a few minutes, may be repeated one after the other. Factors that may trigger the pain include talking, brushing teeth, touching the face, chewing or swallowing, shaving, washing the face, wind hitting the face, and temperature changes. The attacks may come and go throughout the day and last for days, weeks, or months at a time, and then a remission occurs causing the pain to disappear for months or years until it returns. There is no definitive cause of trigeminal neuralgia, but suggested theories include vascular compression of the nerve root, injury to the nerve, infection of teeth, and trauma to the jaw. The disease is more common in middle age or older adults, with women being affected more often than men are.

NURSING DIAGNOSIS 1

 ACUTE PAIN

Related to:

Injury to fifth cranial nerve

Stimulation to trigger zones on face

Defining Characteristics:

Paroxysmal sharp pain

Pain radiating along nerve path

Unilateral pain on side of face

Grimacing

Muscular contraction in the face (tic)

Complaint of pain

Goal:

The patient states that pain is reduced.

Outcome Criteria

✔ The patient rates pain as < 4 on a 10-point scale following interventions.

✔ The patient has no grimacing.

✔ The patient reports satisfaction with pain relief measures.

NOC *Pain: Disruptive effects*
Pain level
Pain control

INTERVENTIONS	RATIONALES
Assess the patient's pain using a pain rating scale of 1–10 with 10 being the worst pain.	Provides a more objective assessment.
Assess or take history regarding time of onset, location, precipitating factors, relieving factors, and effect on function (such as ability to eat, chew, swallow, loss of sensation).	Obtaining this information will assist in accurate diagnosis and treatment; knowing how pain affects function will provide information needed to assist patient with home care needs. The patient's description of typical characteristic pain is needed for accurate diagnosis.
Determine the effect culture and religion may have on pain perception and relief.	Culture may influence a patient's tolerance for pain and how he or she relieves it.

(continues)

(continued)

INTERVENTIONS	RATIONALES
Have the patient identify triggers for pain and how to avoid them.	By identifying factors that trigger pain, the patient is able to avoid these stimuli and thus avoid initiation of pain, which will help with pain management.
Administer Tegretol (carbamazepine), as ordered.	Tegretol is a sodium channel blocker and is the drug of choice. It exerts its action by inhibiting transmission of pain impulses. It lessens the frequency and duration of painful episodes.
Administer analgesic medications as ordered and monitor for effectiveness and side effects.	Alleviates pain.
Give all medications on a regular dosing schedule rather than prn.	Provides better relief and prevents the pain from getting severe.
Teach relaxation techniques such as music therapy, massage, distraction, and meditation.	These techniques enhance the effect of analgesics and may decrease reliance on medications for complete relief.
Assess the effectiveness of all interventions to control pain.	Helps to determine whether adjustments to pain control strategies need to be revised and to ensure that the pain is tolerable and not interfering with nutrition.
Prepare the patient for surgery (rhizotomy) as ordered or required by agency protocol.	Rhizotomy is the surgical severing of the root of the fifth cranial nerve. This results in decreased pain sensation.
Following surgery, monitor for signs of cranial nerve damage: corneal reflex, eye movement, ability to tighten facial muscles, numbness of face.	During surgery, inadvertent damage to the nerve may occur, and some sensory compromise may be unavoidable.
After surgery, teach the patient the following: — To inspect mouth/teeth for signs of infection — To avoid rubbing the eye on affected side — To note signs of eye irritation or infection	Following surgery, the ability to perceive warning signs of infection or irritation (eye, dental) such as pain decreases; therefore the patient must inspect affected areas for irritation or infection. The corneal reflex is gone and rubbing the eye can cause corneal abrasions.
Assist physician with the injection of alcohol and glycerol, as ordered.	Blocks selected branches of the nerve and relieves pain.

NIC *Simple relaxation therapy*
Analgesic administration
Pain management

Evaluation

Assess the degree to which interventions for pain have been effective. The patient reports pain has been reduced and rates pain as being < 4 on a 10-point scale. For persistent pain, the nurse should investigate additional measures for relief. Determine whether the patient is able to verbalize how to reduce pain.

Community/Home Care

The patient with trigeminal neuralgia is seen as an outpatient unless surgical interventions are instituted or pain is uncontrolled. Two major aspects of the patient's care at home include administration of medications and avoiding factors that trigger a pain episode. The patient must remember to take the ordered medication, Tegretol, as prescribed. The patient should establish a routine in which medication is taken with meals to increase absorption. When therapy with Tegretol is initiated, the patient should be warned to avoid activities that require alertness until his or her response to the medication is known, as common side effects include dizziness and drowsiness. The second focus of teaching for home care centers on avoidance of triggers that stimulate pain. The patient needs to keep a diary of pain episodes and document what he or she was doing at the time of onset. If the patient's home has drafty areas, he or she should avoid these or weatherproof the area, as a cold draft can precipitate the pain. Covering the face when out in the cold or wind is necessary to avoid pain. Wearing ski masks or wrapping the face in a warm scarf may help. When shaving, the patient should use an electric razor, or if the episodes are frequent and severe, the patient may avoid shaving until the medications are effective. Because washing the face may also stimulate pain, the patient may want to avoid this activity until medications have had an opportunity to become effective and then avoid any type rubbing to the affected side. The patient can use a very soft toothbrush and mouthwash for oral care, especially early in the treatment phase when pain episodes are likely to be frequent. A therapeutic regimen that allows for tolerable pain may require an extended period of trial and error as the patient attempts to identify triggers to be avoided or controlled, and which pharmacological and non-pharmacological measures combined are effective. If no measures are effective in relieving the pain, a health care provider should be contacted for discussion of new pain relief measures.

Documentation

As the patient is at home for treatment, be sure that office visits document the specific therapeutic interventions initiated for pain relief. Include in the patient record the patient's verbalized perception of pain and satisfaction with pain control. Document identified triggers in the patient's record as well.

NURSING DIAGNOSIS 2

IMBALANCED NUTRITION: LESS THAN BODY REQUIREMENTS

Related to:

> Facial pain
>
> Decreased jaw movement
>
> Fear of chewing

Defining Characteristics:

> Inability to masticate
>
> Weight loss
>
> Eats < 50 percent of food served
>
> Reports of being unable to eat

Goal:

> The patient is receiving adequate nutritional intake.

Outcome Criteria

✔ The patient is able to eat 75 percent of meals served.

✔ The patient states that it does not hurt to eat.

✔ The patient does not lose weight.

✔ Albumin level, electrolytes, hemoglobin, serum transferrin, and iron are normal.

NOC   *Nutritional status: Nutrient intake*

Nutritional status: Food and fluid intake

Pain control

INTERVENTIONS	RATIONALES
Assess patient's willingness and ability to chew food.	Helps to determine the extent of the difficulty with eating.
Weigh the patient on first contact with the health care system and at regular intervals.	Helps to establish baseline for future comparison, to detect weight loss, and to intervene to prevent wasting.
Arrange dietary consult to ascertain the patient's willingness and ability to take in enough food to meet calorie demand and to determine the patient's likes, dislikes, and preferences within the prescribed diet with consideration to cultural and/or religious preferences.	Patients will be more likely to consume foods or liquids that they like and are accustomed to; the dietician can provide information on meals that are nutritionally balanced, appealing to the patient, and require no chewing. These meals would probably consist of pureed foods, nutritional milk shakes, or fruit shakes, and soft foods that do not require chewing, such as yogurt, ice cream, rice, and soups.
Encourage frequent, small liquid supplements that have rich nutrient content including protein and high calories; soft slippery foods such as custards, pudding, and ice cream are easy to swallow; avoid excessive intake of foods and liquids that have no nutritional value.	Liquid supplements and/or milkshakes are generally easy to consume and provide needed calories and nutrients; the patient does not have to chew. As eating and drinking may trigger pain and limit intake, all substances ingested need to be valuable to the patient's nutrition.
Place food on unaffected side of mouth and encourage the patient to chew on this side.	Decreases the likelihood of pain and promotes intake.
Administer pain medications 30 minutes before meals and Tegretol with meals.	Helps to control pain in the facial area that may interfere with consumption of food or fluid; Tegretol is better absorbed in the presence of food.
Assist the dietician in determining the calorie count and the amount of food or liquid consumed with each meal or between meals.	Monitoring calories and amount of food consumed helps to detect problems early and allows for early interventions to address altered nutrition.
Monitor laboratory results: albumin, electrolytes, hemoglobin, serum transferrin, iron.	These tests are frequently used measures of nutritional status and can be used to determine whether the patient is meeting basic nutritional requirements.
Assess amount of food consumed with each meal.	Helps to determine whether the patient is able to consume sufficient amounts of food.

NIC   *Nutritional monitoring*
          Nutrition management
          Nutrition therapy

Evaluation

Determine whether the outcome criteria have been met for the patient. The patient should be eating meals with high nutritional value. Consumption of at least 75 percent of food and fluids served should be achieved with reports from the patient that he or she can eat without pain or discomfort. The patient should report satisfaction with the changes in consistency of foods offered. The health care provider should frequently assess the patient's ability to eat and willingness to attempt to eat, and revise interventions accordingly. Frequent weights need to be obtained to ensure that the patient is not losing weight. Laboratory results such as serum transferrin, iron, electrolytes, albumin, and hemoglobin should be within normal limits.

Community/Home Care

Ensuring adequate nutrition for the patient with trigeminal neuralgia is a problem in the home setting. The majority of patients who experience the pain of trigeminal neuralgia will need to make some adjustments in the type of foods they consume when they are not in remission. Patients who have the disorder may significantly limit their intake for fear of initiating acute pain. The family can assist the patient by preparing foods that are easy to chew and swallow— foods that the patient likes and that also have nutritional value. Soft slippery items such as mashed potatoes, soft baked potatoes, soups, custards, and ice cream are easy to swallow with minimum chewing. Hard fried meats or other foods should be avoided. Liquid nutritional supplements should be encouraged to add nutrients to the patient's diet such as fruit shakes, milk shakes, or commercially prepared liquid supplements. The patient may need to eat small amounts throughout the day and take analgesics before meals. These interventions are especially crucial during the early periods of the disease when medications have not become effective and the patient has not achieved a remission. A 24-hour diet recall may prove helpful to determine whether the patient is eating enough. The patient will need to obtain a scale and monitor his or her weight on a regular basis to detect significant weight loss. The health care provider has a role in preventing declining nutrition by assessing the patient's ability to eat and performing a nutritional assessment including obtaining a current weight.

Documentation

Document all interventions implemented to address the patient's nutritional status, including pain control. Be sure to include whether the patient has met the outcome criteria, and in instances where the criteria have not been achieved, document necessary revisions to the plan. Chart the patient's weight and the type of diet that the patient is comfortable eating, as well as the percentage of each meal taken. A thorough nutritional assessment of the patient should be made and documented, including information about difficulty chewing or swallowing, foods that create special challenges, and any specific concerns that the patient may have relevant to his or her nutritional status.

CHAPTER 3.50

UNCONSCIOUSNESS

GENERAL INFORMATION

Unconsciousness is a state in which the individual is unable to respond to stimuli from the environment or from internal signals from the brain. This term is also used interchangeably with the term *comatose*. A variety of pathophysiological alterations can contribute to a state of unconsciousness that may be permanent or temporary and have a sudden or gradual onset dependent on the etiology. The possible causes can be classified as structural or metabolic-structural causes such as a stroke or tumor disrupt the pathways of nervous transmission, whereas metabolic causes such as diabetic ketoacidosis or drug overdoses affect the biochemical environment of the brain and alter cellular function (Phipps, Monahan, Sands, Marek, and Neighbors, 2003). Clinical presentations attributed to the unconscious state (not causative etiology) include absence of any response to external stimuli, difficulty maintaining respirations, incontinence of bowel and bladder, absent pain response, inability to swallow, absence of purposeful movement, lack of eye opening, and no verbal response.

NURSING DIAGNOSIS 1

INEFFECTIVE BREATHING PATTERN

Related to:

Neuromuscular impairment

Defining Characteristics:

Dyspnea

Tachypnea

Inability to breathe without assistance

Decreased tidal volume and vital capacity

Arterial blood gases (ABGs) demonstrate hypercapnia and hypoxia

Goal:

The patient has effective patterns of respirations with adequate oxygenation.

Outcome Criteria

✔ Oxygen saturation is > 90 percent.

✔ Arterial blood gases (ABGs) are within normal range.

✔ Respirations are unlabored.

✔ The patient's breathing is maintained (through intubation/tracheostomy and mechanical ventilation if necessary).

NOC **Respiratory status: Ventilation**
Respiratory status: Gas exchange
Vital signs
Mechanical ventilation respiratory: Adult

INTERVENTIONS	RATIONALES
Assess respiratory system by noting respiratory rate, depth, chest expansion, rhythm, breath sounds, oxygen saturation, and skin color (examine lip color and color of mucous membranes for dark-skinned patients).	Many patients who are unconscious have difficulty keeping the airway open and maintaining adequate ventilation. Frequent assessments are needed to gather information on the status of the respiratory system, to establish a baseline for future comparisons, and to assist in determining when and if mechanical ventilation is required. Decreased breath sounds indicate atelectasis; decreased oxygen saturation and abnormal blood gases all indicate an ineffective breathing pattern that affects gas exchange.

(continues)

(continued)

INTERVENTIONS	RATIONALES
Place the patient in side-lying or a semi-Fowler's position.	Maximizes thoracic cavity space, decreases pressure from the diaphragm and abdominal organs, facilitates use of accessory muscles, and prevents aspiration of stomach contents that may be refluxed.
Monitor arterial blood gases (ABGs) and oxygen saturation via pulse oximetry.	Arterial blood gases (ABGs) are the most accurate method for determining oxygenation status; pulse oximetry is a quick, easy assessment of oxygen saturation but cannot provide accurate information related to carbon dioxide levels or general gas exchange.
Give supplemental oxygen, as ordered.	The unconscious patient may lack respirations effective enough to provide adequate oxygen; supplemental administration increases the amount of oxygen available to tissues.
Keep suction apparatus available and suction secretions, as needed.	The patient will be unable to cough to remove secretions. If left alone, the secretions will accumulate and cause airway obstruction.
Assist with placement of the patient on mechanical ventilation with endotracheal intubation/tracheostomy as ordered or according to agency protocol (see nursing care plan "Mechanical Ventilation").	The unconscious patient may not be able to breathe on his or her own. Intubation will become necessary when pCO_2 increases, pO_2 decreases, and vital capacity drops, demonstrating severe hypoventilation.
Turn patient every two hours.	Prevents atelectasis in bases; the unconscious patient cannot reposition him or herself.
Provide chest physiotherapy, as ordered.	Mobilizes secretions that tend to accumulate when immobile and to facilitate that all lung fields are clear.
Monitor for signs and symptoms of respiratory infection: elevated temperature, diaphoresis, thick secretions, coughing, and elevated white blood cell counts.	Respiratory infections are easily acquired due to immobility, use of mechanical ventilation, and decreased movement of respiratory muscles.

NIC *Respiratory monitoring*
Artificial airway

Mechanical ventilation
Ventilation
Positioning

Evaluation

The patient should show indications that breathing patterns are effective in meeting the body's need for oxygen. The rate should preferably be between 12–24 breaths per minute and unlabored. Arterial blood gases (ABGs) should indicate an absence of hypercapnia or hypoxia; normal range should be expected. Oxygen saturation should be > 90 percent. The patient's skin is its usual color.

Community/Home Care

For most patients who remain unconscious, care will be provided in alternative settings, such as extended care, nursing homes, or rehabilitation centers. If the unconscious patient is cared for at home without a ventilator, the family will need to monitor the patient's respiratory status closely. The family will need to be taught how to monitor respiratory rate and depth as well as chest movement changes or other evidence that would indicate ineffective patterns of respiration. These would include limited movement on one side, increased respiratory rate, increased mucous production, abnormal sounds with respiration, and changes in skin color. If these are noted, the family will need to seek health care for the patient quickly. It is important to stress to the caregiver that the patient continues to be at risk for development of respiratory infection due to immobility and compromised neurological status that may prevent effective chest movement. In-home caregivers should be taught symptoms of respiratory infection, including elevated temperature, diaphoresis, increased expectoration of sputum, and abnormal colors to sputum. It is important that the family understand how to prevent upper respiratory infections, particularly through the use of immunizations against influenza and pneumonia but also through aggressive repositioning and good hand hygiene. If family members notes signs of infection, they are to report to a health care provider immediately.

Documentation

Chart the results of a comprehensive assessment of the respiratory system. Note respiratory rate, chest expansion, use of any accessory muscles, breath sounds, skin color, and results of pulse oximetry. If the patient expectorates, document the amount, color, and consistency. Document any family teaching completed. Include in the patient's chart all interventions employed to address ineffective breathing pattern and the patient's response to the interventions, indicating whether the problem has been resolved. If the patient is placed on mechanical ventilation, document this according to agency protocol along with the assessment findings that provided evidence for its need.

NURSING DIAGNOSIS 2

 ### RISK FOR IMPAIRED SKIN INTEGRITY

Related to:

> Immobility
>
> Incontinence
>
> Decreased sensory perception

Defining Characteristics:

> None

Goal:

> Impaired skin integrity will not occur.

Outcome Criteria

✔ The patient's skin will have no redness or other discoloration.

✔ The patient's skin will remain intact.

NOC *Immobility consequences: Physiological*

Risk control

Risk detection

INTERVENTIONS	RATIONALES
Complete a thorough skin assessment every shift noting areas of redness/discoloration, pallor, edema, and any denuded or open areas, with particular attention to sacrum/coccyx, heels, ears, hips, inner aspects of knees, back of the head, and elbows.	A thorough assessment establishes a baseline; areas subject to pressure are at higher risk for breakdown, and these include most bony prominences.
Use the Braden Risk Assessment Scale.	This is an objective method of assessing the patient's risk for skin breakdown and includes parameters such as sensory perception, moisture, activity, mobility, nutrition, friction, and shear. Information from this assessment adds to the general assessment and allows for planning to resolve causative factors.
Turn the patient every 2 hours using turn sheets and acceptable patient-handling techniques, avoiding friction and shearing force.	Unconscious patients are unable to sense the pressure on prone areas, and immobility prevents self-repositioning; pressure causes vasculature to be compressed and unable to provide nutrients to the high-risk areas; friction and shearing damage the skin and underlying vasculature.
Post a turning schedule at the patient's bedside.	Ensures that all health care workers are aware of the need for turning; the schedule prevents the patient from being repositioned in a particular position too often.
Apply heel and elbow protectors bilaterally.	Prevents excoriation to bony areas.
Place thin pillows between the patient's knees.	Prevents bony areas of knees from rubbing against one another and causing breakdown.
Keep the patient clean and dry by washing well (avoiding friction) with warm water after each incontinent episode of urine or stool; change the sheets if the patient is diaphoretic; apply protective ointment after cleansing.	Enzymes and chemicals found in urine and feces can irritate tissues, as can the moisture from urine. Hot water should be avoided as it causes dryness of the skin. Friction causes trauma to sensitive at risk skin. Cleansing is required after each episode to clean the irritants away from skin.
Institute use of special mattresses (air, water, or other), as ordered.	Special mattresses are intended to relieve pressure to high-risk areas, especially the sacrum and coccyx.
Avoid massaging over bony prominences.	Pressure from massage increases the risk for ulcer formation due to excessive friction on areas already at risk.
Provide topical moisturizing agents, as ordered.	Skin that is dry and flaky is more likely to experience breakdown.

(continues)

(continued)

INTERVENTIONS	RATIONALES
Assess the patient's hydration and nutritional status.	An adequate diet and hydration are necessary for healthy skin.
Teach the family members or other caregivers how to recognize skin breakdown and techniques for preventing skin breakdown.	If the family is planning to care for the unconsciousness patient at home, they will need to be able to recognize the early signs of skin breakdown and how to prevent.

NIC   *Pressure ulcer prevention*
Skin surveillance
Positioning

Evaluation

Determine that the patient has met the outcome criteria. The patient's skin will remain intact with no areas of redness or other discoloration or excoriation. The skin will be warm and its color will be normal. In addition, the patient's risk for breakdown will be minimized.

Community/Home Care

If the unconscious patient is cared for in the home, great attention should be given to teaching the family strategies to prevent skin breakdown. Because of alterations in sensory perception, nutrition status, elimination patterns, and hydration, the patient remains at high risk for breakdown. The family will need to implement strategies identified in the interventions section with emphasis placed on turning and positioning the patient and maintaining cleanliness of the skin. Often, when completely dependent patients are discharged home, the family does not have a realistic perception of what total patient care involves. The nurse needs to enlist the family members to participate in the care while the patient is still hospitalized so that they may perform tasks while nurses are available to answer questions and provide assistance. The most critical aspects of care in the home will be turning the patient unfailingly every 2 hours to relieve pressure on high-risk areas. A schedule that outlines which position the patient should be in at specific times will be helpful, particularly if there will be multiple caregivers. It is also crucial that the family learn how to use bed pillows or possibly a small rolled throw to support the patient in the side-lying position and smaller, semi-flat pillows between the knees to prevent rubbing of the bony inner aspects against each other. The family can also use a pillow or a smooth texture blanket to place beneath the feet to keep heels off of the bed. The second area of emphasis in the home is handling incontinence. All too often, when patients experience urinary incontinence, caregivers remove soiled incontinence pads and replace with a clean one, but never cleanse the skin. The harsh components of urine can continue to irritate the skin, contributing to breakdown. Family caregivers must be diligent in cleansing the skin well after each episode of incontinence (urine and stool) with mild soap and warm water. There are many commercial barrier products on the market, but they can be expensive. Good, inexpensive substitutes that act as barriers, especially to urine, include petroleum jelly and zinc oxide paste. Even though the patient has on incontinent briefs, he or she should still be checked at least every 2 hours for wetness, and caregivers can check for wetness or stool at the same time they reposition the patient. In addition, the family will need to learn the signs of beginning skin breakdown, such as redness or other discolorations, pallor, warmth, or any open area. Nutritional needs are generally prescribed to be given via tube feedings of some sort, and the family will need to maintain the prescribed feedings to ensure adequate nutrients needed for tissue maintenance. If the family detects any change in the skin, a health care provider must be notified and a visit from a visiting nurse may be warranted.

Documentation

Chart the results of a thorough assessment of the patient's skin, including the results of the Braden Risk Assessment Scale. If any signs of impaired skin integrity are noted, chart these along with the interventions implemented to address them. Document all actions employed to prevent skin impairment, including instruction to caregivers.

NURSING DIAGNOSIS 3

 IMPAIRED PHYSICAL MOBILITY

Related to:

Decreased cognition

Altered cerebral function

Defining Characteristics:

No purposeful movement in extremities

No response to external stimuli

Muscle atrophy and paresis

Goal:

No contractures occur.

Outcome Criteria

✔ The patient's arms and hands will be able to move through range of motion.

✔ The patient's lower extremities will be able to move through range of motion.

✔ Complications of immobility do not occur (pneumonia, skin breakdown).

NOC *Immobility consequences: Physiological*

Mobility

INTERVENTIONS	RATIONALES
Assess the patient for abnormal findings: reflexes, complications of immobility such as contractures, decreased muscle mass, decerebrate posturing, and decorticate posturing.	A baseline of function needs to be established. These abnormal findings are common in patients who are unconscious.
Arrange for physical therapy consultation for methods/ therapies to improve or preserve function for as long as possible.	The physical therapist can implement a plan for improvement of weakness and for preservation of muscle and prevention of contractures.
Encourage range of motion exercises at least three times a day.	Prevents contractures.
Reposition patient every 2 hours, or as requested, using a turn schedule. Provide trochanter rolls and pillow supports.	Maintains positions of function and comfort. Proper positioning helps to prevent contractures.
Assess patient skin for redness/discoloration or skin breakdown every 2 hours when repositioning and implement strategies for prevention (see nursing diagnosis "Risk for Impaired Skin Integrity")	Pressure from immobility compresses blood vessels in high-risk areas, depriving them of nutrients and oxygenation which leads to skin death.
Teach the family turning and lifting/moving techniques, correct body alignment, use of assistive devices, and how to perform range of motion.	Helps to maintain function and prevent contractures. Even though a physical therapist may come into the home to work with the patient, family members will be required to move and position the patient.
For patients discharged home, give printed instructions on exercise (range of motion).	Even though teaching has been carried out, the family may need written instructions to refer to at home for review and to reinforce what was taught.

NIC *Exercise therapy: Joint mobility*

Positioning

Evaluation

The patient has met all stated outcome criteria. The patient maintains full range of motion of all extremities with no contractures. Skin breakdown and pneumonia do not occur because of immobility.

Community/Home Care

Unconscious patients at home are completely dependent for mobility. The family should receive thorough information regarding the underlying disease that caused the state of unconsciousness and subsequent immobility. The patient has no motor response, and thus others must exercise all four extremities in an attempt to preserve some muscle tone and prevent contractures. Other interventions, such as the use of special braces and splints, should be initiated by the caregiver to prevent contractures that may develop quickly (1 week). Range of motion exercises must be aggressive and frequent, administered at least every 2 hours to prevent complications. Turning and repositioning are required to prevent skin breakdown and pneumonia, especially if the patient shows no signs of recovery or improvement and remains on bedrest. The physical therapist has a role in providing teaching to the family on correct techniques for range of motion and proper turning and positioning using pillows or other devices. The family can also use a turning schedule in the home as a reminder to turn the patient. Providing care for a completely dependent patient can prove challenging to family members and necessitate a change in their routines; thus, it is important that family members are supported in their caregiving. A visiting nurse can assess how the patient is progressing, troubleshoot with the family, and assist in reducing anxiety that may be present. The family will need to be equipped with coping strategies that are successful during stressful times of physical and mental exhaustion. Caregivers will need to understand that it is okay to ask for and accept assistance in the caregiving role.

Documentation

Chart the findings from an assessment of motor function and muscle strength, giving an accurate description of the patient's capacity for motor activity. If the patient is able to ambulate or move, detail the extent of his or her capabilities and participation. Document all interventions implemented to address the issue of immobility, including instruction to the caregiver. Chart any complications of immobility in accordance with agency protocol.

NURSING DIAGNOSIS 4

IMBALANCED NUTRITION: LESS THAN BODY REQUIREMENTS

Related to:

Inability to ingest food or liquids orally

Defining Characteristics:

Loss of weight

No oral intake

Decreased albumin levels

Decreased iron and hemoglobin

Dry flaky skin

Loss of muscle mass

Goal:

Nutritional status is maintained.

Outcome Criteria

✔ The patient does not lose weight.

✔ The patient tolerates tube feedings without vomiting or diarrhea.

✔ Albumin, iron, and hemoglobin are within normal limits.

✔ The family verbalizes an understanding of nutritional needs of the patient, including artificial means of delivering nutrition.

✔ The family demonstrates proper techniques for administering nutrition to the patient.

NOC *Nutritional status:*
Food and fluid intake
Weight: Body mass

INTERVENTIONS	RATIONALES
Assess the patient's laboratory results: transferrin, BUN, albumin, iron, hemoglobin, and hematocrit.	These give clues to nutritional status when combined with history and other indices. If the BUN is elevated with a normal creatinine, it can indicate dehydration; decreased levels may indicate overhydration or inadequate dietary protein. Decreased levels of albumin occur in malnutrition but may not be evident for 21 days. A decrease in hemoglobin indicates iron deficiency as well as possible deficiencies in folate, vitamin B_{12}, or protein. Transferrin can be measured to assess for anemia and iron transport ability of hemoglobin.
Conduct a thorough nutritional assessment, noting condition of skin, hair and nails, mucous membranes; condition of mouth and tongue; muscle wasting; bowel sounds, diarrhea, or constipation.	These give clues to current status. In states of imbalanced nutrition, the patient may have dry flaky skin, dry mucous membranes, hair that comes out easily, and brittle, ridged nails. The corners and inside of mouth may crack and tongue may become edematous and dry. Muscles waste. The patient may experience diarrhea or constipation, and bowel sounds may range from hyperactive to hypoactive.
Weigh patient using bed scales on admission and regularly afterwards.	Establishes a baseline weight and provides for future comparisons to determine whether nutritional status stabilizes and weight loss is prevented.
Assist with ordered alternative means of providing nutrition according to agency protocol, such as enteral tube feedings via nasogastric or gastrostomy tubes.	If the patient does not regain consciousness and the ability to eat within a short time, a means of offering nutrition and fluids artificially will need to be explored with the family by the physician.
If tube feedings are initiated, offer water with each bolus feeding, or every 4 hours for continuous feedings, or as ordered by the physician.	Many tube-feeding solutions are metabolized easily but leave very little free water, causing the patient to experience dehydration. Because many

INTERVENTIONS	RATIONALES
	solutions are also high in protein, water is needed to protect the kidneys.
Follow agency protocol for administration of tube feedings, in general: — Check placement of tube (aspirate stomach contents). — Keep the patient elevated at least 30 degrees during feedings. — Flush the tube at least every 4 fours. — Check residual prior to each bolus feed or every 8 hours for continuous feedings. — Hold tube feedings for specified amount of residuals as ordered (~ 150 cc). — For patients on continuous feeds, discard administration bag every 24 hours or according to agency protocol; refill feeding bag every 4 hours with only enough formula for a 4-hour period. — Monitor response to feedings, noting any diarrhea or vomiting.	These are all accepted standards of care for patients receiving tube feedings. Tube placement is assured by aspirating stomach contents and not auscultating for injected air; keeping the patient elevated prevents aspiration; flushing the tube maintains patency, especially if the tube is being used for medication administration; large amounts of residual indicate a lack of absorption or digestion of feedings, necessitating a slower rate; administration bags that hang longer than 24 hours become a medium for bacteria growth; placing only enough tube-feed solution in the bag for 4 hours decreases the chance of proliferation of bacteria. Vomiting and/or diarrhea indicate intolerance, and feeding solution may need to be diluted initially and the strength gradually increased.
Provide oral care to the patient using commercial preparations or gauze pads saturated with warm water.	Minimizes drying of oral mucous membranes and promotes comfort; lemon glycerin swabs, though frequently used, often cause more drying than do other methods.
Provide information to the family or significant other on recommended strategies for providing artificial nutrition, and support them in decisions regarding whether to allow implementation.	The family will need sufficient information in order to make an informed decision regarding the need and desire for artificial nutrition. Families may decide to forego artificial nutrition based on a variety of factors, including the patient's expressed desire, patient prognosis, cultural practices, and anticipated quality of life.
If the patient is to be discharged home, teach family members or other caregivers how to administer tube feedings.	This is a skill that the family will need to demonstrate to health care providers prior to taking the patient home. It requires teaching and reinforcements.

NIC *Nutritional monitoring*
Enteral tube feeding
Nutrition therapy

Evaluation

Determine whether the patient has met the stated outcome criteria. The patient should have a means of receiving nutritional intake and fluids. Weight loss is prevented and laboratory results indicate a stable nutritional status. Family members indicate an understanding of the nutritional needs of the patient and are supported in decisions regarding artificial means of delivering nutrition.

Community/Home Care

The unconscious patient has continued nutritional needs if discharged home. Family members must learn how to administer tube feedings, most likely via a gastrostomy tube, as nasogastric tubes usually are not used for long-term feedings. Family members or caregivers will need to have a realistic view of what administering tube feedings in the home will entail. Included in the teaching should be equipment to be used (syringe for bolus feedings, pumps and bags for continuous feedings, and syringes for checking for residual), type of solution used, as well as complications to anticipate (occlusion, diarrhea, constipation, excess residual) and how to correct them. Of utmost importance is positioning of the patient to prevent aspiration. A hospital bed is desirable if one can be obtained and afforded because it is easily elevated to a Fowler's or semi-Fowler's position. A nurse should be in the home the first time the family does the procedure, even if the family has demonstrated the procedure in the hospital. There is a certain level of comfort in performing tasks with nursing staff standing by at the bedside for support or assistance; however, it is very different to undertake the task at home with no health care personnel present and possibly with a different set of equipment. Someone should be on call to answer questions and troubleshoot for the family in case problems occur. The family will need to understand how to clean equipment and store it when not in use, particularly syringes used in the feeding procedure. Cleansing syringes in hot soapy water, rinsing well, and storing in the refrigerator should decrease bacteria count, but syringes should be replaced on a regular basis as both bulb and plunger types lose their ability to suction or operate smoothly with repeated use. The syringes can be placed in an airtight freezer bag for storage. It is important that the family understand the need for water as well as the feeding solution and be given specific instructions for the amount to be given and how often. In case of emergency, such as running out of feeding solution, teach the family what types of substances can be substituted on a temporary basis—juices, sugar water, whole milk (unless contraindicated)—but first verify these with the physician. A backup provider of nutrition needs to be available in case the main caregiver becomes ill or for some other reason is unable to render the service. The family should be given written instructions that outline the procedure; give pointers for common trouble areas; state clearly the solution, amount to be given, and frequency; and state the amount of water to be given and how often. This document should be made in duplicate and laminated so that it does not tear or soil resulting in an unreadable document. The services of a social worker should be utilized to obtain equipment needed in the home for administration of feedings, such as pumps and bags for the solution.

Evaluation

Determine whether the patient has met the proposed outcome criteria. The patient's lab values indicate a stable nutritional status with iron, transferrin, albumin, hemoglobin, and hematocrit within normal ranges. The patient tolerates tube feedings and has not lost any weight during hospitalization. The family will understand what is required to maintain an adequate nutritional status and has learned how to implement tube feedings in the home if necessary.

Documentation

Document all strategies implemented for nutritional support. Include in the patient record assessments of nutritional status such as weight, condition of skin and hair, and hydration status. Chart feedings given according to agency protocol, including amount of residual. Also record any untoward effects of tube feedings, such as diarrhea or vomiting. Document all teaching and the family's verbalization of understanding. If the patient is going home with tube feedings, have the family demonstrate correct technique for performing the feedings. If the family foregoes implementation of artificial nutrition, include this in a note in the patient's record. Record all referrals made.

NURSING DIAGNOSIS 5

BOWEL INCONTINENCE AND TOTAL URINARY INCONTINENCE

Related to:
　　Impaired ability to perceive bladder cues
　　Lack of voluntary sphincter control

Defining Characteristics:
　　Involuntary passage of stool
　　Involuntary passage of urine

Goal:
　　Complications of incontinence will be prevented.

Outcome Criteria

✔ The patient will be clean, dry, and without odor.
✔ The patient will have no skin breakdown.
✔ The patient evacuates stool every 3 days.

NOC *Bowel continence*
　　　Urinary continence
　　　Urinary elimination
　　　Bowel elimination

INTERVENTIONS	RATIONALES
Monitor intake and output every shift.	Ensures that the patient is taking in adequate amounts of fluid to promote urinary elimination and softening of stool.
Monitor bowel elimination for amount, consistency, and frequency.	Assures regular evacuation of stool in order to prevent constipation and to intervene accordingly. Monitoring consistency helps note tendencies towards constipation and/or diarrhea, as these may be a side effect of tube feedings.
Restrict fluids after 6 p.m., with the exception of ordered tube feedings.	Fluids after 6 p.m. add to nighttime incontinent episodes.
Check patient at least every 2 hours.	Allows for early detection of incontinent episodes in order to minimize the time that irritants are on the skin.

INTERVENTIONS	RATIONALES
Cleanse perineal area with warm, soapy water after each incontinent episode, whether stool or urine.	Irritants in stool and urine can cause skin breakdown; meticulous attention needs to be given to skin.
Apply protective barrier to skin following cleansing: petroleum jelly or zinc oxide, or others as ordered.	These agents provide a protection to the skin that protects against moisture and irritants.
Place protective incontinent briefs on the patient following baths.	Protects the skin from moisture.
If no stool after three days, give laxative, as ordered.	Promotes adequate evacuation of the bowel and prevents severe constipation/impaction.

NIC *Urinary incontinence care*
Bowel incontinence care
Perineal care

Evaluation

Determine that the outcome criteria have been met. The patient should be kept dry for at least 2 of every 4 hours. There should be no odor or hint of urine or stool on the patient's skin. In addition, the patient has been checked for wetness and stool at least every 2 hours; if these are noted, cleanse skin well and apply ointment as a barrier to wetness and stool. The patient acquires no skin breakdown.

Community/Home Care

The family or caregiver will need to be taught the above interventions for addressing incontinence in the unconscious patient. Learning how to change incontinent briefs on an immobile patient may prove to be a challenge as the patient cannot turn or assist in any way. Family members will need to be diligent in their care in order to prevent skin breakdown due to bowel and stool incontinence. Stress to the family the importance of not just changing the incontinent brief but also washing the perineal area after each episode of stool and urine incontinence. Early morning baths and perineal care may require more attention as the patient may have been wet for longer periods of time during the night, creating a stronger odor of ammonia from the urine. It would be easy for the patient to be bathed with application of incontinent brief and not checked again for several hours; however, the caregiver must remember to check and change pads at least every 2 hours. If fluids are restricted after 6 p.m., the family may discover that the patient will void less during the night. The family should keep a log of when bowel movements occur so that constipation can be avoided by early interventions. A single subject spiral bound notebook would work for this and can be kept at the patient's bedside. Inexpensive ointments that act as barriers include petroleum jelly (Vaseline) and can be purchased in large sizes. Incontinent briefs can be very expensive and this should be discussed with a social worker to determine if some assistance is available.

Documentation

Chart the number of incontinent episodes that the patient experiences throughout each shift. Include all interventions employed to address the issue such as cleansing, checking for skin breakdown, and use of incontinent briefs. An assessment of the urine should also be made to include odor, color, and amount (large, moderate, or small). If a more accurate measurement of urine output is necessary, the incontinent brief or pad can be weighed. Always chart bowel movements when they occur, noting amount, consistency, and color. Include in the patient chart teaching done to the family regarding incontinence care.

UNIT 4
MUSCULOSKELETAL SYSTEM

CHAPTER 4.51

AMPUTATION: LOWER LIMB (TRAUMATIC/SURGICAL)

GENERAL INFORMATION

An amputation is a separation of a part of the body from the main part of the body. Amputation is most frequently seen in digits, extremities, or other protruding body parts, such as noses, ears, or penises. Lower extremities are the most common surgically amputated body parts. Surgical amputation most frequently occurs when digits or a limb are no longer being perfused and therefore no longer viable; the necrosis that may result may cause severe systemic poisoning if the extremity is not removed. Traumatic amputations occur when the limb is severed accidentally. The most common cause of traumatic amputation is machinery: farm or industrial. Other causes of traumatic amputations are motor vehicle crashes, battlefield explosions, or incidents in the home, most commonly involving lawn mowers or saws. Traumatic amputation requires immediate attention to assure that hemorrhage has been stopped, and to control anxiety in the patient. Of utmost importance is to locate the amputated part whenever it is possible, so that the part can be reattached.

NURSING DIAGNOSIS 1

 IMPAIRED PHYSICAL MOBILITY

Related to:

Loss of extremity

Defining Characteristics:

Inability to move

Reluctance to participate in prescribed activities

Hesitance to increase activity level

Anxiety regarding use of prosthetic device

Physical restriction

Goal:

The patient achieves an optimal level of physical mobility.

Outcome Criteria

✔ The patient demonstrates gradual improvement in muscle tone, strength, and control.

✔ The patient can use adjunctive devices to assist mobility (e.g., wheelchair, prosthetic device).

✔ The patient verbalizes an understanding of required conditioning and physical therapy, and expresses a willingness to participate in physical therapy as prescribed.

NOC *Balance*
Mobility

INTERVENTIONS	RATIONALES
Maintain proper alignment and positioning. During the first 24 hours after surgery, the stump is elevated on pillows to reduce edema; after this period patients with below-the-knee amputation should not have pillows placed beneath the calf. Place trochanter rolls or blankets on outer aspect of the limb. Patients should be prone 3–4 times daily for 30 minutes; assume low Fowler's or flat position for above-the-knee amputation.	Proper alignment and positioning prevents contractures and promotes maximum neurological and vascular function. Pillows are not used because they can cause hip and knee contractures; rolls or blankets on the outer aspect prevents external rotation that would cause a hip contracture.
Perform range of motion exercises for all joints.	Prevents contractures and preserves mobility.
Provide physical therapy consult as ordered for ambulation.	Helps to maintain maximum range of motion and muscle function and to assess the

INTERVENTIONS	RATIONALES
	patient's ability to move and beliefs about mobility following amputation. The loss of a limb causes a distortion in center of gravity, and the physical therapist needs to be involved in assisting the patient to adapt.
Encourage early ambulation and/or mobility as directed by the orthopedic surgeon and physical therapist, and reduce length of bedrest; encourage active range of motion of unaffected limb.	Early mobilization will prevent complications of immobility including pneumonia, skin breakdown, urinary tract infection, thrombophlebitis, and deep vein thrombosis (DVT). Exercising the unaffected extremity helps prevent complications of immobility and maintains strength.
Condition the stump for future prosthesis: Wrap the limb with compression bandage, as ordered, and keep in place unless bathing or as directed by physical therapy; reapply when the bandage becomes loose or wrinkled.	Fosters the shaping of the stump for proper prosthetic fitting, reduces edema, supports tissues, and shrinks the residual limb.
Assess neurovascular status of affected limb: pulses proximal to amputation site, color, and temperature.	Neurovascular compromise may occur due to edema, surgical intervention, and wrapping of extremity.
Instruct the patient on proper use of assistive devices, such as trapeze bars, and encourage their use.	This maintains some independence with movement in bed and allows for some exercise.
Assist with or reinforce teaching regarding mobility and future prosthesis.	Many patients have questions regarding the prosthesis and positioning; answering their questions and addressing their concerns decreases anxiety and enhances compliance.
Administer pain medications before physical therapy (see nursing diagnosis "Acute Pain").	The patient will be more likely to participate if pain-free.
Teach the patient about activity restrictions, activity requirements for rehabilitation, wrapping of stump, and conditioning of stump for prosthesis fitting.	An informed patient is more likely to be compliant with recommendations; the patient will need to be responsible for activity and mobility at home; the physical therapist's instruction can enhance the patient's ability to be independent.

Check results of diagnostic tests: x-rays, angiographic studies, Doppler flowmetry studies, and computed tomography (CT) scan.	These exams provide information regarding circulation, bone structure, and tissue trauma.
Assess the need for extended nursing care for rehabilitation; consult before surgery, or immediately after surgery if amputation was traumatic.	An early rehabilitation consult should discuss post-operative expectations, plan for physical activity, and fitting and molding for the prosthesis; a short stay in an extended care facility or rehabilitation center may be required until the patient is able to resume self-care activities.
Arrange for prosthetic consultation.	Experts in prosthetic options and fittings will be able to answer specific questions regarding the prosthetic device.

NIC *Amputation care*
Positioning
Exercise therapy: Ambulation
Teaching: Prescribed activity/exercise

Evaluation

Evaluate the degree to which the patient has achieved the stated outcome criteria. The patient should verbalize an understanding of interventions utilized to maintain mobility. Evaluate whether the patient understands rehabilitation needs and methods to condition stump for prosthesis fitting. Mobility is maximized through use of assistive devices or physical therapy. The patient participates in ordered physical therapy and maintains strength and control of all extremities. No deformities occur secondary to immobility.

Community/Home Care

The patient who has had an amputation of the lower limb will require some adaptations in performance of activities once at home. Safety will be an issue for the patient who has to use a walker or crutches to maneuver about the home as amputations of lower extremities create an imbalance of weight on one side and make ambulation difficult at first. Even though crutches may be available, use of them will require some trial and error, during which time the patient is at higher risk for falling. The environment will need to be assessed to determine how the patient can maneuver safely and whether doorways and passageways in the home can accommodate a wheelchair. Look for factors such as presence of steps and excessive furniture or clutter that pose a risk. Be sure that the patient knows how to wrap the stump to continue shrinkage and conditioning for future prosthesis application. The patient and family should demonstrate the proper wrapping of the stump to the nursing staff prior to discharge. Nursing care may not be necessary, but physical therapy may be of assistance in ensuring that the patient can implement strategies to remain mobile and prevent complications or deformities due to disuse or improper positioning. Prior to discharge from the hospital, the patient should be questioned regarding ability to function in the home in terms of self-care requirements in order for health care providers to determine whether in-home physical therapy is indicated.

The patient and family will need instruction on the use of crutches and other assistive devices as well as signs and symptoms of wound infection, improper healing of the wound, and DVT. The patient will need to understand the critical importance of following prescribed instructions for exercise, ambulation, use of crutches, walkers, and any other physical therapy. Prior to discharge the patient should demonstrate mobility techniques such as moving from chair to bed, and bed to chair. For the patient who is a candidate for a prosthesis, stress the importance of stump conditioning—shrinkage and healing. Once healing has occurred and the limb is molded, the patient can begin the process of prosthesis fitting. Although many patients want a prosthesis, the motivation to use one may not be present. Ambulating with a prosthesis requires a significant amount of energy expenditure, especially for above-the-knee amputees. A professional prosthetist fits the prosthesis by making molds of the limb and assisting in determining an appropriate stocking to wear over the stump. Once the prosthesis is complete and all necessary accessories provided, the patient will require physical therapy for instruction on ambulating with and care for the prosthesis. The patient needs to understand that shoes that fit properly and are in good condition willl help to achieve a good gait with the prosthesis. The patient and family will need to understand that some difficulties and frustrations are likely but over time will improve through trial and error.

Follow-up care to monitor progress of amputation and patient adaptation will be required. If in-home care is not possible, referrals to a rehabilitation center or extended care facility may be needed for ambulation and transfer training.

Documentation

Chart an assessment of the stump, including type of dressing present and neurovascular status (pulses, color, and skin temperature). Include teaching done on how to wrap the stump and the patient or family's return demonstration of the procedure. If the patient uses any assistive devices, such as trapeze bar, crutches, or walker, document this. Document all interventions employed and the patient's response to them. Document any complaints that the patient verbalizes and include interventions employed to correct the problem. Rely on the physical therapist to document implementation of physical therapy activities, but document any other relevant activity or follow-up reinforcement of physical therapy teachings.

NURSING DIAGNOSIS 2

 ACUTE PAIN

Related to:
> Surgical amputation
> Traumatic amputation

Defining Characteristics:
> Patient complaints of pain
> Obvious signs of trauma
> Grimacing and moaning

Goal:
> The patient's pain is relieved.

Outcome Criteria

✔ The patient will verbalize that pain has been relieved 30 minutes after interventions.

✔ The patient will verbalize an understanding of what causes pain.

NOC *Pain level*
Pain control
Comfort level

INTERVENTIONS	RATIONALES
Assess for location, intensity, quality, and precipitating factors.	Identifying these will assist in accurate diagnosis and treatment; most patients who experience amputations experience some pain, especially with movement.
Have the patient rate pain intensity using a pain rating scale.	Provides a more objective description of level of pain.
Assess status of affected extremity, including pain at amputation site, tenderness to touch, temperature, and edema.	These assessments are needed for early detection of signs of neurovascular dysfunction, patients with extremity amputations are at risk for impaired circulation and altered innervation to the extremity.
Administer analgesics as ordered on a regular schedule, not allowing pain to get intense; narcotics via patient-controlled analgesia (PCA) may be required for during the early post-operative period.	Decreased pain will improve the patient's ability to participate in physical therapy activities required for improved function; use of a PCA gives the patient control of pain management.
Move the patient's extremity gently and cautiously.	Movement of affected extremity causes pain, and careful movement provides support for the painful area.
Elevate stump on pillows for first 24 hours after surgery.	Improves venous return, which decreases edema that can contribute to pain.
Implement strategies to reduce anxiety such as staying with the patient, using relaxation techniques, and playing soft music.	Anxiety often intensifies the pain experience.
Investigate the use of diversional activities.	Decreases the attention or focus on the pain.
Encourage the patient to change position.	Improves circulation and reduces pressure points.
Administer muscle relaxants, as ordered.	Relaxes muscles (decreasing muscle spasms) and reduces pain.
Vigilantly monitor patient for sudden onset of chest pain or limb pain.	The sudden onset of pain may be indicative of another process, such as infection, pulmonary embolus, fat embolus, or compartment syndrome.
Assess effectiveness of interventions to relieve pain.	Determines whether interventions have been effective in relieving pain or

whether new strategies need to be employed.

Monitor the patient for phantom pain and phantom limb sensations, and assure the patient that these sensations are normal.	The exact cause of phantom pain is unknown, but the sensation is real for the patient and he or she may become anxious knowing that the limb is gone; the patient needs reassurance that these feelings are to be expected.

NIC *Pain management*
Analgesic administration
Anxiety reduction

Evaluation

The patient reports that the pain has been reduced or alleviated following interventions. The degree to which the patient is able to assist in the management of the pain through anxiety reduction and relaxation techniques is assessed. The patient should appear calm and have no observable signs of discomfort. If the pain is controlled, the patient will be able to participate in mobility activities prescribed and implemented by physical therapy.

Community/Home Care

The patient's pain should decrease once healing is achieved, but some type of pain management program will still be needed when he or she is discharged home. Pain at home is usually managed with mild analgesics, and the duration of pain should be short. Instruction should be undertaken to give the patient the information needed to manage pain, as pain control will be crucial to the patient's willingness and motivation to participate in rehabilitation programs for ambulation. The patient needs to monitor response to pain medications and be able to identify those factors or positions that increase pain. Encourage the patient to use assistive devices such as walkers and crutches to relieve pressure on the affected site. The patient should be instructed to notify a health care provider if sudden onset of calf pain or chest pain occurs as these may signal complications of DVT or pulmonary embolus. In the home, the patient may find comfort in elevating the extremity when sitting if not contraindicated. If the recommended analgesics are not working, the patient should seek follow-up care with the health care provider.

Documentation

Document in the patient's own words the description of the pain and rating of the level of pain. Chart all interventions employed and the patient's response. Include in the documentation assessments made relevant to the pain. Indicate all instruction in the patient record, including the patient's level of understanding. Document whether the patient reports phantom sensations and phantom pain.

NURSING DIAGNOSIS 3

IMPAIRED SKIN INTEGRITY

Related to:

> Surgical procedure of amputation
>
> Presence of drainage tubes
>
> Traumatic amputation

Defining Characteristics:

> Presence of surgical incisions
>
> Wound from traumatic amputation
>
> Sutures/staples
>
> Redness or other discoloration
>
> Edema
>
> Pain

Goal:

> Incision heals without complications.
>
> Infection is prevented or eliminated.

Outcome Criteria

✔ The patient's surgical site has no redness or other discoloration or purulent drainage, and is not hot.

✔ The patient remains afebrile.

✔ White blood cell count remains within normal limits.

✔ The stump is adequately prepared for a prosthetic device.

NOC *Wound healing:*
                Primary intention

INTERVENTIONS	RATIONALES
Monitor surgical site for color, temperature, and pulses.	Helps to detect any signs of infection or neurovascular compromise of amputated site.
Monitor surgical site and drainage tube/device insertion sites for signs and symptoms of infection: redness or other discoloration, swelling, purulent drainage, or increased heat.	Early identification of infection can expedite treatment and prevent irreparable damage to site; infection of the site will postpone prosthesis fitting.
Maintain patency of drainage devices and assess drainage from Hemovac or Jackson Pratt® drains or other drainage tubes for amount, color, and consistency.	The drainage device helps prevent edema at the site; if not draining properly, the drainage may build up within the wound and impede venous drainage from the site; drainage may be bloody initially, but should become serosanguineous.
Take temperature every 4 hours.	Detects signs of infection.
Change dressings as ordered and clean area using sterile technique, cleansing site of drainage devices last.	Maintenance of a clean incisional site or wound decreases number of organisms, reduces chance of infection, and promotes wound healing.
Wrap the stump using proper technique.	Molds the stump in preparation for a prosthetic device.
Teach the patient and family care of the incision and care of the stump.	Prevents infection, promotes wound healing, and molds the stump in preparation for a prosthetic device.
Administer antipyretics (acetaminophen [Tylenol]) as ordered.	Reduces fever.
Administer antibiotics, as ordered, IV (intravenously) or PO (by mouth).	Reduces the number of infective organisms and eliminates or prevents infection.
Encourage adequate nutritional intake with intake of protein, vitamin C, and iron.	Adequate nutrient intake, especially of vitamin C, protein, and iron, is required for healing and tissue repair.

NIC *Incision site care*
                Infection control
                Nutrition management
                Wound care
                Wound care:
                    Closed drainage

Evaluation

Evaluate the degree to which the outcome criteria have been met. The surgical site should be intact and healing by primary intention with incision well approximated. Redness or other discoloration, swelling, purulent drainage, and heat should be absent from the site. Drainage from the drainage devices should be serosanguineous and decreasing in amount. The patient should be afebrile, and white blood cell counts should return to normal.

Community/Home Care

The need for in-home nursing services depends on the patient's ability for self-care. The status of the surgical site may remain problematic after the patient has been discharged home. The risk for infection remains after discharge, and the patient and family will need to know what symptoms may signal the onset of infection. The amputation site will also need to be examined for proper closure of the wound and indications that neurovascular status is not compromised. If the patient or family members detect any abnormalities, they should write them down and notify the health care provider. Dressing changes, including wrapping the stump with an Ace® wrap, are usually required for a period of time, and the patient and family may need to perform these or the services of a nurse may be utilized. The health care provider should ensure that the patient or family members are performing the dressing change correctly, whether prior to discharge or in the home setting. Supplies required for wound care/dressing changes can be kept in a closed air-tight plastic storage box in the bedroom. The importance of good handwashing and cleanliness of supplies in the home should be stressed. If a prosthesis fitting is to be done, healing of the skin without complication is even more crucial, as any delay in healing will delay the fitting and subsequent use of the prosthesis. The patient will need to understand the importance of good nutrition in complete wound healing. Nutritious meals should be prepared with attention to protein consumption and adequate amounts of zinc, iron, and vitamin C. Completing any ordered medications such as antibiotics once at home should be stressed. The patient will need to return to the health care provider for removal of staples or sutures. If any evidence of infection, circulatory compromise, or wound opening should occur, the patient should be instructed to contact the health care provider.

Documentation

Document assessment findings of the wound to include color, approximation, drainage, etc., being sure to note any sign of infection or circulatory compromise. Chart the status of drainage devices or tubes indicating the color, amount, and consistency of drainage. Document vital signs according to agency protocol, as ordered, for post-operative patients. Chart all interventions, particularly dressing changes, medications for elevated temperature, and instruction regarding incision care.

NURSING DIAGNOSIS 4

 DISTURBED BODY IMAGE

Related to:

Loss of limb

Defining Characteristics:

Depression

Anger

Expressions about not feeling whole/like a whole person

Fixation on pre-injury condition

Denial ("if I don't look, it won't be real")

Withdrawal

Social isolation

Depression

Negative statements about physical appearance

Attempts to cover amputated limb when visitors are present

Goal:

The patient accepts the change in physical appearance and continues social activities and interpersonal relationships.

Outcome Criteria

✔ The patient states willingness to look at and touch surgical site.

✔ The patient learns and participates in care of the amputated limb.

✔ The patient verbalizes a satisfaction with body appearance.

NOC   *Body image*

INTERVENTIONS	RATIONALES
Provide assurance that feelings are very normal after surgery.	Stops the patient from thinking that his or her feelings are abnormal.
Encourage patient to face reality.	Helping the patient to focus on the truth about the loss of the limb will bring the patient one step closer to accepting reality.
Encourage the patient to express feelings of sadness, concerns about inability to fulfill family role, concerns about possible loss of income, grief over loss of body part, concern about sexual relations given new body image, fear of rejection, and fear of further loss, and allow the patient/family to grieve the loss of normal functioning.	It is appropriate to grieve for loss of function of body parts that are vital to everyday life; supporting the family and patient will enhance healthy adaptation.
Engage patient in discussions about how this event will change his or her lifestyle.	These discussions will lead to further discussions about adjustment, lifestyle, etc., and assist with coping with the change.
Arrange for a visit by an amputee who has made a successful adjustment.	Being able to see someone who has been through a similar circumstance and who has achieved success will provide more encouragement than numerous discussions with care providers.
Allow the patient privacy when bathing, dressing, or at dressing changes, if possible.	Gives the patient time to adjust to appearance without concern for how others react.
Encourage the patient to communicate feelings about changes in physical appearance.	Talking about the changes may sometimes be the beginning of acceptance.
Teach the patient methods to care for the amputated limb.	Involvement in care of the limb promotes self-care and assists with acceptance.
Teach the patient to do range of motion exercises three times a day on unaffected limbs and to participate in prescribed physical therapy activities in preparation for the prosthesis.	Preparing for prosthesis fitting gives the patient something positive to focus on and may help with acceptance of body change; maintaining strength of the unaffected extremity will assist with ambulation later.
Monitor the patient's feelings about him or herself, interpersonal relationships with family members and friends, withdrawal, social isolation, anxiety, embarrassment by appearance, fear that appearance will frighten loved ones, and desire to be alone.	Helps to detect early alterations in social functioning, prevent unhealthy behaviors, and intervene early through referral to counseling.
Encourage the patient to participate in at least one outside/public activity each week once health status permits.	Prevents the patient from isolating him or herself from others.
Identify the effects of the patient's culture or religion on body image.	A patient's culture and religion often help define his or her reactions to changes in body image and self-worth.
Identify community support groups, if available.	Discussions with other amputees may be helpful as they will afford the patient the opportunity to share thoughts with and hear thoughts from those who understand what they are going through; it also provides the patient with the support and courage to move forward in terms of acceptance of the change.
Assist the patient in identifying coping strategies and diversionary activities.	Provides diversionary activities so that not all thoughts are on disfigurement.
Arrange for psychosocial counseling if needed.	Provides psychological assistance to the patient and psychosocial evaluation.

NIC   *Body image enhancement*
Emotional support
Support group
Socialization enhancement

Evaluation

The patient is able and willing to learn about the care of the amputated leg and begins to participate in self-care. Time is required for the patient to assimilate the change in body appearance into his or her self-perception completely. It is crucial that the nurse evaluates to what degree the patient is beginning to do this. Look for behaviors such as touching the site, looking at the amputated limb, or asking appropriate questions regarding rehabilitation and possible use of the prosthesis. Communication of feelings and concerns relevant to the change in appearance should be taken as a positive sign that progress towards meeting outcome criteria is being made.

Community/Home Care

At home, continued monitoring of the patient's body image is necessary. The nurse or physical therapist who visits will need to be alert to subtle hints that may indicate that the patient has not completely adapted to the change in body appearance. Open discussions regarding this change and interventions to prevent social isolation and withdrawal should continue with patient and family. Involvement in self-care activities and in care of the limb should be undertaken by the patient to enhance acceptance of the body-structure change. The possibility of use of a prosthesis, which allows for better mobility, may provide the patient with hope for the possible return to some degree of normalcy of function. This may be enough to keep the patient from becoming depressed and isolating him or herself. Loss of a limb also has financial implications due to the possible loss of ability to work, especially if the patient was previously employed in manual labor, such as mill work, construction work, etc. Inability to fulfill the role of providing income may compound negative body image and decrease self-esteem. Community support groups should be explored.

Documentation

Chart any specific behaviors or verbalizations that may indicate an altered body image. Include all interventions employed to address this issue and the patient's response. Note when and if the patient begins to ask questions and participate in care. Document all referrals in the patient record.

NURSING DIAGNOSIS 5

DEFICIENT KNOWLEDGE

Related to:

Care of stump

Use of prosthesis

Transfer techniques

Defining Characteristics:

Asks many or no questions

Verbalizes a lack of knowledge/understanding

Unable to perform new procedures for care

Goal:

The patient or family member will know how to perform stump care and use prosthesis.

Outcome Criteria

✔ The patient indicates a desire to learn necessary information.

✔ The patient knows the purpose of compression wrap of the stump.

✔ The patient and/or family demonstrates proper wrapping of the stump.

✔ The patient expresses an understanding of the care required at home.

✔ The patient demonstrates proper transfer techniques.

✔ The patient verbalizes an understanding of follow-up physical therapy care required and expresses a willingness to comply.

NOC *Ambulation*

Ambulation: Wheelchair

Knowledge: Treatment regimen

Knowledge: Health resources

Body positioning: Self-initiated

INTERVENTIONS	RATIONALES
Assess the patient's current knowledge and ability and readiness to learn.	The teacher needs to ascertain what the patient already knows and build on this; if the patient is not capable of learning or is not ready to learn due to disinterest or inability to understand, teaching will not be effective.
Start with the simplest information and move to complex information.	Patients can understand simple concepts easily and then can build on those to understand concepts that are more complex.
Teach or collaborate with a physician and physical therapist	Knowledge of how to care for stump and improve transfer

(continues)

(continued)

INTERVENTIONS	RATIONALES
to teach the patient and family members: — Purpose of compression wrapping: shapes and molds extremity for proper fitting of prosthesis; reduces edema; minimizes pain. — Reapply wrap several times daily, whenever it becomes loose. — Keep wrap clean and dry. — Prosthesis: time until fitting, requirements for proper fit, types of prostheses, physical therapy required; once fitted for the prosthesis, how to apply and remove, and how to ambulate using the prosthesis. — Transfer techniques: how to transfer from bed to chair and back without a prosthesis; how to adjust to imbalance caused by missing limb; how to use crutches or walker. — Surgical incision or wound skin care: keep clean and dry, inspect for drainage and redness/discoloration; prevention of skin breakdown on stump when using prosthesis. — Signs and symptoms of complications that would indicate a need to seek health care.	empowers the patient to take control and be compliant.
Provide explanation and rationales for each concept or step in a skill taught.	Explanations, theoretical bases, and rationales for the information and steps increases understanding.
Allow adequate time for task mastery and have the patient or family member demonstrate wrapping the stump, transferring, and use of the prosthesis as often as required for them to become comfortable with procedure, performing the skills one step at a time.	The person performing the care should feel comfortable performing the procedure before discharge home, and the nurse needs to know that the patient can correctly perform this activity prior to discharge.
Teach the patient and family measures to prevent infection: good handwashing, especially when working with the surgical incision on the stump; keeping	Infections in the incision of the stump can delay prosthesis fitting and healing; vigilance is required to prevent wound infection.

the incision clean and dry; protecting from trauma; adequate fluid intake; adequate balanced nutrition.	
Teach the patient the importance of adequate nutrition for wound healing.	At home, without monitoring by the nursing staff, the patient may experience alterations in nutrition or lose interest in food. Stressing the importance of nutrition to family and patient will increase the possibility that the patient will be compliant with requirements.
Assess the patient's and family's understanding of all teaching by encouraging them to repeat information, demonstrate all skills, and ask questions as needed.	This allows the nurse to hear in the patient's own words what was taught and makes it easier to know what information may need to be reinforced.
Give the patient or family printed material outlining procedures and all information presented.	Printed materials can serve as a backup when the patient is at home and needs review or reinforcement.
Refer the patient to home health nursing and in-home physical therapy for follow-up and reinforcement of teaching related to transfer techniques, exercises, prosthesis use, and stump care once the patient is at home.	Once at home, the patient and family may have questions about the teaching and self-care that require reinforcement; the nurse and physical therapist also need to be sure that procedures are being performed correctly.
Establish that the patient has all care supplies required to be compliant.	If needed resources such as finances and transportation to follow-up appointments are not available, the patient cannot be compliant; the nurse will need to make necessary referrals.

NIC *Learning readiness enhancement*
Learning facilitation
Teaching: Psychomotor skill

Evaluation

Evaluate the degree to which the patient has achieved the outcome criteria relevant to the teaching sessions. The patient should verbalize an understanding of content presented by repeating the information. It is crucial that the patient or family demonstrate correct performance of all psychomotor skills such as wound care, wrapping of stump, and transfer activities. The nurse must determine whether the patient is capable of being compliant with the recommended regimen. If further teaching is required at time of discharge, the appropriate referrals should be made to continue education.

Community/Home Care

The patient will need to implement the medical regimen in the home setting over an extended period. The success of this implementation will depend upon the degree to which the patient has received adequate teaching and has subsequently understood and internalized it, and the motivation to participate in self-care, particularly transfer activities and physical therapy recommendations. Crucial to successful in-home care are the patient's and family's ability to perform stump wrapping and transfer from bed to chair and back, wound care, and activities relevant to use of prosthesis. A home nurse should follow up with the family and patient to ensure that all procedures are carried out comfortably in the home; the nurse may actually want to plan to be present the first time wound care and wrapping of the stump is done. The physical therapist should visit the home to monitor the patient's progress toward becoming independent with transfer and preparation for use of the prosthesis. Even though a professional prosthetist fits the device, the physical therapist will need to follow up in the home to assure that the patient is comfortable with ambulation activities. Depression and withdrawal are common in patients who have

had amputations, especially those who are not candidates for a prosthesis, but these psychological changes may not be seen until the patient is at home. Psychological changes may manifest in the patient's refusal to learn self-care activities, participate in physical therapy, or transfer self in and out of bed. Adequate teaching may make the family and/or patient comfortable with what is required and give them some sense of control that may assist them to move from a state of grief and denial to one of self-sufficiency and hope.

Documentation

Document the specific content taught and the titles of any printed materials given to the patient. Include in the chart the patient's degree of understanding of the content and the methods used to teach and evaluate learning. Document the patient's ability to perform the psychomotor skills required for incisional care, stump care, and use of prosthesis (when initiated). Even though the physical therapist and other health care providers document their teaching according to protocol, the nurse has a role in follow-up and should document visits by other disciplines when possible. Any areas that need to be reinforced should be documented to ensure appropriate follow-up. If family members are present for the teaching sessions, document this in the chart, and always document any referrals made. Include information regarding the patient's and family's feelings, concerns, and fears about performing care in the home.

CHAPTER 4.52

DISLOCATION: SHOULDER/KNEE/HIP

GENERAL INFORMATION

A dislocation occurs when the joint exceeds its range of motion, causing soft tissue to tear and bones to move out of their normal alignment so that the joint's surfaces are no longer intact and functional. The result is a major amount of soft tissue injury in the joint capsule itself and in the surrounding ligaments. Although dislocated joints are not generally considered life threatening, the patient will experience a considerable amount of pain and immobility. Edema occurs, along with the possibility of disruption and/or permanent damage to veins, arteries, and nerves. Joint dislocations are more common in persons aged 18–41 years and are frequently caused by sports injuries. The most common dislocations are of the hip and shoulder.

Shoulder dislocation is the most common joint dislocation and occurs often among younger persons, particularly young males involved in contact sports. It usually results from a fall on an extended arm in abduction and external rotation resulting in an anterior dislocation. Posterior dislocation is rare and is usually the result of abduction and internal rotation during seizure activity or from a direct blow anteriorly. Clinical manifestations include severe pain in the affected shoulder that is worse with attempted movement, decreased range of motion, and the patient holding the arm in slight abduction.

Knee dislocation occurs most often following hyperextension or a force injury to the proximal tibia, and in some instances occurs due a fall on a flexed knee. Knee dislocation can be severely debilitating if not relocated immediately due to the possibility of perineal and posterior tibial nerve damage or popliteal artery damage. Following relocation of a dislocated knee, Doppler studies and/or arteriograms should be done to assess for arterial disruption. Clinical manifestations of a dislocated knee include intense pain at the site and an obvious deformity of the knee. Patellar dislocation is a very common athletic injury that results from direct trauma to the patella or rotation of the leg when the foot is fixed. It is usually easy to diagnose as the knee is usually in a fixed position and cannot be extended and the patella is located to one side.

Hip dislocations occur most often as a result of automobile accidents where there is a major force impact on an extended leg or on impact when the knee hits the dashboard. Falls from ladders are another cause of hip dislocation. Posterior dislocation that causes the head of the femur to be pushed out and back is the most common type of hip dislocation. Clinical manifestations of hip dislocation will depend on the type: posterior or anterior. In posterior hip dislocation, the hip is in flexion with internal rotation and a noticeable shortening of the extremity when compared with the other extremity. In anterior hip dislocation, the patient will usually have the hip in extension with the leg externally rotated. In both types of dislocation, there is serious pain and decreased range of motion of the extremity. Because hip dislocation is most often caused by traumatic, forcible injury, there is a high likelihood for disruption of blood supply to the femoral head and damage to the sciatic nerve. In order to preserve function of the extremity, special attention should be paid to neurovascular assessment of this patient. It is essential to relocate the femoral head into the joint socket to avoid femoral head necrosis due to femoral artery disruption and sciatic and femoral nerve damage.

NURSING DIAGNOSIS 1

 ### ACUTE PAIN

Related to:

Dislocation of joint

Defining Characteristics:

Complains of severe pain

Pain on attempts at movement of limb

Grimacing

Moaning

Goal:

The patient's pain is relieved or reduced.

Outcome Criteria

✔ The patient will verbalize that pain has been relieved 30 minutes after interventions.

✔ The patient will verbalize an understanding of what causes pain.

✔ The patient is able to identify factors that precipitate pain and understands how to modify behaviors accordingly.

NOC *Pain level*

Pain control

Comfort level

INTERVENTIONS	RATIONALES
Assess for location, intensity, quality, and other signs of pain such as inability to move joint, grimacing, facial expressions, audible expressions of pain, and guarding of injured area.	Identifying these will assist in accurate diagnosis and treatment; most patients who experience dislocations experience some pain, especially with movement.
Have the patient rate pain intensity using a pain rating scale.	Provides a more objective description of level of pain.
Assess status of affected extremity (hip, shoulder, knee), including pain at injury site, tenderness to touch, temperature, edema, peripheral pulses, and color.	Helps to note early signs of neurovascular dysfunction; patients with dislocations are at risk for neurovascular compromise (see nursing diagnosis "Risk for Peripheral Vascular Dysfunction").
Administer analgesics as ordered on a regular schedule, not allowing pain to intensify.	Analgesics decrease pain by altering perception of pain. Decreased pain will improve the patient's ability to tolerate immobilization and reduction of dislocation in the most acute phase and to participate in physical therapy activities required for improved mobility in later phases.

INTERVENTIONS	RATIONALES
Move patient's extremity gently and cautiously.	Movement of affected extremity causes pain, and careful movement provides support for the painful area.
Maintain traction as ordered (see nursing diagnosis "Impaired Physical Mobility").	Maintains the stability of the dislocated joint and decreases muscle spasms.
For shoulder dislocation, assist with efforts to reduce the dislocation and place in a sling.	The shoulder must be put back into place by a physician; the sling immobilizes the shoulder, which helps to relieve pain and will reduce edema.
For hip dislocation without fracture, assist with preparation of the patient for immediate relocation of the hip using manual traction.	Immediate relocation is necessary to prevent necrosis of the head of the femur and injury to nerves.
For hip dislocation, place patient on bedrest and assist with physical therapy activity as required or ordered, including use of assistive devices.	The patient with hip dislocation may be placed on bedrest for a short period until weight bearing is allowed and edema or impaired tissue at the site is improved, which improves pain.
Apply ice packs, 20 minutes on, 20 minutes off for the first 48 hours, especially to the injured knee.	Ice reduces swelling through vasoconstriction and reduces pain.
Implement strategies to reduce anxiety, such as staying with the patient, using relaxation techniques, playing soft music.	Anxiety often intensifies the pain experience.
Investigate the use of diversional activities.	Decreases the attention or focus on the pain.
Administer muscle relaxants, as ordered.	Relaxes muscles and reduces pain.
Assess effectiveness of interventions to relieve pain.	Helps to determine whether interventions have been effective in relieving pain or whether new strategies need to be employed.

NIC *Pain management*

Analgesic administration

Anxiety reduction

Evaluation

The patient reports that the pain has been reduced or alleviated following interventions. The degree to which the patient is able to assist in the management of the pain through anxiety reduction and relaxation techniques is assessed. The patient should appear calm and have no observable signs of being uncomfortable. If the pain is controlled, the patient is able to participate in mobility activities prescribed and implemented by physical therapy. The patient can identify factors that precipitate pain and modify behavior to minimize them.

Community/Home Care

The patient's pain should decrease once the dislocation has been repaired either manually or, in the case of hip dislocation, through surgery or traction, and should completely resolve quickly. Because dislocations that do not require surgery or traction may be treated on an outpatient basis, instruction should be undertaken to give the patient the information needed to manage pain. Pain at home is usually managed with mild analgesics, and the duration of pain should be short. The patient needs to monitor response to pain medications and be able to identify those factors or positions that increase pain. Encourage the patient to use assistive devices such as slings, braces, or crutches to immobilize the affected joint, be it the hip, shoulder, or knee. In the home, the patient may find comfort in elevating the extremity when sitting, if not contraindicated. If the recommended analgesics are not working, the patient should seek follow-up care with the health care provider.

Documentation

Document in the patient's own words the description of the pain and rating of the level of pain. Chart all interventions employed and the patient's responses. Include in the documentation assessments made relevant to the pain. Document all teaching in the patient record with an indication of the patient's level of understanding.

NURSING DIAGNOSIS 2

 ## IMPAIRED PHYSICAL MOBILITY

Related to:

Dislocation of hip, knee, or shoulder

Extreme pain at joint area

Traction

Defining Characteristics:

Physical restriction

Inability to move

Decreased range of motion

Decreased or no movement of extremity

Unable and unwilling to move affected extremity

Goal:

The patient obtains physical mobility to the highest permissible level.

Outcome Criteria

✔ The patient demonstrates gradual improvement in movement in the shoulder, knee, or hip.

✔ The patient can safely use adjunctive devices to assist mobility.

✔ The patient verbalizes a willingness to participate in physical therapy as prescribed.

✔ The patient states ways to prevent reoccurrence.

INTERVENTIONS	RATIONALES
Support and immobilize extremity, including joint above and below the dislocation site: use splint, sling, brace, or other immobilizing materials.	Immobilization will prevent further damage to soft tissue of the joints.
Maintain proper alignment.	Proper alignment promotes maximum neurological and vascular function and minimizes pain.
Check results of diagnostic tests: x-rays, computed tomography (CT) scan, magnetic resonance imaging (MRI), Doppler studies, arteriogram.	These exams confirm the diagnosis, exact location, and severity of injury.
For hip dislocation, assist with immediate relocation by assisting with intravenous sedation and manual traction (closed reduction), as ordered.	Prompt treatment is required to prevent vascular damage to the head of the femur, reduction also decreases pain and restores range of motion.
For hip dislocation not repaired by external relocation: assist with traction set up as ordered and maintain according to protocol. In general, assess for correct alignment, keep appropriate weights attached as ordered, seek assistance from physical therapy as required, and assess neurovascular status	Traction returns the dislocated hip to correct alignment, provides stabilization until internal relocation can occur, and helps to decrease muscle spasms; skin traction is used for short term (48–72 hours).

INTERVENTIONS	RATIONALES
of extremity (see nursing diagnosis "Risk for Peripheral Neurovascular Dysfunction").	
For shoulder dislocation, assist with relocation as required and apply a sling.	The shoulder is usually externally relocated manually; relocation is done immediately, before swelling, inflammation, and spasm of muscles occur.
For knee dislocation, assist with immediate reduction/relocation externally, perform a thorough assessment for vascular injury, and splint the joint or prepare patient for surgical reduction as ordered.	Relocation is necessary to reduce pain and return range of motion; immediate relocation is required due to the danger of damage to nerves and blood vessels (~ 53 percent of patients with knee injury also have popliteal artery injury); arteriograms are generally ordered following repair to evaluate arterial blood flow.
After reduction, keep the affected knee elevated, apply ice to the site, and apply splints or braces, as ordered.	These measures decrease swelling and pain and promote healing.
Provide physical therapy consult for rehabilitation and teaching regarding activity restrictions and use of assistive devices.	Maintains maximum range of motion and muscle function; educates the patient on activity needs, especially following discharge from the acute care setting.
Encourage early ambulation and/or mobility as directed by the physical therapist and reduce length of bedrest.	Early mobilization will prevent complications of immobility in hip and knee dislocations, particularly thrombophlebitis and deep vein thrombosis (DVT).
Assess for neurovascular complications (see nursing diagnosis "Risk for Peripheral Neurovascular Dysfunction").	Neurovascular compromise may occur due to constriction of the extremity by edema or by damage to nerves and blood vessels caused by the injury.
Keep head of bed no higher than 30 degrees if in traction.	Elevating higher than this minimizes the pull of the traction, decreasing its ability to stabilize or realign the bone.
Encourage the patient to exercise unaffected extremities by doing range of motion exercises as directed by physical therapist.	Exercising the unaffected extremity helps prevent complications of immobility and maintains strength.
Instruct the patient on the proper use of assistive devices such as splints, slings, braces,	Maintains some independence with movement; and the patient needs to know how to properly
crutches, etc., and encourage their use.	use assistive devices at home.
Administer pain medications before physical therapy activities if the patient remains in the hospital.	The patient will be more likely to participate if pain-free.
Prepare the patient for operative procedures according to agency procedures as ordered (open relocation or reduction, especially with knees and hips).	Some dislocations may require surgical repair due to the extent of soft tissue damage or because external reduction efforts have been unsuccessful.
Following surgery, implement measures to promote activity as ordered or prescribed in collaboration with physical therapy.	The patient will need assistance with mobility to prevent injury, to repaired extremity, and to promote return to normal function without complications.
Assess the patient's understanding of injury, necessary therapeutic interventions, and hazards that caused the injury, and instruct as appropriate.	The patient needs to know about the possibility of future injuries and mobility with activities, as some dislocations leave the patient with less than usual functioning; gives the patient a realistic picture.

NIC   *Traction/immobilization care*
Positioning
Exercise therapy: Ambulation
Exercise therapy: Joint mobility
Teaching: Prescribed activity/exercise

Evaluation

Evaluate the degree to which the patient has achieved the stated outcome criteria. The patient should verbalize an understanding of interventions utilized to achieve repair of the dislocation and how to prevent a reoccurrence. Mobility is maximized through use of assistive devices or physical therapy. The patient participates in ordered physical therapy and maintains strength and control of all extremities. Gradual improvement in mobility is seen in the patient. No deformities occur and no symptoms of neurovascular compromise are noted secondary to the dislocation.

Community/Home Care

The patient who has suffered dislocation will require some adaptations in performance of activities once at home. For the patient who has a knee or hip injury, safety at home may be an issue because ambulation with canes, splints, or braces can create difficulty with ambulation. Braces tend to create a filling of imbalance because of their weight, to which the patient must adapt. Even though crutches may be available, use of them will require some trial and error in the home, during which time the patient is at higher risk for falling. The environment will need to be assessed to determine how the patient can maneuver safely. Look for factors such as type of flooring (carpet, wood, or tile), distance to bathroom, presence of steps, and excessive furniture or clutter that pose a risk. Steps may be problematic, and the patient and family may need to arrange sleeping quarters in a downstairs room if the patient is unable to climb stairs. Be sure that the patient knows how to use any assistive devices such as slings, braces, or special shoes for walking. Nursing care may not be needed, but physical therapy may be of assistance in ensuring that the patient can implement strategies to remain mobile, perform activities of daily living (ADLs), and prevent complications or deformities due to disuse. The challenges are substantial for younger patients who will need to return to school or college environments, because the school or college environment is not always user-friendly to those with mobility issues. Investigation should be undertaken to determine if assistance will be needed to carry books or take notes, or in the case of knee injuries, how to get from one point to another. Disability services may be of assistance in this situation, and special shuttles may be available. In most instances of knee and hip dislocations, physical therapy is required as an outpatient to regain complete function of the extremity; the importance of this needs to be stressed to the patient and appropriate referrals and appointments made. In addition to use of crutches and other assistive devices, the patient and family will need instruction on signs and symptoms of DVT and neurovascular compromise if the hip or knee has been dislocated. For those patients who have sustained a knee dislocation, the patient and family should understand that full function of the knee to its previous state may not occur and the patient may experience long-term effects, such as pain, instability of the joint, and stiffness. For athletes, this may mean the end to intense sports activities such as football, and for the sports enthusiast this may be a difficult reality. For patients with shoulder dislocation, the sling will be needed for approximately 3 weeks, and for younger patients, compliance may be difficult. The shoulder should be kept in a midrange position, and a general guide

offered by sports medicine to help patients remember this is to keep the arm and hand within the line of vision. Another aspect of home care for the patient with a dislocated shoulder includes teaching how to prevent recurrence. For younger patients, the recurrence rate is high and estimated at some to be almost 90 percent in teenagers. For this reason, the patient will need to understand the critical importance of following prescribed instructions for exercise and physical therapy, particularly strengthening exercises for those with shoulder dislocations. It may be difficult for younger patients to adjust to the limitations that a dislocated shoulder may have on the ability to play sports at the same level as before the injury, especially when the shoulder used extensively (as by quarterbacks, wide receivers, or pitchers), which may necessitate identification of other forms of activity. Follow-up care, including x-rays to determine healing, will be necessary.

Documentation

Chart the presence and correct functioning of all devices used for stabilization of the joint such as traction, splints, slings, and braces. Include in the patient record the results of a thorough assessment of the affected joint/extremity, including activity and neurovascular status. Document all interventions employed to correct the dislocation and the patient's responses to them. Any complaints that the patient verbalizes should be documented, including interventions employed to correct the problem. If the patient is scheduled for surgery, document pre-operative and post-operative assessments according to agency protocol. Rely on the physical therapist to document implementation of physical therapy activities, but document any other relevant activity or follow-up reinforcement of physical therapy teachings.

NURSING DIAGNOSIS 3

RISK FOR PERIPHERAL NEUROVASCULAR DYSFUNCTION

Related to:

Damage to the nerves

Trauma to the popliteal nerve

Edema in area of injury

Defining Characteristics:

None

Goal:

Neurovascular function is maintained.

Outcome Criteria

✔ Peripheral pulses in extremity are palpable.

✔ Extremity is warm with capillary refill brisk at < 3 seconds.

✔ The patient's extremity remains at normal color.

✔ The patient reports absence of severe pain.

✔ The patient has usual sensation in extremity.

NOC *Circulation status*
Mobility
Tissue perfusion: Peripheral

INTERVENTIONS	RATIONALES
Assess neurovascular status of both extremities every 1–2 hours or as ordered: pulses, sensation, temperature, capillary refill, and movement.	Establishes a baseline and detects early any complications that may occur due to surgery, relocation, edema, traction, or initial injury.
Assess for signs and symptoms of blood vessel and nerve damage, especially with knee dislocation: severe pain, diminished or absent pulses, cool extremity, diminished or absent sensation in the extremity, loss of normal color or pallor, decreased capillary refill, or decreased movement.	The above signs and symptoms are indicative of nerve damage pain and impaired blood flow to the extremity. These need to be brought to the attention of the physician for immediate attention to preserve extremity function; early detection by frequent assessments leads to early identification and early treatment.
Elevate extremity if not contraindicated.	Elevation assists with venous return that reduces edema.
Assist with preparation for testing to detect or rule out blood vessel or nerve damage.	Arteriograms, Doppler studies, or other diagnostic tests are often ordered to assess for damage to nerves and blood vessels, especially the popliteal artery in knee dislocation and the sciatic nerve in hip dislocation.
Teach the patient and family signs and symptoms of neurovascular compromise.	Allows for early detection and prompt reporting.

NIC *Peripheral sensation management*
Positioning: Neurologic
Circulatory precautions

Evaluation

No evidence of neurovascular compromise is present. The patient should be evaluated to determine whether neurovascular status is maintained. Evaluate whether physiological indicators such as peripheral pulses, skin color, temperature, sensation, and capillary refill are normal. Assess the patient for undue pain that seems too severe for the injury and is unrelieved by analgesics.

Community/Home Care

Neurovascular problems usually occur during the early stages of injury to the extremity but can occur later. This is especially true for dislocations treated with external relocation with the patient discharged home quickly from the emergency department, when inadequate attention might be given to assessing for the possibility of blood vessel and nerve damage. It is important that the patient understand how to relieve and prevent edema in the extremity. Ambulation and participation in physical therapy as ordered should be stressed. A nurse may not be required, but follow-up visits with a health care provider are needed to be sure that the extremity is healing appropriately and that there are no long-term neurovascular alterations.

Documentation

Chart findings from a thorough neurovascular assessment, including peripheral pulses, extremity color, sensation, pain, and capillary refill. Document the specific content included in teaching sessions. Always include nursing interventions implemented to prevent neurovascular compromise, and chart interventions initiated for treatment. Include in the patient chart the patient's response to all interventions and any specific concerns verbalized.

CHAPTER 4.53

FACIAL TRAUMA

GENERAL INFORMATION

Facial trauma, such as soft tissue, cartilage, and bone trauma to the face or fracture of the bones of the face, most frequently occurs as a result of unrestrained drivers or passengers in motor vehicle crashes, from direct blows or blunt trauma to the face, or from collisions in contact sports. The most critical concern following facial injuries is the possibility of airway obstructions. Facial injuries often occur concurrently with cervical spine injuries that require immediate attention. After the patient has been stabilized, assessment of the face and oral cavity should be undertaken; however, damage to the soft tissue of the face may make accurate assessments difficult to perform. Additional areas of concern include injury to the eye and inside the mouth, nose, and ears. Clinical manifestations of facial trauma or bone fracture depend upon the site and amount of soft tissue trauma but could include mouth bleeding, facial asymmetry, epistaxis, diplopia, bulging or sunken eyes, edema of the face, malocclusion of the teeth, movement of the dental arch if the nose is manipulated, facial bone movement with nasal manipulation, and alterations in airway patency.

NURSING DIAGNOSIS 1

 INEFFECTIVE AIRWAY CLEARANCE

Related to:

Facial trauma

Fracture(s) of the face

Airway obstruction, mechanical or physiologic, causing hypoxia

Edema

Defining Characteristics:

Inability to handle secretions, bleeding

Verbalizations of sensation of choking

Cyanosis

Tachycardia

Nasal flaring

Wheezing

Stridor

Dyspnea

Holding throat and attempting to communicate

Goal:

The patient's airway is patent.

Outcome Criteria

✔ The patient will have normal respirations without stridor, wheezing, nasal flaring, or dyspnea.

✔ The patient will have clear breath sounds.

✔ The patient will have no cyanosis.

✔ The patient will be alert.

NOC *Respiratory status: Airway patency*
Respiratory status: Ventilation

INTERVENTIONS	RATIONALES
Assess respiratory status: respiratory rate, rhythm, depth, changes in respiratory rate (tachypnea), oxygen saturation, dyspnea; monitor for specific indicators of obstructed patient airway (possible obstruction due to edema, blood, debris, fracture displacement) such as swallowing blood, presence of cyanosis, retractions, use of accessory muscles, flaring of nostrils, (decreasing) level of consciousness, pupillary changes, and sleepiness.	Absence of breath sounds may be noted; abnormal breathing patterns may signal worsening of condition; change in level of consciousness, pupillary changes, retractions, stridor, and flaring of nostrils indicate a significant decline in respiratory status and airway patency; establishes baseline and helps to monitor response to interventions.

INTERVENTIONS	RATIONALES
Create a patent and clear airway through suctioning.	Blood and emesis can be removed via suctioning; often, in facial trauma, problems occur with airway management due to an altered level of consciousness and airway obstruction by the tongue, a physical or mechanical obstruction, or bleeding.
Maintain open airway through airway adjuncts, endotracheal intubation, or surgical airway, as ordered.	The use of appropriate airway adjuncts, endotracheal intubation to open and protect the airway, or the surgical creation of an airway (via cricothyrotomy or tracheostomy) to bypass an obstruction may be necessary.
Monitor patient's diagnostic tests: x-rays, computed tomography (CT) scan, MRI.	These will document the injury and give an accurate diagnosis of exact extent of the injury/trauma.
If surgical intervention is required for a cricothyrotomy or tracheostomy, prepare the patient according to agency protocol and assist as ordered.	Cricothyrotomy provides a temporary airway in an emergency situation, and tracheostomy provides a more permanent airway.
Assess mental status during period when airway is obstructed and immediately following.	Lack of oxygen for even short periods can affect cerebral oxygenation, resulting in changes in mental status and level of consciousness.
Monitor arterial blood gases (ABGs) and oxygen saturation, as ordered.	ABG analysis will reveal respiratory acidosis as the lungs are unable to expel carbon dioxide, and oxygen levels will be low as the lungs are unable to take in oxygen and exchange gases.
Assess for anxiety and reassure the patient with presence.	Inability to breathe causes anxiety and fear, which increases the demand for oxygen; a calming presence can decrease anxiety.
Provide humidified oxygen, as ordered, to maintain oxygen saturation at > 90 percent.	Restores oxygenation to tissues.
Establish intravenous access.	Ensures a route for rapid-acting medications; following trauma there may be undiscovered injuries that require emergency intervention.
Place patient in high Fowler's position if not contraindicated due to cervical injury or other trauma.	Maximizes chest excursion and subsequent movement of air.
Perform frequent respiratory assessments following reestablishment of airway: oxygen saturations, respiratory rate, rhythm, depth, color, and breath sounds.	Detects improvements in oxygenation status.
Monitor patient for signs of aspiration of blood into lungs: abnormal breath sounds, fever, or increased secretions.	When foreign substances are in the airway, some particles may be aspirated into lungs and may cause aspiration pneumonia; detects early symptoms that may require further treatment.
Assist with preparation for surgery as ordered or required by agency protocol.	Some facial fractures, such as mandibular fractures, require immobilization by use of wires, screws, and plates, or in some instances when teeth are missing, metal arch bars are placed in the mouth; these provide stabilization to the fractured bones to allow healing.
Keep suction apparatus at the bedside pre- and post-operatively.	To be used in the event of obstructed airway due to bleeding or vomiting.
For the post-operative patient who has wires or bands placed for stabilization of fractures, keep wire cutters and scissors at bedside and be sure to send with the patient if the patient leaves the area.	To cut the wires or rubber bands in case of emergencies, such as respiratory or cardiac distress caused by airway obstruction.

NIC *Airway management*
Presence
Respiratory monitoring

Evaluation

Assess the client to determine the extent to which the outcome criteria have been met. Assessments of the respiratory system should reveal that acute symptoms of airway obstruction have been resolved. The patient's airway should be clear, the patient should be able to speak, and the patient should be breathing easy. Breath sounds should be present, and even though there may be some discomfort with respirations, no respiratory distress should be noted. ABGs and oxygen saturation should indicate adequate oxygenation, and there should be no cyanosis. The patient should be alert and back at a normal level of consciousness.

Community/Home Care

For the patient who has experienced airway obstruction due to facial trauma, in-home care may not be required except as it relates to follow-up for the specific injuries. By the time of discharge, facial edema should have subsided and the dangers of bleeding into the airway have been eliminated. However, the patient and family should still be aware of the signs and symptoms of airway obstruction and what to do in the event that they should occur once at home. If the wires are still in place at time of discharge, the patient and a family member or significant other will need to know how to cut the wires and which wires to cut if an emergency should arise. In addition, the wire cutters will need to carried by the patient when outside the home. Swallowing may be difficult due to prostheses, pain, and limited movement of the jaw; difficulty swallowing places a patient at risk for aspiration or airway problems (see nursing diagnosis "Imbalanced Nutrition: Less Than Body Requirements").

Documentation

Document a comprehensive respiratory assessment to include respiratory status during obstruction and the patient's status once the problem has been resolved. Of particular note should be breath sounds, color, oxygenation status, respiratory rate, depth, and any nonverbal signs that the patient is having difficulty breathing. Include in the patient record interventions carried out to relieve the obstruction and the patient's responses. Note specifically changes in breath sounds in response to interventions and the patient's emotional state. Document vital signs according to agency protocol. Always include in the documentation the patient's progress towards achievement of the stated outcome criteria.

NURSING DIAGNOSIS 2

 IMBALANCED NUTRITION: LESS THAN BODY REQUIREMENTS

Related to:

Facial fractures

Edema

Pain in facial area

Inability to eat solid food

Defining Characteristics:

Expressed feelings of hunger

Weight loss

Eats < 50 percent of food served

Reports of being unable to eat

Goal:

The patient is receiving adequate nutritional intake.

Outcome Criteria

✔ The patient is able to eat 75 percent of meals served.

✔ The patient states that it does not hurt to eat.

✔ The patient does not lose weight.

✔ The patient's albumin level, electrolytes, hemoglobin, serum transferrin, and iron are normal.

NOC *Nutritional status:*
            Nutrient intake

         Nutritional status:
            Food and fluid intake

INTERVENTIONS	RATIONALES
Assess the patient's ability to swallow food and liquid.	Determines the extent of difficulty swallowing.
Weigh patient on admission and at regular intervals.	Establishes baseline for future comparison, detects weight loss, and allows intervention to prevent wasting.
Arrange dietary consult to ascertain the patient's ability to take in enough food to meet calorie demand and to determine the patient's likes, dislikes, and preferences within the prescribed diet with consideration to cultural and/or religious preferences.	Patients will be more likely to consume foods or liquids that they like and are accustomed to; arrangements must be made for processing of foods or liquid that the patient can tolerate; the patient is more likely to attempt foods he or she likes.
Administer pain medications 30 minutes before meals.	Controls pain in the facial area that may interfere with consumption of food or fluid.
Encourage frequent, small liquid supplements that have rich nutrient content including protein and high calories; soft slippery foods such as custards, pudding, and ice cream are easy to swallow.	Liquid supplements and/or milkshakes are generally easy to consume and provide needed calories and nutrients.

INTERVENTIONS	RATIONALES
Remain with the patient the first time he or she attempts to eat.	Helps to assess the ability to eat or drink and to intervene if difficulties occur. The first attempt at eating following injury may prove anxiety-provoking for the patient, and the nurse needs to be present to assess ability to eat.
Allow extended periods of time for meals and assure the patient that this is okay.	The patient may take longer due to structural changes both to the face and in the mouth.
Investigate possible methods of ingesting food: use of straws, spoons, or feeding syringes.	It may be easier for some patients to take liquids via straws, spoons, or syringes. Use of metal spoons may cause pain. The nurse must assist the patient to experiment with these.
Assist the dietician in determining the calorie count and the amount of food or liquid consumed with each meal or between meals.	Detects early problems with adequate calories and nutrients to sustain nutritional status; allows for early interventions to address altered nutrition.
Monitor patient for aspiration and implement necessary measures to control if it occurs.	When difficulty swallowing occurs, the patient may cough or gag when unable to swallow or expectorate.
Monitor laboratory results: albumin, electrolytes, hemoglobin, serum transferrin, and iron.	These tests are frequently used measures of nutritional status and can be used to determine whether the patient is meeting basic nutritional requirements.

NIC *Nutritional monitoring*
Nutrition management
Nutrition therapy

Evaluation

Determine whether the outcome criteria have been met for the patient. The patient should be eating meals with high nutritional value. Consumption of at least 75 percent of food and fluids served should be achieved, with reports from the patient that he or she can eat without pain or discomfort. The patient should report satisfaction with dietary restrictions and the foods offered. The nurse should frequently assess the patient's ability to eat and willingness to attempt to eat, and revise interventions accordingly. Frequent weights need to be obtained to ensure that the patient is not losing weight. Laboratory results

such as serum transferrin, iron, electrolytes, albumin, and hemoglobin should be within normal limits.

Community/Home Care

Nutrition will continue to be a problem in the home setting. The majority of patients who experience facial trauma will need some adjustments with the type of foods they consume. Patients who have had facial fractures may be limited for a significant period to liquids due to pain and surgical repairs of the trauma. Baby food can be used as an alternative to regular food; it is easy to consume, the flavor is generally good, and it provides needed nutrients. The use of straws for all intake tires the patient and he or she may also lack motivation to work at eating enough to maintain nutritional status. The use of a spoon also poses a challenge as attempts to open the mouth wide enough for a spoon may create pain, and the patient's use of a spoon may be slow and laborious. The meal preparer could use a food processor or blender to make the food prepared for other family members the correct consistency for the patient. It is crucial for the nurse to visit in the home to assess the patient's ability to cope with these changes and to perform a nutritional assessment including obtaining a current weight. A 24-hour diet recall may prove helpful to determine whether the patient is eating enough. The family can assist the patient by preparing foods that are easy to chew and swallow, that the patient likes, and that also have nutritional value. The patient will need encouragement to eat and even at home may prefer privacy for meals because of the difficulty with chewing and swallowing. Vitamins can be taken to supplement the diet. Oral care is important especially if wires and bands that can trap food particles are present inside the mouth. Gentle rinsing of the mouth not only cleans away food particles but can also enhance healing of damaged oral tissues. Depending on the patient's weight and ability to eat, a referral for alternative means of obtaining nutrition may be needed.

Documentation

Document all interventions implemented to address the patient's nutritional status. Be sure to include whether the patient has met the outcome criteria, and in instances where the criteria have not been achieved, necessary revisions to the plan. Chart the patient's weight and the type of diet that the patient is comfortable eating, as well as the percentage of each meal taken. If special devices such as syringes are used for eating, document this in the patient record. A thorough nutritional assessment of the patient should be made and documented, including difficulty chewing or swallowing, foods that create special challenges, and any specific concerns that the patient may have relevant to nutritional status.

NURSING DIAGNOSIS 3

 ### DISTURBED BODY IMAGE

Related to:

Facial deformities

Surgical repairs

Defining Characteristics:

Withdrawal

Social isolation

Depression

Negative statements about physical appearance

Attempts to cover face when visitors are present

Goal:

The patient accepts the change in physical appearance and continues social activities and interpersonal relationships.

Outcome Criteria

✔ The patient states willingness to look at and touch surgical site.

✔ The patient verbalizes a satisfaction with body appearance.

✔ The patient verbalizes an understanding of appliances, wires, and prostheses, whether temporary or permanent.

NOC *Body image*

INTERVENTIONS	RATIONALES
Provide assurance that feelings are very normal following traumatic injury and after surgery.	Stops the patient from thinking that his or her feelings are abnormal.
Encourage the patient to look at self in mirror while hospitalized.	Allows the patient time to adjust to appearance without concern for how others react.
Encourage the patient to communicate feelings about changes in physical appearance.	Talking about the changes may sometimes be the beginning of acceptance.
Teach the patient and family how to care for any wounds or surgical sites.	If the patient is comfortable with self-care, that comfort level may translate into acceptance for the change in appearance and incorporation of body appearance change into a positive self-image.
Monitor the patient's feelings about self, interpersonal relationships, withdrawal, social isolation, anxiety, embarrassment by appearance, fear that appearance will frighten loved ones, and desire to be alone.	Detects early alterations in social functioning, prevents unhealthy behaviors, and allows early intervention through referral to counseling.
Encourage the patient to participate in at least one outside/public activity each week once health status permits.	Prevents the patient from isolating him or herself from others.
Identify the effects of the patient's culture or religion on perceived body image.	A patient's culture and religion often help define reactions to changes in body image and self-worth.
Assist the patient in identifying coping strategies/diversionary activities.	Provides diversion so that not all thoughts are on disfigurement.
Arrange for psychosocial counseling if required.	Provides psychological assistance to the patient and psychosocial evaluation.
Provide reassurance.	Explain that deformity appears greater closer to the injury event due to swelling and discoloration. As days pass, edema will subside and discoloration will resolve.
In collaboration with the physician, arrange consultation with a plastic surgeon.	A plastic surgeon can explain procedures that can be done in the near or distant future to reduce disfigurement. It is often helpful for the patient to see "before" and "after" photos of other patients with similar deformities who have had plastic surgery intervention.

NIC *Body image enhancement*
Emotional support
Socialization enhancement

Evaluation

The patient is able and willing to learn about care required following the trauma and adaptations required for eating. Time is required for the patient to assimilate the change in body appearance into their self-perception completely. It is crucial that the nurse evaluates to what degree the patient is beginning to do so. Look for behaviors such as touching the site, looking at the disfigurement in the mirror, or asking appropriate questions. Communication of feelings and concerns relevant to the change in appearance should be taken as a positive sign that progress towards meeting outcome criteria is being made.

Community/Home Care

At home, continued monitoring of the patient's body image is needed. For the patient with facial disfigurement, the changes may only be temporary, but during this time the patient may be self-conscious about how others view him or her. Once initial wounds have healed, the patient must be encouraged, supported, and assisted to venture outside the home on a regular basis to prevent social isolation, which can worsen negative feelings about appearance. The patient can start with activities such as taking a walk or visiting friendly, familiar people (who are less likely to stare) and places where the patient feels comfortable. If the patient attends civic or religious activities, these may also be a source of comfort. The patient should look in the mirror daily and touch the site of disfigurement to become more accustomed to its appearance and feeling. The nurse who visits will need to be alert to subtle hints that may indicate that the patient has not completely adapted to the change in body appearance. Open discussions regarding this change and interventions to prevent social isolation and withdrawal should continue with patient and family. Discussions with health care providers regarding future reconstructive/plastic surgery should be encouraged.

Documentation

Chart any specific behaviors or verbalizations that may indicate an altered body image. Include all interventions employed to address this issue and the patient's responses. Note when and if the patient begins to ask questions and participate in care. Document all referrals made.

CHAPTER 4.54

FAT EMBOLISM

GENERAL INFORMATION

A fat embolism occurs when a bolus of fat or fat globules are released from the bone marrow of an injured bone then enter the vascular system and progress to obstruct the vasculature of other organs, primarily the lungs. These fat particles travel through the venous circulation to the small blood vessels of the lung, causing obstruction. These foreign substances initiate a cascade of pathophysiological events that cause destruction of lung tissue resulting in hypoxemia, clotting disorders, and altered cerebral blood flow. Fat emboli commonly come from fracture sites of long bones, particularly the tibia and the femur, and from fractures of the pelvis and following hip replacement surgery. In patients who experience a fat embolism the embolism occurs within 24 to 48 hours after the injury/surgery in 46 percent of the cases and within 72 hours in 91 percent of the cases (Phipps, Monahan, Sands, Marek, and Neighbors, 2003). The earliest clinical manifestation may be a change in mental status, such as confusion and restlessness. Other clinical manifestations include hypoxemia, rapid respirations, increased pulse, chest pain, and the classic petechiae on the neck, chest, and axilla (this occurs in approximately 50 percent of cases). The patient may appear apprehensive and have a feeling of doom. A fat embolism is a life-threatening event that often results in death.

NURSING DIAGNOSIS 1

IMPAIRED GAS EXCHANGE

Related to:

Obstruction of pulmonary vasculature

Defining Characteristics:

Tachypnea

Decreased arterial pO_2

Decreased or normal pCO_2

Cyanosis

Petechiae

Severe dyspnea

Agitation

Decreased oxygen saturation

Goal:

Gas exchange is adequate.

Outcome Criteria

✔ ABGs return to baseline or normal and oxygen saturation is > 90 percent.

✔ The patient's skin color returns to normal baseline color.

✔ Respiratory rate is within baseline (12–24).

✔ The patient reports no dyspnea/shortness of breath.

✔ The patient exhibits no agitation or restlessness.

NOC *Respiratory status: Ventilation*
Respiratory status: Gas exchange
Vital signs

INTERVENTIONS	RATIONALES
Assess respiratory status: respiratory rate, rhythm, depth, oxygen saturation, dyspnea, panic/air hunger, breath sounds, quality, and effort.	Establishes baseline information about respiratory function.
Perform cardiovascular assessment: cardiac rate, presence of petechiae, vital signs, skin color/cyanosis, and peripheral perfusion (pedal pulses, capillary refill).	Establishes a baseline and determines what effects the fat emboli and impaired gas exchange have on cardiac function.

INTERVENTIONS	RATIONALES
Perform a neurological assessment: note decreasing level of consciousness, restlessness, anxiety, confusion, and agitation.	Establishes a baseline and determines effects on cerebral function; often, changes in mental status are early indicators of fat emboli, indicating decreased oxygenation of cerebral tissues.
Assess oxygen saturation using pulse oximetry and arterial blood gases (ABGs), as ordered.	Determines status of oxygen to tissues and allows monitoring for respiratory acidosis.
Monitor ordered laboratory tests: hematocrit and hemoglobin, platelets, serum triglycerides, ABGs, sputum for fat globules, urinalysis (free fat in urine), and chest x-ray.	In fat emboli, hemoglobin decreases with sequestration of red blood cells in fat; platelets decrease to < 150,000 due to hemodilution and because of platelet aggregation at the site of fat emboli. These changes in hemoglobin and platelets indicate a positive diagnosis for fat emboli. Fat cells may be present in the blood, urine, and sputum. ABGs will reveal decreased oxygen levels, often as low as 60. Chest x-ray will demonstrate atelectasis and pulmonary infiltrates.
Provide supplemental high flow oxygen via non-rebreather mask, as ordered; monitor for improvement, and if none noted, consider endotracheal intubation and mechanical ventilation.	Maximizes oxygen saturation and relieves hypoxemia and shortness of breath.
Place in high Fowler's position.	This position allows for better chest expansion and subsequent air exchange.
Establish intravenous access and administer fluids as ordered.	Intravenous access is required to administer corticosteroids and in case of emergency; fluid resuscitation may also need to be implemented; due to the clotting disorders caused by decreased circulating platelets, the patient may need blood products.
Give medications, such as corticosteroids, as ordered.	Decreases inflammation that occurs with the presence of foreign substances in the lungs.
Have patient perform coughing and deep breathing if able.	Enhances gas exchange and opening of alveoli.
Limit movement and repositioning if affected bone has not been stabilized or immobilized.	Frequent movement could dislodge additional fat globules into the circulatory system.
Provide for bedrest and assist with activities as needed.	Conserves oxygen reserves and prevents exacerbation of hypoxemia.
Implement strategies to decrease anxiety, such as controlled deep breathing, playing soft music, therapeutic touch, presence of family, staying with patient during crisis, and spiritual consult.	The patient feels a sense of doom and with dyspnea may begin to panic; the patient needs to relax to decrease oxygen demands.

NIC *Oxygen therapy*
Respiratory monitoring
Acid/base management:
*   Respiratory acidosis*
Positioning

Evaluation

Evaluate the status of outcome criteria. The patient should have indicators of good gas exchange such as even, easy respirations, good skin color, and an oxygen saturation of at least 90 percent. Blood gas analyses should indicate an absence of respiratory acidosis and oxygen levels between 80–100 percent. The patient should report an absence of shortness of breath and respirations should be within baseline. Mental status should return to baseline levels and the patient should not be restless or agitated. Skin changes of petechiae are resolved.

Community/Home Care

For patients who have experienced fat emboli, impaired gas exchange is resolved during acute hospitalization with no long-term effects. Typically, no follow-up care is required once the respiratory problem has been resolved except as it relates to the initial bone injury event. At home, the patient may notice some activity intolerance as a result of being hospitalized, but this should resolve quickly. The patient should be encouraged to pace activities and take rest periods to conserve energy until usual level of energy or stamina have returned. If fatigue or any shortness of breath persists, the patient should contact a health care provider.

Documentation

Include in the documentation a complete respiratory assessment with specific attention to skin color, effort of breathing, breath sounds, neurological changes, presence of petechiae, and patient's level of comfort with breathing. Chart all interventions and the patient's specific response in terms of respiratory status. Results of oxygen saturation readings and ABGs should be documented as they represent the best measure of gas exchange. If the patient still has indicators of impaired gas exchange, these should be specifically noted along with the planned revisions to the plan of care.

NURSING DIAGNOSIS 2

 ## ANXIETY

Related to:

Severe shortness of breath

Severity of illness

Feeling of doom

Defining Characteristics:

Restlessness

Verbalization of anxiety

Verbalization of fear

Goal:

Anxiety is relieved.

Outcome Criteria

✔ The patient verbalizes that anxiety has been reduced.

✔ The patient reports feeling relaxed.

✔ The patient has no physiological signs of anxiety.

NOC *Anxiety control*

INTERVENTIONS	RATIONALES
Have the patient rate anxiety on a numerical scale if possible.	Allows for a more objective measure of anxiety level.
Provide oxygen, as ordered.	With assistance to breathe easier, the patient faces less physical stress (physical stress can lead to anxiety).
Implement strategies to manage respiratory status (see nursing diagnosis "Impaired Gas Exchange").	Correction of the alterations in respiratory status will help to reduce anxiety level.
Reassure the patient by explaining what is happening and treatments that are being implemented to correct the problem.	Inability to breathe contributes to anxiety because of the fear that interventions may not work quickly enough; knowing what to expect helps the patient maintain control.
Encourage the patient to verbalize concerns.	Verbalizing concerns can help patient cope with anxiety and avoid negative feelings.
Stay with patient during the crisis event and until respiratory status has improved, and use a calm manner.	Allows the nurse to offer comfort, care, and assurances that help is available, which can reduce anxiety and fear.
Allow family or significant other to visit liberally if the patient so desires.	Family and significant other may provide emotional support that calms the patient and promotes a sense of comfort.
Teach the patient relaxation techniques (such as guided imagery, playing soft music) and encourage their use.	Reduces anxiety and creates a feeling of comfort.
Provide spiritual consult as requested.	A chaplain may be able to provide spiritual comfort and reduce anxiety.
Administer anti-anxiety medications as ordered.	If non-pharmacological measures do not work, medications may be needed to reduce anxiety and decrease oxygen demands during the crisis period.

NIC *Anxiety reduction*
Calming technique
Emotional support
Presence

Evaluation

Assess the extent to which the patient is free of anxiety. The patient should verbalize that anxiety is reduced and that he or she feels comfortable. Assess the patient for physiological signs of anxiety, such as increased pulse and sweating. During evaluation, be sure to inquire about the use of relaxation techniques. The patient will also need to report that he or she understands what is happening in terms of his or her current respiratory status and the fat embolus.

Community/Home Care

Once the patient's acute respiratory status improves, the anxiety should resolve. However, in some instances the patient may be fearful that a fat embolus may occur again. The patient needs to understand the pathophysiological process that caused the emboli and the sequelae of events that followed. It is important that health care providers equip the patient with this knowledge so that the patient feels in control when discharged home. Encourage the use of simple relaxation techniques at home, such as taking a walk, reading, using guided imagery, and deep breathing. Meditation can also be used in the home to slow breathing and create a sense of peace; having the patient rest in an easy chair with eyes closed and drift away mentally is a method of meditation that can calm and soothe. The issue of anxiety should only be temporary.

Documentation

Document the degree of anxiety experienced by the patient. Using some type of numerical rating scale similar to the pain scale will provide health care providers with a more objective measure of the degree of anxiety the patient is experiencing. Document any physiological or observable signs of anxiety, such as restlessness, tachycardia, or diaphoresis. Interventions implemented to treat these should be documented along with subsequent assessments to determine their effectiveness.

NURSING DIAGNOSIS 3

ACUTE PAIN

Related to:

Occlusion of pulmonary vasculature

Defining Characteristics:

Complaint of sharp chest pain

Increased pain with respirations

Grimacing and moaning

Goal:

Pain has been relieved.

Outcome Criteria

✔ The patient will verbalize that pain has been relieved 30 minutes after interventions.

✔ The patient will verbalize an understanding of what causes pain.

NOC   *Pain level*
         Pain control
         Comfort level

INTERVENTIONS	RATIONALES
Assess for location, intensity, quality, and precipitating factors.	Identifying these will assist in accurate diagnosis and treatment; not all patients who experience a fat embolus will have pain, but many will due to the infarction of the pulmonary circulation and as the lungs progressively are unable to oxygenate.
Have the patient rate pain intensity using a pain rating scale.	Provides a more objective description of level of pain.
Assess respiratory status, including breath sounds and respiratory rate.	Helps to monitor for early signs of respiratory complications; atelectasis and pneumonitis may occur due to inflammation of lung tissue secondary to presence of fat molecules; respiratory rate is increased due to the emboli but may increase further in the presence of pain.
Administer analgesics, such as morphine, as ordered.	Narcotics may be used not only for pain control but also to decrease respiratory rate, anxiety, and oxygen demand.
Implement strategies to improve respiratory status (see nursing diagnosis "Impaired Gas Exchange").	Treating the underlying cause will alleviate the pain.
Implement strategies to reduce anxiety (see nursing diagnosis "Anxiety").	Anxiety often intensifies the pain experience.
Assess effectiveness of interventions to relieve pain.	Helps to determine whether interventions have been effective in relieving pain or whether new strategies need to be employed.

NIC   *Pain management*
       Analgesic administration
       Anxiety reduction

Evaluation

The patient is able to report that the pain has been reduced or alleviated following interventions. The degree to which the patient is able to assist in the management of the pain through anxiety reduction and relaxation techniques is assessed. The patient should appear calm and have no observable signs of being uncomfortable.

Community/Home Care

The patient's pain should be temporary and be resolved once respiratory function improves. Home care is not required for pain except as it relates to the initial injury (fracture, surgery, etc.). It is important that the patient understand why he or she experienced the pain. Reassurances by the health care provider that the pain should not recur need to be given prior to discharge. Mild analgesics may be taken, but the need for them should resolve quickly. The patient, however, will need to know what type of respiratory symptoms or new types of pain manifestations would require him or her to return to the physician.

Documentation

Document in the patient's own words the description of the pain and rating of the level of pain. Chart all interventions (pharmacological and non-pharmacological) employed and the patient's response. Include in the documentation assessments made relevant to the pain and to the respiratory system.

CHAPTER 4.55

FRACTURE: LIMB

GENERAL INFORMATION

A fracture is a disruption or break of a bone usually caused by a traumatic event, such as a motor vehicle crash, a sports injury, or a fall. The bone breaks due to direct or indirect force or stress applied to the bone that the bone is not able to tolerate. Fractures are divided into two major categories: closed or simple fractures (no skin disruption) and open or compound fractures (skin is disrupted). Open fractures have the added risk of infection due to the open traumatic wound. In addition, there are nine types of fractures: transverse (from an angulation force or direct blunt trauma), oblique (from a severe twisting force), spiral (from a twisting force with a planted distal part), comminuted (from severe direct trauma or impact trauma), impacted (from a force that jams the bone), compression (severe force from an injury forces the bone segments to be wedged against each other), greenstick (compression force that causes partial fracture), avulsion (when muscle contracts forcefully, bone is torn away near the area of muscle insertion), and depression (from blunt trauma to a flat bone). Severity of clinical manifestations is determined by the location and type of fracture sustained; manifestations may include pain, loss of mobility of the affected extremity, swelling at the site, deformity of the extremity, warmth over the site, crepitus over area when moved, and possible loss of feeling.

NURSING DIAGNOSIS 1

 IMPAIRED PHYSICAL MOBILITY

Related to:

Fracture

Pain

Casts

Traction

Defining Characteristics:

Physical restriction

Inability to move

Decreased range of motion

Instability of fractured extremity

Goal:

The patient obtains physical mobility to the highest possible level.

Outcome Criteria

✔ The patient demonstrates gradual improvement in muscle tone, strength, and control.

✔ The patient can use adjunctive devices to assist mobility.

✔ The patient verbalizes a willingness to participate in physical therapy as prescribed.

INTERVENTIONS	RATIONALES
Support and immobilize extremity, including joint above and below the fracture site: use a splint or other immobilizing materials.	Immobilization will prevent further damage that would occur if bony ends were allowed to move freely or were inadvertently moved by a caregiver; decreases movement of fractured bone ends and prevents tissue trauma.
Maintain proper alignment.	Proper alignment promotes maximum neurological and vascular function.
Check results of diagnostic tests: x-rays, computed tomography (CT) scan, MRI (magnetic resonance imaging).	These exams confirm the diagnosis, exact location, and severity of injury.
Assist with traction set-up as ordered, and maintain according to protocol, but in general keep appropriate weights attached as ordered and	Traction returns the fractured extremity to correct alignment, provides stabilization until surgery or casting can occur, and helps to decrease muscle

(continues)

399

(continued)

INTERVENTIONS	RATIONALES
seek assistance from physical therapy as required: — Skeletal traction: Assess skin at pin or wire insertion site for redness, drainage, and increased tenderness; perform pin or wire care according to agency protocol; maintain weights at 10–30 lbs as ordered. — Skin traction: Assess skin for pressure points; for lower extremities keep heel of foot off bed to prevent skin breakdown; maintain weights (5–10 lbs) off floor. — Be sure that ropes are in center of pulleys. — Keep the patient in center of the bed. — Encourage the patient to shift weight every 2 hours to prevent skin breakdown. — Be sure weights hang free and do not touch floor. — Assess neurovascular status of extremity (see nursing diagnosis "Risk for Peripheral Neurovascular Dysfunction).	spasms: skeletal traction is indicated for long-term stabilization (several weeks); skin traction is used for shorter terms (48–72 hours).
Assist with cast or splint application as ordered or according to agency protocol.	Following fracture reduction (if necessary), maintains alignment and promotes bone healing. Splints are used when edema is anticipated or present to prevent neuromuscular compromise.
For patients in casts, implement the following and teach patient and family: — Keep cast dry. — If itching occurs, use a hair dryer on cool setting to blow air into the cast; inform patient not to attempt to scratch under cast by using objects placed into the cast. — Perform neurovascular checks every 4 hours (see nursing diagnosis "Risk for Peripheral Neurovascular Dysfunction"). — Wet casts: Allow cast to dry completely before touching or palpating; if it is necessary	These interventions allow for proper functioning of casts, prevent complications, and promote patient comfort.
to move before drying, use palm of hands rather than fingertips, which could cause indentations; do not cover wet cast with covers (prevents air circulation and causes increased heat inside cast); inform patient that extremity and cast will feel warm during the drying process. — Petal cast (application of waterproof strips/tape to protect skin) once dry to avoid skin irritation from rough edges. — Assist with or reinforce teaching by physical therapist on crutch walking.	
Assess for neurovascular complications (see nursing diagnosis "Risk for Peripheral Neurovascular Dysfunction").	Neurovascular compromise may occur due to constriction of the extremity by edema or by casts, taping, or supportive devices.
Provide physical therapy consult for physical and occupational therapy.	Helps to assess the patient's ability and to maintain maximum range of motion and muscle function.
Maintain positions of function using hand rolls, splints, leg rolls (trochanter rolls), foot board.	Maintains maximum positions of function and prevents foot drop.
Encourage early ambulation and/or mobility as directed by the physical therapist and reduce length of bedrest.	Early mobilization will prevent complications of immobility, including pneumonia, skin breakdown, urinary tract infection, thrombophlebitis, and deep vein thrombosis (DVT).
Keep head of bed no higher than 30 degrees if in traction.	Elevating higher than this minimizes the pull of the traction, decreasing its ability to stabilize or realign the bone.
Encourage the patient to exercise unaffected extremities by doing range of motion and isometric exercises as directed by physical therapy.	Exercising the unaffected extremity helps prevent complications of immobility and maintains strength.
Instruct on proper use of assistive devices, such as trapeze bars, and encourage their use.	Maintains some independence with movement in bed.
Assist with or reinforce teaching regarding traction.	Many patients have questions about what they can and cannot do when in traction; answering their questions and addressing their concerns decreases anxiety and enhances compliance.

INTERVENTIONS	RATIONALES
Administer pain medications before physical therapy.	The patient will be more likely to participate if pain-free.
Prepare patient for operative procedures as ordered (open reduction with internal fixations).	Some fractures will require surgical interventions to repair broken bones with pins, screws, or plates.
Following surgery, implement measures to promote activity as ordered or prescribed in collaboration with physical therapy.	The patient will need assistance with mobility to prevent injury to repaired extremity and to promote return to normal function without complications.
Assess patient for signs and symptoms of fat embolus, such as agitation, restlessness, petechiae, shortness of breath, or rapid respirations (see nursing care plan "Fat Embolism").	Patients with long bone fractures are at risk for the release of fat molecules from the marrow of the bone into the circulation. These travel to small vessels in the lung, causing symptoms of respiratory distress, and may also go to microvessels of the brain where they impair cerebral oxygenation, producing changes in mental status.
Teach the patient about activity restrictions, activity requirements for rehabilitation, and cast care.	An informed patient is more likely to be compliant with recommendations; the patient will need to be responsible for activity and mobility at home, and teaching by the physical therapist can enhance ability to be independent.

NIC   *Cast care: Wet*

Cast care: Maintenance

Traction/immobilization care

Positioning

Exercise therapy: Ambulation

Exercise therapy: Joint mobility

Teaching: Prescribed
activity/exercise

Evaluation

Evaluate the degree to which the patient has achieved the stated outcome criteria. The patient should verbalize an understanding of interventions utilized to achieve stabilization of the fracture. Mobility is maximized through use of assistive devices or physical therapy. The patient participates in ordered physical therapy and maintains strength and control of all extremities. No deformities occur secondary to immobility.

Community/Home Care

The patient who has sustained a fracture will require some adaptations in performance of activities once at home. For the patient who has a cast, safety at home will be an issue as casts create an imbalance of weight on one side, making ambulation difficult at first. Even though crutches may be available, their use will require some trial and error, during which time the patient is at higher risk for falling. The environment will need to be assessed to determine how the patient can maneuver safely. Look for factors such as distance to bathroom, presence of steps, and excessive furniture or clutter that may pose a risk. Be sure that the patient knows how to use any assistive devices, such as slings. Nursing care may not be necessary, but physical therapy may be of assistance in ensuring that the patient can implement strategies to remain mobile, perform activities of daily living (ADLs), and prevent complications or deformities due to disuse. At home, the patient may need to alter clothing to accommodate the presence of a cast. Women can wear skirts or dresses for easy dressing. Some pajama pants and scrubs have wider legs than regular pants and will be easier to manipulate. Athletic shorts are another option. Prior to discharge from the hospital or emergency room, the patient should be questioned about ability to function in the home in terms of self-care requirements in order to determine whether in-home physical therapy may be indicated. The patient and family will need instruction on the use of crutches and other assistive devices as well as signs and symptoms of infection, DVT, and compartment syndrome. The patient will need to understand the critical importance of following prescribed instructions for exercise and physical therapy. Follow-up care for x-rays to determine healing will be necessary.

Documentation

Chart the presence and correct functioning of all devices used for stabilization of the joint, such as traction and casts. Document all interventions employed and the patient's responses to them. Include in the patient chart the findings from a thorough assessment of the patient's musculoskeletal functioning, particularly with respect to neurovascular function (see also nursing care plan "Fat Embolism"). Any complaints that the patient verbalizes should be documented to include interventions employed to correct the problem. If the patient is scheduled for surgery, document pre- and post-operative assessments and preparations according to agency protocol. Rely on the physical therapist to document implementation of physical therapy activities, but document any other relevant activity or follow-up reinforcement of physical therapy teachings.

NURSING DIAGNOSIS 2

 ### ACUTE PAIN

Related to:

Fracture of bone

Bone fragment movement

Fracture ends grating (crepitus)

Muscle spasms

Orthopedic appliances

Defining Characteristics:

Complaints of pain

Obvious signs of trauma

Grimacing and moaning

Goal:

The patient's pain is relieved.

Outcome Criteria

✔ The patient will verbalize that pain has been relieved 30 minutes after interventions.

✔ The patient will verbalize an understanding of what is causing the pain.

NOC *Pain level*

Pain control

Comfort level

INTERVENTIONS	RATIONALES
Assess for location, intensity, quality, and precipitating factors.	Identifying these will assist in accurate diagnosis and treatment; most patients who experience fractures experience some pain, especially with movement.
Have the patient rate pain intensity using a pain rating scale.	Provides a more objective description of the level of pain.
Assess status of affected extremity, including pain at injury site, tenderness to touch, temperature, and edema.	Allows detection of early signs of neurovascular dysfunction; patients with fractures are at risk for impaired circulation and altered nervous innervation to the extremity (see nursing diagnosis "Risk for Peripheral Vascular Dysfunction").
Administer analgesics as ordered on a regular schedule; do not allow pain to get intense; narcotics via patient-controlled analgesia (PCA) may be required for a period of time.	Decreased pain will improve the patient's ability to participate in physical therapy activities required for improved mobility.
Move the patient's extremity gently and cautiously.	Movement of affected extremity causes pain; careful movement provides support for the painful area.
Maintain traction as ordered (see nursing diagnosis "Impaired Physical Mobility").	Maintains stability of the fractured joint and decreases muscle spasms.
Elevate fractured extremity.	Elevation will reduce edema.
Apply ice packs: 20 minutes on, 20 minutes off for first 48 hours.	Ice reduces swelling through vasoconstriction and reduces pain.
Assess for pressure points in cast, splint, and traction; pad or alleviate pressure points to reduce pain.	Treating the underlying cause will alleviate the pain.
Implement strategies to reduce anxiety, such as staying with the patient, using relaxation techniques, playing soft music.	Anxiety often intensifies the pain experience.
Investigate the use of diversional activities.	Decreases the attention or focus on the pain.
Encourage the patient to change position.	Improves circulation; reduces pressure points.
Administer muscle relaxants, as ordered.	Relaxes muscles and reduces pain.
Vigilantly monitor patient for sudden onset of chest pain or limb pain.	The sudden onset of pain may be indicative of another process, such as infection, pulmonary embolus, fat embolus, or compartment syndrome.
Assess effectiveness of interventions to relieve pain.	Helps to determine whether interventions have been effective in relieving pain or whether new strategies need to be employed.

NIC *Pain management*
       Analgesic administration
       Anxiety reduction

Evaluation

The patient is able to report that the pain has been reduced or alleviated following interventions. The degree to which the patient is able to assist in the management of the pain through anxiety reduction and relaxation techniques is assessed. The patient should appear calm and have no observable signs of discomfort. If pain is controlled, the patient is able to participate in mobility activities prescribed and implemented by physical therapy.

Community/Home Care

The patient's pain should decrease once the fracture has been stabilized and realigned by surgery, casting, or traction and should completely resolve once fractures heal. Because simpler fractures that do not require surgery or traction may be treated on an outpatient basis, teaching should be done to give the patient the information needed to manage pain. Pain is usually managed with mild to moderate analgesics given orally, and the length of time the patient has pain will vary. The patient can use non-pharmacological measures to enhance the effect of the analgesics. The patient needs to monitor response to pain medications and be able to identify those factors or positions that increase pain. If the patient is receiving physical therapy, it should be suggested that he or she take analgesics prior to therapy. Encourage the patient to use assistive devices such as splints and crutches to relieve pressure on the affected site. The patient should be instructed to notify a health care provider if sudden onset of calf pain or chest pain occurs as these may signal complications of DVT, fat embolus, or pulmonary embolus. The patient may find comfort in elevating the extremity when sitting if not contraindicated. If the recommended analgesics are not working, the patient should seek follow-up care with the health care provider.

Documentation

Document in the patient's own words the description of the pain, the exact location, and the patient's rating of the level of pain. In addition, record exactly what the patient was doing before the onset of pain. Chart all interventions employed and the patient's responses. Include in the documentation assessments made relevant to the pain.

NURSING DIAGNOSIS 3

RISK FOR PERIPHERAL NEUROVASCULAR DYSFUNCTION

Related to:

   Possible constriction and pressure due to edema

   Nerve damage due to instability of fractured limb

   Excess pressure within a cast

Defining Characteristics:

   None

Goal:

   Neurovascular function is maintained.

Outcome Criteria

✔ Peripheral pulses in extremity are palpable.

✔ Extremity is warm with capillary refill brisk at < 3 seconds.

✔ The patient's extremity remains at normal color.

✔ The patient experiences no severe pain at injury site.

NOC *Circulation status*
        Mobility
        Tissue perfusion: Peripheral

INTERVENTIONS	RATIONALES
Assess neurovascular status of both extremities every 1–2 hours or as ordered: pulses, sensation, temperature, capillary refill, and movement.	Establishes a baseline and then detects early any complications that may occur due to surgery, casting, edema, traction, or initial injury; if pallor, paresthesia, or coolness to touch are found on assessment, these are indicators of decreased nuerovascular funtion
Assess for signs and symptoms of compartment syndrome: severe pain unrelieved by usual	Unrelenting pain not relieved by usual analgesic is the early classic sign of compartment

(continues)

(continued)

INTERVENTIONS	RATIONALES
analgesic, diminished or absent pulses, cool extremity, decreased or absent sensation in the extremity, loss of normal color, and decreased capillary refill.	syndrome; later symptoms, such as absence or diminished pulses, pallor, coolness, and slow capillary refill, usually indicate irreparable damage. The patient may report a change in sensation that could range from numbness to a feeling of pins and needles as nerves become compressed. Early attention to prevention of compartment syndrome is critical to preserve extremity function; early detection by frequent assessments leads to early identification and early treatment.
Monitor vital signs with particular attention to blood pressure readings.	A patient must maintain sufficient blood pressure in order to maintain perfusion to the affected extremity compartments.
Assist with invasive monitoring procedures such as compartmental pressure readings, as ordered or required by agency protocol.	Helps to obtain an accurate measurement of pressures within the compartments of the affected extremity and to allow for early detection and treatment; this is especially useful in unconscious patients who are unable to report or verbalize complaints that would point to compartment syndrome. Normal compartment pressures are 0–10 mm of Hg, and when elevated pressures of 30–40 mm of Hg persist, compartment syndrome is likely to occur.
Maintain cast and check for tightness.	Casts that are too tight may lead to compartment syndrome by causing undue pressure on the compartments of the extremity.
Check extremity for excess edema or tightness; ask patient about feeling of constriction.	Edema that is unrelieved through elevation could lead to compartment syndrome due to a poor venous system that is unable to handle the outflow of excess of fluid; as the fluid continues to accumulate, pressure is applied to nerves in the extremity.
If compartment syndrome does develop, implement strategies or assist with strategies to relieve pressure as ordered. These include cast cutting and fasciotomy (surgical interventions).	Casts are removed, cut, or bivalved by the physician to relieve pressure, following which interventions to maintain stability of fracture, such as splints, are employed until the cast can be reapplied. If the compartment syndrome is caused by pressures within the extremity due to edema, a fasciotomy is performed, which cuts the fascia of the extremity to allow for pressure release. The wound is left open and requires sterile dressing changes with sterile normal saline.
Elevate extremity if not contraindicated.	Elevation assists with venous return that reduces edema.

NIC *Peripheral sensation management*
Positioning: Neurologic
Cast care maintenance
Circulatory precautions

Evaluation

The patient should be evaluated to determine whether neurovascular status is maintained. Evaluate whether physiological indicators such as peripheral pulse, skin color, temperature, sensation, and capillary refill are normal. Assess the patient for undue pain that seems too severe for the injury and is unrelieved by analgesics. All patient parameters relevant to the status of the injured extremity should be normal or near normal.

Community/Home Care

Neurovascular problems usually occur during the early stages of injury to the extremity but can be recurring. The patient and family need to be able to recognize signs and symptoms that would indicate the possibility of compartment syndrome that would necessitate a return for emergency follow-up care. It is important that the patient understand how to relieve and prevent edema in the extremity. The patient is taught to change positions frequently and elevate the extremity when sitting in a chair unless contraindicated. Inspection of the cast, skin above the cast, and the toes or fingers should be done daily. Ambulation and participation in physical therapy as ordered once at home should be stressed. A nurse may not be required, but follow-up visits with a health care provider are necessary to be sure that the extremity is healing properly and that there are no long-term neurovascular alterations.

Documentation

Chart findings from a thorough neurovascular assessment, including peripheral pulses, extremity color, sensation, pain, and capillary refill. Always include nursing interventions implemented to prevent compartment syndrome, and if the syndrome occurs, chart interventions initiated for treatment. Include in the patient's chart the patient's responses to all interventions and any specific concerns verbalized.

NURSING DIAGNOSIS 4

IMPAIRED SKIN INTEGRITY

Related to:

> Open wound that occurred at the time of injury
>
> Pressure points from splint, cast, traction, bedrest
>
> Skeletal traction appliance insertion sites
>
> Surgical incision site(s)

Defining Characteristics:

> Reddened, sore, or broken-down areas
>
> Broken skin over injury site
>
> Surgical incisions
>
> History of dirty wound
>
> Major crash injury and soft tissue trauma
>
> Decreased sensation/movement
>
> Foul smell
>
> Elevated white blood count
>
> Complaint of pain, pressure, numbness

Goal:

> The patient's skin will heal, and infection is prevented.

Outcome Criteria

✔ The patient's skin is intact.

✔ Skin pressure point signs are gone.

✔ The patient's wounds/incisions show no signs of infection, such as redness or other discoloration, odor, excessive pain, or purulent drainage.

NOC   *Wound healing: Primary intention*

INTERVENTIONS	RATIONALES
Monitor wounds and pressure points.	Detects signs of skin breakdown and infections.
Monitor surgical site and any drainage apparatus insertion sites for signs and symptoms of infection: redness or other discoloration, swelling, purulent drainage.	Early identification of infection can expedite treatment.
Maintain patency of drainage devices and assess drainage from Hemovac drains or other drainage tubes for amount, color, and consistency.	The drainage device helps drain secretions from surgical area; if not draining properly, the drainage may build up providing an excellent medium for bacteria growth.
Take temperature every 4 hours.	Detects signs of infection.
Monitor results of white blood cell counts.	White blood cells elevate in the presence of active infection.
Change dressings as ordered and clean area using sterile technique, cleansing site of drainage devices last.	Maintenance of a clean incisional site decreases number of organisms and reduces chance of infection.
Administer antipyretics (acetaminophen [Tylenol]) as ordered.	Reduces fever.
Administer antibiotics, as ordered via IV or PO (by mouth).	Prevents or treats infection by reducing number of infective organisms.
Administer NSAIDs, as ordered.	Reduces local inflammation; increases immune response.
Avoid pressure points whenever possible by frequently repositioning the patient.	Repositioning will remove pressure from specific areas of the body.
Keep cast/splint dry and non-frayed: bivalve or replace.	Use hair dryer or room air to keep casting/splinting materials dry. Petal cast edges and repair frayed cast edges to prevent tissue breakdown/necrosis.
Provide proper care at skin traction site: carefully wash, dry, and apply antibiotic ointment as ordered.	Prevents infection.

(continues)

(continued)

INTERVENTIONS	RATIONALES
Encourage adequate nutritional intake of protein, vitamin C, and iron, whether orally, parenterally, or enterally.	Adequate nutrient intake, especially of vitamin C, protein, and iron, is required for healing and tissue repair.

NIC   *Incision site care*

        Infection control

        Nutrition management

        Wound care

        Wound care: Closed drainage

Evaluation

Evaluate the degree to which the outcome criteria have been met. The surgical site should be intact, healing by primary intention with incision well approximated. Redness or other discoloration, swelling, purulent drainage, and heat should be absent from the site. Drainage from the drainage devices should be serosanguineous and decreasing in amount. The patient should be afebrile, and white blood cell counts should return to normal. There should be no odor or increased pain in affected limbs, especially areas beneath casts.

Community/Home Care

The status of the surgical site or wound injury may remain a problem after the patient has been discharged home. The risk for infection remains, and the family will need to know what symptoms may signal the onset of infection. The family will need to inspect the injury sites for redness or other discoloration, drainage, heat at the site, a wound that opens, or edema. Health care providers need to ensure that the family and/or patient know how to take a temperature and should be encouraged to do so if the patient feels unusually warm. Whether the patient has a cast or has had open reduction and internal fixation, he or she will need to be taught how to care for it, especially how to properly cover when showering/bathing. The patient will need to understand the importance of good nutrition in complete wound and bone healing. Completing any ordered medications, such as antibiotics, should be stressed. The patient should be instructed to contact the health care provider immediately if the wound opens, if pain significantly increases, or if any evidence of infection occurs.

Documentation

Document assessment findings from the wound, including color, approximation, temperature, and pulses, being sure to note any sign of infection. Chart the status of drainage devices or tubes indicating the color, amount, and consistency of drainage. Document vital signs according to agency protocol as ordered for post-operative patients. If antipyretics are given, chart these according to protocol, and document follow-up temperatures when obtained. Include the patient's and family's understanding of the signs and symptoms of infection in the patient record.

CHAPTER 4.56

FRACTURE: PELVIS

GENERAL INFORMATION

A fracture is a disruption or break of a bone usually caused by a traumatic event, such as a motor vehicle crash, a sports injury, or a fall. The bone breaks due to direct or indirect force or stress applied to the bone that the bone is not able to tolerate. Fractures are divided into two major categories: closed or simple fractures (no skin disruption) and open or compound fractures (skin is disrupted). Open fractures have the added risk of infection due to the open traumatic wound. Severity of clinical manifestations are determined by the location and type of fracture sustained and may include pain, loss of mobility of the affected extremity, swelling at the site, deformity of the extremity, and warmth over the site. Pelvic fractures usually occur because of motor vehicle crashes (including motorcycles), crush injuries, or falls (from a height). Pelvic fracture is the most common orthopedic injury because of multiple trauma. There are several common locations of pelvic fractures: the iliac wings, the inferior pubic rami, and the superior pubic rami, and combinations of these. A major concern with pelvic fractures is the possibility of hemorrhage, which is the leading cause of death for those who sustain a pelvic fracture leading to death. This occurs due to the shearing force of the injury that damages internal structures and ruptures blood vessels. Clinical manifestations include swelling at the site, redness on the abdomen, pain in the back or abdominal area, and leg length abnormality. Trauma to internal organs may manifest itself as blood in the urine, bruising on the abdominal wall or around the scrotum, or blood in the stool.

NURSING DIAGNOSIS 1

 IMPAIRED PHYSICAL MOBILITY

Related to:

Fracture

Pain

Casts

Traction

Defining Characteristics:

Physical restriction

Inability to move

Decreased range of motion

Instability of fractured pelvis

Goal:

The patient obtains physical mobility to the highest permissible level.

Outcome Criteria

✔ The patient demonstrates gradual improvement in muscle tone, strength, and control.

✔ The patient can use adjunctive devices to assist mobility.

✔ The patient verbalizes a willingness to participate in physical therapy as prescribed.

✔ The patient demonstrates correct technique for mobility with splint, cast, or traction.

✔ The patient has no signs of complications from fracture such as hemorrhage, fat emboli, or compartment syndrome.

INTERVENTIONS	RATIONALES
For stable pelvic fractures, implement activity as ordered; bedrest on a firm mattress for a few days may be ordered.	Immobilization will prevent further damage that would occur if bone fragments were loose.
Maintain proper alignment and stabilize fracture with use of external fixator or pelvic sling.	Proper alignment promotes maximum neurological and vascular function.
Check results of diagnostic tests: x-rays, computed tomography (CT) scan, MRI (magnetic resonance imaging).	These exams confirm the diagnosis, exact location, and severity of injury.

(continues)

(continued)

INTERVENTIONS	RATIONALES
Assist with external fixation/traction set-up as ordered, and maintain according to protocol, but in general keep appropriate weights attached as ordered and seek assistance from physical therapy as required: — Skeletal traction: Assess skin at pin or wire insertion site for redness, drainage, and increased tenderness; perform pin or wire care according to agency protocol; maintain weights at 10–30 lbs as ordered. — Skin traction: Assess skin for pressure points; maintain weights (5–10 lbs) off floor. — Be sure that ropes are in center of pulleys. — Keep the patient in center of the bed. — Encourage the patient to shift weight every 2 hours to prevent skin breakdown. — Be sure weights hang free and do not touch floor. — Assess neurovascular status of extremities for any indications of compartment syndrome secondary to cast (see nursing diagnosis "Risk for Peripheral Neurovascular Dysfunction").	Traction returns the fractured pelvis to correct alignment, provides stabilization until surgery or casting can occur, helps to decrease muscle spasms: skeletal traction is indicated for long-term stabilization (several weeks); skin traction is used for shorter terms (48–72 hours).
Provide physical therapy consult for physical and occupational therapy.	Helps to assess the patient's ability and to maintain maximum range of motion and muscle function.
Turn the patient every two hours only if ordered by physician, handling the patient gently using logrolling technique.	To prevent pressure points, careful handling is needed to prevent injury to tissues from displaced fragments; logrolling is the most comfortable for changing positions.
Encourage early ambulation and/or mobility with crutches or walkers for patients with nondisplaced fractures as directed by the physical therapist.	Early mobilization will prevent complications of immobility including pneumonia, skin breakdown, urinary tract infection, thrombophlebitis, and deep vein thrombosis (DVT).

INTERVENTIONS	RATIONALES
Assist with spica cast application, traction set-up, or pelvic sling use as ordered or according to agency protocol.	Maintains alignment and promotes healing. Pelvic slings are used when the patient is not able to go to surgery for repair and stabilizes the pelvis allowing for movement in bed; spica casts immobilize the trunk.
For patients in casts, implement and teach the patient and family the following: — Keep cast dry. — If itching occurs, use a hairdryer on cool setting to blow air into the cast; inform patient not to attempt to scratch under cast by using objects placed into the cast. — Perform neurovascular checks every 4 hours (see nursing diagnosis "Risk for Peripheral Neurovascular Dysfunction"). — Wet casts: Allow cast to dry completely before touching or palpating; if it is necessary to move before drying, use palms of hands rather than fingertips, which could cause indentations; do not cover wet cast with covers (prevents air circulation and causes increased heat inside cast); inform patient that extremity and cast will feel warm during the drying process. — Petal cast (application of waterproof strips/tape to protect skin) once dry to avoid skin irritation from rough edges. — If in a double hip spica cast, the support bar on the cast should not be used for assisting in turning. — Assess the patient for indications that the cast might be too tight or compressing the abdominal cavity (abdominal pain, abdominal pressure, nausea, vomiting, decreased bowel sounds).	These interventions will allow for proper functioning of casts, prevent complications or provide for early detection of complications, and promote patient comfort.
Maintain proper patient positioning while in traction.	Maximizes proper bone alignment.

INTERVENTIONS	RATIONALES
Assess for neurovascular complications (see nursing diagnosis "Risk for Peripheral Neurovascular Dysfunction").	Neurovascular compromise may occur due to constriction of the pelvis by edema, internal bleeding, or by casts.
Keep head of bed no higher than 30 degrees if in traction.	Elevating higher than this minimizes the pull of the traction, decreasing its ability to stabilize or realign the bone.
Assist with or reinforce teaching regarding traction and casts.	Many patients have questions regarding what they can and cannot do when in traction; answering their questions and addressing their concerns decreases anxiety and enhances compliance.
Administer pain medications liberally.	Pain can be moderate to severe depending on the extent of injury, and pain relief is required to promote patient comfort and willingness to participate in prescribed activities.
Prepare the patient for operative procedures as ordered (open reduction with internal fixations).	Some fractures will require surgical interventions to repair broken bones with pins, screws, or plates.
Following surgery, implement measures to promote activity as ordered or prescribed in collaboration with physical therapy; weight bearing will usually be limited with the use of crutches or walkers until healing has occurred.	The patient will need assistance with mobility to prevent injury to repaired fracture and to promote return to normal function without complications.
Assess the patient for signs and symptoms of fat embolus, such as agitation, restlessness, petechiae, shortness of breath, or rapid respirations (see nursing care plan "Fat Embolism").	Patients with pelvic fractures are at risk for the release of fat molecules from the marrow of the bone into the circulation. These travel to small vessels in the lung, causing symptoms of respiratory distress, and may also go to micro-vessels of the brain where they impair cerebral oxygenation, producing changes in mental status.
Teach the patient about activity restrictions, activity requirements for rehabilitation, and cast care.	An informed patient is more likely to be compliant with recommendations; the patient will need to be responsible for activity and mobility at home; instruction from the physical therapist can enhance ability to be independent.

Monitor the patient for signs of hemorrhage following admission (decreased blood pressure, elevated pulse, ecchymosis on abdomen, abdominal distention, abdominal pain, blood in urine); if noted, notify physician immediately.	Pelvic fractures can result in rupture of blood vessels and injury to abdominal structures including the bladder, urethra, and colon. Bleeding into the peritoneal space may become massive before it is detected because of the attention to treatment of obvious injuries. Mortality from hemorrhage is the most common cause of death in those with pelvic fractures, and attention to early detection is crucial.

NIC ***Cast care: Wet***
Cast care: Maintenance
Traction/immobilization care
Positioning
Exercise therapy: Ambulation
Exercise therapy: Joint mobility
Teaching: Prescribed
  activity/exercise

Evaluation

Evaluate the degree to which the patient has achieved the stated outcome criteria. The patient should verbalize an understanding of interventions utilized to achieve stabilization of the fracture, including use of traction, casts, and surgery. Mobility is maximized through use of assistive devices or physical therapy. The patient participates in ordered physical therapy and maintains strength and control of all extremities. No complications are noted due to the fracture or treatments implemented. The patient is able to report an understanding of required treatment modalities.

Community/Home Care

The patient who has sustained a pelvic fracture will require some adaptations in performance of activities once at home. For the patient who has a cast, safety at home will be an issue as casts create an imbalance of weight, making ambulation difficult at first. Patients treated by surgery or external fixators will need to use crutches at home but their use will require some trial and error, during which time the patient is at higher risk for falling. The environment will need to be assessed to determine how the patient can maneuver safely. Look for factors such as distance to bathroom, presence of steps, and excessive furniture or clutter that may pose a risk. Furniture may need to be rearranged so that the patient can ambulate freely with crutches or walker. Creativity is required when determining how the patient can get into the tub/shower without rails, as installation of handrails may not be desired for this temporary situation. Be sure that the patient knows how to use any assistive devices such as walkers and crutches. Nursing care may not be necessary, but physical therapy will be required to ensure that the patient can implement strategies to remain mobile and prevent complications or deformities due to disuse. For the patient who has had surgery, the status of the surgical wound will need to be monitored. Particular attention is given to the prevention and early detection of infection. Prior to discharge from the hospital or emergency room, the patient should be questioned regarding ability to function in the home in terms of self-care requirements to determine whether in-home physical therapy is indicated. The patient and family will need instruction on the use of crutches and other assistive devices as well as signs and symptoms of DVT. The patient will need to understand the critical importance of following prescribed instructions for exercise and physical therapy. Follow-up care for x-rays to determine healing will be necessary.

Documentation

Chart the presence and correct functioning of all devices used for stabilization of the pelvis such as traction/external fixators and casts. Document all interventions employed and the patient's responses to them. Include in the patient's chart the findings from a thorough assessment of the patient's musculoskeletal functioning with attention to assessments for decreased neurovascular functioning and signs and symptoms of fat embolus. Document any complaints that the patient verbalizes, including interventions employed to correct the problem. If the patient is scheduled for surgery, document pre-operative and post-operative assessments according to agency protocol. Rely on the physical therapist to document implementation of physical therapy activities, but document any other relevant activity or follow-up reinforcement of physical therapy teachings.

NURSING DIAGNOSIS 2

 ACUTE PAIN

Related to:
    Bone fragment movement
    Muscle spasms
    Orthopedic appliances

Defining Characteristics:
    Complaints of pain
    Obvious signs of trauma
    Grimacing and moaning

Goal:
    The patient's pain is relieved.

Outcome Criteria

✔ The patient will verbalize that pain has been relieved 30 minutes after interventions.
✔ The patient will verbalize an understanding of what causes pain.

NOC *Pain level*
       Pain control
       Comfort level

INTERVENTIONS	RATIONALES
Assess for location, intensity, quality, and precipitating factors.	Identifying these will assist in accurate diagnosis and treatment; most patients who experience fractures experience some pain, especially with movement.
Have the patient rate pain intensity using a pain rating scale.	Provides a more objective description of level of pain.
Assess status of affected extremity, including pain at injury site, tenderness to touch, color, temperature, edema, and pulses.	Allows for early detection of signs of neurovascular dysfunction; patients with fractures are at risk for impaired circulation and altered nervous innervation to the extremity (see nursing diagnosis "Risk for Peripheral Vascular Dysfunction").

INTERVENTIONS	RATIONALES
Administer analgesics as ordered on a regular schedule; do not allow pain to become intense; narcotics via patient-controlled analgesia (PCA) may be required for a period of time.	Decreased pain will improve patient's ability to participate in physical therapy activities required for improved mobility.
Move patient gently and cautiously.	Movement causes pain and careful movement provides support for the painful area.
Maintain traction as ordered (see nursing diagnosis "Impaired Physical Mobility").	Maintains stability of the fractured pelvis.
Assess for pressure points in cast, sling, or traction and pad as allowed.	Treating the underlying cause (pressure points) will alleviate the pain.
Implement strategies to reduce anxiety, such as staying with the patient, using relaxation techniques, or playing soft music.	Anxiety often intensifies the pain experience.
Investigate the use of diversional activities.	Decreases the attention or focus on the pain.
Encourage the patient to change position if allowed.	Improves circulation; reduces pressure points.
Administer muscle relaxants, as ordered.	Relaxes muscles and reduces pain.
Vigilantly monitor patient for sudden onset of chest pain, pelvic/abdominal pain, or limb pain.	The sudden onset of pain may be indicative of another process, such as infection, pulmonary embolus, fat embolus, or compartment syndrome.
Assess effectiveness of interventions to relieve pain.	Helps to determine whether interventions have been effective in relieving pain or whether new strategies need to be employed.

NIC   *Pain management*
   Analgesic administration
   Anxiety reduction

Evaluation

The patient reports that pain has been reduced or alleviated following interventions. The degree to which the patient is able to assist in the management of the pain through anxiety reduction and relaxation techniques is assessed. The patient should appear calm and have no observable signs of discomfort. If the pain is controlled, the patient is able to participate in mobility activities prescribed and implemented by physical therapy.

Community/Home Care

The patient's pain should decrease once the pelvic fracture has been stabilized and realigned by surgery, casting, or traction, and should completely resolve once fractures heal. Because simpler pelvic fractures that do not require surgery or traction may be treated on an outpatient basis, the patient should be given the information needed to manage pain. Pain is usually managed with mild to moderate analgesics, and the duration of pain should be short. The patient needs to monitor responses to pain medications and be able to identify those factors or positions that increase pain. Encourage the patient to use assistive devices such as pelvic slings, walkers, and crutches to relieve pressure on the affected site. The patient should be instructed to notify a health care provider if sudden onset of calf pain or chest pain occurs, as these may signal complications of DVT or pulmonary embolus. If the recommended analgesics are not working, the patient should seek follow-up care with the health care provider.

Documentation

Document in the patient's own words the description of the pain and the rating of the level of pain. Chart all interventions employed and the patient's responses. Include in the documentation assessments made relevant to the pain and to the musculoskeletal system. Indicate all teaching in the patient record with an indication of the patient's level of understanding.

NURSING DIAGNOSIS 3

RISK FOR PERIPHERAL NEUROVASCULAR DYSFUNCTION

Related to:
   Possible constriction and pressure due to edema
   Nerve damage due to instability of fractured segments
   Excess pressure within a cast

Defining Characteristics:
   None

Goal:

Neurovascular function is maintained.

Outcome Criteria

✔ Peripheral pulses in extremities are palpable.

✔ Extremity is warm with capillary refill brisk at < 3 seconds.

✔ The patient's extremity remains at normal color.

✔ The patient does not experience severe pain at injury site.

NOC *Circulation status*
Mobility
Tissue perfusion: Peripheral

INTERVENTIONS	RATIONALES
Assess neurovascular status of both extremities every 1–2 hours or as ordered: pulses, sensation, temperature, capillary refill, and movement.	Establishes a baseline and allows early detection of any complications that may occur due to surgery, casting, edema, traction, or initial injury.
If a cast has been applied, assess for signs and symptoms of compartment syndrome: severe pain unrelieved by usual analgesic, diminished or absent pulses, cool extremities, decreased or absent sensation in the extremity, loss of normal color, decreased capillary refill.	Unrelenting pain not relieved by usual analgesic is the early classic sign of compartment syndrome; later symptoms such as absence or diminished pulses, pallor, coolness, and slow capillary refill, if noted, usually indicate irreparable damage. The patient may report a change in sensation that could range from numbness to a feeling of pins and needles as nerves become compressed. Early attention to prevention of compartment syndrome is critical to preserve extremity function; early detection through frequent assessment leads to early identification and treatment.
Maintain cast and check for tightness.	Casts that are too tight may lead to compartment syndrome by causing undue pressure on the compartments of the extremity.
Check extremities for excess edema or tightness; ask patient about feeling of constriction.	Edema that is unrelieved through elevation could lead to compartment syndrome due to a poor venous system that is unable to handle the outflow of

excess of fluid; as the fluid continues to accumulate, pressure is applied to nerves in the extremity or pelvic area.

If compartment syndrome does develop, implement strategies or assist with strategies to relieve pressure, as ordered, such as cast cutting and fasciotomy (surgical interventions).	Casts are removed, cut, or bivalved by the physician to relieve pressure, following which interventions to maintain stability of fracture, such as splints, are employed until the cast can be reapplied. If the compartment syndrome is caused by pressures within the extremity due to edema, a fasciotomy is performed, which cuts the fascia of the extremity to allow for pressure release. The wound is left open and requires sterile dressing changes with sterile normal saline.

NIC *Peripheral sensation management*
Positioning: Neurologic
Cast care maintenance
Circulatory precautions

Evaluation

The patient should be evaluated to determine whether neurovascular status is maintained. Evaluate whether physiological indicators such as peripheral pulse, skin color, temperature, sensation, and capillary refill are normal. Assess the patient for undue pain that seems too severe for the injury and is unrelieved by analgesics. All patient parameters relevant to the status of the fractured pelvis should be normal or near normal.

Community/Home Care

Neurovascular problems usually occur during the early stages of injury to the pelvis but can be recurring. The patient and family need to be able to recognize signs and symptoms that would indicate the possibility of neurovascular compromise, particularly compartment syndrome (for patients with a cast), that would necessitate a return for emergency follow-up care. It is important that the patient understand how to relieve and prevent edema in the extremities. Ambulation and participation in physical therapy as ordered once at home should be stressed. A nurse may not be required, but follow-up visits with a health care provider are needed to be sure that the pelvic fracture is healing appropriately and that there are no long-term neurovascular alterations.

Documentation

Chart findings from a thorough neurovascular assessment, including peripheral pulses, extremity color, sensation, pain, and capillary refill. Document the specific content included in discharge teaching sessions. Always include nursing interventions implemented to prevent compartment syndrome and if the syndrome occurs, chart interventions initiated for treatment. Include in the patient chart the patient's responses to all interventions and any specific concerns verbalized.

NURSING DIAGNOSIS 4

 ## IMPAIRED TISSUE INTEGRITY

Related to:

Open wound that occurred at the time of injury

Pressure points from splint, cast, traction, bedrest

Traction appliance insertion sites

Surgical incision site(s)

Defining Characteristics:

Reddened, sore, or broken-down areas

Broken skin at injury site

History of dirty wound

Major crash injury and soft tissue trauma

Decreased sensation/movement

Foul smell

Elevated white blood count

Complaint of pain, pressure, numbness

Goal:

The patient's skin will heal, and infection is prevented.

Outcome Criteria

✔ The skin will be intact.

✔ Skin pressure point signs are gone.

✔ The patient's wounds/incisions show no signs of infection such as redness, odor, excessive pain, or purulent drainage.

NOC *Wound healing: Primary intention*

INTERVENTIONS	RATIONALES
Monitor wounds and pressure points.	Helps to detect signs of skin breakdown and infections.
Monitor surgical site and any drainage apparatus insertion sites for signs and symptoms of infection: redness or other discoloration, swelling, purulent drainage.	Early identification of infection can expedite treatment.
Maintain patency of drainage devices and assess drainage from Hemovac drains or other drainage tubes for amount, color, and consistency.	The drainage device helps drain secretions from surgical area; if not draining properly, the drainage may build up providing an excellent medium for bacteria growth.
Take temperature every 4 hours.	Helps to detect signs of infection.
Monitor results of white blood cell counts.	White blood cells elevate in the presence of active infection.
Change dressings as ordered and clean area using sterile technique, cleansing site of drainage devices last.	Maintenance of a clean incisional site decreases number of organisms and reduces chance of infection.
Administer antipyretics (acetaminophen [Tylenol]), as ordered.	Reduces fever.
Administer antibiotics, as ordered, via IV (intravenously) or PO (by mouth).	Reduces number of infective organisms and eliminates or prevents infection.
Administer NSAIDs, as ordered.	Reduces local inflammation; increases immune response.
Reposition the patient, or have the patient shift weight.	Repositioning will remove pressure from specific areas of the body.
Keep cast dry and non-frayed: bivalve or replace.	Use hair dryer or room air to keep casting materials dry. Petal cast edges and repair frayed cast edges to prevent tissue breakdown/necrosis.
Provide proper care at skin traction site.	Carefully wash, dry, and apply antibiotic ointment as ordered to prevent complications.
Encourage adequate nutritional intake orally, parenterally or enterally, especially of protein, vitamin C, and iron.	Adequate nutrient intake, especially of vitamin C, protein, and iron, is required for healing and tissue repair.

NIC   *Incision site care*
Infection control
Nutrition management
Wound care
Wound care: Closed drainage

Evaluation

Evaluate the degree to which the outcome criteria have been met. The surgical site should be intact, healing by primary intention with incision well approximated. Redness or other discoloration, swelling, purulent drainage, and heat should be absent from the site. Drainage from the drainage devices should be serosanguineous and decreasing in amount. The patient should be afebrile, and white blood cell counts should return to normal. There should be no odor or increased pain in areas beneath the cast.

Community/Home Care

The status of the surgical site or wound injury may remain a problem after the patient has been discharged home. The risk for infection remains, and the family will need to know what symptoms may signal the onset of infection. Whether the patient has a cast or pelvic sling, or has had open reduction and internal fixation, he or she will need to be taught how to care for the wound with attention to how to properly cover when showering/bathing. The proper technique for washing hands should be demonstrated by the patient, as this will be an important strategy in preventing infection. If dressing changes are needed, a nurse may be required to either change the dressing or watch the patient perform the first change. The patient will need to understand the importance of good nutrition in complete wound and bone healing, as well as of completing any ordered medications such as antibiotics. If any evidence of infection occurs, the patient should be instructed to contact the health care provider.

Documentation

Document assessment findings from the wound, including color, approximation, drainage, etc., being sure to note any sign of infection. Chart the status of drainage devices or tubes indicating the color, amount, and consistency of drainage. Document vital signs according to agency protocol as ordered for post-operative patients but at least every 4 hours. If antipyretics are given, chart these according to protocol, and document follow-up temperatures when obtained. Include the patient's and family's understanding of the signs and symptoms of infection in the patient record.

CHAPTER 4.57

FRACTURES: RIB/FLAIL CHEST/BLUNT INJURY

GENERAL INFORMATION

The most common type of chest injury is a simple rib fracture. The most common ribs fractured are the fifth and tenth ribs on the right side overlying the liver and the fifth and ninth ribs on the left side, with the ninth rib overlying the spleen. A first rib fracture (the first rib is located under the clavicle and the subclavian artery and vein run between the two) is a very serious fracture producing a 15 percent mortality rate due to undetected hemorrhage. First, second, and third rib fractures often cause injury to the underlying aorta and tracheobronchial tree. The presence of multiple rib fractures usually indicates the possibility of severe injuries. Fracture of two or more adjacent ribs in two or more places or a detached sternum produces a flail chest. The detached segment responds directly to intrathoracic pressure changes rather than retaining continuity with the chest wall. When negative intrathoracic pressure increases, causing the lungs to inflate, the flail segment will be drawn inward. When negative pressure decreases, causing exhalation, the flail segment pushes outward. If the flail segment is large enough, respiratory distress will occur. This movement of the flail segment opposite what the rest of the chest wall is doing is known as paradoxical movement. Rib fractures occur more frequently in the elderly. Clinical manifestations include pain on inspiration, rapid shallow respirations, and decreased breath sounds on the affected side. Patients with flail chest present with dyspnea, pain on inspiration, unequal chest expansion, crackles, and decreased breath sounds.

NURSING DIAGNOSIS 1

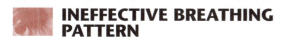

INEFFECTIVE BREATHING PATTERN

Related to:

    Severe chest pain

    Trauma to chest wall

Defining Characteristics:

    Shallow respirations

    Tachypnea

    Use of accessory muscles of respiration

    Decreased oxygen saturation

    Abnormal arterial blood gases (ABGs), primarily decreased pO_2 (hypoxia) and increased pCO_2 (due to incomplete respiratory excursion)

    Absent or diminished breath sounds over affected lung

    Paradoxical movement of affected side (flail chest)

    Pain on inspiration

    Inability to breathe deeply

    Unequal chest expansion

    Anxiety

Goal:

    The patient's respirations are regular.

    Adequate gas exchange is restored.

Outcome Criteria

✔ Breath sounds are present over affected area.

✔ Oxygen saturation is > 90 percent.

✔ ABGs are normal.

✔ Respiratory rate is between 12–24 per minute.

NOC   **Respiratory status: Ventilation**

      Respiratory status: Gas exchange

INTERVENTIONS	RATIONALES
Assess respiratory system and note abnormalities such as patient splinting chest wall, presence of crepitus over fracture site, paradoxical motion of chest wall, respiratory distress, pain on inspiration, inability to deep breathe, shallow breaths because of pain on movement, respiratory rate, depth, unequal chest expansion, and diminished breath sounds with crackles.	Establishes a baseline for comparison for early detection of complications or worsening condition.
Assess the patient's mental status for lethargy, restlessness, confusion, or agitation.	These are early indicators of decreased cerebral tissue oxygenation because of poor pulmonary function.
Assess cardiac status.	In serious chest injury, there may be cardiac manifestations such as distended neck veins, increased pulse, and decreased blood pressure (shock) if flail movement is not stabilized; early detection can prevent mortality.
Monitor results of ABGs and oxygen saturation.	Helps to evaluate respiratory adequacy, to determine oxygen needs, and to monitor response to treatments.
Administer oxygen, as ordered.	Improves oxygenation and decreases hypoxia.
Assist patient in assuming a semi- or high Fowler's position.	Maximizes intrathoracic space.
Implement strategies to alleviate pain (see nursing diagnosis "Acute Pain").	Pain with chest wall movement contributes to inadequate gas exchange and ineffective breathing pattern.
If hemothorax or pneumothorax occurs following chest trauma, assist with insertion of chest tube into intrathoracic space as directed; connect to water seal drainage system; implement strategies to maintain chest tubes and drainage system.	Relieves air, re-establishes negative pressure, and re-expands the lung; in the case of hemothorax, removes blood from pleural space (see nursing care plan "Pneumothorax/Hemothorax").
If time permits, administer analgesic prior to insertion of chest tube.	Chest tube insertion can be uncomfortable, and in the case of hemothorax, a larger tube is required to remove blood, which causes more discomfort.
Encourage the patient to cough and deep breathe every 2 hours and use incentive spirometry.	Maximizes ventilation and minimizes risk of atelectasis.
Teach the patient how to splint the affected side of the chest with a pillow when moving or coughing.	Splinting provides support for the injury and decreases pain with movement or coughing.
Monitor chest x-ray reports.	Helps to assess improvement or worsening of fractured ribs/flail chest.
Assist with endotracheal tube placement and mechanical ventilation set-up as required for patients with flail chest.	If respiratory distress is severe in flail chest, and ABGs do not reveal gas exchange improvement with oxygen therapy, mechanical ventilation is required to maintain adequate gas exchange.
For patients unresponsive to general interventions to correct gas exchange, prepare to assist with hemodynamic monitoring in an intensive care unit (central venous pressure, pulmonary artery pressures, etc.).	Patients whose ABGs do not reveal correction or improvement in gas exchange will need invasive monitoring and care in an intensive care unit (ICU) once on a ventilator.
For patients experiencing flail chest, assist with preparation for surgery to stabilize the flail chest, as ordered.	Helps to improve pulmonary function and prevent complications.
Monitor patient for signs and symptoms of pneumonia, such as sputum production, chills, fever, and decreased breath sounds in affected lung.	Shallow respirations due to pain lead to inadequate gas exchange and stasis of secretions in the base of the affected lung, predisposing the patient to bacterial growth.

NIC *Respiratory monitoring*
Oxygen therapy
Tube care: Chest
Positioning

Evaluation

The patient should return to a baseline respiratory function or see improvement in respiratory status. Diminished breath sounds over the affected lung should return to normal. If the fractured rib is accompanied with hemothorax or pneumothorax, the patient should show indications that the lung has re-expanded and respiratory status is improving. Respirations should be easy, with equal chest expansion bilaterally and a rate of 12–24 per minute. If a chest tube was required due to hemo-thorax/pneumothorax, drainage from the chest tube should have decreased or stopped. ABGs and oxygen saturation results should provide evidence that breathing patterns are able to achieve adequate gas exchange.

Community/Home Care

At time of discharge, the patient should have gas exchange resolved. Simple rib fractures generally heal spontaneously without long-term complications or concerns necessitating special in-home care. However, patients who experience flail chest may have some alterations in pulmonary function. Once at home, the patient may continue to have some soreness in the affected lung area and require mild analgesics. The patient will need to experiment with positioning to determine the position of comfort. It is crucial that the patient continue to deep breathe and use incentive spirometry to open airways and prevent stasis of secretions since pneumonia remains a threat. The nurse can make the patient a schedule for deep breathing and using the spirometry and ask him or her to document adherence to the schedule. The patient will need to limit activities for a short time until healing is complete and soreness abates, especially activities involving lifting or quick movements of the upper body. If the patient has spent time in the ICU on a ventilator, fatigue may be an issue at home following discharge, and the patient should be taught how to progress activities to build stamina and energy. Teaching should include how to avoid chest wall injuries, particularly those resulting from seat belt use, as a majority of rib fractures are secondary to motor vehicle accidents. The patient will need to be aware of respiratory symptoms that warrant a return to the physician, such as worsening shortness of breath, sudden onset of chest pain, or blood in sputum. Although a visiting nurse may not be required, the patient should be encouraged to return for a follow-up appointment with a health care provider.

Documentation

Document respiratory assessment findings, including breath sounds, respiratory rate, effort of breathing, and chest expansion. Include in the documentation any evidence of respiratory distress that would indicate worsening of oxygenation status, with particular attention to oxygen saturation levels. If there are chest wall wounds, document a thorough assessment of them as well. Include in the patient record the presence of any chest tubes and equipment for drainage, amount of output from the tube every shift, and a description of the drainage. Always document all interventions carried out, and the patient's responses to them, if any. If the patient verbalizes concerns about health status or treatments, include this in the documentation as well. Chart discharge instructions and the patient's verbalization of understanding.

NURSING DIAGNOSIS 2

 ACUTE PAIN

Related to:

Rib fractures

Defining Characteristics:

Complaints of pain

Obvious signs of trauma

Grimacing and moaning

Pain with inspiration

Goal:

The patient's pain is relieved.

Outcome Criteria

✔ The patient will verbalize that pain has been relieved 30 minutes after interventions.

✔ The patient will verbalize an understanding of what causes the pain.

NOC *Pain level*

Pain control

Comfort level

INTERVENTIONS	RATIONALES
Assess for location, intensity, quality, and precipitating factors.	Identifying these will assist in accurate diagnosis and treatment; most patients who experience fractured ribs experience some pain, especially with inhalation.

(continues)

(continued)

INTERVENTIONS	RATIONALES
Have the patient rate pain intensity using a pain rating scale.	Provides a more objective description of level of pain.
Assess respiratory status, including breath sounds, respiratory rate, depth, quality, presence of paradoxical movements, and oxygen saturation.	Allows detection of early signs of respiratory complications; patients with fractured ribs tend to breathe shallowly due to the pain associated with inspiration, this compromises respiratory function, which may lead to atelectasis and pneumonia; paradoxical movements are noted as the loose segments of rib or sternum move freely and in opposition.
Administer analgesics, as ordered, on a regular schedule, not allowing pain to get intense.	Decreased pain will improve the patient's respiratory efforts, especially inspiration, assuring adequate oxygenation, ventilation, and complete expansion of the lungs (preventing atelectasis). Narcotics may be used not only for pain control but also to decrease respiratory rate and anxiety and decrease oxygen demand.
Teach the patient to splint chest with a pillow when moving or coughing.	Splinting provides support for the painful area and allows the patient to participate in coughing and deep breathing more comfortably.
Administer oxygen, as ordered.	Improves oxygenation until pain control is achieved and patient respiratory effort has improved.
Implement strategies to improve respiratory status (see nursing diagnosis "Ineffective Breathing Pattern").	Treating the underlying cause will alleviate the pain.
Implement strategies to reduce anxiety, such as staying with the patient, using relaxation techniques, and playing soft music.	Anxiety often intensifies the pain experience.
Assess effectiveness of interventions to relieve pain.	Helps to determine whether interventions have been effective in relieving pain or whether new strategies need to be employed.

NIC *Pain management*
     Analgesic administration
     Anxiety reduction

Evaluation

The patient reports that the pain has been reduced or alleviated following interventions. The degree to which the patient is able to assist in the management of the pain through anxiety reduction and relaxation techniques is assessed. Determine whether the patient demonstrates equal chest expansion and can breathe easily without holding chest or grimacing. The patient should appear calm and have no observable signs of discomfort.

Community/Home Care

The patient's pain should be temporary and resolve once fractures heal and respiratory function improves. Because simple rib fractures may be treated on an outpatient basis, teaching should be done to give the patient the information needed to manage pain. Pain is usually managed with mild analgesics, and the duration of pain should be short. The nurse should stress to the patient that weak respiratory efforts resulting from pain could cause more serious respiratory problems, such as pneumonia. Encourage the patient to use splinting when moving or coughing at home and to immediately report any new onset chest pain. Once at home, patients may be tempted to apply binders, wraps, or even tape to the chest wall to help pain, not realizing that this could cause complications by restricting chest movement. The health care provider needs to be clear in explaining why this simple action should be avoided. If the recommended analgesics are not working, the patient should seek follow-up care with the health care provider.

Documentation

Document in the patient's own words the description of the pain and rating of the level of pain. Chart all interventions employed and the patient's responses. Include in the documentation assessments made relevant to the pain and to the respiratory system, particularly breath sounds and chest excursion. Document all teaching in the patient record with an indication of the patient's level of understanding.

NURSING DIAGNOSIS 3

 DEFICIENT KNOWLEDGE

Related to:

New onset injury

Lack of information

Anxiety

Defining Characteristics:

Many or no questions

Verbalizes a lack of knowledge/understanding

Goal:

The patient verbalizes an understanding of the injury that caused rib fractures.

Outcome Criteria

✔ The patient verbalizes a willingness and desire to learn the necessary information.

✔ The patient verbalizes an understanding of the injury and interventions required.

NOC   *Knowledge: Disease process*
Knowledge: Health behavior
Treatment behavior: Illness or injury

INTERVENTIONS	RATIONALES
Assess readiness of client to learn (motivation, cognitive level, physiological status).	Patient must be motivated to learn, have the capability to learn the content, and be free of distractions to learning, such as pain and shortness of breath.
Assess what the patient already knows.	The patient may have some knowledge about rib fracture injury and its treatment, and teaching should begin with what the patient already knows.
Create a quiet environment conducive to learning.	Environmental noise can prevent the learner from focusing on the content taught.
Teach the learners about the pathophysiology of rib fractures.	Understanding of pathophysiology assists the learners to understand rationales for therapeutic interventions.
Teach the patient deep breathing and coughing exercises.	Maximizes ventilatory excursion and reduces the likelihood of atelectasis and pneumonia.
Review pain control measures.	Provides information so that the patient can anticipate and/or reduce pain response.
If chest tubes are in place, teach the patient about the chest tube and drainage system functioning.	Understanding the rationale for these interventions will enhance the patient's willingness to comply with limitations.
Demonstrate to the patient how to splint chest to reduce pain.	Many patients express apprehension about the presence of pain when breathing or moving and tend to limit their movement, not realizing that immobility can contribute to more complications such as pneumonia. Demonstration will allow the patient to feel comfortable with activity.
Teach the patient which signs and symptoms to report to a health care provider (signs and symptoms of pneumonia, sudden onset chest pain, blood in sputum).	Monitoring for signs and symptoms early can prevent a crisis that requires hospitalization.
Teach the patient the importance of implementing safety measures to prevent injury, such as wearing seat belts, and general in-home safety. Safety measures are particularly important for elderly patients.	Most rib fractures occur due to motor vehicle accidents and may be attributed to not wearing seat belts; rib fractures due to falls are common in the elderly due to decreased bone density, osteoporosis, and other changes in the musculoskeletal system due to aging.
Evaluate the patient's understanding of all content covered by asking questions.	Helps to identify areas that require more teaching and to ensure that the patient has enough information to be compliant.
Give the patient written information.	Provides reference at a later time, and for review.

NIC   *Teaching: Disease process*
Teaching: Individual
Positioning
Fall prevention

Evaluation

The patient is able to repeat all information for the nurse and asks questions about the rib fractures and flail chest, and if pneumothorax or hemothorax were present, asks questions specifically about the chest tube. The patient is able to demonstrate to the nurse how to splint the chest when breathing and moving and how to perform deep breathing exercises; he or she identifies measures to relieve pain and states the importance of wearing seat belts. The patient should be able to identify for the nurse clinical manifestations that would indicate a need to seek health care assistance, and should specifically be aware of indications of worsening respiratory status and respiratory infection.

Community/Home Care

For patients who have experienced a fractured rib/flail chest the problem will probably still exist at time of discharge, but follow-up care in the home is rarely required. The patient will need to monitor him or herself for respiratory complications such as pneumonia by observing any sputum for color, odor, and amount, and by keeping track of temperature changes. As the patient resumes more normal activity, he or she may discover that some activities cause shortness of breath, but this should be resolve with time. Considerations for the prevention of future injury should be reinforced to the family and patient. Follow-up care with a health care provider focuses on assurance that respiratory function has returned and ribs have healed adequately, and that the patient or family understands the content taught.

Documentation

Document all content taught, especially information related to injury prevention and the patient's understanding. If the patient had a chest tube due to pneumothorax or hemothorax, include in the documentation the patient's ability to demonstrate the proper method of ambulation and mobility with chest tube system. Clearly indicate any area that requires further teaching in the record. Chart any questions or concerns that the patient has verbalized. Always include the names of any printed literature given to the patient for reinforcement.

CHAPTER 4.58

JOINT REPLACEMENT (HIP AND KNEE)

GENERAL INFORMATION

Joint replacement surgery (arthroplasty) is the surgical replacement of a joint that has been damaged so severely that mobility is extremely limited. Damage can occur due to osteoarthritis, rheumatoid arthritis, dislocation, degeneration of the bone that is congenital or traumatic, fractures that can cause necrosis, or other deformities. Replacements are indicated when the joints are the source of chronic pain with poor control and produce limited mobility of the extremity. The most common joint replacements are the knee and hip. The prosthetic joint implant may be composed of synthetic material or metal. During the surgical procedure, the entire damaged joint is replaced with a prosthetic joint.

NURSING DIAGNOSIS 1

IMPAIRED PHYSICAL MOBILITY

Related to:

Activity restrictions imposed by surgery

Pain at surgical site

Anxiety regarding movement of affected extremity

Defining Characteristics:

Moves slowly

Refuses to move

Reports extremity is stiff

Limited ability to move

Goal:

The patient will regain mobility to the highest possible level.

Outcome Criteria

✔ The patient will be able to ambulate 10 feet.

✔ The patient verbalizes a willingness to participate in prescribed physical therapy activities.

✔ The patient reports the absence of joint stiffness.

✔ The patient demonstrates gradual improvement in muscle tone, strength, and control.

✔ The patient can use adjunctive devices to assist mobility.

INTERVENTIONS	RATIONALES
Assess patient's ability to assist with movement, ability to carry out range of motion, and any concerns or fears about movement.	The first time activity is attempted, the patient may be anxious due to fear of injury or pain. Discussing this with the patient before activities can provide assurance and enhance willingness to participate.
Assess neurovascular status of extremity (color, temperature, capillary refill, edema, sensory perception, pulses, and pain); assess for signs and symptoms of compartment syndrome: severe pain unrelieved by usual analgesic, diminished or absent pulses, cool extremity, decreased or absent sensation in the extremity, loss of normal color, decreased capillary refill.	Joint surgery places the patient at risk for altered nerve function and blood supply to the extremity; assessment of neurovascular status is required to be sure that no complications are present. Extremity should be warm, have palpable pulses, and have a capillary refill < 3 seconds; some pain or discomfort is normal, but sensations of numbness or pins and needles are abnormal; edema should be minimal.
Assist physical therapist as needed for ambulation and transfers.	Physical therapists generally implement the prescribed activity protocols following joint replacements.
Encourage early ambulation and/or mobility with restrictions as ordered and as directed by the physical therapist; these may include the following: — Hip: Prevent flexion of > 90 degrees, avoid adduction of the affected leg beyond midline; no lying on operative	Prescribed activity will restore strength and early mobilization will prevent complications of immobility, including thrombophlebitis and deep vein thrombosis (DVT); correct positioning prevents dislocation of joint prosthesis or injury to prosthesis.

(continues)

(continued)

INTERVENTIONS	RATIONALES
side; avoid crossing legs or bending from waist; practice active dorsiflexion/plantar flexion exercise of the ankles and quadriceps, as ordered, to prevent thrombophlebitis and increase muscle tone; observe weight-bearing restrictions as ordered by the physician with assistance of physical therapy; use an abduction splint or pillow to maintain position when in bed; use assistive devices such as walkers, crutches, or canes.	
— Knee: Elevate leg on pillows beneath calf and avoid passive flexion; allow weight bearing, as ordered, usually on the first post-operative day, with assistive devices such as walkers; assist with performance of active dorsoplantar flexion, quadriceps setting exercises, and straight leg raises during period of limited ambulation; observe weight-bearing restrictions as ordered by the physician with assistance of physical therapy.	
Administer analgesics prior to physical therapy or nurse-assisted ambulation and transfers.	If the patient is fearful of pain with movement, he or she will be hesitant to participate in activity.
Apply continuous passive motion device for knee replacement surgery and use for 8–12 hours per day or as ordered.	Prevents venous stasis that could lead to the development of thrombophlebitis.
Administer anticoagulants as ordered (low molecular weight heparin, heparin, or warfarin), and monitor for side effects of bleeding; monitor activated partial thromboplastin time (APTT), international normalized ratio (INR), or prothrombin time (PT).	Joint replacement surgery carries a high risk for development of DVT, and this is especially true for knee replacements because of the surgical technique. Anticoagulants are given prophylactically to prevent thrombus formation, and APTT, INR, or PT give data relevant to coagulability of the blood.
Instruct on proper use of assistive devices, such as trapeze bars, and encourage their use.	This maintains some independence with movement in bed.
Assist with or reinforce teaching regarding activity, position	Many patients have questions regarding what they can and

restrictions, weight-bearing restrictions, and assistive devices.	cannot do following joint replacement surgery; answering their questions and addressing their concerns decreases anxiety and enhances compliance.
Assess patient for signs and symptoms of fat embolus, such as agitation, restlessness, petechiae, shortness of breath, and rapid respirations (see nursing care plan "Fat Embolism").	Patients with joint replacement are at risk for the release of fat molecules from the marrow of the bone into the circulation. These travel to small vessels in the lung, causing symptoms of respiratory distress, and may also go to micro-vessels of the brain, where they impair cerebral oxygenation, producing changes in mental status.
Assess the patient for signs and symptoms of deep vein thrombus/thrombophlebitis, such as positive Homan's sign, redness in calf, swelling, or tenderness in calf, and if noted, report immediately.	Patients having joint replacement surgery are at high risk for thrombus formation due to surgical technique, length of surgery, and immobility of the extremity.
Assess the patient for signs and symptoms of pulmonary embolism, such as rapid respi-rations, sudden onset of chest pain, anxiety, or hemoptysis.	Pulmonary emboli may occur because of undetected DVT, and symptoms may occur without warning; if detected, report immediately.
Teach or reinforce teaching regarding activity and position restrictions, activity requirements for rehabilitation, signs of dislocation of prosthesis, use of assistive devices, and signs of complications.	An informed patient is more likely to be compliant with recommendations. The patient will need to be responsible for activity and mobility at home, and teaching by the physical therapist can enhance the patient's ability to be independent.

NIC *Positioning*
      Exercise therapy: Ambulation
      Exercise therapy: Joint mobility
      Teaching: Prescribed
        activity/exercise

Evaluation

Evaluate the degree to which the patient has achieved the stated outcome criteria. The patient should verbalize an understanding of interventions utilized and required to achieve mobility. Mobility following joint replacement surgery is maximized through the use of assistive devices and physical therapy assistance, especially during the first few post-operative days. The patient participates in ordered physical therapy and maintains strength and control of affected extremities.

Community/Home Care

The patient who has had joint replacement surgery will require some adaptations in performance of activities once at home. For the patient who has activity restrictions, safety at home will be an issue, as assistive devices such as walkers, crutches, and canes can create a sensation of imbalance, making ambulation difficult. Use of these devices will require some trial and error, during which time the patient is at higher risk for falling. The environment will need to be assessed to determine how the patient can maneuver safely. Look for factors such as area rugs, distance to bathroom, presence of steps, and excessive furniture or clutter that may pose a risk. Nursing care may not be needed for mobility issues, but physical therapy referrals are crucial for ensuring that the patient can implement strategies to remain mobile and prevent complications or deformities due to disuse. Weight bearing will continue to be restricted for up to 2 months following discharge, and the physical therapist must ensure that the patient understands how to achieve this. Prior to discharge from the hospital, the patient should be questioned about ability to function in the home in terms of self-care requirements. Elevated toilet seats for home toilets are usually needed for hip replacement patients to avoid flexion. The patient and family will need instruction on the use of assistive devices as well as on signs and symptoms of dislocation of joint prosthesis, wound infection, and DVT, and what manifestations would dictate a need to return to the physician. The patient should understand that the presence of metal prostheses may activate metal detectors. The patient will need to understand the critical importance of following prescribed instructions for exercise and physical therapy. Follow-up care for assessment of wounds and x-rays to determine healing will be necessary.

Documentation

Document all interventions employed to address mobility and the patient's responses to them. Include in the patient's chart the findings from a thorough assessment of the patient's musculoskeletal functioning and neurovascular status. Document any complaints that the patient verbalizes, including those about interventions employed to correct the problem. Document participation in physical therapy activities and the patient's response to activity. Rely on the physical therapist to document implementation of physical therapy activities, but document any other relevant activity or follow-up reinforcement of physical therapy teachings.

NURSING DIAGNOSIS 2

ACUTE PAIN

Related to:

Surgical intervention

Orthopedic appliances

Defining Characteristics:

Complaints of pain

Grimacing and moaning

Goal:

The patient's pain is relieved.

Outcome Criteria

✔ The patient will verbalize that pain has been relieved 30 minutes after interventions.

✔ The patient will verbalize an understanding of what causes pain.

NOC *Pain level*

Pain control

Comfort level

INTERVENTIONS	RATIONALES
Assess for location, intensity, quality, and precipitating factors.	Identifying these will assist in accurate diagnosis and treatment; most patients who experience fractures experience some pain, especially with movement.
Have the patient rate pain intensity using a pain rating scale.	Provides a more objective description of level of pain.
Assess the status of affected extremity, including pain at	Detects early signs of neurovascular dysfunction;

(continues)

(continued)

INTERVENTIONS	RATIONALES
operative site, tenderness to touch, temperature, and edema.	patients with joint replacements are at risk for impaired circulation and altered nervous innervation to the extremity.
Administer analgesics, as ordered, on a regular schedule, not allowing pain to get intense; narcotics via patient-controlled analgesia (PCA) may be required for a period of time.	Decreased pain will improve the patient's ability to participate in physical therapy activities required for improved mobility.
Move the patient's extremity gently and cautiously.	Movement of affected extremity causes pain, and careful movement provides support for the painful area.
For knee replacement surgery, elevate the extremity.	Elevation will reduce edema.
Apply ice pack for 20 minutes.	Ice reduces swelling and reduces pain.
Implement strategies to reduce anxiety, such as staying with the patient, using relaxation techniques, and playing soft music.	Anxiety often intensifies the pain experience.
Investigate the use of diversional activities.	Decreases the attention or focus on the pain.
Administer muscle relaxants, as ordered.	Relaxes muscles and reduces pain.
Vigilantly monitor patient for sudden onset of chest pain or limb pain.	The sudden onset of pain may be indicative of another process, such as infection, pulmonary embolus, fat embolus, or compartment syndrome.
Assess effectiveness of interventions to relieve pain.	Determines whether interventions have been effective in relieving pain or whether new strategies need to be employed.

NIC   *Pain management*
      Analgesic administration
      Anxiety reduction

Evaluation

The patient is able to report that the pain has been reduced or alleviated following interventions. The degree to which the patient is able to assist in the management of the pain through anxiety reduction and relaxation techniques is assessed. The patient

should appear calm and have no observable signs of discomfort. If the pain is controlled, the patient is able to participate in mobility activities prescribed and implemented by physical therapy.

Community/Home Care

The patient's pain should be decreased once the surgical site has begun to heal. Teaching should be done to give the patient the information needed to manage pain. Pain is usually managed with mild analgesics, and the duration of pain should be short. The patient should take analgesics prior to any physical therapy visits in the home to increase the likelihood that he or she can participate fully in the planned activity. The patient needs to monitor responses to pain medications and be able to identify those factors or positions that increase pain. Encourage the patient to use assistive devices such as walkers, canes, and crutches to relieve pressure on the affected site. The patient should be instructed to notify a health care provider if sudden onset of calf pain or chest pain occurs, as these may signal complications of DVT or pulmonary embolus. The patient should not take over-the-counter medications containing aspirin for pain if also on anticoagulants. If pain intensity increases as activity level increases, the patient should incorporate more rest periods in the day. In the home, the patient may find comfort in elevating the extremity when sitting, if not contraindicated. If the recommended analgesics are not working, the patient should seek follow-up care with the primary health care provider.

Documentation

Document in the patient's own words the description of the pain and rating of the level of pain. Chart all interventions employed and the patient's responses. Include in the documentation assessments made relevant to the pain and to the musculoskeletal system. Document all teaching in the patient record, with an indication of the patient's level of understanding.

NURSING DIAGNOSIS 3

 IMPAIRED SKIN INTEGRITY

Related to:
   Surgical intervention

Defining Characteristics:

> Surgical incision
>
> Presence of staples or sutures
>
> Presence of drainage device

Goal:

> The patient's incision will heal and infection is prevented.

Outcome Criteria

✔ Incisions show no signs of infection such as redness, odor, excessive pain, or purulent drainage.

✔ Incision will be approximated with sutures or staples intact.

✔ Incision will be clean and dry.

NOC *Wound healing: Primary intention*

INTERVENTIONS	RATIONALES
Monitor surgical site and any drainage apparatus insertion sites for signs and symptoms of infection: redness, swelling, purulent drainage.	Early identification of infection can expedite treatment.
Maintain patency of drainage devices and assess drainage from Hemovac drains or other drainage tubes for amount, color, and consistency.	The drainage device helps drain secretions from surgical area; if not draining properly, the drainage may accumulate in the surgical site, providing an excellent medium for bacteria growth.
Take temperature every 4 hours.	Detects signs of infection.
Monitor results of white blood cell counts.	White blood cells elevate in the presence of active infection.
Change dressings as ordered and clean area using sterile technique, cleansing site of drainage devices last.	Maintenance of a clean incisional site decreases the number of organisms and reduces chance of infection.
Administer antipyretics (acetaminophen [Tylenol]), as ordered.	Reduces fever.
Administer antibiotics, as ordered IV (intravenously) or PO (by mouth).	Reduces the number of infective organisms and eliminates or prevents infection.
Encourage adequate nutritional intake orally, parenterally, or enterally, especially intake of protein, vitamin C, and iron.	Adequate nutrient intake, especially of vitamin C, protein, and iron, is required for healing and tissue repair.

NIC *Incision site care*
Infection control
Nutrition management
Wound care: Closed drainage

Evaluation

Evaluate the degree to which the outcome criteria have been met. The surgical site should be intact healing by primary intention with incision well approximated. Signs of infection such as odor, increased pain, redness, swelling, purulent drainage, and heat should be absent from the site. Drainage from the drainage devices should be serosanguineous and decreasing in amount. The patient should be afebrile, and white blood cell counts should return to normal.

Community/Home Care

The status of the surgical site may remain a concern after the patient has been discharged home, as the length of stay for joint replacement is between 3 and 5 days. Teaching relevant to the incision will need to be provided with attention to preventing infection, promoting healing, and properly covering the site when showering/bathing. The patient needs written information describing the symptoms that signal an infection or problem with wound healing for later reference. Good handwashing should be stressed as a means of preventing infection, especially if the incision is left open to air. If a dressing is required, be sure that the patient or a family member knows how to change the dressing and that they have necessary resources to purchase supplies. Items needed for the dressing change can be kept in a heavy plastic storage box with a lid. The patient will need to understand the importance of good nutrition in complete wound and bone healing, especially inclusion of vitamin C, zinc, and protein in the diet. The importance of completing any ordered medications such as antibiotics should be stressed. In case any evidence of infection occurs, the patient should be instructed to contact the health care provider.

Documentation

Document assessment findings from the wound, including color, approximation, drainage, etc., being sure to note any sign of infection. Chart the status of drainage devices or tubes, indicating the color, amount, and consistency of drainage. Document vital signs according to agency protocol, as ordered, for post-operative patients. If antipyretics are given, chart these according to protocol and document when follow-up temperatures are obtained. The patient's and family's understanding of the signs and symptoms of infection should be included in the patient record.

NURSING DIAGNOSIS 4

RISK FOR INEFFECTIVE MANAGEMENT OF THERAPEUTIC REGIMEN

Related to:

Insufficient knowledge of activity requirements

Noncompliance with therapeutic regimen due to lack of understanding

Complexity of prescribed activity restrictions

Defining Characteristics:

Asks many or no questions

Verbalizes a lack of knowledge/understanding

Goal:

The patient verbalizes an understanding of prescribed activity.

Outcome Criteria

✔ The patient verbalizes a desire to learn necessary information.

✔ The patient verbalizes a willingness to keep appointments and follow prescribed regimen.

✔ The patient demonstrates knowledge of joint replacement.

✔ The patient demonstrates knowledge of use of assistive devices for ambulation and understands activity restrictions.

NOC *Knowledge: Infection control*
Knowledge: Prescribed activity
Knowledge: Treatment regimen
Compliance behavior

INTERVENTIONS	RATIONALES
Assess the patient's current knowledge and ability to learn, readiness to learn, and risk for noncompliance.	Teachings need to be tailored to the patient's ability and willingness to learn for maximum effectiveness; assessment of the patient for likelihood of noncompliance will allow the nurse to intervene early.
Identify a family member or significant other who will also learn the content and assist the patient with compliance.	This person can reinforce the teaching and assist with implementation if the client becomes incapable of follow-through.
Create a quiet environment conducive to learning.	Environmental noise and distractions can prevent the learner from focusing on the content being taught.
Teach the learners the following information about joint replacement surgery: — Surgical procedure and wound care — Prescribed activity, restrictions, and proper use of assistive devices (see nursing diagnosis "Impaired Physical Mobility") — Importance of good nutrition in healing — Signs and symptoms of complications (DVT, infection) to be reported (see nursing diagnosis "Impaired Physical Mobility") — Importance of complying with follow-up appointments	Knowledge of surgical procedure and wound care, prescribed physical therapy, and signs of complications will assist the patient in assuming control of own rehabilitation. Stressing the adherence to the regimen as prescribed will prevent complications.
Assess the patient's understanding of the discharge instructions by asking the patient to repeat information and ask questions as needed.	This allows the nurse to hear in the patient's own words what was taught, making it easier to know what information may need to be reinforced.
Establish that the patient has the resources required to be compliant, including availability and affordability of physical therapy services.	If needed resources such as finances, transportation, and psychosocial support are not available, the patient cannot be compliant.
Refer to appropriate disciplines as needed (physical therapy, social worker, home health nurse, etc.).	These disciplines can provide additional services to help patient be compliant with the prescribed regimen.
Give the patient printed version of the information covered in the teaching session.	The patient may be more comfortable at home knowing that there is printed material for future reference.

NIC *Teaching: Prescribed
　　　activity/exercise
　Learning readiness enhancement
　Learning facilitation*

Evaluation

Evaluate the degree to which the patient has achieved the expected outcomes. The patient verbalizes an understanding of the therapeutic regimen, particularly the prescribed, including use of assistive devices, and activity restrictions. The patient is able to repeat all information for the nurse and asks questions about the information that has been taught and is able to demonstrate the use of walkers, crutches, or canes, as prescribed. The patient should be able to inform the nurse about signs and symptoms that would necessitate contact with a health-care provider. The nurse must determine that the patient is capable of being compliant, and it should also be ascertained whether the patient expresses a willingness to comply with the activity recommendations. Once this is established, it is crucial to determine that the patient has the necessary information to manage rehabilitation at home.

Community/Home Care

For patients who have had joint replacement surgery, home care focuses on activity and maintenance of functional mobility. Home environments may pose a safety risk for the patient as he or she attempts to ambulate using walkers, crutches, and canes around furniture and other obstacles common to homes. Once at home, the patient may limit ambulation due to fear of falling or lack of motivation to be aggressive with prescribed regimen. Successful management will depend on the patient's understanding of the information provided in teaching sessions and the internal motivation to continue with physical therapy recommendations for activity. The patient will need to implement strategies to monitor for complications, such as joint deformities and DVT. Follow-up by a community health nurse may be required once the patient is at home to monitor the status of the surgical incision, and the physical therapist will be needed for reinforcement and follow-up on the most critical aspect of home care, continued participation in prescribed physical activities. Nutrition will be important so that healing can be enhanced and strength returned.

Documentation

Document the specific content taught and the titles of printed materials given to the patient or family. Chart the patient's and family's understanding of the content and the methods used to evaluate learning. The nurse must clearly indicate areas that need to be reinforced. After the teaching session is complete, the nurse should assess to determine whether the patient indicates a willingness to comply with health care recommendations. If the teaching includes a family member or significant other, indicate this in the documentation. In addition, document any referrals made in the patient record.

CHAPTER 4.59

LYME DISEASE

GENERAL INFORMATION

Lyme disease is an inflammatory disease caused by the spirochete *Borrelia burgdorferi*, which is transmitted by the Ixodes tick. It is transmitted in nymphal form (very difficult to see), and the bite is painless, often going unnoticed. Deer ticks account for 95 percent of cases, but Lyme disease can arise from ticks from other animals including dogs, cats, raccoons, cows, etc. Incubation is from 3 to 32 days but usually occurs 7 to 10 days after exposure. The disease manifests itself in three phases; however, not all phases necessarily appear in all patients. In the first stage (early Lyme disease), an expanding, non-pruritic circular red rash (erythema migrans) appears at the bite site and clears spontaneously. Often the patient will have flu-like symptoms of fatigue, arthralgias, myalgias, and fever. The rash resolves without treatment in 2 weeks, but the other symptoms may last up to 2 months. Normally serology is negative at this point. Stage two (early disseminated Lyme disease) begins 1 to 2 months after the tick bite. It may manifest itself with cardiac symptoms that include dyspnea, heart block, palpitations, symptoms of heart failure, and dysrhythmias. Characteristic neurological findings include a stiff neck and headache. Stage three (late disseminated Lyme disease) may last from 2 months to 2 or more years. In this stage, the patient usually demonstrates symptoms of chronic arthritis, dermatologic changes consisting of bluish-red lesions known as acrodermatitis chronica atrophicans, ataxia, spastic paresis, and memory loss (Phipps, Monahan, Sands, Marek, and Neighbors, 2003). Due to its vague and varied symptomatology, Lyme disease is often misdiagnosed. It most commonly occurs between the months of June and October with most of the reported cases (90 percent) in the Northeastern and Midwestern states. The disease is a CDC notifiable disease, and the goal of the CDC is disease prevention.

NURSING DIAGNOSIS 1

INFECTION (ACTUAL)*

Related to:

Invasion of host by *B. burgdorferi* spirochete

Defining Characteristics:

Fever

Chills

Myalgias

Arthralgias

Headache

Cardiopathies

Goal:

Infection is resolved.

Outcome Criteria

✔ The patient is afebrile.

✔ The patient verbalizes no complaints of muscle or joint discomfort.

✔ The patient verbalizes an absence of headache.

✔ The patient's skin will be free of rashes, lesions, or discoloration.

✔ The patient reports symptoms of the disease have improved.

NOC *Infection severity*
Risk control

INTERVENTIONS	RATIONALES
Monitor results of laboratory tests: enzyme-linked immunosorbent assay, Western blot, or indirect immunofluorescence assay to detect antibodies to *B. burgdorferi*.	Allows confirmation of diagnosis; in stage one, only 50 percent of people have antibodies; in stage two, 70 to 90 percent have antibodies.

INTERVENTIONS	RATIONALES
Administer antibiotics, as ordered: amoxicillin, vibramycin, rocephin, ceftin, tetracycline, or erythromycin.	All of these antibiotics are specific for *B. burgdorferi* spirochete.
Instruct patient to take the entire course of antibiotics, and monitor for side effects.	Therapy may continue for as long as 1 month, and the patient may stop taking the antibiotics when feeling better; the patient needs to be aware of side effects to report to the health care provider.
Give NSAIDs (aspirin, etc.), as ordered.	Reduces inflammation and relieves arthritic symptoms.
Splint any affected joints, and if knee is affected, restrict weight bearing.	Helps to rest joint; knees are commonly affected by arthritic changes, with immune complexes being deposited in the synovium.
Take temperature every 4 hours.	Allows detection of elevations and monitoring of response to treatment.
Monitor for development of cardiac complications that would compromise cardiac output: palpitations, irregular rhythm, congestion, abnormal heart sounds, chest pain, results of EKG.	Patients with Lyme disease may experience cardiac manifestations during stage two of the disease, including tachydysrhythmias, PVCs, and heart blocks, all detected by EKG; early detection provides for early intervention to prevent a cardiac crisis and to maintain cardiac output.
Monitor for development of neurological complications: assess for headache and stiff neck in stage two; memory loss, ataxia, and spastic paresis in stage three.	Detection of these changes provides for early treatment to promote patient safety and prevent worsening.
Assess for dermatologic changes.	In stage one, a flat or slightly raised red area that expands with a clear central area occurs at site of bite; in stage 3, there is a bluish-red lesion noted; these are characteristic findings, and in stage one the skin change resolves spontaneously. Noting their presence supports the diagnosis.
Teach the patient and family how to prevent the disease: — Wear protective clothing such as long pants and long-sleeved	Prevention of disease through education is the best approach to controlling the number of cases.

shirts when outdoors/in the woods.
— Pull socks up over pants legs and tuck shirt in.
— Use tick repellant.
— Check self for ticks daily.
— Wash sites of bites with soap and water and follow with antiseptic solution, such as alcohol.
— If symptoms develop, contact a physician.

Provide printed materials regarding Lyme disease.	The patient and family can review materials when they are ready to absorb the information. This will provide a review and perhaps answer some questions that were not asked.

NIC *Infection protection*
Medication prescribing
Skin surveillance
Infection control

Evaluation

Determine the degree to which the outcome criteria have been achieved. The patient's infection is controlled and symptoms are relieved. The patient should be afebrile and report no complaint that would indicate complications of Lyme disease.

Community/Home Care

The patient with Lyme disease is treated at home as an outpatient unless there are complications that warrant hospitalization. Teaching should include symptoms of cardiac disease and neurological manifestations that should be reported to the health care provider. The patient may continue to experience fatigue for a while and should implement strategies to conserve energy (see nursing diagnosis "Fatigue"). Treatment regimens are typically a success if the patient has received early treatment; however, for some patients there are long-term effects of the disease. The patient can take NSAIDs or other mild analgesics for the aches that accompany the disease. It may prove beneficial to take these early in the day to enhance the patient's ability to be active during the day. Because development of the disease does not achieve immunity, the patient will need to implement strategies to prevent tick bites in the future. It is crucial that the patient use tick/insect repellant when outdoors, especially in areas frequented by deer. The patient may need to have another person check the back of the body for tick bites or stand in front of a mirror and use a hand-held mirror to see his or her back. There usually is no need for in-home visits from a nurse, but follow-up care to monitor progress is required.

Documentation

Whether the patient is seen in the hospital, at a health care provider's office, or in an emergency room, the nurse should chart the findings from a thorough assessment of the musculoskeletal, cardiac, and neurological systems. Document all strategies that have been implemented to treat the disease and the patient's responses. Always include in the patient's chart whether the outcome criteria have been achieved. Chart the temperature, pulse, blood pressure, heart sounds, and breath sounds. Any specific patient complaints of joint pain and aches should be specified along with relief measures employed. An assessment of the skin, including the presence of lesions typical of those seen in stages one or three, should be noted. Teaching relevant to prevention of Lyme disease should be documented with an indication of the patient's understanding.

NURSING DIAGNOSIS 2

 FATIGUE

Related to:

Infectious process (Lyme disease)

Fever

Defining Characteristics:

Verbalization of tiredness

States a lack of energy

Inability to carry out normal activities

Goal:

Fatigue will be relieved.

Outcome Criteria

✔ The patient is able to perform activities of daily living.

✔ The patient verbalizes that fatigue has improved or been eliminated.

NOC *Activity tolerance*
Endurance
Energy conservation
Nutritional status: Energy

INTERVENTIONS	RATIONALES
Obtain subjective data regarding normal activities and limitations.	Helps to determine the effect fatigue has on normal functioning.
Monitor patient for signs of excessive physical and emotional fatigue.	Provides a guideline for adjusting activity.
Encourage periods of rest and activity.	Conserves oxygen and prevents undue fatigue.
Schedule activities so that excessive demands for oxygen and energy are avoided; for example, space planned activities away from meal times.	Digestion requires energy and oxygen; participation in activities close to meals will cause increased fatigue because of insufficient energy reserves.
Gradually increase activity as tolerated.	Use the results to indicate when activity may be increased or decreased.
Limit visitors during acute illness.	Socialization for long periods may cause fatigue.
Increase intake of high-energy foods such as meat (especially organ meats), poultry, dried beans and peas, whole grains, and foods high in vitamin C.	These foods increase oxygen-carrying capacity, and provide ready sources of energy needed in hypermetabolic states such as infection and fever.
Encourage the patient to plan activities when he or she has the most energy, usually early in the day.	Prevents fatigue.

NIC *Energy management*

Evaluation

Obtain subjective information from the patient regarding the presence of fatigue. The patient should gradually report the ability to participate in activities of daily living and other normal activities with no fatigue.

Community/Home Health

Patients with Lyme disease should understand that fatigue may persist until the infectious process is resolved. The patient must understand how to adjust activity in response to feelings of fatigue, possibly even arranging for rest or nap periods in the afternoon. Attention to good nutrition should continue with intake of foods that are good sources of iron, vitamin C, and protein. Early in the disease, when fatigue is greatest, the patient may benefit from having some assistance with household chores. For those who work outside the home, several days off work or a shortened workday may be needed until the fatigue improves. If fatigue persists for extended periods, the patient may need to seek health care to investigate the possibility of other causes of the fatigue.

Documentation

Chart the specific complaint of fatigue, including what activities the patient has been performing. Document interventions implemented to address fatigue, being sure to document food intake. An assessment of the patient's sleep patterns should also be documented.

CHAPTER 4.60

OSTEOARTHRITIS

GENERAL INFORMATION

Osteoarthritis (OA), often referred to as degenerative joint disease, is a degeneration or loss of articular cartilage in synovial joints. As joint cartilage deteriorates, bone begins to become involved and may begin to deteriorate due to physical stressors directly on the bone ends. Ligaments and tendons become less pliable as they begin to increase in density, causing stiffness and decreased mobility of the joint. Inflammation is not a characteristic finding in OA, but it may occur in the form of synovitis in response to tissue destruction. OA most frequently affects fingers, hip joints, knees, ulnar collateral ligaments, thoracic and lumbar vertebrae, and the pelvis at the sacrum and iliac junction. OA can be primary idiopathic associated with aging, which is the most common type. Secondary OA is caused by wear and tear on the joint or by trauma to the joints such as that seen with repetitive strains and sprains. This is often seen in athletes (frequently gymnasts who hyperextend joints and football players) and certain occupations, such as carpet installers. The onset is gradual with a slow progression. Some sources estimate that 90 percent of all adults are affected with some degree of OA by the age of 40 (Lewis, Heitkemper, and Dirksen, 2004). OA generally occurs in persons older than 50 years, and its incidence increases with age. Women are affected more often than men, and after age 50, the incidence in women is twice that of men. This is thought to be attributed to decreased estrogen levels after menopause.

NURSING DIAGNOSIS 1

 CHRONIC PAIN

Related to:

Joint deterioration

Loss of articular cartilage

Defining Characteristics:

Pain in one or more joints especially on movement

Decreased physical activity

Stiffness in large joints in morning lasting 30 minutes

Pain resolution with rest

Goal:

Pain is decreased and mobility improved.

Outcome Criteria

✔ The patient states that pain is decreased 1 hour after intervention.

✔ The patient verbalizes methods to reduce early morning pain.

NOC *Pain: Disruptive effects*
Pain level
Pain control

INTERVENTIONS	RATIONALES
Assess the patient's pain using a pain rating scale.	Provides a more objective assessment.
Assess or take history regarding time of pain onset, location, precipitating factors, relieving factors, and effect on function; complaint of localized pain upon joint extension; joint pain, especially after sleeping or increased physical activity.	These will assist in accurate diagnosis and treatment; knowing how pain affects function will provide information needed to assist patient with home care needs.
Administer first-line analgesic medications as ordered (such as acetaminophen) and monitor for side effects.	Large doses of acetaminophen are required for pain relief and are usually considered first; baseline hepatic function studies should be done as well as regular checks, because adverse side effects include hepatic toxicity.

432

INTERVENTIONS	RATIONALES
Administer nonsteroidal anti-inflammatory drugs (NSAIDs) (such as ibuprofen, Indocin®, Feldene®, naproxen), as ordered; assess effectiveness and monitor for side effects.	Decreases pain and discomfort; even though the inflammatory response is small in OA, these medications are still suggested for their pain relief qualities. There are numerous NSAIDs available, and they are usually recommended if the patient's pain is not controlled with acetaminophen. Common side effects include gastrointestinal (GI) upset and bleeding; monitor body fluids for blood and patient for nausea.
Administer COX-2 inhibitors, as ordered; assess for effectiveness and monitor for side effects.	Used for analgesic properties; inhibits prostaglandin synthesis by inhibiting COX-2; also an anti-inflammatory agent.
Administer salicylates (aspirin) PO (by mouth), as ordered; assess effectiveness and monitor for side effects.	Aspirin may be given if acetaminophen is contraindicated or is not effective to decrease pain response and joint inflammation; inhibits prostaglandin production; must be monitored for GI bleeding, hypersensitivity, tinnitus, and fullness in ears.
Give all medications on a regular dosing schedule rather than prn.	Provides better relief.
Assist with injection of corticosteroid agents into the joint (intra-articularly).	Combined with an anesthetic and injected into the joint space, this decreases joint pain.
Apply moist heat packs.	Aids muscle relaxation and decreases pain; moist heat is able to penetrate deeper.
Arrange for physical therapy consult to consider ultrasound, hydrotherapy, diathermy, ambulatory assistive devices, etc.	The physical therapy consult may provide therapies to loosen the joint, decrease pain, and increase flexibility.
Encourage the patient to lose weight.	Obesity is a risk factor for OA, especially of the knee, because it places more stress on the weight-bearing joints.
Implement strategies to protect joints (see nursing diagnosis "Deficient Knowledge").	By minimizing stress on the joints, function can be preserved for a longer time and self-care enhanced.
Instruct the patient to exercise on a regular basis as prescribed by health care providers. Swimming, water exercises, and walking are helpful.	Maintains and restores function; these exercises are low impact and decrease stress on affected joints.
Teach relaxation techniques such as music therapy, massage, distraction, and meditation.	These techniques enhance the effect of analgesics and may decrease reliance on medications for complete relief.

NIC *Simple relaxation therapy*
Heat/cold application
Analgesic administration
Pain management

Evaluation

Assess the degree to which the patient reports pain has been relieved by interventions. For persistent pain, the nurse should investigate additional measures to relieve pain. Determine whether the patient is able to verbalize how to reduce pain.

Community/Home Care

The patient with osteoarthritis is typically treated as an outpatient. A cornerstone of care is the management of painful joints. A therapeutic regimen that allows for tolerable pain may require an extended period of trial and error with a variety of pharmacological and non-pharmacological measures. If able, the patient needs to learn how to implement relaxation techniques that relax joints and provide some relief of pain. The patient needs to understand the need for rest and schedule rest periods throughout the day to relieve stress on joints that could aggravate pain. Simple changes in routine, such as doing household chores incrementally over the course of the week rather than having a "cleaning day" could contribute to joint rest and thus decreased pain. If the home has stairs, the patient may need to limit the number of times he or she goes up and down, as climbing stairs can aggravate the pain. Cold packs may help the pain; a bag of frozen peas or mixed vegetables that molds easily to the contour of a joint, especially knees and hands, can be used. Health care providers should follow up to determine if the pain prevents the patient from performing activities of daily living. If so, a change in regimen should be undertaken. The patient will need to understand the side effects of all medications as many of them are significant, such as GI bleeding, ototoxicity, and hepatic dysfunction. An often overlooked side effect with some NSAIDs is the decreased effectiveness of some antihypertensive medications when taken concurrently with NSAIDs, particularly

ACE inhibitors and beta blockers such as atenolol. Be sure that the patient knows what symptoms are to be reported to a health care provider.

Documentation

Because the patient is at home for treatment, be sure that office visits document the specific therapeutic interventions prescribed for pain. Include in the patient record the patient's verbalized perception of pain control.

NURSING DIAGNOSIS 2

 IMPAIRED PHYSICAL MOBILITY

Related to:

Deterioration of joint cartilage and other joint tissue and bone

Pain

Stiffness in large joints

Defining Characteristics:

Limited range of motion, moves slowly

Decreased joint space on x-ray

Bony enlargements of distal interphalangeal joints (Heberden's nodes)

Bony enlargements of proximal interphalangeal joints (Bouchard's nodes)

Crepitus when joint is put through range of motion

Goal:

The patient has improved physical mobility.

Outcome Criteria

✔ The patient is able to ambulate without pain in joints.

✔ The patient is able to perform activities of daily living.

✔ The patient reports stiffness of joints has dissipated 30 minutes after awakening.

NOC *Mobility*

Joint movement: Knee

Joint movement: Hip

Joint movement: Wrist

INTERVENTIONS	RATIONALES
Assess patient's current range of motion in affected joints as well as ability to walk with correct posture, to get up and down from chairs, and to perform activities of daily living.	Helps to determine functional ability and to plan for appropriate interventions.
Obtain history from patient about occupation, nature of work, trauma, sports in the past or present, or obesity past or present.	Helps to determine whether adaptations in lifestyle will need to be made and whether lifestyle is a contributing factor.
Monitor results of ordered tests: synovial fluid evaluation, joint x-rays, complete blood count (CBC), erythrocyte sedimentation rate (ESR), rheumatoid factor, renal, and hepatic studies.	X-rays are used to confirm a diagnosis and will show narrowing of joint space; synovial joint fluid is analyzed to allow for differentiation between various types of inflammatory processes in the joint; CBC is usually done for baseline comparisons and to rule out infectious processes. ESR is often done along with rheumatoid factor analysis to rule out rheumatoid arthritis. The ESR would be only slightly elevated if acute synovitis were present; tests of renal and hepatic function are done to establish a baseline before medication therapy is begun.
Have patient take analgesics upon awakening in the morning.	Alleviating the pain will allow for better mobility.
Have patient perform range of motion exercises in bed before arising.	Helps patient to decrease stiffness before attempting ambulation.
Encourage regular exercises such as walking on level surfaces, swimming, or water exercises specifically designed for patients with arthritis.	Exercise helps maintain and restore function, maintains muscle tone and mobility, and prevents contractures.
Arrange for physical therapy consultation for methods/ therapies to improve mobility (moist heat, ultrasound, hydrotherapy, gentle exercise, massage, and ambulatory assistive devices).	Improves physical mobility by relaxing the joint, relieving pain, and improving range of motion.
Encourage the patient to use assistive devices as prescribed (canes, walkers, etc.).	Helps relieve stress on joints when moving.

INTERVENTIONS	RATIONALES
Have patient avoid stairs if possible.	The act of climbing or descending causes undue stress on knee joints and can cause more irritation.
Teach patient good posture, correct body mechanics, and body alignment.	Protects the joint and reduces stress on affected joints.
Implement strategies to reduce pain (see nursing diagnosis "Chronic Pain").	If pain is alleviated, the patient is able to move better.
Teach the patient how to protect joints: use palms rather than fingers; slide objects; change positions frequently; avoid repetitious movements; when performing household chores avoid stress on joints— for example, sit down when performing tasks rather than standing; rest between tasks; and perform household duties incrementally throughout the week.	These strategies protect joints by alleviating stress on them while maintaining optimum function.
Assess home environment for safety and help the patient identify needs for items such as handrails, grab bars in bathrooms, and stationary pieces of furniture that can be used to assist movement; remove hazards such as throw rugs.	The patient with impaired physical mobility is at risk for injury, and the home should be assessed and changes made that decrease the risk for injury. Many of the changes can be made at a low cost.
Investigate the need for assistive devices such as long-handled tools to grab or pick up objects, bigger zippers for clothing, jar openers, and larger buttons. If necessary, teach patient how to use properly.	These items prevent stress on joints and make it easier for patients to remain self-sufficient.
Prepare patient for arthrodesis/ fusion or muscle release. (Arthrodesis is the surgical immobilization of a joint and can only be performed on joints where movement is not essential, such as certain vertebral joints or digit joints).	Reduces movement and controls pain; relieves restriction.
Prepare patient for arthroscopy, as ordered.	Arthroscopy will provide access to the joint for debridement of devitalized, thickened tissue and can also be used to repair tissue, if possible. Arthroscopy is also used as a diagnostic tool.
Prepare patient for joint replacement surgery (see nursing care plan "Joint Replacement: Hip/Knee").	In joint replacement surgery, the affected joint is removed and replaced with an artificial joint.
Teach patient how to cope with chronic pain through use of medications and non-pharmacological measures.	Many patients become dependent and focus on what they cannot do rather than taking control of the disease. Patients must learn how to cope with pain on a daily basis and maintain optimum function.
Teach the patient about the disease process and effect on mobility.	Knowledge of the disease and how it affects the body will give the patient a sense of control and allows for a better understanding of the role of prescribed therapeutic interventions.
Make referrals to arthritis support groups.	Support groups can offer emotional support as well as helpful tips on how to live with arthritis.

Evaluation

Determine the degree to which the patient is achieving the established outcomes. The patient should report to the health care provider that he or she is able to perform routine household chores and activities of daily living. The extent to which the patient is able to ambulate without pain as well as the effectiveness of interventions to enhance mobility should be assessed.

Community/Home Care

Osteoarthritis is a disorder that is treated almost exclusively in the home environment. In the early stages of the disease, the patient may require no in-home assistance or adaptations in environment or lifestyles, but simply control the pain with analgesics and exercise. As the joint continues to deteriorate, the health care provider will need to more closely monitor the effect that chronic pain and limited mobility have on effective functioning. Assessments of the patient's feelings about limitations in mobility, any social isolation, and future disability, as well as feelings of depression, should be made. Concerns and needs may focus on household chores such as laundry and cleaning, or on self-care needs such as bathing, dressing, and receiving adequate nutrition. An assessment of the home is required in order to make suggestions for changes in the environment that promote independence and safety. Issues to be addressed include ability to get in or out of the shower or tub, ability to reach for objects on kitchen shelves, ability to clean the home, ability to cook meals, ability to manipulate the fasteners on clothing (zippers, hooks, buttons), and ability and willingness to ambulate around the home rather than remaining stationary for long periods. It is crucial that the patient understand the strategies required to maintain optional functioning of affected joints (see "Interventions/Rationales"). Referrals to physical therapy for a period of time will be important to the patient's health maintenance so that appropriate exercises and instructions on the use of assistive devices can be completed. For as long as the status of the disease allows, the patient should exercise daily. The physical therapist can develop an exercise regimen with the patient that is realistic. Walking is most often recommended and the patient can do this in his or her neighborhood or go to a local mall. If the patient does not desire to go out, he or she can develop simple exercises that can be done in the comfort of the home. The patient who undertakes walking should invest in a good pair of walking shoes that can provide adequate support and cushioning. Encourage the patient and significant other to utilize community resources such as Meals on Wheels or arthritis support groups. Arthritis support groups or organizations may also know where the patient can purchase assistive devices, such as "reach-it" handles or jar openers, as well as share strategies for managing simple tasks that members have discovered through trial and error.

Documentation

Document a thorough assessment of the patient's functional mobility. Include in the patient record all interventions that have been recommended to the patient to address the problem of mobility. Record all teaching. A report of the patient's perception of the ability to be mobile should be included. The effectiveness of all interventions, particularly those implemented for control of joint pain, should be clearly documented for all members of the health care team. This documentation will most likely be in a record in a physician's office or a home health agency and should be completed according to the agency protocol.

CHAPTER 4.61

RHEUMATOID ARTHRITIS

GENERAL INFORMATION

Rheumatoid arthritis (RA) is a chronic, autoimmune disease of the connective tissue where synovial membranes are destroyed, causing destruction of body joints, immobilization of joints, and joint deformity. It is characterized by inflammation of the connective tissue. Even though no specific cause has been identified for RA, a commonly accepted theory includes initiation of an autoimmune response due to Epstein-Barr virus or other bacteria. The body produces an abnormal immunoglobin G (IgG), and then production of antibodies (RF Factor) against this abnormal IgG occurs. This triggers an extensive inflammatory response beginning with the deposition of immune complexes on synovial membranes or articular cartilage in the joints. Once inflammation is present, neutrophils travel to the site and begin proteolytic activity that further damages the joint cartilage and synovial lining. There may also be a genetic component to the development of RA.

As a systemic disease, RA can affect a single joint or the entire body. The progression of the disease is atypical with remissions and exacerbations. Patient complaints include joint pain that increases with activity; stiffness in the morning lasting longer than 1 hour; limited range of motion; and inflammation of affected joints evidenced by redness, swelling, heat, and a spongelike feeling when palpated. Joint involvement is symmetrical and bilateral, with involvement of smaller joints: proximal interphalangeal (PIPs), metacarpophalangeal (MCPs), and metatarsophalangeal (MTPs) joints first. Other nonspecific complaints include fatigue, anorexia, weight loss, and discomfort. The disease is seen two to three times more often in women than in men, with onset beginning most often between the ages of 20 and 40. The incidence of the disease increases with age. Other syndromes seen in the disease are Sjögren's syndrome, which is seen late in the disease with symptoms of dry eyes, dry mouth, and dry vagina due to destruction of secretory ducts and glands. The patient may complain of eyes feeling gritty due to lack of normal tearing and mouth being dry and sticky. RA patients are said to have Felty's syndrome if in addition to the RA there is also evidence of hepatosplenomegaly and leucopenia.

NURSING DIAGNOSIS 1

 CHRONIC PAIN

Related to:

Joint destruction

Joint effusion

Swelling

Inflammation

Defining Characteristics:

Erythema and edema of joint

Body joint destruction

Complaints of pain with movement

Morning stiffness in joints lasting more than 1 hour

Goal:

Pain is decreased and mobility improved.

Outcome Criteria

✔ The patient states that pain is decreased 1 hour after intervention.

✔ The patient verbalizes methods to reduce pain.

NOC *Pain: Disruptive effects*

Pain level

Pain control

INTERVENTIONS	RATIONALES
Assess the patient's pain using a pain rating scale.	Provides a more objective assessment.
Assess or take history regarding time of pain onset, location, precipitating factors, relieving factors, and effect on function; complaint of localized pain upon joint extension; joint pain, especially after sleeping or increased physical activity.	These will assist in accurate diagnosis and treatment; knowing how pain affects function will provide information needed to assist patient with home care needs.
Monitor results of laboratory and diagnostic tests: rheumatoid factor, erythrocyte sedimentation rate (ESR), white blood cell (WBC) count, antinuclear antibody (ANA), serum electrophoresis, and x-rays of affected joints.	These tests are used to validate diagnosis and guide treatment; rheumatoid factor indicates the presence of unusual antibodies of the IgG and IgM type in 60 percent of patients with RA; ESR elevates in RA and is increased in 85 percent of patients; WBC may be elevated due to inflammation; ANA demonstrates a high titer for unusual antibodies, and the higher the value the more active the disease; serum electrophoresis demonstrates the presence of elevated levels of gamma globulin; x-ray may reveal soft tissue swelling and later in the disease may show narrowing of the joint space, destruction of articular cartilage, erosion, and the presence of deformities.
Administer first line analgesic and anti-inflammatory medications (e.g., aspirin) as ordered, and monitor for effectiveness and side effects; monitor for gastrointestinal (GI) bleeding, alterations in clotting times, hypersensitivity, tinnitus, and fullness in ears.	Large doses of aspirin may be required for pain relief and are usually considered first; aspirin inhibits prostaglandin production and provides anti-inflammatory effects along with pain relief.
Administer nonsteroidal anti-inflammatory (NSAIDs) drugs, such as ibuprofen (Motrin®, Advil®), indomethacin (Indocin), piroxicam (Feldene), naproxen (Naprosyn®, Aleve®), as ordered, and assess effectiveness and monitor for common side effects including GI upset and bleeding; an often overlooked side effect is hypertension with a decrease in effectiveness of antihypertensive agents such as beta blockers and ACE inhibitors.	To decrease pain and discomfort, NSAIDs also inhibit prostaglandin production; these medications are suggested for their double effect of pain relief and anti-inflammatory qualities. NSAIDs are usually recommended if the patient's pain is not controlled with aspirin.
Administer COX-2 inhibitors as ordered; assess for effectiveness and monitor for common side effects, which include GI disturbances such as abdominal pain, diarrhea, dyspepsia, nausea, and hepatic dysfunction.	Used for analgesic and antipyretic properties; inhibit prostaglandin synthesis by inhibiting COX-2; also an anti-inflammatory agent.
Administer disease modifying anti-rheumatic drugs (such as Plaquenil®, methotrexate, penicillamine, gold compounds, minocycline), as ordered, and monitor for effectiveness and side effects. — Plaquenil: antimalarial agent that requires 3 to 6 months of therapy with side effects of pigmentary retinitis and loss of vision; baseline vision testing and regular vision checks at least every 6 months are required — Methotrexate: cytotoxic agent given if no response to NSAIDs; effects are seen in 2 to 4 weeks; side effects include headache, mouth ulcers, bone marrow suppression, liver inflammation, and thrombocytopenia (monitor for easy bruising, petechiae); perform lab tests to check for side effects—CBC, liver enzymes — Penicillamine: action is unclear but thought to be related to inhibition of collagen formation; used for patients who for whatever reason fail to respond to usual therapy; toxic reactions are common and severe, and include proteinuria, bone marrow suppression with agranulocytosis, hemolytic anemia, and aplastic anemia; other less severe effects are loss of taste, especially for salt and sweet, anorexia and nausea, generalized pruritus and rashes — Gold salts: relieve pain and may arrest degeneration, but take 4 to 6 months to develop therapeutic effects, so concurrent treatment with NSAIDs is required; can be	These medications demonstrate the ability to provide clinical improvement and decrease progression of the disease activity.

INTERVENTIONS	RATIONALES
given orally (PO) and intramuscularly (IM), but oral is less effective; injections are initially taken weekly and then reduced to maintain therapeutic effects; it is thought that gold acts to suppress the immune response and suppress lysosome release; with oral gold, diarrhea, nausea, and abdominal pain are common; other common side effects include intense pruritus, rashes, and stomatitis; one of the more severe side effects is renal toxicity in the form of proteinuria, which occurs frequently — Minocycline: a form of tetracycline; has an unknown mechanism of action, but a large number of patients treated with this drug demonstrate marked improvements after 3 years of treatment; has antimicrobial and anti-inflammatory effects; inhibits certain chemicals like collagenase and metalloproteinase that cause bone damage; there is a low incidence of side effects but when present they include dizziness, nausea, candida, and sun sensitivity	
Give all medications on a regular dosing schedule rather than prn.	Provides better relief.
Give corticosteroids, as ordered, and/or assist with injection of corticosteroid agents into the joint (intra-articularly), and monitor for side effects, including elevations of blood sugar levels, water retention, hypertension, and osteoporosis.	These medications are given to relieve joint pain and inflammation temporarily while awaiting the therapeutic effects of other treatments; steroidal preparations are used during acute exacerbations, but long-term daily use is contraindicated due to the serious side effects.
Apply moist heat or cold.	Aids muscle relaxation and decreases pain; moist heat is able to penetrate deeper; if pain intensifies during acute inflammation, cold can be used for analgesia properties as well. If commercial heat packs are not available, the patient can use showers or baths.
Arrange for a physical therapy consult to consider ultrasound, hydrotherapy, diathermy, ambulatory assistive devices, etc.	The physical consult may provide therapies to loosen the joint, decrease pain, and increase flexibility.
Implement strategies to protect joints (see nursing diagnosis "Impaired Physical Mobility").	By minimizing stress on the joints, function can be preserved for a longer time and self-care enhanced.
Exercise on a regular basis as prescribed by health care providers, such as swimming, water exercises, and walking, are helpful.	Maintains and restores function; these exercises are low impact and decrease stress on affected joints.
Teach relaxation techniques such as music therapy, massage, distraction, and meditation.	These techniques enhance the effect of analgesics and may decrease reliance on medications for complete relief.

NIC *Simple relaxation therapy*
Heat/cold application
Analgesic administration
Pain management

Evaluation

Assess the degree to which the patient reports pain has been relieved by interventions. For persistent pain, the nurse should investigate additional pain relief measures. Determine whether the patient is able to verbalize how to reduce pain.

Community/Home Care

The patient with RA is typically treated as an outpatient unless there are systemic effects or complications. A cornerstone of care is the management of painful, swollen joints. A therapeutic regimen that allows for tolerable pain may require an extended period of trial and error with a variety of pharmacological and non-pharmacological measures. If able, the patient needs to learn how to implement relaxation techniques that relax joints and provide some relief of pain. The patient needs to understand the necessity of rest, and schedule rest periods throughout the day to relieve stress on joints that could aggravate pain. Small suggestions such as having the patient do household chores incrementally over the course of the week rather than having a "cleaning day" could contribute to joint rest and thus decreased pain. Sitting to fold laundry and while cooking are also strategies to be considered. Elevating the affected extremity (hand, arm, or leg) may also provide some relief of pain, and pillows or small ottomans or stools can be used. Health care providers should follow up to determine if the pain prevents the patient from performing activities of daily living. If so, a change in regimen should be undertaken. Encourage the patient to take the medications upon arising, which can help with stiffness and function during the day. If the patient does not have an ice collar, packages of frozen vegetables, such as peas, that mold easily can be wrapped in a towel and used for cold application to painful joints. Warm compresses can be made by placing a washcloth soaked in warm water on the joint and then wrapping it in plastic wrap. The patient will need to understand the side effects of all medications, as many of them are significant, such as GI bleeding, ototoxicity, nephrotoxicity, and hepatic dysfunction. In addition, an often overlooked side effect of some NSAIDs is the decreased effectiveness of some antihypertensive medications when taken concurrently, particularly ACE inhibitors and beta blockers such as atenolol. Be sure that the patient knows what symptoms need to be reported to a health care provider. Because of the debilitating nature of RA, home care providers should be attuned to the possibility of frustration, depression, and altered body image in the patient (see nursing diagnosis "Disturbed Body Image").

Documentation

Because the patient is at home for treatment, be sure that office visits document the specific therapeutic interventions prescribed for pain. Include in the patient record the patient's verbalized perception of pain control.

NURSING DIAGNOSIS 2

IMPAIRED PHYSICAL MOBILITY

Related to:

Tender, swollen, warm joints

Deterioration of joint cartilage and other joint tissue and bone

Pain with movement

Stiffness

Deformities in joints

Defining Characteristics:

Limited range of motion

Moves slowly

Unable to perform normal tasks requiring movement of hands and wrists

Rheumatoid nodules (firm, non-tender masses over bony prominences)

Goal:

The patient has improved physical mobility.

Outcome Criteria

✔ The patient is able to ambulate without pain in joints.

✔ The patient is able to perform activities of daily living.

✔ The patient reports stiffness of joints has been relieved 30 minutes after awakening.

NOC *Mobility*
Joint movement: Knee
Joint movement: Hip
Joint movement: Wrist

INTERVENTIONS	RATIONALES
Assess patient's current range of motion in affected joints as well as ability to walk with good posture, to get up and down from chairs, and to perform activities of daily living.	Determines functional ability and allows planning for appropriate interventions.
Examine results of diagnostic studies: synovial fluid analysis and x-rays.	Synovial fluid will demonstrate changes consistent with inflammation, including cloudiness, increased protein, and elevated WBCs; x-rays show joint space narrowing, soft tissue swelling, and joint effusion and bone deformities (see nursing diagnosis "Chronic Pain," third Intervention/Rationale for other diagnostic tests.)
Obtain history from the patient about occupation, nature of work, trauma, sports in the past or present, or obesity past or present.	Helps to determine whether adaptations in lifestyle will need to be made and to decide if lifestyle is a contributing factor.

INTERVENTIONS	RATIONALES
Arrange for physical therapy consultation for methods/ therapies to improve mobility (moist heat, ultrasound, hydrotherapy, gentle exercise, massage, ambulatory assistive devices).	Improves physical mobility by relaxing the joint, relieving pain, and improving range of motion.
Have the patient take analgesics upon awakening in the morning.	Alleviating the pain will allow for better mobility.
Have patient perform range of motion exercises in bed before arising.	Decreases stiffness before attempting ambulation.
Encourage regular exercises, such as walking on level surfaces, swimming, or water exercises specifically designed for patients with arthritis.	Exercise helps to maintain and restore function; maintains muscle tone and mobility, and prevents contractures.
Encourage patient to use assistive devices as prescribed (canes, walkers, splints, and braces, etc.).	Helps relieve stress on joint when moving; braces and splints keep joints in proper alignment.
Teach the patient how to balance rest and activity with a realistic regimen that is part of a routine.	Regular rest periods at different times during the day can benefit the patient by decreasing the inflammatory response; patients tend to limit activities due to pain, thus putting themselves at more risk for impaired mobility due to the loss of function; the more routinized the activity recommendations are, the more likely the patient is to be compliant.
Teach the patient good posture, as well as correct body mechanics and body alignment.	Helps to protect the joint and reduce stress on affected joints.
Implement strategies to reduce pain (see nursing diagnosis "Chronic Pain").	If pain is alleviated, the patient is able to move better.
Teach the patient how to protect joints: use palms rather than fingers; slide objects; change positions frequently; avoid repetitive movements; when performing household chores avoid stress on joints, e.g., sit down when performing tasks rather than standing, rest between tasks, and perform household duties incrementally throughout the week.	These strategies protect joints by alleviating stress on them while maintaining optimum function.
Assess home environment for safety and help the patient identify the need for items such as handrails, grab bars in bathrooms, and stationary pieces of furniture that can be used to assist movement; remove hazards such as throw rugs or clutter.	The patient with impaired physical mobility is at risk for injury, and the home should be assessed and changes made to decrease the risk for injury. Many of the changes can be made at a low cost.
Investigate the need for assistive devices, such as long-handled tools to grab or pick up objects, larger zippers and buttons for clothing, jar openers, and elevated toilet seats. If needed, assist the patient in locating available places for purchase and teach patient how to use properly.	These items prevent stress on the joints and make it easier for patients to remain self-sufficient (see nursing diagnosis "Self-Care Deficit").
Prepare patient for arthrodesis/ fusion or muscle release. (Arthrodesis is the surgical immobilization of a joint and can only be performed on joints where movement is not essential, such as certain vertebral joints or digit joints.)	Reduces movement and controls pain; relieves restriction.
Prepare patient for arthroscopy.	Arthroscopy will provide access to the joint for debridement of devitalized, thickened tissue and for repair of tissue, if possible. Arthroscopy is also used as a diagnostic tool.
Prepare patient for joint replacement surgery (see nursing care plan "Joint Replacement: Hip and Knee").	In joint replacement surgery, the affected joint is removed and replaced with an artificial joint.
Teach patient how to cope with chronic pain through use of medications and non- pharmacological measures.	Many patients become dependent and focus on what they cannot do rather than taking control of the disease. Patients must learn how to cope with pain on a daily basis and maintain optimum function.
Teach the patient about disease process and effect on mobility.	Knowledge about the disease and its effect on the body will give the patient a sense of control and allows for a better understanding of the role of prescribed therapeutic interventions.
Make referrals to arthritis support groups.	Support groups can offer emotional support as well as helpful tips on how to live with arthritis.

Evaluation

Determine the degree to which the patient is achieving the established outcomes. The patient should report to the health care provider that he or she is able to perform routine household chores and activities of daily living. Assess the extent to which the patient is able to ambulate without pain as well as the effectiveness of interventions to enhance mobility.

Community/Home Care

RA is treated almost exclusively in the home environment unless there are systemic complications. In the early stages of the disease, the patient may require no in-home assistance or adaptations in environment or lifestyle, but simply control the pain with analgesics and exercise. As the joint continues to deteriorate, the health care provider will need to more closely monitor the effect that chronic pain and limited mobility have on effective functioning. Assessments of the patient's feelings concerning limitations in mobility, any social isolation, and possible future disability, as well as feelings of depression, should be made. Social isolation may become an issue as the deformities in the hands appear and become disfiguring. These movement-limiting deformities also make performance of everyday tasks a challenge. It is at this point that in-home assistance may be required. Concerns and needs may be centered on household chores such as laundry and cleaning, or self-care needs such as bathing, dressing, and receiving adequate nutrition. Issues to be addressed include ability to get in or out of the shower or tub, to reach for objects on kitchen shelves, to clean the home, to cook meals, and to manipulate the fasteners on clothing (zippers, hooks, buttons), as well as the ability and willingness to ambulate around the home rather than remain stationary for long periods. It is crucial that the patient understand the strategies required to maintain optimal functioning of affected joints (see Interventions/Rationales). The patient will need to establish a routine for some type of exercise as long as mobility permits. Simple walking on level surfaces may prove helpful. Even though water exercises have proven to be beneficial, the availability of swimming facilities may be limited in rural areas or due to financial constraints. Referrals to physical therapy will be important to the patient's health maintenance so that appropriate exercises and instructions on the use of assistive devices can be completed. Encourage the patient, family members, and/or significant other to utilize community resources such as Meals on Wheels or arthritis support groups.

Documentation

Document a thorough assessment of the patient's functional mobility as well as the presence of obvious deformities in joints. Include in the patient record and all interventions that have been recommended to the patient to address the problem of mobility. Include a report of the patient's perception of the ability to be mobile and a psychosocial assessment. Document clearly the effectiveness of all interventions for all members of the health care team. This documentation will most likely be in a record in a physician's office or a home health agency and should be completed according to the agency protocol.

NURSING DIAGNOSIS 3

 ### SELF-CARE DEFICIT

Related to:
>   Impaired physical mobility
>   Chronic pain
>   Joint deformities
>   Lack of fine motor control

Defining Characteristics:
>   Unable to bathe or dress self
>   Difficulty preparing meals and eating
>   Difficulty with self-care

Goal:
>   The patient's self-care needs are met.

Outcome Criteria

✔ The patient reports being able to bathe and clothe self.

✔ The patient reports being able to obtain nutrition and feed self.

✔ The patient is able to perform household chores or reports having resources available for assistance.

NOC *Self-care: Instrumental activities of daily living*

Self-care: Activities of daily living

INTERVENTIONS	RATIONALES
Obtain a home assessment to determine functionality, need for assistive devices, financial abilities, community, and family support system.	Before arranging for professional help, the nurse needs to know what is available or what could be available to the patient.
Assess patient's ability to perform activities of daily living as well as normal household tasks, chores, and responsibilities.	Helps to determine the patient's current ability and what the specific needs may be.
Contact the social worker for referral to a home health nurse for home visits and planning so that the patient's and family's needs are met. The home health nurse can coordinate all other professional and nonprofessional consults/help.	The home health nurse is familiar with planning and mobilizing community resources.
With the assistance of the patient and/or family, arrange personal care items so that they are easily accessible, and be sure that items can be opened easily. For example, place specific hygiene items together in a large shower pail placed on a waist-level table or shower caddy.	Having items readily available enhances the patient's ability to use them.
Establish a routine for self-care activities.	Patients respond better to a routine, ritualistic method of performing tasks and will incorporate this into their lives.
Have patient pace activities throughout the day and do the most important ones early.	Helps to avoid fatigue and decrease the likelihood of pain.
Implement strategies to enhance/maintain mobility and decrease pain.	The patient is more likely to participate in self-care activities and activities of maintaining a household if joints are mobile and pain-free (see nursing diagnoses "Chronic Pain" and "Impaired Physical Mobility").
Delegate household chores to other family members if possible or investigate outside assistance.	A change in role performance may be required to maintain optimal functioning and prevent exacerbations; requesting the assistance of family members should be seen as a necessary part of the plan of care.
Place clothing in a readily accessible place and investigate whether drawers or closet doors open easily.	Some restructuring may be required to make storage areas more user-friendly. Older drawers often wear away,

INTERVENTIONS	RATIONALES
	making them difficult to open; the patient with RA may lack the necessary dexterity and strength to open stubborn drawers. Clothing on high shelves or extremely low shelves of closets may need to be rearranged so that the patient neither reaches nor bends excessively.
Investigate special devices that assist with dressing, eating, toileting, bathing, and other chores. Such devices include hooks that can pull a zipper up or down, brushes with long handles, special large buttons, a long-handle helper to reach items in cabinets, eating utensils and cups with special easy-to-grip handles, devices to assist with opening jars, shower chairs, elevated toilet seats, and bedside commodes. Consider a consult with an occupational therapist for development of individualized assistive devices. Encourage clothing that has elastic waists and no back zippers, as well as shoes that are easy to put on.	These special devices assist the patient to maintain optimal functioning and prevent dependence; they are used when the patient cannot close the hand around normal items, when items are out of reach, or just for the ease on the joint; long-handled items used for reaching are also useful when the patient has limited hip flexion. The twisting motion required to open jars creates tension and stress on the joints of the wrist and hand.
Teach patient to purchase food items that can be opened easily with easy-tear opening instructions requiring scissors or little physical strength, and if possible, to avoid purchasing food items in difficult-to-open packages, such as frozen vegetables and other items encased in heavy plastic.	Attempting to open thick plastic without the benefit of an easy-tear strip can irritate joints of the hand and wrist because of the motion required.
Teach the patient to use the larger and stronger joints when performing tasks.	Protects the small joints and distributes stress of work better.
Instead of carrying items in arms around the home, place them in a tote bag with shoulder straps to move from place to place or on a rolling cart.	Protects joints.
Perform ongoing assessments to determine how the patient is managing self-care by making home visits or inquiring at follow-up appointments.	The patient may need assistance while going through periods of trial and error with special devices, and as the disease progresses the patient may need additional assistance.

(continues)

(continued)

INTERVENTIONS	RATIONALES
Provide a means for emotional support for the patient, such as referral to support groups.	The patient may need support to maintain functioning and for general mental well-being as he or she adapts to a change in functional status.

NIC *Self-care deficit: Bathing/hygiene*

Self-care deficit: Dressing/grooming

Self-care deficit: Feeding

Environmental management

Evaluation

Determine to what extent the patient has reported the ability to take care of own needs. Examine closely patient reports of satisfaction with adjustments made in activities to accommodate functional status. The outcome criteria should be met, and if not, revisions should be made and new ways to assist the patient to be self-sufficient in activities of daily living (ADLs) and household chores should be identified.

Community/Home Care

An assessment of the home environment to determine what adaptations can be made to make the home easier for the patient to function in is a first step towards enhancing independence. Appropriate education on ways to adapt self-care and household activities for the patient with RA is paramount. Many patients will eventually require some assistance with at least some of their routine activities, such as cleaning and preparing food. Alterations in the home, such as installing an elevated toilet seat or placing frequently used items on lower shelves, are simple but can improve the patient's functioning greatly. Teaching the patient about available resources for assistive devices before they are needed allows the patient to adapt better rather than try to assimilate this information when joints are painful and mobility limited. A heads-up plan that includes family members and the patient is important as the presence of family members can serve as a source of assistance and emotional support. A history should be obtained from the patient regarding his or her usual routine for ADLs and household chores so that individualized interventions can be implemented

(see "Interventions/Rationales" for suggested ways to modify tasks). Attention to what the patient normally does and how the patient wants to make adaptations can only enhance compliance. The nurse must remain aware of cultural background that may influence a patient's perception of and adaptation to perceived dependency on others. As the disease progresses, the health care provider will need ongoing assessments of the patient's ability to function independently and need for other resources.

Documentation

Chart a plan for the patient's self-care needs according to agency protocol. Include all interventions recommended to address self-care deficits and findings from a follow-up with the patient to determine whether they have been effective. Also include in the documentation any referrals made, teaching completed, and especially any special devices that have been obtained for the patient.

NURSING DIAGNOSIS 4

 DISTURBED BODY IMAGE

Related to:

Physical deformities of hands, wrists

Immobility

Dependence

Defining Characteristics:

Withdrawal

Social isolation

Depression

Negative statements about physical appearance

Patient's attempts to cover hands in the presence of others

Goal:

The patient accepts the change in physical appearance and continues social activities and interpersonal relationships.

Outcome Criteria

✔ The patient states a willingness to look at and touch hands.

✔ The patient does not verbalize negative feelings toward self.

NOC *Body image*

INTERVENTIONS	RATIONALES
Encourage the patient to get his or her feelings out in the open and assure the patient that these feelings are normal.	The patient should understand that his or her emotions are real and should be expected.
Encourage the patient to communicate feelings about changes in physical appearance.	Talking about the changes may sometimes be the beginning of acceptance.
Teach the patient methods to care for hands to slow the process of development of deformities.	Protecting the joints from trauma and stress can slow the inflammation process.
Teach patient and family how to maintain optimal self-care functioning.	If the patient is able to remain independent with self-care activities and common household tasks, that comfort level may translate into acceptance of the change in appearance and incorporation of body appearance change into a positive self-image.
Monitor the patient's feelings about him or herself, interpersonal relationships, withdrawal, social isolation, fear, anxiety, and embarrassment by appearance of hands.	Allows early detection of alterations in social functioning and early interventions to prevent unhealthy behaviors.
Encourage the patient to participate in at least one outside/public activity each week once health status permits.	Prevents the patient from isolating him or herself from others.
Identify the effects of the patient's culture or religion on body image.	A patient's culture and religion often help define their reactions to changes in body image and self-worth.
Identify community support groups, such as Arthritis Foundation and arthritis support groups, if available.	Discussions with other patients in similar situations is good for the patient as it will allow him or her to share experiences with others who understand what he or she is going through; provides the patient with support and the courage to move forward in terms of acceptance of the change.
Assist the patient in identifying coping devices/diversionary activities.	Provides diversion so that not all thoughts are on disfigurement.
Arrange for psychosocial counseling, as ordered.	Provides psychological assistance to and psychosocial evaluation of the patient.

NIC *Body image enhancement*
Emotional support
Support group
Socialization enhancement

Evaluation

The patient should be able and willing to learn about the strategies to improve functioning and manage own activities to the extent possible. Determine whether the patient is able to verbalize feelings regarding the deformities and the impact they will have on role performance. Time is required for the patient to assimilate the change in body appearance into his or her self-perception completely. It is crucial that the nurse evaluate to what degree the patient is beginning to do this. Communication of feelings and concerns relevant to the change in appearance should be taken as a positive sign that progress towards meeting outcome criteria is being made.

Community/Home Care

At home, continued monitoring of the patient's body image is needed. The nurse who visits will need to be alert to subtle hints that may indicate that the patient has not completely adapted to the change in body appearance. Open discussions regarding this change and interventions to prevent social isolation and withdrawal should continue with patient and family. In some instances, the patient may choose to wear gloves on hands to prevent others from seeing them. Encourage the patient in the home to express feelings openly and honestly with health care providers and family/significant others. Community support groups should be explored.

Documentation

Chart any specific behaviors or verbalizations that may indicate an altered body image. Include all interventions employed to address this issue and the patient's responses. Note when and if the patient begins to verbalize feelings regarding the deformities of the joints and extremities. Document all referrals in the patient record.

CHAPTER 4.62

SYSTEMIC LUPUS ERYTHEMATOSUS (SLE)

GENERAL INFORMATION

Systemic lupus erythematosus (SLE) is an autoimmune disease affecting many body organs/systems and characterized by inflammation that results in a varied clinical picture. The exact etiology of SLE is unknown, but several popular theories have been suggested. It is believed that environmental, genetic, and hormonal factors play a role in the development of SLE. The most prominent etiologic theory is that SLE patients have immune systems that are incapable of regulating immune responses due to abnormalities of both B cells and T cells. Once the body is exposed to the offending factor, it produces autoantibodies against normal constituents of the body, frequently nucleic acids. These SLE autoantibodies then react with their antigens to form immune complexes that become deposited in connective tissues throughout the body. These deposits then initiate an inflammatory response that causes additional damage to the tissue. A common site of involvement is the renal system, but other organs such as the brain, heart, and lungs can also be affected. Medications such as procainamide, isoniazid, and Apresoline can cause a syndrome similar to SLE, but symptoms abate once the medication is discontinued and completely metabolized or eliminated from the body. Other etiologic theories are sensitivities to light, drug sensitivities, vitamin deficiencies, or viral invasion. Even though clinical manifestations vary from person to person, in the early stage of disease diagnosis the patient generally presents with signs and symptoms mimicking RA. These include multiple arthralgias, fatigue, malaise, weight loss, fever, and symmetrical joint involvement. Later in the disease other clinical manifestations include a classic area of erythema on the face in a butterfly pattern, photosensitivity manifested by skin rashes when exposed to light, round raised lesions on the skin with a red rim, ulcers in mouth or nose, and alopecia (however the hair grows back). The disease is not predictable and is characterized by exacerbations and remissions. It is more prevalent in females than males (a 9:1 ratio) with African American women having the highest incidence. Native Americans, Chinese, and Asians living in Hawaii have higher incidences than Caucasians (Phipps, Monahan, Sands, Marek, and Neighbors, 2003). SLE can occur at any age, but its highest incidence is during the childbearing years.

NURSING DIAGNOSIS 1

 IMPAIRED PHYSICAL MOBILITY

Related to:

Joint stiffness

Joint pain

Fatigue

Defining Characteristics:

Difficulty changing positions from lying to sitting, sitting to standing

Difficulty ambulating

Limited range of motion, moves slowly

Goal:

The patient has improved physical mobility.

Outcome Criteria

✔ The patient is able to ambulate without pain in joints.

✔ The patient is able to perform activities of daily living.

✔ The patient reports stiffness of joints has dissipated.

NOC *Mobility*

Joint movement: Knee

Joint movement: Hip

Joint movement: Wrist

INTERVENTIONS	RATIONALES
Assess the patient's current range of motion in affected joints as well as ability to walk with erect posture, to get up and down from chairs, and to perform activities of daily living.	Helps to determine functional ability and to plan for appropriate interventions.
Obtain history from the patient about mobility limitations and effect on ability to remain functional.	Determines if adaptations in lifestyle will need to be made and severity of mobility limitations.
Have patient take analgesics as prescribed (see nursing diagnosis "Acute Pain").	Patients with SLE experience arthritic pain and arthralgias that may impede ability to lead an active life; thus, alleviating the pain will allow for better mobility, improving independence.
Have patient perform range of motion exercises in bed before arising.	Decreases stiffness before the patient attempts ambulation.
Encourage regular exercises, such as walking on level surfaces, swimming, or water exercises specifically designed for patients with arthritis or arthritis-related diseases.	Exercise helps maintain and restore function, maintains muscle tone and mobility, and prevents contractures.
Teach the patient how to balance rest and activity with a realistic regimen that is part of a routine.	Regular rest periods at different times during the day can benefit the patient by decreasing the inflammatory response; patients tend to limit activities due to pain, thus putting themselves at more risk for impaired mobility due to loss of function, but the more routinized the activity recommendations are, the more likely the patient is to be compliant.
Arrange for physical therapy consultation for methods/therapies to improve mobility (moist heat, ultrasound, hydrotherapy, gentle exercise, massage, and ambulatory assistive devices).	Improves physical mobility by relaxing the joint, relieving pain, and improving range of motion.
Teach the patient good posture, correct body mechanics, and body alignment.	Protects joints and reduces stress on affected joints.
Implement strategies to reduce pain (see nursing diagnosis "Acute Pain").	If pain is alleviated, the patient is able to move better.
Teach the patient how to protect joints: use palms rather than fingers; slide objects; change positions frequently; avoid repetitious movements; when performing household chores, avoid stress on joints, e.g., sit down when performing tasks rather than standing, rest between tasks, and perform household duties incrementally over the week.	These strategies protect joints by alleviating stress on them while maintaining optimum function.
Assess the home environment for safety and help the patient identify needs for items such as handrails, grab bars in bathrooms, and stationary pieces of furniture that can be used to assist movement; remove hazards.	The patient with impaired physical mobility is at risk for injury, and the home should be assessed and changes made that decrease risk. Many of the changes can be made at a low cost. Items such as scatter or throw rugs should be removed.
Investigate the need for assistive devices, such as long-handled tools to grab or pick up objects, larger zippers and buttons clothing, jar openers, elevated toilet seats. If needed, assist the patient in locating available places for purchase and teach patient how to use properly.	These items prevent stress on joints and make it easier for patients to remain self-sufficient.
Teach the patient how to cope with pain through the use of medications and non-pharmacological measures.	Many patients become dependent and focus on what they cannot do rather than taking control of the disease. Patients must learn how to cope with joint pain and stiffness on a daily basis and maintain optimum function.
Teach the patient about disease process and effect on mobility.	Knowledge about disease and its effect on the body will give the patient a sense of control and allows for a better understanding of the role of prescribed therapeutic interventions.
Make referrals to support groups.	Support groups can offer emotional support as well as helpful tips on how to live with SLE.

Evaluation

Determine the degree to which the patient is achieving the established outcomes. The patient should report to the health care provider that he or she is able to perform routine household chores and activities of daily living. Assess the extent to which the patient is able to ambulate without pain as well as the effectiveness of interventions to enhance mobility. The patient should report that joint stiffness has been minimized.

Community/Home Care

SLE is a disorder that is treated both at home and in the hospital setting in the initial stages, dependent upon the severity of symptoms. In the early stages of the disease, patient teaching is crucial to allow the patient to understand the disease and the possible pathophysiological events that are possible (see nursing diagnosis "Deficient Knowledge"). The patient may require no in-home assistance or adaptations in environment or lifestyles, but will simply need to control the joint stiffness and pain with mild analgesics. Because SLE has an unpredictable course, the patient needs to be able to recognize all of the possible complications that can occur, especially signs of exacerbations and renal disease. Follow-up with a health care provider is crucial so that progression of the disease can be monitored. The health care provider will need to more closely monitor the effect that limited mobility has on effective functioning. Assessments of the patient's feelings concerning limitations in mobility, any social isolation, concerns about future disability, and feelings of depression should be made. The performance of everyday tasks may prove to be a challenge during exacerbations and at this point assistance may be required from family or others. Even though deformities of joints may not be present and limitations on movement may not be as pronounced as in rheumatoid arthritis, concerns and needs centered around household chores such as laundry and cleaning or self-care needs may still exist. Issues to be addressed include ability to get in or out of the shower or tub, ability to clean the home, and ability to cook meals. It is crucial that the patient understand the strategies required to maintain optimal functioning of affected joints (see interventions).

Documentation

Document a thorough assessment of the patient's functional mobility as well as the presence of stiffness or pain with movement. Include in the patient record all interventions that have been recommended to the patient to address the problem of mobility. All teaching should be recorded. A report of the patient's perception of the ability to be

mobile and a psychosocial assessment should be included. The effectiveness of all interventions should be clearly documented for all members of the healthcare team.

NURSING DIAGNOSIS 2

ACUTE PAIN

Related to:

Swelling

Inflammation

Deposit of immune complexes into joints

Defining Characteristics:

Complaints of pain with movement

Stiffness in joints

Facial grimace

Goal:

Pain is decreased and mobility improved

Outcome Criteria

✔ The patient states that pain is decreased 1 hour after intervention.

✔ The patient verbalizes an ability to ambulate without pain.

✔ The patient verbalizes methods to reduce pain.

NOC *Pain: Disruptive effects*
 Pain level
 Pain control

INTERVENTIONS	RATIONALES
Assess the patient's pain using a pain rating scale.	Provides a more objective assessment.
Assess or take history regarding time of onset, location, precipitating factors, relieving factors, and effect on function; complaint of localized pain upon joint extension; and joint pain, especially after sleeping or increased physical activity.	These will assist in accurate diagnosis and treatment, knowing how pain affects function will provide information needed to assist patient with home care needs.
Monitor results of laboratory and diagnostic tests: anti-DNA	The anti-DNA test is used to confirm the diagnosis SLE by

INTERVENTIONS	RATIONALES
antibody, LE cell prep, anti-nuclear antibody tests (ANA), CBC, x-rays of affected joints.	identifying antibodies to single-stranded or double-stranded DNA (found in 60 to 70 percent of patients with SLE); in patients with SLE, the value will be elevated. LE cell prep is a measure of LE cells that resulted from immunological activity that altered the nucleus of leukocytes. An elevated value supports a diagnosis but is not conclusive and is less sensitive than the ANA test; the ANA test is used to detect SLE and to monitor the effectiveness of treatment, it indicates the presence of the anti-tissue antibodies and in SLE patients, the value will be elevated. Complete blood cell (CBC) count may reveal thrombocytopenia, leukopenia or lymphocytopenia, and anemia. X-rays of joints determine extent of involvement.
Apply moist heat or cold.	Aids muscle relaxation and decreases pain; moist heat is able to penetrate deeper; if pain intensifies during acute inflammation, cold can be used for analgesia properties as well. If commercial heat packs are not available, the patient can use showers (15 minutes) or baths.
Administer first-line analgesic and anti-inflammatory medications as ordered (aspirin) and monitor for effectiveness and side effects, including for gastrointestinal (GI) bleeding, alterations in clotting times, hypersensitivity, tinnitus, and fullness in ears.	Large doses of aspirin may be required for pain relief and are usually considered first; aspirin inhibits prostaglandin production and provides anti-inflammatory effects along with pain relief.
Administer nonsteroidal anti-inflammatory drugs (NSAIDs) as ordered and assess effectiveness; monitor for common side effects that include GI upset and bleeding. An often overlooked side effect is hypertension with a decrease in effectiveness of antihypertensive agents such as beta blockers and ACE inhibitors.	Decreases pain and discomfort and inhibits prostaglandin production; these medications are suggested for their combined effect of pain relief and anti-inflammatory properties.
Administer disease-modifying drugs (e.g., Plaquenil, methotrexate), as ordered, and monitor for effectiveness and side effects: — Plaquenil: antimalarial agent that requires 3 to 6 months of therapy with side effects of pigmentary retinitis and loss of vision; baseline vision testing and regular vision checks at least every 6 months are required. — Methotrexate: cytotoxic agent given if the patient does not respond to NSAIDs; sometimes used instead of steroids or to lower dose of steroidal preparations; side effects include headache, mouth ulcers, bone marrow suppression, liver inflammation, and thrombocytopenia (monitor for easy bruising, petechiae). Perform lab tests to check for side effects: CBC, liver enzymes.	These medications demonstrate ability to provide clinical improvement and decrease progression of the disease activity.
Give all pain medications on a regular dosing schedule rather than prn.	Provides better relief.
Give corticosteroids (such as prednisone), as ordered, and monitor for side effects that include elevations of blood sugar levels, water retention, hypertension, and cushingoid face.	These medications are given to decrease inflammation during exacerbations; also used for patients with severe disease.
Arrange for physical therapy consult to consider ultrasound, hydrotherapy, diathermy, ambulatory assistive devices, etc., during periods of joint inflammation.	The physical therapist may provide therapies to loosen the joint, decrease pain, and increase flexibility.
Implement strategies to improve mobility (see nursing diagnosis "Impaired Physical Mobility").	By improving mobility and minimizing stress on the joints, joint pain and stiffness may be resolved.
Exercise on a regular basis as prescribed by health care providers; swimming, water exercises, and walking are helpful.	Maintains and restores function; these exercises are low impact and decrease stress on affected joints.
Teach relaxation techniques such as music therapy, massage, distraction, and meditation.	These techniques enhance the effect of analgesics and may decrease reliance on medications for complete relief.

NIC *Simple relaxation therapy*
Heat/cold application
Analgesic administration
Pain management

Evaluation

Assess the degree to which the patient reports pain has been relieved by interventions. For persistent pain, the nurse should investigate additional pain relief measures. Determine whether the patient is able to verbalize how to reduce pain.

Community/Home Care

The patient with SLE is typically treated as an outpatient unless there are systemic effects or complications. A cornerstone of care is the management of symptoms, including joint stiffness and pain. A therapeutic regimen that allows for tolerable pain may require an extended period of trial and error with a variety of pharmacological and non-pharmacological measures. If able, the patient needs to learn how to implement relaxation techniques that relax joints and provide some relief of pain. Learning distraction techniques or guided imagery can create a sense of calm and relaxation that can enhance the effects of analgesics. It may be helpful for the patient to keep a pain diary in which to record onset of pain, duration of pain, time of day pain occurs, and pain relieving measures. This can be used to help tailor a plan for pain relief and can be shared with the health care provider. The patient needs to understand the need for rest and schedule rest periods throughout the day to relieve stress on joints that could aggravate pain. Simple strategies, such as having the patient do household chores incrementally over the course of the week rather than having a "cleaning day," could contribute to joint rest and thus decreased pain. Health care providers should follow up to determine if the joint pain prevents the patient from performing activities of daily living. The patient will need to understand the side effects of all medications, as many of them, such as GI bleeding, are significant. In addition, an often overlooked side effect of some NSAIDs is the decreased effectiveness of some antihypertensive medications, particularly ACE inhibitors and beta-blockers such as atenolol, when taken concurrently with NSAIDs. Be sure that the patient knows what symptoms need to be reported to a health care provider. Because of the chronic nature of SLE and the unpredictable course of SLE, home care providers should be attuned to the possibility of frustration, depression, and altered body image in the patient (see nursing diagnosis "Disturbed Body Image").

Documentation

Document any complaints of joint pain and or stiffness. Be sure to include in the documentation at the health care provider's office or in the hospital setting the specific therapeutic interventions prescribed for pain. Include in the patient record the patient's verbalized perception of pain control.

NURSING DIAGNOSIS 3

 FATIGUE

Related to:
   Arthralgias, myalgias
   Anemia

Defining Characteristics:
   Verbalization of being tired
   Reports a lack of energy
   Inability to carry out normal activities

Goal:
   Fatigue will be relieved.

Outcome Criteria

✔ The patient is able to perform activities of daily living.
✔ The patient verbalizes that fatigue has improved or been eliminated.

NOC *Activity tolerance*
Endurance
Energy conservation
Nutritional status: Energy

INTERVENTIONS	RATIONALES
Obtain subjective data regarding normal activities, limitations, and nighttime sleep patterns.	Helps to determine the effect fatigue has on normal functioning. Adequate sleep is required for restoration of the body.

INTERVENTIONS	RATIONALES
Monitor patient for signs of excessive physical and emotional fatigue.	Use as a guideline for adjusting activity.
Encourage periods of rest and activity, and gradually increase activities as tolerated.	Conserves oxygen and prevents undue fatigue. The patient with SLE often has anemia that adds to fatigue because of decreased amounts of oxygen-carrying hemoglobin. SLE patients often require 10 hours of sleep in order to feel rested.
Schedule activities so that excessive demands for oxygen and energy are avoided, e.g., space planned activities away from meal times.	Digestion requires energy and oxygen; participation in activities close to meals will cause increased fatigue because of insufficient energy reserves.
Limit visitors during exacerbations or acute illness.	Socialization for long periods may cause fatigue.
Increase intake of high-energy foods such as meat (especially organ meats), poultry, dried beans and peas, whole grains, and foods high in vitamin C.	These foods enhance energy metabolism, increase oxygen carrying capacity, and provide ready sources of energy needed in hypermetabolic states such as infection and fever.
Encourage patients to plan activities when they have the most energy, usually early in the day.	Prevents fatigue.

NIC *Energy management*

Evaluation

Obtain subjective information from the patient regarding the presence of fatigue. The patient should gradually report the ability to participate in activities of daily living and other normal activities with no fatigue.

Community/Home Care

Patients with SLE should understand that at home, fatigue may persist and actually worsen during times of exacerbation or infections. Appropriate education on ways to adapt self-care and household activities when the SLE patient is fatigued is paramount. A history should be obtained from the patient regarding his or her usual routine for activities of daily living (ADLs) and household chores, so that individualized interventions can be implemented. Attention to what the patient normally does and how the patient wants to make adaptations can only enhance

compliance. The nurse must remain aware of cultural backgrounds that may influence a patient's perception of and adaptation to perceived dependency on others. The patient must understand how to adjust activity in response to feelings of fatigue, possibly even arranging for rest or nap periods in the afternoon. This may not be a realistic recommendation for some people whose occupations may preclude them from napping or even resting during the day. Strategies to enhance nighttime sleep should be implemented so that the patient can get adequate rest. Attention to good nutrition should continue with intake of foods that are good sources of iron, vitamin C, and protein. If fatigue persists for extended periods, the patient may need to seek health care to investigate the possibility of other causes of the fatigue and more aggressive methods to address the problem.

Documentation

Chart the specific complaint of fatigue to include what activities the patient has been performing. Document interventions implemented to address fatigue, being sure to document food intake. An assessment of the patient's sleep patterns should also be documented.

NURSING DIAGNOSIS 4

 IMPAIRED SKIN INTEGRITY

Related to:

    Inflammation

    Autoimmune reactions

Defining Characteristics:

    Butterfly rash on face

    Skin rash on any part of body

    Sensitivity to light

    Ulcers in mouth or nose

    Skin lesions

    Alopecia

Goal:

    The patient's skin will remain intact.

Outcome Criteria

✔ Skin lesions will heal and not become infected.

✔ Butterfly rash will dissipate following treatment and control of disease.

✔ The patient will verbalize care required for skin.
✔ Ulcers will heal within 1 week.

NOC *Tissue integrity: Skin and mucous membranes*
Knowledge: Treatment regimen

INTERVENTIONS	RATIONALES
Assess the patient's and family's knowledge regarding skin changes that occur with SLE.	Gives the nurse a starting point for recommending strategies and implementing teaching.
Assess the patient's skin well to include mouth and nose for ulcers, remainder of body for rashes, and face for butterfly rash.	Establishes a baseline for comparison and to make recommendations for care.
Encourage the patient to avoid exposure to sun, use sunblock (SPF 15 or higher), remain inside during the hottest parts of the day, and wear protective clothing and hats when outdoors.	Sunlight can cause skin manifestations and also lead to an acute exacerbation of the disease.
Avoid the use of perfumed lotions, ointments, or cosmetics; try instead unscented dermatologist-recommended products such as Eucerin for dry skin.	These products tend to cause drying due to alcohol content and may irritate sensitive skin.
Arrange consult with dermatologist or skin care specialist for cosmetic products to cover rash.	The presence of a facial rash affects body image and appropriate cosmetics can prevent disturbed body image; specially prepared cosmetics need to be used to prevent further skin impairment.
Administer or encourage patient to take medications for disease control as prescribed.	These medications control the disease and decrease inflammation and likelihood of rash development.
For oral ulcers, keep mouth clean by rinsing with solutions as ordered (such as antiseptic mouthwash, half-strength peroxide, and normal saline).	Keeps the mouth clean and decreases bacteria count.
For oral ulcers, avoid foods that are irritating such as citrus juices, tomato-based sauces, hot seasonings, and spicy food.	These foods contain irritating substances such as acid that can further impair tissue integrity.
Encourage a nutritious diet.	Promotes healing.

Assess for scalp lesions, excoriations, and degree of hair loss.	Establishes a baseline.
Have patient avoid harsh hair products (alcohol-based shampoos, relaxers, and dyes) and hot curling irons, especially during acute exacerbations. Implement strategies to address hair loss (see nursing diagnosis "Disturbed Body Image").	Many hair care products contain chemicals that are caustic to sensitive skin on the scalp; intense heat applied close to the scalp can cause irritation. The patient may be more prone to develop scalp lesions and lose hair during acute exacerbations. Some of the medications used to treat SLE cause hair loss (corticosteroids, immunosuppressants).
Inform patient that hair will grow back, though often with a different texture.	This may provide some assurance to the patient that body changes are temporary, making it somewhat easier to adapt to the change and protect body image.
Assess effectiveness of interventions through a thorough assessment of lesions, ulcers, and rashes.	Helps to determine whether revisions to the plan need to be made.

NIC *Skin care: Topical treatments*
Skin surveillance

Evaluation

Determine the degree to which the patient has achieved the stated outcome criteria. If skin rashes or ulcers are present, they should be free of infections and show signs of healing. The patient should be able to verbalize the care required for the skin changes and be willing to comply.

Community/Home Care

The patient with SLE will need to implement strategies for skin care in the home setting. Because of the potential for altered body image due to these physical changes, it is important for the nurse to be sure that the patient has received adequate teaching regarding what is required. At home, the patient should make skin assessment a routine part of daily personal care, especially inspecting the nose and mouth for lesions. A small mirror similar to that used by dentists to inspect the mouth can be purchased at a drug store. For some patients who may have previously enjoyed a day in the sun at the beach or working in the yard, changes to routine must be made. Time outside will need to be limited, and when in sunshine at home, aggressive measures to protect the skin will need to be implemented. Protective lightweight clothing that covers the skin and a wide-brim hat can protect the patient and should be worn. The patient can also use an umbrella to shield him or herself from the sun. If the patient normally seeks profressional hair care, he or she will need to inform the hairdresser of the special requirements for hair and scalp care and in some instances may need to provide the hairdresser with products obtained from a dermatologist. The hairdresser may also be a resource in terms of where to purchase fashionable wigs that are hypoallergenic and for inspecting the scalp for lesions. Some larger, upscale department stores may carry special cosmetics that can be used to cover facial rashes, but the patient should consult with a dermatologist or other physician to be sure of its appropriateness for SLE-impaired skin. The butterfly rash may disappear once the disease is controlled, but other rashes or skin impairments may appear from time to time, necessitating attention to skin care. Any type of scented soap, perfume, or other personal care items should be used with caution. Milder soaps may need to be used for daily hygiene as common deodorant soaps may be too strong for the skin. During follow-up visits, assessment of the patient's body image should be made, and if problems are present, attention should be given to their resolution. Support groups may be helpful to the patient in this area as other patients can offer suggestions for skin care that have worked for them or recommend safe products. The patient will need to be aware of changes in the skin that would warrant a return visit to the health care provider.

Documentation

Document the results of a thorough assessment of the patient's skin, particularly the presence and description of any rashes, ulcers, or skin lesions. Chart all nursing interventions implemented to address the problem, including any attention given to psychosocial needs, such as disturbed body image. Include in the patient record all teaching implemented and the patient's understanding, as well as referrals to a dermatologist. Document whether the outcome criteria have been achieved.

NURSING DIAGNOSIS 5

DISTURBED BODY IMAGE

Related to:

Skin lesions on face

Facial rash (butterfly rash)

Alopecia

Body rashes

Defining Characteristics:

Withdrawal

Social isolation

Depression

Negative statements about physical appearance

Attempts to cover face or head in the presence of others

Goal:

The patient accepts the change in physical appearance and continues social activities and interpersonal relationships.

Outcome Criteria

✔ The patient states willingness to look at face.

✔ The patient does not verbalize negative feelings toward self.

✔ The patient verbalizes a satisfaction with body appearance.

NOC *Body image*

INTERVENTIONS	RATIONALES
Encourage patient to communicate feelings about changes in physical appearance and assure the patient that his or her feelings are normal.	Talking about the changes may sometimes be the beginning of acceptance, and the patient should understand that his or her emotions are real and should be expected.
Allow the patient privacy when bathing or dressing unless assistance is requested.	Allows patient time to adjust to appearance without concern for how others will react.
Teach the patient methods to care for skin to prevent disfigurement and complications (see nursing diagnosis "Impaired Skin Integrity").	Protecting the skin from light and chemical agents that worsen lesions and rashes can improve appearance and prevent further problems.

(continues)

(continued)

INTERVENTIONS	RATIONALES
Investigate the use of wigs or hairpieces if alopecia is present. If the patient is conscientious about hair loss, arrange for a specialist in wigs to visit the patient so that the patient can pick out a wig in the style and color of his or her choice.	Loss of hair can cause serious problems with body image, most often the hair will grow back, making the wig a temporary strategy.
Monitor patient's feelings about him or herself, interpersonal relationships with family members and friends, withdrawal, social isolation, fear, anxiety, embarrassment by appearance, and desire to be alone.	Helps to detect early alterations in social functioning, prevent unhealthy behaviors and intervene early through referral to counseling.
Encourage patient to participate in at least one outside/public activity each week once health status permits.	Prevents patient from isolating self from others.
Identify the effects of the patient's culture or religion in terms of body image.	A patient's culture and religion often help define reactions to changes in body image and self-worth.
Identify community support groups if available, such as Arthritis Foundation or Lupus Foundation, or other support groups.	Discussions with other patients in a similar situation are good for the patient; provides the patient with support and the courage to move forward in terms of acceptance of the change.
Assist the patient in identifying coping strategies/diversionary activities.	Provides diversionary activities so that not all thoughts are on disfigurement.
Arrange for psychosocial counseling.	Provides psychological assistance to the patient and psychosocial evaluation.

NIC   *Body image enhancement*
       Emotional support
       Support group
       Socialization enhancement

Evaluation

The patient is able and willing to learn about the strategies to improve psychosocial health. Determine whether the patient is able to verbalize feelings regarding hair loss and skin changes and the impact it will have on role performance. Time is required for the patient to assimilate the change in body appearance into his or her self-perception completely. It is crucial that the nurse evaluate the degree to which the patient is beginning to do this. Communication of feelings and concerns relevant to the change in appearance should be taken as a positive sign that the patient is making progress towards meeting outcome criteria.

Community/Home Care

At home, continued monitoring of the patient's body image is necessary. The nurse who visits will need to be alert to subtle hints indicating that the patient has not completely adapted to the change in body appearance. Hair should begin to grow back while the patient is being followed at home. A nice wig that resembles the patient's own hair may improve body image. In addition, skin changes may be resolved or masked with dermatologist-approved cosmetics and other simple strategies for protection (see nursing diagnosis "Impaired Skin Integrity"). Both of these should enhance body image. Open discussions regarding physical changes and interventions to prevent social isolation and withdrawal should continue with patient and family. Have the patient look at him or herself in the mirror daily as a way to gain positive feelings and perceptions about appearance. Encourage the patient to participate in public activities with familiar people, such as religious or civic events. Community support groups should be explored.

Documentation

Chart any specific behaviors or verbalizations that may indicate an altered body image. Include all interventions that have been employed to address this issue and the patient's responses. Note when and if the patient begins to verbalize feelings regarding the skin changes and hair loss. Document all referrals in the patient record.

NURSING DIAGNOSIS 6

DEFICIENT KNOWLEDGE

Related to:

New onset of disease

Numerous diagnostic tests for diagnosis

Lack of information about disease and treatment

Defining Characteristics:

Ask many or no questions

Verbalizes a lack of knowledge/ understanding

Goal:

The patient will receive and understand information relevant to SLE.

Outcome Criteria

✔ The patient and family will verbalize a need for information regarding SLE and its treatment.

✔ The patient and family verbalize an understanding of medication regimen.

✔ The patient and family verbalize an understanding of possible disease progression.

✔ The patient will verbalize how to prevent exacerbations.

✔ The patient and family member or significant other verbalize a desire to learn necessary information.

✔ The patient verbalizes an understanding of follow-up care required and expresses a willingness to comply.

NOC *Knowledge: Medication*
Knowledge: Disease process
Knowledge: Treatment regimen
Compliance behavior

INTERVENTIONS	RATIONALES
Assess the patient's current knowledge as well as his or her ability and readiness to learn.	The nurse needs to ascertain what the patient already knows and build on this; if the patient is not capable of learning or is not ready to learn, teaching will not be effective due to disinterest or inability to understand.
Start with the simplest information and move to complex information.	Patients can understand simple concepts easily and then can build on those to understand concepts that are more complex.

Collaborate with physician to teach patient, family members, and significant others:

— Disease process of SLE, which can be mild and chronic or virulent with multi-system involvement

— Early clinical manifestations: fatigue, joint stiffness, joint pain, arthralgias, skin rashes (butterfly rash over bridge of nose), skin lesions, mouth ulcers, hair loss, and photosensitivity

— Chronic, long-term possibilities: renal impairment (edema, decreased urine output, increased weight), infections (elevated temperature, malaise), anemia, thrombocytopenia, anorexia and nausea, Raynaud's phenomenon (change in color of fingers and toes in response to cold—blanching, cyanosis, redness), and changes in cerebral function

— Strategies to prevent infection: good hand hygiene, avoiding crowds, avoiding people with upper respiratory infections, good nutrition, receiving appropriate vaccinations (influenza)

— Seek health care for any signs of chronic, long-term complications

— Strategies to prevent infections as well as signs and symptoms of infection

Teaching decreases anxiety and prepares the patient for what to expect. Knowledge of disease and long-term complications empowers the patient to take control and be compliant.

Instruct patient regarding possible drug treatments required:

— Aspirin for arthralgias and to prevent platelet aggregation to help prevent thrombosis; side effects to monitor for include GI bleeding

— NSAIDs for pain relief

— Antimalarial agents such as Plaquenil (hydroxychloroquine) to reduce episodes of exacerbations; side effects include retinal changes; patient should have regular eye exams

— Corticosteroids such as prednisone to reduce inflammatory responses and

Knowledge of the possibilities of the disease (both short-term and long-term) allows the patient to cope with the disease better and be better prepared to comply with recommendations. A polypharmacy approach to treatment may be required to achieve adequate disease control and teaching relevant to the medications is crucial.

(continues)

(continued)

INTERVENTIONS	RATIONALES
prevent damage to organs; side effects include weight gain, GI upset, hyperglycemia, hypertension, cushingoid effects such as moon face; patient should take medication with food and should not stop taking the medicine abruptly — Immunosuppressive drugs such as Cytoxan are used to suppress the immune system, decreasing progression of the disease; common side effects include increased risk for infection, nausea, vomiting, and neutropenia; the patient should implement strategies to prevent infection (avoiding crowds, good handwashing. etc.) and monitor for fever	
Provide the patient with information about skin impairments and recommendations for care (see nursing diagnosis "Impaired Skin Integrity").	Knowing what to expect in terms of skin changes can help the patient cope or minimize frustrations with alterations in appearance.
Teach the patient strategies to control or cope with fatigue (see nursing diagnosis "Fatigue").	Fatigue is a common complaint of the patient with SLE, especially during the early phases.
Provide patient and family with information on Lupus Foundation of America.	This agency can assist with information, support, and other services.
Assess the patient's and family's understanding of all teaching by encouraging them to repeat information and ask questions as needed.	This allows the nurse to hear in the patient's own words what was taught and makes it easier to know what information may need reinforcement.
Provide the patient and family with written information on content taught.	Provides reference at a later time.
Establish that the patient has the resources required to be compliant, such as transportation to appointments and finances to buy medications.	If needed resources such as finances and transportation to follow-up appointments are not available, the patient cannot be compliant; the nurse will need to make necessary referrals. This may be a real problem for patients in remote and rural areas, especially if family support is not available.

NIC   *Learning readiness enhancement*
Learning facilitation
Teaching: Disease process
Teaching: Prescribed medication

Evaluation

Evaluate the degree to which the patient has achieved the outcome criteria relevant to the teaching sessions. The patient should verbalize an understanding of content presented by repeating the information, particularly the disease process of SLE, along with the possible long-term complications, pharmacological treatments, and side effects of medications. The nurse must determine whether the patient is capable of being compliant with the recommended regimen. If further teaching is required, the appropriate referrals should be made to continue patient education.

Community/Home Care

The patient and family will need to implement the medical regimen in the home setting over an extended period of time. The success of this implementation will depend upon the degree to which the patient has received adequate teaching and has subsequently understood and internalized it. Because of the potential effects of SLE on all body systems, compliance with treatments and follow-up appointments should be monitored. In most instances, the patient will need to have frequent follow-up visits with a health care provider to monitor progression of disease and response to therapy (both positive outcomes and side effects). As indicated in the preceding interventions, there are many facets of care that the patient and family need to understand. The patient with lupus frequently has long-term effects from the disease, and early detection of these will allow for early intervention. Control of joint stiffness, arthralgias, and fatigue is a big part of home care and will require frequent follow-up to ensure patient satisfaction.

Documentation

Document the specific content taught and the titles of any printed documents given to the patient. Include in the chart the patient's degree of understanding of the content and the methods used to evaluate learning. Document any areas that need reinforcement to ensure appropriate follow-up. If family members are present for the teaching sessions, document this in the chart, and always document any referrals made.

UNIT 5

RENAL SYSTEM

CHAPTER 5.63

RENAL FAILURE: ACUTE

GENERAL INFORMATION

Acute renal failure (ARF) usually has a rapid onset and is accompanied by electrolyte imbalances and evidence of azotemia with extremely high blood urea nitrogen (BUN) and a significantly elevated creatinine. The numerous causes of ARF are categorized into three types: prerenal, intrarenal, and postrenal. Prerenal causes of acute kidney failure are those causes that affect renal blood flow and perfusion, including any disease entity that causes hypovolemia (i.e., hemorrhage, burns), decreased cardiac output (i.e., congestive heart failure, myocardial infarction), systemic vasodilation (i.e., sepsis, anaphylaxis), and hypotension/hypoperfusion (i.e., shock). Prerenal causes of ARF accounts for 55 to 70 percent of all ARF cases (Lemone and Burke, 2004; Phipps, et. al, 2003). Intrarenal causes of ARF are those factors that cause damage to the renal tissue and structures including the nephrons. The most common intrarenal cause is acute tubular necrosis, which can be attributed to a variety of factors: antibiotics such as aminoglycosides, heavy metals, chemicals, radioactive dyes, and other drugs. Other intrarenal causes include glomerulonephritis, malignant hypertension, vascular disorders, and rhabdomyolysis. Intrarenal causes of ARF account for approximately 25 to 40 percent of all cases. Postrenal causes of ARF only account for approximately 5 percent of all cases; these cause renal failure through obstruction of urine flow and include benign prostatic hyperplasia (most common), renal calculi, tumors, or any other obstructive process.

Sources differ in their classification of ARF, but it is generally accepted that there are distinct physiological phases to the progression of the renal failure: an initiating event, oliguria, diuresis, and recovery. During the initiation or onset stage, the precipitating event occurs with subsequent damage to the kidney. The patient often has no recognizable symptoms at this time. During the oliguric phase, the kidneys are unable to maintain their normal excretory function. If urine output is < 400 ml/24 hours, waste products begin to build up in the blood and the BUN level rises with a concomitant elevation in creatinine, which indicates impaired nephron functioning. At this point, the patient begins to have periods of confusion and drowsiness as the waste products interfere with cerebral oxygenation. When the oliguria reaches < 30 ml/24 hours, the patient is unable to maintain homeostasis. The most pronounced changes include hyperkalemia, hyperphosphatemia, hyponatremia, hypocalcemia, and metabolic acidosis. Other abnormal laboratory findings include decreased red blood cells, leukopenia, platelet abnormalities, and increased specific gravity as waste products continue to build in the bloodstream. The kidneys are unable to excrete fluids, causing fluid overload in the circulating volume, and dialysis is indicated to remove both fluids and waste products. The third phase is the diuretic phase. During this period, large amounts of fluids and electrolytes (especially potassium) are excreted, but the renal tubules are unable to concentrate the urine. As much as 4000 milliliters per day may be lost. The patient may demonstrate hypotension; signs and symptoms of dehydration, such as dry skin and dry mucous membranes; as well as weight loss due to fluid loss. Signs of positive outcomes include resolution of some fatigue and an increasing mental status (more alert, no confusion). The final phase of ARF is the recovery stage, which may last for up to one year. During this time, kidney function returns to normal and the renal tubules begin to concentrate urine and excrete waste products as evidenced by renal function studies (creatinine, specific gravity, and BUN) that progress to normal. However, for some patients, residual impairment may continue. For some critically ill, unstable patients who develop ARF, hemodialysis cannot be tolerated. In this case continuous veno-venous hemodialysis (CVVHD) is implemented with a slow removal of fluids over a 24-hour period rather than the traditional 3-hour period of hemodialysis during which large amounts of fluid are exchanged.

NURSING DIAGNOSIS 1

 IMPAIRED URINARY ELIMINATION

Related to:

Structural damage to kidney tissue

Decreased function of nephrons

Impaired function of glomeruli

Defining Characteristics:

Oliguria (initial stage)

Polyuria (recovery stage)

Increased creatinine

Increased BUN

Lethargy/fatigue

Weakness

Goal:

Urinary elimination will return to baseline.

Outcome Criteria

✔ The patient will void no < 30 ml/hour.

✔ The patient will not experience frequency of urination.

✔ The patient's kidney function studies (creatinine, BUN, specific gravity) will return to normal.

NOC *Urinary elimination*

Kidney function

Systemic toxin clearance: Dialysis

INTERVENTIONS	RATIONALES
Monitor amount of output during each phase of ARF.	In ARF, absolute cessation of urine may not occur. The patient may be oliguric but not anuric. The amount of output may give clues to the extent of kidney function. As the acute process is treated and kidney function resumes, output will proceed to polyuria before returning to normal.
Monitor frequency, consistency, color, and odor of urine.	During the early phase of ARF, the small amount of urine excreted may be dark and highly concentrated as the kidneys continue to try to excrete waste products; in the recovery phase, the kidneys can excrete urine but not concentrate it with waste products, making the urine very pale yellow and in some instances almost colorless.
Monitor results of laboratory tests: urinalysis (specific gravity, proteinuria, red blood cells), BUN, creatinine, electrolytes, arterial blood gases (ABGs), red blood cells, hemoglobin, and hematocrit.	The urinalysis will reveal a specific gravity that is low and eventually fixes at a level equal to that of the patient's plasma as the kidneys are unable to concentrate urine; the presence of red blood cells and protein in the urine suggest damage to glomeruli; BUN (end product of protein metabolism) will be elevated and can rise as much as 30 mg/dl per day as the kidneys can no longer rid the blood of this waste product; creatinine is an end product of muscle energy that is excreted by the kidneys, and as kidney function deteriorates, the creatinine rises; potassium is normally excreted via a process of ion exchange by the nephron, but due to the limited numbers of functioning nephrons in ARF, potassium cannot be excreted, leading to dangerously high levels; sodium levels are low due to increased amounts of circulating volume secondary to inability to excrete fluids; phosphorous levels are high due to inability of kidneys to excrete phosphate; calcium levels are low due to decreased levels of ionized calcium in the circulating volume secondary to increased levels of phosphorous; ABGs reveal metabolic acidosis due to inability of the kidneys to excrete hydrogen ions and produce bicarbonate ions; red blood cells, hemoglobin, and hematocrit are all low. Red blood cells are more fragile in the waste-ridden circulating volume

(continues)

(continued)

INTERVENTIONS	RATIONALES
	and erythropoietin secretion is decreased; hemoglobin drops as not enough mature red blood cells are available for oxygen transport; hematocrit levels are decreased.
Assess cardiovascular and respiratory systems: breath sounds, respiratory rate and depth, heart sounds, blood pressure, pulse, skin color, and peripheral pulses; note abnormalities of orthostatic hypotension, or edema.	The presence of excess fluids and electrolyte imbalances (especially potassium) may contribute to cardiac dysrhythmias and fluid accumulation in the respiratory system. Weak distal pulses may be detected along with generalized and dependent edema. Kussmaul respirations may be noted due to metabolic acidosis, and the breath may have an ammonia-like odor. Elevated blood pressure and tachycardia occur due to excess circulating volume. Heart sounds may reveal abnormal sounds such as S_3 and S_4 due to increased volume. Early detection of these symptoms allows for early interventions to prevent complications (see nursing diagnoses "Decreased Cardiac Output" and "Excess Fluid Volume").
Assess neurological and musculoskeletal systems for abnormalities: weakness, decreased level of consciousness (memory loss, confusion, lethargy), muscle twitching, seizures, headache, difficulty focusing, and muscle cramps.	Increased amounts of toxins and waste products in the blood interfere with normal functioning of nervous tissue and impair oxygen uptake by cerebral tissues. Electrolyte imbalances and the presence of waste products in the blood also contribute to impaired innervation of muscles required for function. Twitching and muscle weakness may be noted due to decreases in calcium and increases in potassium.
Treat the underlying cause of ARF.	Acute renal failure can be caused by a variety of factors including sepsis, myocardial infarction, hypovolemia, hypotension, etc.
Prepare the patient for dialysis and assist as required by agency protocol (insertion of central line, femoral lines, access ports, etc.).	Patients who develop ARF need a means to remove waste products, excess fluids, and toxins from the blood,

and restore homeostasis. Hemodialysis is accomplished through a central Multilumen catheter. Once a route for dialysis is established and functional, the preparation for dialysis is dependent upon agency requirements but generally includes withholding antihypertensive medications but allowing meals. Dialysis will remove waste products, toxins, and excess fluid from the body. For patients who are critically ill and unstable, CVVHD may be required, allowing for slow removal of fluids, as the rapid removal can disrupt cardiac output due to decreases in blood pressure.

Monitor patient for side effects of dialysis treatment: decreased blood pressure, dizziness, fatigue, and hypothermia (as a result of CVVHD).	Recognizing side effects will protect the patient from physiological and physical injury and allow for early intervention.
Apply warm covers or thermal blankets if hypothermia occurs.	Hypothermia causes increased metabolic rates and oxygen demand that results in more waste products to be excreted by the kidneys; keeping the patient warm decreases oxygen demand and cardiac workload, thereby decreasing work required of the failing kidneys.
Administer medications as ordered: sodium bicarbonate, diuretics, vasodilators, and antihypertensives.	Sodium bicarbonate treats acidosis; diuretics increase fluid loss; vasodilators enhance renal blood flow and promote fluid excretion; antihypertensives decrease elevated blood pressure caused by sodium and water retention.
Maintain central line dialysis site according to agency protocol: change dressing using sterile technique as ordered, flush unused lumens with heparin according to agency protocol, assess site for infection every shift (redness or other discoloration, heat, pain, drainage), do not use the dialysis lines for medications or intravenous fluids.	Central line care is crucial to maintaining function of the access site. Because this is the patient's lifeline, health care providers must assure that the site is functional by preventing infection and clotting off of the lumens. Heparin is used to maintain patency.

INTERVENTIONS	RATIONALES
Assist with implementation of dietary restrictions, as ordered.	Restriction of proteins is necessary to decrease waste products, and fluid restrictions may be required until volume excess is resolved and kidney function is restored (see nursing diagnosis "Imbalanced Nutrition: Less than Body Requirements").
Teach the patient and family about ARF: all interventions required including the process of dialysis, in-home care required, and symptoms that indicate need for return to a health care provider.	Keeping the patient informed can decrease anxiety; the patient needs to understand the disease, treatments, and prognosis.

NIC *Hemodialysis therapy*
Fluid monitoring

Evaluation

The patient has a urine output of at least 30 ml/hour. The urine is clear yellow with no evidence of sediment and a normal specific gravity. Creatinine level is the most accurate measure of kidney function, and it should return to normal, as should the BUN following a period of treatment with or without dialysis. Urinary elimination patterns return to baseline, and the patient has no urinary frequency.

Community/Home Care

The patient who has been acutely ill due to ARF and its cause will require monitoring in the home setting due to residual effects. Once at home, the patient may continue to experience some feelings of general malaise and fatigue that will prevent him or her from performing usual routines. Gradual resumption of activities will assist the patient to return to usual activity patterns without complications as stamina and endurance improves. The nurse should determine that the patient has the assistance required for performance of activities of daily living (ADLs) and household chores, and if not, alternative care environments should be explored. The patient should limit what he or she does in the early phase of recovery as the more active the patient is, the more waste products produced require excretion by the kidneys. Diet recommendations (protein restrictions) are important at home to allow for decreased work by the recovering kidneys. Protein and fluid restrictions should continue for a period of time for this reason (see nursing diagnosis "Imbalanced Nutrition: Less than Body Requirements"). Continued monitoring of kidney function will be necessary to ensure that kidney function returns to normal. Symptoms that the patient should note include decreasing urine volume, rapid weight gain, changes in alertness, headache, muscle twitching, and/or muscle cramps. The patient can obtain a measuring container from the hospital to use at home to monitor amount of urinary output. A simple scale purchased at a retail store can be placed in the bathroom so that the patient can weigh self regularly. The nurse can prepare an informational booklet for the patient that contains vital information so that the patient has a reference document. If any untoward symptoms occur, the patient should contact a health care provider. At follow-up appointments, the health care provider will determine specific indicators of kidney function, such as creatinine, specific gravity, and BUN.

Documentation

Document findings from all assessments: genitourinary, cardiovascular, and respiratory. Include all interventions implemented to address the impaired patterns of urinary elimination along with the patient's responses. Document the placement of central lines or other access devices for dialysis and the type of dialysis employed. Document all vital signs, noting any changes from baseline and interventions initiated to address hypertension or hypotension, temperature elevations, and increased respirations. Intake and output are documented according to agency protocol, noting specifically polyuria or oliguria.

NURSING DIAGNOSIS 2

 EXCESS FLUID VOLUME

Related to:

Inability to excrete water

Renal failure that causes sodium and water retention

Defining Characteristics:

Weight gain

Lethargy

Hypertension

Lung congestion/crackles

Dyspnea

Jugular vein distention

Urine output < 30 ml/hr

Edema

S_3 heart sound

Goal:

The patient's fluid and electrolyte imbalances are corrected.

The patient's vital signs return to normal.

Outcome Criteria

✔ The patient will have no edema, crackles in lungs, abnormal heart sounds, or jugular vein distention.

✔ The patient will lose weight during treatment.

✔ The patient will have urine output > 30 ml/hour.

✔ Electrolytes will return to normal ranges.

✔ Blood pressure and pulse will return to patient baseline.

NOC *Fluid balance*

Electrolyte and acid/base balance

Fluid overload severity

INTERVENTIONS	RATIONALES
Assess location and extent of edema particularly in extremities.	Helps to assess severity of the fluid excess.
Assess breath sounds for crackles.	When the kidneys are unable to excrete fluids, circulating volume becomes excessive; monitoring breath sounds provides for early detection of left heart failure; crackles are an indicator of fluid in the lungs and should be monitored for worsening or improvement as an indicator of disease status and response to interventions.
Place the patient in high Fowler's position.	Minimizes cardiac workload and decreases fluid return to the heart.
Assess vital signs every 4 hours or as ordered.	In the presence of renal failure, the blood pressure elevates, as does the pulse in response to the increased fluid volume; respiratory rate and depth may increase secondary to metabolic acidosis as the lungs attempt to blow off more carbon dioxide to create acid/base balance.
Administer oxygen, as ordered, if the patient experiences shortness of breath.	Improves oxygenation and peripheral perfusion.
Weigh patient daily at the same time on the same scale, in the morning before breakfast and after voiding. The patient should wear similar clothing each time he or she is weighed.	The most accurate method of determining fluid volume loss is through daily weights; 1 kilogram of weight loss = 1 liter of fluid lost. Morning weights are a better reflection of true weights as most people accumulate fluid as the day progresses. On the days that the patient undergoes dialysis, weights will be obtained before and after dialysis to detect fluid gain and to determine how much fluid should be drawn off during the procedure.
Implement a renal diet low in sodium, potassium, and protein, as ordered.	Sodium increases fluid retention; thus, decreasing the amount of dietary sodium intake will decrease the amount of retained fluid. Salty foods also increase the thirst sensation, which increases the desire for more oral fluid. A low-potassium diet is necessary because of the elevated potassium levels resulting from the kidneys' inability to excrete potassium; proteins create waste products that the kidneys cannot excrete.
Implement fluid restrictions, as ordered, and inform all other health care providers of the specific amount allowed on each shift; inform the patient of restrictions.	Restricting fluid intake can assist in decreasing circulating volume, thereby decreasing cardiac workload.
Obtain accurate intake and output information, noting color of urine.	Helps to monitor the balance between fluid consumed and urinary output, and to detect the return of kidney function. Polyuria indicates that the kidneys are able to make large amounts of urine, but urine may be extremely pale in color due to an inability to concentrate urine in the early phase of recovery.

INTERVENTIONS	RATIONALES
Monitor electrolytes (especially potassium, phosphorous, sodium, and calcium).	In ARF, the kidneys are unable to excrete potassium; calcium decreases as the kidneys are unable to excrete phosphorous or activate vitamin D; sodium levels decrease due to increased fluid volume (hyperdilution).
Implement strategies to lower potassium levels, as ordered, such as by giving Kayexalate® PO (orally) or via enema; administer regular insulin, 50 percent dextrose, and calcium gluconate IV, as ordered.	In renal failure, the kidneys are unable to excrete adequate amounts of potassium; high potassium levels may produce life-threatening dysrhythmias and need to be addressed. Kayexalate is a cation exchange resin that exchanges sodium ions for potassium ions in the bowel, allowing for excretion of potassium via stools. Insulin is given to cause a movement of potassium into the intracellular spaces; glucose is given to counteract the hypoglycemic effects of the insulin; calcium gluconate is given to protect the myocardium from effects of potassium.
Implement strategies to lower phosphorous and elevate calcium levels, such as administering phosphorous binding/lowering agents such as calcium acetate (PhosLo®) or aluminum hydroxide agents (Basaljel®).	The kidneys are unable to excrete phosphorous and as serum levels rise, calcium levels drop (inverse relation of phosphorous levels to calcium levels); ALWAYS give phosphorous-lowering agents with meals in order to enhance the binding effects and also to decrease further absorption of calcium; aluminum hydroxide agents bind dietary phosphorous, prohibiting phosphorous absorption, and phosphate is then excreted via stool. Calcium products raise the serum level of calcium.
Monitor for side effects of electrolyte imbalance: muscle weakness, cardiac dysrhythmias, tingling and numbness in extremities, muscular twitching.	Patients with renal failure have accompanying electrolyte imbalances that may never return to normal levels. However, dangerously low or high alterations need to be treated in order to maintain homeostasis and prevent impaired muscle function or other organ damage. Early detection of symptoms allows for prompt treatment.
Monitor ABGs for metabolic acidosis.	In ARF, metabolic acidosis is common as the kidneys are no longer able to perform their buffering function by excreting hydrogen ions and conserving bicarbonate. This should improve as ARF is corrected.
Protect edematous skin in extremities and sacrum.	Fluid inhibits adequate circulation to the tissue, predisposing the patient to skin breakdown.

NIC *Fluid management*
Electrolyte monitoring

Evaluation

Patient has no symptoms of fluid excess. Urine output is at least 30 ml/hour. Breath sounds are clear and weight loss has been demonstrated. Edema is absent or decreasing, with no pitting edema. Skin in edematous-dependent areas should be intact. Jugular vein distention has been alleviated, and blood pressure and pulse return to baseline.

Community/Home Care

Ensure that the patient at home understands the importance of monitoring fluid status. Weighing daily at home will allow the patient to notice subtle changes in fluid retention. If the patient still requires dialysis at the time of discharge, the patient should ask that the dialysis team provide his or her weight on dialysis days for comparison. In addition, the patient should be taught how to assess for excessive fluid retention, such as by noting clothing that becomes too tight in a short period or a rapid weight gain in 24 hours. These could indicate heart failure, which could lead to more health care complications for the patient. At home, the patient needs to limit the intake of sodium-rich foods and table salt to reduce the risk of further fluid excess. Teach the patient how to read food labels for sodium content, especially on the types of food the patient normally purchases; this can be reinforced once at home by having the nurse or dietician visit and simply pull foods from the cupboard and discuss them with the patient or caregiver. An important aspect of dietary management for the patient with renal failure is avoidance of potassium-rich foods, such as cantaloupe, oranges, orange juice, and broccoli, or consuming them in moderation until renal function has been restored. Because of the restriction on sodium, many patients may want to use salt substitutes; however, most of these are high in potassium and should also be avoided. Dietary instructions for the home should consider the patient's normal diet and any cultural or religious preferences and restrictions. Have the patient keep a log of food and fluid intake as well as weights. Assist the patient in developing a schedule for taking any prescribed medications that is mindful of his or her lifestyle and daily routine. The patient can discuss concerns with a visiting nurse, or if dialysis treatments continue, after discharge, at dialysis treatments. Noncompliance with dietary and fluid restrictions during the recovery phase may occur, causing the patient to be hospitalized for respiratory symptoms or congestive heart failure due to the excess fluid volume. Instruction about preventing these complications should be reinforced by all health care providers, and assistance of in-home caregivers should be sought for ensuring compliance with recommended therapies. The patient may experience some distress or ineffective coping when faced with the need for dialysis, even on a temporary basis. If this happens, the patient may need counseling and assistance with spiritual distress. As the renal function returns, the patient should be aware of the signs and symptoms to note, including polyuria and a return of energy levels. When this happens, the patient should note the color of urine, looking for a return to a normal yellow. Teaching should result in the patient's understanding of symptoms that would indicate a need to return to the health care provider (these may include increasing shortness of breath, rapid weight gain, edema, etc.). Stress the need for keeping all appointments for follow-up care by a primary health care provider.

Documentation

Always document the extent to which the outcome criteria have been achieved. Record intake and output, blood pressure, pulse, weights, breath sounds, and the patient's understanding of the therapies for eliminating fluid excess. Document all therapeutic interventions employed to address fluid excess and include specifically dietary restrictions. If edema persists, document location and whether it is pitting. For the patient on dialysis, document the status of access sites/central lines, response to dialysis, and an assessment of level of consciousness or mental status.

NURSING DIAGNOSIS 3

DECREASED CARDIAC OUTPUT

Related to:
> Effects of hyperkalemia
> Fluid volume excess
> Elevated blood pressure

Defining Characteristics:
> Increased heart rate
> Blood pressure higher than patient baseline
> Diminished peripheral pulses
> Peripheral edema
> Shortness of breath with activity
> Neck vein distention

Goal:
> Cardiac output will be maintained.

Outcome Criteria

✔ The patient achieves adequate cardiac output as demonstrated by pulse and blood pressure at patient's baseline.
✔ The patient's breath sounds will be clear.
✔ The patient will have no peripheral edema or neck vein distention.
✔ The patient's skin will be warm and peripheral pulses will be palpable.
✔ The patient will be alert.

NOC *Cardiac pump effectiveness*
Circulation status
Respiratory status: Gas exchange

INTERVENTIONS	RATIONALES
Assess for abnormal heart and lung sounds, along with rate, rhythm, and depth of respirations, every 4 hours or as ordered.	Helps to detect the presence of pulmonary congestion that may occur with renal failure patients due to fluid volume excess, as the diseased kidneys are unable to excrete water. A third heart

INTERVENTIONS	RATIONALES
	sound may develop as the heart tries to fill a distended ventricle and the left ventricle becomes less compliant; distant heart sounds coupled with a pericardial friction rub can be an indicator of pericarditis, which is caused by retained toxins (this is rare when renal failure is treated early); crackles indicate the presence of fluid in the lungs.
Monitor blood pressure and pulse; note dysrhythmias and irregularities.	Patients with renal failure are most often hypertensive, which is attributable to the excess fluid and the initiation of the rennin-angiotensin mechanism; heart rate increases as a compensatory mechanism to increase the effectiveness of the heart in handling the excess fluid, but also to compensate for decreased oxygenation to tissues caused by anemia. Dysrhythmias may occur due to electrolyte imbalance (particularly potassium and calcium), acid/base imbalance, anemia, and the altered internal environment in general.
Assess neurological status, particularly level of consciousness.	The accumulation of waste products in the bloodstream impairs oxygen transport and uptake by cerebral tissues, which may manifest as confusion, lethargy, and altered thought processes. Immediately prior to dialysis, the patient may be more lethargic.
Assess the patient's skin temperature and peripheral pulses.	Decreased perfusion and oxygenation of tissues secondary to anemia and pump ineffectiveness may lead to decreased skin temperature and peripheral pulses that are diminished and difficult to palpate.
Monitor results of laboratory and diagnostic tests (chest x-ray, electrocardiogram, BUN, electrolytes, creatinine).	Results of these tests provide clues to cardiac status, renal system status, and response to treatments; BUN and creatinine will be elevated, potassium and phosphorous are generally elevated, and calcium and

INTERVENTIONS	RATIONALES
	sodium will be decreased; EKG will be able to identify changes in the electrical activity of the myocardium due to electrolyte imbalances; chest x-ray will identify congestion.
Monitor oxygen saturation and ABGs.	Provides information regarding heart's ability to perfuse distal tissues with oxygenated blood; also identifies the presence or severity of metabolic acidosis.
Give oxygen as indicated by patient symptoms, oxygen saturation, and ABGs.	Makes more oxygen available for gas exchange, assisting to alleviate signs of hypoxia and subsequent activity intolerance.
Prepare the patient for dialysis, as ordered or required by agency protocol.	Dialysis is indicated in ARF for the removal of fluid, toxins, and potassium, which can contribute to disturbances in cardiac function.
Implement strategies to treat fluid and electrolyte imbalances (see nursing diagnosis "Excess Fluid Volume").	Decreases the risk for development of decreased cardiac output due to imbalances.
Administer inotropic/cardiac glycoside agents (digitalis preparations) as ordered for signs of left-sided failure, and monitor for toxicity (nausea/vomiting, visual impairments). Count pulse for a full minute and hold medication if pulse is < 60 beats per minute.	Digitalis has a positive inotropic effect on the myocardium that strengthens contractility, thus improving cardiac output.
Administer ACE inhibitors as ordered.	Prevents the vasoconstrictive action of angiotensin II, which results in lowered peripheral vascular resistance, vasodilation, and subsequent improvement in cardiac output.
Encourage periods of rest and assist with all activities.	Reduces cardiac workload and minimizes myocardial oxygen consumption; also reduces the amount of waste products of metabolism that accumulate in the bloodstream.
Assist the patient in assuming a high Fowler's position.	Allows for better chest expansion, thereby improving pulmonary capacity.
Teach the patient about the relationship of ARF to cardiac symptoms, treatments, prognosis, and required home care.	Provides patient with needed information for management of cardiac symptoms and for compliance.

NIC *Oxygen therapy*
Cardiac care: Acute
Hemodynamic regulation
Vital signs monitoring

Evaluation

Patient's cardiac output is improved. Examine the extent to which the stated outcome criteria have been achieved. Patient's lungs are clear to auscultation; there is no edema or jugular vein distention. Skin is warm and peripheral pulses are present. The patient's blood pressure and pulse return to patient's baseline, and the patient has no symptoms of altered mental status.

Community/Home Care

Patients who experience decreased cardiac output due to ARF may not require follow-up by a health care provider in the home, but will need to return to the health care provider for follow-up care to ensure that they are making progress towards returning to their previous state of health. During recovery at home, the patient will need to be cognizant of the signs and symptoms of heart failure and decreased cardiac output. The patient will need to be attuned to subtle changes in health status that may indicate a cardiac problem, such as rapid weight gain, shortness of breath, and even mild edema. Prevention of cardiac complications will need to be accomplished through adherence to recommendations given for controlling fluid excess (see nursing diagnosis "Excess Fluid Volume"). A critical piece of those recommendations is diet and fluid restrictions. Even though the patient may not need fluid, potassium, or sodium restriction, once renal function has returned to normal, the restrictions may still be needed early in the recovery period. In addition to informing the patient of common foods that are high in sodium and potassium, the dietician or nurse should specifically inquire about what the patient normally eats or drinks and examine these foods for sodium and potassium content. Provide the patient with a list of acceptable foods and drinks to post in the kitchen for reference. Be sure that the patient and family know how to read food labels as well. The patient, family members, or significant other should be taught how to take a pulse and encouraged to do so daily and in response to activity. The patient can also keep a log of blood pressure and pulse to help in determining the baseline. Once the patient is able, he or she can go to places such as drugstores or health departments where free screenings are offered. Monitoring responses (pronounced shortness of breath, increased respiratory rate, exertional syncope, or increased pulse) to routine activities will provide clues to cardiac function and the need to seek health care. All of this can be recorded in the log and shared with the primary health care provider. The patient will need to understand that it may take a significant amount of time to return to the level of function that he or she experienced prior to a diagnosis of ARF. Such things as work schedules, diets, religion, social support systems, and beliefs about health may influence adherence to recommendations for enhanced cardiac output. It is not uncommon for patients to experience denial.

Documentation

Always document the status of achievement of outcome criteria with specific patient behaviors. Chart the blood pressure, pulse, heart sounds, breath sounds, assessments relevant to edema, distended neck veins, output, and the patient's tolerance for activity. All interventions and teaching should be a part of the documentation. Include in the patient record his or her understanding of any teaching and responses to the therapeutic interventions.

NURSING DIAGNOSIS 4

IMBALANCED NUTRITION: LESS THAN BODY REQUIREMENTS

Related to:

Anorexia

Dietary restrictions

Defining Characteristics:

Weight loss

"Food tastes bad"

Vomiting

Anorexia

Decreased intake

Goal:

The patient's nutritional status is restored.

Outcome Criteria

✔ The patient reports that anorexia has decreased and appetite has increased.

✔ The patient consumes 75 percent of meals served.

NOC *Nutritional status: Food and fluid intake*

Nutritional status: Nutrient intake

INTERVENTIONS	RATIONALES
Refer to a dietician or perform a dietary/nutrition assessment: 24-hour recall, usual diet prior to illness, food likes and dislikes, weight, and condition of skin.	Establishes a baseline and a starting point for education regarding foods allowed during ARF, and allows development of a nutritional plan that is likely to be consumed, as the patient is more likely to eat foods that he or she likes.
Administer anti-emetics, as ordered, and give prophylactically prior to meals.	Reduces nausea and vomiting, and improves likelihood of ingestion of meals.
Provide good mouth care before meals.	A fresh mouth can enhance the flavor of foods.
Create an environment for meals that is pleasant and free of odors.	Pleasant environments can enhance intake; odors may prevent patient from eating and may cause nausea.
Arrange for small, frequent meals that are high in calories and fiber but low in protein, and that are appealing to the patient.	The patient may find small meals decrease feelings of anorexia. The small meals should provide adequate dietary needs without causing bloating. Protein is restricted until kidney function has been restored, usually during the recovery phase.
When food arrives at the room, remove the cover before bringing food into the room.	Removal of a cover from a plate of food that has been covered for a period of time releases a strong aroma that may be overpowering for a patient who has experienced nausea.
Encourage PO fluids within prescribed restrictions.	Ensures hydration and reduces dry mucous in mouth. Offering fluids throughout the day in small amounts is better for maintaining moisture of mucous membranes than giving large amounts less frequently.
Provide nutritious between-meal snacks within prescribed restrictions.	Adds calories and nutrients.
Weigh patient daily.	Helps to monitor for non-fluid loss that may indicate a need for more aggressive nutritional management.
Teach the patient about fluid and dietary (sodium, potassium, and protein) restrictions required due to renal failure, with consideration for usual food types consumed and cultural and religious preferences.	The patient needs to maintain adequate nutrition but also stay within the restrictions of protein, sodium, and fluid. The patient is more likely to adhere to diet restrictions that take his or her usual dietary practices into consideration.

NIC *Nutritional monitoring*

Nutritional management

Evaluation

Determine that the patient has not lost weight. The patient should report absence of nausea, anorexia, and vomiting. The patient eats at least 75 percent of meals served or is making progress towards that goal. Monitor other indicators of nutrition, such as total protein, albumin, iron, hemoglobin, and electrolytes.

Community/Home Care

The patient should have progressed to an adequate nutritional status by time of discharge home. At home, the patient needs to be cognizant of foods that may be toxic to the recovering kidneys, such as large amounts of protein. Because fatigue may persist, the patient may continue to consume foods that provide energy and are high in iron, such as green vegetables, cereals, and organ meat within any protein restriction. If the patient is experiencing fatigue, small meals with nutritious snacks may be indicated, as they require less energy to consume and also give the patient a sense of accomplishment. As the ARF is resolved, the patient's nausea, anorexia, or vomiting should resolve as well, allowing the patient to consume foods without incident. It is crucial that the meal preparer be included in dietary instructions and be willing to comply with recommendations. As with all nutritional instructions, education should consider any cultural or religious restrictions. A list of acceptable foods and fluids can be prepared for the patient to use that also includes instructions on how to determine serving sizes, especially for meat portions. Scales can be used to weigh the meat, or simply draw a picture that is the approximate size of the recommended portion. At follow-up visits, the health care provider needs to obtain history from the patient regarding intake and determine whether laboratory tests are needed for a more accurate assessment.

Documentation

Document the patient's intake (fluid and percentage of meal) following each meal and any complaints about the type of food served. If a diet history is obtained, chart this according to agency protocol. Chart the patient's weight on the appropriate flow sheet. Record any reports of nausea or vomiting along with interventions implemented to resolve them, such as administration of anti-emetics. Document the effectiveness of the interventions in follow-up notes. Include in the patient record any nutritional education given to the patient and whether family members and/or a significant other are present. Document any referrals to nutritionists or dieticians.

NURSING DIAGNOSIS 5

 ANXIETY

Related to:

    Change in health status

    Threat to lifestyle

    Fear of unknown

Defining Characteristics:

    Anxiety, restlessness

    Distraction, decreased concentration

    Expressions of fear

Goal:

    Anxiety is relieved.

Outcome Criteria

✔ The patient verbalizes that anxiety has been reduced.

✔ The patient states that he or she is relaxed.

✔ The patient has no physiological signs of anxiety (diaphoresis, tachycardia, restlessness, difficulty breathing).

✔ The patient and/or family/significant other ask appropriate questions about ARF.

NOC *Anxiety control*
      Acceptance: Health status

INTERVENTIONS	RATIONALES
Have patient rate anxiety on a numerical scale if able.	Allows for a more objective measure of anxiety level.
Assess the patient for physiological signs of anxiety, such as tachycardia, restlessness, difficulty breathing, and diaphoresis.	Moderate to severe anxiety often produces physiological symptoms due to a sympathetic nervous system response and will vary from patient to patient.
Encourage the patient to verbalize concerns about health status.	Verbalizing concerns can help the patient deal with issues and avoid negative feelings.
Stay with patient during acute episodes of anxiety and use a calm manner.	Allows the nurse to offer comfort, care, and assurances to reduce anxiety and fear.
Implement strategies to manage ARF (see nursing diagnosis "Impaired Urinary Elimination").	New onset of diseases cause anxiety because of the unknown and unfamiliarity with requirements for treatment; correction of the alteration in renal function will help to reduce anxiety level as the patient sees progress towards optimal health.
Reassure the patient by explaining ARF and treatments that are being implemented to correct the problem that caused the kidneys to fail.	Being unable to produce urine contributes to anxiety because of the fear that interventions may not work and long-term dialysis may be required; knowing what to expect helps the patient maintain a sense of control.
Administer anti-anxiety medication, as ordered.	Calms patient and promotes rest.
Ensure quiet, calm environment.	Reducing the amount of stimuli may help to decrease patient's stress and anxiety.
Assist patient with identification/development of coping mechanisms.	Coping mechanisms may help reduce anxiety.
Provide diversions, such as TV, music, books on tape, and visual imagery.	These types of activities can help divert the patient's attention from the disease and thus reduce anxiety.
Allow family to visit liberally if the patient so desires.	Family may provide emotional support that calms the patient and promotes a sense of comfort.
Teach the patient relaxation techniques (such as slow, purposeful breathing) and encourage their use.	Reduces anxiety and creates a feeling of comfort.

NIC *Anxiety reduction*
Calming technique
Emotional support
Presence

Evaluation

Assess the patient for the extent that he or she is free of anxiety. The patient should verbalize that anxiety is reduced and that he or she feels comfortable. Assess the patient for physiological signs of anxiety, such as increased pulse, restlessness, difficulty breathing, and sweating. During evaluation, be sure to inquire about the use of relaxation techniques. The patient will also need to report that he or she understands the disease process that has changed his or her health status.

Community/Home Care

The patient will need to know how to control anxiety in the home setting. It is crucial that health care providers provide adequate education so that the patient feels in control of his or her health. Once the ARF has been resolved, anxiety may also resolve. However, some patients may continue to be anxious with the thought that their kidneys may not recover and long-term dialysis may be required, which is always a possibility. For this reason, one of the most important interventions that needs to be carried out before discharge is educating the patient about what caused ARF, with a clear explanation of current status and prognosis. By ensuring that the patient understands the health care regimen and knows what to do if acute symptoms develop, the health care provider may prevent unnecessary concern and worry regarding health status. Simple strategies that may prove helpful in anxiety reduction in the home include reading, meditating, involvement in religious rituals (if patient participates in organized religion), watching favorite television programs, or taking short walks in a natural setting. If the patient experiences pronounced anxiety at home, he or she should notify the health care provider for more aggressive interventions or for referral to counseling.

Documentation

Document the degree of anxiety experienced by the patient. Using some type of numerical rating scale similar to the pain scale will provide health care providers with a more objective measure of the degree of anxiety the patient is experiencing. Document any physiological or observable signs of anxiety, such as restlessness, tachycardia, or diaphoresis. Interventions implemented to treat anxiety should be documented along with subsequent assessments to determine their effectiveness. Document content of all teaching done.

NURSING DIAGNOSIS 6

 INEFFECTIVE PROTECTION

Related to:

Decreased red blood cell production due to lack of erythropoietin

Shortened life span of red blood cells due to uremia

Poor absorption of iron from the gastrointestinal tract

Altered platelet function

Leukopenia

Decreased calcium and vitamin D

Altered immune function

Defining Characteristics:

Fatigue

Decreased hemoglobin and hematocrit

Easy bruising

Prolonged bleeding

Blood in stool or emesis

Decreased red blood cell count

Falls

Dizziness

Goal:

The patient will sustain no injury.

The patient will be protected from physiological injury.

Outcome Criteria

✔ The patient will not experience bleeding or bruising.

✔ The patient will not fall.

✔ The patient will have no signs or symptoms of infections (urinary, respiratory, central access sites, skin areas).

✔ The patient will verbalize an understanding of the necessary precautions needed to prevent bleeding, infection, and injury.

NOC *Blood coagulation*
Immune status
Knowledge: Infection control
Risk control

INTERVENTIONS	RATIONALES
Monitor red blood cells (RBC), hemoglobin (Hgb), hematocrit (Hct), iron, platelets, prothrombin time (PT), and partial thromboplastin time (PTT), as ordered.	Helps to detect abnormalities that put the patient at risk for injury, and protects against injury. Anemia is common in ARF and measures of RBC, Hgb, and Hct indicate severity. RBCs are more fragile with a shortened lifespan; fewer RBCs are produced due to a lack of or decreased production of erythropoietin. Platelets are decreased, and Ptt and Pt are altered, placing the patient at high risk for bleeding.
Assess for fatigue, weakness, shortness of breath, and any alteration in mental status.	These symptoms occur due to the body's inability to transport enough oxygen to tissues secondary to decreased RBC and iron. In addition, waste products (uremia) in the blood interfere with the transport and exchange of oxygen in cerebral tissue; early manifestations include change in mentation (confusion, fatigue, lethargy, difficulty concentrating).
Assess skin color.	Skin may become pale due to impaired perfusion.
Monitor for indicators of bleeding abnormalities: bruising, easy bleeding, blood in emesis or stool, petechiae, bleeding gums, nosebleed, and purpura.	These indicate that the body is unable to clot effectively, and further examination and interventions may be warranted to prevent complications.
Test any emesis or stool for blood.	Helps to detect bleeding not recognizable through observation.
Assess patient closely for side effects of drugs secondary to decreased excretion.	Due to the impaired kidney function, many medications cannot be excreted effectively, increasing the risk for drug toxicity.

Monitor for signs of infection: redness/discoloration, drainage or heat at any wound or IV access insertion site, elevated temperature, cough with expectoration of sputum, or pulmonary congestion.	With bone marrow suppression, there are fewer white blood cells, placing the patient at higher risk for infection.
Assist the patient with careful ambulation and other activities.	Due to dizziness, weakness, and fatigue the patient is at higher risk for falls; providing assistance decreases that risk. Due to decreased calcium levels and subsequent resorption of calcium from bones, the patient's bones may be fragile and prone to pathological fractures.
Apply pressure to all puncture sites.	Helps to effectively stop bleeding.
Brush teeth with a soft bristle toothbrush.	Decreases bleeding from gums; gums tend to bleed easily due to altered clotting factors.
Administer Epogen® as ordered and monitor for side effects and therapeutic effects.	Stimulates the bone marrow production of red blood cells and raises the hematocrit level.
Practice good hand hygiene.	Handwashing is one of the best ways to stop the transmission of infection.
Limit visitors in the hospital, and have patient avoid crowds after discharge home.	Visitors who mean well often transmit organisms that can make immunocompromised patients ill; being in crowds increases the risk of acquiring respiratory infections.
Increase iron-rich foods in diet within renal diet restrictions.	Increases the oxygen-carrying capacity of RBCs.
If dialysis is done via a central line catheter, change dressing in accordance with agency protocol using strict sterile technique.	Central lines are an easy port for entry of organisms. Strict sterile technique is required to reduce risk for infection.
Teach the patient all safety precautions required related to falls, bleeding, and infection.	The patient needs to be well informed in order to practice health promotion behaviors.

NIC *Bleeding precautions*
Risk identification
Self-care assistance
Surveillance

Evaluation

Evaluate whether the outcome criteria have been met. The patient should have no bleeding; any bleeding that does occur is detected and treated early. Infections have been prevented, as demonstrated by the absence of signs of infection, such as elevated temperature, pulmonary congestion, and sputum production and expectoration. The patient ambulates without injury with assistance. At time of discharge, the patient is able to verbalize safety precautions required.

Community/Home Care

The patient with ARF will continue to be at risk for ineffective protection until kidney function has been adequately restored, which takes from 3 months to 1 year. Once at home, the patient will need to continue to practice safety-enhancing behaviors for bleeding, physical injury, and infections. The patient must be vigilant in preventing or controlling bleeding promptly if it occurs, as well as preventing falls. Implementing strategies to protect self from injury, such as bumping into objects that may cause bruising or disruption of skin, is important. This may include rearranging furniture or removing rugs to make walking areas clear. Because the patient is prone to dizziness and fatigue due to loss of large amounts of fluid during the diuretic phase of recovery, assistance with ambulation and household activities may be required. Dietary interventions that can assist the patient with energy levels can prevent some of the fatigue and dizziness caused by decreased RBC and subsequent impaired oxygen transport. Foods rich in iron should be encouraged, taking into consideration the patient's likes/dislikes, culture, religion, and dietary restrictions. If bleeding is noted in stools or emesis, the health care provider should be notified for treatment. The patient who has experienced ARF may want to avoid large crowds or other activities that may increase risk for infection. Handshaking is a common expression of greeting but can also be the source of transmission of organisms from well-intending persons. Practicing good handwashing techniques can minimize the risk of infections and should be stressed. It is recommended that patients with young children or grandchildren avoid them if possible when they are sick with colds or the flu. At the first sign of infection, the patient should return to a health care provider for further assistance.

Documentation

Include in the documentation findings from a thorough assessment of the patient for evidence of bleeding such as bruises, bleeding gums, bleeding from access sites, etc. Also document the patient's activity level and response to activity (fatigue, dizziness, shortness of breath). If the patient has any signs of infection, even minor ones, document them in the patient record. Chart all interventions implemented to address safety, bleeding, and prevention or treatment of infections. If teaching is implemented, include who the learners were and their level of understanding.

CHAPTER 5.64

RENAL FAILURE: CHRONIC (CRF)

GENERAL INFORMATION

Chronic renal failure (CRF) occurs due to insults to the kidney structures from a variety of causes that over time yield the kidneys unable to function. This disorder is most often characterized by a gradual loss of functioning of a majority of the kidney's nephrons. Diabetes mellitus and hypertension are the most common causes of CRF, accounting for approximately 70 percent of all cases. Other causes of CRF include obstruction of the urinary system, chronic glomerulonephritis, chronic pyelonephritis, and systemic lupus erythematosus (SLE). Although the disease is categorized into four stages—decreased kidney reserve, kidney insufficiency, kidney failure, end-stage renal disease—for most patients 50 percent of nephrons are destroyed before any signs of renal impairment are recognized (Phipps, Monahan, Sands, Marek, and Neighbors, 2003). During the early stages, the functioning kidneys are able to compensate by increasing the filtration rate; however, after 75 percent of the nephrons are destroyed, compensation cannot be sustained. As a result, the kidneys are no longer able to maintain homeostasis through the normal mechanisms of waste, toxins, and fluid excretion and regulation of electrolytes and acid/base balance with subsequent effects on all body systems. Noticeable symptoms do not occur until the glomerular filtration rate falls to < 60 ml/minute. Clinical manifestations vary, but common ones seen in most patients include edema, decreased urine output, nausea and vomiting, anorexia, weakness, lethargy, and hypertension at various points in the disease. In addition to the laboratory tests directly related to kidney function (blood urea nitrogen, creatinine, creatinine clearance, specific gravity), there are numerous other abnormalities. Electrolyte imbalance accompanies CRF with elevated potassium, magnesium, and phosphorous, and decreased levels of sodium and calcium. Erythropoietin, the hormone that regulates red blood cell (RBC) production, cannot be produced in adequate amounts by the failing kidneys, contributing to a low RBC count. In addition, the increased amount of waste products in the bloodstream makes the RBC fragile with a shortened lifespan that also contributes to the low RBC count and anemia.

NURSING DIAGNOSIS 1

EXCESS FLUID VOLUME

Related to:

Inability of the kidneys to produce and eliminate urine

Defining Characteristics:

Crackles

Shortness of breath

Edema

Decreased urine output

Elevated blood pressure

Weight gain

Electrolyte imbalances

Goal:

Fluid volume excess is decreased.

Outcome Criteria

✔ The patient will demonstrate weight loss following dialysis.

✔ Blood pressure will return to patient's baseline prior to onset of renal failure.

✔ The patient's edema will be absent or decreased.

✔ The patient will have no distended neck veins.

✔ The patient's breath sounds will be clear.

✔ The patient's electrolytes will be normal or at baseline.

Systemic toxin clearance: Dialysis
Kidney function
Fluid balance
Electrolyte and acid/base balance
Fluid overload severity

INTERVENTIONS	RATIONALES
Assess location and extent of edema, particularly in extremities.	Helps to assess severity of the fluid excess.
Assess breath sounds for crackles.	Helps to detect early any signs of left heart failure; crackles are an indicator of fluid in the lungs and should be monitored for worsening or improvement as an indicator of disease status and response to interventions.
Place patient in high Fowler's position.	Minimizes cardiac workload and decreases fluid return to the heart.
Assess vital signs.	In the presence of renal failure, the blood pressure elevates, as does the pulse, in response to the increased fluid volume; respiratory rate and depth may increase secondary to metabolic acidosis as the lungs attempt to blow off more carbon dioxide to create acid/base balance.
Administer oxygen, as ordered, if the patient experiences shortness of breath.	Improves oxygenation and peripheral perfusion.
Weigh patient daily at the same time, on the same scale, in similar clothes, in the morning before breakfast, after voiding.	The most accurate method of determining fluid volume loss is through daily weights: 1 kilogram of weight loss = 1 liter of fluid lost. Morning weights are a better reflection of true weights because most people accumulate fluid as the day progresses. On the days that the patient undergoes dialysis, weights will be obtained before and after dialysis to detect fluid gain between visits and to determine how much fluid should be drawn off during the procedure.
Implement a renal diet: low in sodium, potassium, and protein.	Sodium increases fluid retention; thus, decreasing the amount of dietary sodium intake will decrease the amount of retained fluid. Salty foods also increase the thirst sensation, which increases the desire for more oral fluid. A low-potassium diet is necessary because of the elevated potassium levels due to inability of the kidneys to excrete potassium; proteins create waste products that the kidneys cannot excrete.
Implement fluid restrictions, as ordered.	Restricting fluid intake can assist in decreasing circulating volume, thereby decreasing cardiac workload.
Accurate intake and output.	To monitor the balance between fluid consumed and urinary output, some patients who have a few functioning nephrons may have urinary output on dialysis days.
Monitor renal function studies (creatinine, BUN, creatinine clearance) and electrolytes (especially potassium, phosphorous, sodium, and calcium).	Creatinine is an end-product of muscle energy excreted by the kidneys, and as kidney function deteriorates, the creatinine rises because the kidneys are unable to function. BUN, an end-product of protein metabolism, will be elevated as the kidneys can no longer rid the blood of this waste product; the creatinine clearance measures the glomerular filtration rate and is decreased to < 5 percent of normal due to the loss of function of the glomeruli; in CRF, the kidneys are unable to excrete potassium; calcium decreases as the kidneys are unable to excrete phosphorous or activate vitamin D, sodium levels are decreased due to increased fluid volume (hyperdilution).
Implement strategies to lower potassium levels, as ordered, such as giving Kayexalate PO (orally) or via enema; administer regular insulin, 50 percent dextrose, and calcium gluconate IV, as ordered.	In CRF, the kidneys are unable to excrete adequate amounts of potassium; high potassium levels may produce life-threatening dysrhythmias and need to be addressed. Kayexalate is a cation exchange resin that exchanges sodium ions for potassium ions in the bowel where it is then excreted. Insulin is given to cause a movement of potassium

(continues)

(continued)

INTERVENTIONS	RATIONALES
	into the intracellular spaces; glucose is given to counteract the hypoglycemic effects of the insulin; calcium gluconate is given to protect the myocardium from effects of potassium.
Implement strategies to lower phosphorous and elevate calcium levels, such as administering phosphorous-binding/lowering agents such as calcium acetate (PhosLo) or aluminum hydroxide agents (Basaljel).	The kidneys are unable to excrete phosphorous, and as serum levels rise, calcium levels drop (inverse relation of phosphorous levels to calcium levels); aluminum hydroxide agents bind dietary phosphorous, prohibiting phosphorous absorption, and phosphate is then excreted via stool. ALWAYS give phosphorous-lowering agents with meals in order to enhance the binding effects and also to decrease further absorption of calcium.
Monitor for side effects of electrolyte imbalance: muscle weakness, cardiac dysrhythmias, tingling and numbness in extremities, and muscular twitching.	Patients with renal failure have accompanying electrolyte imbalances that may never return to normal levels. However, dangerously low or high alterations need to be treated in order to maintain homeostasis and prevent impaired muscle function or other organ damage. Early detection of symptoms allows for prompt treatment.
Monitor arterial blood gases (ABGs) for metabolic acidosis.	In CRF, metabolic acidosis is common, as the kidneys are no longer able to perform their buffering function by excreting hydrogen ions and conserving bicarbonate.
Administer sodium bicarbonate as ordered.	Corrects metabolic acidosis.
Assess for gastrointestinal (GI) symptoms: vomiting, anorexia, nausea, gastric reflux, and hiccups.	Nausea, vomiting, and anorexia are common in renal failure patients and can be caused by electrolyte imbalances and the build-up of waste products in the body. Fatigue can also contribute to anorexia. Hiccups are also common and often difficult to control.

INTERVENTIONS	RATIONALES
Implement strategies to treat GI symptoms: offer the patient small meals that require less time to consume, give anti-emetics before meals, and treat hiccups, as ordered.	Small meals may be preferable because the patient may be unable to consume large meals due to anorexia and fatigue; fear of vomiting may prevent the patient from eating, so giving anti-emetic medications prior to meals can enhance intake. Hiccups prevent intake and are annoying to most patients, treatment is attempted to enhance intake.
Protect edematous skin in extremities and sacrum (see nursing diagnosis "Impaired Skin Integrity").	Fluid in tissue inhibits adequate circulation to the tissue, predisposing the patient to skin breakdown.
Prepare the patient for hemodialysis or peritoneal dialysis as ordered or required by agency protocol; assist with insertion of central line or peritoneal catheter or assist with preparation for surgery for creation of arteriovenous shunt (see nursing diagnosis "Deficient Knowledge").	Patients who have CRF need a means to remove waste products, excess fluids, and toxins from the blood. Hemodialysis is accomplished through a central multilumen catheter or via a surgically created arteriovenous shunt/fistula. Peritoneal dialysis is accomplished through a catheter inserted into the peritoneal cavity where the peritoneal membrane is the dialyzing area. Once either is functioning, the preparation for dialysis is dependent upon agency requirements but generally includes withholding antihypertensive medications but allowing meals and other medications.
Maintain central line dialysis site according to agency protocol: change dressing using sterile technique as ordered, flush unused lumens with heparin according to agency protocol, assess site for infection every shift (see nursing diagnosis "Ineffective Protection").	Central line care is crucial to maintaining function of the access site. Given that this is the patient's lifeline, health care providers must assure that the site is functional by preventing infection and clotting off of the lumens. Heparin is used to maintain patency.
Ensure patency of AV fistula by feeling for a palpable thrill and auscultating for bruit at shunt site every shift.	Created fistulas have a thrill felt by gently palpating the site; the rush of blood through the large created vessel is transmitted to the surface; the abnormally large vessel created through merger of vein and artery allows for the swooshing

INTERVENTIONS	RATIONALES
	sound (bruit) to be easily heard. The absence of either or both indicates a problem in the fistula, possibly clotting.
Post signs at the patient bedside indicating that the patient has an AV fistula and in which arm it is located.	Cautions other health care providers against using the arm that contains the AV fistula; venipuncture and blood pressures are prohibited in the arm that is the site of an AV fistula due to risk of clotting or injury to the arm causing it to be unsuitable for continued use.

NIC *Fluid management*
       Electrolyte monitoring

Evaluation

The patient has no symptoms of fluid excess. Breath sounds are clear, no dyspnea is present, and weight loss has been demonstrated. Edema is absent or decreasing, with no pitting edema. Skin in edematous-dependent areas should be intact. Jugular vein distention has been alleviated and blood pressure and pulse return to baseline.

Community/Home Care

Ensure that the patient at home understands the importance of monitoring fluid status. Weighing daily at home will allow the patient to notice subtle changes in fluid retention. The patient should ask that the dialysis team provide his or her weight on dialysis days for comparison. In addition, the patient should be taught how to assess him or herself for excessive fluid retention by noticing signs such as clothing that becomes too tight in a short period or a rapid weight gain in 24 hours. These could indicate heart failure that could lead to more health complications for the patient. At home the patient needs to limit the intake of sodium-rich foods and table salt to reduce the risk of further fluid excess. The patient should be taught how to read food labels for sodium content, ideally using the food that the patient normally purchases. A visiting nurse or dietician can reinforce this at home by pulling foods from the cupboard and discussing them with the patient or caregiver. An important aspect of dietary management for the patient with CRF is avoidance of potassium-rich foods such as cantaloupe, oranges, orange juice, and broccoli or consuming them in moderation. Because of the restriction on sodium, many patients may want to use salt substitutes; however, most of these are high in potassium and should also be avoided. Proteins are also restricted in the renal diet. As many people get a majority of their protein from meat sources, it is important that the patient or family member understand how to measure serving portions of meat. The patient can invest in a food scale or the dietician can draw pictures of meats that reflect what a serving size should be. Diet instructions for home should consider the patient's normal diet and any cultural or religious preferences and restrictions. Have the patient keep a log of food and fluid intake as well as weights. Assist the patient to develop a schedule for taking any prescribed medications that is mindful of his or her lifestyle and daily routines. The patient can discuss concerns at dialysis treatments.

Noncompliance with dietary and fluid restrictions may occur, causing the patient to have periodic hospitalizations for respiratory symptoms or congestive heart failure due to the excess fluid volume. Instruction about how to prevent noncompliance should be reinforced by all health care providers, and assistance of in-home caregivers should be sought for ensuring compliance with recommended therapies. The patient may experience some distress or ineffective coping when faced with the need for dialysis. This intervention drastically changes a person's life and influences every aspect of day-to-day existence. Patients often become depressed, going through a period of denial and anger that manifests itself as noncompliance with dietary recommendations and refusal to attend dialysis. For these reasons, it is strongly recommended that all CRF patients be seen in the home in the initial stages of diagnosis and treatment for a thorough psychosocial assessment not only of the patient but also of the family. The patient may experience spiritual distress and may benefit from professional counseling or visits from religious leaders as indicated.

Support groups, if available, may also be helpful. Stress the need to keep all appointments for dialysis and follow-up care by a primary health care provider. Prior to discharge from the health care agency, the nurse or social worker should be sure that the patient has required resources for compliance, particularly transportation to dialysis treatments.

Documentation

Always document the extent to which the outcome criteria have been achieved. Record intake and output, blood pressure, pulse, weights, breath sounds, and the patient's understanding of the therapies for eliminating fluid excess. Document all therapeutic interventions employed to address fluid excess and specifically include dietary restrictions. If edema persists, document location and whether it is pitting. For the patient on dialysis, document the status of access sites or fistulas, response to dialysis, and an assessment of level of consciousness or mental status.

NURSING DIAGNOSIS 2

 ## DECREASED CARDIAC OUTPUT

Related to:

Effects of hyperkalemia

Fluid volume excess

Elevated blood pressure

Defining Characteristics:

Increased heart rate

Crackles in lungs

Elevated blood pressure

Diminished peripheral pulses

Pale skin

Cool extremities

Peripheral edema

Shortness of breath with activity

Neck vein distention

Lethargy

Goal:

Cardiac output will be maintained.

Outcome Criteria

✔ The patient's blood pressure and pulse are at baseline.

✔ The patient will have absence of or reduced peripheral edema and no neck vein distention.

✔ The patient's breath sounds will be clear, and there will be no shortness of breath.

✔ The patient's skin will be warm, and peripheral pulses will be palpable.

✔ The patient will be alert.

NOC *Cardiac pump effectiveness*
        Circulation status
        Respiratory status:
           Gas exchange

INTERVENTIONS	RATIONALES
Assess for abnormal heart and lung sounds, along with rate, rhythm, and depth of respirations.	Allows detection of left-sided heart failure that may occur with chronic renal failure patients due to fluid volume excess as the diseased kidneys are unable to excrete water. Even though fluid is removed during dialysis, some patients may skip days or may not adhere to sodium restrictions in the diet which will lead to further fluid retention. A third heart sound may develop as the heart tries to fill a distended ventricle and the left ventricle becomes less compliant; distant heart sounds coupled with a pericardial friction rub can be an indicator of pericarditis, which is caused by retained toxins (pericarditis is rare when CRF is treated early); crackles indicate the presence of fluid in the lungs.
Monitor blood pressure and pulse, note dysrhythmias and irregularities, and notify physician if these occur.	Patients with renal failure are most often hypertensive, which is attributable to excess fluid and the initiation of the renin-angiotensin mechanism; heart rate increases as a compensatory mechanism to increase the effectiveness of the heart in handling the excess fluid but also to compensate for decreased oxygenation to tissues caused by anemia. Dysrhythmias may occur due to electrolyte imbalance (particularly potassium and calcium), acid/base imbalance, and anemia.

INTERVENTIONS	RATIONALES
Assess mental status and level of consciousness.	The accumulation of waste products in the bloodstream impairs oxygen transport and uptake by cerebral tissues, which may manifest itself as confusion, lethargy, and altered consciousness. Just prior to dialysis, the patient may be more lethargic.
Assess the patient's skin temperature and peripheral pulses.	Decreased perfusion and oxygenation of tissues secondary to anemia and pump ineffectiveness may lead to decreased skin temperature and peripheral pulses that are diminished and difficult to palpate.
Monitor results of laboratory and diagnostic tests (chest x-ray, electrocardiogram [EKG], BUN, electrolytes, and creatinine).	Results of these tests provide clues to the status of the disease and response to treatments; BUN and creatinine will be elevated; EKG will be able to identify changes in the electrical activity of the myocardium due to electrolyte imbalances; the chest x-ray is useful in identifying congestive heart failure.
Monitor oxygen saturation and ABGs.	Provides information regarding the heart's ability to perfuse distal tissues with oxygenated blood; also identifies the presence or severity of metabolic acidosis.
Give oxygen as indicated by patient symptoms, oxygen saturation, and ABGs.	Makes more oxygen available for gas exchange, assisting to alleviate signs of hypoxia and subsequent activity intolerance.
Prepare the patient for dialysis as ordered or required by agency protocol.	Dialysis is indicated for the removal of fluid, toxins, and potassium, which all contribute to disturbances in cardiac function.
Implement strategies to treat fluid and electrolyte imbalances (see nursing diagnosis "Excess Fluid Volume").	Decreases the risk for development of decreased cardiac output due to imbalances.
Administer inotropic/cardiac glycoside agents (digitalis preparations), as ordered, for signs of left-sided failure, and monitor for toxicity	Digitalis has a positive inotropic effect on the myocardium that strengthens contractility, thus improving cardiac output.

(nausea/vomiting, visual impairments, elevated serum drug levels). Count pulse for a full minute and hold medication if pulse is < 60 beats per minute	
Administer ACE inhibitors, as ordered.	Lowers blood pressure; prevents the vasoconstrictive action of angiotensin II, which results in lowered peripheral vascular resistance, vasodilation, and subsequent improvement in cardiac output.
Encourage periods of rest and assist with all activities.	Reduces cardiac workload and minimizes myocardial oxygen consumption; also reduces the amount of waste products from metabolism that then accumulate in the bloodstream.
Assist the patient in assuming a high Fowler's position.	Allows for better chest expansion, thereby improving pulmonary capacity.
Teach the patient pathophysiology of disease, treatment (dialysis), medications, prognosis, and required home care.	Provides the patient with needed information for management of disease and for compliance.

NIC *Oxygen therapy*
Cardiac care: Acute
Hemodynamic regulation
Vital signs monitoring

Evaluation

Examine the extent to which the stated outcome criteria have been achieved. The patient's peripheral edema has decreased or been alleviated and lungs are clear to auscultation. Skin is warm, peripheral pulses are present, and there is no neck vein distention. The patient's blood pressure and pulse return to patient's baseline and the patient has no symptoms of altered mental status.

Community/Home Care

Patients with decreased cardiac output due to CRF will require follow-up by a health care provider to monitor the effects of renal failure on the cardiac system. At home, the patient will need to be cognizant of the signs and symptoms of heart failure and decreased cardiac output. Because many of the symptoms of heart failure (edema, shortness of breath, fatigue) are also constantly present in the patient with CRF, the patient will need to be attuned to subtle changes in health status that may indicate a cardiac problem. Instruction of the family and patient about necessary interventions at home should be planned, detailed, and reinforced in writing. Prevention of cardiac complications will need to be accomplished through adherence to recommendations given for controlling fluid excess (see nursing diagnosis "Excess Fluid Volume"). A critical piece of those recommendations is diet and fluid restrictions. In addition to informing the patient of common foods that are high in potassium, sodium, and protein, the dietician should specifically inquire about what the patient normally eats or drinks and examine these foods for protein, sodium, and potassium content. This should be the starting place for education. Ensuring that the patient knows how to read food and drink labels is crucial, as is ensuring that he or she is able to implement fluid restrictions. The patient on dialysis can also keep a log of blood pressure and pulse to help in determining his or her baseline. On days when the patient has dialysis, the nurse can give the readings to the patient, and on other days, the patient (if able) can go to places such drugstores or health departments where free screenings are offered. By recording both readings, the patient is able to make comparisons and get a better idea of what the normal baseline is. Monitoring responses (pronounced shortness of breath, increased respiratory rate, exertional syncope, or increased pulse) to routine activities will provide clues to cardiac function and the need to seek health care. The patient with chronic renal disease may actually have an underlying cardiac disease that is complicated by the renal failure. In any case, the patient will need to understand that he or she may never return to the normal level of cardiac function that he or she experienced prior to a diagnosis of CRF and initiation of dialysis. Adherence to recommendations for enhanced cardiac output may be influenced by such things as work schedules, diets, religion, social support systems, and beliefs about health.

Documentation

Always document the status of achievement of outcome criteria with specific patient behaviors. Chart the blood pressure, pulse, heart sounds, breath sounds, assessments relevant to edema, distended neck veins, output, and the patient's tolerance for activity. All interventions and teaching should be a part of the documentation. Include in the patient record the patient's understanding of any teaching and response to the therapeutic interventions.

NURSING DIAGNOSIS 3

INEFFECTIVE PROTECTION

Related to:

Decreased RBC production due to lack of erythropoietin

Shortened life span of RBCs due to uremia

Poor absorption of iron from the GI tract

Altered platelet function

Bone marrow suppression

Decreased calcium and vitamin D

Chronic bone loss

Defining Characteristics:

Fatigue

Decreased hemoglobin and hematocrit

Easy bruising

Prolonged bleeding

Blood in stool or emesis

Decreased RBC count

Falls

Dizziness

Outcome Criteria

✔ The patient will not experience bleeding or bruising.

✔ The patient will not fall.

✔ The patient will not sustain a pathological fracture.

✔ The patient will have no signs or symptoms of infections (urinary, respiratory, central access sites, skin areas).

✔ The patient will verbalize an understanding of the necessary precautions needed to prevent bleeding, infection, and injury.

NOC *Blood coagulation*

Immune status

Knowledge: Infection control

Risk control

INTERVENTIONS	RATIONALES
Monitor red blood cells (RBCs), hemoglobin (Hgb), hematocrit (Hct), iron, platelets, calcium, partial thromboplastin time (PTT), prothrombin time (PT), as ordered.	Allows detection of abnormalities that place the patient at risk for injury and protects against injury. Anemia is common in CRF, and measures of RBC, Hgb, and Hct are indicators of severity. RBCs are more fragile with a shortened lifespan; fewer RBCs are produced due a lack of or decreased production of erythropoietin. Platelets are decreased, and PTT and PT are altered, placing the patient at high risk for bleeding.
Assess for fatigue, weakness, shortness of breath, and any alteration in mental status.	These symptoms occur due to the body's inability to transport enough oxygen to tissues secondary to decreased RBC and iron. In addition, waste products (uremia) in the blood interfere with the transport and exchange of oxygen in cerebral tissue, which may result in change in mentation (confusion, fatigue, lethargy, difficulty concentrating).
Assess skin color.	Skin may become pale due to impaired perfusion; in darker-skinned patients, the skin may take on an ashen color. Most patients who have been on dialysis for an extended time experience changes in skin color, which usually becomes darker.
Monitor for indicators of bleeding abnormalities: bruising, easy bleeding, blood in emesis or stool, petechiae, bleeding gums, nose bleed, purpura.	These indicate that the body is unable to clot effectively, and further examination and interventions may be warranted to prevent complications.
Test any emesis or stool for blood.	Allows detection of bleeding not recognizable through observation.
Assess patient closely for drug toxicity.	Due to the impaired kidney function, many medications cannot be excreted effectively, increasing the risk for drug toxicity.
Monitor for signs of infection: elevated white blood cells; redness or other discoloration; drainage or heat at any wound or IV-access insertion site.	With bone marrow suppression, there are decreased numbers of white blood cells (WBCs), placing the patient at higher risk for infection.
Assist patient with careful ambulation and other activities.	Due to dizziness, weakness, and fatigue the patient is at higher risk for falls; providing assistance decreases that risk. Due to decreased calcium levels and subsequent resorption of calcium from bones, the patient's bones may be fragile and prone to pathological fractures.
Apply pressure to all puncture sites.	Helps to stop bleeding.
Brush teeth with soft bristle toothbrush.	Decreases bleeding from gums that could occur with firm toothbrushes; gums tend to bleed easily due to altered clotting factors.
Administer Epogen as ordered, and monitor for side effects and therapeutic effects.	Epogen stimulates the bone marrow production of RBCs and raises the Hct level.
Practice good hand hygiene.	Handwashing is one of the best ways to stop the transmission of infection.
Have the patient avoid crowds.	Being in crowds increases the risk of acquiring respiratory infections.
When the patient is in the hospital, place a notice over the bed to alert health care providers of safety precautions needed for AV fistula (no IVs, venipunctures, or blood pressures in affected extremity).	Simple procedures such as taking blood pressure or venipuncture can cause damage, usually occlusion to the AV fistula site. The site needs to be protected since this is the patient's "lifeline."
Increase iron-rich foods in diet within renal diet restrictions.	Increases oxygen-carrying capacity of RBCs.
If dialysis is done via a central line catheter, change dressing in accordance with agency protocol using strict sterile technique.	Central lines are an easy portal for entry of organisms. Strict sterile technique is required to reduce risk for infection.
Teach patient all safety precautions required related to falls, bleeding, and infection.	The patient needs to be informed in order to practice health-promoting behaviors.

NIC   *Bleeding precautions*
Risk identification
Self-care assistance
Surveillance

Evaluation

Evaluate whether outcome criteria have been met. The patient should have no bleeding; if bleeding does occur, it is detected and treated early. Infections have been prevented, as demonstrated by the absence of signs and symptoms of infection, such as elevated temperature, pulmonary congestion, and sputum production and expectoration. The patient ambulates with assistance and no injury occurs. At time of discharge from the health care agency, the patient is able to verbalize safety precautions required.

Community/Home Care

The patient with CRF will always be at risk for ineffective protection, as kidney function is not expected to return. Once at home, the patient will need to continue to practice safety-enhancing behaviors to avoid bleeding, physical injury, and infections. The patient must be vigilant in preventing or controlling bleeding promptly, if it occurs, as well as preventing falls. Implementing strategies to avoid injuries from bumping into objects that may cause bruising or disruption of skin is important; these may include rearranging furniture or removing rugs to make walking areas clear. Because the patient is prone to be dizzy and fatigued, assistance with ambulation or activities requiring mental alertness, such as operating machinery or driving, may need to be restricted. A fall in the home may result in hip fractures or fractures of other extremities due to the loss of calcium. Dietary interventions that can assist the patient with energy levels can prevent some of the fatigue and dizziness caused by decreased RBCs and subsequent impaired oxygen transport. Foods rich in iron should be encouraged; diet should take into consideration the patient's likes and dislikes as well as culture, religion, and dietary restrictions. Because the renal diet is quite restrictive and lends itself to noncompliance, it is crucial that the dietician make dietary recommendations only after a thorough consult with the patient and, if applicable, significant other. The patient should always protect the arm that has the AV fistula and avoid using it for lifting or long periods of activity. If bleeding is noted in stools or emesis, the health care provider should be notified for treatment. The patient with renal failure may want to avoid large crowds or other activities that may increase risk for infection. Handshaking is a common expression of greeting but can also be the source of transmission of organisms. Practicing good handwashing techniques can minimize the risk of acquiring infection from others. If possible, routine handwashing in the home should be undertaken with liquid soap as bar soap used by other members of the home may harbor bacteria. Patients with young children or grandchildren should avoid them if possible when they are sick with colds or the flu. At the first sign of infection, the patient should return to a health care provider for further assistance.

Documentation

Include in the documentation findings from a thorough assessment of the patient for evidence of bleeding such as bruises, bleeding gums, bleeding from access sites, etc. Also document the patient's activity level and response to activity (fatigue, dizzy). If the patient has any signs of infection, even minor ones, document this in the patient record. Chart all interventions implemented to address safety, bleeding, and prevention of infections. If teaching is implemented, include who the learners were and their level of understanding.

NURSING DIAGNOSIS 4

 IMPAIRED SKIN INTEGRITY

Related to:
> Elevated uric acid levels
> Hyperpigmentation
> Uremia
> Edema

Defining Characteristics:
> Pruritus
> Skin color changes
> Uremic frost
> Dry, scaly skin
> Bruising

Goal:
> The patient's skin will remain intact.

Outcome Criteria

✔ The patient's skin will have no areas of breakdown.

✔ Itching will be relieved.

✔ Skin will be moist.

NOC *Hemodialysis access*
Tissue integrity: Skin & mucous membranes

INTERVENTIONS	RATIONALES
Perform a thorough skin assessment noting especially edematous areas, open areas, bruising, and color changes.	In patients suffering from renal failure, edematous skin increases the risk for development of skin breakdown; the skin often darkens, or in fairer-skinned patients may take on a yellowish hue.
Keep any open or excoriated areas clean and treat as ordered.	Prompt treatment of any open areas can prevent further deterioration in skin integrity. Skin needs to be kept clean to prevent infection.
Assess the patient for itching and ask patient to describe itching if it is present.	Most patients with CRF experience itching that can be attributed to increased levels of phosphorous and in some cases the deposition of waste products/toxins on the skin (uremic frost). The itching may be described as intense and deep.
Discourage the patient from vigorous scratching and encourage him or her to keep nails short.	Scratching can cause disruption to the skin that can lead to lesions that are difficult to heal.
Apply moisturizing products to the skin: oil-based lotions, petroleum jelly, oatmeal, or oil-based shower gels or lotions. Avoid products containing alcohol and deodorant soaps.	These products add moisture back to the skin and ease the itching. Alcohol-based products and most deodorant soaps cause further drying of the skin.
Instruct patient to bathe in tepid rather than hot water.	Hot water increases pruritus.
Instruct the patient to apply lotions before completely drying the skin following a shower or bath.	Vigorous rubbing or drying of the skin following a bath closes skin pores, rendering emollients ineffective.
Lower room temperature, especially at night.	Excessive warmth increases itching.
Administer Benadryl or Atarax®, as ordered.	Both medications relieve itching.
Administer phosphorous-binding agents, as ordered.	Increased levels of phosphorous contribute to itching, and these agents decrease phosphorous levels.
Encourage the use of distraction or relaxation therapy.	These will help change the perception of the discomfort of itching.
Elevate feet slightly if edematous.	Promotes venous return; however, if the patient has acute symptoms of excess fluid volume, refrain from elevation.
Teach the patient and family strategies to treat itching and prevent skin breakdown.	Itching is a common chronic problem of patients with CRF, and the patient will need to know how to treat it once at home.

NIC *Skin care: Topical treatments*
Skin surveillance

Evaluation

Determine whether the stated outcome criteria have been achieved. The patient should report decrease in or absence of itching. No skin breakdown has occurred, and the skin is moist without scaliness.

Community/Home Care

In the home setting, the patient will continue implementation of the interventions initiated by the nursing staff. The intensity of the pruritus will vary from time to time, often dependent upon the amount of toxins present in the blood and the levels of phosphorous. The patient will need to experiment with a number of measures or products to relieve the itching. It is important that the patient pay attention to environmental factors at home that may contribute to itching such as temperature in the home (cool is better than warm or hot), types of linens used (coarse cotton sheets may increase itching, whereas flannel sheets may feel better), and simple items such as dishwashing detergent, household cleaning products, and hand soaps, which all can worsen the condition. Hot water for baths may intensify the itching, so tepid baths are encouraged. The patient or significant other should inspect the skin for open areas, edema, or bruising on a regular basis, so that early treatment can be instituted. The patient should be clear on when to take medications for itching and be aware that medicines such as Benadryl may cause drowsiness that limits the ability to engage in activities requiring alertness. The patient may find it helpful to take medicines for itching at night if itching prevents adequate sleep.

Documentation

Chart any complaints of itching and interventions employed to treat it. If medications are given, document them on the medication record according to agency protocol, with follow-up documentation regarding the patient's response. Document assessment findings of any abnormalities in the skin, including discoloration of the skin. Document education provided regarding skin impairment and suggested treatments.

NURSING DIAGNOSIS 5

 FATIGUE

Related to:

Disease process

Anemia

Uremia

Defining Characteristics:

Verbalization of being tired

States a lack of energy

Inability to carry out normal activities

Goal:

Fatigue will be relieved.

Outcome Criteria

✔ The patient is able to perform activities of daily living without fatigue.

✔ The patient verbalizes that fatigue has improved or been eliminated.

NOC *Activity tolerance*

Endurance

Energy conservation

Nutritional status: Energy

INTERVENTIONS	RATIONALES
Obtain subjective data regarding normal activities, limitations, and nighttime sleep patterns.	Helps to determine the effect fatigue has on normal functioning. Adequate sleep is required for restoration of the body.
Monitor the patient for signs of excessive physical and emotional fatigue.	Helps to determine when the patient is ready for activity or needs extended periods of rest; use as a guideline for adjusting activity.
Gradually increase activity, as tolerated.	Use the results to indicate when activity may be increased or decreased.
Encourage periods of rest and activity.	Conserves oxygen and prevents undue fatigue. The patient with CRF has anemia, which adds to fatigue because of decreased amounts of oxygen-carrying Hgb. CRF patients often require extended periods of rest or sleep in order to feel rested.
Schedule activities so that excessive demands for oxygen and energy are avoided; for example, space planned activities away from meal times.	Digestion requires energy and oxygen; participation in activities close to meals will cause increased fatigue because of insufficient energy reserves.
Limit visitors during any periods of acute illness or on dialysis days.	Socialization for long periods may cause fatigue; patients frequently report feeling tired following dialysis.
Within the restrictions of the renal diet, increase the intake of high energy foods such as poultry, dried beans and peas, whole grains and foods high in vitamin C.	These foods enhance energy metabolism, increase oxygen-carrying capacity, and provide ready sources of energy needed in hypermetabolic states such as as infection and fever.
Encourage the patient to plan activities for times when he or she has the most energy, usually early in the day.	Prevents fatigue.

NIC *Energy management*

Evaluation

Obtain subjective information from the patient regarding the presence of fatigue. The patient should gradually report the ability to participate in activities of daily living and other normal activities with limited fatigue.

Community/Home Care

Patients with CRF should understand that fatigue may persist and actually be more pronounced on dialysis days or immediately before dialysis. Appropriate education on adapting self-care and household activities during times of fatigue is paramount. A history should be obtained from the patient regarding his or her usual routine for activities of daily living (ADLs) and household chores, so that individualized interventions can be implemented. Attention to what the patient normally does and how the patient wants to make adaptations can only enhance compliance. The nurse must remain aware of cultural backgrounds that may influence a patient's perception of and adaptation to perceived dependency on others. The patient must understand how to adjust activity in response to feelings of fatigue, possibly even arranging for rest or nap periods in the afternoon. This may not be a realistic recommendation for some people who continue to work and whose occupations preclude them from napping or even resting during the day. Household chores should be performed over several days rather than all on one day. Another strategy may be for the patient to attend to activities such as shopping on the day following dialysis, when the patient is likely to be more energetic. Strategies to enhance nighttime sleep should be implemented so that the patient can get adequate rest. Attention to good nutrition should continue with intake of foods that are good sources of iron, vitamin C, and protein within dietary restrictions. If fatigue persists for extended periods, the patient may need to seek health care to investigate the possibility of other causes of the fatigue or new treatments.

Documentation

Chart the specific complaint of fatigue, including what activities the patient has been performing. Document interventions implemented to address fatigue, being sure to document food intake. Include in the record the patient's particular verbalization of the degree of fatigue and response to treatment. Document an assessment of the patient's sleep patterns.

NURSING DIAGNOSIS 6

DEFICIENT KNOWLEDGE

Related to:

New disease: CRF

Complicated treatment regimen: Dialysis

Dietary restrictions

Defining Characteristics:

Asks no questions

Has many questions

Verbalizes a misunderstanding or lack of knowledge related to CRF

Goal:

The patient understands the therapeutic regimen as prescribed.

Outcome Criteria

✔ The patient verbalizes an understanding of CRF and the need for follow-up health care.

✔ The patient verbalizes an understanding of all aspects of the treatments prescribed, especially dialysis.

✔ The patient verbalizes an understanding of a renal diet and is able to identify foods allowed from a list.

NOC *Knowledge: Disease process*
Knowledge: Diet
Knowledge: Illness care

INTERVENTIONS	RATIONALES
Assess patient's learning readiness (motivation, cognitive level, and physiological status).	The patient must be motivated to learn, have the capability to learn, and be free from distractions to learning such as pain, anxiety, itching, fatigue, and shortness of breath.
Identify a family member or significant other who will also learn the content and assist the patient with compliance.	This person can reinforce the teaching and assist with implementation if the patient becomes incapable of follow-through.
Create a quiet environment conducive to learning.	Environmental noise can prevent the learner from focusing on what is being taught.
Teach the learners about the pathophysiology of CRF in the initial teaching session.	Patient must understand what the disease is and how it affects the body before understanding the rationale for treatments.
Teach the learners about the prescribed diet to include fluid, sodium, potassium, and protein restrictions,	Understanding the rationale for these interventions will enhance compliance, and considering cultural/religious

(continues)

(continued)

INTERVENTIONS	RATIONALES
taking into consideration the patient's normal diet and any cultural or religious preferences.	preferences will increase the likelihood that the prescribed changes will be assimilated into the patient's routine.
Teach the learners about prescribed medications to include action, side effects, and dosing schedule (phosphorous binders, antihypertensives, Epogen, etc.).	Knowledge of why the medication is necessary and how it works will focus the importance of the medication. Identification of side effects will minimize anxiety if these occur.
Provide the patient and family information regarding dialysis: — Purpose of dialysis (to replace the loss of function of the kidneys, which is to remove waste products, toxins, and fluids from the body) — Process of dialysis (frequency, equipment, side effects, complications, establishing access, and requirements from the patient) — Types of dialysis (hemodialysis and peritoneal dialysis) — Resources available for assistance (financial, transportation, etc.)	Providing the patient with this information allows him or her to make an informed decision about dialysis. This information also gives the patient the rationale for treatment.
Teach learners how to balance rest and activity and how to monitor responses, understanding that some preferred activities may need to be eliminated due to fatigue. Instruct the patient to eliminate any activity that produces dizziness or severe shortness of breath.	Fatigue is a persistent problem for patients on dialysis, and the patient needs to understand that this is normal; educating the patient in ways to conserve energy and prevent fatigue can prevent anxiety.
If the patient is to perform peritoneal dialysis in the home, refer him or her to the dialysis nurse or appropriate educator for instruction on how to perform the procedure. Include information on what peritoneal dialysis is, how to access the catheter, care of the access site and catheter, signs of peritonitis, how to perform the dialysis treatment, and care of the equipment.	A specialist needs to teach the patient and family how to perform this specialized skill, and the patient needs thorough teaching with return demonstration.
Teach the patient which signs and symptoms to report to a health care provider	Monitoring for signs and symptoms early can prevent a crisis that requires emergency

— Signs and symptoms of infection (respiratory, access site, etc.) — Persistent swelling or color changes at site of AV fistula — Chest pain — Shortness of breath not relieved by rest — Rapid weight gain or edema — Bleeding from access site	room visits or hospitalization. All of these symptoms represent complications, such as heart failure, angina, bleeding abnormalities following dialysis secondary to heparin or lost clotting factors, and acquired infections.
Teach the patient how to protect dialysis access sites (no heavy lifting with arm used for AV fistula; do not allow others to take blood pressures or do venipuncture in affected arm), preventing infection in IV central line access sites or peritoneal dialysis catheter insertion site (keep dressing intact; use aseptic technique when working around site; monitor for drainage, redness or discoloration, heat at site).	The site of the AV fistula must always be protected to prevent clotting of the fistula or physical damage to the fistula; central line access sites must be protected from entry of organisms.
Evaluate the patient's understanding of all content covered by asking questions.	Helps to identify areas that require more teaching and to ensure that the patient has enough information to ensure compliance.
Give the patient written information.	Provides reference at a later time, and for review.
Assess the patient's and family's ability to carry out the therapeutic regimen.	The patient and family must be able and willing to carry out recommended regimens. Because of the complexity of the regimens, some obstacles, such as transportation, work requirements, resources, etc., may need to be addressed.
Refer to necessary disciplines for assistance (visiting nurse, social worker, support groups).	These disciplines can assist in locating resources available for dialysis patients and provide emotional support needed to cope with change in lifestyle. A nurse is needed for follow-up in the home.

NIC *Teaching: Prescribed diet*
Teaching: Disease process
Teaching: Prescribed medication
Teaching: Psychomotor skill

Evaluation

The patient or family is able to verbalize an understanding of all information presented and asks questions about the prescribed regimen (activity, diet, disease process, dialysis). Following teaching sessions, the patient is able to identify allowed and prohibited foods from a list. The patient can identify all medications by name and report the common side effects as well as the dosing schedule. The patient states a willingness to comply with dialysis requirements. If the patient is doing in-home peritoneal dialysis, he or she is able to demonstrate the correct procedure prior to discharge. The patient should be able to inform the nurse of signs and symptoms (shortness of breath, weight gain, edema, signs of infection etc.) that require immediate attention from a health care provider.

Community/Home Care

For patients with CRF, home care may prove challenging, especially at the time dialysis is initiated. Even though the patient may not need hands-on nursing care, follow-up visits by a nurse are warranted to assess the patient's willingness and ability to carry out the medical regimen, including dialysis, and what financial resources may be required. Adhering to the renal diet with its restrictions of protein, potassium, and sodium may prove to be the greatest challenge to the patient. The dietician can initiate teaching, but the health care provider involved in follow-up must monitor the patient's ability to adhere to the diet. Methods that enhance compliance include consideration of the foods that the patient normally eats, cultural influences, inclusion of family members in teaching, and having other family members eat some of the same foods so that the patient does not feel so "different." In some instances, the dialysis team may allow the patient to have a day during which he or she can eat freely, for some this is the day prior to a dialysis treatment. Having the patient keep a diet history will allow the health care provider the opportunity to examine the foods the patient eats and determine whether reinforcement is required. When hospitalized patients are told they need dialysis, they may agree to the intervention, but once at home the patient may decide to forego dialysis because of other chronic illnesses and decreased quality of life. The health care providers must be prepared to accept the patient's decisions and intervene in a supportive manner by identifying what the patient's needs are if dialysis is not undertaken.

For the patient who does undergo hemodialysis, the nurse should determine that the patient has the necessary resources, which usually centers on transportation to dialysis centers, particularly when the patient lives in a remote rural area far from the nearest center. In addition, the nurse should be sure that the patient understands how to protect and care for the access site (fistula or central line). If family members or significant others are providing transportation, alternative plans should be arranged for transportation to the dialysis site in case of car trouble or illness of the primary driver. Alternatives may include volunteers from religious or civic organizations, or special medical transport vans. If the patient is to perform peritoneal dialysis, the home environment should be assessed to determine where to store equipment and what if any adaptations need to be made. The first few times that the patient initiates peritoneal dialysis, a nurse should be present to decrease anxiety and ensure that the patient or family can carry out the procedure. The visiting nurse should ascertain that the equipment is properly stored and that the patient understands how to care for it. The patient on peritoneal dialysis should have clear instructions about what to do if problems such as catheter occlusion or severe abdominal pain or distention arise. Prior teaching should be reinforced in the home with attention to prevention of infection (peritonitis). The period in which the patient needs further education or monitoring for compliance will vary depending on internal motivation and available support persons for assistance. Follow-up care for patients on peritoneal dialysis should be frequent, and for those on hemodialysis, the dialysis staff should question the patient regarding management of the regimen.

Documentation

Document the exact information taught to the patient. Include the names of any printed materials given to the patient and his or her understanding of the content. If significant others or family members were present during the teaching sessions, include this in the documentation. Chart the patient's willingness to comply with the recommended regimen and referrals made to assist the patient. Also include in the record the patient's demonstration of correct techniques for peritoneal dialysis.

NURSING DIAGNOSIS 7

 SEXUAL DYSFUNCTION

Related to:

Altered nervous function

Fatigue

Defining Characteristics:

Reports decreased libido

Reports erectile dysfunction

Reports being too tired to engage in sexual activity

Goal:

The patient will report satisfaction with sexual ability.

Outcome Criteria

✔ The patient reports ability to be sexually active.

✔ The patient discusses concerns and fears regarding sexual dysfunction.

✔ The patient identifies at least one medical intervention that may assist with sexual function.

NOC *Sexual functioning*

INTERVENTIONS	RATIONALES
Complete a sexual assessment.	Helps to determine the nature of any problem.
Encourage the patient to discuss concerns openly with health care provider.	Recognizing that there is a problem is the first step towards dealing with a problem.
Implement strategies to decrease fatigue.	Fatigue often contributes to the inability to engage in sexual activity.
Encourage the patient to discuss medical options with a physician (medications, implants, etc.).	Advances in treatment of sexual dysfunction have made several methods for enhancement available to patients.
Encourage patient to discuss concerns openly with partner/significant other.	Honest sharing of concerns with loved ones can decrease anxiety regarding sexual activity and open the doors for creative solutions.
Refer the patient to appropriate resources, such as counselors or sex therapists.	These disciplines are trained to assist the patient in this area.

For women in childbearing years, collaborate with physician to refer to medical practitioners who can determine fertility and assist in identifying alternative ways to become parents (artificial insemination, adoptions, in vitro fertilization, etc.).

The patient may want to have children and should be informed about acceptable alternatives to usual methods of becoming a parent.

NIC *Sexual counseling*
Role enhancement

Evaluation

The patient reports ability to engage in sexually satisfying activities. The patient verbalizes concerns and anxiety with health care providers. Counseling has been recommended, and the patient is able to identify medical solutions to the problem.

Community/Home Care

At home, this problem may continue. Dialysis is required for all patients who have CRF, and almost always carries with it decreased sexual function. Fatigue worsens the problem, and often the patient simply does not feel like engaging in sexual activities. Open, frank discussions are required so that the patient can confront concerns and anxiety and move forward to solutions. Sexual enhancement drugs may be an option for the patient but require a thorough physical examination by a physician who can determine whether such treatments are acceptable for the CRF patient. Those patients with erectile dysfunction secondary to diabetes and CRF may be candidates for penile implants. At home, the patient must be monitored for the psychological impact that decreased sexual functioning has on self-esteem. This is particularly true for younger patients who may still be in the childbearing years. Referrals to social workers, counselors, or professionals who are specifically trained in this area are beneficial to the patient.

Documentation

Chart the results of the sexual assessment, including any of the patient's stated concerns, verbatim. Document any referrals made and the suggested recommendations for resolution. Include in the record any other indicators of decreased self-esteem or disturbed body image related to sexual dysfunction.

CHAPTER 5.65

HYPERCALCEMIA (EXCESSIVE CALCIUM)

GENERAL INFORMATION

Hypercalcemia is an electrolyte imbalance that occurs when serum calcium levels increase above 10.5 mg/dl. Normally, 99 percent of calcium is in the bones and the remaining one percent of calcium is in the blood. When total serum calcium levels are measured, it is this 1 percent of calcium that is assessed. Approximately 50 percent of the total serum calcium is transported on serum albumin. The remainder of the serum calcium that is unbound is classified as the ionized calcium; it is this ionized calcium that is physiologically active and most important. Calcium regulation is normally balanced through dietary intake of calcium-rich foods and the influence of parathormone, calcitonin, vitamin D, and phosphate. Parathormone is a hormone produced by the parathyroid glands, facilitating calcium absorption from the intestines, calcium resorption from bone, and increasing serum calcium levels. Calcitonin is a hormone produced by the thyroid gland that has an opposite effect on calcium levels, causing calcium to be reabsorbed by bone and decreasing serum calcium levels. Phosphate regulation is intimately and inversely related to calcium levels: when phosphate levels elevate, calcium levels decrease, and when phosphate levels decrease calcium levels elevate. There are many causes of hypercalcemia, but most instances are caused by malignancies and primary hyperparathyroidism. Parathyroid tumors can cause hypercalcemia by increasing parathormone production. Ectopic hormone production of parathormone also occurs with some malignancies. Another cause of hypercalcemia is bone cancer, or metastatic cancer that spreads to the bone, resulting in lytic lesions that allow calcium to move from bones into the blood. Hypercalcemia can be caused by increased ingestion of calcium or vitamin D-rich foods or by increased intake of calcium supplements or antacids such as calcium carbonate. Patients with osteoporosis or osteomalacia may also lose bone calcium into the blood. Prolonged bedrest may result in bone demineralization and hypercalcemia. It can also occur with the use of thiazide diuretics and lithium, and as a complication of certain diseases such as hyperthyroidism, hyperparathyroidism, hypervitaminosis A or D, hyperproteinemia, tuberculosis, or Addison's disease. Clinical manifestations of hypercalcemia include muscle weakness, anorexia, nausea/vomiting, constipation due to decreased motility, bradycardia, mental status changes if excess is severe, polyuria, and thirst. Because of the increased amount of calcium in the circulating volume, the patient is at high risk for development of kidney stones due to the calcium precipitates. Although hypercalcemia is not usually a life-threatening condition, with the exception of hypercalcemic crisis, the electrolyte imbalance should be corrected.

NURSING DIAGNOSIS 1

IMBALANCED NUTRITION: MORE THAN BODY REQUIREMENTS

Related to:

Malignancy

Excessive use of calcium-containing antacids

Excessive use of calcium supplements

Ingestion of large amounts of foods rich in calcium and vitamin D

Inability of kidneys to excrete calcium

Loss of calcium from bones

Defining Characteristics:

Elevated serum calcium levels

Muscular weakness

Constipation

Nausea/vomiting

Anorexia

Goal:

Calcium levels will decrease.

Outcome Criteria

✔ The patient will report no muscular weakness.

✔ Gastrointestinal (GI) symptoms (nausea, vomiting, constipation, anorexia), if present, will abate.

✔ Serum calcium levels will return to normal.

✔ The patient verbalizes understanding of the cause of hypercalcemia and interventions required for treatment.

NOC *Electrolyte and acid/base balance*
Fluid balance

INTERVENTIONS	RATIONALES
Complete a GI assessment, including history of constipation, nausea, vomiting, and anorexia.	These are common symptoms that occur with hypercalcemia.
Take a nutritional history, including ingestion of antacids (type, amount, how long), usual diet intake, and use of dairy products.	Helps to determine whether eating habits could be a cause of hypercalcemia. In some cases, hypercalcemia may be caused by the excessive use of antacids and consumption of dairy products, such as milk and cheese.
Monitor serum calcium levels and serum parathyroid hormone (PTH) levels.	Allows determination of the extent of the problem and monitoring of response to treatment; the PTH level is measured to rule out hyperparathyroidism as the cause of the hypercalcemia.
Administer fluids intravenously (severe hypercalcemia) or orally (3000 ml), as ordered.	Promotes excretion of calcium by the renal system.
Administer phosphate preparations, such as Neutra-phos, as ordered.	Oral phosphate preparations inhibit intestinal absorption of calcium and raise the phosphorous level, thereby decreasing calcium levels.
Administer bone metabolism regulators/synthetic hormones, such as calcitonin, as ordered.	These agents oppose the effects of PTH, inhibiting the resorption of calcium by bones and increasing the kidneys' excretion of calcium to decrease the circulating serum calcium.
Administer anti-neoplastic agents, such as mithramycin, as ordered.	This medication decreases serum levels of calcium by inhibiting PTH effect on osteoclasts, preventing bone resorption.
Administer sodium bicarbonate, as ordered.	Causes alkalosis, which will decrease ionization of calcium.
Administer diuretics, as ordered.	Promotes urinary excretion of calcium.
Restrict milk and other calcium-rich dairy products and green leafy vegetables.	Reduction of oral intake of excess calcium will assist in reducing this electrolyte imbalance.
Restrict the use of antacids containing calcium or calcium supplements and administer non-calcium antacids if required and ordered.	Excessive calcium intake through these products can contribute to hypercalcemia and should be restricted to correct the problem. Tums® is a common antacid that contains calcium.
Teach the patient causes of hypercalcemia, contents of antacids, calcium-rich foods to avoid, importance of fluid intake, and signs and symptoms of hypercalcemia.	Information is needed for the patient to understand the electrolyte imbalance, comply with recommendations, and assume responsibility for health-promoting behaviors.
Monitor reports of all diagnostic and laboratory tests to identify other possible causes of hypercalcemia and other electrolyte imbalances.	Although treatment of hypercalcemia always involves nutritional interventions, most cases are caused by malignancies or parathyroidism, and the nurse should be aware of these. When the calcium levels are elevated, the phosphorous levels will be decreased.

NIC *Electrolyte monitoring*
Electrolyte management:
   Hypercalcemia
Nutrition monitoring
Nutrition management
Nutrition counseling

Evaluation

Determine the extent to which the outcome criteria have been met. The patient should be able to report the causative factors for hypercalcemia. Calcium supplements and calcium-rich foods have been eliminated from the current diet. Serum calcium levels return to normal, and the patient has no symptoms of calcium excess, such as muscle weakness, nausea/vomiting, and anorexia.

Community/Home Care

Once the causative factor has been identified, it must be eliminated if possible. However, attention is still given to nutritional interventions that can lower the serum calcium level. The patient will need to receive instruction about calcium-rich foods to avoid. Many patients can identify milk and cheese, but few can identify other foods that may contain calcium, such as broccoli, collards, turnip greens, spinach, fortified orange juice, sardines, and canned salmon. Any instruction regarding diet should include attention to normal dietary habits (types of food eaten), as well as cultural and religious practices that impact diet. The patient will need to establish a plan to drink large amounts of fluid to increase renal excretion of calcium, but must be careful not to ingest liquids that contain calcium. The patient can keep a water bottle close by at all times to remind him or her to drink water throughout the day. The patient will need to be mindful of returning for a follow-up visit to have a serum calcium level done.

Documentation

Chart the results of a GI assessment and nutrition history. Document all therapeutic interventions and the patient's response to treatments in the patient record. Chart medications given to lower the serum levels of calcium according to the agency guidelines. Record any patient complaints, such as nausea and muscle weakness, as the patient verbalizes them, along with actions taken to resolve the complaint.

NURSING DIAGNOSIS 2

DECREASED CARDIAC OUTPUT

Related to:

Alteration in myocardial muscle function

Dysrhythmias

Defining Characteristics:

Bradycardia

Electrocardiogram (EKG) changes: Shortened ST segment

Decreased capillary refill

Elevated blood pressure

Goal:

The patient's cardiac output will return to normal.

Outcome Criteria

✔ Pulse will be strong, regular, and > 60 beats per minute.

✔ The patient's EKG will demonstrate normal sinus rhythm.

✔ The patient's blood pressure will return to baseline.

NOC *Electrolyte and acid/base balance*
Cardiac pump effectiveness
Circulation status

INTERVENTIONS	RATIONALES
Assess cardiac system, including pulse rate and rhythm and blood pressure; check pulse and blood pressure sitting and standing.	Abnormal heart rate or irregular rhythm may be an indication of dysrhythmias caused by hypercalcemia.
Monitor for EKG changes, and notify physician immediately if noted.	Hypercalcemia may cause shortened ST segments and dysrhythmias.
Assess peripheral perfusion: capillary refill, peripheral pulses, skin temperature, and color.	When cardiac output decreases, perfusion may also decrease, resulting in diminished peripheral pulses, capillary refill > 2 seconds, cool skin temperature, and decrease in normal color.
Assess for causative factors of hypercalcemia such as malignancy, parathyroid disease, medication use, dietary factors, and osteoporosis, and collaborate with physician about the feasibility of eliminating causes.	Obtaining a good history from the patient regarding medication history, dietary practices, and possible causes can provide clues to needed therapeutic interventions.
Monitor laboratory results: calcium and other serum electrolytes, blood urea nitrogen (BUN), and creatinine.	Identifies the current serum level, and after treatment is initiated, allows monitoring of response to treatment; when one electrolyte is abnormal, others may be as well; BUN and creatinine give clues to renal function. Hypercalcemia can cause life-threatening cardiac dysrhythmias requiring immediate attention.

(continues)

(continued)

INTERVENTIONS	RATIONALES
Restrict calcium intake in the diet and through medications (see nursing diagnosis "Imbalanced Nutrition: More Than Body Requirements").	Corrects hypercalcemia and prevents cardiac dysrhythmias in order to prevent decreased cardiac output.
Administer fluids intravenously (via IV) or orally (PO), as ordered.	Increases calcium excretion by the kidneys.
Implement strategies to reduce calcium levels (see nursing diagnosis "Imbalanced Nutrition: More Than Body Requirements").	Decreases serum calcium levels in order to prevent cardiac complications.

NIC *Electrolyte management: Hypercalcemia*
Cardiac precautions
Dysrhythmia management
Electrolyte monitoring

Evaluation

Note the degree to which outcome criteria have been achieved. There are no changes in the EKG, such as dysrhythmias or shortened ST segment. The patient should demonstrate adequate cardiac output as demonstrated by normal peripheral pulses and warm skin. The pulse and blood pressure should be within the patient's baseline. Calcium levels return to normal.

Community/Home Care

Patients who have experienced decreased cardiac output due to hypercalcemia will need to know how to prevent this electrolyte imbalance in the future. Once at home, the patient should be attuned to the symptoms of increased calcium levels, such as weakness in the legs, tiredness, constipation, nausea, and vomiting. In most situations, home care by a nurse is not specifically required because hypercalcemia is an acute problem easily corrected within hours to a few days. With the elimination of the causative factor, restriction of calcium in the diet, and increase in fluids to promote excretion, the calcium returns to normal, generally without long-term consequences. The patient should be instructed to decrease the intake of calcium-rich foods such as broccoli, spinach, milk, and cheese. In most patients, once electrolyte balance is reestablished, cardiac output is restored and

no further interventions are required in the home. However, a follow-up appointment is necessary to be sure that the patient's calcium level is normal.

Documentation

Chart the results of all assessments made, particularly of the musculoskeletal and cardiac systems. Document all interventions implemented to treat hypercalcemia (medications, fluids, dietary restrictions), and the patient's responses to the interventions. Include vital signs in the chart according to agency guidelines. Document the specific content of all teaching sessions.

NURSING DIAGNOSIS 3

 DEFICIENT FLUID VOLUME

Related to:
Polyuria
Nausea and vomiting

Defining Characteristics:
Constipation
Vomiting
Output > intake
Thirst
Poor skin turgor
Dry mucous membranes
Hypotension

Goal:
Fluid balance is restored.

Outcome Criteria

✔ The patient will have good skin turgor (skin returns to original position when pinched in fewer than 3 seconds).
✔ Mucous membranes are moist.
✔ Blood pressure is within baseline.
✔ Serum calcium levels are within normal range.

NOC *Electrolyte and acid/base balance*
Hydration
Fluid balance

INTERVENTIONS	RATIONALES
Assess the patient's hydration status: skin turgor, mucous membranes, intake/output, skin temperature, blood pressure, and capillary refill.	Helps to determine current status and to monitor response to treatment. Patients with elevated levels of calcium often have disturbances in renal tubular function that causes polyuria and polydipsia with an inability to concentrate urine.
Administer fluids via IV or PO, as ordered.	Restores fluid balance, rehydrates the patient, and assists with mobilization and excretion of excess calcium via kidneys; reduces risk of renal calculi formation.
Encourage PO fluid intake of 3 to 4 liters/day, including those containing a balanced salt solution and some acid-ash solutions, such as cranberry juice; avoid fluids high in calcium, such as milk and cocoa.	A patient able to take PO fluids should do so to supplement IV fluids. Increased fluid intake promotes excretion of calcium. Acid-ash solutions will reduce the risk of renal calculi formation.
Ensure dietary bulk in patient's diet.	Facilitates normal bowel movements; dehydration and loss of normal GI motility may lead to constipation.
Implement strategies to decrease serum calcium levels (see nursing diagnosis "Imbalanced Nutrition: More Than Body Requirements").	Lowers serum calcium levels and protects the body from untoward effects.
Monitor patient for signs and symptoms of kidney stones (colicky pain especially with urination), and strain all urine.	Kidney stones may occur due to calcium precipitates in the kidney; however, such occurrences are rare in cases of acute hypercalcemia. Pain is a sign of stone passage in the urine. Straining the urine allows visualization of the stone. Detecting the stone early allows for initiation of prompt treatment.

NIC *Electrolyte management:*
      Hypercalcemia
      Electrolyte monitoring
      Fluid management
      Fluid monitoring

Evaluation

The patient's hydration status is normal. The skin is warm and dry with good turgor. In addition, the patient's blood pressure has returned to baseline.

Intake and output are balanced, with intake of at least 3000 ml per day. Serum calcium levels return to normal, and no kidney stones have developed.

Community/Home Care

The patient at home will need to continue to take fluids generously to prevent a recurrence of hypercalcemia. The patient may find it helpful to make a schedule for drinking fluids so that fluids can be easily consumed throughout the day. Keeping a water bottle at work or at home to sip on can greatly enhance the amount of water consumed, as it serves as a constant reminder of the need. The nurse or dietician should instruct the patient about calcium-rich foods to be avoided. In addition, the patient should monitor self for signs of hypercalcemia, such as muscle weakness and fatigue, constipation, and a general feeling of fatigue that may be attributed to a slowed pulse. The patient should be instructed to notify a health care provider if he or she notes these signs.

Documentation

Always include the results of a thorough assessment of fluid status, including skin turgor, skin temperature, status of mucous membranes, and blood pressure. Chart the patient's intake and output in the record, along with vital signs, according to agency guidelines. Include in the patient record the types of fluid taken by the patient and the patient's understanding of the need for fluids. Document any complaints or concerns as the patient states them, as well as all interventions employed to address the problem of fluid volume deficits and the patient's response.

NURSING DIAGNOSIS 4

 FATIGUE

Related to:
      Reduced neuromuscular excitability

Defining Characteristics:
      Verbal report of fatigue and weakness
      Muscle weakness
      Depressed deep tendon reflexes
      Abnormal heart rate or blood pressure in response to activity

Goal:
      The patient's normal activity level will return.

Outcome Criteria

✔ The patient reports that fatigue is improved or relieved.

✔ The patient reports no muscle weakness in extremities.

✔ Pulse and blood pressure return to baseline in response to activity.

NOC *Activity tolerance*
Electrolyte and acid/base balance

INTERVENTIONS	RATIONALES
Complete a neuromuscular assessment, including abnormalities of muscle weakness, decreased strength, and decreased deep tendon reflexes.	Helps to determine the effects of hypercalcemia on the muscles; increased levels of calcium usually cause a reduction of neuromuscular excitability resulting in muscle weakness.
Assess the patient's ability to perform activities without complications by assessing heart rate, blood pressure, and respiratory effort before and after each activity.	Activity intolerance can result in vital sign changes after activity, and responses should be monitored.
Implement strategies to lower calcium levels (see nursing diagnosis "Imbalanced Nutrition: More Than Body Requirements").	Returns calcium to normal and reverses effects of muscular weakness.
Assist the patient with activities.	Hypercalcemia influences the excitability of nerves and acts as a sedative at the myoneural junction, causing muscle weakness and fatigue, making normal activity tiring, and increasing the risk for injury from falls.
Help the patient to prioritize activities.	Allows the patient to conserve energy and decreases the chance of adverse effects.
Assist the patient with activities of daily living (ADLs), as required.	The muscle weakness and fatigue caused by hypercalcemia may prevent the patient from participating in self-care.
Provide a quiet environment.	Promotes rest.
Monitor calcium levels.	Helps to monitor response to treatment and to determine when activity intolerance may resolve.

NIC *Electrolyte monitoring*
Energy management
Electrolyte management: Hypercalcemia

Evaluation

The patient states that fatigue has been relieved and is able to participate in self-care. Muscle weakness is absent in all extremities. Elevated levels of calcium decrease and return to normal. The patient reports no exertional dyspnea, and vital signs return to normal.

Community/Home Care

In-home care required is minimal for the patient who has experienced fatigue and activity intolerance secondary to hypercalcemia unless the elevated calcium was caused by an underlying disease. The patient may need to increase activities gradually until the calcium's effects on the muscles have resolved. The patient will need to plan rest periods throughout the day, and return to work may be delayed. Once calcium levels are normal, the patient may experience normal energy levels but find that with strenuous activities the legs are still weak. Because of the treatment for hypercalcemia, the danger always exists that the patient will become hypocalcemic or borderline low; then, when dietary restriction of calcium is implemented at home, the patient experiences alterations in activity tolerance and muscle performance because of low calcium, thus the importance of doing a serum calcium level as part of the follow-up plan.

Documentation

Document an assessment of the neuromuscular system, including any complaints of weakness or fatigue. In addition, chart the findings from an assessment of the respiratory system, including any complaints about difficulty breathing or exertional dyspnea. Include in the record interventions implemented to assist the patient, including assistance with ADLs.

CHAPTER 5.66

HYPERKALEMIA

GENERAL INFORMATION

Hyperkalemia is defined as a serum potassium level that exceeds 5 mg/liter. Potassium regulation is normally balanced through dietary intake of potassium-rich foods and beverages and potassium excretion by the kidneys. Elevated levels of potassium are caused by excessive potassium intake from the diet or from potassium supplements; however, in most instances of hyperkalemia there is some degree of renal impairment that inhibits the kidneys from regulating the excretion of the excess. In cases of acidosis, hydrogen ions move into the cells, resulting in potassium movement out of cells. Potassium may also shift from the intracellular spaces to the extracellular spaces when the cell walls are damaged, such as in trauma, burns, untreated hyperglycemia, rhabdomyolysis, and extreme hemolysis. Other causes of potassium excess include retention of potassium by the kidneys in kidney dysfunction, massive blood transfusions, Addison's disease, use of nonsteroidal anti-inflammatory agents (NSAIDs), and hypovolemic states. A hyperkalemic state increases the cell membranes' excitation threshold, causing cells to become less excitable. The biggest concern with hyperkalemia is the effect on the cardiac tissue, as the cardiac conduction system is affected first, and in the event of severe hyperkalemia the strength of myocardial contraction decreases. Clinical manifestations of potassium excess include bradycardia, electrocardiogram (EKG) changes (vary dependent on severity of hyperkalemia, but always include peaked T wave), dysrhythmias, abdominal cramps, muscle twitching and tremors, and muscle weakness that begins in the legs.

NURSING DIAGNOSIS 1

 DECREASED CARDIAC OUTPUT

Related to:

Decreased strength of myocardial contraction
Dysrhythmias

Defining Characteristics:

Bradycardia or tachycardia

EKG changes: peaked T wave, prolongation of PR interval, depression of ST segment, widened QRS interval, and loss of the P wave

Irregular pulse

Hypotension

Decreased capillary refill

Goal:

The patient's cardiac output will return to normal.

Outcome Criteria

✔ Pulse will be regular and the rate will return to the patient's baseline.

✔ EKG changes will return to normal and the patient will have a normal sinus rhythm.

✔ The patient's blood pressure will return to baseline.

NOC *Electrolyte and acid/base balance*
Cardiac pump effectiveness
Circulation status

INTERVENTIONS	RATIONALES
Assess cardiac system, including pulse rate and rhythm, and blood pressure.	Abnormal heart rate or irregular rhythm may be an indication of dysrhythmias caused by hyperkalemia. The patient may be bradycardic or tachycardic. Hypotension results from decreased cardiac output in the presence of cardiac dysrhythmias.
Monitor for EKG changes, and notify physician immediately if noted.	Hyperkalemia may cause peaked T waves (very common), widened QRS complex, short QT interval, ST segment depression, and

(continues)

493

(continued)

INTERVENTIONS	RATIONALES
	dysrhythmias: sinus bradycardia, 1st degree and 3rd degree heart block, and ventricular fibrillation. Medical intervention is needed.
Assess peripheral perfusion: capillary refill, peripheral pulses, skin temperature, and color.	When cardiac output decreases, perfusion may also decrease, resulting in diminished peripheral pulses, capillary refill > 2 seconds, cool skin temperature, and decrease in normal skin color.
Administer calcium gluconate or calcium chloride IV, slowly, as ordered.	Calcium gluconate and calcium chloride both are given as an emergency measure to protect the myocardium from the toxic effects of potassium while other measures to reduce the potassium level are implemented and take effect. The calcium is rapid-acting and enhances cellular uptake of potassium.
Administer regular insulin and 10 to 50 percent glucose, as ordered.	Insulin promotes cellular uptake of potassium, and the glucose prevents hypoglycemia in the patient; begins action in 30 minutes; lasts 4 to 6 hours.
Administer sodium bicarbonate IV, slowly, as ordered.	Raises the pH, which promotes cellular uptake of potassium; onset of action is 15 to 30 minutes, with a duration of 1 to 2 hours.
Administer Kayexalate via enema (25 g followed by 15 ml 70 percent sorbitol) or by mouth (PO), as ordered.	Kayexalate is a cation exchange resin that exchanges sodium ions for potassium ions in the large intestine, and the sorbitol promotes excretion of the potassium through stool; it takes about 2 hours to work.
Give loop diuretics such as Lasix (furosemide), as ordered.	Loop diuretics cause a wasting of potassium by the kidneys.
Restrict potassium intake (diet and medications).	Assists in correcting the hyperkalemia; prevents complications of cardiac system and muscle function. Salt substitutes should be eliminated from the diet, as these are high in potassium. Potassium-rich foods include oranges, baked potatoes, cantaloupes, and bananas.
Administer antidysrhythmic agents, as ordered.	Decreases myocardial irritability and corrects dysrhythmias.
Prepare for dialysis.	Dialysis is used in cases of severe hyperkalemia to eliminate potassium, especially when the threat of life-threatening dysrhythmias is present.
Monitor laboratory results: potassium and other serum electrolytes, blood urea nitrogen (BUN), and creatinine.	Frequent laboratory assessments of potassium are done to monitor response to treatment. In most cases, treatment of potassium excess may cause other electrolytes to become abnormal. BUN and creatinine levels give clues to status of renal function that could be a contributing cause of the hyperkalemia.

NIC *Electrolyte management: Hyperkalemia*
Cardiac precautions
Dysrhythmia management
Electrolyte monitoring

Evaluation

Note the degree to which outcome criteria have been achieved. There are no changes in the EKG, such as dysrhythmias or fibrillation. The patient should demonstrate adequate cardiac output as demonstrated by normal peripheral pulses and warm skin. If cardiac output is normal, perfusion to the kidneys should be adequate, with the patient producing at least 30 ml of urine per hour on average. The pulse and blood pressure should be within the patient's baseline. Potassium levels return to normal levels.

Community/Home Care

Patients who have experienced decreased cardiac output due to hyperkalemia will need to know how to prevent hyperkalemia in the future. Once at home, the patient should be attuned to the symptoms of increased potassium, such as palpitations, fatigue, etc. Home care is not required because hyperkalemia is a very acute problem corrected in a matter of hours with no long-term consequences. The patient should be instructed to limit the intake of high-potassium foods, such as baked potatoes, cantaloupes, bananas, salt substitutes, and orange juice. For most patients, once electrolyte balance is re-established, cardiac output is restored and no further interventions are required in the home.

However, a follow-up appointment is necessary to be sure that the patient's potassium level is normal.

Documentation

Chart the results of all assessments made, particularly musculoskeletal, respiratory, and cardiac. All interventions should be documented in a timely fashion with the patient's specific response to the intervention. Chart all interventions implemented to treat hyperkalemia (diuretics, diet restrictions, Kayexalate, calcium, insulin, sodium bicarbonate, glucose) and the patient's response to the interventions. Particularly with Kayexalate, specifically chart stools, noting amount and consistency. Include vital signs in the chart and any patient complaints.

NURSING DIAGNOSIS 2

ACTIVITY INTOLERANCE

Related to:

Neuromuscular fatigability

Defining Characteristics:

Verbal report of fatigue/weakness

Muscle twitching and tremors (early manifestation)

Muscle weakness (as level rises)

Exertional discomfort or dyspnea

Abnormal heart rate or blood pressure in response to activity

Goal:

The patient's normal activity level will return.

Outcome Criteria

✔ The patient reports that fatigue is improved or relieved.

✔ The patient reports no muscle twitching or tremors in extremities.

✔ There is no report of exertional discomfort or dyspnea.

NOC *Activity tolerance*

Electrolyte and acid/base balance

INTERVENTIONS	RATIONALES
Complete a neuromuscular assessment, noting abnormalities of muscle twitching, tremors, muscle cramps, flaccid paralysis (progressive/ascending), seizures, lethargy, decreased deep tendon reflexes, and paresthesias.	The above abnormalities occur with hyperkalemia; muscle twitching and tremors are common.
Assess respiratory status, including rate and depth of respirations, and reports of shortness of breath with activity.	Hyperkalemia can also weaken respiratory muscles.
Implement strategies to reduce potassium levels (see nursing diagnosis "Decreased Cardiac Output").	Returns potassium to normal and reverses effects on musculoskeletal system.
Assess heart rate, blood pressure, and respiratory effort before and after each activity.	Helps to monitor response; activity intolerance can result in vital sign changes after activity.
Assist the patient when engaging in activities to prevent injury.	Hyperkalemia causes decreased muscle excitability and ability to contract; legs become weak, making normal activity tiring. The risk for falls increases.
Help the patient prioritize activities to conserve energy.	Hyperkalemia causes muscle twitching and tremors; eventually as the potassium level rises, muscular weakness occurs that could lead to flaccid paralysis, limiting the degree to which the patient can participate in usual activities.
Assist the patient with activities of daily living (ADLs), as required.	The muscle weakness and fatigue caused by hyperkalemia may prevent the patient from participating in self-care.
Monitor potassium levels.	Allows for detection of elevated levels, early treatment, and monitoring of response to treatment.

NIC *Electrolyte monitoring*

Electrolyte management: Hyperkalemia

Evaluation

The patient is able to participate in self-care, and states that fatigue has been relieved. Function of muscles in lower extremities has returned to normal. The patient reports that muscle twitching, weakness, and tremors are absent in the lower extremities. The patient reports no exertional dyspnea.

Community/Home Care

The patient who has had activity intolerance secondary to hyperkalemia requires very little in the way of home care, unless the elevated potassium was caused by an underlying disease. The patient may need to increase activities gradually until the effects of the potassium on the muscles has resolved. The patient will need to plan rest periods throughout the day, and return to work may be delayed. Once potassium levels are normal, the patient may experience normal energy levels but find that with strenuous activities, the legs are still weak and cramping may occur. Because of the aggressive nature of treatment for hyperkalemia, the danger always exists that the patient becomes hypokalemic or borderline normal. As a consequence, when dietary restrictions are implemented at home, the patient experiences alterations in activity tolerance and muscle cramping because of low potassium; thus, it is important for the patient to have a serum potassium level done shortly after discharge.

Documentation

Document an assessment of the neuromuscular system to include any complaints of weakness, tremors, cramping, or twitching, particularly in the lower extremities. In addition, chart findings from an assessment of the respiratory system, including any complaints of difficulty breathing or exertional dyspnea. Include in the record interventions implemented to assist the patient, including assistance with activities of daily living. Be sure to document the patient's response to activity. Record interventions implemented to lower the potassium and the patient behaviors that provide evidence for effectiveness.

CHAPTER 5.67

HYPERMAGNESEMIA (EXCESSIVE MAGNESIUM)

GENERAL INFORMATION

When serum magnesium increases above 2.5 mEq/L, the condition is classified as hypermagnesemia. Of the magnesium in our bodies, 50 to 60 percent is in bones, 30 to 45 percent is in cells, and approximately 1 percent is in the blood. When serum magnesium levels are measured, it is this 1 percent of magnesium that is assessed. Approximately one-third of the serum magnesium is transported on serum albumin. The remainder is unbound in an ionized state; it is this ionized magnesium that is physiologically active and most important physiologically. Magnesium influences neuromuscular irritability and contractility and is an important co-factor for enzyme systems involved with carbohydrate metabolism, protein synthesis, and the sodium potassium pump. Magnesium regulation is normally balanced through dietary intake of magnesium-rich foods, absorption in the small intestine, and excretion by the kidneys. Alcohol interferes with magnesium absorption, and diuresis commonly causes magnesium losses. Magnesium abnormalities commonly parallel calcium and potassium imbalances. Causes of hypermagnesemia include increased intake of magnesium-rich foods or administration of excessive antacids, laxatives, or nutritional supplements containing magnesium. Decreased renal excretion of magnesium occurs with chronic renal failure. Hypermagnesemia is also seen in patients with diabetic ketoacidosis, hyperparathyroidism, adrenal insufficiency, aldosterone deficiency, Addison's disease, viral hepatitis, lithium overdoses, near-drowning (salt water), chronic diarrhea, hypothermia, and shock. Ninety percent of patients with increased or decreased magnesium levels do not demonstrate clinical signs and symptoms. When they are present, clinical manifestations at lower elevations include sweating, a feeling of warmth, and facial flushing. With increasing levels of magnesium, central nervous system involvement is evident, with neuromuscular depression resulting in weakness, lethargy, drowsiness, or depressed deep tendon reflexes. In severe cases, respiratory depression may occur and cardiac function is affected, resulting in brady-dysrhythmias, hypotension, heart block, or cardiac arrest. Gastrointestinal (GI) effects include nausea and vomiting.

NURSING DIAGNOSIS 1

 IMBALANCED NUTRITION: MORE THAN BODY REQUIREMENTS

Related to:

Excessive use of antacids and laxatives containing magnesium

Inability of kidneys to excrete magnesium

Defining Characteristics:

Elevated magnesium levels

Nausea/vomiting

Lethargy

Sweating

Feeling warm

Weak or absent deep tendon reflexes

Goal:

Magnesium levels will decrease.

Outcome Criteria

✔ The patient will report no muscular weakness.

✔ GI symptoms (nausea and vomiting), if present, will abate.

✔ The patient will be alert.

✔ Serum magnesium levels will return to normal.

✔ The patient verbalizes understanding of the cause of hypermagnesemia and interventions required for treatment.

NOC   *Electrolyte and acid/base balance*
Fluid balance

INTERVENTIONS	RATIONALES
Complete a gastrointestinal assessment, including history of constipation, nausea, and vomiting.	Nausea and vomiting are common symptoms that occur with hypermagnesemia, and a history of constipation may imply the use of magnesium laxatives for treatment.
Take a nutritional history, including ingestion of antacids and laxatives (type, amount, how long) and usual diet intake.	Helps to determine whether eating habits could be a cause of hypermagnesemia. In some cases, hypermagnesemia may be caused by the excessive use of antacids and laxatives. Common laxatives that can cause elevated magnesium levels include milk of magnesia, Haley's M-O®, Epsom salts, and magnesium oxide. Common antacids containing magnesium include Maalox®, Maalox Plus®, Riopan®, Mylanta®, and Gelusil®.
Monitor serum magnesium levels.	Helps to determine the extent of the problem and monitor response to treatment.
Restrict the intake of magnesium-rich foods.	Lowers the magnesium level. Foods to be avoided include leafy green vegetables, citrus fruits, seafood, meats, and milk products.
Restrict intake of magnesium-based antacids or laxatives.	Magnesium is a component of commonly prescribed antacids and laxatives that can cause hypermagnesemia. Excessive magnesium intake through these products should be restricted to correct the problem.
As ordered, administer calcium chloride or calcium gluconate.	If magnesium levels are greater than 5 mEq/L, calcium chloride or calcium gluconate should be given to counteract the effect of magnesium on myocardial muscle and to bind excess magnesium (calcium chloride antagonizes magnesium).
Administer thiazide diuretics, as ordered.	Thiazide diuretics enhance the renal clearance of magnesium.
Teach the patient causes of hypermagnesemia, contents of antacids and laxatives, and signs and symptoms of hypermagnesemia.	Information is needed in order for the patient to understand the electrolyte imbalance, comply with recommendations, and assume responsibility for health-promoting behaviors.
Monitor reports of all diagnostic and laboratory tests to identify other possible causes of hypermagnesemia and other electrolyte imbalances.	Although treatment of hypermagnesemia always involves nutritional interventions, other causes should be investigated. Examining all laboratory and diagnostic tests will give clues to other causes of hypermagnesemia and guide accurate treatment.

NIC   *Electrolyte monitoring*
Electrolyte management:
Hypermagnesemia
Nutrition monitoring
Nutrition management
Nutrition counseling

Evaluation

Determine the extent to which the outcome criteria have been met. Deep tendon reflexes have returned, nausea and vomiting are relieved, and the patient has no muscular weakness. The patient should be able to report the causative factors for hypermagnesemia. The patient verbalizes an understanding of the causes of hypermagnesemia and the treatment required. Medications containing magnesium (laxatives, antacids) and magnesium-rich foods have been eliminated from the current diet. Serum magnesium levels will return to normal.

Community/Home Care

Once the causative factor has been identified, it must be eliminated. However, attention is still given to nutritional interventions that can lower the serum magnesium level. The patient will need to receive instruction on foods to avoid that are high in magnesium. Most people have limited or no knowledge about what foods in the diet contain magnesium; however, many can name laxatives that contain magnesium. Magnesium-rich foods to be avoided until the serum level returns to normal include leafy green vegetables, seafood, meat, legumes, bananas, and citrus fruits. Common medications to be avoided include antacids—Maalox, Mylanta, Riopan, Maalox Plus—and laxatives—milk of magnesia, Haley's M-O, magnesium citrate, and Epsom salts. Any instruction about diet should include attention to normal dietary habits (types of food eaten), as well as cultural and religious practices that affect diet. For those patients who use (and in some cases, misuse) antacids and laxatives on a regular basis, teaching should include safer alternatives for treating constipation or GI problems. The patient should have a thorough review of medical conditions and all medications currently being taken to determine what a safe alternative may be. The patient will need to remember to return for a follow-up visit to have a serum magnesium level done.

Documentation

Document the extent to which outcome criteria have been met. Chart the results of a GI assessment and nutrition history, including the use of antacids or laxatives. Document all therapeutic interventions carried out in the patient record and the patient's responses to treatments. Record any patient complaints as the patient verbalizes them, along with actions taken to resolve the complaints.

NURSING DIAGNOSIS 2

ACTIVITY INTOLERANCE

Related to:

Neuromuscular fatigability

Central nervous system depression

Defining Characteristics:

Verbal report of fatigue or weakness

Exertional discomfort or dyspnea

Weak or absent deep tendon reflexes

Hypotension

Goal:

The patient's normal activity level will return.

Outcome Criteria

✔ The patient reports that muscle weakness is relieved.

✔ The patient verbalizes no complaints of feeling tired, drowsy, or lethargic.

✔ Pulse and blood pressure return to baseline response with activity.

✔ The patient reports no exertional discomfort or dyspnea.

NOC *Activity tolerance*
Electrolyte and acid/base balance

INTERVENTIONS	RATIONALES
Complete a neuromuscular assessment, noting abnormalities of muscle weakness and decreased deep tendon reflexes.	Helps to determine the effects of hypermagnesemia on the muscles.
Complete a respiratory assessment, noting rate, rhythm, effort, depth, and any complaints of shortness of breath. If changes in respiratory status are noted, notify physician immediately and support ventilation, as ordered.	If hypermagnesemia progresses and becomes severe, respiratory depression may occur. Routine respiratory assessments can detect beginning changes in respiratory status that may signal a problem, and allow for early treatment. Respiratory assessments also assist in determining the patient's ability to perform activities.
Assess the patient's energy level and ability to perform activities without complications by assessing heart rate, blood pressure, and respiratory effort before and after each activity.	Helps to ascertain baseline energy and performance level and to monitor response to activity; intolerance can result in vital sign changes after activity, especially because the patient with hypermagnesemia frequently has hypotension.
Implement strategies to decrease magnesium levels, particularly restricting magnesium intake (see nursing diagnosis "Imbalanced Nutrition: More Than Body Requirements").	Helps to return magnesium to normal and reverse effects of muscular weakness, feeling tired, etc.
Assist the patient with activities.	Hypermagnesemia interferes with normal neurotransmission and results in muscle weakness and lethargy that may impair the patient's ability to perform activities.

(continues)

(continued)

INTERVENTIONS	RATIONALES
Assist the patient to prioritize activities, and encourage the patient to alternate periods of activity with periods of rest.	Conserves energy and minimizes adverse effects from hypermagnesemia.
Monitor magnesium levels.	Helps to detect response to treatment.

NIC   *Electrolyte monitoring*
      Electrolyte management:
          Hypermagnesemia
      Energy management

Evaluation

Magnesium levels decrease and return to normal. The patient states that muscle weakness and feelings of tiredness have been relieved and he or she is able to participate in self-care. No injuries due to fatigue or muscle weakness occur, and the patient performs activities as desired. The patient reports no exertional dyspnea, and vital signs return to normal.

Community/Home Care

In-home care required for the patient who has had activity intolerance and fatigue secondary to hypermagnesemia is minimal unless the high magnesium was caused by an underlying disease. The patient may need to increase activities gradually until the effects of the high magnesium on the muscles have resolved. The patient will need to plan rest periods throughout the day, and return to work may be delayed. Interventions to return the magnesium level to normal should continue at home through dietary restrictions and restrictions of medications that contain magnesium (see nursing diagnosis "Imbalanced Nutrition: More than Body Requirements"). Once magnesium levels are normal, the patient may experience normal energy levels but find that with strenuous activities the legs are weak. Because of the treatment for hypermagnesemia, the danger always exists that the patient becomes hypomagnesemic or borderline low; then, when dietary magnesium is decreased, the patient experiences alterations in activity tolerance and muscle performance because of low magnesium. This is why it is important for the patient to have a serum magnesium level done as part of the follow-up plan.

Documentation

Document an assessment of the neuromuscular system, including any complaints of weakness, weak or absent deep tendon reflexes, or fatigue. In addition, chart the findings from an assessment of the respiratory and cardiac system, including any complaints from the patient of difficulty breathing or exertional dyspnea. Include in the record interventions implemented to assist the patient, including assistance with activities of daily living (ADLs).

NURSING DIAGNOSIS 3

 DECREASED CARDIAC OUTPUT

Related to:
> Alteration in myocardial muscle function
> Magnesium's direct effect on the myocardial muscle causing decreased inotropy, contractility, and dysrhythmias

Defining Characteristics:
> Cardiac dysrhythmias
> Hypotension
> Bradycardia
> Diminished peripheral pulses

Goal:
> The patient's cardiac output improves.

Outcome Criteria

✔ The patient will have a normal sinus rhythm.

✔ The patient's blood pressure returns to baseline.

✔ The patient's pulse will be > 60 beats per minute.

NOC   *Electrolyte and acid/base balance*
      Cardiac pump effectiveness
      Circulation status

INTERVENTIONS	RATIONALES
Assess cardiac system, including pulse rate and rhythm, blood pressure (sitting and	Abnormal heart rate or irregular rhythm may be an indication of dysrhythmias caused by

INTERVENTIONS	RATIONALES
standing), flushed/red skin, and diaphoresis. Note changes consistent with level of increase: mild (3 to 5 mEq/L): bradycardia, hypotension, red, and warm skin; moderate (5 to 15 mEq/L): prolonged P–R interval, QRS complex, and QT interval; severe (> 15 mEq/L): third-degree heart block and asystole.	hypermagnesemia; patients with elevated levels of magnesium also experience changes in skin such as red flushing to face and diaphoresis.
Monitor for electrocardiogram (EKG) changes and notify physician immediately if noted.	Hypermagnesemia may cause bradycardia, prolonged PR interval, QRS complex, QT intervals, and dysrhythmias; severe elevations in the magnesium level can cause life-threatening alterations in cardiac function, such as third-degree block and asystole that require immediate attention.
Assess peripheral perfusion: capillary refill, peripheral pulses, skin temperature, and color.	When cardiac output decreases, perfusion may also decrease, resulting in diminished peripheral pulse, capillary refill > 2 seconds, cool skin temperature, and decrease in normal color.
Assess for causative factors of hypermagnesemia, such as excessive use of laxatives and antacids, and collaborate with physician about the feasibility of eliminating causes.	Obtaining a good history from the patient regarding medication history, dietary practices, and possible causes can provide clues to needed therapeutic interventions.
Monitor laboratory results: magnesium levels and other serum electrolytes.	Helps to identify the current serum level; after treatment is initiated, examine results to monitor response to treatment; usually when one electrolyte is abnormal others may be also. Hypermagnesemia can cause life-threatening cardiac dysrhythmias requiring immediate attention.
Restrict magnesium intake in the diet and in medications (see nursing diagnosis "Imbalanced Nutrition: More than Body Requirements").	Helps to correct hypermagnesemia and prevent cardiac dysrhythmias in order to prevent decreased cardiac output.
Administer fluids as ordered, intravenously (via IV) or orally (PO).	Increases magnesium excretion.
Administer diuretics, as ordered.	Promotes urinary excretion of magnesium to decrease serum magnesium levels in order to prevent cardiac complications.
Teach the patient the effect of high magnesium levels on the cardiac system, role of antacids and laxatives in causing high magnesium levels, and alternative ways to relieve constipation and GI upset.	Providing the patient with this information allows him or her to understand the rationales for interventions and play a role in managing health and preventing recurrences of high magnesium level.

NIC *Electrolyte management:*
      Hypermagnesemia
  Cardiac precautions
  Dysrhythmia management
  Electrolyte monitoring

Evaluation

Note the degree to which the outcome criteria have been achieved. The patient has a normal sinus rhythm with no bradycardia, and the blood pressure returns to patient's baseline. The patient should demonstrate adequate cardiac output as demonstrated by normal peripheral pulses, warm skin, and the absence of facial flushing. If cardiac output is normal, perfusion to the kidneys should be adequate, with the patient producing at least 30 ml of urine per hour on average. Magnesium levels return to normal levels.

Community/Home Care

Patients who have experienced decreased cardiac output due to hypermagnesemia will need to know how to prevent this electrolyte imbalance in the future. Once the patient is at home, he or she should be attuned to the symptoms of increased magnesium, such as weakness in the legs, tiredness, nausea and vomiting, etc. In most situations, home care by a nurse is not required specifically for hypermagnesemia as it is an acute problem easily corrected within hours to a few days. With the elimination of the causative factor (when possible), restriction of the magnesium in the diet and in medications such as laxatives and antacids, and increasing fluids to promote excretion, the magnesium level returns to normal with generally no long-term consequences. The patient should be instructed to decrease the intake of high magnesium foods such as leafy green vegetables, meat, seafood, legumes, citrus fruit, bananas, etc. Alternative means of achieving bowel regularity and relief from GI upset should be investigated for the patient who uses laxatives and antacids for this purpose. Be sure that instruction about dietary changes considers religious, cultural, and usual diet practices. In most patients, once electrolyte balance is re-established, cardiac output is restored, and no further interventions are required in the home. However, a follow-up appointment is necessary to be sure that the patient's magnesium level is normal, bradycardia is corrected, and blood pressure is no longer in the hypotensive range.

Documentation

Chart the results of all assessments made, particularly the cardiac and neuromuscular systems. All interventions implemented to treat hypermagnesemia (medication restrictions, fluids, dietary restrictions) and the patient's responses to the interventions should be documented in a timely fashion with the patient's specific response to the intervention. Include vital signs in the chart according to agency guidelines. Document teaching implemented relevant to need for elimination of magnesium-rich foods and avoidance of antacids and laxatives containing magnesium.

CHAPTER 5.68

HYPERNATREMIA

GENERAL INFORMATION

When serum sodium increases above 145 mEq/L, the condition is classified as hypernatremia. Sodium is a major extracellular cation and is the key determinant of serum osmolality. Serum sodium levels are influenced by antidiuretic hormone (ADH), aldosterone, and natriuretic hormone. ADH is produced by the hypothalamus, stored in the posterior pituitary gland, and released when serum osmolality increases. Hypernatremia is rare in persons with intact thirst mechanisms. When it does occur, the causes include body fluid losses comprised of relatively large amounts of sodium, such as that which occurs with diaphoresis, diarrhea, wound drainage, gastric suction, vomiting, and burns; fluid intake consisting of an inadequate volume of water; diabetes insipidus (DI) where decreased/absent secretion of ADH causes water excretion in the kidneys, resulting in elevated serum sodium levels; excessive administration of hypertonic fluids; excessive ingestion of salt; and seawater near-drowning. Clinical manifestations directly related to the hypernatremia result from cellular dehydration that can result in thirst from shrunken osmoreceptors and cerebral hemorrhage from shrunken brain cells; these manifestations include seizures, restlessness, irritability, headache, and intense thirst. The degree of change in mental status (level of consciousness) is related not only to actual sodium level but also to the rate of development; the more rapid the development of hypernatremia, the more serious the change in level of consciousness. Patients with hypernatremia secondary to volume deficits may exhibit decreased blood pressure and urine output, dry skin and mucous membranes, and poor skin turgor. Other general clinical manifestations that may occur include dry and sticky mucous membranes and elevated body temperature.

NURSING DIAGNOSIS 1

 DEFICIENT FLUID VOLUME

Related to:

Vomiting

Diarrhea

Diaphoresis

Wound drainage

Gastric suction

Burns

Inadequate water intake

Diuresis

Decreased ADH production resulting in excessive water loss in urine (diabetes insipidus)

Defining Characteristics:

Dry mucous membranes

Decreased skin turgor

Hypotension

Tachycardia

Prolonged capillary refill

Decreased urine output of < 30 ml/hour

Serum sodium > 145 mEq/L

Goal:

The patient will have adequate fluid volume restored.

Sodium level returns to normal.

Outcome Criteria

✔ Mucous membranes will be moist.

✔ Skin turgor will be resilient (pinched skin returns to normal position in < 3 seconds).

✔ Blood pressure and pulse will return to patient's baseline.

✔ Urine output will be > 30 ml/hour.

✔ Serum sodium will be within normal range of 135 to 145 mEq/L.

NOC   *Fluid balance*

         Electrolyte and acid/base balance

         Vital signs

INTERVENTIONS	RATIONALES
Assess for signs of dehydration: decreased blood pressure, increased pulse, dry mucous membranes, poor skin turgor, and decreased urinary output.	Helps to determine the seriousness of the problem, to guide treatment, and to assess effectiveness of treatments.
Monitor intake and output, and conduct an assessment of usual dietary habits.	Allows assessment of fluid balance; a contributing factor in high sodium levels could be the excessive intake of high-sodium foods.
Monitor serum electrolytes, especially serum sodium and serum osmolality.	Helps to determine fluid and electrolyte replacement needs.
Administer hypotonic intravenous fluids, such as 5 percent dextrose in water or 0.45 percent sodium chloride, as ordered.	Helps to attain fluid and electrolyte balance. Correction should be slow, and attempts to normalize the sodium level should occur over 48 hours to prevent brain edema.
Encourage at least 3000 ml/day fluid intake if tolerating oral liquids, unless contraindicated.	Helps to increase body fluids and restore fluid balance.
Encourage intake of water.	Helps to re-establish fluid and electrolyte balance.
Administer antidiarrheal or anti-emetic medication, as ordered.	Slows intestinal peristalsis and raises fluid uptake; decreases fluid loss from vomiting.
Teach the patient about causes of increased sodium level, treatments required, and prevention of recurrence.	Enhances compliance with recommendations and promotes patient control of health.

NIC   *Fluid monitoring*

         Fluid management

         Fluid and electrolyte management

         Electrolyte management:

            Hypernatremia

Evaluation

Assess the patient for return of normal fluid volume. The patient's blood pressure and pulse should return to baseline with the pulse strong and regular. Skin should be warm, and color should return to the patient's normal appearance. There should be no signs of neurological involvement due to sodium excess. Renal function should not be impaired, with an hourly output on the average of 30 ml/hour. The cause of the increased sodium has been determined and treated, and serum sodium levels should be within normal range.

Community/Home Care

Patients treated for deficient fluid volume and hypernatremia should have normal fluid status restored prior to discharge home. Patients experiencing the deficit secondary to loss of fluid from vomiting or diarrhea should receive education about prevention of complications of these entities and the need to seek medical assistance in a timely manner. For those who lose large amounts of fluid through profuse diaphoresis, instruction should include methods of replacing electrolytes. The patient should continue to drink adequate amounts of fluid, but may need to temporarily restrict the intake of sodium in the diet. The patient requires instruction about which foods to avoid and should understand how to read food labels for sodium content. A list of appropriate beverages and foods will provide the patient with a handy reference. Encourage the patient to keep a filled water bottle at work and at home to enhance the likelihood of adequate fluid intake. The patient may not require any follow-up, as this is an acute situation that generally has no long-term complications. Fatigue may be an issue because volume deficit and its causes create a sense of weakness, even if the deficit is mild. This can be handled simply by instructing the patient to perform activities as tolerated until stamina/endurance is re-established. The health care provider may want the patient to return for a follow-up appointment to ensure that parameters such as serum sodium have returned to normal.

Documentation

In this situation, document initial assessment findings such as blood pressure, pulse, respirations, temperature, skin status (turgor, mucous membranes), and mental status. Be sure to document the patient's intake and output every shift. Document all interventions such as intravenous catheter insertion, fluids initiated (type, rate), urine output (amount, color), and dietary modifications such as sodium restrictions. Be specific when charting patient responses to treatment so that other health care providers can clearly determine improvement or deterioration.

NURSING DIAGNOSIS 2

IMBALANCED NUTRITION: MORE THAN BODY REQUIREMENTS

Related to:

Increased intake of sodium-rich foods

Increased intake of sodium-rich medications

Defining Characteristics:

Elevated serum sodium levels

Thirst

Lethargy

Weakness

Dry, sticky mucous membranes

Headache

Goal:

Sodium levels will decrease.

Outcome Criteria

✔ The patient will report no sensations of intense thirst.

✔ Neurological symptoms, if present, will abate (restlessness, irritability, headache).

✔ Mucous membranes will be moist.

✔ Serum sodium levels will return to normal.

✔ The patient verbalizes an understanding of the cause of hypernatremia and interventions required for treatment, including dietary restrictions.

NOC *Electrolyte and acid/base balance*
Fluid balance

INTERVENTIONS	RATIONALES
Complete a neurological assessment, including history of intense thirst, headache, restlessness, and irritability.	These are common symptoms of hypernatremia.
Take a nutritional history, including ingestion of medications (type, amount, how long), usual diet intake, and consumption of sodium-rich foods.	Helps to determine whether eating habits could be a cause of hypernatremia. In some cases, hypernatremia may be caused by the excessive use of salt and ingestion of sodium-rich foods.
Monitor serum sodium levels.	Helps to determine the extent of the problem and monitor response to treatment.
Restrict intake of sodium-rich foods, such as seafood, canned foods, processed grains, processed luncheon meats, dried fruits, spinach, and snack foods such as potato chips, etc.	Ingestion of sodium-rich foods contributes to hypernatremia.
Restrict the addition of salt to food.	Adding salt to food can cause hypernatremia and should be avoided.
Encourage the use of salt substitutes and herbs to season food.	Helps to decrease the use of salt and decrease serum sodium.
Consult with dietician for instruction about low-sodium foods and cooking without salt.	This information is necessary in order for the patient to be compliant with recommendations and assume responsibility for health-promoting behaviors.

NIC *Electrolyte monitoring*
Electrolyte management:
   Hypernatremia
Nutrition monitoring
Nutrition management
Nutrition counseling

Evaluation

Determine the extent to which the outcome criteria have been met. The patient has no signs of neurological impairments due to increased sodium levels, such as headache, intense thirst, weakness, or restlessness. The patient verbalizes an understanding of dietary restrictions required for controlling sodium levels. Foods rich in sodium have been eliminated from the current diet. Serum sodium levels will return to normal.

Community/Home Care

Once the causative factor has been identified and eliminated, the serum sodium level is returned to normal. However, attention is still given to nutritional interventions that can lower the serum sodium level. The patient will need instruction about high-sodium foods to avoid. For many, common snack foods such as potato chips and peanuts can be identified as culprits, but few can identify other foods that may be high in sodium. Sodium-rich foods to be avoided until the sodium level returns to normal include canned foods, seafood, canned meats, processed luncheon meats, spinach, processed grains, and dried fruit. Any instruction about diet should include attention to normal dietary habits (types of food eaten), as well as cultural and religious practices that impact diet. The patient will need to establish a plan to drink adequate amounts of fluid to maintain fluid balance and promote normal renal excretion of sodium, but must be careful not to ingest liquids that contain sodium. The patient will need to remember to return for a follow-up visit to have serum sodium level assessed.

Documentation

Chart the results of a neurological assessment and nutrition history. Document all therapeutic interventions carried out in the patient record with an indication of the patient's responses. Implement dietary restrictions along with indications of instruction about sodium restrictions. Record any patient complaints as the patient verbalizes them, along with actions taken to resolve the complaint.

NURSING DIAGNOSIS 3

 RISK FOR INJURY

Related to:

     Shrinkage of cerebral cells

     Seizures

     Altered levels of consciousness

     Lethargy

     Confusion

     Slowed problem solving

     Serum sodium level is > 145 mEq/L

Defining Characteristics:

     None

Goal:

     The patient will sustain no injury.

Outcome Criteria

✔ The patient will have no injuries.

✔ The patient will have no traumatic injury secondary to seizures.

✔ The patient's skin will be free from traumatic injuries.

✔ The patient will not fall.

NOC   *Fall prevention behavior*
        Physical injury severity
        Risk control
        Seizure control
        Risk detection

INTERVENTIONS	RATIONALES
Assess environment for safety hazards.	Detecting unsafe environmental factors facilitates arranging a safe environment.
Arrange environment for safety.	Decreases injury risk.
Monitor serum sodium level.	Hypernatremia places the patient at risk for seizures; monitoring the level allows for early detection and treatment.
Conduct a neurological assessment: monitor for changes in level of consciousness, seizures, headache, lethargy, confusion, weakness, and muscle twitching.	Patients with neurologic manifestations related to hypernatremia are at increased risk for injury and seizures.
Maintain bed in low position with side rails elevated.	Decreases the risk of falls if the patient becomes confused or is lethargic; decreases fall distance should the patient fall out of bed.
Implement seizure precautions and treat seizures as ordered (see nursing care plan "Seizures").	If sodium levels are uncorrected and continue to rise, seizures and other alterations in cerebral function are likely.
Place call bell within easy reach.	Facilitates communication from patient to nurse if the patient needs assistance.
Do not leave bedside if a seizure occurs.	Patients need to be monitored during a seizure.
Notify physician immediately when a seizure occurs.	Seizures can be life-threatening, and medical intervention is required.

INTERVENTIONS	RATIONALES
Provide a quiet environment.	A calm and quiet environment reduces stimuli that could excite the central nervous system.

NIC *Electrolyte management: Hypernatremia*

Surveillance

Risk identification

Neurologic monitoring

Seizure precautions

Seizure management

Evaluation

Determine that the outcome criteria have been met. The patient should be protected from injury that might occur due to altered neurological function. No traumatic injury occurs to the skin during seizures, or due to falls. If a seizure occurs, the patient is protected and sustains no injury.

Community/Home Care

When discharged home, the patient's risk for injury has already been resolved because the sodium levels should have returned to normal or close to normal ranges. No special in-home care is required to address risk for injury unless the problem recurs. However, the patient will need to continue interventions to maintain sodium levels at normal range, and this includes diet restrictions. Diet instructions about sodium intake should be clear to the patient and should take into consideration the patient's cultural and religious practices, as well as usual dietary preferences. If the increased sodium was caused by preventable factors, the patient should be taught how to prevent or treat these occurrences. The patient should be able to identify the signs and symptoms of hypernatremia, and, if noted, decrease dietary intake of sodium-rich foods and liquids.

Documentation

Document any complications that occur due to increased sodium levels. If seizures occur, document interventions; a description of the seizure; duration; patient status following the seizure, including mental status (alert, lethargic) and vital signs. Chart results of an assessment of the neurological system, and note any injuries sustained. Document all interventions implemented to treat any problems that occur and to treat the high sodium levels. Chart any medications administered according to agency protocol.

NURSING DIAGNOSIS 4

 FATIGUE

Related to:

Muscular weakness

Altered level of consciousness

Hypernatremia

Defining Characteristics:

Lack of energy

Lethargy

Drowsiness

Feeling tired

Difficulty performing activities of daily living

Goal:

The patient will be able to perform activities.

Outcome Criteria

✔ The patient will verbalize no complaints of fatigue or drowsiness.

✔ The patient will perform activities of daily living (ADLs) without assistance.

NOC *Energy conservation*

Endurance

Activity tolerance

INTERVENTIONS	RATIONALES
Assess level of energy and ability to perform ADLs.	Helps to ascertain baseline energy and performance level.
Provide a private, quiet environment.	Promotes rest.
Assess and correct abnormal fluid and electrolyte status (see nursing diagnoses "Deficient Fluid Volume" and "Imbalanced Nutrition: More Than Body Requirements")	Increased serum sodium level is a cause of fatigue; correcting the fluid imbalance resolves the electrolyte imbalance, resulting in increased stamina.

(continues)

(continued)

INTERVENTIONS	RATIONALES
Restrict sodium intake.	Corrects hypernatremia and improves energy levels.
Encourage water intake.	Corrects the water deficit and subsequently lowers sodium level by diluting the elevated sodium.
Assist the patient as needed with activities.	Due to fatigue, the patient may be unable to complete all ADLs.
Provide for uninterrupted rest periods during the day.	Promotes rest and endurance, allowing the patient to perform activities.

 NIC   *Energy management*
Electrolyte monitoring
Electrolyte management:
Hypernatremia

Evaluation

No evidence of lasting effects of high sodium such as fatigue exists. The patient reports that fatigue has resolved and the patient is not drowsy. Performance of ADLs is accomplished without complaints of feeling tired. The patient has serum sodium levels that return to normal.

Community/Home Care

No specific in-home follow-up care is required for the problem of fatigue. The patient may have some mild residual tiredness initially; this is handled simply by pacing activities and gradually increasing them until maximum activity level is achieved. It may be necessary for the patient to schedule rest periods during the day for several days until stamina has returned. If the patient does not like returning to bed for naps or rest periods, a favorite easy chair can be used for the rest period. It is not necessarily sleep that is needed, but rest. The patient will need to implement strategies to prevent a recurrence of hypernatremia if possible, which will include drinking water and avoiding foods and fluids with high sodium content. If the fatigue does not resolve, the patient should contact a health care provider for follow-up.

Documentation

Chart the results of a thorough assessment of the patient's ability to perform activities with pulse and respirations taken after any activity. Include the patient's verbalization of any fatigue is in the patient record. Chart whether the patient requires assistance with ADLs or performs them independently. Chart interventions to treat increased sodium levels.

CHAPTER 5.69

HYPOCALCEMIA (LOW CALCIUM)

GENERAL INFORMATION

When total serum calcium decreases below 8.5 mg/dl, the condition is classified as hypocalcemia. Normally, 99 percent of calcium is in the bones, and the remaining 1 percent in the blood. When total serum calcium levels are measured, it is this 1 percent of calcium that is assessed. Approximately 50 percent of the total serum calcium is transported on serum albumin. The remainder of the serum calcium that is unbound is classified as the ionized calcium; it is this ionized calcium that is physiologically active and most important. Calcium regulation is normally balanced through dietary intake of calcium-rich foods and the influence of parathormone, calcitonin, vitamin D, and phosphate. Parathormone is a hormone produced by the parathyroid glands, facilitating calcium absorption from the gut, calcium resorption from bone, and increasing serum calcium levels. Calcitonin is a hormone produced by the thyroid gland that has an opposite effect on calcium levels, causing calcium to be reabsorbed by bone and decreasing serum calcium levels. Phosphate regulation is intimately and inversely related to calcium levels: when phosphate levels elevate, calcium levels decrease, and when phosphate levels decrease, calcium levels elevate. Causes of hypocalcemia include poor dietary practices, septically decreased intake of calcium-rich foods and vitamin D, or decreased exposure to sunlight. Hypocalcemia can be a chronic condition caused by parathyroid hormone (PTH) deficiency or impaired PTH caused by inadvertent removal of excess parathyroid tissue during thyroidectomy surgery. Renal failure/disease is a common cause of hypocalcemia in which kidneys not only lose the ability to activate vitamin D but also the ability to excrete phosphate. Hypoalbuminemia results in a decreased ability to transport calcium in the blood. Massive transfusion of blood decreases serum calcium levels because the preservative citrate binds with calcium, taking it out of circulation. Other causes of hypocalcemia include intestinal malabsorption, peritonitis, severe diarrhea, alcohol abuse, malignancies with bone involvement, or chronic use of laxatives or enemas that contain phosphates. Commonly prescribed medications that can cause hypocalcemia include loop diuretics, corticosteroids, heparin, anticonvulsants, and antibiotics, such as gentamicin. Patients with pancreatitis may develop hypocalcemia because calcium may sequester in areas of fat necrosis triggered by pancreatic lipase activation. Finally, calcium ionization decreases with high pH levels as occurs with alkalosis. Clinical manifestations of hypocalcemia include paresthesias (numbness and tingling around the mouth and in the hands and feet), muscle spasms of the face and extremities, hyperactivity of reflexes, serious neuromuscular dysfunction that may be indicative of tetany (tonic muscular spasms), laryngospasm, and seizures. Because of the effect of hypocalcemia on the neuromuscular system, the patient demonstrates a Trousseau's sign, a carpal spasm demonstrated by the fingers curling upward when a blood pressure cuff is inflated above the patient's systolic pressure. Trousseau's sign is not specific to hypocalcemia, and it is negative in a significant number of patients who actually have tetany. Chvostek's sign is elicited when the face is tapped at the site of the facial nerve in front of the ear and ipsilateral facial muscle contraction occurs. Effects on cardiac function are significant due to the effect calcium has on cardiac muscle contraction; these effects include decreased cardiac output evidenced by hypotension, ventricular dysrhythmias, bradycardia, and prolongation of the QT interval.

NURSING DIAGNOSIS 1

IMBALANCED NUTRITION: LESS THAN BODY REQUIREMENTS

Related to:

Inadequate intake of calcium-rich foods

Lack of exposure to sunlight

Use of loop diuretics

Renal failure

Low serum albumin levels

Defining Characteristics:

Decreased serum calcium levels

Muscular spasms

Positive Trousseau's sign

Positive Chvostek's sign

Abdominal cramping

Diarrhea

Goal:

Calcium levels will increase.

Outcome Criteria

✔ The patient will report no muscular spasm.

✔ Signs of tetany will not be present.

✔ Serum calcium levels will return to normal.

✔ The patient verbalizes an understanding of the cause of hypocalcemia and interventions required for treatment.

NOC *Electrolyte and acid/base balance*
Fluid balance

INTERVENTIONS	RATIONALES
Complete a gastrointestinal (GI) assessment, including history of diarrhea and abdominal cramping.	These are common symptoms that occur with hypocalcemia.
Take a nutritional history, including ingestion of antacids (type, amount, how long), usual diet intake, and amount of calcium-rich foods consumed in normal diet.	Helps to determine whether eating habits could be a cause of hypocalcemia. In some cases, hypocalcemia may be caused by the excessive use of antacids that contain phosphorous, such as Amphojel®, and a lack of dairy products, such as milk and cheese.
Monitor serum calcium levels.	Helps to determine the extent of the problem and monitor response to treatment.
Assess serum albumin levels.	Hypoalbuminemia results in decreased calcium-carrying capacity in the blood, causing hypocalcemia.
Monitor other electrolytes, especially phosphorous.	There is an inverse relationship between calcium and phosphorous. To correct calcium imbalance, the phosphorous levels need to be restored to normal.
Encourage the patient to eat calcium-rich foods such as milk, cheese, yogurt, rhubarb, broccoli, collard greens, spinach, tofu, and fortified orange juice.	Increasing the amount of calcium-rich foods in the diet will raise the calcium levels.
Administer calcium supplements intravenously (via IV) or orally (PO), as ordered.	Replaces calcium and decreases risk of tetany.
Administer vitamin D supplements, as ordered.	Vitamin D facilitates calcium absorption in the intestine.
Teach the patient causes of hypocalcemia, medications used to treat it, medications that contribute to its development, importance of adequate intake of foods rich in calcium, and signs and symptoms of hypocalcemia.	Information is needed in order for the patient to understand the electrolyte imbalance, enhance compliance with recommendations, and assume responsibility for health-promoting behaviors.
Monitor reports of all diagnostic and laboratory tests to identify other possible causes of hypocalcemia and other electrolyte imbalances.	Although treatment of hypocalcemia always involves nutritional interventions, in some instances, the causes are unrelated to diet, and the nurse should be aware of these. When the calcium levels are decreased, the phosphorous levels will be increased.

NIC *Electrolyte monitoring*
Electrolyte management:
Hypocalcemia
Nutrition monitoring
Nutrition management
Nutrition counseling

Evaluation

Determine the extent to which the outcome criteria have been met. The patient should be able to report the causative factors for hypocalcemia and ways to treat hypocalcemia. Calcium supplements and foods rich in calcium and vitamin D have been added to the current diet. The patient has no muscle spasms or signs of tetany. Serum calcium levels will return to normal.

Community/Home Care

Once the causative factor has been identified, every attempt should be made to eliminate it. However, attention is still given to nutritional interventions that can raise the serum calcium level. The patient will need to receive instruction on foods to consume that are high in calcium. Many people can identify milk and cheese as good foods to eat, but few can identify other foods that may contain calcium. Calcium-rich foods that can be added to the diet include broccoli, collards, turnip greens, spinach, fortified orange juice, sardines, and canned salmon. A written list of foods may be helpful to the patient for reference once at home. In addition, the patient can be encouraged to spend time in the sunlight, which can increase the absorption of calcium through the effects of vitamin D. Any instruction about diet should include attention to normal dietary habits (types of food eaten), as well as cultural and religious practices that affect diet. The patient needs to be aware of the signs and symptoms of neuromuscular involvement that predispose him or her to injury. If the calcium level is not at normal at the time of discharge from the health care institution, the patient may need to limit activities until muscle spasm and numbness are alleviated (see nursing diagnosis "Risk for Injury"). The patient will need to be mindful of returning for a follow-up visit to have serum calcium level assessed.

Documentation

Chart the results of a GI assessment and nutrition history. Document all therapeutic interventions carried out and the patient's response to treatment in the patient record. Chart medications given to raise the serum levels of calcium according to the agency guidelines. Record any patient complaints as the patient verbalizes them, along with actions taken to resolve the complaints.

NURSING DIAGNOSIS 2

RISK FOR INJURY

Related to:

Muscle spasms

Laryngospasm

Convulsions

Tetany

Paresthesias

Verbal report of shakiness or tremors

Hyperactive deep tendon reflexes

Defining Characteristics:

None

Goal:

The patient sustains no injury.

Outcome Criteria

✔ The patient will have no injuries due to paresthesias or spasms.

✔ The patient will demonstrate effective breathing patterns.

✔ The patient will have no traumatic injury secondary to seizures.

✔ The patient's skin will be free from traumatic injuries.

✔ The patient will not sustain a fall injury (head injury, fractures, etc.).

NOC   *Fall-prevention behavior*

Physical injury severity

Risk control

Seizure control

Risk detection

INTERVENTIONS	RATIONALES
Assess environment for safety hazards.	Detecting unsafe environmental factors facilitates arranging a safe environment.
In collaboration with the patient, arrange the environment for safety.	Decreases injury risk.

(continues)

(continued)

INTERVENTIONS	RATIONALES
Perform respiratory assessments every 4 hours, or as ordered, to note respiratory rate, depth, breath sounds, effort, and airway.	Laryngospasms can occur with hypocalcemia due to neuromuscular dysfunction and lowered threshold for excitability. The presence of stridor (high-pitched whistling sounds on inspiration) indicates upper airway obstruction.
If laryngospasms occur, administer high-flow oxygen, as ordered.	Maximizes oxygen delivery until condition can be corrected.
If not relieved spontaneously, consider emergency cricothyrotomy or elective tracheostomy.	When laryngeal stridor/spasms are present, the upper airway may become obstructed. Emergency surgical airway intervention may be necessary to gain access to the airway and provide oxygen.
Assess cardiac status: pulse rate, blood pressure, rhythm, and peripheral pulses. Notify physician of abnormalities and treat as ordered (see nursing diagnosis "Decreased Cardiac Output").	Decreased levels of calcium lessen cardiac muscle contractions that may lead to decreased cardiac output reflected as hypotension, bradycardia, or ventricular dysrhythmias.
Assess for numbness, tingling, hyperactive reflexes, muscle tremors, and spasms.	These are symptoms of low calcium levels and predispose the patient to injury.
Administer calcium replacements via IV or PO, as ordered.	Corrects the underlying cause and eliminates hypocalcemic symptoms.
Implement seizure precautions (see nursing care plan "Seizures").	As the calcium levels decrease, the risk for tetany and seizures rises. Precautions are necessary to decrease risk of head or extremity trauma during seizure.
Monitor patient during seizure activity, and do not leave the patient alone.	Patients need to be monitored during a seizure to protect them and to be able to describe the seizure and patient's response.
Notify physician immediately when a seizure occurs.	Seizures can be life-threatening, and medical intervention is required.
Inspect feet, hands, and other skin daily for injury.	Due to paresthesias (numbness) and uncontrollable spasms, the patient may not sense injuries.
Assist the patient when engaging in activities.	Hypocalcemia influences the excitability of nerves; threshold for excitation is lowered, causing the nerves to be more excitable

	and leading to paresthesias and muscle spasms; also predisposes the patient to seizures and increases the risk for injury from falls (see nursing diagnosis "Risk for Injury").
Assist patient with activities of daily living (ADLs), as required.	The muscle spasms and paresthesias of hypocalcemia may make the patient hesitant to participate in self-care.
Provide a quiet environment.	A calm and quiet environment reduces stimuli that could excite the central nervous system.

NIC   *Surveillance*
Risk identification
Respiratory monitoring
Neurologic monitoring
Seizure precautions

Evaluation

Determine that the outcome criteria have been met. The patient should be protected from injury in the event a seizure occurs. Seizures are prevented, and no signs or symptoms of decreased cardiac output exist. Muscle spasms and tremors are resolved, and no injury occurs. Respiratory function is not compromised due to laryngospasms, and the patient's respiratory status is stable.

Community/Home Care

When discharged home, the patient's risk for injury has already been resolved because the calcium levels should have returned to normal ranges. No special in-home care is required to address risk for injury unless the problem recurs. However, the patient will need to continue interventions to maintain calcium levels at normal range, and this includes supplements and diet practices. Diet instructions regarding calcium intake should be made clear to the patient, with consideration to cultural/religious practices and the patient's usual diet preferences. The patient should be able to identify the signs and symptoms of hypocalcemia; if these are noted, the patient should increase dietary intake of calcium and calcium supplements. If the calcium is still low, the patient will need to implement strategies to prevent injury in the home. Inspection of the skin, especially on the feet, will remain important, as paresthesias may prevent the patient from recognizing injury. Hypotension and bradycardia predispose the patient to fall. Thus, caution with ambulation is undertaken, including rising slowly, seeking assistance if dizziness occurs, and clearing pathways. If signs of hypocalcemia such as muscle tremors, numbness, and tingling continue or worsen, the patient should seek immediate medical attention. It may be helpful to give the patient written information that outlines the symptoms that would necessitate a return to the health care provider.

Documentation

Document any complications that occur due to decreased calcium levels. Chart results of an assessment of neuromuscular, cardiovascular, and respiratory systems. Document all interventions implemented to treat any problems that occur and to treat the low calcium levels. Chart any medications administered according to agency protocol. If seizures occur, document a description of the seizure, duration, and patient status following the seizure including mental status (alert, lethargic, vital signs). Note any injuries sustained during ambulation or seizures, or due to trauma.

NURSING DIAGNOSIS 3

 DECREASED CARDIAC OUTPUT

Related to:

Decreased myocardial muscle contraction

Dysrhythmias

Defining Characteristics:

Bradycardia

Hypotension

Electrocardiogram (EKG) changes: Prolongation of QT interval

Decreased capillary refill

Ventricular dysrhythmias

Goal:

The patient's cardiac output will return to normal.

Outcome Criteria

✔ Pulse will be strong and regular.

✔ The patient's EKG will demonstrate normal sinus rhythm and rate.

✔ The patient's blood pressure will return to baseline.

✔ The patient will have warm skin, strong peripheral pulses, and urinary output > 30 ml/hour.

NOC *Electrolyte and acid/base balance*
Cardiac pump effectiveness
Circulation status

INTERVENTIONS	RATIONALES
Assess cardiac system every 4 hours or as ordered, including pulse rate and rhythm and blood pressure; check pulse and blood pressure sitting and standing.	Low calcium levels cause a decrease in effective myocardial muscle contraction; abnormal heart rate or irregular rhythm may be an indication of dysrhythmia caused by hypocalcemia.
Monitor for EKG changes, and notify physician immediately if noted.	Hypocalcemia may cause prolongation of QT interval and ventricular dysrhythmias; can also cause bradycardia and ventricular dysrhythmias requiring immediate attention.
Assess peripheral perfusion: capillary refill, peripheral pulses, skin temperature, and color.	When cardiac output decreases, perfusion may also decrease, resulting in diminished peripheral pulses, capillary refill > 2 seconds, cool skin temperature, and decrease in normal skin color.
Assess for causative factors of hypocalcemia such as bone disease, decreased intake of calcium in the diet, end-stage renal disease, medications, or alkalosis, and collaborate with the physician about the feasibility of eliminating causes.	Obtaining a good history from the patient about medication history, dietary practices, and possible causes can provide clues to necessary therapeutic interventions.
Monitor laboratory results: calcium and other serum electrolytes, blood urea nitrogen (BUN), and creatinine.	Identifies the current serum level; after treatment is initiated, examine results to monitor response to treatment; when one electrolyte is abnormal, others may be also, and hyperphosphatemia can be a cause of hypocalcemia; BUN and creatinine give clues to renal function.

(continues)

(continued)

INTERVENTIONS	RATIONALES
Increase calcium intake in the diet and give calcium supplements, as ordered (see nursing diagnosis "Imbalanced Nutrition: Less Than Body Requirements").	To correct hypocalcemia and prevent effects on cardiac muscle function in order to prevent decreased cardiac output.
Implement strategies to increase calcium levels (see nursing diagnosis "Imbalanced Nutrition: Less than Body Requirements").	Increase serum calcium levels in order to prevent cardiac complications.

NIC *Electrolyte management:*
   Hypocalcemia
Cardiac precautions
Dysrhythmia management
Electrolyte monitoring

Evaluation

Note the degree to which outcome criteria have been achieved. There are no changes in the EKG, such as dysrhythmias or prolonged QT interval. The patient should demonstrate adequate cardiac output as demonstrated by normal peripheral pulses and warm skin. If cardiac output is normal, perfusion to the kidneys should be adequate, with the patient producing at least 30 ml of urine per hour on average. The pulse and blood pressure should be within the patient's baseline. Calcium levels return to normal levels.

Community/Home Care

Patients who have experienced decreased cardiac output due to hypocalcemia will need to know how to prevent this electrolyte imbalance in the future. Once at home, the patient should be attuned to the symptoms of decreased calcium, such as numbness and tingling around the mouth and in the hands and feet, muscle spasms of the face and extremities, diarrhea, and feeling that the pulse is too slow. The patient should know how to check pulse, so that if bradycardia is suspected, he or she will know how to accurately count the pulse. In most situations, home care by a nurse is not required specifically for hypocalcemia because it is an acute problem that is easily corrected within hours to a few days. After the elimination of the causative factor (when possible), increasing the calcium and vitamin D in the diet and taking calcium supplements will return the calcium to normal, generally without long-term consequences. The patient should be instructed to increase the intake of high-calcium foods such as broccoli, spinach, milk, cheese, etc. In most patients, once electrolyte balance is re-established, cardiac output is restored, and no further interventions are required in the home. However, a follow-up appointment is necessary to be sure that the patient's calcium level is normal.

Documentation

Chart the results of all assessments made, particularly assessments relevant to the cardiac system. Document all interventions implemented to treat hypocalcemia (medications, fluids, dietary enhancements) and the patient's responses to the interventions. Include vital signs in the chart according to agency guidelines. Document teaching implemented relevant to the need for calcium-rich foods.

CHAPTER 5.70

HYPOKALEMIA

GENERAL INFORMATION

When serum potassium decreases below 3 mg/dl, the condition is known as hypokalemia. Potassium regulation is normally balanced through dietary intake of potassium-rich foods and beverages and excretion by the kidneys. Body fluids such as urine, stool, and emesis each have a variable amount of potassium. The two major causes of hypokalemia are decreased intake of potassium or increased loss of potassium. Decreased intake of potassium may occur in patients who are anorexic, nauseated, and vomiting or those who are NPO ("nothing by mouth"). Simply put, these patients are unable to ingest or unwillingly refrain from ingesting foods and liquids containing potassium. The most common cause of increased potassium loss is potassium-wasting diuretics, such as furosemide (Lasix). Additional causes of losses include vomiting, diarrhea, and nasogastric suction (gastric juices are rich in potassium) due to the loss of body fluids. A deficiency of potassium may also be due to malabsorption of potassium or a concurrent magnesium deficiency, if present. Hypokalemia can also occur in patients with alkalosis because hydrogen ions move out of cells, resulting in potassium movement into cells. Consequently, serum potassium levels decrease. Another cause of a potassium deficit is hyperaldosteronism because aldosterone increases sodium and water conservation but also increases potassium excretion. Clinical manifestations include nausea/vomiting, anorexia, muscle weakness, leg cramps, decreased breath sounds, electrocardiogram (EKG) changes, fatigue, flattened ST segment, increased risk of dysrhythmias, and slow peristalsis. Severe hypokalemia causes rhabdomyolysis and decreased ability to concentrate urine.

NURSING DIAGNOSIS 1

DECREASED CARDIAC OUTPUT

Related to:

Decreased strength of myocardial contraction

Dysrhythmias

Defining Characteristics:

Orthostatic hypotension

Weak and thready pulse

Bradycardia

Diminished peripheral pulses

EKG changes: flattened or inverted T wave, presence of U waves, depression of ST segment

Goal:

The patient's cardiac output will return to normal.

Outcome Criteria

✔ Pulse will be strong and regular.

✔ The patient's EKG will demonstrate normal sinus rhythm with resolution of abnormal changes.

✔ The patient will not be hypotensive.

✔ The patient will have no symptoms of decreased cardiac output (skin cool and pale, diminished peripheral pulses, decreased output, weak pulse).

NOC *Electrolyte and acid/base balance*
Cardiac pump effectiveness
Circulation status

INTERVENTIONS	RATIONALES
Assess cardiac system, including pulse rate and rhythm and blood pressure; check pulse and blood pressure sitting and standing.	Abnormal heart rate or irregular rhythm may be an indication of dysrhythmias caused by hypokalemia; orthostatic hypotension is common in states of hypokalemia.

(continues)

(continued)

INTERVENTIONS	RATIONALES
Monitor for EKG changes and notify physician immediately if noted.	Hypokalemia may cause flattened T waves, ST segment depression, dysrhythmias, and the presence of a U wave. Medical intervention is necessary.
Assess peripheral perfusion: capillary refill, peripheral pulses, skin temperature, and color.	When cardiac output decreases, perfusion may also decrease resulting in diminished peripheral pulse, capillary refill > 2 seconds, cool skin temperature, and decrease in normal color.
Assess for causative factors such as nasogastric suction, diarrhea, vomiting, or excessive fluid loss through diuretics and cathartics, and collaborate with physician about the feasibility or possibility of eliminating causes.	Obtaining a good history from the patient regarding medication history and loss of fluids can provide clues to needed therapeutic interventions. Patients who suffer anorexia nervosa or bulimia are at high risk of hypokalemia because of the use of cathartics and diuretics for purging.
Determine if the patient is taking digitalis and assess for toxicity: nausea, vomiting, confusion, yellow halos around objects, diplopia.	Patients who have hypokalemia due to diuretics may also be taking digitalis preparations; hypokalemic states predispose the patient to digitalis toxicity. Potassium ions normally compete with digoxin for binding to Na^+, K^+-ATPase, and in states of hypokalemia bonding of digoxin to Na^+, K^+ ATPase increases so that the serum level of digoxin is increased and toxicity occurs.
Monitor laboratory results: potassium and other serum electrolytes, blood urea nitrogen (BUN), creatinine, arterial blood gases (ABGs).	Helps to identify the current serum level, and after treatment is initiated, frequent laboratory assessments of potassium are done to monitor response to treatment; when one electrolyte is abnormal others may be also; the renal system is responsible for excreting potassium, and the BUN and creatinine are done to establish adequate renal function; ABGs show metabolic alkalosis (increased bicarbonate).
Administer potassium supplements as ordered intravenously (IV) via a primary infusion or IV piggyback	Replacement of potassium is required to bring serum levels to within normal and protect the

or orally (PO). If given IV, ensure that the IV site is free of complications such as phlebitis or infiltration prior to administration, and administer only with an infusion pump.	muscles from continued effects. Potassium is irritating to veins, and a pump is required to ensure proper flow rate. Potassium is never given via IV push directly into the vein.
Implement strategies to replace lost fluid volume (IV or PO) as ordered.	Loss of fluid is a frequent cause of potassium loss.
Assess the patient's diet.	Determines whether the diet lacks potassium-rich foods.
Give foods and fluids that are rich in potassium: cantaloupes, baked potatoes, bananas, orange juice, raisins, dried fruits, green leafy vegetables, etc. Consider the patient's normal eating habits and any cultural or religious dietary restrictions.	Eating a diet that contains potassium-rich foods increases levels of serum potassium.
Teach the patient: — Causes of hypokalemia with particular attention to cathartics and diuretics — Effects of hypokalemia on the body, especially muscles in lower legs and heart — Signs and symptoms of hypokalemia — Potassium-rich foods	This information can assist the patient to prevent a recurrence.

NIC *Electrolyte management: Hypokalemia*
Cardiac precautions
Dysrhythmia management
Electrolyte monitoring

Evaluation

Note the degree to which outcome criteria have been achieved. There are no changes in the EKG, such as dysrhythmias or flattened T waves, U waves, or ST segment depression. The patient should demonstrate adequate cardiac output as evidenced by normal peripheral pulses and warm skin. If cardiac output is normal, perfusion to the kidneys should be adequate with the patient producing at least 30 ml of urine per hour on average. The pulse and blood pressure should be within the patient's baseline. Potassium levels return to normal levels.

Community/Home Care

Patients who have experienced decreased cardiac output due to hypokalemia will need to know how to prevent hypokalemia in the future. Once at home, the patient should be attuned to the symptoms of decreased potassium, such as cramping of the muscles in the leg, feeling tired, etc. Home care by a nurse is not required because hypokalemia is an acute problem that is easily corrected with the elimination of the causative factor when possible or by giving the patient supplemental potassium, and there are generally no long-term consequences. The patient should be instructed to increase the intake of high-potassium foods such as baked potatoes, cantaloupes, bananas, and orange juice. The person teaching dietary needs must ask specifically about the use of salt substitutes as most are high in potassium and when added with potassium supplements may cause hyperkalemia. For example, one teaspoon of a particular brand of salt substitute has 72 meq of potassium. When suggesting foods for inclusion in the diet, the nurse must be cognizant of the patient's ability to purchase them and whether they are part of the patient's usual diet. If the patient is taking diuretics, there is a real possibility of a recurrence, and the patient needs to make a conscious effort to ingest foods rich in potassium or take a daily supplement, as prescribed. Patients on digoxin preparations need to take note of signs and symptoms of digoxin toxicity and know to call the physician if they occur. For most patients, once electrolyte balance is reestablished, cardiac output is restored, and no further interventions are required in the home. However, a follow-up appointment is needed to be sure that the patient's potassium level is normal.

Documentation

Chart the results of all assessments made, particularly of the musculoskeletal and cardiac systems. Document all interventions in a timely fashion, along with the patient's specific response to the intervention. Chart all interventions implemented to treat hypokalemia (oral and intravenous potassium supplements) and the patient's responses to the interventions. Include vital signs in the chart with a sitting and standing blood pressure according to agency guidelines. Document all teaching implemented with an indication of who the learners were and their willingness and ability to comply.

NURSING DIAGNOSIS 2

 ## ACTIVITY INTOLERANCE

Related to:
> Neuromuscular fatigability

Defining Characteristics:
> Verbal report of fatigue and weakness
> Abnormal heart rate or blood pressure in response to activity

Goal:
> The patient's normal activity level will return.

Outcome Criteria

✔ The patient reports that fatigue is improved or relieved.

✔ The patient reports no muscle weakness in extremities.

✔ Pulse and blood pressure return to baseline following activity.

NOC *Activity tolerance*
Electrolyte and acid/base balance

INTERVENTIONS	RATIONALES
Complete a neuromuscular assessment, noting abnormalities of muscle weakness, poor muscle tone, muscle cramps, and paresthesias.	Determine the effects of hypokalemia on the muscles.
Assess the patient's ability to perform activities without complications by assessing heart rate, blood pressure, and respiratory effort before and after each activity.	Helps to monitor response to activity; activity intolerance can result in vital sign changes after activity.
Administer potassium supplements as ordered and encourage intake of potassium-rich foods.	Restores potassium to normal and reverses effects of decreased potassium on muscles.
Help the patient to prioritize activities, and assist with activities of daily living (ADLs) or other activities as needed.	Hypokalemia influences the transmission of nerve impulses, eventually causing skeletal muscle weakness, with the muscles of the legs affected first, and making normal activities tiring. The risk for falls increases.

(continues)

(continued)

INTERVENTIONS	RATIONALES
Provide a quiet environment.	Promotes rest.
Monitor potassium levels.	Helps to detect decreased levels and monitor response to treatment.

NIC   *Electrolyte monitoring*

Electrolyte management:
Hypokalemia

Evaluation

The patient states that fatigue has been relieved and that he or she is able to participate in self-care. Muscle weakness is absent in the lower extremities. Pulse and blood pressure return to the patient's baseline.

Community/Home Care

The patient who has had activity intolerance secondary to hypokalemia requires very little in the way of home care, unless the decreased potassium was caused by an underlying disease. The patient may need to increase activities gradually until the effects of the potassium on the muscles has resolved. The patient will need to plan rest periods throughout the day, and return to work may be delayed. Once potassium levels are normal, the patient may experience normal energy levels but find that with strenuous activities, the legs still are weak and cramping may occur. The patient should include potassium-rich foods and fluids in his or her diet. A laminated list of these foods can be provided to the patient to be used as a reference at home. Because of the treatment for hypokalemia, the danger always exists that the patient becomes hyperkalemic or borderline high as the deficit is overcorrected with dietary supplements or potassium-rich foods. This is why it is important for the patient to have a serum potassium level done as part of the follow-up plan.

Documentation

Document an assessment of the neuromuscular system, including any complaints of weakness, cramping, or fatigue. Also, chart the findings from an assessment of the respiratory system, including any complaints from the patient regarding difficulty breathing or exertional dyspnea. Include in the record interventions implemented to assist the patient, including assistance with ADLs. Chart all medications given to correct hypokalemia according to agency protocol.

CHAPTER 5.71

HYPOMAGNESEMIA (LOW MAGNESIUM)

GENERAL INFORMATION

When serum magnesium decreases below 1.5 mEq/L the condition is classified as hypomagnesemia. Of the magnesium in our bodies, 50 to 60 percent is in bones, and 30 to 45 percent is in cells, while approximately 1 percent of magnesium is in the blood. When serum magnesium levels are measured, it is this 1 percent that is assessed. Approximately one-third of the serum magnesium is transported on albumin, while the remainder is unbound in an ionized state. It is the ionized magnesium that is physiologically active and most important to physiological functioning. Magnesium regulation is normally balanced through dietary intake of magnesium-rich foods, absorption in the small intestine, and excretion by the kidneys. Alcohol interferes with magnesium absorption, and diuresis commonly causes magnesium losses. Hypomagnesemia is most often accompanied by hypokalemia and hypocalcemia. Magnesium influences neuromuscular irritability and contractility. Neural transmission in the central nervous system is mediated when ATP is activated in the presence of magnesium, controlling muscle contraction. Magnesium is important in that it enhances potassium and sodium transport across the cellular membrane, enhances parathyroid hormone secretion, and plays a role in both carbohydrate metabolism and the synthesis of fats, nucleic acid, and proteins. Magnesium also activates enzymes that are responsible for oxidative phosphorylation. The most common cause of hypomagnesemia in the United States is chronic alcohol use or alcoholism. Hypomagnesemia states also commonly occur as a result of poor dietary intake and loss of fluids from the gastrointestinal (GI) tract, especially through diarrhea, but also with GI suctioning. Other causes of low magnesium levels include an increased requirement for magnesium that is not provided (such as in pregnancy, lactation, and the normal growth of children); malabsorption syndrome; ileostomy drainage; pancreatitis; renal losses; parathyroid disease; hyperthyroid condition; losses through use of diuretics; kidney disease; in the treatment process of diabetic ketoacidosis; during/following massive transfusions with citrated blood; or following the cardiopulmonary bypass procedure. Clinical manifestations of hypomagnesemia include anorexia, nausea, vomiting, diarrhea, neuromuscular dysfunction such as spasticity, muscle weakness, hyperactive reflexes, tremors, or seizures. Manifestations that indicate an accompanying hypocalcemia are tetany, Chvostek's sign, Trousseau's sign, and paresthesias. Central nervous system effects include confusion and mood changes. The effects on the cardiovascular system are increased heart rate and ventricular dysrhythmias, particularly if the hypomagnesemia occurs with hypokalemia. The electrocardiogram (EKG) will show a prolonged PR interval, widened QRS complex, and depression of the ST segment with T wave inversion.

NURSING DIAGNOSIS 1

 IMBALANCED NUTRITION: LESS THAN BODY REQUIREMENTS

Related to:

Inadequate intake of magnesium-rich foods

Use of loop diuretics

Renal failure

Low serum albumin levels

Diarrhea

Excess ileostomy drainage

Excess alcohol intake

Defining Characteristics:

Decreased serum magnesium levels

Anorexia

Nausea/vomiting

Tremors

Muscle weakness

Positive Trousseau's sign

Positive Chvostek's sign

Confusion

Hyperactive reflexes

Goal:

Magnesium levels will increase.

Outcome Criteria

✔ The patient will report no muscular weakness or tremors.

✔ Signs of tetany will not be present.

✔ Serum magnesium levels will return to normal.

✔ The patient verbalizes understanding of the cause of hypomagnesemia and interventions required for treatment.

NOC *Electrolyte and acid/base balance*
Fluid balance

INTERVENTIONS	RATIONALES
Complete a gastrointestinal assessment, including history of diarrhea and vomiting.	These are common causes of hypomagnesemia.
Complete a neuromuscular assessment to detect alterations secondary to hypocalcemia: tetany, Chvostek's sign, and Trousseau's sign.	Detects serious symptoms of hypocalcemia that accompany hypomagnesemia and allows early treatment.
Take a nutritional history, including history of vomiting, diarrhea, gastric suctioning, usual diet intake, amount of magnesium-rich foods consumed in normal diet, and alcohol use.	Helps to determine whether vomiting or diarrhea have contributed to the decreased magnesium or if eating habits could be a cause of hypomagnesemia. The most common cause of hypomagnesemia is the chronic intake of alcohol, and hypocalcemia may be caused by the excessive use of antacids

	that contain phosphorous, such as Amphojel.
Monitor serum magnesium.	Allows determination of the extent of the problem and monitoring of response to treatment.
Assess serum albumin levels.	Hypoalbuminemia results in decreased magnesium-carrying capacity in the blood, resulting in hypomagnesemia.
Monitor other electrolytes, especially potassium and calcium.	Hypomagnesemia is usually accompanied by hypokalemia and hypocalcemia.
Encourage the patient to eat magnesium-rich foods, such as leafy green vegetables, seafood, meat, legumes, bananas, oranges, chocolate, milk, and wheat grain.	Increasing the amount of magnesium-rich foods in the diet will raise the magnesium levels.
Encourage the patient to eat protein-rich foods.	Increasing protein amplifies the magnesium-carrying capacity of albumin by augmenting albumin levels and should raise serum magnesium levels.
Administer magnesium sulfate, intravenously (IV) or deep intramuscularly (IM), as ordered according to agency protocol and special procedures for administration.	Restores magnesium levels to normal.
Administer magnesium hydroxide orally (PO) (if non-emergency condition), as ordered.	Restores magnesium level to normal.
Avoid alcohol intake.	Alcohol interferes with intestinal absorption of magnesium.
Teach the patient causes of hypomagnesemia, medications used to treat it, risk factors that contribute to its development, importance of adequate intake of magnesium-rich foods, and signs and symptoms of hypomagnesemia.	Information is needed in order for the patient to understand the electrolyte imbalance, comply with recommendations, and assume responsibility for health-promoting behaviors.
Monitor reports of all diagnostic and laboratory tests to identify other possible causes of hypomagnesemia and other electrolyte imbalances.	While treatment of hypomagnesemia always involves nutritional interventions, in some instances the causes are not related to diet, and the nurse should be aware of these. When the magnesium levels are decreased, potassium and calcium levels are also frequently decreased.

NIC *Electrolyte monitoring*

Electrolyte management: Hypomagnesemia

Nutrition monitoring

Nutrition management

Nutrition counseling

Evaluation

Determine the extent to which the outcome criteria have been met. There is no muscle tremor or complaints of weakness and tetany has not occurred. The patient should be able to report the causative factors for hypomagnesemia. Magnesium supplements and magnesium-rich foods, calcium, and protein have been added to the current diet. Serum magnesium levels will return to normal.

Community/Home Care

Once the causative factor has been identified, every attempt should be made to eliminate it. However, attention is still given to nutritional interventions that can raise the serum magnesium level. The patient will need to receive instruction on magnesium-rich foods to consume. For most people, this will be new knowledge, and they will be unable to name any food that is a good source of magnesium. Magnesium-rich foods include leafy green vegetables, meat, citrus fruits, bananas, and seafood. Patients should include protein-rich foods in the diet to improve albumin levels, which enhances magnesium-carrying ability of the blood. A written list of foods may be helpful to the patient for reference at home. In addition, the patient must be encouraged to avoid alcohol intake, which alters magnesium levels through intestinal losses, malabsorption, and decreased nutritional status. Any teaching regarding diet should include attention to normal dietary habits (types of food eaten), and cultural and religious practices that affect diet. The dietician or nurse needs to be cognizant of alternative sources of protein for vegetarians and people who eat little meat or restrict their intake of meat (for example, those who do not eat red meat or pork). For alcoholic patients, the nurse collaborates with the patient to establish long-term goals for resolution of the drinking problem. A referral to social workers or community support groups may be beneficial. The patient who has magnesium deficiency due to GI losses resulting from diarrhea will need to learn methods to control losses and replace electrolytes. Intake of foods and liquids that are electrolyte-rich will be crucial for this patient. Teaching the patient how to monitor the amount and consistency of stools each day and to keep a record will assist him or her to intervene before imbalances become symptomatic and problematic. The patient needs to be aware of the signs and symptoms of neuromuscular involvement that may predispose him or her to injury. The patient will need to be mindful of returning for a follow-up visit to have a serum magnesium level done.

Documentation

Chart the results of GI and neurovascular assessments and a nutrition history. Document all therapeutic interventions carried out in the patient record. Document the patient's response to treatments by noting the serum magnesium levels. Chart medications given to raise the serum levels of magnesium according to the agency guidelines. Record any patient complaints verbatim, along with actions taken to resolve the complaint. Document the specific content of teaching sessions along with an indication of the patient's understanding of the content and any areas for reinforcement.

NURSING DIAGNOSIS 2

 DECREASED CARDIAC OUTPUT

Related to:

Irritability of myocardial muscle cells

Dysrhythmias

Defining Characteristics:

Tachycardia

Hypertension

EKG changes: Prolongation of PR interval, widened QRS complex, depression of ST segment with T wave inversion

Goal:

The patient's cardiac output will return to normal.

Outcome Criteria

✔ The patient's pulse will decrease to baseline and be strong and regular.

✔ The patient's EKG will demonstrate normal sinus rhythm and rate.

✔ The patient's blood pressure will decrease and return to baseline.

✔ The patient will have no symptoms of decreased cardiac output (decreased capillary refill, cool skin, decreased urine output).

NOC *Electrolyte and acid/base balance*
Cardiac pump effectiveness
Circulation status

INTERVENTIONS	RATIONALES
Assess cardiac system, including pulse rate and rhythm and blood pressure; check pulse and blood pressure sitting and standing.	Abnormal heart rate or irregular rhythm may be an indication of dysrhythmias caused by hypomagnesemia and hypokalemia. Hypertension is common in patients with chronic hypomagnesemia, such as alcoholics.
Monitor for EKG changes, and notify physician immediately if noted.	Hypomagnesemia may cause changes in the EKG tracing dysrhythmias, as well as tachycardia that require immediate attention. In the presence of hypocalcemia and hypokalemia, these changes are more likely to occur.
Assess peripheral perfusion: capillary refill, peripheral pulses, skin temperature, and color.	When cardiac output decreases, perfusion may also decrease resulting in diminished peripheral pulses, capillary refill > 2 seconds, cool skin temperature, and decrease in normal color.
Assess for causative factors of hypomagnesemia such as diarrhea; vomiting; decreased intake of magnesium in the diet, especially in patients who are malnourished, such as alcoholics; renal disease; medications (diuretics, certain antibiotics); and rapid administration of blood; and collaborate with physician about the feasibility of eliminating causes.	Obtaining a good history from the patient regarding medications, dietary practices, and possible causes can provide clues to needed therapeutic interventions.
Monitor laboratory results: magnesium, calcium, potassium, and albumin. Notify physician immediately of low magnesium level.	Helps to identify the current serum level and, after treatment is initiated, to examine results to monitor response to treatment; when one electrolyte

is abnormal, others may be also; albumin levels give indicators of nutritional status, and protein deficits contribute to a low magnesium level. Hypomagnesemia can cause life-threatening cardiac dysrhythmias and seizures, making early detection necessary to ensure patient safety.

Increase magnesium intake in the diet and give magnesium supplements as ordered (see nursing diagnosis "Imbalanced Nutrition: Less than Body Requirements").	Corrects hypomagnesemia and prevents effects on cardiac muscle function in order to prevent decreased cardiac output.
If the patient is taking digitalis products, monitor for digitalis toxicity: nausea and vomiting, blurred vision, halos, yellow lights, dysrhythmias, heart blocks, and digoxin levels.	Hypomagnesemia increases the risk of digitalis toxicity.

NIC *Electrolyte management:*
     Hypomagnesemia
Cardiac precautions
Dysrhythmia management
Electrolyte monitoring

Evaluation

Note the degree to which outcome criteria have been achieved. There are no changes in the EKG, such as dysrhythmias or prolonged PR interval. The patient should demonstrate adequate cardiac output as demonstrated by normal peripheral pulses and warm skin. Urinary output should be adequate, with the patient producing at least 30 ml of urine per hour on average. The pulse and blood pressure should be within the patient's baseline. Magnesium levels return to normal levels.

Community/Home Care

Patients who have experienced decreased cardiac output due to hypomagnesemia will need to know how to prevent this electrolyte imbalance in the future. Once at home, the patient should be attuned to the symptoms of decreased magnesium such as tremors, muscle weakness, numbness and tingling, and feeling that the pulse is too fast or the heart is racing. The patient should be aware of the signs of digitalis toxicity that should be reported to a health care provider. In most situations, home care by a nurse is not required specifically for hypomagnesemia as it is an acute problem easily corrected within hours to a few days. The patient should be instructed to increase the intake of high magnesium foods such as leafy green vegetables, seafood, meat, legumes, citrus fruit, bananas, chocolate, wheat grain, and milk. By eliminating the causative factor (when possible), increasing the magnesium in the diet, and taking any prescribed magnesium supplements, the magnesium returns to normal with generally no long-term complications. Alcoholic patients may pose a challenge for the health care provider because they frequently suffer from malnutrition, and alcohol consumption decreases the absorption of magnesium that is consumed. Assistance of family members or significant others may be required to enhance compliance with recommendations for dietary intake and alcohol abstinence. For most patients, once electrolyte balance is re-established, cardiac output is restored and no further interventions are required in the home. However, a follow-up appointment is needed to be sure that the patient's magnesium level is normal.

Documentation

Chart the results of all assessments made, particularly those in regard to the neuromuscular and cardiac systems. Chart all interventions implemented to treat hypomagnesemia (medications, fluids, dietary enhancements) and the patient's responses to the interventions. Include vital signs in the chart according to agency guidelines, especially blood pressure and pulse. Document teaching implemented relevant to the need for magnesium-rich foods.

NURSING DIAGNOSIS 3

 RISK FOR INJURY

Related to:

Neuromuscular excitability

Verbal report of shakiness or tremors

Muscle tremors

Muscle weakness

Paresthesias

Abnormal heart rate or blood pressure in response to activity

Defining Characteristics:

None

Goal:

The patient will not be injured.

Outcome Criteria

✔ The patient does not fall.

✔ The patient sustains no traumatic injuries.

✔ The patient reports that muscle tremors are relieved.

✔ The patient reports no muscle weakness in extremities.

✔ Pulse and blood pressure return to baseline following activity.

NOC *Fall prevention behavior*

Risk detection

Electrolyte and acid/base balance

INTERVENTIONS	RATIONALES
Complete a neuromuscular assessment, including noting abnormalities of muscle tremors, muscle weakness, hyperactive reflexes, tingling, and numbness in feet.	Helps to determine the effects of hypomagnesemia and hypocalcemia on the muscles; decreased levels of magnesium are frequently accompanied by hypocalcemia, which may cause an increase in neuromuscular excitability.
Assess the patient's ability to perform activities safely and without complications by assessing heart rate, blood pressure, and respiratory effort before and after each activity.	Helps to monitor response; activity intolerance can result in vital sign changes after activity, especially given that the patient with hypomagnesemia frequently has hypertension.
Implement strategies to raise magnesium levels: administer magnesium supplements and magnesium-rich foods.	Returns magnesium to normal and reverses effects of muscular tremors, weakness, etc., that predispose the patient to injury.
Assist the patient to prioritize activities and assist the patient with all activities, as needed.	Hypomagnesemia influences the excitability of nerves and results in muscle tremors and weakness; because of the

(continues)

(continued)

INTERVENTIONS	RATIONALES
	possibility of low calcium levels the patient is at risk for seizures and for falls.
Implement seizure precautions (see nursing care plan "Seizures").	Low magnesium levels lead to nervous excitability that increases the risk for seizures. Precautions are necessary to decrease risk of head or extremity trauma during seizure.
Monitor patient during seizure activity and do not leave alone.	During a seizure, patients need to be monitored by someone who can protect them and describe the seizure and patient response.
Notify physician immediately when a seizure occurs.	Seizures can be life-threatening, and medical intervention is required.
Monitor magnesium levels.	Establishes decreased levels and monitors response to treatment.

NIC   *Seizure precautions*
          Surveillance
          Electrolyte monitoring
          Electrolyte management:
             Hypomagnesemia

Evaluation

The patient sustained no injury. The patient is able to participate in self-care and states that muscle weakness or any paresthesias have been relieved. Decreased levels of magnesium increase and return to normal. No seizures occur, and the patient performs activities without injury. The patient reports no exertional dyspnea, and vital signs return to the patient's baseline.

Community/Home Care

In-home care required for the patient who has been at risk for injury secondary to hypomagnesemia is minimal, unless the low magnesium level was caused by an underlying disease. The patient may need to gradually increase activities at home until the effects of the low magnesium on the muscles has resolved to decrease the risk for injury. Interventions to return the magnesium level to normal should continue at home through dietary intake or oral supplements (see nursing diagnosis "Imbalanced Nutrition: Less than Body Requirements"). Once magnesium levels are normal, the patient may experience normal energy levels but find that with strenuous activities the legs are weak. The patient will need to anticipate this by seeking assistance with strenuous activities until the magnesium level has returned to normal. Family members should be aware of interventions required if the patient has a seizure. It is important for the patient to have a follow up plan that includes assessment of the serum magnesium level.

Documentation

Document an assessment of the neuromuscular system, including any complaints of weakness, muscle tremors, paresthesias, or fatigue. Chart the patient's ability to perform self-care activities. Include in the record interventions implemented to assist the patient including assistance with activities of daily living. Include in the patient record all content that has been taught to the family and patient. If the patient falls, document this according to the agency guidelines with an assessment for injuries. Likewise, if seizures occur, chart a description of the seizure activity, interventions to protect the patient, duration of the seizure, interventions to treat the patient, and the patient's behavior following the seizure. Chart all medications given to the patient according to agency protocol.

CHAPTER 5.72

HYPONATREMIA

GENERAL INFORMATION

When serum sodium decreases below 135 mEq/L, the condition is classified as hyponatremia. Sodium is a major extracellular cation and is the key determinant of serum osmolality. Serum sodium levels are influenced by antidiuretic hormone (ADH), aldosterone, and natriuretic hormone. ADH is produced by the hypothalamus, stored in the posterior pituitary gland, and released when serum osmolality increases. ADH causes water reabsorption in the kidneys that dilutes and lowers serum sodium levels. Aldosterone is produced by the adrenal cortex and released when sodium, volume, or blood pressure are sensed to be low. Aldosterone causes sodium and water reabsorption in the kidneys that increases serum sodium levels and conserves fluid volume. Atrial natriuretic factor (ANF) is produced by atrial muscle in response to increased blood volume that causes increased sodium and water excretion by the kidneys. Lowered serum sodium levels are caused by an actual loss of sodium or by dilution of sodium in the serum due to excess fluid. Hyponatremia may occur with fluid losses comprised of relatively large amounts of sodium, such as diaphoresis, diarrhea, wound drainage, gastric suction, vomiting, diuresis from diuretics, and burns. Third spacing of plasma that contains sodium may occur with peritonitis, bowel obstruction, or following bowel surgery. In the syndrome of inappropriate ADH secretion (SIADH) increased secretion of ADH causes water reabsorption in the kidneys that dilutes serum sodium levels. Excessive administration of hypotonic fluids, such as 5 percent dextrose in water, can contribute to hyponatremia. Congestive heart failure, cirrhosis of the liver, and renal disease can contribute to low sodium levels due to the excessive fluid volume that occurs. Clinical manifestations directly related to hyponatremia result from cellular swelling and consequent alterations in the abilities of cells to depolarize and repolarize. Specific manifestations include muscle cramps, weakness, fatigue, depressed deep tendon reflexes, muscle twitching, tremors, abdominal cramping, nausea/vomiting, headache, confusion, seizures, or coma. The extent of the clinical symptoms is dependent upon the rate of onset/development of hyponatremia.

NURSING DIAGNOSIS 1

 ### EXCESS FLUID VOLUME

Related to:

Excessive fluid intake

Administration of hypotonic intravenous (IV) fluids

Excessive water drinking

Syndrome of inappropriate ADH (SIADH)

Stimulation of ADH secretion by head injury/trauma/infection, CHF, or cirrhosis

Defining Characteristics:

Decreased serum sodium below 135 mEq/L

Decreased urine sodium

Edema

Crackles in lungs

Elevated blood pressure

Goal:

No signs of fluid volume excess are noted, and electrolyte balance is achieved.

Outcome Criteria

✔ Sodium levels will return to normal range of 135–145 mEq/L.

✔ The patient will lose excess fluid as demonstrated by weight loss.

✔ Lungs will be clear to auscultation.

✔ The patient will have no edema.

NOC *Fluid balance*
Fluid overload severity
Electrolyte and acid/base balance
Vital signs

INTERVENTIONS	RATIONALES
Assess for signs of fluid volume excess such as edema, hypertension, and crackles in lungs.	Clinical manifestations such as these must be detected early to initiate treatment and prevent complications.
Monitor vital signs.	Blood pressure and pulse will be elevated with excess volume.
Monitor intake and output.	Helps to determine fluid balance.
Monitor serum sodium, other electrolytes, and serum osmolality.	Helps to determine sodium or other electrolyte replacement needs. In the presence of fluid volume excess, there may not be a true sodium deficit, but the low sodium is due to dilution.
Weigh patient daily at same time (before breakfast, after voiding) on the same scale; have patient wear similar clothes for each weighing.	Weight is the best determinant of fluid loss or retention: 1kg of weight loss = 1L of fluid loss. It is important to weigh the patient under similar conditions for accuracy.
Restrict fluid intake to 1000–2000 ml/day; spread out intake of fluids over the course of the day, ensuring that fluids served with meals and needed for medications are included. Scheduling a certain amount for 8-hour intervals will help keep the patient compliant.	Decreases total body water and risk of CHF or increased intracranial pressure development.
Administer loop diuretics (with concurrent electrolyte replacement), as ordered.	Decreases total body water and corrects electrolyte imbalance. Loop diuretics induce isotonic diuresis and fluid volume loss, which will raise the serum concentration of sodium.
Assess for signs and symptoms of SIADH: decreased urine output, concentrated urine, edema, hyponatremia.	SIADH is a possible cause of excessive fluid volume.

NIC *Electrolyte management: Hyponatremia*
Fluid monitoring
Fluid management

Evaluation

Determine the extent to which the outcome criteria have been achieved. Serum sodium levels are within normal range. The patient should have a resolution of fluid volume excess as demonstrated by absence of edema and clear breath sounds. The patient's blood pressure and pulse are at baseline. The patient will demonstrate a weight loss indicative of fluid loss.

Community/Home Care

Ensure that the patient at home understands the importance of monitoring fluid status. The patient should have a reliable scale that is calibrated and easily accessible. Weighing daily at home will allow the patient to notice subtle changes in fluid retention that may indicate a recurrence of the problem. Patients should be instructed to take note of clothing that becomes too tight in a short period, which is an indicator of fluid retention. The patient who has decreased sodium levels due to fluid volume excess that has diluted the sodium may need to restrict sodium intake once the fluid excess is corrected. At home, the patient needs to limit the intake of salt and sodium-rich foods. Teaching the patient how to read food labels for sodium content should be undertaken. Diet instructions for home should consider the patient's normal diet and any cultural or religious preferences and restrictions. Have the patient keep a log of food and fluid intake as well as weights. Help the patient develop a schedule for taking prescribed diuretics that is mindful of his or her lifestyle and daily routines. Stress the need for follow-up care to assess sodium levels.

Documentation

Always document the extent to which the outcome criteria have been achieved. An assessment of fluid status should be noted that includes intake and output, blood pressure, pulse, weights, and breath sounds. Document medications administered for excess fluid volume in the medication administration record, and indicate the amount of fluid the patient lost in response. Chart the patient's understanding of the therapies for eliminating fluid excess.

NURSING DIAGNOSIS 2

DEFICIENT FLUID VOLUME

Related to:

Vomiting

Diarrhea

Diaphoresis

Wound drainage, gastric suction

Burns

Third spacing of plasma that contains sodium

Fluid replacement with inadequate volume of 5 percent dextrose in water

Defining Characteristics:

Dry mucous membranes

Decreased skin turgor

Hypotension

Tachycardia

Prolonged capillary refill

Decreased urine output of < 30 ml/hour

Serum sodium < 135 mEq/L

Goal:

The patient will have adequate fluid volume restored.

Outcome Criteria

✔ Mucous membranes will be moist.

✔ Skin turgor will be resilient.

✔ Blood pressure and pulse will return to patient's baseline.

✔ Urine output will be > 30 ml/hour.

✔ Serum sodium will be within normal range of 135–145 mEq/L.

NOC *Fluid balance*

Electrolyte and acid/base balance

Vital signs

INTERVENTIONS	RATIONALES
Assess for signs of dehydration/volume excess: decreased blood pressure, increased pulse, dry mucous membranes, poor skin turgor, and decreased urinary output.	Helps to determine the seriousness of dehydration in order to guide treatment and assess effectiveness of treatments.
Monitor intake and output, and conduct an assessment of usual dietary habits.	Helps to assess fluid balance; contributing factors to low sodium levels could be the intake of low sodium foods, diuretic use, intake of large amounts of water, or anorexia.
Monitor serum electrolytes, especially serum sodium and serum osmolality.	Helps to determine fluid and electrolyte replacement needs.
Administer IV fluids containing sodium (0.9 percent sodium chloride) as ordered.	Replaces fluid and corrects deficient sodium level.
Encourage at least 3000 ml/day fluid intake if tolerating oral liquids unless contraindicated.	Increases body fluids and restores fluid balance.
Encourage intake of electrolyte-rich fluids and diet, avoiding free water.	Helps to maintain electrolyte balance.
In mild hyponatremia, give sodium-rich foods, such as canned foods, meat and fish, tomato products, dried fruit, and spinach.	In mild hyponatremia, diet alone may correct the low serum sodium.
Administer antidiarrheal medication, as ordered.	Slows intestinal peristalsis, raises fluid uptake, and prevents sodium loss from diarrhea.
Administer anti-emetics as ordered.	Decreases losses from vomiting.

NIC *Electrolyte management: Hyponatremia*

Fluid monitoring

Fluid management

Fluid and electrolyte management

Evaluation

Assess the patient for return of normal fluid volume and electrolyte balance. Serum sodium levels should be within normal range. The patient's blood pressure and pulse should return to baseline. The pulse should be strong and regular and at the patient's baseline or only slightly increased. Skin should be warm, and color should return to the patient's normal appearance. Renal function should not be impaired, with an hourly output on the average of 30 ml/hour.

Community/Home Care

Patients treated for deficient fluid volume and hyponatremia should have normal fluid status restored prior to discharge home. Patients experiencing the deficit secondary to vomiting or diarrhea should receive education regarding prevention of complications of these entities and the need to seek medical assistance in a timely manner. For those who lose large amounts of sodium through diaphoresis, instruction should include attention to methods of replacing electrolytes and avoiding large volumes of free water. The patient should continue to drink adequate amounts of fluid and pay attention to the intake of adequate amounts of sodium in the diet. Providing the patient with a list of drinks and foods that are appropriate will provide a handy reference. Encourage the patient to keep a water bottle filled with electrolyte liquids with him or her at all times to enhance the likelihood of adequate intake of fluids. The patient may not require any follow-up, as this is an acute situation that for the most part has no long-term complications. Fatigue may need to be addressed, as true decreases in sodium often produce a sense of weakness, even if the deficit is mild. The patient can handle fatigue by performing activities as tolerated until stamina/endurance is re-established. The health care provider may want the patient to return for a follow-up appointment to ensure that parameters such as serum sodium have returned to normal.

Documentation

In this situation, document initial assessment findings such as blood pressure, pulse, respirations, temperature, skin status (turgor, mucous membranes), and mental status. Be sure to document the patient's intake and output every shift. Document all interventions such as intravenous catheter insertion, fluids initiated (type, rate), urine output (amount, color), and dietary modifications such as sodium-rich foods or liquids. Be specific when charting patient responses to treatment so that other health care providers can clearly determine improvement or deterioration.

NURSING DIAGNOSIS 3

FATIGUE

Related to:

Alterations in cellular depolarization and repolarization

Cellular swelling

Hyponatremia

Defining Characteristics:

Lack of energy

Lethargy

Drowsiness

Feeling tired

Difficulty performing activities of daily living (ADLs)

Goal:

The patient will be able to perform activities.

Outcome Criteria

✔ The patient will verbalize no complaints of fatigue or drowsiness.

✔ The patient will perform activities of daily living without assistance.

NOC   *Energy conservation*
      Endurance
      Activity tolerance

INTERVENTIONS	RATIONALES
Assess level of energy and abilities to perform ADLs.	Helps to ascertain baseline energy and performance level.
Provide a private, quiet environment.	Promotes rest.
Assess and correct abnormal fluid and electrolyte status (see nursing diagnosis "Deficient Fluid Volume").	Decreased serum sodium level is a cause of fatigue; correcting the fluid imbalance corrects the electrolyte imbalance resulting in increased stamina.
Encourage sodium intake.	Corrects hyponatremia and improves energy levels.
Administer sodium supplements as ordered.	Corrects hyponatremia and improves energy levels.
Avoid free water.	Free water dilutes serum sodium and can cause further drops in sodium levels.
Assist the patient as needed with activities.	Due to fatigue, the patient may not be able to complete all ADLs.
Provide for uninterrupted rest periods during the day.	Promotes rest and endurance, allowing the patient to perform activities.

NIC *Energy management*
Electrolyte monitoring
Electrolyte management:
Hyponatremia

Evaluation

The patient has serum sodium levels that return to normal. No evidence exists of lasting effects of low sodium, such as fatigue. The patient reports that he or she is not drowsy and fatigue has resolved. Performance of ADLs is accomplished without complaints of feeling tired.

Community/Home Care

No specific in-home follow-up care is required for the problem of fatigue. The patient may have some mild residual tiredness initially. The patient can resolve this by pacing activities and gradually increasing them until maximum activity level is achieved. It may be necessary for the patient to schedule rest periods during the day for several days until stamina has returned. If the patient does not like returning to bed for naps or rest periods, a favorite easy chair can be used for the rest period. It is not necessarily sleep that is needed, but rest. The patient will need to implement strategies to prevent a recurrence of hyponatremia, if possible, which will include drinking electrolyte-rich liquids and consuming some foods with sodium content. If the fatigue does not resolve, the patient should contact a health care provider for follow-up.

Documentation

Chart the results of a thorough assessment of the patient's ability to perform activities, with pulse and respirations taken after any activity. The patient's verbalization of any fatigue or feelings of fatigue are included in the patient record. Chart whether the patient requires assistance with ADLs or whether they are performed independently. Chart interventions to treat decreased sodium levels.

NURSING DIAGNOSIS 4

RISK FOR INJURY

Related to:

Altered levels of consciousness
Lethargy

Confusion
Seizures
Hyperreflexia
Slowed problem solving
Serum sodium level is < 135 mEq/L

Defining Characteristics:

None

Goal:

The patient will sustain no injury.

Outcome Criteria

✔ The patient will have no injuries.
✔ The patient will have no traumatic injury secondary to seizures.
✔ The patient's skin will be free from traumatic injuries.
✔ The patient will not fall.

NOC *Fall prevention behavior*
Physical injury severity
Risk control
Seizure control
Risk detection

INTERVENTIONS	RATIONALES
Assess environment for safety hazards and arrange as needed for safety.	Detecting unsafe environmental factors facilitates arranging a safe environment to decrease risk for injury.
Conduct a neurological assessment: monitor for changes in level of consciousness, confusion, personality changes, muscle twitching, hyperreflexia, seizures, headache, and lethargy.	Patients with neurological manifestations related to hyponatremia may be at increased risk for injury and seizures.
Assess serum electrolytes.	Hyponatremia places the patient at risk for seizures due to excitability of cerebral tissue.
Maintain bed in low position with side rails elevated.	Decreases the risk of falls if the patient becomes confused or is lethargic; decreases fall distance should the patient fall out of bed.

(continues)

(continued)

INTERVENTIONS	RATIONALES
Implement seizure precautions and treat seizures as ordered (see nursing care plan "Seizures"); remain in room and monitor patient during seizures; notify physician immediately when a seizure occurs.	If sodium levels are uncorrected and continue to drop to levels at or below 120 mEq/L, seizures are likely; seizures can be life-threatening, and the nurse needs to remain with the patient in order to protect the patient; physician needs to be notified for medical intervention.
Place call bell within easy reach.	Facilitates communication from patient to nurse.
Administer IV fluids or dietary sodium as ordered.	Corrects the underlying cause.
Provide a quiet environment.	A calm and quiet environment reduces stimuli that could excite the central nervous system.

NIC *Electrolyte management:*
   Hyponatremia
 Surveillance
 Risk identification
 Neurologic monitoring
 Seizure precautions
 Seizure management

Evaluation

Determine that the outcome criteria have been met. The patient should be protected from injury due to altered neurological function. If a seizure occurs, the patient is protected and sustains no injury. Neurological status returns to normal as the sodium level returns to normal range.

Community/Home Care

When discharged home, the patient's risk for injury has already been resolved as the sodium levels should have returned to normal or close to normal ranges. No special in-home care is required to address risk for injury unless the problem recurs. However, the patient will need to continue interventions to maintain sodium levels at a normal range, including taking supplements and modifying diet. Diet instructions regarding sodium intake should be clear to the patient, with consideration given to cultural/religious practices and the patient's usual diet preferences. Muscle weakness may persist for several days. When attempting ambulation, the patient should implement strategies to decrease the risk of falling, such as sitting on the side of bed before standing. This is especially true for the elderly. If the decreased sodium was caused by preventable factors such as diarrhea or severe vomiting the patient should be instructed on how to prevent or treat these occurrences. The patient should be able to identify the signs and symptoms of hyponatremia and, if noted, to increase dietary intake of sodium-rich foods and liquids.

Documentation

Chart results of an assessment of the neuromuscular system, describing any patient complaints of muscle weakness. Note any injuries sustained. If seizures occur, document a description of the seizure, duration, and patient status following the seizure, including mental status (alert, lethargic) and vital signs. Document all interventions implemented to treat any problems that occur and to treat the low sodium levels. Chart any medications administered according to agency protocol.

CHAPTER 5.73

METABOLIC ACIDOSIS

GENERAL INFORMATION

Metabolic acidosis is an acid/base disorder involving an increase in metabolic acids or a decrease in base bicarbonate in the blood resulting in bicarbonate levels diminishing below 22 mEq/dl and causing the arterial blood pH to decrease below 7.35 (normal range is 7.35 to 7.45). The carbonic acid buffering system is activated when metabolic acidosis occurs, resulting in decreased carbonic acid retention in the form of partial pressure of carbon dioxide in the arterial blood (pCO_2). The pCO_2 decreases through increased ventilatory rated and depth, causing the arterial blood pH to rise to normal levels. Respiratory buffering can be effective in normalizing the pH within minutes if the patient can support the increased ventilatory effort and if the magnitude of the metabolic acidosis is not too severe. Metabolic acidosis causes electrolyte imbalance, especially hyperkalemia. In metabolic acidosis, there is increased movement of hydrogen ions into the cells causing potassium to shift out of the cells and accumulate in the blood. There are numerous causes of metabolic acidosis. It can occur with dieting or starvation as fats are broken down into ketoacids or with diabetic ketoacidosis (DKA) because of the increases in ketoacids produced during insulin deficiency. In end-stage renal disease, metabolic acidosis occurs as the kidneys lose the ability to alkalinize the blood through bicarbonate production and reabsorption. Lactic acidosis causes metabolic acidosis during increases in anaerobic metabolism such as occurs with cardiac failure, shock, strenuous prolonged exercise, or pulmonary failure. Diarrhea can cause metabolic acidosis through increased loss of bicarbonate from intestinal secretions. Other possible causes include aspirin toxicity, intestinal fistulas, and renal tubular acidosis. Clinical manifestations of metabolic acidosis include headaches and Kussmaul's respirations as the lungs try to blow off more carbon dioxide to reduce the pH; later, if the acidosis is uncorrected disorientation, warm flushed skin and potassium excess may occur.

NURSING DIAGNOSIS 1

DEFICIENT FLUID VOLUME

Related to:

Compensatory mechanisms that attempt to reduce acid content (rapid respirations, increased urine output)

Polyuria

Diarrhea

Defining Characteristics:

Dry mucous membrane

Decreased skin turgor

Capillary refill > 3 seconds

Concentrated urine

Low blood pressure

Arterial blood gases (ABGs) reveal pH < 7.35 and $HCO_3 < 22$ mEq/L

Goal:

Fluid balance is restored.

Outcome Criteria

✔ Patient will have good skin turgor (skin returns to original position when pinched in < 3 seconds).

✔ Mucous membranes are moist.

✔ Urine output will be > 30 ml/hour.

✔ Blood pressure is within baseline.

NOC *Electrolyte and acid/base balance*
Hydration
Fluid balance

INTERVENTIONS	RATIONALES
Assess patient's hydration status: skin turgor, mucous membranes, intake/output, skin temperature, blood pressure, pulse, capillary refill, and color of urine.	Helps to determine current hydration status, monitor response to treatment, and assess fluid balance.
Assess electrolytes.	Electrolyte abnormalities commonly accompany fluid deficits with metabolic acidosis.
Administer fluids intravenously (IV) or orally (PO) as ordered.	Restores fluid balance, rehydrates the patient, and maintains electrolyte balance; replaces losses from diarrhea or polyuria; restores circulating volume.
Correct acid/base imbalance, as ordered. If acidosis is severe (< 7.2), sodium bicarbonate should be given via IV in small amounts to move pH closer to normal gradually. (Too much sodium bicarbonate can lead to metabolic alkalosis, which is very difficult to correct and dangerous for the patient.)	A severely acidotic pH will cause the patient to seize, go into a coma, and possibly experience cardiorespiratory arrest.
Collaborate with the physician to correct the underlying condition.	If the underlying condition is corrected, the acid/base balance will usually also improve.
Encourage PO fluid intake of 3L/day if able to take orally.	Helps to maintain fluid and electrolyte balance, replace losses from diarrhea or polyuria, and restore circulating volume.
Ensure dietary bulk in the patient's diet.	Facilitates normal bowel movements; dehydration and loss of normal gastrointestinal (GI) motility may lead to constipation.

NIC *Electrolyte monitoring*
     Fluid management
     Fluid monitoring

Evaluation

The patient's hydration status is normal. The skin is warm and dry with good turgor. In addition, the patient's blood pressure has returned to baseline. Intake and output reveal a balanced intake and output with at least 3000 ml of intake per 24 hours. No electrolyte imbalances have occurred.

Community/Home Care

The patient at home will need to continue to take fluids generously to prevent a recurrence of fluid volume deficit. This is especially true for those patients who have experienced metabolic acidosis due to diabetes, as recurrence is possible if the blood sugar rises too high again. The patient with renal failure may not experience fluid volume deficits due to metabolic acidosis, but for all others, this is a common problem. The patient may find it helpful to make a schedule for drinking fluids so that fluids can be easily consumed throughout the day. Keeping a water bottle nearby at all times to sip on can greatly enhance the amount consumed, as it serves as a constant reminder of the need. The diabetic patient will need to adhere to dietary restrictions and limit fluids to those allowed in his or her diet; water is the best choice. The patient can be taught how to assess for dehydration by looking for excess skin dryness, poor turgor, and dark, concentrated urine. Information on ways to prevent dehydration in the home setting should be given to the patient and includes drinking while exercising, controlling insensible loss when outside in hot weather, controlling diarrhea, and replenishing electrolytes.

Documentation

Always include the results of a thorough assessment of fluid status, including skin turgor, skin temperature, status of mucous membranes, and blood pressure. Chart the patient's intake and output on the record along with vital signs according to agency guidelines. Include in the patient record the types of fluid taken by the patient and the patient's understanding of the need for fluids. Document any patient complaints or concerns, as the patient states them. Document all interventions employed to address the problem of fluid volume deficiency, including the patient's responses.

NURSING DIAGNOSIS 2

DECREASED CARDIAC OUTPUT

Related to:

Abnormal potassium levels secondary to metabolic acidosis

Decreased strength of myocardial contraction

Dysrhythmias

Defining Characteristics:

Hypotension

Thready peripheral pulses

Bradycardia

Pale, cool skin

Possible electrocardiogram (EKG) changes

Goal:

The patient's cardiac output will return to normal.

Outcome Criteria

✔ Pulse will be strong and regular.

✔ The patient's EKG will demonstrate normal sinus rhythm.

✔ The patient will not be hypotensive.

✔ Any EKG changes will return to normal.

✔ The patient will demonstrate good peripheral perfusion.

NOC *Electrolyte and acid/base balance*
Cardiac pump effectiveness
Circulation status

INTERVENTIONS	RATIONALES
Assess cardiac system, including pulse rate and rhythm and blood pressure; check pulse and blood pressure sitting and standing.	Abnormal heart rate or irregular rhythm may be an indication of dysrhythmias caused by abnormal serum potassium levels. Orthostatic hypotension is common in states of hypokalemia and decreased cardiac output.
Monitor for EKG changes and notify physician immediately if noted.	Potassium imbalances that accompany metabolic acidosis may cause EKG changes. Medical intervention may be needed.
Assess peripheral perfusion: capillary refill, peripheral pulses, skin temperature, and color.	When cardiac output decreases, perfusion may also decrease resulting in diminished peripheral pulse, capillary refill > 2 seconds, cool skin temperature, and decrease in normal color.
Assess for causative factors such as aspirin toxicity, renal failure, diabetes, starvation, severe diarrhea, or alcoholism, and collaborate with physician about the feasibility of eliminating causes.	Obtaining a good history from the patient regarding medication history and loss of fluids can provide clues to needed therapeutic interventions.
Assess serum potassium levels and notify physician immediately if abnormalities are detected.	Abnormal serum potassium levels can cause life-threatening cardiac dysrhythmias that require immediate attention; in metabolic acidosis, potassium levels may be high initially as potassium is forced out of cells as hydrogen ions enter; however, as the acidosis is corrected, the potassium re-enters the cells and some is excreted, and the patient may actually experience hypokalemia.
Treat hyperkalemia during metabolic acidosis development by restricting potassium intake (diet and medications) and administering any ordered medications to lower the potassium (sodium bicarbonate or insulin).	Restricting the intake of potassium will help lower the level; insulin and sodium bicarbonate cause the extracellular potassium to move intracellularly and resolve the hyperkalemia; sodium bicarbonate raises the pH, which promotes cellular uptake of potassium.
If potassium is high, administer calcium gluconate solution via IV, slowly, as ordered.	Calcium gluconate is given as an emergency measure to protect the myocardium from the toxic effects of potassium while other measures to reduce the potassium level are implemented and take effect. The calcium is rapid-acting and enhances cellular uptake of potassium.
Once treatment for metabolic acidosis has begun, monitor decreasing potassium levels.	Potassium returns to cells when acidosis resolves, which can result in hypokalemia.
Administer potassium supplements PO or IV, as ordered, if potassium drops below normal.	Corrects hypokalemia and prevents cardiac dysrhythmias.
Assess for headache and give mild analgesics as ordered or required.	Headache is a common complaint of patients with metabolic acidosis, but is usually corrected with correction of the acidosis. Only mild analgesics are required. The headache could be due to neurological alterations or vascular alterations caused by the lowered pH.

NIC *Electrolyte management:*
        Hypokalemia

Electrolyte management:
        Hyperkalemia

Electrolyte monitoring

Cardiac precautions

Evaluation

Note the degree to which outcome criteria have been achieved. There are no changes in the EKG that indicate decreased output, and there is a normal sinus rhythm. The patient should demonstrate adequate cardiac output as demonstrated by normal peripheral pulses and warm skin. If cardiac output is normal, perfusion to the kidneys should be adequate with the patient producing at least 30 ml of urine per hour on average. The pulse and blood pressure should be within the patient's baseline. Potassium levels return to normal levels.

Community/Home Care

Patients who have experienced decreased cardiac output due to metabolic acidosis and potassium imbalances will need to know how to prevent this in the future. Metabolic acidosis is an acute event that is totally corrected by time of discharge. Decreased cardiac output occurs secondary to the potassium imbalances that occur with metabolic acidosis, so home care is minimal. The patient will need to understand how to prevent metabolic acidosis. For patients who are diabetic, this includes maintaining blood sugars at baseline levels through exercise, diet, and medications. For the patient with renal failure, this means complying with dialysis and dietary recommendations. Other causes of metabolic acidosis must be addressed, including the dangers of

prolonged strenuous exercise that predisposes the development of lactic acid due to anaerobic metabolism. For patients who have been dieting or for other reasons starved, adequate nutrition is stressed to avoid breakdown of fat for energy that has as a by-product lactate, and subsequently lactic acid. Once at home, the patient should be attuned to the symptoms of decreased potassium and increased potassium in order to implement the necessary strategies for correction. In addition, if the patient detects that respirations are changing and becoming more labored and deep, he or she should also seek health care, as this may be the beginning of Kussmaul's respirations, which signals metabolic acidosis. Home care by a nurse is not required as metabolic acidosis is an acute problem easily corrected with the elimination of the causative factor (when possible) and there are generally no long-term consequences. For most patients, once acid/base and electrolyte balance are re-established, cardiac output is restored and no further interventions are required in the home. However, a follow-up appointment is needed to be sure that the patient's blood gases and potassium level are normal.

Documentation

Chart the results of all assessments made, particularly that of the cardiac and respiratory systems. Document all interventions in a timely fashion, along with the patient's specific response to the intervention. If cardiac monitoring is initiated, document rhythm according to agency protocol. Chart all interventions implemented to treat metabolic acidosis, hypokalemia, and/or hyperkalemia, and the patient's responses to the interventions. Include vital signs in the chart with a sitting and standing blood pressure according to agency guidelines. Chart medications according to agency guidelines.

CHAPTER 5.74

METABOLIC ALKALOSIS (BICARBONATE EXCESS)

GENERAL INFORMATION

Metabolic alkalosis is a disorder involving a decrease in metabolic acids or an increase in base bicarbonate in the blood, resulting in bicarbonate levels increasing above 26 mEq/L and causing the arterial blood pH to increase above 7.45. The carbonic acid buffering system is activated when metabolic alkalosis occurs, resulting in increased carbonic acid retention in the form of partial pressure of carbon dioxide in the arterial blood (pCO_2). The pCO_2 increases through decreased ventilatory rate and depth, causing the arterial blood pH to decrease to 7.45. Respiratory buffering can be effective in normalizing the pH within minutes, but hypoventilation can dangerously affect oxygenation. The respiratory system depresses its efforts at respiration because of a need to conserve acid products to decrease the pH, which could lead to impaired gas exchange. Electrolyte imbalances, particularly of calcium and potassium, may also occur. In alkalosis, more calcium combines with serum proteins, which decreases the amount of ionized calcium in the blood. In metabolic alkalosis, the potassium becomes low because of the shift of hydrogen ions out of the cells and into the blood, which then causes potassium to shift into the cells. Metabolic alkalosis can also occur because of hypokalemia and gastric suction or intractable vomiting because of hydrochloric acid loss. Excessive bicarbonate administration can cause metabolic alkalosis during treatment of peptic ulcer disease with bicarbonate containing antacids or treatment of metabolic acidosis with bicarbonate. Certain chemotherapy protocols for cancer treatment include continuous intravenous (IV) administration of bicarbonate containing fluids in order to cause a metabolic alkalosis therapeutically for hepato-protective effects. Decreased calcium levels contribute to the clinical manifestations of metabolic alkalosis, including numbness and tingling, especially in toes and fingers; Trousseau's sign; Chvostek's sign; muscle spasms; and abdominal cramping.

NURSING DIAGNOSIS 1

IMPAIRED GAS EXCHANGE

Related to:

Pulmonary systems attempt to retain CO_2 to maintain homeostasis

Respiratory depression secondary to CO_2 retention

Defining Characteristics:

Hypoventilation

Hypoxemia

Cyanosis

Decreased pO_2

Oxygen saturations < 90 percent

Arterial blood gas (ABG): pH is increased > 7.45, HCO_3 is elevated > 26 mEq/L

Goal:

The patient's acid/base balance returns to normal.

Outcome Criteria

✔ The pH level will return to normal range (7.35–7.45).

✔ Carbon dioxide levels will be within normal limits (35–45 mm/Hg).

✔ Bicarbonate levels will be within normal levels (22–26 mEq/L).

✔ Oxygen saturation will be > 93 percent (chronic CO_2 retainers O_2 sat: 88–92 percent).

✔ Respiratory rate will be 12 to 20 breaths per minute

NOC   *Electrolyte and acid/base balance*
Respiratory status: Ventilation
Respiratory status: Gas exchange
Vital signs

INTERVENTIONS	RATIONALES
Assess respiratory system, including rate, depth, effort, rhythm, any cyanosis, skin color, and mental status.	Helps to determine a baseline in order to evaluate response to treatment. In metabolic alkalosis, the respiratory system attempts to compensate by decreasing the respiratory rate and effort to retain carbon dioxide. This hypoventilation occurs as a part of the body's compensatory mechanism to return acid/base balance back to normal. The patient needs to be monitored for parameters that may signal serious respiratory depression. Cyanosis around the mouth and oral mucous membranes indicates significant hypoxemia and the need for oxygen. Changes in mental status, such as restlessness, are an early indication of oxygen deprivation.
Assess ABGs, particularly pH, bicarbonate, and oxygen, and report as required.	Helps to determine current acid/base status, determine treatment, and monitor for improvement. The pH and bicarbonate will be higher than normal. As the respiratory system compensates for the alkalotic state, the ABGs may reveal an elevated carbon dioxide.
Assess oxygen saturation and report abnormalities.	Detects hypoxemia and allows for early treatment.
Assist patient to semi-Fowler's or Fowler's position.	Sitting upright allows diaphragm to descend, resulting in easier breathing and improved gas exchange.
Administer oxygen, as ordered, to maintain oxygen saturation > 93 percent (chronic CO_2 retainers O_2 sat: 88–92 percent).	Promotes tissue oxygenation.

Encourage periods of rest.	Decreases need for oxygen.
Assist the patient with activities as required.	Due to decreased oxygen levels, the patient may be unable to complete activities without fatigue or dyspnea.

NIC   *Acid/base monitoring*
Acid/base management
Respiratory monitoring
Airway management

Evaluation

Evaluate the status of outcome criteria. The patient should have indicators of effective gas exchange, such as even, easy respirations and an oxygen saturation of at least 90 percent. Blood gas analyses should indicate an absence of metabolic alkalosis by a return of pH and bicarbonate levels to normal levels or show compensation and oxygen levels between 80 to 100 percent. Respiratory rate should return to the patient's baseline.

Community/Home Care

In most patients, metabolic alkalosis is corrected quickly by treating the cause and is not a problem in the home environment unless the patient has a chronic metabolic condition. If vomiting has contributed to the problem, teaching the patient how to replace acid will be helpful in preventing future events. In addition, the patient needs to be able to identify antacids that contain large amounts of bicarbonate in order to avoid them as well as to refrain from using baking soda as an antacid on a regular basis. If the patient takes high doses of diuretics that promote the excretion of potassium, sodium, and chloride, measures should be implemented at home to restore these through the diet. The patient needs to know the signs of metabolic alkalosis (see nursing diagnosis "Deficient Fluid Volume"). The patient should verbalize an understanding of the signs of respiratory complications and report what needs to be done if they are noticed. At home, the patient should continue to engage in periods of rest and monitor response to activity. If weakness or shallow effortless respirations persist over time, the patient should contact the health care provider.

Documentation

Included in the documentation should be a complete respiratory assessment with specific attention to a description of skin color, how the patient is breathing, and whether the patient feels comfortable with breathing. Chart all interventions employed to address respiratory status and hypoventilation, and the patient's specific response. Results of oxygen saturation readings and ABGs should be documented, as they represent the best measure of gas exchange. If the patient still has indicators of altered acid/base balance (increased pH and increased bicarbonate) these should be specifically noted along with needed revisions to the plan of care.

NURSING DIAGNOSIS 2

DEFICIENT FLUID VOLUME

Related to:

Gastric suction

Vomiting

Polyuria secondary to diuretics

Defining Characteristics:

Thirst

Poor skin turgor

Dry mucous membranes

Hypotension

Tachycardia

Goal:

Fluid balance is restored.

Outcome Criteria

✔ The patient will have good skin turgor (skin returns to original position when pinched < 3 seconds).

✔ Mucous membranes are moist.

✔ Blood pressure is within baseline.

✔ Serum calcium levels are within normal range.

✔ Urine output will be > 30 ml/hour.

NOC   *Electrolyte and acid/base balance*
    Hydration
    Fluid balance

INTERVENTIONS	RATIONALES
Assess patient's hydration status: skin turgor, mucous membranes, intake/output, skin temperature, blood pressure, capillary refill.	Helps to determine current status and monitor response to treatment.
Assess serum electrolyte values, especially calcium.	Electrolyte abnormalities commonly accompany fluid deficits with metabolic alkalosis; clinical manifestations of metabolic alkalosis are indicative of decreased calcium levels. Hypokalemia is often present as well, occurring because of diuretic use or shifting of hydrogen ions out of the cells, causing potassium to shift into the cells.
Take history regarding causative factors: nasogastric suctioning, vomiting, use of diuretics.	This information can guide correction of the underlying cause.
Administer intravenous (IV) fluids as ordered.	Restores fluid balance and rehydrates the patient.
Encourage oral (PO) fluid intake of 3–4 L/day; liquids should be rich in calcium and potassium.	A patient able to take PO fluids should do so to supplement IV fluids. Increased fluid intake promotes a return to normal hydration.
Implement strategies to increase serum calcium and potassium levels as ordered (see nursing care plans "Hypocalcemia" and "Hypokalemia").	Loss of potassium can contribute to alkalosis and needs to be corrected to resolve metabolic alkalosis; calcium levels are decreased in metabolic alkalosis due to increased binding with serum proteins. Most of the symptoms of metabolic alkalosis are those of hypocalcemia; these need to be treated to protect the patient from injury.
Administer anti-emetics, as ordered.	Decreases loss of hydrochloric acid from the upper GI tract.

NIC   *Acid/base management:*
    Metabolic alkalosis
    Electrolyte management:
    Hypocalcemia
    Electrolyte management:
    Hypokalemia
    Electrolyte monitoring
    Fluid management
    Fluid monitoring

Evaluation

The patient's hydration status is normal. The skin is warm and dry with good turgor. In addition, the patient's blood pressure has returned to baseline. Intake and output reveal a balanced intake and output with at least 3000 ml per 24 hours. Serum calcium and potassium levels return to normal, and ABGs indicate a resolution of metabolic alkalosis.

Community/Home Care

Metabolic alkalosis is treated promptly by eliminating the underlying cause, leaving most patients with no residual effects when returning home. However, it may be recommended that the patient at home continue to take fluids generously to prevent a recurrence of metabolic alkalosis. The patient may find it helpful to make a schedule for drinking fluids so that fluids can be easily consumed throughout the day. Keeping a water bottle close by at all times can greatly enhance the amount consumed, as it serves as a constant reminder of the need. It is critical that the nurse or dietician instruct the patient on foods that are good sources of calcium and potassium, within any cultural or religious practices. These include cantaloupe, oranges, bananas, and spinach for potassium, and dairy products such as cheese and milk for calcium. In addition, the patient should monitor for signs of hypocalcemia such as muscle weakness and fatigue, muscle tremors and twitching, and numbness and tingling, especially in the hands and feet. The patient should be instructed to contact a health care provider if he or she notes these signs.

Documentation

Always include the results of a thorough assessment of fluid status, including skin turgor, skin temperature, status of mucous membranes, intake/output, pulse, and blood pressure. If the patient has GI suctioning, specify the exact amount of fluids being removed. Chart the patient's intake and output on the record along with vital signs according to agency guidelines. Include in the patient record the types of fluid taken by the patient and the patient's understanding of the need for fluids. Document any complaints or concerns as the patient states them, as well as all interventions employed to address the problem of fluid volume deficiency, including the patient's responses.

DECREASED CARDIAC OUTPUT

Related to:

   Hypokalemia

   Hypocalcemia

   Decreased strength of myocardial contraction

   Dysrhythmias

Defining Characteristics:

   Hypotension

   Thready peripheral pulses

   Bradycardia

   Pale, cool skin

Goal:

   The patient's cardiac output will return to normal.

Outcome Criteria

✔ The patient's pulse will return to baseline rate and be strong and regular.

✔ The patient's electrocardiogram (EKG) will demonstrate normal sinus rhythm.

✔ The patient's blood pressure will return to baseline.

✔ The patient will demonstrate adequate peripheral perfusion (peripheral pulses strong, warm skin, and capillary refill < 3 seconds).

NOC   *Electrolyte and acid/base balance*
   Cardiac pump effectiveness
   Circulation status

INTERVENTIONS	RATIONALES
Assess cardiac system, including pulse rate and rhythm and blood pressure; check pulse and blood pressure sitting and standing; check renal perfusion by noting urinary output.	Abnormal heart rate or irregular rhythm may be an indication of dysrhythmias caused by abnormal serum potassium levels. Orthostatic hypotension is common in states of hypokalemia and decreased cardiac output. If decreased output is sustained, the kidneys will experience decreased perfusion, resulting in decreased output.

INTERVENTIONS	RATIONALES
Monitor for EKG changes and notify physician immediately if noted.	Potassium imbalances that accompany metabolic alkalosis may cause EKG changes.
Assess peripheral perfusion: capillary refill, peripheral pulses, skin temperature, and color.	When cardiac output decreases, perfusion may also decrease resulting in diminished peripheral pulse, capillary refill > 2 seconds, cool skin temperature, and decrease in normal color.
Assess for causative factors of metabolic alkalosis such as nasogastric suction, diarrhea, vomiting, or excessive fluid loss through diuretics and cathartics, and collaborate with physician about the feasibility or possibility of eliminating causes.	Obtaining a good history from the patient regarding medication history and loss of fluids can provide clues to needed therapeutic interventions.
Monitor for decreased potassium levels and notify physician immediately if detected.	Decreased serum potassium levels can cause life-threatening cardiac dysrhythmias that require immediate attention.
Administer potassium supplements PO or IV, as ordered.	Corrects hypokalemia and prevent cardiac dysrhythmias.
Assess for increasing potassium levels after initiation of treatment for metabolic alkalosis and treat as ordered. Restrict potassium intake (diet and medications) and administer any ordered medications to lower the potassium (Kayexalate or insulin).	Potassium exits the cells, accumulates in the blood during treatment for metabolic alkalosis, and may result in hyperkalemia. Restricting the intake of potassium will help lower the level; insulin causes extracellular potassium to shift into the cells lowering the serum potassium level; sodium bicarbonate raises the pH which promotes cellular uptake of potassium; Kayexalate is an exchange resin that exchanges sodium ions for potassium ions in the intestine and is combined with sorbitol to promote rapid excretion of potassium via stools.
If potassium is high, administer calcium gluconate via IV, slowly, as ordered.	Calcium gluconate is given as an emergency measure to protect the myocardium from the toxic effects of potassium while other measures to reduce the potassium level are implemented and take effect. The calcium is rapid-acting and also enhances cellular uptake of potassium.

Administer carbonic anhydrase inhibitors, such as acetazolamide (Diamox®), as directed.	Enhances renal bicarbonate excretion.

NIC *Acid/base management: Metabolic alkalosis*

Electrolyte management: Hypokalemia

Electrolyte management: Hyperkalemia

Electrolyte monitoring

Cardiac precautions

Evaluation

Note the degree to which outcome criteria have been achieved. There are no changes in the EKG that indicate decreased cardiac output; there is a normal sinus rhythm. The patient should demonstrate adequate cardiac output as evidenced by normal peripheral pulses and warm skin. If cardiac output is normal, perfusion to the kidneys should be adequate, with the patient producing at least 30 ml of urine per hour on average. The pulse and blood pressure should be within the patient's baseline. Potassium levels return to normal levels.

Community/Home Care

Home care by a nurse is not required, as metabolic alkalosis is an acute problem that is easily corrected with the elimination of the causative factor when possible, and there are generally no long-term consequences. For most patients, once acid/base and electrolyte balance is re-established, cardiac output is restored and no further interventions are required. However, the patient will need to understand how he or she can prevent metabolic alkalosis or at least treat it promptly. Monitoring fluid loss that occurs with vomiting or prolonged diarrhea and then making efforts to consume electrolyte-rich liquids or foods can help the patient. The nurse or nutritionist can consult with the patient to develop a list of the foods that are consistent with the patient's dietary habits, preferences, and cultural and religious practices. Doing this will enhance the likelihood that the patient will utilize the list if needed. The patient also must be clear on the dangers of misuse of antacids that are alkaline-based, such as baking soda or Alka-Seltzer®. A follow-up appointment is needed to be sure that the patient's blood gases and potassium level are normal.

Documentation

Chart the results of all assessments made, particularly of the cardiac and respiratory systems. If cardiac monitoring is initiated, document rhythm according to agency protocol. Chart all interventions implemented to treat metabolic alkalosis, hypokalemia, and/or hyperkalemia, and the patient's responses to the interventions. Include vital signs in the chart with a sitting and standing blood pressure according to agency guidelines. Chart medications according to agency protocol.

NURSING DIAGNOSIS 4

 RISK FOR INJURY

Related to:

Hypocalcemia secondary to alkalosis

Seizures

Tetany

Paresthesias

Defining Characteristics:

None

Goal:

The patient sustains no injury.

Outcome Criteria

✔ The patient will have no injuries resulting from paresthesias.

✔ The patient will have no traumatic injury secondary to seizures.

✔ The patient's skin will be free from traumatic injuries.

✔ The patient will not fall.

NOC *Fall-prevention behavior*

Physical injury severity

Risk control

Seizure control

Risk detection

INTERVENTIONS	RATIONALES
Assess environment for safety hazards and arrange environment for safety.	Detecting unsafe environmental factors facilitates arranging a safe environment and decreases risk for injury.
Assess for numbness, tingling, hyperactive reflexes, muscle tremors, and spasms.	These are symptoms of low calcium levels and predispose the patient to injury.
Administer calcium replacements IV or PO, as ordered.	Corrects the underlying cause and decreases risk of injury due to neurological impairments caused by hypocalcemia.
Implement seizure precautions and remain with patient during any seizure activity (see nursing care plan "Seizures").	As the calcium levels decrease, the risk for tetany and seizures rises. Precautions are needed to decrease risk of head or extremity trauma during seizure.
Notify physician immediately when a seizure occurs and treat as ordered.	Seizures can be life-threatening, and medical intervention is required.
Inspect feet, hands, and other skin daily for injury.	Due to uncontrollable paresthesias (numbness) and spasms, the patient may not sense injuries.
Provide a quiet environment.	A calm, quiet environment reduces stimuli that could excite the central nervous system.

NIC *Surveillance*

Risk identification

Neurologic monitoring

Seizure precautions

Seizure management

Evaluation

Determine that the outcome criteria have been met. The patient has no injury and is protected from injury during seizure activity. No falls occur and the patient has no injury resulting from paresthesias of feet and hands.

Community/Home Care

Patients who have metabolic alkalosis have symptoms of hypocalcemia and experience neurological deficits similar to those of the patient with hypocalcemia without metabolic alkalosis. When discharged home, the patient's risk for injury has already been resolved, as calcium levels should have returned to normal ranges. No special in-home care is required to address risk for injury unless the problem recurs. However, the patient will need to continue interventions to maintain calcium levels at normal range and this includes supplements and diet practices. Dietary instructions regarding calcium intake should be clear to the patient with consideration to cultural and religious practices and usual diet preferences. In general, the patient should consume calcium-rich foods, such as dairy products, broccoli, spinach, and salmon, etc. The patient should be able to identify the signs and symptoms of hypocalcemia and, if noted, increase dietary intake of calcium and calcium supplements. The patient may be required to return to the health care provider for assessment of his or her calcium level.

Documentation

Chart results of an assessment of neuromuscular and cardiovascular systems, with particular attention to documentation of paresthesias or signs of tetany. Note any injuries sustained. If seizures occur, document a description of the seizure, duration, and patient status following the seizure, including mental status (alert, lethargic, vital signs). Document all interventions implemented to treat any problems that occur and to treat the low calcium levels. Chart any medications administered according to agency protocol.

CHAPTER 5.75

NEPHROTIC SYNDROME

Nephrotic syndrome is a disorder of the glomeruli caused by alterations in the basement membrane of the glomeruli due to a variety of factors, including diseases (systemic lupus erythematosus, hepatitis, diabetes, and sickle cell anemia), allergic reactions (insect bites, pollen, and acute glomerulonephritis), infection (herpes), and drugs (gold, penicillamine). The most common cause of nephrotic syndrome in adults is membranous glomerulonephropathy, in which the glomerular basement membrane thickens but there is no inflammation (Lemone and Burke, 2004). About a third of all cases of nephrotic syndrome in adults can be attributed to systemic diseases. Other types of nephrotic syndrome include focal sclerosis (scarring of glomeruli) and membranoproliferative glomerulonephritis (caused by thickening and proliferation of glomerular basement membrane cells). In all cases, there is damage to the glomeruli that allows proteins to leak from the circulating plasma during filtration with resultant severe proteinuria, with losses of up to 3.5 grams of protein daily. As protein continues to be excreted, serum albumin is decreased, thus lessening the serum osmotic pressure. The capillary hydrostatic fluid pressure in all body tissues becomes greater than the capillary osmotic pressure, and generalized edema occurs. As fluid is lost into the tissues, the plasma volume decreases, stimulating the secretion of aldosterone to retain more water and sodium, which decreases the glomerular filtration rate in order to retain water. This extra fluid that is being retained also passes out of the capillaries into the tissues, leading to more edema.

With the loss of protein in the urine, hypoalbuminemia occurs and the oncotic pressure of the vascular fluids drops, causing a shift of fluids from the vascular compartment to the interstitial spaces, resulting in edema. As the fluid shifts persist, the body's built-in homeostatic mechanism perceives that the body needs fluid and thus responds by activating the renin angiotensin mechanism, which

causes the kidneys to retain fluid. The edema seen in nephrotic syndrome is severe and occurs in dependent areas (lower extremities, sacrum) and the face, with periorbital edema being a common finding. Because of a loss of proteins, the liver is stimulated to increase albumin production and lipoprotein synthesis. As a result, serum triglyceride levels rise, low density lipoprotein levels increase, and levels of lipids in the urine also increase. Thromboemboli are common in nephrotic syndrome and are thought to be caused by a disruption of the coagulation system by the loss of plasma proteins and the loss of clotting and anti-clotting factors. Patients should be watched for pulmonary emboli, deep vein thrombosis (DVT), and renal vein thrombus. Fewer than 50 percent of adults recover fully and many have persistent proteinuria, and 30 percent go on to end-stage renal failure. Clinical manifestations include severe generalized edema (anasarca), pronounced proteinuria, hypoalbuminemia, and hyperlipidemia that develops from increased hepatic production of lipids perhaps from interference of lipid utilization. Urine volume and renal function may be normal or greatly altered dependent upon how much damage has occurred to the glomeruli and symptoms of renal failure may occur as the disorder progresses. Fatigue is also a common finding.

NURSING DIAGNOSIS 1

 ### EXCESS FLUID VOLUME

Related to:

Loss of protein from circulating volume

Decreased oncotic pressure of plasma

Shift of fluid into interstitial space

Defining Characteristics:

Periorbital edema

Generalized edema (severe)

Jugular vein distention

Increased blood pressure

Proteinuria

Fatigue

Goal:

Fluid volume excess is decreased.

Outcome Criteria

✔ The patient will demonstrate weight loss.

✔ The patient's edema will be absent or decreased.

✔ The patient will have no distended neck veins.

✔ Blood pressure returns to patient's baseline.

✔ Proteinuria will decrease or be absent.

NOC *Fluid balance*
Electrolyte and acid/base balance
Fluid overload severity

INTERVENTIONS	RATIONALES
Assess location and extent of edema, particularly in dependent areas (including the sacrum), and note the presence of the classic periorbital edema.	Because of the decreased oncotic pressure of the circulating volume due to loss of proteins, fluid escapes into interstitial spaces. In nephrotic syndrome, a common finding is edema in the face, especially around the orbit of the eye; a thorough assessment of edema is needed to assess severity of the fluid excess.
Assess breath sounds for crackles.	Detects early any signs of left heart failure that may occur if edema is not relieved; crackles indicate fluid in the lungs and should be monitored for worsening or improvement as an indicator of disease status and response to interventions.
Monitor laboratory and diagnostic studies: blood urea nitrogen (BUN), creatinine, 24-hour urine for protein, urinalysis for protein and red blood cells (RBCs), creatinine clearance, serum lipids, total serum protein, albumin, triglycerides, low-density proteins, very low-density lipids,	Disorders such as nephrotic syndrome alter glomeruli function that produce changes in serum indicators of renal function, and changes in lipoprotein synthesis by the liver causes elevations in triglycerides and lipids: BUN elevates due to decreased volume-to-waste product ratio and because the
electrolytes, white blood cells (WBCs), kidney scans, and renal biopsy.	glomeruli are unable to filtrate and excrete urea; creatinine elevates as renal function is impaired; 24-hour urine for protein reveals elevated protein levels; urinalysis will show 3–4+ proteins and the presence of RBCs, which are able to enter the filtrated urine due to damage to the capillary membranes of the glomeruli; if the glomeruli are damaged, the kidneys will be unable to clear creatinine from the blood (decreased creatinine clearance), lipids will be elevated, serum protein and albumin levels will be decreased, triglycerides will be elevated, low-density and very low-density lipids will be increased; electrolytes may be altered—sodium is decreased in nephrotic syndrome, but the other electrolytes may not show imbalances unless there is renal impairment; WBCs may elevate in the presence of infection; kidney scans may reveal a decreased uptake and excretion of radioactive substances; renal biopsy can confirm a diagnosis and discover the extent of damage to the kidneys.
Administer small doses of loop or thiazide diuretics, as ordered.	Inhibits the reabsorption of sodium and chloride, thereby causing an increased fluid output by the kidneys.
Give salt-poor albumin (SPA) as ordered.	Salt-poor albumin is a protein derivative that increases oncotic pressure of the circulating volume, causing fluid to shift from the interstitial space back into the circulating volume.
Administer oral corticosteroids (prednisone) as ordered and monitor for side effects.	The use of corticosteroids is sometimes controversial, but they are often given to induce remission of nephrotic syndrome.
Administer immunosuppressant agents (cyclophosphamide) as ordered.	The exact mechanism of action for nephrotic syndrome is unknown, but it is used to decrease proteinuria and induce remission.
Give ACE inhibitors as ordered.	Helps to reduce protein loss.

(continues)

(continued)

INTERVENTIONS	RATIONALES
Weigh patient daily at the same time on the same scale, in the morning before breakfast, and measure abdominal girth if ascites is present.	The most accurate method of determining fluid volume loss is through daily weighing, 1 kg of weight loss = 1 L of fluid lost. Morning weights are a better reflection of true weights because most people accumulate fluid as the day progresses. Measuring the abdominal girth helps determine fluid loss in the abdominal area.
Implement a diet low in sodium.	Sodium increases fluid retention; thus, decreasing the amount of dietary sodium intake will decrease the amount of retained fluid.
Monitor intake of protein as ordered: intake of protein should be moderate to high depending upon the amount lost in urine. Give complete protein foods (provides all amino acids) that have high nutritional value, such as dairy foods, fish, lean meat, and poultry.	Due to the loss of proteins in the urine, dietary consult is required to ensure that the patient is getting adequate amounts of protein to avoid malnourishment. If azotemia is pronounced, protein is restricted, as the kidneys are responsible for eliminating the waste products of protein metabolism (BUN); protein intake may further elevate BUN, causing worsening azotemia for a compromised renal system that cannot respond by filtering and excreting more protein.
Implement fluid restrictions as ordered.	Restricting fluid intake can assist in decreasing interstitial edema by decreasing the circulating volume.
Obtain accurate intake and output.	Helps to monitor balance between fluid consumed and urinary output; output also gives an indicator of renal perfusion.
Monitor electrolytes (especially sodium and potassium).	Diuretics cause an abnormal excretion of electrolytes.
Provide potassium supplements as ordered.	Replaces urinary potassium loss caused by diuretics.
Protect edematous skin in extremities and sacrum, and reposition every 2 hours.	Fluid in tissue inhibits adequate circulation to the tissue, predisposing the patient to skin breakdown; if edema is unrelieved, pressure within the skin causes the development of small breaks that begin to ooze,

	creating a prime situation for skin ulceration.
Position patient upright if periorbital edema is present.	The upright position promotes fluid drainage from facial area.
Monitor blood pressure and pulse.	Excess fluid causes the heart to work harder, resulting in an elevated blood pressure and pulse; however, if diuretics and ACE inhibitors are used the patient may become hypotensive.
Teach the patient and family pathophysiology, medications and side effects, fluid excess management, dietary requirements, prognosis, and long-term complications.	This information is needed to enhance compliance with recommendations and prevent any complications. Knowledge enhances health-promoting behaviors.

NIC   *Fluid management*
  Electrolyte monitoring
  Skin surveillance

Evaluation

Patient has weight loss and output greater than intake. There is no periorbital or facial edema, and edema in other areas such as the sacrum is absent or decreasing. Skin in edematous dependent areas should be intact. Blood pressure and pulse return to baseline, and breath sounds are clear. Proteinuria is decreasing, and serum protein levels are within normal range.

Community/Home Care

Patients with nephrotic syndrome continue their treatment and recovery for an extended period in the home environment. The nurse must be sure that the patient has received the appropriate instructions regarding fluid excess and how to prevent and treat it. Once at home, the patient should continue to weigh him or herself daily and to notice subtle changes. The patient should be instructed to take note of clothing that becomes too tight in a short period, which could be an early indicator of fluid excess. When teaching the patient, be sure that he or she can identify periorbital edema, especially if the patient has not experienced this before. Pictures from nursing books can be photocopied and given to the patient for this purpose. If fluid excess worsens, the patient will need to contact a health care provider immediately. At home, the patient needs to limit the intake of sodium-rich foods. The patient should be taught how to read food labels for sodium content, as many people do not know how to decipher labels, and often foods thought to be healthy are high in sodium. A dietician should teach the patient about protein content of foods in accordance with physician-ordered requirements. The patient needs to be able to identify protein-rich foods that are a part of his or her usual diet and demonstrate how to determine serving size. Diet instructions for home must consider the patient's normal diet, eating patterns and any cultural or religious preferences and restrictions. Have the patient keep a log of food and fluid intake as well as weights. This information can then be taken to the health care provider for review. Assist the patient to develop a schedule for taking prescribed medications—such as diuretics, corticosteroids, and immunosuppressants—that is mindful of lifestyle, daily routines, and medication interactions. The nurse should write out critical instructions for medications on one sheet of paper. Preprinted medication instructions that are found in many hospital computer information systems tend to be wordy without attention to what is critical for the patient to know. A simple instruction sheet would serve as a quick reference and contain such information as whether to take with food, what over-the-counter medications should be avoided, what symptoms indicate problems, etc. Because nephrotic syndrome can cause long-term damage to kidneys, the need for follow-up care by a health care provider for early detection of any complications should be stressed.

Documentation

Always document the extent to which the outcome criteria have been achieved. Record intake and output, blood pressure, pulse, weights, breath sounds, and the patient's understanding of the therapies for eliminating fluid excess. Document the presence and extent of any edema, particularly facial or periorbital edema and edema that is present in places not easily noticeable. If fluid restrictions are implemented, note this in the record and include the patient's compliance. Document results of protein dipstick readings according to agency protocol and all medications administered according to agency guidelines.

NURSING DIAGNOSIS 2

IMPAIRED SKIN INTEGRITY

Related to:

Edema

Decreased protein

Deposition of toxins on skin

Defining Characteristics:

Sacral edema

Pedal edema

Small open areas due to edema

Goal:

Skin integrity will be maintained.

Outcome Criteria

✔ The patient will have no open areas on skin.

✔ Edema will be relieved.

NOC *Tissue integrity: Skin and mucous membranes*
Risk detection
Risk control

INTERVENTIONS	RATIONALES
Perform a complete skin assessment, with particular attention to edematous areas; utilize the Braden Pressure Ulcer Risk Assessment Tool.	Establishes a baseline; use of a tool can quantify the risk for skin breakdown while considering contributing factors.
Place telfa non-adhesive pads on any oozing areas.	Telfa does not adhere to the skin, thus preventing further disruption of the skin when dressing is removed.
Wash any open areas gently with warm water or normal saline as ordered.	The areas need to be kept clean; soaps may cause irritation.
Elevate edematous extremities on pillows.	Helps to relieve pressure and promote venous return of fluid.
Administer medications prescribed for relief of edema (diuretics, albumin).	Helps to promote elimination of fluid or return to circulating volume.
Turn patient every 2 hours or encourage frequent position changes.	Edema prevents adequate perfusion to the affected skin, increasing the risk of breakdown due to pressure. Frequent repositioning relieves pressure on vulnerable areas that could easily break down in the presence of edema.

Evaluation

Determine the extent to which the outcome criteria have been met. The patient should have no areas of breakdown, and edema is relieved. Any area that opens due to edema is clean and heals without complication.

Community/Home Care

In the home setting, the patient will monitor the status of skin, especially on the lower extremities. If edema persists, meticulous care of the skin will be needed. The patient must be careful to protect the skin from injury, such as that which could be caused by bumping against furniture. Simple incidents that normally are of no concern can easily disrupt the integrity of edematous skin. First aid for minor skin breakdown needs to be taught to the patient and family. If the skin does become open, but does not respond to simple first aid, the patient will need to notify the health care provider for further instructions or follow-up. The patient should be encouraged to get up and move about the home at scheduled intervals rather than remaining sedentary for long periods, which only worsens the edema and increases the risk for breakdown. Adequate amounts of protein will be required to maintain oncotic pressure that will prevent abnormal protein loss. Within the prescribed diet recommendations, the patient will need to make a conscious effort to eat foods with protein content, such as meat, cheese, peanut butter, etc. The dietician or nurse needs to give the patient a list of acceptable foods that meet the dietary requirements and are in keeping with cultural and religious restrictions.

Documentation

Chart the results of a thorough skin assessment, including findings from the Braden Scale. In addition, document all interventions implemented to relieve pressure and edema or to treat any noted areas of breakdown.

NURSING DIAGNOSIS 3

 RISK FOR INFECTION

Related to:

Immunocompromised status secondary to medications: Cytotoxic agents, corticosteroids

Edematous areas of legs

Altered defenses due to abnormal urinary protein losses

Defining Characteristics:

None

NOC   *Knowledge: Infection control*
         Risk detection
         Tissue integrity: Skin and mucous membranes

INTERVENTIONS	RATIONALES
Take vital signs every 4 hours, particularly the temperature.	An elevated temperature may indicate the beginning of an infection; however, due to the effects of immunosuppressants and anti-inflammatory medications, the body may not produce this response. Be suspect of even low-grade temperatures. Tachycardia may be the earliest sign of infection.
Assess IV access sites for infection: redness/discoloration, warmth, drainage, and swelling.	Any break in the skin can serve as an easy source of infection.
Change peripheral IV sites or perform site care for peripheral IV access sites every 48 hours or according to agency policy or protocol using sterile technique.	Changing IV sites and dressings decreases the bacteria count and minimizes the risk for acquiring infection.
Assess skin thoroughly, especially for open lesions in dependent areas, such as legs and sacrum, caused by gross edema.	Edematous skin is more likely to open or break down, becoming an entry port for invasive organisms that could cause infection.
Position the patient to protect the skin from trauma and encourage repositioning every 2 hours.	Helps to relieve pressure and prevent breakdown, which can become a portal for infection.
Monitor for urinary tract infection (UTI): frequency, pain on urination, blood in urine, foul odor of urine, and cloudy urine.	The urinary system may be one of the first places for infection due to the already compromised status of the renal system. By identifying the signs and symptoms of urinary tract infection, treatment can be instituted early.
Monitor laboratory results: WBC or any culture results.	Elevated WBC counts may be an indicator of infection, and cultures will identify the causative organism.

INTERVENTIONS	RATIONALES
Practice good hand hygiene and have the patient wash hands frequently.	Handwashing is one of the most effective means of halting the spread of organisms; with use of corticosteroids and immunosuppressants, the patient with nephrotic syndrome has an altered immune state with a decreased ability to resist even common organisms.
Limit contact with people with respiratory infections, including the common cold, and be cautious of handshaking.	Helps to decrease the risk of acquiring infections from others; organisms can be easily spread via handshaking when others do not practice effective hand hygiene.
Provide adequate nutrition (complete proteins, vitamins, etc.).	Protein loss decreases defenses against infection, and good nutrition is needed to enhance immune system.
Teach the patient and family signs and symptoms of infection and how to prevent infection at home.	The risk for acquiring infection will remain due to the continued use of corticosteroids and immunosuppressants.

NIC *Infection protection*
      Infection control

Evaluation

The patient remains afebrile and heart rate is at baseline. WBC counts are normal, with no evidence of immature WBCs (shift to left). The patient has no signs or symptoms of infection in skin, IV access sites, or the urinary system. In addition, the patient can verbalize an understanding of signs and symptoms of infection and ways to prevent infection.

Community/Home Care

The risk for infection remains a threat for the patient with nephrotic syndrome when at home. In the home, measures should be taken to reduce exposure to organisms in the environment that could cause infections. Avoidance of visitors who have respiratory infections is an important way to decrease the risk for infection. Well-wishers do not always realize the danger that they pose for patients who are immunocompromised, and thus family

should screen everyone. Small children who attend day care centers are a common carrier of infectious organisms, and their contact with adults with nephrotic syndrome should be limited. Practicing handwashing in the home should be undertaken with the same vigor as that practiced in the hospital setting. Harsh abrasive deodorant soaps should be avoided, as they may cause cracking of the skin leaving an easy route for organism invasion. Meticulous protection of edematous skin through repositioning and padding is required if edema persists. It is important for the patient or a family member to be able to identify signs of skin impairment and what measures to implement to prevent infection. Decreasing the risk for UTI is also important and can be achieved through adequate intake of fluid and good nutrition. If symptoms of infection occur, the patient should contact a health care provider for assistance and possibly the initiation of antibiotic therapy.

NURSING DIAGNOSIS 4

 FATIGUE

Related to:
   Loss of protein in urine
   Anemia

Defining Characteristics:
   Verbalization of being tired
   States a lack of energy
   Inability to carry out normal activities

Goal:
   Fatigue will be relieved.

Outcome Criteria

✔ The patient is able to perform activities of daily living (ADLs).
✔ The patient verbalizes that fatigue has improved or been eliminated.

NOC *Activity tolerance*
      Endurance
      Energy conservation
      Nutritional status: Energy

INTERVENTIONS	RATIONALES
Obtain subjective data regarding normal activities and limitations.	Helps to establish a baseline of activity.
Monitor patient for signs of excessive physical and emotional fatigue.	Helps to determine the effect that the disease has on normal functioning and to obtain information to guide interventions.
Encourage periods of rest and activity.	Conserves oxygen and prevents undue fatigue.
Schedule or space activities so that excessive demands for energy are avoided; for example, space planned activities away from meal times.	The patient with nephrotic syndrome lacks energy for extended periods of activity, necessitating the need for spacing; digestion requires energy and oxygen; participation in activities close to meals will cause increased fatigue because of insufficient energy reserves.
Gradually increase activity as tolerated and monitor response.	Helps to allow the patient time to adapt to increased activity; noting the patient's response gives data about when activity may be increased or needs to be decreased.
Limit visitors during acute illness.	Socialization for long periods may cause fatigue.
Increase intake of high-energy, protein-rich foods, such as meat (especially organ meats), poultry, dried beans and peas, and whole grains, as well as foods high in vitamin C.	These foods enhance energy metabolism, increase oxygen-carrying capacity, and provide ready sources of energy needed in hypermetabolic states such as infection and fever. Protein is required in moderate to high amounts to replace protein lost in the urine.
Encourage the patient to plan activities when he or she has the most energy, usually early in the day.	Helps to prevent fatigue.

NIC   *Energy management*

Evaluation

Obtain subjective information from the patient regarding the presence of fatigue. The patient should gradually report the ability to participate in ADLs and other normal activities with no fatigue.

Community/Home Care

The patient with nephrotic syndrome will continue to experience fatigue at home with the continued loss of proteins in the urine. The patient must understand how to adjust activity in response to feelings of fatigue, possibly even arranging for rest or nap periods in the afternoon. Attention to good nutrition should continue with intake of foods that are good sources of iron, vitamin C, and especially protein. The nurse or dietician should consult with the patient about his or her usual dietary practices, including cultural and religious preferences, and then provide the patient with a list of foods that enhance energy. As protein loss lessens and nutrition improves, the fatigue should resolve. If fatigue persists for extended periods, the patient may need to contact a health care provider to investigate the possibility of other causes of the fatigue.

Documentation

Chart types of activities the patient is able to perform. Document specific complaints of fatigue in the patient's own words. In addition, document all interventions implemented to address fatigue, including types of food consumed.

CHAPTER 5.76

RENAL CALCULI

GENERAL INFORMATION

Renal calculi (kidney stones, urolithiasis, and nephrolithiasis) are the most common cause of urologic obstruction. Risk factors for the development of renal calculi include excess calcium intake, genetic predisposition, dehydration, immobility, and frequent urinary tract infections (UTIs). Most kidney stones (75 to 80 percent) are composed of calcium oxylate or calcium phosphate crystals and are attributed to hypercalciuria. Struvite stones are composed of magnesium ammonium phosphate crystals and account for 15 percent of kidney stones. These stones are due to the presence of urea-splitting organisms in alkaline urine that is high in ammonia. A smaller percentage of kidney stones are composed of uric acid (8 percent) and are associated with increased levels of serum uric acid, as seen in patients with gout. Cystine stones (3 percent) are rare and most often are seen in patients with a defect in renal absorption of cystine. Stones usually form in the kidney and then travel through the urinary tract causing obstruction, infection, pain, and bleeding. Kidney stones typically cause severe, intermittent pain in the flank and lower abdomen, associated with ureteral obstruction and spasm. This severe pain is commonly classified as "renal colic." A sympathetic response is commonly triggered by the severe pain, resulting in tachycardia, nausea, vomiting, pallor, and cool, clammy skin. The nausea and vomiting associated with renal colic frequently causes a fluid volume deficit. Kidney stones may pass through the urinary tract or become lodged and obstruct the urinary tract. In severe cases, obstruction can lead to hydronephrosis and acute renal failure. Treatment involves pain management for comfort and generous fluid administration to facilitate passage of the stones and to dilute the concentrated substances that contribute to stone formation. The patient passes a majority of stones spontaneously; however, in some cases kidney stones need to be removed via lithotripsy (crushing stones using shock waves) or surgery (nephrolithotomy, urolithotomy).

The incidence of renal stones varies by geographic region, ethnicity, and family history. The southeastern United States has a higher incidence than other areas of the United States. In general, kidney stones are more common in men, but the incidence of struvite stones is twice as high in women. Kidney stones are rare in African Americans.

NURSING DIAGNOSIS 1

ACUTE PAIN

Related to:

Ureteral obstruction and spasm

Tissue irritation and damage due to presence of stone and attempted passage

Defining Characteristics:

Complaint of severe, intermittent pain in the flank and lower abdomen (especially when voiding)

Grimacing

Moaning

Guarding of painful area

Goal:

The patient's pain will be relieved.

Outcome Criteria

✔ The patient will verbalize that pain has been relieved 30 minutes after intervention.

✔ The patient will report satisfaction with pain control measures.

 NOC *Pain control*

INTERVENTIONS	RATIONALES
Assess pain character, location, severity, onset, and duration; utilize a pain assessment scale.	Pain assessment can provide clues about diagnosis and complications, and provides information from the patient that is needed for effective treatment.
Assist to position of comfort; patients will often be more comfortable with knees drawn up to chest. Encourage ambulation, when not experiencing an attack of renal colic.	Pain from renal colic is worse in the supine position; ambulation can help pass the stone.
Administer analgesics (narcotics) as ordered.	Decreases pain caused by ureteral spasm and tissue damage.
Assess effectiveness of analgesics using a pain rating scale.	Helps to determine if revisions are needed in pain control methods; if desired effects have not occurred, the nurse may use alternative pain relief techniques or contact physician.
Provide alternative methods of relief, including distraction, massage, therapeutic touch, meditation, and music.	These techniques can enhance comfort level and increase effectiveness of analgesics.
Encourage oral fluids freely (if not contraindicated) to 3 liters or more.	Prevents dehydration, promotes urine output, increases likelihood of stone passage, decreases chance of crystals forming new stones.
Administer fluids intravenously (IV) as ordered.	IV fluids may facilitate passage of stones and decrease concentration of stone-causing substances, thereby decreasing new stone formation and subsequent pain.
Assess voiding patterns and urinary output.	Patients with calculi often limit voiding due to perceived pain with elimination.
Assess laboratory and diagnostic tests for abnormalities: blood urea nitrogen (BUN), white blood cells (WBCs), uric acid, calcium, electrolytes, intravenous pyelogram, computed tomography (CT) scan, and KUB (kidneys, ureters, bladder).	Lab and diagnostic tests provide objective data needed to make an accurate diagnosis, to monitor response to treatment, and to monitor for complications.
Strain all urine.	Many stones are passed with urination, and straining is required to detect passage of stone; passage of the stone relieves pain.
Assess urine for hematuria, and crush any clots passed in the urine.	Hematuria is an indicator of irritation that contributes to the pain; clots are crushed because the stone may be embedded in the clot.
Provide information about surgery, lithotripsy, or other invasive procedures.	Keeping patients informed about surgery, lithotripsy, or other invasive procedures can decrease anxiety and help reduce the impact of pain.

NIC　*Pain control*

Evaluation

The patient states that pain is controlled or tolerable. After the stone has passed or been removed, the patient has no further pain. The patient states satisfaction with pain management efforts. If the patient is not satisfied, reassess interventions and collaborate with physician for needed changes.

Documentation

Document an assessment of pain using a pain rating scale. Ask the patient to describe pain and document subjective information. Include in the patient record nonverbal indicators of pain such as guarding, moaning, and frequent position changes. Always document all therapeutic nursing interventions implemented and the patient's response to each. Document medications given for pain on the medication administration record according to agency guidelines, with a follow-up assessment of effectiveness.

Community/Home Care

Patients with renal calculi may be treated at home if pain is not severe, or they may be discharged before the stone has passed, placing them at risk for acute pain. Patients should be taught how to manage their pain at home, utilizing a variety of interventions. The patient should be taught and encouraged to use non-pharmacological pain management strategies that can enhance medications. Have the patient keep a pain diary that documents time of pain, location, rating, interventions attempted, and effectiveness. This documentation assists the patient to review what is effective and what is not. This diary can then be shared with the patient's health care provider during scheduled or prn visits.

NURSING DIAGNOSIS 2

DEFICIENT FLUID VOLUME

Related to:

Nausea and vomiting

Defining Characteristics:

Dry mucous membranes

Decreased skin turgor

Decreased urine output (< 30 ml/hr)

Goal:

The patient will maintain adequate hydration.

Outcome Criteria

✔ The patient will have moist mucous membranes.

✔ The patient will have good skin turgor.

✔ Serum electrolytes are normal.

✔ Kidney stones will pass in the urine.

✔ Urine output will be > 30 ml/hr.

NOC *Fluid balance*

Hydration

Electrolyte and acid/base balance

INTERVENTIONS	RATIONALES
Establish IV access and administer IV fluids as ordered.	Helps to maintain fluid and electrolyte balance, replace losses from vomiting, and facilitate stone passage.
Monitor intake and output.	Helps to assess fluid balance.
Assess heart rate, blood pressure, mucous membranes, skin turgor, and capillary refill.	Helps to determine hydration status.
Obtain history of medication intake.	Some medications (such as antacids with high calcium content, large frequent doses of diuretics) cause decreased volume and predispose the patient to stone development.
Encourage intake of fluids high in acid-ash (when tolerating oral intake) if kidney stones are calcium-based.	Cranberry, grape, and tomato juice can decrease the formation of calcium-based stones.
Discourage the intake of high-calcium fluids if kidney stones are calcium-based.	Milk, milk products, cocoa, and chocolate are high in calcium and can increase stone formation.
Encourage the intake of fluids high in alkaline-ash if kidney stones are uric acid-based (when tolerating oral intake).	Fruit juice (except cranberry, grape, or tomato), milk, and milk products can decrease the formation of uric acid stones.
Discourage the intake of high-oxalate fluids if kidney stones are calcium-oxalate–based.	Beer, cola, chocolate, cocoa, tea, and tomatoes are high in calcium-oxalate and can increase stone formation.
Encourage at least 3000 ml/day fluid intake (when tolerating oral intake).	Regardless of stone type, hydration is recommended to dilute stone-creating substances, to prevent infection, and to assist in the movement of the stone by increasing volume of urine produced.
Assess for nausea, vomiting, and precipitating factors; give anti-emetics as ordered.	Alleviating nausea and subsequent vomiting will prevent fluid loss.
Teach the patient and family about the role of fluids in preventing stone formation.	The patient needs to understand the rationale for increased fluid intake so that he or she can be compliant and prevent future stone development.

NIC *Fluid management*

Fluid/electrolyte management

Evaluation

The patient's blood pressure and pulse return to baseline and capillary refill is normal. The patient's mucous membranes are moist and urine output is > 30 ml/hr. Intake and output are balanced with the patient being well hydrated. Kidney stones pass in the urine.

Community/Home Care

The nurse promotes health by educating the patient about the impact a deficient fluid state has on stone formation. Teach the patient to maintain a high fluid intake to prevent concentrated urine. This is especially true during periods of extreme heat when insensible water loss may be high due to sweating. The patient should be informed to take fluids every 1 to 2 hours during the day. Keeping a water bottle nearby at all times can make intake easier and serves as reminder to drink fluids. Include support persons in teaching and be sure to inform the patient about volume amounts of common containers, such as a standard coffee cup or a can of soda. If the patient has lithotripsy, stress the importance of increased fluid intake at home to allow for flushing of fragments from the urinary system.

Documentation

A thorough assessment of hydration status should be documented in the patient record, including assessment of skin turgor, mucous membranes, vital signs, and accurate intake/output. In addition, patterns of urinary elimination should be documented (i.e. frequency, urgency, and dysuria). Identification of factors that precipitate nausea and vomiting should be documented along with the patient's response to any interventions implemented. If the stone is passed, record a description of the stone and the disposition of the stone.

NURSING DIAGNOSIS 3

RISK FOR INFECTION

Related to:

Presence of stones

Stasis of urine caused by obstruction of urine flow

Invasive procedures of the urinary tract

Disruption of skin integrity by surgical incision

Defining Characteristics:

None

Goal:

The patient will not develop an infection.

Outcome Criteria

✔ The patient's temperature will be normal.

✔ WBC counts will be within normal limits.

✔ Urine will be yellow and clear with no odor.

✔ The patient will have no burning with urination.

✔ The patient will verbalize an understanding of risk factors associated with infection.

NOC *Infection status*
      Knowledge: Infection control

INTERVENTIONS	RATIONALES
Assess for signs of infection: leukocytosis (with shift to left-increased bands), fever, chills, diaphoresis, tachycardia, urinary frequency, burning with urination, abnormal odor to the urine, and redness and drainage from surgical incision.	When infections develop, WBCs and increased immature WBCs (bands) are released from the bone marrow into the blood; assessing the patient for signs of infection will allow for early detection and treatment; in particular, concentrated, dark, cloudy, malodorous urine produced in a pattern of frequent small amounts and associated with burning are symptoms of UTI.
Monitor any urine cultures.	Identifies causative organisms and aids in correct treatment.
Administer antibiotics as ordered.	Helps to reduce and kill bacteria.
Encourage intake of at least 3000 ml/day.	Helps to reduce bacterial numbers through increased urinary output that helps in moving obstructing stones forward.
Ensure urine acidification (vitamin C, cranberry juice, if not contraindicated).	Acidic urine deters bacterial reproduction.
Monitor output from any urinary drainage tubes (indwelling catheters, nephrostomy tubes, ureteral tubes) for blood, mucous, amount of drainage, and color, and insertion sites for redness/discoloration or pain.	These changes may indicate infection.
Monitor any surgical site for redness/discoloration, swelling, heat, or pain.	Detects early signs of infection.

NIC *Infection control*
     Infection protection

Evaluation

Determine that the patient has no signs and symptoms of infection. WBC counts are within normal ranges and the patient is afebrile. The patient's urine is clear, and there are no complaints of pain or frequency. Any surgical incision shows no signs of infection.

Community/Home Care

Whether the patient is being discharged from the hospital or being treated at home, teaching should include the identification of factors that contribute to the development of urinary and incisional infections. The importance of monitoring for signs of infection should be stressed to the patient. Strategies for preventing infection at home include attention to urine color, odor, and whether there is mucous or blood. The patient is likely to forget to do this, as most people are not accustomed to assessing their output. Women will be at higher risk for UTI, and health care providers should reinforce information on proper perineal hygiene. It is crucial that the patient understands that when and if signs of infection occur, the health care provider should be notified. Whether treated at home or hospitalized, the patient who has kidney stones will need to continue to drink large volumes of appropriate liquids at home to prevent stasis of urine. Making a schedule for intake, for example, drinking every hour on even hours, may prove helpful, especially for people unaccustomed to drinking large volumes of fluid.

Documentation

Document assessment findings that would indicate the presence or absence of a UTI or infection of the surgical incision. A description of the patient's urine should always be documented as well as the amount. Drainage from drainage tubes is documented on the intake and output record according to agency guidelines. If the patient demonstrates signs of infection, document any nursing interventions that are implemented, along with the patient's responses. For example, if medications are given for elevated temperatures, document the temperature, medication, and follow-up assessment of temperature. Always include in the documentation information about when cultures are collected and sent to the laboratory.

NURSING DIAGNOSIS 4

DEFICIENT KNOWLEDGE

Related to:

New onset of disease

Lack of information about the disease and treatment

Defining Characteristics:

Asks no questions

Asks many questions

Goal:

The patient's and family's knowledge will increase.

Outcome Criteria

✔ The patient and family will verbalize an understanding of renal calculi, causes, prevention, and treatments.

✔ The patient will verbalize a willingness to follow the therapeutic regimen.

NOC *Knowledge: Disease process*
Knowledge: Diet
Knowledge: Treatment regimen

INTERVENTIONS	RATIONALES
Assess the patient's and family's readiness and ability to learn.	Teaching must be tailored to the patient's and family members' ability and willingness to understand for maximum effectiveness.
Determine what the patient and family already know.	Helps to determine a starting point for education.
Teach incrementally from simple to complex.	The patient and family member will learn and retain knowledge better when information is presented in small segments; must learn simple concepts first.
Instruct the patient/family about — Disease process of renal calculi — Causes — Common signs and symptoms — Need to strain urine and how to strain urine — Treatment options (diet, lithotripsy, and surgery) — Pain control — Signs and symptoms of infection	When the patient and family understand the disease process, treatment, and possible complications, compliance is more likely, complications decrease, and recurrences are reduced.
Assess for religious restrictions, as well as food likes, dislikes, and habits that may be culturally defined.	The patient will be more likely to comply with a new diet if it considers usual eating patterns, habits, and cultural practices.
Teach or reinforce diet teaching: *Calcium stones:* — Intake of a diet high in acid-ash if kidney stones are	Understanding the diet requirements and restrictions leads to compliance and prevention of recurrence.

(continues)

(continued)

INTERVENTIONS	RATIONALES
calcium-based, including cranberry, tomato, grape juices; cheese, eggs, meat, poultry, and whole grains, which can decrease formation of calcium-based stones — Restrict the intake of high-calcium diet: milk, milk products, cocoa, beans, lentils, dried fruits, canned or smoked fish (except tuna), and chocolate are high in calcium and increase stone formation — Restrict the intake of high-oxalate diet if stones are calcium-oxalate–based: beer, cola, chocolate, cocoa, tea, tomatoes, asparagus, cabbage, celery, green beans, and nuts increase stone formation *Uric acid stones:* — Intake of diet high in alkaline-ash, which includes fruit juice (except cranberry, grape or tomato), milk, milk products, green vegetables, legumes, and rhubarb; these foods decrease the formation of uric acid stones — Restrict the intake of purine-rich diet; goose, organ meats, sardines, and venison are high in purine and increase stone formation — Ingest with caution or moderation foods with moderate amounts of purine; beef, chicken crab, pork, salmon, and veal are lower in purines	
Teach the patient the importance of drinking at least 3000 ml of fluid each day.	Regardless of stone type, hydration is recommended to dilute stone-creating substances and aid in elimination of stone.
Teach pre- and post-lithotripsy and surgical care.	Knowing what to expect will help reduce anxiety, and knowledge allows the patient to take control and be self-sufficient.
Ask the patient and family to repeat information.	Helps to assess understanding of information and the need for further teaching.

Give printed information the patient and family can understand.	Once at home, the patient has information for further reference.

NIC *Teaching: Disease process*
Teaching: Prescribed diet

Evaluation

The patient reports the absence of or decreased levels of anxiety about the disease and treatment. The patient is able to discuss the disease process and treatment options. The patient verbalizes an understanding of dietary/fluid considerations to be implemented in order to decrease further stone development. Following teaching sessions, the patient verbalizes a willingness to be compliant with the therapeutic regimen and preventative measures. The patient and family are able to identify signs and symptoms to be reported to a health care provider to allow for early intervention.

Community/Home Care

Verbalization of intentions to follow and comply with the therapeutic regimen is expected. When new diets are to be implemented at home, additional expenditures for groceries may be required, as well as additional expenditures of time by the meal preparer. At home, the patient will continue to implement strategies to prevent new stone formation. Compliance with the regimen in terms of diet will be enhanced if requirements or expectations are consistent with usual dietary customs and cultural practices. For those patients who have had surgery or lithotripsy, post-operative care or post-procedure care should be clear. Keeping incisions clean and free of infection is accomplished by ensuring that the patient understands the importance of good handwashing before touching the incision. If drainage devices are left in place, the nurse should be sure that the patient understands how to empty and in some instances flush them, and the patient or family should demonstrate this before discharge. It is recommended that the first time the patient or family attempt these skills that a nurse is present in the home to ensure that the procedure is carried out correctly. The nurse can at this time reinforce information on how to store supplies, maintain cleanliness of equipment used, and measure the output. Written instructions should be given to the patient, especially about diet instructions. A nice folder can be used to organize the information with color-coding to indicate the different topics so that the patient can easily find the information he or she needs. The patient will need to contact the health care provider if the information previously given is unclear. When teaching patients about renal stones, the nurse must take into consideration whether the patient has the resources to be compliant with the teaching and the new health behaviors required. Follow-up visits with health care providers are an opportune time to re-assess knowledge level and reinforce information.

Documentation

At the completion of each teaching session, document the specific content taught, who was taught (the learner), and the methodology. Always assess the patient's understanding of the content taught and document in the patient record. If further teaching is required, or referrals are made, indicate this in the documentation. Indicate in the record the titles of any printed information given to the patient. In addition, chart the patient's verbalization of a willingness to comply.

CHAPTER 5.77

UROSTOMY/URINARY DIVERSION (POST-OPERATIVE)

GENERAL INFORMATION

Urinary diversions are indicated for a variety of reasons including removal of the bladder or kidneys due to cancer, renal obstructions, incontinence due to neurological damage, chronic pyelonephritis, birth defects, and serious trauma to the urinary tract structures. There are four basic types of urostomies: ureterostomy where the ureters are advanced through the abdominal wall to the outside; ileal conduit in which the ureters are anastomosed to a segment of the ileum and a stoma to the outside is created for the passage of urine; a colonic conduit that is similar to the ileal conduit except the ureters are anastomosed to a portion of the colon; and the continent urostomy, in which the ureters are anastomosed to a section of intestine with the creation of an internal reservoir or pouch with an external stoma from which urine can then be drained with the use of a catheter. The Koch pouch uses the small intestine (ileum) and the Indiana pouch uses the terminal ileum, ascending colon, and cecum with the reservoir formed from the colon and cecum. In both of these, the patient must be willing to perform and capable of performing self-catheterization to empty the reservoir.

NURSING DIAGNOSIS 1

ALTERED PATTERNS OF URINARY ELIMINATION*

Related to:

Surgical interventions (creation of urinary diversion)

Defining Characteristics:

Presence of ostomy on abdominal wall

Presence of continent reservoirs

Presence of stents

Retrograde urine flow

Goal:

Adequate urinary elimination will be maintained.

Outcome Criteria

✔ Urinary output will average at least 30 ml/hour.

✔ Urinary output will be clear/no blood or clots.

NOC *Urinary elimination*
Hydration

INTERVENTIONS	RATIONALES
Monitor output from urinary stents placed in the stoma every hour for first 24 hours after surgery, or as ordered, and be sure that flow is continuous.	In the early post-operative period, stents in the stoma drain into urostomy pouches that may be attached to drainage bags. Urinary output must be monitored to detect early any retention or obstruction that could cause distention and subsequent leakage at the anastomosis site. Output should be at least 30 ml per hour. Sudden cessation of urine flow may indicate an obstruction.
Monitor for edema of stoma.	Edema of the stoma can prevent urine from draining and cause backflow of urine or disturbance of the anastomosis.
Monitor color and consistency of urine.	The color of the urine will be pink but gradually return to a normal yellow color. It is normal to see mucous in the urine for patients who have had an ileal conduit or continent urostomy.

INTERVENTIONS	RATIONALES
Monitor output from other drainage tubes such as Jackson Pratts or pelvic drainage tubes.	These devices are used to drain blood and other surgical fluids from the surgical site. The amount should decrease gradually and cease over the first 72 hours after surgery.
Carefully check stoma for signs of adequate blood flow (pink/red, no dusky discoloration) and area around stoma for skin irritation. After stents are removed, carefully wash and dry area before applying appliance. Ensure proper fit of appliance (see nursing diagnosis "Impaired Skin Integrity").	Dark or dusky color of the stoma indicates a lack of blood flow to area. Excoriation or other signs of irritation may be due to urine leakage or abrasive appliance adhesive.
Encourage the intake of 3000 ml of fluid when allowed and include cranberry juice.	Helps to maintain urine flow and decrease risk of developing urinary tract infection. Cranberry juice is thought to serve two purposes: it acidifies urine decreasing the risk for urinary tract infections (UTIs) and, because of its acidic nature, decreases odor of the urine.
Administer antibiotics, as ordered, as prophylaxis or to treat infection.	Antibiotics may be ordered to prevent infection or to treat a specific organism.
Drain external urostomy collection device prior to its being full.	A full collection device may overflow, become detached, or cause retrograde reflux of urine.
Once reservoir is functioning (stents are removed), drain/empty every 2 to 4 hours.	Helps to prevent overflow or retrograde flow of urine.
Monitor for signs of urinary infection (fever, elevated white blood cell [WBC] count, decreased amount of urine, cloudiness, foul odor to urine).	Infection can occur due to manipulation to the urinary system during surgery as well as because of backflow of urine into the kidney via the ureters.
Teach the patient and family how to care for urinary diversions (pouch or conduit).	The patient and family will eventually need to provide care (see nursing diagnosis "Deficient Knowledge" and "Impaired Skin Integrity").
Examine results of any diagnostic studies: intravenous pyelogram (IVP), computed tomography (CT) scan, cystoscopy, bladder biopsy, or other tests.	These tests monitor urinary system functioning and determine possible metastasis of any cancerous growths if cancer of the bladder was the reason for the urostomy.

NIC *Urinary elimination management*

Evaluation

The patient achieves an output of at least 30 ml per hour. Urine color is clear yellow, and patient has no signs of urinary retention/obstruction or infection. Healing of the stoma occurs without any edema to site.

Community/Home Care

One of the biggest challenges for the patient when discharge is eminent is the uncertainty of managing the new method for urinary elimination (see nursing diagnosis "Deficient Knowledge"). Even though teaching has occurred during hospitalization, at home the patient may experience some anxiety when faced with independently caring for a urinary diversion without a nurse present. Therefore, for most patients home nursing visits are highly desirable to monitor the patient's ability to perform procedures correctly and to enhance comfort level with the urinary diversion. At home, the patient will need to be mindful of the amount of urine output in order to detect early any signs of obstruction. The patient will need to drink adequate amounts of fluid due to the increased risk of UTI. In the absence of cardiac disease, the patient should attempt to drink 2000–3000 ml of fluid daily, avoiding large amounts of caffeine, but including generous amounts of water. Caffeine is an irritant and has natural diuretic properties. The patient can develop a schedule for intake of fluids and keep a water bottle handy at all times as a reminder to drink adequate amounts. In the early stages following discharge from the hospital, the patient should keep a diary or log of intake and output to be sure to consume adequate amounts and that the urine amount is sufficient. If the patient is engaging in social activities outside the home, he or she may want to refrain from consuming large amounts of liquids for the hour preceding leaving the home, to prevent excessive output that would require emptying the reservoir or the urostomy bag while away from home. The patient needs to understand the importance of returning for a follow-up visit which may include having x-rays/scans done to ensure the integrity of the anastomosis and proper functioning of the reservoir. As the patient and family become more comfortable with management of the urinary diversion, the services of the visiting nurse may not be needed, but participation in support groups may be helpful as many times other patients or families may have helpful hints or pointers to make living with the urostomy easier.

Documentation

Document the achievement of stated outcome criteria and all interventions employed by the nurse to achieve them. Chart assessments relevant to the urinary system and the urostomy. Include in the record the amount of urinary drainage every hour or according to the orders or protocol, and include a description of the color of the urine. Note specifically the presence of any retention and strategies to relieve it. Document any patient concerns or complaints.

NURSING DIAGNOSIS 2

IMPAIRED SKIN INTEGRITY

Related to:

> Urine leakage onto skin
>
> Irritation from ostomy bag adhesive
>
> Surgical incisions
>
> Presence of drainage tubes

Defining Characteristics:

> Reddened, bruised, irritated area around stoma
>
> Presence of surgical incisions
>
> Fever
>
> Elevated WBC count
>
> Redness, swelling, drainage around wound or from pelvic area

Goal:

> The area around the stoma is free from irritation or infection.
>
> Incision heals without complications.
>
> Infection is prevented or eliminated.

Outcome Criteria

✔ The patient is able to perform appropriate ostomy skin care.

✔ Skin around stoma remains pink with no discoloration (dusky, dark).

✔ Skin around stoma remains intact.

✔ The patient's surgical site has no redness or other discoloration, purulent drainage, or heat.

✔ The patient is afebrile.

✔ WBC count remains within normal limits.

NOC *Wound healing: Primary intention*

INTERVENTIONS	RATIONALES
Monitor surgical site and any stents/urinary drainage tube insertion sites for signs and symptoms of infection or irritation from urine leakage: redness/discoloration, swelling, purulent drainage, poor approximation, heat, and increased pain.	Urine leakage onto the abdominal wall can reach the surgical incision and cause infection or irritation. Early identification of infection can expedite treatment and prevent irreparable damage to site.
Maintain patency of any drainage devices and assess drainage for amount, color, and consistency.	The drainage device helps prevent accumulation of drainage from surgical site; drainage may be bloody initially, but should become serosanguineous.
Consult with ostomy specialist who can measure stoma, choose an appropriate appliance, and identify appropriate adhesives and skin barriers that are appropriate for the patient.	Assisting the patient in choosing the appropriate products and troubleshooting problem areas or potential problems will allay anxiety and enhance self-care.
Change the ostomy bag 24 to 48 hours after surgery, or as ordered, and assess the stoma for bright pink or red color; change barrier as needed.	The bag placed in the operating room may be soiled, and a clean transparent bag 24 hours after surgery allows for better inspection of the stoma. Bright pink and red color indicates healthy mucous of the stoma.
Measure the stoma carefully with each appliance change. The adhesive opening should be just slightly larger than the base of the stoma. Be sure that the adhesive and skin barrier are free of wrinkles.	There will be post-operative edema. Therefore, the size of the stoma may change due to edema and for 6 to 8 weeks until the stoma shrinkage ceases permanently. It is important to measure the appliance opening carefully to ensure that the opening closely fits the stoma size and that the skin around the stoma is not exposed to the urine coming from the stoma/ostomy. The barrier protects the skin in case there is urine leakage and is gentler to the skin than the adhesive found directly on the pouch. Wrinkles in the barrier or the adhesive can prevent proper fit, causing it to leak; wrinkles can also cause skin irritation.

INTERVENTIONS	RATIONALES
Periodically remove barrier with adhesive remover, wash, and dry area carefully, and then replace with a clean, new barrier.	The barrier can be left in place when the bag is removed, preventing repeated skin irritation. Careful, meticulous skin care is essential to remove residual adhesive and prevent skin breakdown.
Change dressings on surgical incision as ordered and clean area using sterile technique, cleansing the entry site of any drainage devices last. If pelvic drainage tubes are present, give perineal care after each bowel movement, as ordered.	Maintenance of a clean incisional site decreases number of organisms and reduces the chance of infection; incisional infection may occur due to contamination with urine.
Ensure that stents/catheters are properly placed.	Improperly placed stents can irritate the stoma.
Take temperature every 4 hours.	Temperature elevations may indicate infection.
Administer antipyretics (acetaminophen [Tylenol]), as ordered.	Helps to reduce fever.
Administer antibiotics IV (intravenously) or PO (by mouth), as ordered.	Helps to reduce number of infective organisms and eliminate or prevent infection.
Encourage adequate nutritional intake with intake of protein, vitamin C, and iron.	Adequate nutrient intake, especially of vitamin C, protein, and iron, is required for healing and tissue repair.
Teach the patient to turn, cough, and deep breathe, as well as proper use of incentive spirometry, if ordered.	Helps to open airways, improve oxygenation, and prevent atelectasis that could lead to pneumonia.
Monitor for signs and symptoms of UTI and retention.	Patients who have had surgery to create urinary diversions are at risk for urinary infection due to the presence of stents in the ureters, manipulation of anatomical structures of the urinary system, and possible backflow of urine. Symptoms to note include urine that is cloudy, urine with an offensive odor, feeling of fullness in the pelvic area, and distended abdomen.

NIC *Incision site care*
  Infection control
  Nutrition management

Wound care
Wound care: Closed drainage

Evaluation

Evaluate the degree to which the outcome criteria have been met. The surgical site should be intact, and healing by primary intention with incision well approximated. Redness, swelling, purulent drainage, and heat should be absent from the site. Drainage from the drainage devices (if present) should be serosanguineous and should be decreasing in amount. The stoma of the urinary diversion should be bright pink or red. The patient should show no signs of UTI (foul odor to urine, cloudiness, mucous). The patient should be afebrile, and WBC counts should return to normal.

Community/Home Care

The status of the surgical site and stoma may remain a problem after the patient has been discharged home. The risk for infection remains, and the family will need to know what symptoms may signal the onset of infection. Infections of the abdominal surgical site or UTIs may occur once the patient is at home. Incisional care and stoma care will need to be taught to the patient (see nursing diagnosis "Deficient Knowledge"). For the patient with an ureterostomy, ileal, or colonic conduit, the size of the stoma will continue to decrease as healing progresses and post-operative edema subsides, making it necessary for the patient to measure the stoma regularly to adjust the size of the drainage bag. A visiting nurse will need to monitor the patient's ability to do this, as improper fitting of the device can lead to urine leakage and skin irritation. At home, the patient will need to locate a place to keep supplies for easy access, and the bathroom is a logical place. Durable plastic storage boxes in a variety of sizes can be purchased at any retail store that sells household items. The patient can experiment to figure out what works, for example, keeping all bags in one box, adhesives in another, and barriers in a third, or the use of a three-drawer rolling cart or one big box for all items. For the patient who must empty a bag and the patient who must empty the internal reservoir, use of the bathroom rather than the bedroom or other places for these activities helps add a dimension of normalcy. It is crucial that the patient who must drain the internal pouch maintains cleanliness of the catheter. Patients with Koch or Indiana pouches may go through periods of trial and error to determine how often to empty the reservoir. The patient will need to understand the importance of good nutrition in complete wound healing and recovery. The patient should be aware of signs of infection and indications of wound dehiscence. If any evidence of poor wound healing, discoloration of the stoma, irritation of surrounding skin, or infection should occur the patient should be instructed to contact the health care provider. The importance of completing any ordered medications such as antibiotics once at home should be stressed.

Documentation

Document assessment findings from the wound, including skin color and approximation and amount, color, and odor of any drainage, being sure to note any sign of infection. Chart the status of drainage devices or tubes, indicating the color, amount, and consistency of drainage. Document an assessment of the stoma and surrounding skin every shift or every 8 hours, as required. Record vital signs according to agency protocol, as ordered, for post-operative patients. Always include in the documentation all interventions implemented to address skin integrity, including achievement of stated outcome criteria.

NURSING DIAGNOSIS 3

 ### ACUTE PAIN

Related to:
  Surgical interventions

Defining Characteristics:
  Complaints of pain
  Guarding abdomen
  Grimacing and moaning

Goal:
  The patient's pain is relieved.

Outcome Criteria

✔ The patient will verbalize that pain has been relieved 30 minutes after interventions.

✔ The patient will verbalize satisfaction with pain control.

✔ The patient is able to participate in self-care activities without pain.

NOC	*Pain level*
	Pain control
	Comfort level

INTERVENTIONS	RATIONALES
Assess for location, intensity, quality, and precipitating factors.	Identifying these will assist in accurate diagnosis and treatment; most patients who undergo surgical intervention experience some pain.
Have patient rate pain intensity using a pain rating scale.	Provides a more objective description of level of pain.
Assess respiratory status, including breath sounds, respiratory rate, depth, quality, oxygen saturation.	For early signs of respiratory complications; patients who have abdominal incisions tend to breathe shallowly due to the pain associated with inspiration, which compromises respiratory function that may lead to atelectasis and pneumonia.
Administer analgesics on a regular schedule, as ordered, or dosed by direct IV route or via patient-controlled analgesia (PCA).	Narcotic analgesics will promote rest and relaxation and promote pain relief by not allowing pain to get intense; decreased pain will improve patient's respiratory efforts, especially inspiration, assuring adequate oxygenation, ventilation, tissue perfusion, and complete expansion of the lungs (preventing atelectasis); pain relief makes it easier for the patient to participate in coughing and deep breathing.
Implement strategies to enhance effects of pain medication, such as relaxation techniques, soft music, distraction, television, books on tape, backrubs, etc.	Non-pharmacological interventions can assist in reducing pain by affecting the perception of the pain experience.
Teach patient to splint abdomen when moving or coughing with a pillow or rolled bath blanket.	Splinting provides support for the painful area, decreases stress on surgical site that may increase pain. and allows the patient to participate in coughing and deep breathing more comfortably.
Assess effectiveness of interventions to relieve pain.	Helps to determine if interventions have been effective in relieving pain or if new strategies need to be employed.

NIC *Pain management*
      Analgesic administration
      Anxiety reduction

Evaluation

The patient is able to report that the pain has been reduced or alleviated following interventions. The degree to which the patient is able to assist in the management of the pain through anxiety reduction and relaxation techniques is assessed. The patient should have no observable signs of discomfort and reports satisfaction with pain management. The patient is able to participate in prescribed postoperative activities such as ambulation, incentive spirometry, and self-care activities without complaints of pain.

Community/Home Care

The patient's pain should be temporary and be resolved once the surgical wounds heal. Pain at home is usually managed with mild analgesics, and the duration of pain should be short. The nurse should stress to the patient that weak respiratory efforts because of pain can cause respiratory problems such as pneumonia. Encourage the patient to splint the incision with a small pillow when moving or coughing at home. If the pain worsens at home, the patient should contact the health care provider to determine other causes for the pain; most often increased pain signals a wound infection. If the recommended analgesics are not working, the patient should seek follow-up care with the health care provider.

Documentation

Document in the patient's own words the description of the pain and rating of the level of pain. Include in the documentation assessments made relevant to the pain. Chart all interventions employed and the patient's responses. All teaching should be documented in the patient record with an indication of the patient's level of understanding. Document analgesic administration on the medication administration record according to agency guidelines.

NURSING DIAGNOSIS 4

DISTURBED BODY IMAGE

Related to:
    Physical change in body post surgery
    Altered method for elimination

Defining Characteristics:
    Withdrawal
    Social isolation
    Depression
    Negative statements about physical appearance
    Patient attempts to cover stoma

Goal:
    The patient adapts to or accepts the change in physical appearance, and continues social activities and interpersonal relationships.

Outcome Criteria

✔ The patient states a willingness to look at and touch urinary diversion surgical site.

✔ The patient learns and participates in care of ileal/colonic conduit, ureterostomy, or Koch/Indiana pouch.

✔ The patient verbalizes acceptance of body appearance.

NOC *Body image*

INTERVENTIONS	RATIONALES
Provide assurance that any negative feelings are very normal after surgery.	Helps to stop the patient from thinking that his or her feelings are abnormal.
Allow the patient privacy when bathing or dressing.	Helps to allow the patient time to adjust to appearance without concern for how others react.
Encourage the patient to communicate feelings about changes in urinary elimination patterns.	Talking about the changes may sometimes be the beginning of acceptance.
Encourage the patient and significant other or family members to participate in the selection of the type of external drainage bag to be worn (for patient without internal reservoirs).	Participation in decision-making can enhance self-esteem and body image.

(continues)

(continued)

INTERVENTIONS	RATIONALES
Teach the patient and family how to care for the stoma, urinary drainage bag, or internal reservoir.	If the patient is comfortable with self-care, that comfort level may translate into acceptance for the change in appearance and incorporation of body appearance change into a positive self-image (see nursing diagnosis "Deficient Knowledge").
Be with the patient during the initial views of the stoma, initial care of the stoma, and, if desirable, the first time the stoma is viewed by a family member or significant other.	It is important to provide the patient with support and assurance that the stoma is a reality and that stoma care and urine elimination can be controlled by the patient.
Assess patient's feelings about self, interpersonal relationships with family members and friends, withdrawal, social isolation, anxiety, embarrassment by appearance, desire to be alone, or fear that significant other may not want to engage in intimate relations.	Helps to detect early alterations in social functioning, prevent unhealthy behaviors, and intervene early through referral to counseling. Concerns about sexual function are common as it relates to ability to engage in sexual relations, embarrassment about exposure of drainage device, and desirability to partner.
Encourage the patient to participate in at least one outside/public activity each week once health status permits.	Prevents patient from isolating self from others.
Identify the effects of the patient's culture or religion on perception of body image.	A patient's culture and religion often help define reactions to changes in body image and self-worth.
Identify community support groups and patients with similar stoma/device to visit the patient, if available.	Discussions with other patients with similar situations allows the patient the opportunity to share experiences with those who understand what he or she is going through; provides the patient with support and the courage to move forward in terms of acceptance of the change.
Assist the patient in identifying coping strategies and diversionary activities.	Coping strategies are needed to adapt to the changes in the body; diversionary activities are needed so that thoughts do not focus on disfigurement.

Discuss concerns about ability to return to work or engage in recreational activities such as sports, if applicable.	The patient is often concerned about physical activity, and this may be due to fear of the external drainage device becoming loose or leakage of urine if too active. Most patients are able to return to their pre-operative level of physical activity unless contraindicated by underlying disease.
Allow the patient to grieve the loss of normal urinary system functioning; allow the patient/family time and privacy to do this.	It is appropriate to grieve for loss of function of body parts that are vital to everyday life; supporting the family and patient will enhance healthy adaptation.

NIC *Body image enhancement*
Emotional support
Support Group
Socialization enhancement

Evaluation

The patient is able and willing to learn about the care of the urinary diversion—ureterostomy, conduits, or continent reservoirs—or stoma site and begin to participate in self-care. Time is required for the patient to completely assimilate the change in body appearance and function into his or her self-perception. It is crucial that the nurse evaluate the degree to which the patient is beginning to do this. Look for behaviors such as touching the site, looking at the stoma site, and agreeing to assist with the care or asking appropriate questions. Communication of feelings and concerns relevant to the change in appearance should be taken as a positive sign that progress is being made towards meeting outcome criteria.

Community/Home Care

At home, continued assessment of the patient's perception of body image is needed. The nurse who visits will need to be alert to subtle hints that may indicate that the patient has not completely adapted to the change in body appearance and urinary elimination. Open discussions about body changes and interventions to prevent social isolation and withdrawal should continue with patient and family. Many patients are concerned about the possibility of urine leakage and odor. Because of this, they may limit social activities, which will negatively influence body image. Methods of controlling leakage and odor are keys to the success of the patient's ability to sustain a positive body image and remain socially active (see nursing diagnosis "Deficient Knowledge"). The nurse who visits in the home needs to question the patient and family specifically about social isolation and engagement and provide any information required to attend to the patient's concerns. Community support groups should be explored, keeping in mind that such support groups may not be available in rural areas and an alternative activity should be identified.

Documentation

Chart any specific behaviors or verbalizations that may indicate an altered body image. Include all interventions that have been employed to address this issue and the patient's responses. Note when and if the patient begins to ask questions and participate in care. All referrals should be documented in the patient record.

NURSING DIAGNOSIS 5

DEFICIENT KNOWLEDGE

Related to:

Care of urinary diversion devices

Drainage of Koch or Indiana pouches

New medical problem

Defining Characteristics:

Many or no questions

Verbalizes a lack of knowledge/understanding

Unable to perform new procedures for care

Goal:

The patient or significant other will know how to care for urinary diversion devices and internal reservoirs.

Outcome Criteria

✔ The patient indicates a desire to learn necessary information.

✔ The patient verbalizes an understanding of the altered urinary structure.

✔ The patient and or family members demonstrate proper care of urinary diversion: external drainage devices, drainage of continent pouches.

✔ The patient expresses an understanding of the care required at home.

✔ The patient verbalizes an understanding of skin care and how to prevent skin impairment.

✔ The patient verbalizes an understanding of nutritional requirements.

✔ The patient verbalizes an understanding of follow-up care required and expresses a willingness to comply.

NOC *Knowledge: Treatment procedures*
Knowledge: Infection control
Knowledge: Treatment regimen
Knowledge: Health resources

INTERVENTIONS	RATIONALES
Assess the patient's current knowledge as well as ability and readiness to learn.	The nurse needs to ascertain what the patient already knows and build on this; if the patient is not capable of learning or is not ready to learn, teaching will not be effective due to disinterest or inability to understand.
Start with the simplest information and move to complex information.	Patients can understand simple concepts easily and then can build on those to understand more complex concepts.
Teach patient and family members or significant others the following or reinforce teaching by the ostomy nurse: — Anatomy and physiology of newly created urinary diversion — Procedure for draining internal reservoirs: clean catheterization of Koch or Indiana pouches to drain urine, importance of cleaning urine off skin, empty every 2 to 4 hours to avoid overfilling — Procedure for applying new drainage/ostomy bag: measuring the stoma for correct size, applying skin barrier, applying pouch; make opening in drainage bag no larger than 1 to 2 mm wider than outside of stoma; allow no wrinkles in barrier or adhesive part of bag	Knowledge of how to provide self-care, recognition of complications, and prevention of complications empower the patient to take control and be compliant.

(continues)

(continued)

INTERVENTIONS	RATIONALES
— Procedure for emptying drainage/ostomy bag: empty when less than half full to avoid leakage; change pouch first thing in the morning before intake of fluids when urine flow is slowest — Prevention of skin irritation: apply barriers, use plain water or gentle soap to cleanse skin around stoma, being sure to rinse soap off well; cleanse urine from skin promptly to prevent breakdown; inspect skin for breakdown — Prevention of infection by preventing backflow of urine — Surgical incision skin care: keep clean and dry, inspect for drainage and redness/discoloration — Signs and symptoms of complications that would indicate a need to seek health care: decreased urine flow (external drainage devices) or decreased output when internal reservoir is catheterized, fever, bloody or cloudy urine, purulent drainage from incision, sudden change in size or color of stoma, pain in back or in stoma site	
Teach the patient to pat, not rub, the stoma or the surrounding skin when performing care.	Rubbing can cause irritation to already sensitive skin.
When changing external device, place a gauze pad over the stoma.	Helps to absorb flow of urine while appliance is being changed.
Allow adequate time for task mastery; have the patient and a family member return demonstrate all skills and provide rationales for performing each step in a skill.	The person performing the care should feel comfortable performing the procedure before discharge to home, and the nurse needs to know that the patient can correctly perform this activity prior to discharge. Rationales for the steps increase understanding.
Teach the patient and family measures to prevent infection: good handwashing, especially when performing drainage of Koch and Indiana pouches or performing dressing changes.	The patient's first line of defense against organisms into the body is good hand hygiene, and vigilance is required to prevent UTI.
Teach the patient with conduits or ureterostomies to attach ostomy bags to larger drainage bags at night, such as those used with indwelling urinary catheters, by attaching to the emptying valve of the ostomy bag.	Urine production and drainage throughout the course of the night is more than the ostomy bag can hold. Attaching a larger bag allows the patient to sleep through the night rather than awaking to empty the pouch.
Teach the patient to ingest foods rich in vitamin C, protein, and iron. Suggest that the patient avoid asparagus.	These nutrients are necessary for good wound healing; asparagus gives urine a pungent odor. Stressing the importance of nutrition to the family and patient will increase the possibility that the patient will be compliant with requirements.
Teach patient and family to carry supplies needed for care of the urinary diversion in a small travel case kept with them when traveling.	If care supplies are placed in checked luggage, the patient will not have access to them in case of an emergency, and if luggage is lost the patient will need to buy new supplies. It may be difficult to get the identical supplies that are needed.
Assess the patient's and family's understanding of all teaching by encouraging them to repeat information; demonstrate all skills and ask questions as needed.	This allows the nurse to hear in the patient's own words what was taught and makes it easier to know what information may need to be reinforced.
Give the patient or family printed materials outlining the procedure and all information presented; if desired, obtain educational materials from the United Ostomy Association or the Wound, Ostomy, and Continence Nurses Society.	Printed materials can serve as a backup when the patient is at home and needs review or reinforcement; educational materials from these agencies provide updates on care strategies and innovations in care of urinary diversions.
Refer patient to home health or visiting nurse association for follow-up and reinforcement of teaching once the patient is at home.	Once at home, the patient and family may have questions about the care of surgical site, drainage devices, and emptying of internal reservoir; the nurse needs to be sure that care procedures are being performed correctly.
Establish that the patient has means to obtain all care supplies required to be compliant prior to discharge.	If needed resources such as finances and transportation to follow-up appointments are not available, the patient cannot be compliant; the nurse or social worker will need to make necessary referrals.

Learning readiness enhancement
Learning facilitation
Teaching: Psychomotor skill
Teaching: Individual

Evaluation

Evaluate the degree to which the patient has achieved the outcome criteria relevant to the teaching sessions. The patient should verbalize an understanding of content presented by repeating the information. It is crucial that the patient or family demonstrate correct performance of all psychomotor skills such as applying a new ostomy bag and barrier, emptying the drainage device, or inserting the catheter into the internal reservoir. The patient verbalizes an understanding of how to care for skin to prevent irritation. The nurse must determine if the patient is capable of being compliant with the recommended regimen. If further teaching is required at time of discharge, the appropriate referrals should be made to continue education.

Community/Home Care

The success of the patient's ability to implement strategies for self-care will be dependent upon the degree to which the patient has received adequate teaching and has subsequently understood and internalized it, as well as the motivation to participate in self-care. Crucial to successful in-home care is the patient's and family's ability to perform the required psychomotor skills of draining urinary drainage devices and catheterizing the Koch or Indiana pouches. The first time the patient or family changes the ostomy bag or performs the catheterization of the internal reservoir, the presence of a visiting nurse may decrease the uncertainty and anxiety for the patient. There may be some adaptations made in the procedure such as using a paper towel or old washcloth, rather than gauze, to absorb urine when the appliance is changed. Some sources suggest the use of a small tampon for this purpose, but male patients may not find this appealing. Cotton balls should not be used for this purpose because they can deposit lint

into the stoma. Dependent on the location of the stoma and/or drainage device, tight clothing may need to be avoided, and the patient will need to decide through trial and error which clothes will work and which will not. In most instances, loose clothing is more comfortable. Tight-fitting clothes may inhibit free flow of urine that could cause reflux and place the patient at risk for UTI. If the bag is allowed to become more than halfway full, the bag may be noticeable under snug-fitting clothes, as it creates a bulge. A home nurse should follow up with the family and patient to ensure that all procedures are carried out comfortably in the home and may actually want to plan to be present the first time a procedure is done. Depression and withdrawal may occur due to the changes in body appearance and method of elimination. This may not be evident until the patient is at home and may manifest itself in the patient's refusal to participate in self-care activities or isolation. Adequate teaching may make the family and/or patient comfortable with what is required and will give them some sense of control that may assist them to move from a state of denial to one of self-sufficiency. Be sure that the patient has the means to purchase needed supplies.

Documentation

Chart whether the stated outcome criteria have been achieved. Document the specific content taught and the titles of any printed materials given to the patient. Include in the chart the patient's degree of understanding of the content and the methods used to teach and evaluate learning. Documentation of the patient's ability to perform the psychomotor skills required for incisional care, stoma care, drainage of urinary devices, application of drainage pouches, and how to catheterize the internal reservoir should be specified. Any areas that need to be reinforced should be documented to ensure appropriate follow-up. If family members are present for the teaching sessions, document this in the chart, and always document referrals made for in-home assistance. Include information about the patient's and family's feelings, concerns, and fears about performing care in the home.

CHAPTER 5.78

URINARY TRACT INFECTIONS (UTIS)

GENERAL INFORMATION

Urinary tract infections (UTIs) are the most common infections affecting people in the United States and are caused by entry of bacteria into the urinary system. Approximately 90 percent of all UTIs are caused by *Eschericia coli* (commonly found in the lower gastrointestinal [GI] tract, rectum), but can also be caused by a variety of other organisms such as staphylococcus, Klebsiella, and pseudomonas. UTIs are classified as lower-cystitis (bladder), urethritis (urethra), prostatitis (prostate), or as upper-pyelonephritis (renal parenchyma and renal pelvis). Pyelonephritis usually occurs because of bacteria from a lower UTI migrating to the renal tissue. Nosocomial (hospital acquired) UTIs are associated with instrumentation of the urinary system, frequently indwelling catheterization. Women are more likely to acquire a UTI than men due to the short urethra, which allows easy entry of bacteria from the vagina and the rectum. Clinical manifestations vary dependent on the severity of the infection but can include frequency, dysuria, fever, chills, cloudy malodorous urine, and costovertebral tenderness.

NURSING DIAGNOSIS 1

INFECTION (ACTUAL)*

Related to:

Invasion of urinary tract by bacteria

Defining Characteristics:

Positive urine culture

Positive blood culture

Frequency

Dysuria

Fever

Chills

Flank pain and costovertebral angle tenderness

Elevated white blood cell (WBC) count

Blood in urine

Goal:

Infection is resolved.

Outcome Criteria

✔ The patient will have a negative urine culture.

✔ The patient will report no pain on urination.

✔ The patient will be afebrile.

NOC *Infection severity*
Knowledge: Infection control

INTERVENTIONS	RATIONALES
Assess for costovertebral angle tenderness, flank tenderness on palpation, pyuria, hematuria, nausea, urinary frequency with voiding of small amounts, urinary urgency, nocturia, and dysuria.	These are all symptoms of UTI and give clues to severity of the infection; costovertebral angle tenderness and flank tenderness are symptoms of pyelonephritis, indicating infection of the renal tissue.
Obtain urine specimen for routine urinalysis and culture and sensitivity, and send to lab immediately.	Provides a definitive diagnosis and identifies the causative organism, which is necessary for appropriate antibiotic therapy. A colony count of 10^3 organisms per milliliter of urine constitutes a positive culture. Immediate transport to the lab is necessary because if urine is left at room temperature, bacterial count will double every 30 to 40 minutes; routine urinalysis will reveal the presence of casts, white blood cells, and bacteria.

INTERVENTIONS	RATIONALES
Monitor results of other diagnostic tests: WBC count, blood cultures, serum creatinine, blood urea nitrogen (BUN), and intravenous pyelogram (IVP).	These tests give indications of any impaired renal function; blood cultures assist in determining whether bacteremia is present.
Observe urine, noting amount, color, presence of blood, and odor.	Infected urine is usually cloudy, foul smelling, and may contain small amounts of blood due to irritation; amounts at each voiding may be small; monitor for improvement in response to treatment.
Administer antibiotics specific to culture and sensitivity, as ordered, by mouth (PO) or in the case of serious pyelonephritis, intravenously (IV). Often the first choice antibiotic is trimethoprim-sulfamethoxazole (Bactrim®).	Decreases bacteria through bacteriocidal or bacteriostatic action.
Instruct the patient to take medications until the prescribed regimen is complete (see nursing diagnosis "Deficient Knowledge").	Patients often discontinue taking medications when symptoms are relieved, increasing the risk of inadequate resolution of the infection.
Have patient increase fluids to at least 3 to 4 liters per day by mouth if not contraindicated due to cardiac disease.	To dilute urine and decrease burning and irritation of the bladder.
Instruct patient to consume liquids such as cranberry juice or prune juice, and avoid liquids containing caffeine.	Cranberry and prune juice will acidify urine, and bacteria generally do not flourish in acidic urine; caffeine is a bladder irritant and will aggravate symptoms.
Have patient void every 2 hours.	Prevents stasis of urine.
If indwelling catheter is present, remove it prior to treatment.	The indwelling catheter is a frequent source of infection, and treatment cannot be effective if the catheter remains in place, as it provides a good source for continued and new bacterial growth.
Take temperature every 4 hours and administer antipyretics, as ordered.	Helps to monitor for elevations that may occur with UTI; give antipyretics to reduce fever and monitor response.

NIC *Urinary elimination management*
Medication management
Infection control
Fluid management

Evaluation

Assess the patient's overall status in regards to the UTI. Evaluate the degree to which the outcome criteria have been met. The patient should have no evidence of UTI, such as pain, frequency, urgency, fever, or chills. Laboratory results indicate decreased WBC count and a negative urine culture.

Community/Home Care

The patient with lower UTIs will be treated as an outpatient. The most common problem encountered when treating this group is compliance with the antibiotic regimen. Once symptoms dissipate, many people stop taking medications or take them sporadically, increasing the risk for inadequate treatment. For the patients with upper UTI, the same issues are of concern. Even though these patients may have been hospitalized for administration of IV antibiotics, upon discharge they too will probably need oral antibiotics for a period of time. It is crucial to stress the need for taking all medications as prescribed until gone. In the home, the patient needs to plan the intake of 3000 ml of fluids each day, unless contraindicated. The patient can keep water bottles close at hand, whether at home or at work, and keep a record of how much is consumed. Both groups will need instruction about prevention of UTIs and signs and symptoms of infection (see nursing diagnosis "Deficient Knowledge"). The role of fluids in maintaining an aseptic environment in the urinary system needs to be discussed. A follow-up visit with a health care provider should be recommended to ensure that urine cultures are negative. Be sure that the patient has financial means to purchase antibiotics and return to the health care provider for follow-up.

Documentation

Chart the results of all assessments. Urinary elimination patterns should be documented including any complaints of urgency, frequency, dysuria, or burning on urination. In addition, chart a description of the urine, noting color, amount, and whether hematuria is present. Document patient complaints of pain with follow-up assessment following interventions. Document all interventions that have been implemented to address the problem of urinary infection, and the patient's response to treatment. Chart vital signs, especially temperature, in accordance with agency standards. If specimens are sent to the laboratory, note this in the patient's record.

NURSING DIAGNOSIS 2

 ### ACUTE PAIN

Related to:

Renal infection

Irritation of bladder

Defining Characteristics:

Complaint of flank pain

Pain on palpation

Burning on urination

Goal:

The patient's pain is alleviated.

Outcome Criteria

✔ The patient reports that pain has been relieved 1 hour after interventions.

✔ The patient reports an absence of pain on urination.

✔ The patient rates pain < 5 on a pain rating scale.

NOC *Pain level*

Pain control

Comfort level

INTERVENTIONS	RATIONALES
Assess for location, intensity, quality, and precipitating factors.	Identifying these will assist in accurate treatment.
Assess intensity of pain utilizing a pain rating scale.	Allows for a more objective measure of pain.
Administer narcotic (for pyelonephritis) or non-narcotic (lower urinary tract) analgesics, as ordered.	Reduces pain.
Apply moist heat, as ordered, to flank area.	Heat will cause vasodilation and reduced pain response.
Implement strategies to alleviate infection (see nursing diagnosis "Infection").	Infection is the underlying cause of the pain.
Provide forced fluids (at least 3 to 4 liters per day), PO if possible.	Helps to "flush" urinary tract; prevents dehydration.
Implement non-pharmacological measures to relieve pain (guided imagery, distraction, music therapy, and relaxation techniques).	These techniques will enhance the effects of pharmacological interventions.
Assess the effectiveness of all interventions implemented to relieve pain.	Helps to determine if interventions are working and to decide if the nursing care plan should be revised.

NIC *Pain management*

Analgesic administration

Evaluation

The patient reports that the pain has been relieved or alleviated following interventions, and dysuria is absent. The degree to which the patient feels comfortable should be evaluated using the pain rating scale.

Community/Home Care

For the patient with UTI, the pain should gradually resolve as the infection improves. For the patient with upper UTI, the pain may not be resolved before discharge home. In this case, the patient will need to continue to take analgesics for relief and force fluids to 3000 ml per day. Patients with lower UTIs will manage pain at home and will need to implement strategies such as using heating pads, forcing fluids, and taking mild analgesics. In both instances, the patient should report back to a health care provider if pain worsens, which could indicate a worsening of the infection.

Documentation

Chart the patient's description of the pain and rating on the pain scale. All measures implemented to address the problem of pain should be included in the patient record. The patient's response to nursing interventions should be charted, and if the pain is not relieved, document necessary revisions to the plan of care. All teaching relevant to pain control is included in the patient record.

NURSING DIAGNOSIS 3

 ## DEFICIENT KNOWLEDGE

Related to:

Lack of experience with disease

Defining Characteristics:

Asks many questions

Verbalizes lack of understanding about the disease (UTI)

Is non-compliant

Non-compliance results in repeat infections

Goal:

The patient states knowledge of the disease, therapeutic interventions, and preventive measures.

Outcome Criteria

✔ The patient demonstrates knowledge of the disease and its signs and symptoms, and verbalizes the need for follow-up health care.

✔ The patient verbalizes an understanding of medications prescribed, including purpose/action, side effects, dosing schedule, and need to take all of the medicine.

✔ The patient verbalizes an understanding of the need to increase fluids to 3000 ml per day.

NOC *Knowledge: Disease process*
Knowledge: Diet
Knowledge: Medication
Knowledge: Energy conservation

INTERVENTIONS	RATIONALES
Assess patient's readiness to learn (motivation, cognitive level, physiological status).	The patient must be motivated to learn, have the capability to learn the content, and be free of distractions from learning such as pain and a noisy environment.
Identify a family member or significant other who will also learn the content and assist the patient with compliance.	This person can reinforce the teaching and assist with implementation if the patient becomes incapable of follow-through.
Create a quiet environment conducive to learning.	Environmental noise can prevent the learner from focusing on what is being taught.
Teach the learners about the pathophysiology of the disease (UTI) in the initial teaching session, including complications.	The patient must understand what the disease is and how it affects the body before understanding the rationale for treatments.
Teach the learners to increase fluid to 3000 ml per day if tolerated, including acidic liquids such as cranberry juice, and to avoid caffeine and alcohol.	The increased volume of intake prevents stasis of urine and dilutes urine; fluids such as cranberry juice acidify the urine, and bacteria generally do not thrive in acidic environments; understanding the rationale for these interventions will enhance compliance; caffeine and alcohol are irritating to the bladder and could worsen symptoms of infection.
Teach the learners about prescribed medications (antibiotics) including action, side effects, and dosing schedule; instruct patient to take all of the prescribed medications.	Knowledge of why the medication is necessary and how it works will stress the importance of the medication. Identification of side effects will minimize anxiety if these untoward effects should occur.
Teach the patient appropriate hygiene practices: — Take showers rather than tub baths. — Avoid bubble baths, douches, feminine sprays, and powders in the perineal area. — Cleanse from front to back. — Empty bladder every 2 hours while being treated. — Void before and after intercourse.	All of these interventions decrease the chance for introduction of bacteria into the urethra; emptying the bladder frequently prevents stasis of urine, which may serve as a medium for bacteria growth. Bubble baths, douches, and feminine sprays may dry and irritate the perineal area predisposing the patient to bacteria growth, which could migrate to the urinary meatus; powders serve as a source for bacteria growth.
Teach the patient what signs and symptoms need to be reported to the health care provider (worsening pain, continued dysuria and frequency, blood in urine, foul odor to urine).	These are symptoms that would indicate re-infection and a need for further treatment.
Teach the patient the importance of return for follow-up appointments for repeat urine culture.	Only a repeat culture taken 7 to 10 days after completing antibiotic therapy can validate resolution of the infection.

(continues)

(continued)

INTERVENTIONS	RATIONALES
Evaluate the patient's understanding of all content covered by asking questions.	Identifies areas that require more teaching and ensures that the patient has enough information to comply.
Give the patient written information.	Provides reference at a later time, and for review.

NIC   *Teaching: Disease process*
Teaching: Prescribed medication

Evaluation

The patient is able to repeat all information and asks appropriate questions about the prescribed regimen (medications, pain control, fluid intake). The patient can identify all medications by name, report the common side effects as well as the dosing schedule, and state that he or she should take all medications even if feeling better. The patient should be able to inform the nurse when health care assistance should be sought.

Community/Home Care

For patients with UTIs, home care focuses on taking antibiotics and increasing fluid intake. The nurse should determine that the patient understands what is required to resolve the infection and is willing to carry out the recommendations. The patient will need to be mindful of the amount of fluids that are being consumed on a daily basis to ensure that adequate amounts are taken to keep the urine dilute. Keeping a written record of intake and output might be helpful for the patient. At home or work, the patient can keep water in a water bottle and drink throughout the day to improve intake of liquids. Health care providers should be sure that the patient understands the need to return for a follow-up urine culture to validate that the infection has been resolved. Because UTIs often recur, it is important that the patient implement strategies for prevention, and the follow-up appointment is an ideal time to reinforce this information.

Documentation

Chart the results of the assessment of the patient's ability and readiness to learn. Include in the patient record a description of all content covered and titles of any printed material given. Document the patient's understanding of the information taught and their willingness and ability to comply. If the patient has questions, document these in the record to allow for appropriate follow-up. When other family members or significant others are present for the teaching sessions, document this in the patient chart as well.

UNIT 6

GASTROINTESTINAL/ HEPATIC SYSTEMS

CHAPTER 6.79

APPENDICITIS

GENERAL INFORMATION

Acute appendicitis occurs when the appendix, a small tube-like pouch attached to the cecum below the ileocecal valve, becomes acutely inflamed. Inflammation is usually caused by obstruction from hardened feces, a foreign body, a calculus (stone), or, rarely, a tumor. The appendix becomes distended and edematous, which may cause ischemia. Ulceration, infection, gangrene, necrosis, perforation, and peritonitis may develop within 24 to 36 hours if the condition is untreated. Appendicitis is the most common reason for emergency abdominal surgery in the United States (Lemone and Burke, 2004). There are currently two surgical approaches to treating appendicitis. The first is via a traditional open procedure, where an incision is made through the abdominal midline or laterally in the right lower quadrant at McBurney's point. This approach is usually selected when the patient has had previous abdominal surgeries and the likelihood of adhesions is high, when the appendix is found to be posterior lying, or when rupture has already occurred. The second approach is a laparoscopic procedure involving a smaller incision with insertion of a laparoscope facilitating visualization. This approach is chosen when the surgery appears to be a simple uncomplicated procedure. Advantages of this procedure are a short hospital stay (possibly fewer than 24 hours) and fewer postoperative complications.

NURSING DIAGNOSIS 1

ACUTE PAIN

Related to:

Distention

Inflammation of appendix and surrounding tissue

Visceral rupture

Post-operative abdominal incision

Gas from laparoscopy

Defining Characteristics:

Complains of periumbilical pain

Complains of right lower quadrant pain at McBurney's point

Grimace, moaning, guarding, rebound tenderness

Complains of incisional pain

Goal:

The patient's pain will be reduced or eliminated.

Outcome Criteria

✔ The patient states that pain has been relieved 30 minutes after interventions.

✔ The patient reports that pain is less than a 4 on a scale of 1 to 10.

NOC *Pain level*
Pain control
Comfort level

INTERVENTIONS	RATIONALES
Assess for location, intensity, quality, duration, and precipitating factors.	Identifying these will assist in accurate diagnosis and treatment; most patients who have appendicitis have typical pain that begins in the upper abdomen and localizes in the lower right quadrant, around the umbilicus, that is aggravated by movement. Rebound tenderness is described as pain relief when the abdomen is

INTERVENTIONS	RATIONALES
	directly palpated at McBurney's point, but return of pain when palpation ceases is also characteristic.
Have the patient rate pain intensity using a pain rating scale.	Provides a more objective description of pain intensity.
Assess for nausea and vomiting.	Nausea and vomiting are common with appendicitis and can add to a decreased comfort level and pain.
Administer anti-emetics as ordered.	Helps to relieve nausea and vomiting to increase comfort level.
Assist to position of comfort.	Patients will often be more comfortable in side-lying position with knees drawn up to chest.
Withhold analgesics before surgery.	Analgesics may mask symptoms of rupture.
Implement strategies to enhance effects of pain medication, such as relaxation techniques, soft music, distraction, and meditation.	Non-pharmacological interventions can assist in reducing pain by affecting the perception of the pain experience.
Teach the patient about anticipated surgery: type of procedure (laparoscopic, open appendectomy) and post-operative requirements (early ambulation or discharge, nothing by mouth, need for turn, cough, deep breathe [TCDB]).	Keeping patients informed about surgery can decrease anxiety and help reduce the impact of pain. Knowing that surgery will relieve the pain can decrease anxiety and subsequently decrease pain.
Administer analgesics after surgery as ordered on a regular schedule, not allowing pain to get intense.	Decreased pain will improve patient's respiratory efforts, especially inspiration, assuring adequate oxygenation, ventilation, tissue perfusion, and complete expansion of the lungs (preventing atelectasis); makes it easier for patient to participate in coughing and deep breathing.
Post-surgery, assess respiratory status, including breath sounds, respiratory rate, depth, quality, and oxygen saturation.	For early detection of signs of respiratory complications; patients who have had abdominal surgery tend to breathe shallowly due to the pain associated with inspiration, which compromises respiratory function and may lead to atelectasis and pneumonia.
Assess effectiveness of analgesics.	Helps to determine whether a change of medications is required.
Teach the post-operative patient to splint abdomen when moving or coughing with a pillow or rolled bath blanket.	Splinting provides support for the painful area, decreases stress on surgical site that may increase pain, and allows the patient to participate in coughing and deep breathing more comfortably.
For gas pain in patients who have had laparoscopic surgery encourage ambulation, apply heat to shoulder, or massage area.	These measures help gas to dissipate which decreases pain.
Assess effectiveness of all interventions to relieve pain.	Helps to determine whether interventions have been effective in relieving pain or if new strategies need to be employed.

NIC *Pain management*
Analgesic administration
Anxiety reduction

Evaluation

The patient is able to report that the pain has been reduced (is < 4 on a scale of 1 to 10) or alleviated following interventions. Before surgery, the patient reports that the pain is tolerable. The degree to which the patient is able to assist in the management of the pain through anxiety reduction and relaxation techniques is assessed. The patient should be able to participate in activities and have no observable signs of discomfort.

Community/Home Care

The patient's pain should be temporary, and should be resolved once appendicitis is relieved with surgery and the surgical wounds heal. Pain at home is usually managed with mild analgesics, and the duration of pain should be short. Encourage the patient to use splinting when moving or coughing at home. Following surgery, the patient often guards the abdomen and takes shallow breaths because of the pain that may occur with deep respirations. The nurse should stress to the patient that weak respiratory efforts because of pain can cause respiratory problems, such as pneumonia. If the pain worsens at home, the patient should contact the health care provider to determine other causes for the pain. Most often, increased pain signals a wound infection. If the recommended analgesics are not working, the patient should seek follow-up care with the health care provider.

Documentation

Document in the patient's own words the description of the pain and rating of the pain intensity. Include in the documentation assessments made relevant to the pain and to the respiratory system. Chart all interventions employed and the patient's response. Medications are charted on the medication administration record according to the agency guidelines, with follow-up documentation to record the effectiveness of analgesics. Any instruction done about pain management should be indicated in the patient record, along with an indication of the patient's level of understanding.

NURSING DIAGNOSIS 2

 ### IMPAIRED SKIN INTEGRITY

Related to:

> Disruption of skin integrity by the surgical incision (abdominal)
>
> Rupture of appendix with bacteria and feces entry into the peritoneal space

Defining Characteristics:

> Presence of surgical incisions
>
> Staples or sutures
>
> Drainage devices
>
> Presence of puncture wounds
>
> Fever
>
> Chills
>
> Elevated white blood cells (WBCs) (Leukocytosis with shift to left/increased bands)
>
> Redness, swelling, drainage around wound

Goal:

> Incision heals without complications by primary intention.
>
> Infection is prevented.

Outcome Criteria

✔ Incision is well approximated.

✔ The patient's surgical site has no redness/discoloration, purulent drainage, or heat.

✔ The patient remains afebrile.

✔ WBC count remains within normal limits.

NOC *Wound healing: Primary intention*

INTERVENTIONS	RATIONALES
Monitor surgical site and any drainage tube insertion sites for signs and symptoms of infection, such as redness/discoloration, swelling, purulent drainage, poor approximation, heat, and increased pain.	Early identification of infection or poor wound healing can expedite treatment and prevent irreparable damage to site.
Monitor for elevation of WBCs and for increased immature WBCs (bands, known as shift to left).	Infection causes increased WBCs and increased immature WBCs to be released from the bone marrow into the blood.
Take temperature every 4 hours.	Temperature elevations may be indicative of infection.
Assess for abdominal distention and rigidity, decreased or absent bowel sounds.	Distention could signal peritonitis or gas due to decreased peristalsis. Either can cause stress on suture lines, which can cause dehiscence with a greater risk for infection; decreased or absent bowel sounds may signal paralytic ileus after surgery.
Change dressings on incision as ordered and clean area using sterile technique as ordered; if incision has been left open due to rupture of the appendix, pack the wound as ordered and cover with sterile dressing.	Maintenance of a clean incisional site decreases number of organisms and reduces chance of infection; if appendix has ruptured the wound is left open and packed, healing by secondary intention and wound infection is inevitable.
Administer antibiotics, as ordered IV (intravenously) or PO (by mouth).	Helps to reduce number of infective organisms and eliminate or prevent infection.
Administer antipyretics (acetaminophen [Tylenol]), as ordered.	Helps to reduce fever.
Encourage adequate nutritional intake with intake of protein, vitamin C, and iron.	Adequate nutrient intake, especially of vitamin C, protein, and iron, is required for healing and tissue repair.
Teach the patient: — Care of the incision or wound — Signs and symptoms of infection	The patient needs to understand how to care for the incision or wound at home. Patients with abdominal incisions tend to

INTERVENTIONS	RATIONALES
— Role of nutrition in wound healing — Turn, cough, and deep breathe exercises — Use of incentive spirometer (IS)	breathe shallowly due to pain at incision site. TCDB and IS are required to open airways, improve oxygenation, and prevent atelectasis. This knowledge gives the patient a sense of control over health, allows for self-care, and can assist the patient in preventing complications by early detection.

NIC *Incision site care*
Infection control
Nutrition management
Wound care
Wound care: Closed drainage

Evaluation

Evaluate the degree to which the outcome criteria have been met. The surgical site should be intact healing by primary intention with incision well approximated. Redness/discoloration, swelling, purulent drainage, and heat should be absent from the site. Any drainage from the wound should be serosanguineous and should be decreasing in amount. The patient should be afebrile and WBC counts should return to normal.

Community/Home Care

For the patient who has had a laparoscopic procedure, there is little need for wound care, as the wound is generally covered by a band-aid which can be removed the next day, and post-operative complications are rare. However, the risk for infection in the puncture sites is still present if the sites do not close quickly. For patients who have had an open appendectomy, the risk for problems with the surgical site remain a concern after the patient has been discharged home. The risk for infection remains, and the family will need to know what symptoms may signal the onset of infection. Incisional care will need to be taught to the patient, especially if the wound was left open due to a ruptured appendix. This will include packing the wound at least daily and covering with sterile

dressings, and in some instances a visiting nurse may be employed to perform this task. Generally the care for the intact suture or staple line includes rinsing with warm water and keeping covered to prevent irritation from clothes. Wearing loose-fitting clothes over incision lines may be necessary for a period of time to prevent irritation to the site. Regardless of the type of incisional wound, the patient at home must practice good hand hygiene at all times and realize that even normal bacteria can cause infection in open wounds and incision lines. It is crucial that the patient understand that the most important intervention to prevent infection is proper handwashing before touching the incisional site. The patient should be aware of signs of infection as well as indications of wound dehiscence. The patient can use a handheld mirror to get a better view of the incision and should be encouraged to assess the incision daily. The patient will need to understand the importance of good nutrition in complete wound healing and recovery. The patient who has had nausea or vomiting prior to surgery may be hesitant to eat but must be encouraged to do so at home. The importance of completing any ordered medications, such as antibiotics, should be stressed. If any evidence of poor wound healing or infection should occur, the patient should be instructed to contact the health care provider.

Documentation

Document assessment findings from the wound including the presence of sutures or staples, wound approximation, skin color, and amount, color, and odor of any drainage. Be sure to note any sign of infection. Vital signs are documented according to agency protocol, as ordered, for postoperative patients. Include in the patient record all interventions implemented for wound care and the prevention of infections.

NURSING DIAGNOSIS 3

 DEFICIENT FLUID VOLUME

Related to:

Vomiting/nausea

NPO (nothing by mouth) restrictions before and after surgery

Defining Characteristics:

Hypotension

Tachycardia

Delayed capillary refill

Dry mucous membranes

Decreased skin turgor

Decreased urine output

Goal:

Adequate fluid volume is maintained.

Outcome Criteria

✔ Urinary output is > 30 ml per hour on average.

✔ Skin is moist.

✔ Mucous membranes are moist.

✔ Capillary refill is < 3 seconds.

✔ Vital signs return to baseline.

NOC *Fluid balance*

INTERVENTIONS	RATIONALES
Assess the patient's fluid status: intake and output, pulse, blood pressure, mucous membranes, skin turgor, and capillary refill.	In dehydration, output will be greater than intake, pulse elevates as the heart attempts to increase cardiac output, blood pressure drops due to decreased circulating volume in the vessels, mucous membranes are dry due to lack of moisture, skin becomes dry, and capillary refill time increases as the amount of circulating volume is decreased.
Monitor intake and output, noting color of urine.	Helps to assess fluid balance; dark, concentrated urine is a sign of dehydration.
Establish intravenous access and administer intravenous fluids and electrolytes, as ordered.	Helps to maintain fluid and electrolyte balance while NPO.
Maintain NPO status as ordered (before and after surgery).	Patients may be NPO before surgery due to nausea and vomiting; after surgery, NPO is maintained due to general anesthesia that causes cessation of peristalsis (paralytic ileus); liquids/oral intake is resumed with the return of bowel function (bowel sounds, flatulence).
Resume intake of food and fluids by mouth when bowel sounds return, starting with clear liquids and progressing as tolerated.	Helps to restore fluid volume and decrease risk for dehydration.
For the patient who has had laparoscopic surgery, offer food and liquids as ordered or tolerated after surgery.	Once the patient is alert, no dietary restrictions are required, as the intestines have not been manipulated; the patient goes home within 24 hours and is encouraged to drink fluids liberally.

NIC *Fluid management*
Fluid monitoring
Intravenous insertion
Intravenous therapy

Evaluation

Assess the patient for return of normal fluid volume. The patient's blood pressure and pulse should be at baseline. Mucous membranes should be moist and skin should be warm and dry. Renal output should average 30 ml/hour. The patient has no nausea or vomiting.

Community/Home Care

Patients treated for fluid volume deficit secondary to appendicitis have normal fluid status restored prior to discharge home. Patients experiencing the deficit secondary to vomiting should receive education about prevention of fluid deficit through management of nausea and vomiting as well as the need to seek medical assistance in a timely manner. At home, the patient may not require any follow-up, as this is an acute situation that for the most part has no long-term complications. Initially the patient may have some anxiety or fear about the ability to take fluids and foods without vomiting or pain, and may be cautious about intake. For this reason, the patient should start the intake of oral substances with clear liquids and progress as tolerated. This is particularly true for patients undergoing laparoscopic surgery, as they will not be in the hospital setting for monitoring. Fatigue secondary to NPO status and fluid loss may be an issue to be addressed at home, and can be handled simply by instructing the patient to perform activities as tolerated until stamina/endurance is re-established. The health care provider may want the patient to return for a follow-up appointment to ensure that parameters such as hemoglobin, hematocrit, and renal function studies are normal.

Documentation

Findings from an assessment of the patient's fluid status are charted, including blood pressure, pulse, skin turgor, mucous membranes, and intake and output with a description of the urine. Include in the record assessment of bowel sounds and flatus as these provide data to be used in determining when food/fluids are allowed after surgery. Document all interventions implemented to address the problem of fluid volume deficit. If the patient vomits, document this, as well as strategies for relief. Type and amount of IV fluid administered is charted according to agency guidelines. When oral substances are resumed, document the type and the patient's tolerance. Be specific when charting patient responses to treatment so that other health care providers can clearly determine improvement or deterioration.

NURSING DIAGNOSIS 4

INEFFECTIVE BREATHING PATTERN

Related to:

Pain at surgical site

Abdominal incision

Guarding incisional site

Defining Characteristics:

Shallow breathing after surgery

Decreased breath sounds

Adventitious breath sounds

Goal:

The patient will have effective breathing patterns.

Outcome Criteria

✔ Breath sounds will be equal and clear bilaterally.

✔ The patient will have no symptoms of atelectasis (diminished breath sounds in bases).

✔ The patient will have no signs of respiratory infection (elevated temperature, increased sputum production, and shortness of breath).

✔ The patient will demonstrate proper use of IS.

✔ The patient will demonstrate TCDB technique.

NOC *Respiratory status: Gas exchange*
Respiratory status: Ventilation
Pain level

INTERVENTIONS	RATIONALES
Assess respiratory status, including rate, rhythm, effort, depth, and breath sounds.	Helps to obtain a baseline and to detect problems; because of the abdominal incision the patient may take shallow breaths that predispose him or her to atelectasis and subsequently to pneumonia.
Assess for signs of pneumonia or atelectasis every shift.	Atelectasis is common in abdominal surgery patients and is characterized by diminished breath sounds in the bases; pneumonia occurs secondary to atelectasis, and the patient should be monitored for elevated temperature, shortness of breath, and expectoration of sputum.
Teach the patient how to turn, cough, and deep breathe, and encourage to do so every 2 hours while awake.	Helps to stimulate deep breathing; opens the distant airways to prevent atelectasis.
Have the patient splint incision when practicing TCDB exercises.	This provides support for the incision, decreasing pain in the incisional area.
Teach the patient how to use the incentive spirometer and encourage the patient to use it 10 times per hour while awake.	Helps to open distant airways and prevent atelectasis.
Administer pain medications, as needed.	If pain is relieved, the patient can breathe more effectively and is more willing to participate in breathing exercises.

NIC *Respiratory monitoring*
Positioning

Evaluation

Respirations should be easy with equal chest expansion bilaterally and a rate of 12 to 24 per minute. The patient's breath sounds are clear and equal bilaterally in all lobes. IS and TCDB exercises are understood and practiced as requested. The patient does not present with any symptoms of pneumonia. Diminished breath sounds, especially over right lung, should return to normal. Oxygen saturation results should provide evidence that breathing patterns are able to achieve adequate gas exchange.

Community/Home Care

At time of discharge, the patient's breathing patterns should be effective. There should be no long-term concerns that would necessitate special in-home care. Once at home, the patient may continue to have some soreness in the incisional site that may cause continued shallow breathing, but this should not be a problem as the patient should be fully ambulatory. The patient should continue to utilize the IS as directed by the physician, and generally one is sent home with the patient. The patient will need to be aware of symptoms of respiratory infection that warrant a return to the physician, such as fever, shortness of breath, large amounts of sputum, and a cough. Although a visiting nurse may not be required, the patient should be encouraged to return for a follow-up appointment with a health care provider.

Documentation

Document an assessment of the patient's respiratory status, including breath sounds, respiratory rate, and effort. Use of the IS is documented in the patient record as well as TCDB. If the patient expectorates sputum, this is documented by giving a description of the sputum and amount of sputum expectorated. If any abnormalities are noted with the respiratory assessment, document them, including interventions that were implemented to resolve the abnormalities. Record temperature in keeping with agency guidelines.

CHAPTER 6.80

CHOLECYSTITIS/CHOLELITHIASIS

GENERAL INFORMATION

Cholecystitis is inflammation of the gallbladder, which is most often caused by cholelithiasis, the presence of gallstones. Gallstones can be of the cholesterol or pigmented types. Cholesterol gallstones are the most common and result from supersaturation of bile with cholesterol. Risk factors include obesity, high-fat diet, hyperlipidemia, female gender, and Native American heritage. Pigmented gallstones are composed of calcium bilirubinate and are associated with biliary infection or increased amounts of unconjugated bilirubin in the bile. Pigmented gallstones are closely related to cirrhosis, in which the liver loses its ability to conjugate bilirubin. Gallstones may accumulate in the gallbladder or may become lodged in one of the biliary ducts, obstructing bile flow that causes an inflammatory response. Gallstones in the cystic duct cause the gallbladder to distend resulting in severe, cramping, right upper-quadrant (RUQ) abdominal pain classified as "biliary colic." Gallstones in the common bile duct cause bile reflux into the liver, resulting in jaundice, abdominal pain, and liver damage. Gallstones at the ampulla of Vater or pancreatic duct cause obstruction of pancreatic secretions, resulting in severe abdominal pain and pancreatitis. Treatment for gallstones includes pain management, dietary modifications, medications to dissolve the stone, lithotripsy, and surgical removal of the gallbladder called cholecystectomy. Cholecystectomy can be performed laparoscopically or through an abdominal incision (open cholecystectomy). Patients who have laparoscopic surgery are discharged on the day of the procedure, and those with uncomplicated open cholecystectomy have an average length of stay of 3 to 5 days. When the bile ducts are surgically explored for stone removal, a T-tube is commonly placed to facilitate bile drainage until duct inflammation, edema, and spasms subside.

NURSING DIAGNOSIS 1

 ACUTE PAIN

Related to:

Inflammation of gallbladder

Distention of gallbladder

Post-operative abdominal incision

Bile obstruction

Defining Characteristics:

Complaint of severe, cramping, RUQ abdominal pain classified as biliary colic

Epigastric pain

Pain after eating fatty foods

Incisional pain

Grimacing

Goal:

The patient reports pain is reduced or relieved.

Outcome Criteria

✔ The patient will state pain is relieved 30 minutes after interventions.

✔ The patient will state that pain does not occur after eating.

NOC *Pain level*

Pain control

Comfort level

INTERVENTIONS	RATIONALES
Assess pain, character, location, severity, and duration; use a pain rating scale.	Pain assessment can provide clues about diagnosis; used to determine treatment required.

(continues)

(continued)

INTERVENTIONS	RATIONALES
Assist to position of comfort.	Patients will often be more comfortable in side-lying position with knees drawn up to chest.
Administer analgesics, as ordered (before and after surgery), and monitor for side effects.	Narcotics are usually required for pain relief. Meperidine (Demerol®) is considered the drug of choice because morphine may cause sphincter of Oddi spasm in some patients.
Administer anticholinergics.	Helps to reduce bile duct spasms.
Avoid fatty foods.	Fatty foods can precipitate pain by causing gallbladder contraction.
Provide information about surgery and/or lithotripsy.	Keeping the patient informed about treatments can decrease anxiety and help reduce the impact of pain.
Administer analgesics prior to ambulation and turn, cough, deep breathe (TCDB) exercises.	Helps to decrease incisional pain with activity and increase likelihood that the patient will participate in therapies.
Have the patient splint incision when moving.	Helps to provide support to the incision and decrease pain.
Encourage use of alternative methods of pain relief, such as relaxation techniques, music therapy, massage, distraction, and guided imagery.	These strategies can enhance the effectiveness of analgesics.

Evaluation

The patient is able to report that the pain has been reduced or alleviated following interventions. The patient is able to ambulate and participate in breathing exercises and self-care without pain. The degree to which the patient is able to assist in the management of the pain through anxiety reduction and relaxation techniques is assessed. The patient should have no observable signs of discomfort.

Community/Home Care

The patient's pain should be temporary and resolve once medical treatment has been initiated and the surgical wounds heal. Pain is usually managed with mild analgesics, and the duration of pain should be short. Use of non-pharmacological measures such as guided imagery, relaxation techniques, and music should be encouraged. The nurse should stress to the patient that weak respiratory efforts because of pain could cause respiratory problems such as pneumonia. Encourage the patient to use splinting when moving or coughing at home to decrease the discomfort. If the pain worsens at home, the patient should contact the health care provider to determine other causes for the pain; most often increased pain signals a wound infection. If the recommended analgesics are not working, the patient should seek follow-up care with the health care provider.

Documentation

Document in the patient's own words the description of the pain and rating of the level of pain. Chart all interventions employed and the patient's responses, including medication administration according to agency guidelines. Include in the documentation assessments made relevant to the pain and to the respiratory system. Document all instruction in the patient record with an indication of the patient's level of understanding.

NURSING DIAGNOSIS 2

 ### DEFICIENT FLUID VOLUME

Related to:

> Vomiting/nausea
>
> NPO (nothing by mouth) restrictions
>
> Nasogastric tube to suction

Defining Characteristics:

> Hypotension
>
> Tachycardia
>
> Delayed capillary refill
>
> Dry mucous membranes
>
> Decreased skin turgor
>
> Decreased urine output

Goal:

> Adequate fluid volume is maintained.

Outcome Criteria

✔ Urinary output is > 30 ml per hour on average.

✔ Skin is moist.

✔ Mucous membranes are moist.

✔ Capillary refill is < 3 seconds.

✔ Vital signs return to baseline.

NOC *Fluid balance*

INTERVENTIONS	RATIONALES
Assess the patient's fluid status: intake and output, pulse, blood pressure, mucous membranes, skin turgor, and capillary refill.	This information provides data to validate a diagnosis of dehydration.
Monitor intake and output, noting color of urine.	Helps to assess fluid balance; dark, concentrated urine is a sign of dehydration.
Establish intravenous access and administer intravenous fluids and electrolytes as ordered.	Helps to maintain fluid and electrolyte balance while NPO.
Maintain NPO status as ordered (before and after surgery).	Patients may be NPO before treatment due to nausea and vomiting with ingestion of food; post-operatively, NPO is maintained due to general anesthesia that causes cessation of peristalsis.
For open cholecystectomy: maintain nasogastric tube to suction, as ordered.	Helps to keep the stomach free of gastric juices, especially if the patient has been vomiting immediately before the surgery.
Monitor output from any drainage devices: T-tube, Jackson Pratt (JP) drainage device, nasogastric tube and record every 8 hours, or as ordered.	Helps to detect excessive loss of fluid and provide information needed for treatment.
Maintain patency of nasogastric tube by checking for kinks and irrigating, as ordered.	Occluded nasogastric tubes can cause vomiting (due to accumulation of gastric juices in the stomach) that worsens fluid volume status.
Resume intake of food and fluids by mouth when gastrointestinal (GI) function returns, starting with clear liquids and progressing as tolerated.	Helps to restore and maintain fluid volume as soon as possible.

NIC *Fluid management*
Fluid monitoring
Intravenous insertion
Intravenous therapy

Evaluation

Assess the patient for return of normal fluid volume. The patient's blood pressure and pulse should be at baseline. Mucous membranes should be moist, and skin should be warm and dry. Renal output should be an average of 30 ml/hour. The patient has no nausea or vomiting. Output from drainage devices, such as T-tube and JP, as well as nasogastric tube suction, should be minimal.

Community/Home Care

Patients treated for fluid volume deficit secondary to cholecystitis/cholecystectomy have normal fluid status restored prior to discharge home. Patients experiencing the deficit secondary to vomiting should receive education about prevention of fluid deficit through management of nausea and vomiting and the need to seek medical assistance in a timely manner. At home, the patient may not require any follow-up as this is an acute situation that for the most part has no long-term complications. Initially the patient may have some anxiety or fear about the ability to take fluids and foods without vomiting or pain, and may be cautious about intake. For this reason, the patient should start intake of oral substances with clear liquids and progress as tolerated. This is particularly true for patients undergoing laparoscopic surgery, as they will not be in the hospital setting for monitoring. Fatigue secondary to fluid loss should be addressed at home, and can be handled simply by instructing the patient to perform activities as tolerated until stamina/endurance is re-established. The health care provider may want the patient to return for a follow-up appointment to ensure that parameters such as hemoglobin, hematocrit, and renal function studies are normal.

Documentation

Chart findings from an assessment of the patient's fluid status, including blood pressure, pulse, skin turgor, mucous membranes, and intake and output with a description of the urine. Document drainage from T-tube, nasogastric suction, or JP drains in the patient's intake/output record according to agency guidelines. If the patient vomits, document this, as well as strategies for relief. Chart measures to maintain patency of any nasogastric tubes, such as irrigating or relieving kinks, as well as type and amount of IV fluid administered. Document all interventions implemented to address the problem of fluid volume deficit. Be specific when charting patient responses to treatment so that other health care providers can clearly determine improvement or deterioration.

NURSING DIAGNOSIS 3

IMPAIRED SKIN INTEGRITY

Related to:

Surgical procedures (laparoscopic or open cholecystectomy)

Presence of T-tube

Presence of JP drainage device

Defining Characteristics:

Surgical incision with staples or sutures

Puncture wounds from laparoscopic procedure

Fever

Chills

Abdominal distention

Elevated white blood cell (WBC) count

Redness, swelling, drainage around wound or drainage tube insertion sites

Goal:

Incision heals without complications.

Infection is prevented or eliminated.

Outcome Criteria

✔ The patient's surgical site has no redness/discoloration, purulent drainage, or heat.

✔ The patient remains afebrile.

✔ Incision is well approximated.

✔ WBC count remains within normal limits.

NOC *Wound healing: Primary intention*

INTERVENTIONS	RATIONALES
Monitor surgical site and any drainage tube insertion sites for signs and symptoms of infection: redness/discoloration, swelling, purulent drainage, poor approximation, heat, and increased pain.	Early identification of poor wound healing or infection can expedite treatment.
Maintain patency of any drainage devices by monitoring for kinks and assess drainage for amount, color, and consistency.	The drainage device helps prevent accumulation of drainage from surgical site; drainage may be bloody initially, but should become serosanguineous. Yellow, thick drainage may signal infection. Drainage is a medium for bacteria growth.
Monitor for elevation of WBCs and for increased immature WBCs (bands, known as a shift to the left).	Infection causes increased WBCs and increased immature WBCs to be released from the bone marrow into the blood.
Take temperature every 4 hours.	Fever is caused by pyrogens, which are produced by infecting microorganisms, and is a classic indicator of infection.
Assess for abdominal distention and rigidity.	Distention could signal peritonitis or gas due to decreased peristalsis. Either can cause stress on suture lines that can result in dehiscence with a greater risk for infection.
Administer antibiotics, as ordered, IV or PO (orally).	Helps to reduce the number of infective organisms and eliminate or prevent infection; antibiotics may be given prophylactically.
Change dressings on incision and over drainage tube insertion sites or puncture sites, as ordered. Clean area using sterile technique, cleansing site of drainage devices last.	Maintenance of a clean incisional site decreases number of organisms and reduces chance of infection.
Administer antipyretics (acetaminophen [Tylenol]), as ordered.	Helps to reduce fever.
Encourage adequate nutritional intake, especially of protein, vitamin C, and iron.	Adequate nutrient intake, especially of vitamin C, protein, and iron, is required for healing and tissue repair.

NIC *Incision site care*
Infection control
Wound care
Wound care: Closed drainage

Evaluation

Evaluate the degree to which the outcome criteria have been met. The surgical site should be intact healing by primary intention with incision well approximated. Redness, swelling, purulent drainage, and heat should be absent from the site. The puncture sites from a laparoscopic procedure should have no drainage. Drainage from the JP drainage devices (if present) should be serosanguineous, and drainage from T-tube should be green with no cloudiness and decreasing in amount. The patient should be afebrile, and WBC counts should return to normal.

Community/Home Care

The status of the surgical site may remain a problem after the patient has been discharged. The risk for infection remains, and the family will need to know what symptoms may signal the onset of infection. Incisional care will need to be taught to the patient (see nursing diagnosis "Deficient Knowledge"). The puncture sites for the laparoscopic procedure are covered with band-aids and generally require no care; however, the risk for infection is still present if the sites do not heal quickly. The patient must practice good hand hygiene at all times and realize that even normal bacteria can cause infection in open wounds. Wearing loose-fitting clothes over incision lines may be necessary for a period of time to prevent irritation to the site. The patient will need to understand the importance of good nutrition in complete wound healing and recovery. The patient who has had nausea or vomiting prior to surgery may be hesitant to eat but must be encouraged to do so at home. Small meals may be needed initially and the patient will need to experiment with what is tolerated, keeping in mind that some patients may not be able to digest fatty foods. The patient needs to be able to identify foods that are high in fat and gradually add them to the diet. It is key that the patient understand the role nutrition plays in healing. The patient should be aware of signs of infection as well as indications of wound dehiscence. The patient can use a handheld mirror to get a

better view of the incision and should be encouraged to assess the incision daily. The importance of completing any ordered medications, such as antibiotics, should be stressed. If any evidence of poor wound healing or infection should occur, the patient should be instructed to contact the health care provider.

Documentation

Document assessment findings from the wound, including the presence of sutures or staples, wound approximation, skin color, and amount, color, and odor of any drainage. Be sure to note any sign of infection. Chart the status of drainage devices or tubes indicating the color, amount, and consistency of drainage. Vital signs are documented according to agency protocol, as ordered, for post-operative patients. Include in the patient record all interventions implemented for wound care and treatment or prevention of infections.

NURSING DIAGNOSIS 4

INEFFECTIVE BREATHING PATTERN

Related to:

High upper abdominal incision

Pain at surgical site

Defining Characteristics:

Shallow breathing post-operatively

Decreased breath sounds

Adventitious breath sounds

Goal:

The patient will have effective breathing patterns.

Outcome Criteria

✔ Breath sounds will be equal and clear bilaterally.

✔ The patient will have no symptoms of atelectasis (diminished breath sounds in bases) or pneumonia (fever, chills, thick sputum, cough, shortness of breath).

✔ The patient will demonstrate proper use of incentive spirometry (IS).

✔ The patient will demonstrate TCDB technique.

NOC *Respiratory status: Gas exchange*
Respiratory status: Ventilation
Pain level

INTERVENTIONS	RATIONALES
Assess respiratory status to include rate, rhythm, effort, depth, and breath sounds.	Helps to obtain a baseline and to detect problems; because of the RUQ incision, the patient may take shallow breaths that predispose him or her to atelectasis and subsequently to pneumonia.
Assess for signs of pneumonia or atelectasis every shift.	Atelectasis is common in abdominal surgery patients and is characterized by diminished breath sounds in the bases; pneumonia occurs secondary to atelectasis, and the patient should be monitored for elevated temperature, shortness of breath, chills, cough, and expectoration of sputum.
Teach the patient how to turn, cough, and deep breathe, and encourage him or her to do so every 2 hours while awake.	Helps to stimulate deep breathing that can open distant airways and prevent atelectasis.
Have the patient to splint incision when practicing TCDB exercises.	This provides support for the incision, decreasing pain in area.
Teach the patient how to use an IS and encourage the patient to use it 10 times per hour while awake.	Helps to open distant airways and prevent atelectasis.
Administer pain medications, as needed.	If pain is relieved, the patient can breathe more effectively and is more willing to participate in breathing exercises.

NIC *Respiratory monitoring*
Positioning

Evaluation

Respirations should be easy with equal chest expansion bilaterally and a rate of 12 to 24 per minute. The patient's breath sounds are clear and equal bilaterally in all lobes. IS and TCDB exercises are understood and practiced as requested. The patient does not present with any symptoms of pneumonia. Diminished breath sounds, especially over right lung, should return to normal. Oxygen saturation results should provide evidence that breathing patterns are able to achieve adequate gas exchange.

Community/Home Care

At time of discharge the patient's breathing patterns should be effective. There should be no long-term concerns that would necessitate special in-home care. Once at home, the patient may continue to have some soreness in the incisional site that may make shallow breathing continue, but effects of this may be minimized, as the patient should be fully ambulatory. The patient should continue to utilize the IS as directed by the physician, and generally one is sent home with the patient. The patient will need to be aware of respiratory symptoms of infection that warrant a return to the physician, such as fever, shortness of breath, large amounts of sputum, and a cough. Although a visiting nurse may not be required, the patient should be encouraged to return for a follow-up appointment with a health care provider.

NURSING DIAGNOSIS 5

DEFICIENT KNOWLEDGE

Related to:

Post-operative care

Lack of information

Anxiety

Defining Characteristics:

No prior experience with cholecystitis/cholecystectomy

Has many questions

Has no questions

Verbalizes misunderstanding

Goal:

The patient verbalizes an understanding of the operative procedure and prescribed post-operative regimens.

Outcome Criteria

✔ The patient verbalizes a willingness and desire to learn the necessary information.

✔ The patient verbalizes an understanding of the operative procedure (cholecystectomy).

✔ The patient verbalizes an understanding of activity restrictions required during convalescence.

✔ The patient will be able to identify signs and symptoms of wound infection.

✔ The patient verbalizes an understanding of any dietary restrictions prescribed.

NOC *Knowledge: Disease process*
Knowledge: Health behavior
Treatment behavior: Illness or injury

INTERVENTIONS	RATIONALES
Assess readiness of client to learn (motivation, cognitive level, and physiological status).	The patient must be motivated to learn, have the capability to learn the content, and be free of distractions from learning, such as pain and emotional distress.
Assess what the patient already knows.	The patient may have some knowledge about cholecystectomy, and instruction should begin with what the patient already knows.
Create a quiet environment conducive to learning.	Environmental noise can prevent the learner from focusing on what is being taught.
Teach the learners about the pathophysiology of cholecystitis, the normal function of the gallbladder, and what happens when the gallbladder is removed.	Understanding of normal function and pathophysiology assists with rationale for therapeutic interventions.
Teach patient deep breathing and coughing exercises.	Helps to maximize ventilatory excursion and reduce likelihood of atelectasis and pneumonia.
Teach the patient activity restrictions following open cholecystectomy, as ordered: — Do not lift any objects heavier than 5 pounds. — Refrain from strenuous activities such as aerobics, horseback riding, and jogging. — No driving for at least 4 to 6 weeks, or as prescribed by physician. — Ambulate as tolerated. — Splint incision when ambulating.	Helps to protect the surgical site from disruption.
Teach the patient wound care and infection control measures: — Keep incision clean and dry. — If dressing is applied, change using aseptic technique. — Monitor for signs of infection at incision site and drain insertion site: warmth, redness, purulent drainage, and increased pain. — Monitor temperature for elevations. — Report signs and symptoms of infection to a health care provider.	Due to the short hospital stay following cholecystectomy, the patient is at home when postoperative infections occur, so it is crucial that the patient know signs of infection; understanding the rationale for these interventions will enhance the patient's willingness to comply with limitations.
Teach the patient care of drains if discharged with T-tube: — How to empty the drainage bag — Emptying every 8 hours or when half full — Using a measuring device to collect drainage and dispose in toilet — Recording amount of drainage, and report excessive increases or abrupt cessation of drainage	The patient who has an open cholecystectomy may go home with a T-tube in place and will need to know how to manage it. It may take 4 to 6 weeks for proper healing to occur and tube to be removed.
Teach the patient about diet required: high calorie, high protein, and in some instances low fat.	Adequate calories and protein are needed for healing and energy. Physicians instruct patients to eat what they can tolerate after cholecystectomy, but patients may want to start in the early post-operative period with low-fat substances.
Evaluate the patient's understanding of all content covered by asking questions.	Helps to identify areas that require more instruction and to ensure that the patient has enough information to comply.
Give the patient written information.	Provides reference at a later time, and for review.

NIC *Teaching: Disease process*
Teaching: Individual
Positioning

Evaluation

The patient is able to repeat information for the nurse, and asks questions about the operative procedure (cholecystectomy) and possible outcomes. Prior to discharge, the patient verbalizes an understanding of the activity restrictions and agrees to be compliant. The patient is able to demonstrate to the nurse how to splint the incision when breathing and moving, how to perform deep breathing exercise, and how to use the IS, and is able to identify measures to relieve pain. The patient can state signs and symptoms of infection accurately, and is able to demonstrate proper technique for emptying T-tube drainage and recording the amount. The patient should be able to inform the nurse when health care assistance should be sought.

Community/Home Care

For patients who have had a cholecystectomy, the hospital stay is short, which dictates that knowledge deficits be identified early in order to improve the likelihood that the patient will be prepared for self-care and self-monitoring. With the exception of elderly patients, follow-up care in the home is rarely required. Many patients who have had their gallbladders removed are concerned about the ingestion of fatty foods, but most physicians inform the patient to eat what they can tolerate. Some period of trial and error of diet may be required to rule out particular foods. The patient may find it helpful to try fatty foods in small amounts to be sure he or she can ingest them without nausea, vomiting, or reflux. The patient will need to monitor self for onset of wound infections and respiratory complications such as pneumonia. The patient with a T-tube must empty this at least once a day or when half full. Use

of the bathroom for this is ideal. The patient should obtain a measuring receptacle from the hospital to carry home so that drainage can be measured. If this is not done, the patient or a family member can obtain a cheap plastic measuring cup from a retail store to use. The patient should pay attention to excessive increases of drainage or abrupt stoppage to drainage, either of which indicate a problem that should be reported. Outpatient cholangiograms may also be scheduled to determine the patency of the common bile duct prior to removal of the T-tube, and the patient will need to understand this and have an appointment scheduled for this procedure prior to discharge. Follow-up with a health care provider is needed for removal of the T-tube and to ascertain that the wound is healing as expected and no complications have occurred.

Documentation

Document all content taught and the patient's verbalization of understanding. Include in the documentation the patient's willingness and ability to comply with all recommendations made about wound care, T-tube care, and activity restrictions. Any area that requires further instruction should be clearly indicated in the record. Include in the record appointments that have been made for outpatient procedures as well. Chart any questions or concerns that the patient has verbalized. Always include the titles of any printed literature given to the patient for reinforcement.

CHAPTER 6.81

CIRRHOSIS

GENERAL INFORMATION

Cirrhosis is a chronic disease characterized by severe destruction of hepatic cells with replacement of normal tissue with fibrosis that disrupts both the structure and function of the liver. These changes decrease hepatic blood flow and filtration. There are three primary types of cirrhosis: Laënnec's cirrhosis, which accounts for approximately 75 percent of all cases in the United States and is caused by alcoholism or malnutrition; postnecrotic cirrhosis, caused by hepatotoxins, usually hepatitis viruses; and biliary cirrhosis, caused by chronic biliary obstruction or infection. Liver tissue can regenerate, so that in Laënnec's cirrhosis, if alcohol intake is discontinued and nutritional status is corrected, reversal in the condition may occur. However, as the fibrotic tissue continues to develop and extend, the amount of scar tissue exceeds the amount of functional liver tissue so that normal tissue cannot function, and the patient demonstrates signs of liver dysfunction. Clinical manifestations are few in the early stages of the disease, but as the disease progresses the patient has an enlarged liver on palpation, tenderness in the right upper quadrant, anorexia, nausea, vomiting, clay-colored stools, and gynecomastia. Signs that occur later include bleeding tendencies, spider angioma, palmar erythema, jaundice, edema, and neurological deficits (asterixis, constructional apraxia). Major complications of cirrhosis include portal hypertension, esophageal varices, ascites, and hepatic encephalopathy. Mortality from active bleeding of esophageal varices is as high as 50 percent. Hepatic encephalopathy can cause the patient to lapse into a coma quickly, and some cases are irreversible. The disease is seen most often in 45 to 60 year olds and is more common in Caucasian men. Females who consume large amounts of alcohol tend to have disproportionately more serious disease than males who consume the same amount of alcohol.

NURSING DIAGNOSIS 1

 IMBALANCED NUTRITION: LESS THAN BODY REQUIREMENTS

Related to:

Anorexia

Nausea and vomiting

Malabsorption of nutrients from foods

Increased metabolic needs causing increased caloric needs

Abdominal pain

No interest in eating

Defining Characteristics:

Weight loss

Decreased total protein and albumin levels

Decreased hemoglobin

Decreased intake of food

Reports lack of energy

Goal:

The patient's normal nutritional status will be restored.

Outcome Criteria

✔ The patient will not lose weight.

✔ Electrolytes will be within normal limits.

✔ Albumin will return to normal limits.

✔ The patient verbalizes an understanding of the importance of adequate nutrition.

NOC *Nutritional status:*
   Food and fluid intake
   Nutritional status:
   Energy

INTERVENTIONS	RATIONALES
Complete a fluid and nutritional assessment, including assessing for nausea; vomiting; poor skin turgor; dry, pale mucous membranes; fatty stools; change in stool color/context: clay-colored or melena; concentrated, dark, foul-smelling urine; dietary intake; fluid intake and output; weight loss, appetite loss; decreased muscle tone; albumin levels; hemoglobin; iron; and electrolytes.	Patients who experience cirrhosis often have a decreased nutritional status due to malabsorption of nutrients in the gastrointestinal (GI) tract and a feeling of malaise that decreases appetite. Anorexia and nausea add to the problem by preventing the patient from taking in enough nutrients to meet metabolic demands. The stool becomes clay-colored due to the lack of bilirubin from the liver, fat content in the stool increases because of an inability of the liver to metabolize it, and the urine is dark because of increased amounts of bilirubin now excreted via the kidneys. These laboratory results give clues to nutritional status and the effect of cirrhosis on nutrition.
Assess laboratory results: liver function studies: alanine aminotransferase (ALT), alkaline phosphatase (ALP), aspartate aminotransferase (AST) and gamma-glutamyltransferase (GGTP); bilirubin; albumin; total protein; iron; electrolytes; folic acid; thiamine; glucose.	Liver enzymes will be elevated in cirrhosis and give an indication that the liver's ability to function may be impaired; bilirubin will be increased; other lab values will be decreased due to the inability of the patient to eat and absorb adequate amounts of nutrients. Iron, folic acid, and electrolytes decrease as nutritional intake decreases. Hypokalemia is a frequent problem due to increased excretion secondary to increased aldosterone levels. Glucose levels may be low due to the inability of the liver to carry out its function of glycolysis and gluconeogenesis. The liver is unable to produce protein, and in patients with ascites, albumin is lost from the circulating volume to third spacing.
Weigh patient and monitor weight daily or weekly.	Establishes a baseline for comparison and allows evaluation of response to interventions.
Collaborate with the dietician to develop an acceptable diet that considers usual habits, food intake, and any cultural or religious restrictions.	The dietician can discuss with the patient which foods may be digested better with the fewest untoward effects but the best nutritional results.
Encourage the patient to take increased nutrients through high-calorie, high-carbohydrate, and low-sodium diets as ordered, preferably through small meals with between-meal snacks.	Promotes adequate intake of nutrients; for patients with decreased appetite, a small meal is easier to consume and more likely to be ingested and to be seen as desirable. In addition, a small meal will not give a sensation of fullness, and snacks provide needed additional calories. Protein is restricted in the patient with high ammonia levels because of the threat of hepatic encephalopathy (ammonia is a by-product of protein metabolism). Sodium is restricted to prevent edema or ascites.
Give nutritional supplements as ordered: folic acid, thiamine, vitamin B$_{12}$, multivitamins.	Supplements nutrient intake; patients with cirrhosis are likely candidates for malnutrition and need these nutrients. This is especially true for those patients with Laënnec's cirrhosis caused by alcohol use.
Provide between-meal snacks that are flavorful and contain supplemental calories.	These can include such things as pudding, ice cream, candy, fruit, juice, milk, soft drinks, and cookies. These may prove to be more appealing than the food served in normal meals.
Administer anti-emetics, as ordered.	Decreases nausea and vomiting.
Administer antacids, as ordered.	Reduces heartburn, stomach acids, and risk of ulcer formation.
Administer intravenous (IV) fluids with electrolytes and multivitamins, as ordered.	Cirrhosis patients admitted to the hospital for acute care often are malnourished and require IV fluids for hydration as well as electrolytes and multivitamins; these are usually given until the patient can take adequate nutrients by mouth (PO).
Assist with administration of total parenteral nutrition (TPN), as ordered.	TPN may be necessary if the patient is unable to meet daily caloric and vitamin requirements via oral intake, especially during times of acute illness.
Monitor and record intake and output according to agency protocol, being sure to include liquid stools as part of the fluid output.	Allows detection of dehydration and initiation of early treatment.

INTERVENTIONS	RATIONALES
Teach the patient and family about nutritional requirements and the role of the liver in maintenance of nutritional status.	Enhances compliance with diet.
Collaborate with physician to make necessary referrals for programs to assist the patient in efforts to abstain from alcohol intake.	Among patients with Laennec's cirrhosis, a majority of cases are caused by excessive alcohol intake. Refraining from ingestion of alcohol is needed to allow for resolution of cirrhosis.

NIC *Nutritional monitoring*
Nutritional management
Nausea management

Evaluation

The patient's nutritional status is stable as demonstrated by the laboratory values of albumin, total protein, iron, electrolytes, folate, etc., and weight loss. The patient verbalizes an interest in eating and understands the need for increased nutrients due to the malnourished state. No further weight loss occurs, and the patient consumes regular meals.

Community/Home Care

The patient must continue to pay attention to nutrition and the role of the liver in nutrition maintenance. A dietary consultation is crucial in assisting the patient in controlling diet. Patients and family require formal instruction regarding the restrictions that may be imposed due to dysfunction of the liver. Areas of concern include glucose and protein as there is the possibility of complications related to excessive intake of both that would necessitate emergency hospitalization. Glucose levels can drop due to poor intake of adequate amounts in food as well as due to the fact that the liver cannot break down glycogen from its stores or manufacture new glucose. Giving the patient a list of foods that can provide sources of glucose, usually carbohydrates, will be helpful. With this in mind, the patient and family will need to remember the signs and symptoms of a hypoglycemic episode. Even though a diet rich in protein is not advised, the patient will need to have sufficient amounts to maintain oncotic pressure and prevent the escape of fluid from the circulating volume that could contribute to the development of ascites. Excessive protein also adds to the production of ammonia, which is undesirable due to the risk of hepatic encephalopathy. Family members and significant others play a role in implementing strategies to improve nutrition by preparing meals and encouraging the patient to ingest them. Frequent small meals at home should be encouraged in order to increase the likelihood that the patient can ingest enough nutrients. Because the dietary recommendations may be rather complex and easily forgotten, a handy, laminated reference guide should be created and given to the patient or family. This guide could include a list of foods that provide protein, foods that provide glucose, foods that provide iron, foods to avoid, and foods that are acceptable; information about how much of any group to consume; and a schedule for small meals. Supplemental drinks can improve nutritional status during periods when the patient is unable to ingest adequate amounts of nutrition through normal meals due to anorexia, abdominal pain, or malaise. There are numerous products on the market (Boost, Ensure), but the patient may need to experiment to determine which ones are tolerated and consult with the dietician. The patient may need to remain on multivitamins, folic acid, thiamine, electrolyte supplements, and other nutritional supplements for an extended period of time. Teach the patient to monitor nutrition/intake by keeping a log of food intake: what he or she has eaten, when he or she has eaten, and how the food was tolerated. If at any time a particular meal or food product causes pain or subsequent nausea/vomiting, the patient should note this in the log and eliminate this food from their diet. Weights should also be included in the log. Even though the patient may not want to weigh every day, weighing at least every other day is a good way to keep track of weight loss or stabilization. This information can be shared with the health care provider at each follow-up visit to provide data for revision in prescribed therapeutic interventions. Despite aggressive measures by the family and nurse to develop an acceptable plan for nutrition, some patients will not be able to meet nutritional needs and may require parenteral nutrition in the home or hospital. In this instance, referrals are made to appropriate home care agencies or infusion companies that can supply the patient with the resources (human and supplies) needed for infusion therapy. The family and patient will need to be taught how to care for the central line or peripherally inserted catheter (PIC) used for infusion when it is not in use. Priority care involves prevention of infection through strict hand hygiene and protection of the site from injury. The infusion specialist in the home will perform dressing changes. The patient is more likely to have proper nutrition when supported by family and friends. Patient's with Laënnec's cirrhosis caused by alcoholism should be referred for assistance with resolving alcohol abuse. Providing the patient with acceptable coping mechanisms to be used at home can enhance compliance with recommendations to refrain from alcohol intake. Follow-up providers should assess the patient for weight loss and monitor laboratory results for improvement.

Documentation

Chart the results of a nutritional assessment, including a history of usual intake. Document vital signs, weights, and intake and output according to agency protocol at least every shift or every 8 hours. Include in the chart the amount of food the patient consumes at each meal and what if any supplements are taken by the patient. For patients who are taking nutritional supplements (vitamins, liquid supplements, etc.), chart this in the patient record. In most agencies, there are specific guidelines for charting regarding TPN that includes specific nutritional parameters, so the nurse should document accordingly. If the patient has complaints of any type, document these in the record along with accompanying documentation indicating responses to interventions. Always include in the record any referrals made, especially to the dietician.

NURSING DIAGNOSIS 2

IMPAIRED SKIN INTEGRITY

Related to:

Bile duct obstruction causing bile salts to build up under the skin

Decreased production of clotting factors

Increased bleeding times due to decreased absorption of vitamin K

Defining Characteristics:

Jaundice (skin and sclera)

Pruritus

Striae on abdomen

Spider angiomas

Gynecomastia

Dry skin

Goal:

The patient's skin will remain intact and return to normal status.

Outcome Criteria

✔ Itching will be relieved.

✔ Skin will be moist.

✔ The patient's skin will have no areas of breakdown.

✔ Jaundice will resolve.

NOC   *Comfort level*
Tissue integrity: Skin and mucous membranes

INTERVENTIONS	RATIONALES
Perform a thorough skin assessment noting jaundice, open areas, any bruising, petechiae, and color changes; monitor laboratory results of bilirubin, coagulation studies, and vitamin K.	Jaundice occurs because of the inability of the diseased liver to conjugate bilirubin and excrete it through urine and stool. As the bilirubin levels increase, the bile salts are deposited in the skin giving it a yellow appearance and causing irritation. The abnormal itchy skin becomes a high-risk area for breakdown, and frequent skin assessments are critical, especially due to the compromised nutritional state of the patient. Due to the inability of the liver to exert its normal role in the absorption and storage of vitamin K and other clotting factors, patients bruise easily.
Assess patient for itching and ask to describe.	Most patients with cirrhosis experience itching that can be attributed to increased levels of bilirubin and the deposition of bile salts in the skin. The itching may be described as intense and deep.
Administer antihistamines (Benadryl), as ordered.	Helps to alleviate itching due to jaundice.
Ensure that the room is cool and humidified, and that bed clothing is light cotton and loose fitting.	These provide for maximum comfort.

INTERVENTIONS	RATIONALES
Apply cool, moist compresses to areas that itch.	This will reduce itching, frustration level, and annoyance.
Discourage the patient from vigorous scratching and encourage him or her to keep nails short.	Scratching can cause disruption to the skin, leading to lesions that are difficult to heal.
Apply moisturizing products to the skin: oil-based lotions, petroleum jelly, or oatmeal. Avoid products containing alcohol and deodorant soaps.	These products add moisture back to the skin and ease the itching. Alcohol-based products and most deodorant soaps cause further drying of the skin.
Instruct patient to bathe in tepid water.	Hot water increases pruritus.
Instruct the patient to pat dry and apply lotions or ointments before completely drying the skin following a shower or bath.	Vigorous rubbing or drying of the skin following a bath closes skin pores yielding emollients ineffective.
Lower room temperature, especially at night.	Excessive warmth increases itching.
Protect edematous skin in extremities and sacrum by moving gently, using padding, placing on pillows.	Fluid in tissue inhibits adequate circulation to the tissue, predisposing the patient to skin breakdown.
Encourage the use of distraction or relaxation therapy.	These will help change the perception of the itching and discomfort.

NIC *Pruritus management*
Skin Care: Topical treatments
Skin surveillance

Evaluation

Determine whether the stated outcome criteria have been achieved. The patient should report decreased itching, and the skin should be intact. Even though jaundice may still be present, the patient's comfort level should improve. Skin should be moist without scaliness. Bruising or petechiae should be resolved or minimal.

Community/Home Care

In the home setting, the patient will continue implementation of the interventions initiated by the nursing staff. The intensity of the pruritus will vary from time to time, often depending upon the amount of bilirubin present in the blood and being deposited onto the skin. The patient will need to experiment with a number of measures or products to relieve the itching. It is important that the patient pay attention to environmental factors at home that may contribute to itching, such as temperature in the home, types of linens used (coarse cotton sheets may increase itching, whereas flannel sheets may feel better), and common items such as dishwashing detergent, household cleaning products, and hand soaps, which can all worsen the condition. Clothes made of fabrics known to be irritating, such as wool, linen, and synthetics, should be avoided. If the patient cannot resist touching the skin when itching, he or she can place a thin layer of clothing over the itching area and rub it gently using wide circular motions. Remembering to reduce the temperature of bath water to lukewarm or tepid can make a difference in comfort, as can applying cool moist compresses when itching occurs. The patient may find that inexpensive home remedies will often work as well as commercial products and medications. The patient or significant other should inspect the skin for open areas, edema, or bruising on a regular basis so that early treatment can be instituted. The patient should know when to take medications for itching and be aware that medicines such as Benadryl may cause drowsiness that limits the ability to engage in activities requiring alertness.

Documentation

Chart any complaints of itching and interventions employed to treat it. If medications are given, document them on the medication record according to agency protocol, with follow-up documentation regarding the patient's response. Any abnormalities in the skin including discoloration, bruising, or breakdown of the skin should be included in the documented assessment findings. Document education provided regarding skin impairment and suggested treatments.

NURSING DIAGNOSIS 3

EXCESS FLUID VOLUME

Related to:

Portal hypertension

Decreased serum proteins

Hypoalbuminemia

Increased levels of aldosterone

Defining Characteristics:

  Ascites

  Crackles in lung

  Engorged neck veins/jugular vein distention

  Increased respirations

  Increased blood pressure

  Tachycardia

  Spider angiomas

  Bounding pulse

  Dilated veins around umbilicus and on abdomen

  Peripheral edema

Goal:

  Fluid volume excess is decreased.

Outcome Criteria

✔ The patient will demonstrate weight loss.

✔ Ascites will decrease as demonstrated by decreasing abdominal girth.

✔ Lung sounds will be clear bilaterally.

✔ Jugular vein distention will disappear.

✔ Edema will be absent or decreased.

✔ Output will be greater than intake.

NOC *Fluid balance*
       Fluid overload severity
       Electrolyte and acid/base balance

INTERVENTIONS	RATIONALES
Perform a respiratory assessment monitoring respiratory rate, rhythm, depth, tachypnea, dyspnea, thoracic restriction due to abdominal ascites, and breath sounds for crackles.	The ascites can lead to impaired movement of the diaphragm, which can impair respiratory function; crackles are an indicator of fluid in the lungs and should be monitored for worsening.
Measure abdominal girth daily; mark the site where measurement will be taken.	Helps to assess severity of the ascites; measurement will provide a more accurate assessment that can be used as a baseline for comparison.
Monitor results of abdominal ultrasound.	The ultrasound can identify the extent of the ascites.
Administer potassium-sparing diuretics, such as aldactone, as ordered.	Aldactone decreases aldosterone levels, which is one of the causes of ascites; spares the excretion of potassium, which is needed for the cirrhosis patient who is typically hypokalemic; and inhibits the reabsorption of sodium and chloride, thereby causing an increased fluid output by the kidneys. If ascites does not improve with aldactone, then a loop diuretic such as Lasix is instituted.
Administer salt-poor albumin (SPA) intravenously, as ordered.	Albumin changes the oncotic pressure of the vascular space and pulls fluid back to the circulating volume.
Weigh patient daily at the same time, in similar clothing, on the same scale, in the morning before breakfast, and after voiding.	The most accurate method of determining fluid volume loss is through daily weighing, 1 kg of weight loss = 1 L of fluid lost. Morning weights are a better reflection of true weights, as most people accumulate fluid as the day progresses.
Implement a diet low in sodium (usually 2 g or less daily), as ordered.	Sodium increases fluid retention; thus, decreasing the amount of dietary sodium intake will decrease the amount of retained fluid.
Implement fluid restrictions, as ordered, if respiratory symptoms occur—usually 1500 cc over 24 hours is allowed.	Restricting the fluid intake can assist in decreasing the amount of fluid entering the circulating volume, which can make the fluid overload worse as it too enters the abdominal cavity.
Obtain accurate intake and output.	Helps to monitor balance between fluid consumed and urinary output; output also gives an indication of renal perfusion.
Monitor electrolytes (especially potassium).	Diuretics cause an abnormal excretion of electrolytes; cirrhosis patients tend to be hypokalemic.
Provide potassium supplements, as ordered.	Replaces potassium loss due to cirrhosis and urinary potassium loss caused by diuretics if loop diuretics are used.
Monitor blood pressure and pulse.	Blood pressure and pulse may be elevated due to fluid retention, but after therapy is implemented, the patient may become hypotensive secondary to diuretic therapy.

INTERVENTIONS	RATIONALES
If non-invasive measures fail, assist with paracentesis (aspiration of fluid from abdominal cavity) as ordered, including informed consent; weigh the patient, measure abdominal girth, take vital signs, void prior to procedure, and position patient as instructed.	Paracentesis is used when the patient has respiratory symptoms and worsening ascites. The patient should understand the purpose of the procedure as well as the risks involved. Weighing the patient and measuring the abdominal girth will allow for evaluation of the success of the procedure; baseline vital signs are needed for comparison; when large volumes are removed the patient may experience a drop in blood pressure and an increase in pulse. Following the procedure, a dressing is placed over the site and is monitored for oozing of fluid. Vital signs should be monitored post-procedure for indications of volume deficit.
In patients unresponsive to other interventions, assist with preparation of the patient for insertion of LaVeen peritoneo-venous shunt.	This shunt provides a mechanism for the continuous reinfusion of ascitic fluid into the venous circulation (jugular vein or superior vena cava). A valve on the shunt opens when the pressure elevates to a certain level, allowing for the flow of fluid.
Encourage the patient to identify a position of comfort.	Although the high Fowler's position is thought to be the position of choice for patients with ascites due to respiratory problems, it is not always comfortable for the patient due to the pressure on the diaphragm.

NIC   *Fluid management*
  Fluid monitoring
  Electrolyte monitoring

Evaluation

Patient has weight loss and output is greater than intake. Ascites is decreasing as demonstrated by weight lost, decreasing abdominal girth, and the patient verbalizes increased comfort. Blood pressure and pulse return to baseline and breath sounds are clear. Abnormal laboratory results such as albumin and blood urea nitrogen (BUN) return to normal levels. The patient reports the absence of shortness of breath and jugular vein distention has resolved.

Community/Home Care

Ensure that the patient at home understands the importance of monitoring fluid status. The patient should have a reliable scale that is calibrated and easily accessible. Weighing daily at home will allow the patient to notice subtle changes in fluid retention that may indicate a worsening of ascites. Be sure that the patient has a tape measure and have the patient or a family member demonstrate how to measure abdominal girth. Patients should be instructed to take note of clothing that becomes too tight in a short period of time, which is an indicator of fluid retention. The patient with cirrhosis will need to continue to limit the intake of salt and sodium-rich foods. Teach the patient how to read food labels for sodium content. Fluid restrictions may be more challenging than sodium restrictions. Instruct the patient about the volume amounts of common fluids consumed, such as a cup of coffee, a can of soda, or his or her favorite drinking glass. Unless contraindicated, have the patient take medications with the fluids consumed at meals so that these fluids can serve a dual purpose. Diet instructions should consider the patient's normal diet and any cultural or religious preferences and restrictions. Have the patient keep a log of food and fluid intake as well as weights and abdominal girth measurements. Help the patient to develop a schedule for taking prescribed diuretics that is mindful of lifestyle and daily routines. The patient should understand that if the cirrhosis advances, the ascites will become a permanent problem that may necessitate periodic treatments by the health care provider for aspiration of fluid. Stress the need for follow-up care.

Documentation

Always document the extent to which the outcome criteria have been achieved. Record intake and output, blood pressure, pulse, weights, breath sounds, and the patient's understanding of the therapies for eliminating fluid excess. If fluid restrictions have been implemented, include this in the record with specifications for amounts to be administered each shift. Medications administered for excess fluid volume (diuretics, SPA) should be documented on the medication administration record, and the nurse should indicate the amount of fluid the patient lost in response. When a paracentesis is performed, document the amount of fluid removed, its disposition, the patient's response to the procedure, location of dressing or band-aid after the procedure, any leakage of fluid, vital signs before and after the procedure, and weights before and after the procedure. Chart other assessments and information as required by agency guidelines.

NURSING DIAGNOSIS 4

INEFFECTIVE PROTECTION

Related to:

Decreased absorption of vitamin K

Decreased production of clotting factors

Impaired fat metabolism

Rupture of esophageal varices

Increased pressure in portal circulation

Development of collateral blood vessels (esophagus and abdomen)

Defining Characteristics:

Hematemesis

Petechiae

Easy bruising

Prolonged bleeding times

Blood in stool or emesis

Goal:

Bleeding will be controlled.

Outcome Criteria

✔ Any patient bleeding will stop 10 minutes after interventions are implemented.

✔ The patient's vital signs (blood pressure and pulse) will be within patient's normal baseline values.

✔ The patient will not experience bleeding or bruising.

✔ The patient will verbalize an understanding of the necessary precautions to prevent bleeding and prevent injury.

NOC *Blood coagulation*
Immune status
Risk control

INTERVENTIONS	RATIONALES
Monitor results of laboratory and diagnostic tests: endoscopy, activated partial thromboplastin time (APTT), prothrombin time (PT), vitamin K, and platelets.	Endoscopy is used to detect the presence of varices; APTT and PT elevations, decreased Vitamin K, and decreased platelets validate an increased risk for bleeding.
Monitor for indicators of bleeding abnormalities: bruising, petechiae, easy bleeding, spider angiomas, distended abdominal blood vessels, blood in emesis or stool, bleeding gums, nosebleed, and purpura.	These indicate that the body is unable to clot effectively, and further examination and interventions may be warranted to prevent complications. When spider angiomas and distended abdominal vessels are noted, this provides information regarding pressure in portal circulation that can be an indicator that the patient is at higher risk for bleeding from varices.
Take vital signs as ordered or every 4 hours if bleeding occurs.	The patient may exhibit signs of hemorrhagic shock: decreased blood pressure and increased pulse due to loss of volume and compensatory mechanisms.
Test any emesis or stool for blood.	Helps to detect bleeding not recognizable through observation.
Administer vitamin K, as ordered.	There is decreased absorption of vitamin K in cirrhosis, and administration is needed to prevent bleeding.
Administer medications to reduce risk of bleeding, such as beta blockers (propranolol).	These medications reduce the pressure in the portal circulation.
Administer vasopressin intravenously, as ordered.	Vasopressin is a vasoconstrictor that lowers portal pressure.
Assist with ordered medical interventions for bleeding varices: — Injection sclerotherapy: With use of an endoscope to visualize areas of bleeding, a sclerosing agent can be injected into the active bleeding sites. This causes thrombosis and sclerosis of the bleeding vessel, and should result in cessation of bleeding	These procedures are used when patients have not responded to other less invasive measures to control bleeding; both the injection sclerotherapy and esophageal tamponade are used in acute emergencies.

INTERVENTIONS	RATIONALES
in 3 to 5 minutes. Keep the patient NPO (nothing by mouth) for at least 6 hours before procedure, and monitor the patient for signs of aspiration, perforation, and fever over the next few days. — Esophageal tamponade: Use of the Sengstaken-Blakemore tube to apply pressure to bleeding sites via inflation of a balloon (there is an esophageal and gastric balloon), a separate lumen is used for gastric suction. Monitor the patient for signs of airway occlusion, continued bleeding, monitor drainage from suction, keep on bedrest, and monitor vital signs. Keep scissors at bedside; in the event of respiratory distress, the balloon lumens must be cut.	
Assist patient with careful ambulation and other activities.	Due to weakness and fatigue, the patient is at higher risk for falls and bumping into objects, which places the patient at risk for bruising and bleeding due to traumatic injury.
Avoid injections if possible, but if puncture sites are necessary, apply pressure for 5 minutes.	Lack of sufficient clotting factors predisposes the patient to bleeding, even from simple procedures, and pressure is required to stop the bleeding effectively.
Brush teeth with soft bristle toothbrush.	Helps to decrease bleeding from gums; gums are highly vascular and tend to bleed easily due to altered clotting factors.
Administer blood products, as ordered.	Based on laboratory results and estimated amount of blood loss, the patient may require blood products to restore circulating volume and provide red blood cells (RBCs) for oxygen transport.
Teach the patient and family about all interventions employed to control bleeding, particularly the invasive procedures and safety precautions required related to bleeding.	Providing information can decrease anxiety; the patient needs to be informed in order to comply with post-procedure requirements.
Monitor for signs of fluid volume deficit: tachycardia, decreased blood pressure, change in mental status, decreased hemoglobin, and hematocrit (see nursing care plan "Hypovolemic Shock") and report to physician.	If bleeding is profuse, the patient may show signs of cardiac compensation to maintain perfusion to vital organs by increasing heart rate; blood pressure drops because of decreased circulating volume; changes in mental status indicate decreased perfusion to cerebral tissue.
Educate the patient on the etiology of esophageal varices, treatments, and complications.	Knowledge enhances reduction of anxiety and allows the patient to understand health status.

NIC *Bleeding precautions*
Risk identification
Surveillance

Evaluation

Evaluate whether outcome criteria have been met. The patient should have no bleeding; any bleeding that does occur is detected and treated early. Vital signs have returned to the patient's baseline. Any bleeding from varices ceases spontaneously or after interventions. No complications occur following insertion of the Sengstaken-Blakemore tube or injection sclerotherapy. The patient's airway is not obstructed by the tube or blood. Hemoglobin and hematocrit return to normal, petechiae resolve, no injuries occur, and bruising is avoided. The patient ambulates with assistance and without injury. At time of discharge from the health care agency, the patient is able to verbalize safety precautions required.

Community/Home Care

The patient with cirrhosis will always be at risk for ineffective protection unless the disease progression is halted. Once at home, the patient will need to continue to practice safety-enhancing behaviors for bleeding and physical injury. The patient must be vigilant in preventing or controlling bleeding promptly if it occurs, as well as preventing falls. Implementing strategies to protect self from injury that may cause bruising or disruption of skin, such as bumping into objects, is important. This may include rearranging furniture or removing rugs to make walking areas clear. Because the patient with cirrhosis is prone to be dizzy and fatigued due to the effects of the disease, assistance with ambulation or activities requiring mental alertness such as operating machinery or driving may need to be restricted for a period of time. The patient will need to avoid any type of strenuous activities as directed by the physician. Dietary interventions that can assist the patient with energy levels can prevent some of the fatigue caused by blood/RBC loss and subsequent decreased and impaired oxygen transport. Foods rich in iron should be encouraged, considering the patient's likes/dislikes, culture, religion, and dietary restrictions. Because the diet may be rather restricted in protein and lends itself to noncompliance by the patient, it is crucial that the dietician make dietary recommendations only after a thorough consult with the patient and, if possible, a significant other. The patient and family should be taught to eat foods that are rich in vitamin K, such as cabbage, spinach, asparagus, broccoli, liver, and fish. Those treating the patient for cirrhosis should review the patient's medications to ascertain if any could be potentiating the risk for bleeding such as steroidal inhalers, aspirin, or aspirin-containing products, which many people take for cardiovascular prophylaxis or arthritis. All cirrhosis patients should be reminded of simple instructions regarding hygienic practices, including shaving with electric razors, using soft bristled toothbrushes, and using the waxed type of dental floss when flossing. Women should take note of increased bleeding at time of menses each month that can occur due to the loss of clotting factors and impaired absorption of vitamin K. The patient is taught to apply pressure or a bandage to any injury site, regardless of how minor it may appear. If spontaneous bleeding should occur, if bleeding is noted in stools, or if the patient starts to vomit blood, health care assistance should be sought for prompt treatment. The patient with cirrhosis should also inform health care providers such as dentists and podiatrists of the condition so that precautions against bleeding can be taken during any procedures.

Documentation

Include in the chart findings from a thorough assessment of the patient for evidence of bleeding such as bruises, petechiae, bleeding gums, bleeding from access sites, etc. Also chart the presence or absence of bleeding with an estimation of amount. If medical interventions such as esophageal tamponade or injection sclerotherapy are implemented, document these according to agency protocol, as well as all nursing assessments and interventions employed to care for them. Document drainage from any gastric suction, as well as the results of tests for blood done on emesis or stool. All other interventions and patient responses should be included in the patient record as specifically as possible. Blood pressure and pulse readings that indicate cardiac response to bleeding should be documented. Also document the patient's activity level and response to activity (fatigue, dizziness). If teaching is implemented, document who the learners were, what was taught, and their level of understanding.

NURSING DIAGNOSIS 5

DISTURBED THOUGHT PROCESSES (HEPATIC ENCEPHALOPATHY)

Related to:

Buildup of waste products in bloodstream

High levels of serum ammonia

Impaired oxygen diffusion in cerebral tissue

Defining Characteristics:

Confusion

Progressing confusion

Change in level of consciousness

Lethargy

Impaired judgment

Goal:

The patient will be oriented to reality to the extent possible.

Outcome Criteria

✔ The patient will state his or her name.

✔ The patient will state his or her location.

✔ Serum ammonia level will decrease and return to normal.

✔ The patient's cognitive ability will return to baseline.

NOC *Cognition*

Cognitive orientation

Information processing

Decision-making

INTERVENTIONS	RATIONALES
Assess the patient's neurological status and level of cognitive impairment/deficit: level of consciousness, gradually decreasing level of consciousness, lethargy, difficulty speaking (slow), confused, asterixis ("liver flap"), constructional apraxia, irritability, peripheral neuritis, impaired judgment, impaired memory (does not recognize family members), and decreased concentration.	Helps to establish a baseline of the patient's functioning, plan care, and monitor for stabilization or improvement. Patients with high levels of ammonia can progress to hepatic encephalopathy within 24 hours and need to be monitored for subtle changes. Early signs are asterixis (may occur first) and constructional apraxia, personality changes, agitation, difficulty with speech, and restlessness. Confusion occurs as ammonia interferes with oxygen consumption of cerebral tissue and progresses to significant deterioration in orientation.
Refrain from giving medications that are hepatotoxic, such as aspirin, NSAIDs, and acetaminophen.	Helps to preserve as much hepatic function as possible.
Avoid the use of medications that worsen or mask signs of hepatic encephalopathy.	Medications such as narcotics and sedatives are normally detoxified by the liver, but in cirrhosis this process is not effective, leading to increased levels in the blood that can make the condition worse.
Administrator lactulose (Cephulac®), as ordered, three times a day.	Reduces blood ammonia level by drawing ammonia and water from the blood and promoting the excretion of ammonia in stool. Lactulose also changes the fecal flora to organisms that do not produce ammonia from urea. The potassium levels should be monitored because the increased excretion of stool, often in the form of diarrhea, leads to loss of potassium.
Limit protein in the diet.	Ammonia is a by-product of protein metabolism that is normally converted to urea by the liver. With a diseased liver this process is not completed, leading to increased amounts of ammonia. Limiting protein decreases the by-product.
Attempt to orient patient to reality by calling the patient by name and telling him or her where he or she is.	Helps to orient to reality and attempts to prevent confusion.
Maintain consistent caregivers and routines in care, if possible.	Routines enhance the likelihood that the patient will remember what to expect and promote a feeling of security. A consistent caregiver can detect subtle changes in mental status that often go undetected.

NIC *Reality orientation*
Surveillance: Safety

Evaluation

Determine whether the stated outcome criteria have been met. The ammonia level returns to normal, the patient's cognitive function returns to baseline, and the patient returns to usual state of consciousness. The patient should be able to state his or her name and location. Participation in daily activities to maximum capability should be allowed.

Community/Home Care

Once ammonia excretion has occurred and levels return to normal, the patient with cirrhosis will likely have a return to normal cognitive function. During the periods of acute confusion and disorientation, family members may find caring for the patient to be challenging. It is at this time that the family will need to be patient and provide a safe environment for recovery. Making each day routine and creating an environment that is familiar may help the patient's acute confusion. Orienting the patient to reality calmly and firmly will help, but often times it is anxiety-provoking for the patient, as there may be periods of mental clarity during which he or she realizes that "something is not quite right" mentally. The greatest threat to well-being is when the confusion creates issues of safety. Close monitoring of the patient while waiting for resolution of the confusion is required. Family members may need to take turns remaining with the patient or even employ the services of a home health agency. It is crucial that the family continue to administer the lactulose as ordered to reduce the ammonia levels; however, patients frequently want to stop taking the medicine due to the number of stools. The family and significant others will need to remain astute observers in order to detect deteriorating mental alertness and orientation and to implement strategies for immediate return to a health care facility for treatment.

Documentation

Document the findings from a complete neurological/psychological assessment. Include orientation, mental alertness, and neurological deficits, such as asterixis and apraxia or loss of deep tendon reflexes. Be sure to specify what the patient can and cannot do, and the extent of cognitive impairments. Document the administration of lactulose and the patient's response (number of stools). Note all other interventions carried out and improvements in mental state following interventions. Always include in your documentation any teaching done with family or significant others.

NURSING DIAGNOSIS 6

 FATIGUE

Related to:

Disease process

Anemia

Uremia

Defining Characteristics:

Lethargy

Verbalization of tiredness

States a lack of energy

Inability to carry out normal activities without becoming exhausted

Goal:

Fatigue will be relieved.

Outcome Criteria

✔ The patient is able to perform activities of daily living (ADLs).

✔ The patient verbalizes that fatigue has improved or been eliminated.

NOC *Activity tolerance*
Endurance
Energy conservation
Nutritional status:
    Energy

INTERVENTIONS	RATIONALES
Obtain subjective data regarding normal activities, limitations, and nighttime sleep patterns.	Helps to determine the effect fatigue has on normal functioning. Adequate sleep is required for restoration of the body.
Monitor patient for signs of excessive physical and emotional fatigue.	Helps to develop a guideline for adjusting activity.
Encourage periods of rest and activity.	Cirrhosis interferes with synthesis of tissue proteins and utilization of nutrients required for energy; rest is required to decrease metabolic demands and allow for recovery of the liver. Rest conserves oxygen and prevents undue fatigue. Cirrhosis patients often require extended periods of rest or sleep in order to feel rested.
Schedule activities so that excessive demands for oxygen and energy are avoided; for example, space planned activities away from meal times.	Digestion requires energy and oxygen; participation in activities close to meals will cause increased fatigue because of insufficient energy reserves.
Gradually increase activity as tolerated.	The patient will need to progress activity slowly in order to avoid undue demands for oxygen and energy while awaiting a return to normal levels of stamina.
Limit visitors during any periods of acute illness.	Socialization for long periods may cause fatigue.
Increase intake of high-energy foods such as poultry, dried beans and peas, whole grains, and foods high in vitamin C, within restrictions of the recommended diet.	These foods enhance energy metabolism, increase oxygen-carrying capacity, and provide ready sources of energy.
Encourage the patient to plan activities when he or she has the most energy, usually early in the day.	Helps to prevent fatigue.

NIC *Energy management*

Evaluation

Obtain subjective information from the patient regarding the presence of fatigue. The patient should gradually report the ability to participate in ADLs and other normal activities with no fatigue.

Community/Home Care

Patients with cirrhosis should understand that when at home fatigue may persist. Appropriate education on ways to adapt self-care and household activities when the cirrhosis patient is fatigued is paramount. A history should be obtained from the patient regarding the usual routine for ADLs and household chores, so that individualized interventions can be implemented. Attention to what the patient normally does and how the patient wants to make adaptations can only enhance compliance. The nurse must remain aware of cultural backgrounds that may influence a patient's perception of and adaptation to perceived dependency on others. During the period when the liver is attempting to regenerate but is still unable to carry out its detoxification function, fatigue will be more pronounced. The patient must understand how to adjust activity in response to feelings of fatigue, possibly even arranging for rest or nap periods in the afternoon. This may not be a realistic recommendation for some people who may try to continue to work and whose occupations preclude them from napping or even resting during the day. Strategies to enhance nighttime sleep should be implemented so that the patient can get adequate rest. Of particular concern is controlling itching that occurs with jaundice (see nursing diagnosis "Impaired Skin Integrity"). Attention to good nutrition should continue with intake of foods that are good sources of iron, vitamin C, and protein, within dietary restrictions. If fatigue persists for extended periods without the ability to progress activities, the patient may need to seek health care assistance to investigate the possibility of other causes of the fatigue or new treatments.

Documentation

Chart the patient's responses to activities including specific complaints of fatigue and the exact activity the patient was performing when fatigue was noticed. Document interventions implemented to address fatigue, being sure to document food intake. Include in the record the patient's particular verbalization of the degree of fatigue and response to treatment. An assessment of the patient's sleep patterns should also be documented.

CHAPTER 6.82

COLON CANCER

GENERAL INFORMATION

Cancer of the colon is the third most common cancer in the United States and the second most common cause of death from cancer in adults. Most colorectal cancers are slow-growing adenocarcinomas in the epithelial tissue of the colon that develop from adenomatous polyps, and the most common sites are the rectum and sigmoid colon. There are no definitive causes for colon cancer but in addition to polyps, contributing risk factors are thought to be red meat (beef) in the diet, a high-fat diet, a family history of colon cancer (25 percent of cases), and inflammatory bowel disease. Clinical manifestations vary depending upon the location of the tumor. However, the presentation that most often causes the patient to seek health care is rectal bleeding. Other clinical manifestations include a change in stools (diarrhea, constipation, or narrowing of the stool causing narrow pencil-like or ribbon-like stools), cramping, anemia (secondary to blood loss), a palpable mass in the lower right quadrant, and weight loss. Unfortunately, the tumor can grow for a long time before causing noticeable symptoms in the patient. The cancer can spread by direct extension through the bowel mucosa or through the circulatory and lymphatic systems. The most common sites of metastasis are the lungs and the liver. The 5-year survival rate is 90 percent if the disease is detected in its earliest stages; however, for most patients the survival rate is slightly < 50 percent because of late detection. Colon cancer occurs equally among men and women, with 95 percent of cases occurring in people over 50 years of age. The incidence of colon cancer has decreased slightly for white males, but the same decline has not been observed in black males.

NURSING DIAGNOSIS 1

 DEFICIENT KNOWLEDGE

Related to:
New diagnosis of colon cancer
Multiple treatment options
Pre-operative preparation for surgery
Post-operative care
Lack of information

Defining Characteristics:
Asks many questions
Asks no questions
Verbalizes misunderstanding

Goal:
The patient verbalizes an understanding of the operative procedure, pre-operative preparation, and prescribed post-operative regimens.

Outcome Criteria

✔ The patient verbalizes a willingness and desire to learn the necessary information.
✔ The patient verbalizes an understanding of the operative procedure (colon resection).
✔ The patient verbalizes an understanding of chemotherapy and radiation therapy.
✔ The patient verbalizes an understanding of activity restrictions required during convalescence.
✔ The patient will be able to identify signs and symptoms of wound infection.

NOC *Knowledge: Disease process*
Knowledge: Health behavior
Treatment behavior: Illness or injury

INTERVENTIONS	RATIONALES
Assess readiness of the patient to learn (motivation, cognitive level, and physiological status).	The patient must be motivated to learn, have the capability to learn the content, and be free of distractions from learning, such as pain and emotional distress.
Assess what the patient already knows.	The patient may have some knowledge about colon cancer and cancer resection, and teaching should begin with what the patient already knows.
Create a quiet environment conducive to learning.	Environmental noise can prevent the learner from focusing on what is being taught.

Pre-operative:

Collaborate with the physician to teach the patient and family the following information about the disease process of colon cancer and required interventions: — Normal function of the colon — Pathophysiology of colon cancer to include signs and symptoms — Diagnostic tests: carcinoembryonic antigen (CEA) and colonoscopy with biopsy — Staging of the disease — Surgical treatments (first choice): colon resection with or without colostomy — Preparations required for surgery: intravenous (IV) fluids, evacuation of bowel with laxatives or enemas, clear liquids, then nothing orally (NPO) — Chemotherapy and radiation for palliative care or rectal cancer — Complete blood count (CBC) (to detect anemia caused by bleeding) — Computed tomography (CT) scans to locate or rule out metastasis	Understanding of normal function and pathophysiology helps the patient to understand the rationales for therapeutic interventions. Knowledge of diagnostic tests, treatments required, and prevention of complications empowers the patient to take control and be compliant.
Instruct the patient about colonoscopy. — Clear liquid diet the day prior to the exam — Withholding all food and liquid for 8 hours before procedure — Bowel preparation of a strong laxative 12 hours before the	Teaching before the test decreases anxiety and prepares the patient for what to expect.

exam and on the morning of the exam
— Signed informed consent required
— Sedative and intravenous fluids required during the procedure

Instruct patient about radiation: — Method of action — Course/duration of treatment, usually 5 treatments each week for 6 weeks — Skin changes to note include redness, sloughing, and tenderness — Skin care: Do not apply soap, ointments, lotions, creams, or powder to area. Do not rub, scrub or scratch the area; do not try to wash off markings; avoid exposing the treated area to the sun during the treatment and for 1 year following treatments. — Wear loose-fitting clothes; tight-fitting pants and undergarments are uncomfortable and probably should be avoided.	Radiation is used as an adjunct with surgery. It can be used before surgery to shrink the tumors to make resection easier. This is especially true for cancers of the rectum. The radiated skin is sensitive, and lotions, creams, ultraviolet rays, rubbing, etc., may cause burning and skin sloughing, and interfere with radiation. The patient must know how to protect the skin from impairment, and knowing what to expect in terms of radiation helps the patient to be more compliant and feel more in control.
Teach patient and family about chemotherapy and its effects: — Method of action — Specific agents used for treatment — Alopecia: Assist the patient to plan for hair loss by investigating purchasing of wigs (females) or having hair cut short and using hair for a specially made wig or men could shave their heads before the onset of alopecia; find a resource that could teach women how to prepare fashionable head wraps. — Nausea/vomiting: Teach prophylactic use of anti-emetics before meals; avoid foods with strong odors; in the hospital setting, have lids removed from trays outside the room (when lids are removed from food trays the smell is often overwhelming to the gastrointestinal [GI]	Knowledge of what to expect helps the patient cope with untoward side effects and better equips him or her to take responsibility for managing the illness and engaging in self-care.

(continues)

(continued)

INTERVENTIONS	RATIONALES
system and causes nausea); attempt frequent small meals, avoiding spicy foods. — Care of access sites: prevention of infection by use of aseptic techniques and procedures according to agency protocol — Control of fatigue: balance of rest and activity; on chemotherapy days a designated naptime should be scheduled — Prevention of infection: chemotherapy causes a depression of white blood cells (WBCs), predisposing the patient to infection; avoid people with infections and large crowds; practice good hand hygiene; know WBC counts	
Teach the patient how to turn, cough, and deep breathe (TCDB) and how to use the incentive spirometer (IS), if ordered.	Patients with abdominal incisions tend to breathe shallowly due to pain at incision site, TCDB and incentive spirometry are required to open airways, improve oxygenation, and prevent atelectasis; these exercises will be required postoperatively.
Post-operative: Teach the patient activity restrictions following colon resection, as ordered, but in general — Do not lift any objects heavier than 5 pounds. — Refrain from strenuous activities such as hard physical labor, aerobics, horseback riding, jogging. — No driving for at least 4 to 6 weeks, or as prescribed by physician. — Ambulate as tolerated. — Splint incision when coughing, moving, or ambulating.	Helps to protect the surgical site.
Teach the patient basic wound care and infection control measures required during the post-operative periods: — Keep incision clean and dry.	Due to the short hospital stay following colon resection, the patient may be at home when post-operative infections occur, so it is crucial that the patient
— If dressing is applied, change using aseptic technique; wash hands thoroughly before performing incision care or touching the wound. — Monitor for signs of infection at incision site and drain insertion site: warmth, redness/discoloration, purulent drainage, increased pain. — Monitor temperature for elevations. — Report signs and symptoms of infection to health care provider.	know what to look for that would signal onset of infections; understanding the rationale for these interventions will enhance the patient's willingness to comply with limitations.
Teach the patient and family about care of the colostomy, if present.	Some patients with colorectal cancer may be left with a permanent or temporary colostomy. The patient and one other person needs to learn all aspects of care (see nursing care plan "Fecal Diversions/Ostomies").
Teach the patient about diet required: no oral intake until bowel function returns as evidenced by flatulence and bowel sounds, then consume a diet that is high calorie, high protein, and rich in vitamin C.	In the early post-operative period, no oral intake is allowed until bowel function has returned. Once allowed, nutrition should include foods that are high in calories, protein, and vitamin C, which are needed for healing and energy.
If surgery has not been curative, provide patient and family with information on hospice and other community service agencies, such as the American Cancer Society.	These agencies can assist with durable medical equipment, in-home care providers, support, and other services when needed.
Assess the patient's and family's understanding of all teaching by encouraging them to repeat information and ask questions as needed.	This allows the nurse to hear in the patient's own words what was taught and makes it easier to know what information may need to be reinforced to enhance compliance.
Establish that the patient has the resources required to be compliant, such as transportation to follow-up appointments, any chemotherapy treatments, and radiation therapy ordered.	If needed resources such as finances and transportation to follow-up appointments are not available, the patient cannot be compliant; the nurse will need to make necessary referrals. This may be a real problem for patients from remote and rural areas, especially if family support is not available.
Give the patient written information.	Provides reference at a later time, and for review.

NIC *Teaching: Disease process*
Teaching: Individual

Evaluation

The patient is able to repeat the information for the nurse and asks questions about the operative procedure (colon resection), diagnostic tests, other treatment modalities (chemotherapy and radiation), and possible outcomes. Prior to discharge, the patient verbalizes an understanding of the activity restrictions and agrees to be compliant. The patient is able to demonstrate to the nurse how to splint the incision when breathing and moving, how to perform deep-breathing exercises, and how to use the IS, and is able to identify measures to relieve pain. Signs and symptoms of infection can be accurately stated. The patient is able to demonstrate proper techniques for caring for the colostomy if present. The patient should be able to identify signs and symptoms that would indicate a need to seek health care assistance.

Community/Home Care

The possibility for the knowledge deficit to persist following hospitalization is very real due to the large volume of information the patient needs. The patient with colon cancer has pre-operative needs that have been resolved once surgery is complete. However, following treatment for colon cancer with surgery, chemotherapy or radiation follow-up is required. For the patient who is being treated with surgery alone, the in-home care focuses on healing of the surgical wound and preventing post-operative complications, such as pneumonia and deep vein thrombosis (DVT), through early ambulation and activity. In addition, if the patient has a colostomy, in-home follow-up is needed to be sure that the patient or family member is able to care for the colostomy (see nursing care plan "Fecal Diversions/Ostomies"). The patient will need to monitor self for onset of wound infections and respiratory complications such as pneumonia. Evaluation of the patient's knowledge level should be ascertained prior to discharge. The patient may need further teaching once at home, especially as it relates to continuing treatments such as chemotherapy or radiation. The nurse should ensure that the patient understands what has happened during the hospitalization and what to expect once at home. Written literature and instructions should be given to the patient in a colorful, easily identifiable folder or envelope. The patient should be encouraged to place the information in a common, easily accessible place in the home. Follow-up with a health care provider focuses on assurance that no complications have occurred, that wounds are healing as expected, that chemotherapy and radiation are progressing, and that the patient has no complications.

Documentation

Document all content taught and the patient's verbalization of understanding. Specific attention should be given to documentation of any particular concerns that the patient expresses. Include in the documentation the patient's willingness to comply with all recommendations made about chemotherapy, radiation therapy, wound care, colostomy care, and activity restrictions. Any area that requires further teaching should be clearly indicated in the record. Include in the record appointments that have been made for outpatient treatments and procedures as well. Always include the titles of any printed literature given to the patient for reinforcement.

NURSING DIAGNOSIS 2

 ACUTE PAIN

Related to:

Distention of abdomen

Post-operative abdominal incision

Defining Characteristics:

Complaint of abdominal pain

Grimacing

Holding abdomen

Goal:

Pain is reduced or relieved.

Outcome Criteria

✔ The patient will state pain is relieved 30 minutes after interventions.

✔ The patient makes no nonverbal signs of pain, such as grimacing.

NOC *Pain level*
Pain control
Comfort level

INTERVENTIONS	RATIONALES
Assess pain, character, location, severity, and duration; use a pain rating scale.	Pain assessment can provide clues about diagnosis, and be used to determine treatment required.
Assist to position of comfort.	Patients may be more comfortable in a side-lying position.
Administer analgesics as ordered and monitor for side effects.	Narcotics are usually ordered for the early post-operative period for pain relief, and could include meperidine (Demerol) or morphine via patient-controlled analgesia (PCA).
Administer analgesics prior to ambulation and TCDB exercises.	Helps to decrease incisional pain with activity and increase likelihood that the patient will participate in therapies.
Have patient splint incision when moving.	Helps to provide support to the incision and decrease pain.
Encourage use of alternative methods of pain relief such as relaxation techniques, music therapy, massage, distraction, and guided imagery.	These strategies can enhance the effectiveness of analgesics.
Evaluate the effectiveness of all interventions.	Helps to determine patient satisfaction with pain control or whether revisions to the planned interventions are required.

Evaluation

The patient is able to report that the pain has been reduced or alleviated following interventions. The degree to which the patient is able to assist in the management of the pain through anxiety reduction and relaxation techniques is assessed. The patient should have no observable signs of discomfort.

Community/Home Care

The patient's pain should be temporary and resolve following healing of the surgical wound. Pain at home is usually managed with mild analgesics, and the duration of pain should be short. Use of non-pharmacological measures such as guided imagery, relaxation techniques, and music should be encouraged. The nurse should stress to the patient that weak respiratory efforts because of pain could cause respiratory problems such as pneumonia. Encourage the patient to use a small pillow to splint the incision when moving or coughing to decrease the

discomfort. If the pain worsens at home, the patient should contact the health care provider to determine other causes for the pain; most often increased pain signals a wound infection. If the recommended analgesics are not working, the patient should seek follow-up care with the health care provider. For some patients, colon cancer may be advanced at time of diagnosis, and surgery is only palliative, necessitating that a new approach to pain control be taken due to the progressive and persistent nature of cancer pain. In this case, a pain specialist or in-home nurse may be required to assist the patient with pain control.

Documentation

Document in the patient's own words the description of the pain and rating of the level of pain. Chart all interventions employed and the patient's responses, particularly the level of pain following interventions. Include in the documentation assessments made relevant to the pain and to the respiratory system. Chart medications on the medication administration record according to the agency guidelines.

NURSING DIAGNOSIS 3

 IMPAIRED SKIN INTEGRITY

Related to:
   Surgical procedures (colon resection)
   Presence of drains
   Colostomy

Defining Characteristics:
   Surgical incision with staples or sutures
   Puncture wounds for drainage devices
   Excoriation around colostomy

Goal:
   Incision heals without complications.
   Infection is prevented or eliminated.

Outcome Criteria

✔ The incision is well approximated.

✔ The patient's surgical site has no redness/discoloration, purulent drainage, or heat.

✔ Skin around colostomy is not excoriated.

✔ The patient remains afebrile.

✔ White blood cell (WBC) count remains within normal limits.

NOC *Wound healing: Primary intention*

INTERVENTIONS ·	RATIONALES
Monitor surgical site and any drainage tube insertion sites for signs and symptoms of infection: redness/discoloration, swelling, purulent drainage, poor approximation, heat, increased pain.	Early identification of poor wound healing or infection can expedite treatment and prevent damage to surgical site.
Maintain patency of any drainage devices by monitoring for kinks and assess drainage for amount, color, and consistency.	The drainage device helps prevent accumulation of drainage from surgical site; drainage may be bloody initially, but should become serosanguineous. The drainage is a medium for bacteria growth, and yellow, thick drainage may signal infection.
Monitor for elevation of WBCs and for increased immature WBCs (bands, known as a shift to the left).	Infection causes increased WBCs and increased immature WBCs to be released from the bone marrow into the blood.
Take temperature every 4 hours.	Fever is caused by pyrogens, which are produced by infecting microorganisms, and is a classic indicator of infection.
Assess for abdominal distention and rigidity.	Distention could signal peritonitis or gas due to decreased peristalsis. Either can cause stress on suture lines that can cause dehiscence with a greater risk for infection.
Administer antibiotics as ordered, IV or orally (PO).	Helps to reduce the number of infective organisms and eliminate or prevent infection; antibiotics may be given prophylactically.
Change dressings on incision and over drainage tube insertion sites, as ordered. Cleanse area using sterile technique, cleansing site of drainage devices last.	Maintenance of a clean incisional site decreases number of organisms and reduces chance of infection.
If patient has a colostomy, implement strategies to care for skin around the area as directed by enterostomal therapist (see nursing care plan "Fecal Diversions/Ostomies").	Enzymes in stool can be harmful to the skin surrounding a colostomy.
Administer antipyretics (acetaminophen [Tylenol]), as ordered.	Helps to reduce fever.
Encourage adequate nutritional intake, especially of protein, vitamin C, and iron.	Adequate nutrient intake, especially of vitamin C, protein, and iron, is required for healing and tissue repair.

NIC *Incision site care*
Infection control
Nutrition management
Wound care
Wound care: Closed drainage

Evaluation

Evaluate the degree to which the outcome criteria have been met. The surgical site should be intact, healing by primary intention with incision well approximated. Redness, swelling, purulent drainage, and heat should be absent from the site. The puncture sites for any drainage devices are also free of signs and symptoms of infection. Drainage from the drainage devices such as a Jackson Pratt (JP) (if present) should be serosanguineous and should be decreasing in amount. The patient should be afebrile, and WBC counts should return to normal.

Community/Home Care

The status of the surgical site may remain a problem after the patient has been discharged home and will need to be assessed for continued healing. Incisional care will need to be taught to the patient (see nursing diagnosis "Deficient Knowledge"). The patient may need to wear loose-fitting clothes over incision lines for a period of time to prevent irritation to the site. The risk for infection remains, and the family will need to know what symptoms may signal the onset of infection. The patient must practice good hand hygiene at all times and realize that even normal bacteria can cause infection in open wounds. The patient should be aware of signs of infection and indications of wound dehiscence. The patient can use a handheld mirror to get a better view of the incision and should be encouraged to assess the incision daily. The importance of completing any ordered medications, such as antibiotics, once at home should be stressed. If any evidence of poor wound healing or infection should occur, the patient should be instructed to contact the health care provider promptly. The patient will need to understand the importance of good nutrition in complete wound healing and recovery. Small meals may be needed initially, as the patient has a period of no oral intake (NPO), and the patient will need to experiment with what is tolerated, understanding that nutrition plays a critical role in healing.

Documentation

Document assessment findings from the wound, including the presence of sutures or staples, wound approximation, skin color, and amount, color, and odor of any drainage from the wound or drainage devices. Be sure to note any sign of infection. Chart the output from drainage devices in the intake and output record. Vital signs are documented according to agency protocol as ordered for post-operative patients. Include in the patient record all interventions implemented for wound care and prevention of infections.

NURSING DIAGNOSIS 4

IMPAIRED BOWEL ELIMINATION*

Related to:

> Post-operative ileus
>
> Surgical interventions (creation of fecal diversion)
>
> New way of eliminating stool

Defining Characteristics:

> Presence of ostomy on abdominal wall
>
> Absence of bowel sounds or passing of flatulence

Goal:

> Adequate bowel elimination will be maintained.

Outcome Criteria

✔ Bowel elimination will occur daily.

✔ Bowel sounds will be present in all four quadrants of the abdomen.

✔ The patient will pass gas (flatulence).

✔ There will be no constipation or diarrhea (colostomy).

✔ There will be no leakage of liquid stool from collection bag (ileostomy).

NOC *Bowel elimination*

INTERVENTIONS	RATIONALES
Assess for the return of bowel sounds in all quadrants.	The patient who has had surgical interventions for colon cancer may have slowed peristalsis due to anesthesia and manipulation of the intestines. Confirmation that bowel function has resumed is necessary prior to offering oral intake. Bowel sounds indicate a return of peristalsis.
Monitor for the passage of flatus.	Flatus is another indicator of return of bowel function.
Carefully assess for first stool post-operatively.	Occasionally, a paralytic ileus will occur post-operatively. For those patients who have had fecal diversions, it can routinely be expected that an ileostomy will begin to drain within 24 hours and a colostomy will usually discharge feces within 48 hours
Maintain NPO status, as ordered, until bowel function has returned.	Without bowel function/ peristalsis, the bowels are unable to handle food waste products or fluids, and the patient is likely to become nauseated.
If the patient has an ostomy, implement strategies for its care and monitor output from the diversion: color, consistency, and amount (see nursing care plan "Fecal Diversions/Ostomies").	Output must be monitored for early detection of any obstruction that could cause distention and subsequent leakage at the anastomosis site.
Encourage the intake of 1200–1500 ml of oral fluid, when allowed.	Helps to prevent constipation.
Encourage the patient to eat a diet with adequate amounts of fiber and bulk.	The consistency of the stool will be determined by the amount of roughage and fiber in the diet and by the amount of fluid intake; promotes bowel elimination and prevents constipation.
When oral intake is allowed, encourage the patient to avoid foods such as cabbage, beans, carbonated drinks, and dairy products in the early post-operative period.	These foods cause increased flatus that can cause distention of the abdomen and increase pain and stress on incision site.
Ambulate the patient on the first post-operative day, or as ordered.	Activity enhances the return of peristalsis.

Evaluation

The patient achieves bowel elimination through normal routes or the ostomy. The patient has bowel sounds in all four quadrants and is passing flatus. There is no evidence of a paralytic ileus and no constipation or diarrhea occurs. For the patient with an ileostomy, fluid balance is maintained.

Community/Home Care

Establishing the normal pattern of bowel elimination following bowel surgery may remain an issue once at home. Because of manipulation of the bowel, NPO status, and a slow start to taking oral foods, bowel movements may take longer to resume. If no colostomy has been created and the patient requires no further treatment (chemotherapy or radiation) for colon cancer, normal bowel function will return quickly following return of peristalsis. However, the patient needs to consume an adequate diet rich in bulk and fiber to ensure that bowel regularity occurs without straining or the use of laxatives. The patient should include fresh fruit and vegetables in the diet on a daily basis and will need to drink adequate amounts of fluid to promote bowel elimination and prevent constipation. In the absence of cardiac disease, the patient should attempt to drink 1200–1500 ml of fluid per day, avoiding large amounts of caffeine but including generous amounts of water. Drinking prune juice or apple juice, especially with breakfast, may also be enough to stimulate evacuation. The patient needs to be attentive to how often he or she is having bowel movements so that constipation can be prevented. Constipation may cause distention in a tender post-operative abdomen that can place stress on the suture line. For the patient who has a colostomy, one of the biggest challenges for the patient when discharge is eminent is the uncertainty of managing the new method for bowel elimination (see nursing care plan "Fecal Diversions/Ostomies"). Even though teaching has occurred during hospitalization, the patient may experience some anxiety when faced with independently caring for the colostomy. Therefore, for most patients in-home nursing visits are highly desirable to monitor the patient's ability to perform procedures correctly and to enhance the comfort level with the fecal diversion. At home, the patient will need to be mindful of amount of output from the colostomy in order to detect early any signs of obstruction. The patient needs to understand the importance of returning for a follow-up visit that may include having x-rays/scans done to rule out metastasis and, for patients with a fecal diversion, to ensure the integrity of the anastomosis and proper functioning of the ostomy.

Documentation

Chart the achievement of stated outcome criteria and all interventions employed by the nurse to achieve them. Document the status of any drainage devices as well as the color, amount, and consistency of drainage. Always chart when the colostomy or ileostomy begins to function, and describe the color and amount of the stool. Any referrals made are included in the patient record. Visits by the wound or ostomy nurse are documented.

NURSING DIAGNOSIS 5

INEFFECTIVE COPING

Related to:

> Diagnosis of colon cancer
>
> Fear of dying
>
> Fear of poor prognosis

Defining Characteristics:

> Anger
>
> Expressions of fear
>
> Restlessness and anxiety
>
> Crying
>
> Expresses distress at potential loss
>
> Tachycardia
>
> Numerous questions

Goal:

> Anxiety is decreased or alleviated.

Outcome Criteria

✔ The patient identifies one coping mechanism to be used.

✔ The patient verbalizes fears and concerns.

✔ The patient reports being less anxious.

✔ The patient demonstrates no outward signs of anxiety, such as restlessness or agitation.

NOC *Grief resolution*
Anxiety control
Comfort level
Coping

INTERVENTIONS	RATIONALES
Assess level of anxiety (mild, moderate, severe); have patient rate on a scale of 1 to 10, with 10 being the greatest.	Gives the nurse an objective measure of the extent of any anxiety.
Assess the patient to determine feelings about the diagnosis of colon cancer and the patient's prognosis, and support the patient and family as appropriate by answering questions and making referrals.	Assisting the patient and family to deal with the diagnosis and prognosis will enhance their ability to cope with serious illness.
In collaboration with the physician, engage patient and family in an open dialogue about options for treatment and care.	Discussion of treatment options with the patient and family allows the patient to make informed decisions. It also allows the patient to deal with reality. If the disease is in an advanced stage, the family and patient need to begin to discuss the projected outcomes and care required in the final stages of disease. Discussing this early allows the patient to exert more control and gives him or her a sense of empowerment that may assist in coping with the disease.
Keep the patient informed of all that is going on, including information about diagnostic tests, planned treatments (surgery, chemotherapy, radiation in advanced disease), and therapeutic interventions.	Being knowledgeable about care and treatment may help to relieve fear and anxiety.
Use a calm, reassuring manner with the patient, recognizing that anger and misplaced feelings are common.	Gives the patient a sense of well-being.
Encourage the patient to verbalize fears, concerns, and expressions of grief; listen attentively.	Verbalization of fears contributes to dealing with concerns; being attentive relays empathy to the patient.
Encourage the patient to identify one successful coping strategy previously used and encourage its use, or have the patient to engage in relaxation techniques such as guided imagery, music therapy, or meditation. Teach new strategies as required.	The patient needs to utilize methods to relax and reduce anxiety that will assist in coping with a diagnosis of colon cancer. When the patient is newly diagnosed with serious illness, new, more intensive coping strategies may need to be learned and implemented.
Control multiple sources of stimuli that could cause sensory overload.	Overstimulation can worsen anxiety, and in many instances, the patient needs quiet time to think about what has been said in order to decrease anxiety.
Recognize the role of culture in the patient's method of coping, grieving a loss, and verbalization of fears and concerns.	Culture often dictates how a person grieves, and the nurse must recognize this in order to support the patient in a successful grief or loss process.
Seek spiritual consult as needed or requested by the patient and or family.	Meeting the patient's spiritual needs helps him or her to deal with fears through use of spiritual or religious rituals.
Provide the patient and family with information about advance directives and support decisions made.	Allows the patient and family the opportunity to plan for the patient's wishes in the event he or she becomes incompetent to make own decisions.

NIC *Anxiety reduction*
Grief work facilitation
Coping enhancement
Emotional support
Spiritual support

Evaluation

Evaluate the extent to which the outcome criteria have been achieved. The patient should be assessed for behaviors that would indicate adjustment to the diagnosis of colon cancer. The patient should verbalize fears and concerns and be able to identify one way to cope with the diagnosis of cancer. The extent to which the patient displays successful coping behaviors should be noted. In addition, the patient is able to discuss the planned treatment options. If the patient is unable to talk about the diagnosis and communicate concerns, the nurse should explore further interventions to assist the patient.

Community/Home Care

Nurses should assess which coping mechanisms work for the patient and encourage their use by the patient at home. If the patient has had surgery with a full cure anticipated, anxiety may resolve once the surgery is complete and the prognosis validated. However, for the patient with advanced disease at time of diagnosis, problems with anxiety and grieving may continue for a long period of time, and follow-up by a health care provider can detect ineffective coping. The family should be taught to recognize acceptable and non-acceptable strategies for coping. Extreme self-isolation and depression sometimes occur and should be noted and reported to a health care provider. It is crucial that the nurse and family support the patient as needed to foster a healthy psychological state, recognizing that anger and denial are common. As the disease progresses, the patient may require new strategies for coping with the disease and the anticipated loss of life. The patient's culture may dictate how he or she handles anxiety-provoking situations and grieves, and with whom he or she shares this process. For many patients and families, spiritual/religious rituals provide a means of coping with difficult stressful situations. The patient may benefit from quiet periods of meditation during the day. Support to other family members in the home will be important, as they too need to be supported in a grief process. For colon cancer patients in the later stages of uncured disease, hospice can play an important role in the home situation through provision of counselors, chaplains, and in-home care providers. If questions should arise at home about the patient's health status or prescribed regimen, the patient should have a means of contact with a health care provider for answers.

Documentation

The degree to which the patient has developed and utilized effective coping strategies should be documented in the patient record. Chart the degree of anxiety the patient is experiencing. A rating system provides an objective way to relay to others the extent of the anxiety. Document whether the patient is able to discuss feelings about a diagnosis of colon cancer and its treatment. Chart the patient's verbalizations as stated, and include in the record findings from an assessment of the patient's psychological state, including any indicators of depression, anger, crying, or sadness. Document any referrals made to hospice or religious leaders.

CHAPTER 6.83

ENDOSCOPY: ESOPHAGOGASTRODUODENOSCOPY (EGD), ENDOSCOPIC RETROGRADE CHOLANGIOPANCREATOGRAPHY (ERCP), COLONOSCOPY

GENERAL INFORMATION

Endoscopy is a procedure that allows for the direct visualization of certain gastrointestinal (GI) structures for diagnostic and treatment purposes via a flexible lighted scope. Some of its uses include routine screenings for cancer, obtaining specimens for biopsy, diagnosis of cancer or other GI diseases, removal of polyps, control of GI bleeding, removal of stones, and dilation of the esophagus. The scope is passed through the mouth as far as the duodenum, and in the case of the endoscopic retrograde cholangiopancreatography (ERCP), a special scope can be used to reach as far as the ampulla of Vater. A colonoscopy involves passing of the scope through the rectum for examination of the entire colon. Patient preparation for these tests will vary slightly, depending on specific physician and agency requirements, but in general all patients are kept NPO (nothing by mouth) for at least 8 hours prior to the tests, require cleansing with laxatives and/or enemas and a clear liquid diet the day before the exam. The test requires a signed consent form, and during the test, the patient is given conscious sedation.

NURSING DIAGNOSIS 1

 DEFICIENT KNOWLEDGE

Related to:

GI diagnostic tests

Defining Characteristics:

Preparation required for diagnostic tests

Asks many questions

Asks no questions

Verbalizes unfamiliarity with procedure (EGD, ERCP, or colonoscopy)

Goal:

The patient verbalizes an understanding of the diagnostic procedure.

Outcome Criteria

✔ The patient will state the purpose of the procedure.

✔ The patient will verbalize an understanding of the preparation required for the procedure (EGD, ERCP, colonoscopy).

✔ The patient will verbalize an understanding of the interventions required following the procedures.

NOC *Knowledge: Health behavior*

INTERVENTIONS	RATIONALES
Assess the readiness and willingness of the patient to learn (motivation, cognitive level, and physiological status).	The patient must be motivated to learn, have the capability to learn the content, and be free of distractions from learning, such as pain and emotional distress.
Create a quiet environment for learning.	Environmental noise can prevent the learner from focusing on what is being taught.
Assess what the patient already knows.	The patient may have some knowledge about the procedures, and teaching should begin with what the patient already knows.

INTERVENTIONS	RATIONALES
Start with the simplest information first and proceed to more complex information.	Presenting simple concepts as a building block makes more difficult concepts easier to understand.
Teach the patient the following information about EGD and ERCP: **Pre-procedure** — No food or liquids can be taken after midnight the day before the examination (a minimum of 8 hours without food is required). — Intravenous (IV) access will be initiated. — Conscious sedation (such as Versed®, Valium) will be given IV. — Informed consent is required. — Test will last approximately 30 minutes. — The patient may have a feeling of fullness during the procedure. **Post-procedure** — No food or fluid is permitted until gag reflex has returned (approximately 2–4 hours). — Throat lozenges can be taken for sore throat. — Vital signs will be taken every 15 minutes for an hour and then as ordered by physician; blood pressure may be lower than baseline. — Gas or burping is normal.	The patient needs to understand what to expect before, during, and after the procedure. This helps allay anxiety and enhances compliance with restrictions.
Teach the patient the following information about colonoscopy: **Pre-procedure** — Signed informed consent required. — Clear liquid diet is required the day prior to the exam. — Do not take blood thinners, aspirin, or NSAIDs containing aspirin for 1 week prior to the test. — Withhold all food and liquid for 8 hours before procedure. — Bowel preparation of a strong laxative (Fleet® Phospho®-soda) is needed 12 hours before the exam, or between 7 p.m. and 10 p.m., as instructed by the physician. Place in cool water or other clear liquid. Repeat on the morning of the exam,	Teaching before the test decreases anxiety and prepares the patient for what to expect before, during, and after the test.

usually 4 hours before the scheduled time of the procedure, as instructed. Supplement with water, as instructed by physician.
— Sedative will be given before the test, and IV fluids are required during the procedure.
— Arrange for someone to transport the patient home following the procedure.
Post-procedure
— Assess vital signs every 15 minutes immediately following procedure, or as ordered.
— Passing of gas will occur.
— The patient may have mild abdominal pain.
— Cramping may occur.
— If biopsy obtained or polyps removed, the patient may have slight rectal bleeding for approximately 2 days.
— Have patient observe self for excessive bleeding (stool or free bleeding).
— Patient may not operate machinery or drive following the procedure, as instructed.

Encourage the patient to ask questions about the procedures.	The patient needs the opportunity to have all questions answered prior to the test and after the completion of the exam.
Teach the patient the signs and symptoms of complications. For colonoscopy, observe for bleeding, severe abdominal pain or cramping, rigid abdomen, abdominal distention, fever, and pain in rectal area; for EGD, observe for vomiting of blood, epigastric pain, abdominal pain, shortness of breath, difficulty swallowing, and persistent hoarseness; for ERCP, monitor for the same signs as for EGD, as well as nausea and vomiting.	These symptoms could signal perforation of a portion of the GI tract, damage to the bronchial tree, or damage to muscles required for swallowing. Following ERCP, pancreatitis may occur, manifested by abdominal pain accompanied by nausea and vomiting.
Assess the patient's and family's understanding of the content taught by encouraging them to ask questions and to repeat the information.	Helps to determine whether the patient has sufficient information to be compliant, and allows the nurse to hear in the patient's own words what was taught and makes it easier to know what information to reinforce.

(continues)

(continued)

INTERVENTIONS	RATIONALES
Give the patient written information.	Provides reference as the patient prepares for the test and following the procedure.

NIC   *Learning readiness enhancement*
Learning facilitation
Teaching: Individual

Evaluation

Determine whether outcome criteria have been met. The patient can state the purpose of the scheduled test. In addition, the patient or family should verbalize an understanding of the preparation required for the test (colonoscopy, EGD, or ERCP) and care required following the procedure.

Community/Home Care

Many patients have endoscopy procedures performed on an outpatient basis and are responsible for their own care before and after the procedure. Following the procedure, in-home care focuses on being able to recognize signs and symptoms of complications such as perforations or pancreatitis (ERCP). The patient should be instructed to report severe abdominal pain or cramping to a health care provider immediately, as this may signal a perforation. Some slight bleeding from the rectal area is expected for a couple of days if the patient has had a biopsy or removal of polyps, but any free bleeding that becomes excessive needs immediate attention. For this reason, all stools should be observed for the presence of blood, as this could indicate perforation in the colon. If the patient experiences hoarseness or a sore throat, he or she can use a saltwater preparation, or commercial lozenges or anesthetic mouth washes, for relief. Driving is prohibited immediately following the procedure due the effects of the sedative or other medications, but is allowed on the next day. If no complications are noted, the patient can resume all activities within 24 hours. The patient should have written instructions about what signs and symptoms to report and whom to call in the event of an emergency.

Documentation

Document the specific content taught and the patient's and family's verbalization of understanding.

If the patient has any concerns, include these in the patient record with an indication that the patient is willing to carry out the instructions as given. Chart in the patient's record the scheduled appointment and titles of any written instructions given to the patient.

NURSING DIAGNOSIS 2

 RISK FOR ASPIRATION

Related to:
    Application of anesthetic to back of throat
    Conscious sedation
    Absence of gag reflex
    Inability to swallow easily

Defining Characteristics:
    None

Goal:
    The patient will not aspirate.

Outcome Criteria

✔ The patient will not cough during eating or drinking.
✔ Breath sounds will be clear.
✔ The patient will verbalize an understanding of the need to be NPO for 2–4 hours.

NOC   *Aspiration control*

INTERVENTIONS	RATIONALES
Following EGD or ERCP, place patient in a position with head slightly elevated or in semi-Fowler's position.	Helps to promote comfort and to prevent aspiration of natural secretions.
Keep patient NPO for 2–4 hours, or as ordered.	Anesthetics used during the procedure take away the natural gag reflex and swallowing mechanism.
Assess for the return of the gag reflex by swabbing the side of the mouth or back of the throat with a tongue blade or asking the patient to swallow.	Anesthetics used to numb the throat alleviate the gag reflex and swallowing mechanism.

INTERVENTIONS	RATIONALES
Assess respiratory status, including breath sounds, respiratory rate, depth, quality, and oxygen saturation.	Medications used for conscious sedation can cause respiratory depression, especially for patients who have had an EGD or ERCP. This delays the return of the gag reflex or cough mechanism.
Monitor patient for return of usual state of consciousness.	Sedatives are given IV and cause the patient to remain drowsy in the immediate post-procedure period. The patient needs to be fully awake prior to taking food or fluids.
When the gag reflex returns, offer clear liquids first, followed by soft foods.	Helps to ensure that the patient can swallow prior to initiating solid foods; soft foods provide for easy swallowing, especially if the patient has a sore throat.
Monitor for dysphagia.	Difficulty swallowing may predispose the patient to aspiration and could signal complications of the procedure.
Encourage the patient to expectorate fluids that accumulate in the oral cavity.	Helps to prevent aspiration of secretions during the time the gag reflex is diminished.

NIC *Aspiration precautions*

Evaluation

Following an EGD or ERCP, the patient has no aspiration. The gag reflex returns within 2–4 hours, and the patient is able to resume oral liquids without coughing or experiencing difficulty swallowing. Breath sounds remain clear to auscultation.

Community/Home Care

If the patient is hospitalized when the procedure is performed, there will be no lasting effects to necessitate special in-home care for risk for aspiration. When the procedure is done as an outpatient, prior to discharge from the outpatient center the patient must receive instruction on what to expect in terms of resuming intake (see nursing diagnosis "Deficient Knowledge"). The patient will need to maintain the NPO status until able to swallow easily, usually within 4 hours. At this point, the patient should start with clear liquids and progress to soft foods that are easy to swallow. The patient is instructed to stop all intake if he or she coughs or has any difficulty at

all with swallowing. Warm fluids or soft foods are more palatable and will be tolerated better, especially if the patient has complaints of a sore throat. Once at home, if the patient has continued difficulty swallowing and is unable to resume oral intake, the health care provider should be contacted.

Documentation

Chart the results of an assessment following the EGD or ERCP procedure. Document the presence or absence of the gag reflex and the patient's ability to swallow. Any complaints about the ability to swallow are also charted. When the patient takes fluid for the first time, document this in the record. The specific content of any teaching done with the patient on home care should be charted.

NURSING DIAGNOSIS 3

 ACUTE PAIN

Related to:
> Passage of scope for EGD or ERCP
> Passage of scope and insertion of air during colonoscopy
> Complications of perforation

Defining Characteristics:
> Complaints of abdominal pain
> Complaints of abdominal cramping
> Abdominal distention
> Firm rigid appearance to abdomen
> Complaints of sore throat
> Complaints of sore anal area

Goal:
> The patient's pain will be relieved.

Outcome Criteria

✔ The patient will report no abdominal pain or cramping.
✔ The patient will state that the throat is not sore.
✔ The patient will report relief from anal discomfort.
✔ The patient will verbalize an understanding of the need to report severe pain following procedures.
✔ The patient verbalizes relief of discomfort 30 minutes following interventions.

NOC *Pain level*
Pain control
Comfort level

INTERVENTIONS	RATIONALES
Assess for location, intensity, quality, and duration of pain.	Identifying these will assist in accurate diagnosis and treatment; most patients who have endoscopy procedures experience very little pain. Severe pain or persistent pain may signal a perforation.
Have patient rate pain or discomfort intensity using a pain rating scale.	Provides a more objective description of level of pain.
Assess for a distended, rigid abdomen.	A distended, rigid abdomen accompanied by abdominal pain may indicate a perforation.
Administer mild analgesics, as ordered.	Helps to relieve discomfort.
Assist to position of comfort.	Patients will often be more comfortable in a side-lying position with the head of the bed elevated (to relieve pressure on the abdomen).
Implement non-pharmacological strategies to relieve pain and discomfort, such as relaxation techniques, soft music, distraction, or meditation.	Non-pharmacological interventions can assist in reducing pain by affecting the perception of the pain experience.
If abdominal distention occurs due to post-colonoscopy distention syndrome, implement strategies to relieve the bowel of air: insert rectal tube; encourage ambulation with assistance.	The air injected into the bowel during a colonoscopy can cause abdominal discomfort as it becomes trapped in the bowel; simple measures such as ambulation or rectal tubes usually offer quick relief. The patient requires assistance with ambulation due to the effects of the medication.
Assess effectiveness of all interventions.	Helps to determine whether other interventions are required.
Assess for excessive bleeding from rectal area (colonoscopy patients), especially in patients with complaints of pain.	Some slight bleeding is expected for about 2 days if polyps have been removed; however, excessive bleeding or free flow of blood may indicate

a perforation of the bowel, and the patient who is experiencing continued pain should always have stool checked for bleeding.

NIC *Pain management*
Analgesic administration
Anxiety reduction

Evaluation

The patient is able to report that the pain has been reduced (is < a 4 on a scale of 1–10) or alleviated following interventions. The patient should have no observable signs of discomfort, and no abdominal distention, cramping, or severe pain occurs. The degree to which the patient is able to assist in the management of the discomfort through anxiety reduction and relaxation techniques is assessed.

Community/Home Care

The patient's discomfort should be minimal and not an issue once at home in most instances. If discomfort continues in the home setting, it can usually be managed with mild analgesics and ambulation (to help pass the air from a colonoscopy) with a very short duration. For patients who have had an EGD or ERCP, throat discomfort due to the passage of the scope may last for 1 to 2 days but is easily relieved with lozenges or anesthetic mouthwashes such as Chloraseptic or Listerine. The patient can also make a preparation of saltwater to use. If the patient experiences severe pain in the abdomen or rectal area, he or she should contact the health care provider for immediate attention, as this may signal a perforation. If the recommended mild analgesics are not working, the patient should seek follow-up care with the health care provider.

Documentation

Document in the patient's own words the description of the pain and rating of the level of pain. Include in the documentation assessments made relevant to the pain. Chart all interventions employed for pain relief and the patient's responses. All teaching should be indicated in the patient record with an indication of the patient's level of understanding.

CHAPTER 6.84

FECAL DIVERSION/OSTOMY (POST-OPERATIVE)

GENERAL INFORMATION

Fecal diversions are surgically created openings for the elimination of feces, located on the abdominal wall. There are two basic types: an ileostomy and a colostomy. An ileostomy is an opening created from the ileum, resulting in a constant flow of liquid stools, as water is not absorbed from gastrointestinal (GI) products until it reaches the colon. The most common reason for creation of an ileostomy is to re-route fecal material because of colitis, but it can also be used in cases of colon cancer high in the colon, trauma, and congenital problems. A colostomy is a portal into the ascending, transverse, or sigmoid sections of the colon. A colostomy is created as a portal through which fecal material can pass; it is created for a number of reasons, most commonly because of cancer. Stool from a colostomy can be semi-solid or solid depending upon the area of the colon affected. A colostomy may be temporary (to permit the colon to heal), as in the case of diverticulitis, or permanent.

NURSING DIAGNOSIS 1

 ACUTE PAIN

Related to:

Surgical interventions

Defining Characteristics:

Complaints of pain

Guarding affected area

Grimacing and moaning

Goal:

The patient's pain is relieved.

Outcome Criteria

✔ The patient will verbalize that pain has been relieved 30 minutes after interventions.

✔ The patient will verbalize satisfaction with pain management.

NOC *Pain level*
Pain control
Comfort level

INTERVENTIONS	RATIONALES
Assess for location, intensity, quality, and precipitating factors.	Identifying these will assist in accurate diagnosis and treatment; most patients who undergo surgical intervention experience some pain.
Have patient rate pain intensity using a pain rating scale.	Provides a more objective description of level of pain.
Assess respiratory status, including breath sounds, respiratory rate, depth, quality, and oxygen saturation.	Patients who have abdominal incisions tend to breathe shallowly due to the pain associated with inspiration, which compromises respiratory function that may lead to atelectasis and pneumonia; assessment of respiratory status allows for early detection.
Administer analgesics on a regular schedule, as ordered, or dosed by direct intravenous (IV) route or via patient-controlled analgesia (PCA).	Narcotic analgesics will promote rest and relaxation and promote pain relief, preventing pain from becoming intense; decreased pain will improve patient's respiratory efforts, especially inspiration, assuring adequate oxygenation, ventilation, tissue perfusion, and complete

(continues)

(continued)

INTERVENTIONS	RATIONALES
	expansion of the lungs (preventing atelectasis); makes it easier for patient to participate in coughing and deep breathing.
Implement strategies to enhance effects of pain medication, such as relaxation techniques, soft music, distraction, television, books on tape, backrubs, etc.	Non-pharmacological interventions can assist in reducing pain by affecting the perception of the pain experience.
Teach patient to splint abdomen with a pillow or rolled bath blanket when moving or coughing.	Splinting provides support for the painful area, decreases stress on surgical site that may increase pain, and allows the patient to participate in coughing and deep breathing more comfortably.
Assess effectiveness of interventions to relieve pain.	Helps to determine if interventions have been effective in relieving pain or if new strategies need to be employed.

NIC   *Pain management*

      Analgesic administration

      Anxiety reduction

Evaluation

The patient is able to report that the pain has been reduced or alleviated following interventions. The degree to which the patient is able to participate in prescribed activities or activities of daily living is assessed. The patient should have no observable signs of discomfort. Satisfaction with pain management is expressed.

Community/Home Care

The patient's pain should be temporary and resolve once the surgical wounds heal. Pain at home is usually managed with mild analgesics, and the duration of pain should be short. The patient should take the medication at home before the pain becomes severe. The nurse should stress to the patient that weak respiratory efforts because of pain could cause respiratory problems such as pneumonia. Encourage the patient to use a pillow for splinting when moving or coughing at home. If the pain worsens at home, the patient should contact the health care provider to determine other causes for

the pain and be aware that most often increased pain signals a wound infection. If the recommended analgesics are not working, the patient should seek follow-up care with the health care provider.

Documentation

Document in the patient's own words the description of the pain and rating of the level of pain. Chart all interventions employed and the patient's responses. Include in the documentation assessments made relevant to the pain and to the respiratory system. Document analgesics on the medication administration according to agency protocol.

NURSING DIAGNOSIS 2

 ALTERED BOWEL ELIMINATION*

Related to:

     Surgical interventions (creation of fecal diversion)

     New way of eliminating stool

Defining Characteristics:

     Presence of ostomy on abdominal wall

Goal:

     Adequate bowel elimination will be maintained.

Outcome Criteria

✔ Bowel elimination will occur daily.

✔ There will be no constipation or diarrhea (colostomy).

✔ There will be no leakage of liquid stool from collection bag (ileostomy).

NOC   *Bowel elimination*

INTERVENTIONS	RATIONALES
Carefully assess for first effluent post-operatively.	Occasionally, a paralytic ileus will occur post-operatively. It can be expected that an ileostomy will begin to drain within 24 hours, and a colostomy will usually discharge feces within 48 hours.

INTERVENTIONS	RATIONALES
Monitor output from colostomy and ileostomy (color, consistency, amount).	Output must be monitored to detect early any obstruction that could cause distention and subsequent leakage at the anastomosis site.
Monitor for edema of stoma.	Edema of the stoma can prevent proper functioning or disturbance of the anastomosis.
Monitor output from other drainage tubes such as Jackson Pratts (JPs) in the immediate post-operative period.	These devices are used to drain blood and other surgical fluids from the surgical site. The amount should decrease gradually and cease over the first 72 hours post-surgery.
Carefully check stoma for signs of adequate blood flow (pink/ red, no dusky discoloration) and area around stoma for skin irritation. Carefully wash and dry the area before applying colostomy appliance. Ensure proper fit of appliance (see nursing diagnosis "Impaired Skin Integrity").	Dark or dusky color of the stoma indicates a lack of blood flow to area. Excoriation or other signs of irritation may be due to leakage or abrasive appliance adhesive.
Encourage the intake of 1200–1500 ml of fluid, when allowed.	Helps to prevent constipation.
Encourage patient to avoid foods that cause odor (beans, cabbage, eggs, onions, asparagus) and gas (beans, cabbage, carbonated drinks, dairy products).	Gas production causes the bag to fill with air and cause abdominal discomfort for the patient.
Encourage patient to eat a diet with adequate amounts of fiber and bulk.	The consistency of the stool will be determined by the amount of roughage and fiber in the diet, and by the amount of fluid intake; promotes bowel elimination and prevents constipation.
Drain colostomy bag prior to its being half full.	A full collection device may overflow and become detached. It should not be allowed to get more than half full.
Teach patient and family how to care for colostomy.	Patient and family will eventually need to provide care (see nursing diagnosis "Deficient Knowledge" and "Impaired Skin Integrity").

NIC *Bowel elimination*

Evaluation

The patient achieves bowel elimination through the colostomy, and the stoma is healthy in appearance. Healing of the stoma occurs without any edema to site. No constipation or diarrhea occurs. For the patient with an ileostomy, fluid balance is maintained.

Community/Home Care

One of the biggest challenges for the patient when discharge is eminent is the uncertainty of managing the new method for bowel elimination (see nursing diagnosis "Deficient Knowledge"). Even though teaching has occurred during hospitalization, at home the patient may experience some anxiety when faced with independently caring for the ostomy without a nurse present. Therefore, for most patients in-home nursing visits are highly desirable to monitor the patient's ability to perform procedures correctly and to enhance the comfort level with the fecal diversion. At home the patient will need to be mindful of amount of output from the colostomy/ileostomy in order to detect early any signs of obstruction. The patient will need to drink adequate amounts of fluid to promote bowel elimination and prevent constipation. In the absence of cardiac disease, the patient should attempt to drink 1200–1500 milliliters of fluid, avoiding large amounts of caffeine, but including generous amounts of water. If the patient is engaging in social activities outside the home, he or she may want to refrain from consuming foods that cause gas and odor so that embarrassment does not occur. In addition, the gas fills up the bag, which may then become noticeable under clothing. The patient needs to understand the importance of returning for a follow-up visit that may include having x-rays/ scans done to ensure the integrity of the anastomosis and proper functioning of the ostomy. As the patient and family become more comfortable with management of the fecal diversion, the services of the visiting nurse may not be needed, but participation in support groups may be helpful as many times other patients or families may have helpful hints or pointers to make living with the ostomy easier.

Documentation

Document the status of any drainage devices as well as the color, amount, and consistency of drainage. Always chart when the ostomy begins to function and describe the consistency, color, and amount of the stool. Chart the achievement of stated outcome criteria and all interventions employed by the nurse to achieve them. Any referrals made are included in the patient record. Visits by the wound or ostomy nurse are documented.

NURSING DIAGNOSIS 3

 IMPAIRED SKIN INTEGRITY

Related to:

Leakage of stool onto skin

Irritation from ostomy bag adhesive

Surgical incisions

Presence of drainage tubes

Infection

Defining Characteristics:

Reddened/discolored, bruised, irritated area around stoma

Presence of surgical incisions

Fever

Elevated white blood cell (WBC) count

Redness/discoloration, swelling, drainage around wound

Infection in incision

Goal:

The area around the stoma is free from irritation.

Incision heals without complications.

Infection is prevented or eliminated.

Outcome Criteria

✔ The patient is able to perform appropriate ostomy skin care.

✔ Skin around stoma remains pink with no discoloration (dusky, dark).

✔ Skin around stoma remains intact.

✔ The patient's surgical site has no redness/discoloration, purulent drainage, or heat.

✔ The patient remains afebrile.

✔ WBC count remains within normal limits.

NOC *Wound healing: Primary intention*

INTERVENTIONS	RATIONALES
Monitor surgical site for signs and symptoms of infection or irritation from fecal leakage: redness, swelling, purulent drainage, poor approximation, heat, or increased pain.	Fecal leakage onto the abdominal wall can reach the surgical incision and cause infection or irritation. Early identification of infection can expedite treatment.
Maintain patency of any drainage devices and assess drainage for amount, color, and consistency.	The drainage device helps prevent accumulation of drainage at the surgical site; drainage may be bloody initially, but should become serosanguineous.
Consult with ostomy specialist who can measure stoma, choose appropriate appliance, and identify appropriate adhesives and skin barriers.	Much attention must be given to teaching the patient about ostomy care, assisting the patient in choosing the appropriate products, and troubleshooting problem areas or potential problems. The ostomy specialist is an expert and should be used for education, if possible.
Change the ostomy bag 24 to 48 hours after surgery or as ordered and assess the stoma for bright pink or red color.	The bag placed in the operating room may be soiled, and a clean transparent bag 24 hours after surgery allows for better inspection of the stoma.
Measure the stoma carefully with each appliance change. The adhesive opening should be just slightly larger (approximately 1/4 inch) than the base of the stoma. Be sure that the adhesive and skin barrier are free of wrinkles.	There will be post-operative edema. Therefore, the size of the stoma may continue to change until all edema subsides. It is important to measure the appliance opening carefully to ensure that the opening closely fits the stoma size and that the skin around the stoma is not exposed to the stool coming from the ostomy, especially for patients with an ileostomy, which is rich in gastric enzymes. The size may continue to change for 6 to 8 weeks. Wrinkles in the barrier or the adhesive can prevent proper fit, causing it to leak; also, wrinkles can cause skin irritation.
With the assistance of the ostomy expert, select the skin barrier type that is appropriate for the patient.	The barrier protects the skin in case there is stool leakage and is gentler to the skin than the adhesive found directly on the pouch. The barrier can be left in place when the pouch is removed, preventing repeated skin irritation.

INTERVENTIONS	RATIONALES
When the barrier is periodically removed, remove with adhesive remover, wash and dry area carefully, and then replace with a clean, new barrier.	Frequent removal of the barrier is not necessary, but careful, meticulous skin care is essential.
Take temperature every 4 hours.	Temperature elevations may be indicative of infection.
Change dressings on surgical incision as ordered and clean area using sterile technique, cleansing the entry site of any drainage devices last.	Maintenance of a clean incisional site decreases number of organisms and reduces chance of infection; infection may occur due to contamination with stool.
Administer antipyretics (such as acetaminophen [Tylenol]), as ordered.	Helps to reduce fever.
Administer antibiotics, as ordered IV or PO (by mouth).	Helps to reduce number of infective organisms and eliminate or prevent infection.
Encourage adequate nutritional intake, especially of protein, vitamin C, and iron.	Adequate nutrient intake, especially of vitamin C, protein, and iron, is required for healing and tissue repair.

NIC *Incision site care*
      Infection control
      Nutrition management
      Wound care
      Wound care: Closed drainage

Evaluation

Evaluate the degree to which the outcome criteria have been met. The surgical site should be intact healing by primary intention with incision well approximated. Redness/discoloration, swelling, purulent drainage, and heat should be absent from the site. Drainage from the drainage devices (if present) should be serosanguineous and decreasing in amount. The stoma of the fecal diversion should be bright pink or red. The patient should be afebrile, and WBC counts should return to normal.

Community/Home Care

The status of the surgical site and stoma may remain a problem after the patient has been discharged home. Infections of the abdominal surgical site are still possible once the patient is at home, and the family will need to know what symptoms may signal the onset of infection. Not only should the patient be aware of signs of infection, but indications of wound dehiscence should also be made clear to the patient. Incisional care, skin care, and stoma care will need to be taught to the patient (see nursing diagnosis "Deficient Knowledge"). The size of the stoma will continue to decrease as healing progresses and post-operative edema subsides, making it necessary for the patient to measure the stoma regularly to adjust the size of the colostomy bag. A variety of commercial products to protect the skin are available, and the patient, in consultation with the ostomy specialist, will need to experiment with which work best. A visiting nurse will need to monitor the patient's ability to do this, as improper fitting of the device can lead to stool leakage and skin irritation. At home, the patient will need to locate a place to keep supplies for easy access, and the bathroom is a logical place. Durable plastic storage boxes in a variety of sizes can be purchased at any retail store that sells household items. The patient can experiment with what works: keeping all bags in one box, adhesives in another, and barriers in another; or the use of a three-drawer rolling cart; or one big box for all items. For the patient who must empty the bag, use of the bathroom rather than the bedroom for these activities helps add a dimension of normalcy to the process. The patient will need to understand the importance of good nutrition in complete wound healing and recovery. The importance of completing any ordered medications such as antibiotics once at home should be stressed. If any evidence of poor wound healing, discoloration of the stoma, irritation of surrounding skin, or infection should occur, the patient should be instructed to contact the health care provider.

Documentation

Document assessment findings from the wound, including skin color and approximation, and amount, color, and odor of any drainage, being sure to note any sign of infection. Chart the status of drainage devices or tubes indicating the color, amount, and consistency of drainage. An assessment of the stoma and surrounding skin is documented every shift or every 8 hours as required. Document in the chart when the ostomy bag is changed. Vital signs are documented according to agency protocol, as ordered, for post-operative patients. Always include in the documentation all interventions implemented to address skin integrity, including achievement of stated outcome criteria.

NURSING DIAGNOSIS 4

 ## DISTURBED BODY IMAGE

Related to:

Physical change in body appearance post-surgery

Different means for bowel elimination

Defining Characteristics:

Withdrawal

Social isolation

Depression

Negative statements about physical appearance

Patient's attempt to cover stoma

Goal:

The patient accepts the change in physical appearance and continues social activities and interpersonal relationships.

Outcome Criteria

✔ The patient states a willingness to look at and touch fecal diversion surgical site.

✔ The patient learns and participates in care of colostomy.

✔ The patient accepts the change in body appearance.

NOC *Body image*

INTERVENTIONS	RATIONALES
Provide assurance that any negative feelings are very normal post-operatively.	Helps to stop the patient from thinking that his or her feelings are abnormal.
Allow the patient privacy when bathing or dressing.	Helps to allow the patient time to adjust to appearance without concern for how others react.
Encourage the patient to communicate feelings about changes in bowel elimination patterns.	Talking about the changes may sometimes be the beginning of acceptance.
Encourage the patient and significant other or family member to participate in the selection of the type of external collection device to be worn, if possible.	Participation in decision-making can enhance self-esteem and body image.
Teach patient and family how to care for the stoma and ostomy bag.	If the patient is comfortable with self-care, that comfort level may translate into acceptance for the change in appearance and incorporation of body appearance change into a positive self-image (see nursing diagnosis "Deficient Knowledge").
Be with the patient during the initial views of the stoma, initial care of the stoma, and, if desirable, the first time the stoma is viewed by a family member or significant other.	It is important to provide the patient with support and assurance that the stoma is a reality and that stoma care can be controlled by the patient.
Assess the patient's feelings about self, interpersonal relationships with family members and friends, withdrawal, social isolation, anxiety, embarrassment by appearance, desire to be alone, and fear that spouse or significant other may not want to engage in intimate relations.	Helps to detect early alterations in social functioning; prevents unhealthy behaviors and intervenes early through referral to counseling. Concerns about sexual function are common as they relate to the ability to engage in sexual relations, embarrassment about exposure of ostomy bag, and desirability of self to partner.
Encourage the patient to participate in at least one outside/public activity each week once health status permits.	Prevents the patient from isolating self from others.
Identify the effects the patient's culture or religion plays in perception of body image.	A patient's culture and religion often help define reactions to changes in body image and self-worth.
Identify community support groups as well as patients with similar stoma/device that can visit the patient.	Discussions with other patients with similar situations may be beneficial for the patient, allowing him or her to share thoughts with and hear thoughts from those who understand what the patient is going through; provides the patient with support and the courage to move forward in terms of acceptance of the change.
Assist the patient in identifying coping strategies and diversionary activities.	Coping strategies are needed to adapt to the changes in the body and provide diversion so that thoughts do not focus on the ostomy.
Discuss concerns about ability to return to work or engage in recreational activities such as sports, if applicable.	The patient is often concerned about physical activity, and this may be due to fear of the ostomy bag becoming loose or

INTERVENTIONS	RATIONALES
	leakage of stool if too active. Most patients are able to return to their pre-operative level of physical activity unless contraindicated by underlying disease.
Allow the patient/family to grieve the loss of normal bowel functioning; allow the patient/family time and privacy to do this.	It is appropriate to grieve for loss of function of body parts that are vital to everyday life, supporting the family and patient will enhance healthy adaptation.

NIC *Body image enhancement*
Emotional support
Support group
Socialization enhancement

Evaluation

The patient is able to willingly learn about the care of the colostomy/ileostomy or stoma site and begins to participate in self-care. Time is required for the patient to completely assimilate the change in body appearance and function into his or her self-perception. It is crucial that the nurse evaluate the degree to which the patient is beginning to do this. Look for behaviors such as touching the site, looking at the stoma site, agreeing to assist with the care, or asking appropriate questions. Communication of feelings and concerns relevant to the change in appearance should be taken as a positive sign that progress is being made towards meeting outcome criteria.

Community/Home Care

At home, continued monitoring of the patient's perception of body image is needed. The nurse who visits will need to be alert to subtle hints that may indicate that the patient has not completely adapted to the change in body appearance and bowel function. Open discussions about body changes and interventions to prevent social isolation and withdrawal should continue with patient and family. Many patients are concerned about the possibility of stool leakage, the bag coming off, and odor. As a result, the patient may limit social activities, which in turn will further negatively influence body image. Methods of controlling leakage

and odor are key to the success of the patient's ability to sustain a positive body image and remain socially active (see nursing diagnosis "Deficient Knowledge"). Once at home, the patient should experiment with a variety of types of clothing to determine which ones fit best without putting pressure on the ostomy bag or without the bulge of the bag showing. Until the patient feels comfortable that the bag generally will not rupture or come off, loose-fitting clothes may be used to provide some psychological comfort that flow of output will not be impeded. However, the patient should be encouraged to wear his or her usual clothes in an effort to enhance body image. The nurse who visits in the home needs to question specifically about social isolation and engagement in outside activities, and provide any information required to address the patients concerns. Community support groups should be explored, keeping in mind that such support groups may not be available in rural areas, in which case an alternative activity should be identified.

Documentation

Chart any specific behaviors or verbalizations that may indicate an altered body image. Include all interventions that have been employed to address this issue and the patient's response. Note when and if the patient begins to ask questions and participate in care. Specifically note when the patient looks at the ostomy site for the first time and his or her reactions. All referrals should be documented in the patient record.

NURSING DIAGNOSIS 5

DEFICIENT KNOWLEDGE

Related to:

Care of fecal diversion devices

Care of stoma

New medical problem

Defining Characteristics:

Many or no questions

Verbalizes a lack of knowledge/understanding

Unable to perform new procedures for care (ostomy care)

Goal:

The patient or significant other will know how to care for fecal diversion devices.

Outcome Criteria

✔ The patient indicates a desire to learn necessary information.

✔ The patient verbalizes an understanding of the altered colon structure.

✔ The patient and/or family demonstrate proper care of the ostomy bag: emptying, application of new bag, application of barriers.

✔ The patient expresses an understanding of the care required at home.

✔ The patient verbalizes an understanding of skin care and preventing skin impairment.

✔ The patient verbalizes an understanding of nutritional requirements.

✔ The patient verbalizes an understanding of follow-up care required and expresses a willingness to comply.

NOC   *Knowledge: Treatment procedures*
Knowledge: Infection control
Knowledge: Treatment regimen
Knowledge: Health resources

INTERVENTIONS	RATIONALES
Assess the patient's current knowledge as well as ability and readiness to learn.	The nurse needs to ascertain what the patient already knows and build on this; if the patient is not capable of learning or is not ready to learn, teaching will not be effective due to disinterest or inability to understand.
Start with the simplest information and move to complex information.	Patients can understand simple concepts easily and then can build on those to understand concepts that are more complex.
Assess dexterity in the hands to determine if the patient can maneuver clamp on bag.	Patients may not be able to manipulate the clamp that closes the bottom of the ostomy bag if dexterity in hands is poor, especially in those with arthritis.
Teach the patient and significant others the following or reinforce	Knowledge of how to provide self-care, recognition of

teaching by the ostomy nurse:

— Anatomy and physiology of newly created fecal diversion

— Procedure for applying new pouch: measuring the stoma for correct size, applying skin barrier, applying bag, making opening in drainage bag no larger than 1–2 mm wider than outside of stoma, allowing no wrinkles in barrier or adhesive part of bag

— Procedure for emptying drainage bag: empty when less than half full to avoid leakage or pulling away from skin; if the patient is emptying bag, place opening pointing straight down to allow emptying into commode; how to securely fasten clamp on bag opening; how to rinse the bag

— Procedure for regulating bowel evacuation through irrigation for ostomies in the lower colon (sigmoid colostomy)

— Prevention of skin irritation: apply barriers; use plain water or gentle soap to cleanse skin around stoma, being sure to rinse soap off well; cleanse any stool from skin promptly to prevent breakdown; inspect skin for breakdown

— Teach patient to pat (not rub) the stoma or the surrounding skin when performing care; rubbing can cause irritation to already sensitive skin

— Surgical incision skin care: keep clean and dry; inspect for drainage and redness/discoloration

— Signs and symptoms of complications that would indicate a need to seek health care: lack of stool, fever, bloody stool, purulent drainage from incision, sudden change in size or color of stoma, pain in back or in stoma site

When changing external device, place a gauze pad over the stoma.	Helps to absorb any leakage of stool while appliance is being changed.

complications, and prevention of complications empowers the patient to take control and be compliant.

INTERVENTIONS	RATIONALES
Allow adequate time for task mastery; have the patient and a family member return demonstrate all skills, and provide rationales for performing each step in a skill.	The person performing the care should feel comfortable performing the procedure before discharge to home, and the nurse needs to know that the patient can correctly perform this activity prior to discharge. Rationales for the steps increase understanding.
Teach the patient and family measures to prevent infection, especially good handwashing when performing dressing changes.	The patient's first line of defense against organisms into the body is good hand hygiene, and vigilance is required.
Teach the patient to ingest foods rich in vitamin C, protein, and iron. Suggest that the patient avoid foods that cause gas and odor, such as beans, asparagus, cabbage, etc.	These nutrients are necessary for good wound healing. Stressing the importance of nutrition to family and patient will increase the possibility that the patient will be compliant with requirements. Gas inflates the ostomy bag and causes abdominal discomfort.
Teach the patient and family to carry supplies needed for care of the fecal diversion in a small travel case kept with them when traveling.	If care supplies are placed in checked luggage, the patient will not have access to them in case of an emergency, and if luggage is lost the patient will need to buy new supplies. It may be difficult to get identical supplies if needed.
Assess the patient's and family's understanding of all teaching by encouraging them to repeat information, demonstrate all skills, and ask questions as needed.	This allows the nurse to hear in the patient's own words what was taught and makes it easier to know what information may need to be reinforced.
Give the patient or family printed material that outlines the procedure and all information presented; if desired, obtain educational materials from the United Ostomy Association or the Wound, Ostomy, and Continence Nurses Society.	Printed materials can serve as a backup when the patient is at home and needs review or reinforcement; educational materials from these agencies provide updates on care strategies and innovations in care of fecal diversions.
Refer the patient to home health or visiting nurse agencies for follow-up and reinforcement of teaching once the patient is at home.	Once at home, the patient and family may have questions about the care of surgical site, stoma care, and application of ostomy bag; the nurse also needs to be sure that care procedures are being performed correctly.

Establish prior to discharge that the patient has a means to obtain all care supplies required to be compliant.	If needed resources such as finances and transportation to follow-up appointments are not available, the patient cannot be compliant; the nurse will need to make necessary referrals.

NIC *Learning readiness enhancement*
Learning facilitation
Teaching: Psychomotor skill

Evaluation

Evaluate the degree to which the patient has achieved the outcome criteria relevant to the teaching sessions. The patient should verbalize an understanding of content presented by repeating the information. It is crucial that the patient or family demonstrate correct performance of all psychomotor skills such as emptying and changing the ostomy bag. The patient verbalizes an understanding of how to care for skin to prevent irritation. The nurse must determine if the patient is capable of being compliant with the recommended regimen. If further teaching is required at time of discharge, the appropriate referrals should be made to continue education.

Community/Home Care

The success of the patient's ability to implement strategies for self-care will depend upon the degree to which the patient has received adequate teaching, has subsequently understood and internalized it, and has the motivation to participate in self-care. Crucial to successful in-home care is the ability of the patient or family members to perform the required psychomotor skills of draining the ostomy bag, changing the bag, and applying the protective barrier. For patients with impaired dexterity, alternatives to use of the clamp to close the bottom of the bag will need to be identified. The first time the patient or family changes the bag, the presence of a visiting nurse may decrease the uncertainty and anxiety for the patient. Some adaptations may be necessary in the procedure, such as using a paper towel or old washcloth to absorb stool leakage when the appliance is changed, especially with an ileostomy. Some sources suggest the use of a small tampon for this purpose, but male patients may not find this appealing. Cotton balls should not be used on the stoma because they can deposit lint into the stoma. Depending on the location of the stoma and/or drainage bag, tight clothing may need to be avoided, and the patient will need to decide through trial and error which clothes will work and which will not. In most instances loose clothing is more comfortable. If the bag is allowed to get more than half full, the bag may be noticeable under snug-fitting clothes, as it makes a bulge. Even though it is not recommended that bags be changed daily due to costs, some patients make the decision to apply a new bag each day because of the perception of cleanliness. Storage of supplies in the bathroom or bedroom is desirable for ready access, and as previously discussed, plastic storage boxes work well for this. The patient should take an inventory of supplies at set intervals to ensure that they do not run out. A home nurse should follow up with the family and patient to ensure that all procedures are carried out comfortably in the home, and the nurse may actually want to plan to be present the first time a procedure is done. Depression and withdrawal may occur due to the changes in body appearance and in the different way to eliminate. This may not be evident until the patient is at home, and may manifest itself in the patient's refusal to participate in self-care activities. Adequate teaching may help to make the family and/or patient comfortable with what is required and will give them some sense of control that may assist them to move from a state of denial to one of self-sufficiency. Be sure that the patient has the means to purchase needed supplies. The patient should understand when to contact the health care provider, such as when pain or burning at stoma site, change in appearance in stoma site, blood in stool, or absence of stool in bag occur.

Documentation

Chart whether the stated outcome criteria have been achieved. Document the specific content taught and the titles of any printed materials given to the patient. Include in the chart the patient's degree of understanding of the content and the methods used to teach and evaluate learning. Documentation of the patient's ability to perform the psychomotor skills required for incisional care, stoma care, drainage of ostomy bags, application of drainage bags, and irrigation of the colostomy should be specified. Any areas that need to be reinforced should be documented to ensure appropriate follow-up. If family members are present for the teaching sessions, document this in the chart, and always document referrals made for in-home assistance. Include information regarding the patient's and family's feelings, concerns, and fears about performing care in the home.

CHAPTER 6.85

GASTROENTEROCOLITIS/ENTEROCOLITIS

GENERAL INFORMATION

Gastroenterocolitis is an inflammation of the bowel mucosa characterized by severe diarrhea. In most cases, it affects the small intestine and can be attributed to bacterial or viral causes. Some distinct pathophysiological changes occur. Exotoxins are produced by the offending bacteria and are released in the gastrointestinal (GI) tract, where they damage the surrounding tissue, resulting in impaired absorption of water and electrolytes with subsequent movement of both into the large intestines. Some bacteria exert their action directly on the mucosa on the intestine, causing ulceration that results in bleeding, loss of water, and electrolytes. Bacteria responsible for causing gastroenterocolitis include salmonella, *Clostridium perfringens*, shigella, *Staphylococcus aureus*, and *Escherichia coli (E. coli)*. Viral gastroenterocolitis agents include rotavirus (groups A, B, and C), adenovirus, and Norwalk virus. These organisms are most often transmitted via contaminated food and/ or water. Specific disease entities include traveler's diarrhea (*E. coli*), staphylococcal food poisoning, hemorrhagic colitis (*E. coli*), salmonellosis/food poisoning (salmonella), and dysentery (shigella). Clinical manifestations vary depending on the causative organism, but general findings include frequent watery diarrhea, abdominal cramping, hyperactive loud bowel sounds (borborygmi), vomiting, blood in stool from mucosal bleeding, nausea, and abdominal pain. As a result of the fluid loss, the patient will demonstrate signs of dehydration, such as dry skin, poor skin turgor, dry mucous membranes, thirst, weakness, headache, tachycardia, orthostatic hypotension, and decreased blood pressure.

NURSING DIAGNOSIS 1

 DEFICIENT FLUID VOLUME

Related to:

    Severe diarrhea

    Vomiting

    Impaired absorption of water

Defining Characteristics:

    Poor skin turgor

    Dry mucous membranes

    Severe thirst

    Increased urine-specific gravity

    Electrolyte imbalance

    Tachycardia

    Decreased blood pressure

Goal:

    Fluid and electrolyte status return to normal.

Outcome Criteria

✔ The patient's vital signs return to baseline.

✔ The patient reports that thirst has diminished.

✔ Stools will become formed.

✔ Vomiting will be relieved.

✔ Mucous membranes will become moist.

✔ Skin turgor improves (skin, when pinched, returns to original position in < 3 seconds).

NOC *Fluid balance*

       Electrolyte and acid/base balance

       Vital signs

INTERVENTIONS	RATIONALES
Assess the stool history: frequency, color, amount, odor, and presence of blood.	Helps to determine the extent of the problem, identify causative factors, and guide treatment.

(continues)

(continued)

INTERVENTIONS	RATIONALES
Assess for signs of dehydration/volume deficit: decreased blood pressure, increased pulse, dry mucous membranes, poor skin turgor, and decreased urinary output.	Helps to determine the seriousness of the problem, to guide treatment, and to assess effectiveness of treatments.
Take a history of the patient's recent food intake, including visits to any restaurants or picnics, etc.	Sources of contamination include food handlers in restaurants as well as food that has been improperly stored, such as foods containing mayonnaise at picnics.
Monitor intake and output.	Helps to assess fluid balance.
Monitor serum electrolytes, especially serum potassium and serum osmolality.	Helps to determine fluid and electrolyte replacement needs.
Obtain stool specimen as ordered for gram stain, culture, ova and parasites, *Clostridium difficile (C. difficile),* electron microscopy and immunoassay, and toxins.	Stool cultures will identify causative organisms; gram stain will reveal the presence of cells consistent with a diagnosis of shigellosis and campylobacter. With some organisms, the toxins emitted can be isolated in the stool. Some stool cultures need to be sent to state laboratories, and the process for culturing can take up to 6 weeks. In most instances, physicians treat the patient based on history and symptoms.
Institute fluid replacement intravenously: 0.5 normal saline, Ringer's lactate, or others, as ordered.	This is an isotonic solution to replace lost fluid volume.
Administer antibiotics, as ordered, after cultures have been obtained.	Helps to relieve the infection by bacteria.
Administer potassium replacement intravenously (IV), as ordered.	Potassium is rich in the GI tract, and diarrhea and vomiting cause decreases in serum levels, necessitating potassium replacement.
Encourage oral electrolyte solutions, as ordered or tolerated.	Helps to replace electrolytes lost.
Encourage at least 3000 ml/day fluid intake if tolerating oral liquids, unless contraindicated.	Helps to increase body fluids and restore fluid balance; caution is used in patients with cardiac disease.

Administer antidiarrheal medication, as ordered.	Helps to slow intestinal peristalsis and raise fluid uptake.
Administer anti-emetic medications.	Helps to relieve nausea or vomiting that accompanies gastroenterocolitis.
Advance diet as tolerated, offering saltine crackers or toast, and avoiding caffeinated beverages. In addition, adding yogurt to the diet can restore normal bacterial flora to the intestinal tract.	Most patients can advance their diet after 24 hours but should start with easily digestible, bland substances.
Teach the patient proper handwashing techniques and the importance of good hand hygiene after each bowel movement.	Proper handwashing is crucial to stopping the spread of infection.
During the acute process, teach the patient and family not to share eating utensils and items used for drinking. Also, inform family members to wipe toilet seats prior to using.	Gastroenterocolitis is easily transmitted to others through sharing of eating utensils and sharing toilets.

 NIC *Fluid monitoring*
   Electrolyte monitoring
   Fluid/electrolyte management

Evaluation

Assess the patient for return of normal fluid volume. The patient's blood pressure and pulse should return to baseline. The pulse should be strong and regular and at the patient's baseline or only slightly increased. Skin should be warm, and color should return to the patient's normal appearance. The number of stools will decrease and stools will return to normal consistency. Renal function should not be impaired, with an hourly output on the average of 30 ml/hour. Serum electrolytes should be within normal range.

Community/Home Care

Patients treated for deficient fluid volume due to gastroenterocolitis should have normal fluid status restored within a short period of time. The disease is for the most part self-limiting, resolving within 24 to 72 hours; thus, with the exception of the most severe cases, the patient is treated as an outpatient. The patient and family should receive education about prevention of this disease through thorough handwashing, proper food storage, and proper food handling. The patient should be cautious about eating raw foods, foods not cooked thoroughly, foods containing mayonnaise, and eggs. This is extremely important for picnicgoers who keep food unrefrigerated for extended periods of time outside in warm weather. Meat that is not cooked to adequate doneness or temperature can also be an offending source, especially hamburger, which is a source of certain strains of *E. coli*. Encourage the patient to cook hamburger until no redness remains. For some types of gastroenterocolitis transmitted via fecal-oral routes, the patient needs education about prevention of transmission through good hand hygiene. If the home has more than one bathroom, the patient should be limited to the use of a specific toilet, and other family members should be restricted from this bathroom. For those homes with only one toilet, others using the bathroom should wipe the toilet seat with a strong antiseptic solution such as diluted Clorox or Lysol before using the toilet. Commercial wipes containing these substances are available for convenience, but they tend to be expensive. The patient needs to have a specific set of utensils for drinking and eating that are kept separate from others. Attention to methods of replacing electrolytes is important, as the patient almost always loses potassium. Encourage the intake of frequent small amounts of clear liquid electrolyte solutions, such as Gatorade or Pedialyte. Plain water should be avoided, as it makes nausea worse for some, but more importantly, it contains no electrolytes. Providing the patient with a list of drinks and foods that are appropriate will be helpful so that the patient has a handy reference. Encourage the patient to keep a water bottle filled with clear liquids at all times to enhance the likelihood of drinking adequate amounts of fluid. Fatigue may be an issue, as volume deficit create a sense of weakness, even when the deficit is mild. This can be handled simply by informing the patient to perform activities as tolerated until stamina/endurance is re-established (see nursing diagnosis "Fatigue"). The health care provider may want the patient to return for a follow-up appointment to ensure that electrolytes have returned to normal.

Documentation

The patient is treated at home in most instances. Whether the patient is being seen in the health care provider's office, or in the acute care setting, always make a note of the number, consistency, color, odor, and amount of any stools. If antidiarrheals are administered, document this according to agency protocol, with a follow-up note about effectiveness. Document initial assessment findings relevant to fluid status such as blood pressure, pulse, respirations, temperature, and skin status (turgor, mucous membranes). Be sure to document the patient's intake and output every shift. Document all interventions, such as intravenous catheter insertion, fluids initiated (type, rate), urine output (amount, color), and dietary modifications, such as clear liquids. Be specific when charting patient responses to treatment so that other health care providers can clearly determine improvement or deterioration.

NURSING DIAGNOSIS 2

FATIGUE

Related to:
    Loss of electrolytes due to diarrhea
    Loss of fluids due to diarrhea
    Lack of nutrients required for energy

Defining Characteristics:
    Lethargy
    Drowsiness
    Feeling tired
    Difficulty performing activities of daily living (ADLs)

Goal:
    Fatigue will be eliminated or controlled.

Outcome Criteria

✔ The patient will verbalize no complaints of fatigue or drowsiness.

✔ The patient will perform ADLs without assistance.

NOC *Energy conservation*
    Endurance
    Activity tolerance

INTERVENTIONS	RATIONALES
Assess level of energy and ability to perform ADLs.	Helps to ascertain baseline energy and performance level.
Provide a private, quiet environment.	Helps to promote rest.
Assess for and correct fluid volume deficit and electrolyte imbalance (see nursing diagnosis "Deficient Fluid Volume").	Decreased electrolytes, especially serum potassium level, is a cause of fatigue; correcting the fluid imbalance corrects the electrolyte imbalance, resulting in increased stamina.
Encourage potassium intake in the diet through potassium-rich foods and liquids when oral foods are tolerated.	Potassium is low in patients with gastroenterocolitis due to loss from the GI tract in stools, and intake is needed to correct decreased potassium levels and improve energy levels and muscle weakness.
Assist the patient as needed with activities.	Due to fatigue, the patient may not be able to complete ADLs.
Provide for uninterrupted rest periods during the day.	Helps to promote rest and endurance, allowing the patient to perform activities.

NIC   *Energy management*
Electrolyte monitoring
Fluid monitoring

Evaluation

No evidence of lasting effects of deficient fluid volume such as fatigue exists. The patient reports that fatigue has resolved and is not lethargic. Performance of ADLs is accomplished without complaints of feeling tired. Electrolyte levels return to normal.

Community/Home Care

No specific in home follow-up care is required for the problem of fatigue. The patient may find that he or she has some mild residual tiredness initially. This is handled simply by pacing activities and gradually increasing them until maximum activity level is achieved. It may be necessary for the patient to schedule rest periods during the day for several days until stamina has returned. If the patient dislikes returning to bed for naps or rest periods, an easy chair can be used for the rest period. It is not necessarily sleep that is needed, but rest. The patient will need to implement strategies to prevent a recurrence of deficient fluid volume and electrolyte imbalance, if possible; these strategies include prevention of gastroenterocolitis, drinking electrolyte-rich liquids, and consuming foods with potassium content. If the fatigue does not resolve, the patient should contact a health care provider for follow-up.

Documentation

Chart the results of a thorough assessment of the patient's ability to perform activities, with pulse and respirations taken after any activity. The patient's verbalization of any fatigue or feelings of tiredness are included in the patient record. Chart whether the patient requires assistance with ADLs or whether they are performed independently. Document interventions to treat fluid volume deficit.

NURSING DIAGNOSIS 3

 ACUTE PAIN

Related to:
Severe diarrhea
Increased strength of peristalsis
Excoriation of rectal area due to frequency of stools
Irritation by gastrointestinal enzymes in stool

Defining Characteristics:
Complaint of pain
Verbalization of cramping with stools
Complaints of feeling raw in rectal area

Goal:
The patient's pain and discomfort diminishes.
Intestinal motility/peristalsis slow.

Outcome Criteria

✔ The patient reports that the pain has been resolved.
✔ The patient states that abdominal cramping has decreased or been alleviated.
✔ The patient reports that the skin in area of rectum is not painful.

NOC   *Comfort level*
Pain control

INTERVENTIONS	RATIONALES
Assess level of pain or discomfort using a pain rating scale.	Helps to determine the degree of pain or discomfort the patient is experiencing. The rating scale is an objective way to assess the patient's pain.
Encourage the patient to lie on side in fetal position with knees flexed.	This position will take the tension off abdominal wall and omentum.
Apply heating pad or hot packs to abdomen.	Helps to relax muscles and decrease contractions and cramping.
Apply ointments such as petroleum jelly or A & D ointment to rectal area.	These substances are soothing and provide comfort to an area excoriated due to frequent wiping following stools and action of enzymes in stools.
Provide clear liquid diet, avoiding caffeine.	Helps to avoid gastric and colonic distention; caffeine is a gastric stimulant.
Be sure patient avoids foods that will increase intestinal peristalsis/motility.	Severe abdominal cramping can be caused by caffeine, fatty foods, roughage, and particularly hot and cold foods.
Administer antidiarrheal medications, as ordered.	Helps to alleviate the cause of the pain.
Assess the effectiveness of all interventions.	Helps to determine resolution of the problem or to determine whether revisions to the plan are required.

NIC *Pain management*

Evaluation

Determine the extent to which the patient reports that abdominal cramping has resolved. The patient should have no cramping with or without stool. In addition, any excoriation in the rectal area should be resolving or completely relieved as the diarrhea is treated.

Community/Home Care

At home, the patient will need to implement strategies to relieve diarrhea, which should subsequently resolve the abdominal cramping and the rectal discomfort. Simple non-pharmacological strategies are usually sufficient for relief of discomfort. By controlling the diarrhea, the patient is also treating the discomfort. It is important that the patient understand which liquids might stimulate peristalsis to the point of cramping. Although health care providers recommend clear liquids, coffee and tea, which are both clear liquids, should nevertheless be avoided, as they are stimulants that can add to diarrhea. The patient will need to experiment with positions to determine which is the most comfortable. Generally if the patient is lying down, the fetal position is best. Sitting in a tub of warm water for 10 to 15 minutes several times a day may relieve the discomfort in the rectal area. Application of petroleum jelly, A+D ointment, or preparations such as witch hazel pads can provide a soothing relief when the patient is experiencing frequent stools.

Documentation

If the patient is hospitalized, chart the results of a pain assessment, including exact location of the pain and the patient's description of the pain, as well as all interventions implemented. If the patient has complaints of discomfort other than pain, include these in the record. Be specific about the interventions carried out specifically to treat the diarrhea, such as type and amount of IV fluids given, any medications for diarrhea or pain, and the patient's responses.

CHAPTER 6.86

GASTROINTESTINAL BLEEDING: UPPER AND LOWER

GENERAL INFORMATION

Gastrointestinal (GI) bleeding is bleeding that occurs in either the lower or upper parts of the GI tract and can be caused by a variety of factors. Bleeding from any part is serious and requires immediate medical attention to prevent significant fluid losses and resulting hypovolemia. Most cases of GI bleeding occur without any accompanying symptoms. Lower GI bleeding is considered any bleeding from the GI tract that occurs below the level of the stomach. This bleeding usually occurs in the large bowel or the rectum. The cause of the bleeding may be due to inflammatory bowel disease (IBD) (Crohn's disease or ulcerative colitis), ruptured diverticulae, cecal ulcers, cancer/tumors, ruptured hemorrhoids, or bleeding polyps. The bleeding may manifest itself as bright red blood in the stool, which is an indicator of bleeding from the lower colon or rectum, or as occult blood not noticed by the individual but detected during routine screening of stool for occult blood. Upper GI bleeding occurs from the GI tract in the stomach and above, including the esophagus. The most common cause of upper GI bleeding is peptic ulcer disease, which accounts for at least 50 percent of all cases. Other causative factors include acute gastritis (often caused by medications such as aspirin and NSAIDs) and esophageal varices. In upper GI bleeding the patient may have occult blood in the stool or have dark black stools, vomit bright red blood, or vomit gastric contents that resemble coffee ground substances, which indicates that the blood has been in the stomach long enough to undergo alterations by gastric enzymes and hydrochloric acid. Any other symptoms that the patient experiences can be attributed to the causative factor, not the bleeding. The care plan addresses the patient who is hospitalized for GI bleeding.

NURSING DIAGNOSIS 1

DEFICIENT FLUID VOLUME

Related to:

Loss of blood

Defining Characteristics:

Restlessness, agitation

Tachycardia

Hypotension

Delayed capillary refill (> 2 seconds)

Cool, clammy skin

Decreased urinary output

Goal:

Adequate fluid volume will be restored.

Outcome Criteria

✔ The patient's skin will be warm and dry.
✔ Mucous membranes will be moist.
✔ The patient will have blood pressure and pulse at baseline.
✔ Urinary output will be ≥ 30 ml/hour.

NOC *Fluid balance*
Blood coagulation

INTERVENTIONS	RATIONALES
Monitor cardiac status: blood pressure, pulse (quality and rate), pulse pressure, capillary refill, and skin temperature and color.	Changes in blood pressure and pulse give information relevant to degree of volume depletion. The blood pressure may be normal to slightly decreased due to compensatory mechanisms.

INTERVENTIONS	RATIONALES
	If the volume depletion is not corrected, the blood pressure will decrease further; the pulse will become rapid and thready. Capillary refill is an indicator of perfusion; with significant fluid deficits it may be > 2 seconds. Pale, cool, clammy skin indicates decreased perfusion.
Establish two intravenous (IV) access sites with large bore catheters (18 gauge or larger).	IV access is crucial to treatment in acute blood loss; large gauge catheters allow for fluids to be given quickly, and blood products will run best in large catheters; the second site can be used for administration of medications.
Administer IV fluid replacement, as ordered: isotonic crystalloids such as 0.9 percent sodium chloride or lactated ringers are often used. For rapid volume expansion, human serum albumin may be given.	Helps to restore circulating volume and prevent further decreases in blood pressure. Albumin changes oncotic pressure, keeps fluid in the circulating volume, and pulls fluid from extravascular spaces.
Administer blood as ordered: whole blood or packed red blood cells (RBCs).	Acute blood loss from GI bleeding requires replacement; blood can be replaced at a 1:1 ratio as it remains in the intravascular volume; helps to increase oxygen-carrying capacity particularly if hemoglobin (Hgb) is < 12.
Question the patient regarding use of offending substances such as aspirin, NSAIDs, and steroids.	These substances can cause upper GI bleeding by irritating the mucosa of the GI tract, particularly the stomach.
Monitor results of laboratory studies: RBCs, Hgb and hematocrit (Hct), blood urea nitrogen (BUN), electrolytes, PT (prothrombin time), and APTT (activated partial thromboplastin time).	RBCs may be decreased due to loss of cells in blood; Hct fluctuates in response to fluid status; severe absolute loss from volume would produce a decrease in Hct with further drops during aggressive fluid resuscitation due to hemodilution; Hgb is usually decreased due to loss of RBCs; BUN and electrolytes would give indicators of renal function; BUN may be elevated initially, but decrease due to hemodilution of fluid replacement. PT and APTT will indicate the status of

INTERVENTIONS	RATIONALES
	ability to clot. For patients with liver disease, such as those with bleeding due to esophageal varices, the ability of the liver to produce clotting factors contributes to bleeding.
Prepare patient for invasive diagnostic tests: colonoscopy for lower GI bleeding and esophagogastroduodenoscopy (EGD) for upper GI bleeding (see nursing care plan "Endoscopy"). Generally this involves having the patient sign consent, take nothing by mouth (NPO), and, for the colonoscopy, cleanse the lower GI tract through use of cathartics and/or enemas.	Direct visualization of the GI tract through EGD and colonoscopy provides an accurate and quick diagnosis that allows for prompt treatment.
Monitor results of diagnostic tests specific for diagnosing cause of bleeding: abdominal computed tomography (CT) scan, abdominal MRI (magnetic resonance imaging), colonoscopy, EGD, and stool for guaiac.	Stool for guaiac confirms that bleeding has occurred; EGD and colonoscopy provide a definitive diagnosis. CT scans and MRIs can demonstrate the presence of bleeding sites or tumors.
If the patient is actively bleeding, prepare him or her for invasive procedures to control bleeding, as ordered or required.	Stopping the source of the bleeding in the GI system is necessary to stabilize the patient. In the case of lower bleeding in the colon, cauterization of bleeding sites or polyps can be done during a colonoscopy. For upper GI bleeding, thermal coagulation may be attempted, as well as injection therapy using epinephrine or other agents that constrict the bleeding vessel or sites in both the esophagus and the stomach.
For upper GI bleed (stomach), insert nasogastric (NG) tube and perform gastric lavage with room temperature normal saline as ordered until returns are clear.	Nasogastric tube allows for evacuating the stomach of blood; it also provides a means of lavage, which also clears blood and clots from the stomach.
Document returns from gastric lavage and keep a record of intake and output.	Helps to determine extent of bleeding.

(continues)

(continued)

INTERVENTIONS	RATIONALES
Instruct patient to save any emesis or stool for observation by the nurse; note color, amount, and consistency; test all stool and emesis for occult blood.	Assessment of the stool or emesis is required to assess extent of bleeding, site of bleeding, and response to treatment.
If blood is administered, monitor for transfusion reaction (see nursing care plan "Transfusion").	Transfusion reactions may occur due to allergenic response or immune response and need to be treated promptly.
Keep patient NPO as ordered.	For patients with upper GI bleeding, the stomach must be kept empty until bleeding has ceased to prevent further irritation; in patients with esophageal bleeding, food particles may adhere to areas of bleeding.
Administer vitamin K as ordered.	Helps to enhance clotting; especially for patients with esophageal varices.

NIC *Bleeding reduction:*
    Gastrointestinal
Fluid management
Fluid monitoring
Hypovolemia management
Intravenous insertion
Blood products administration
Intravenous therapy

Evaluation

Assess the patient for return of normal fluid volume. The patient's blood pressure and pulse should return to baseline or be only slightly abnormal. The pulse should be strong and regular. Skin should be warm, and color should return to normal appearance. Renal function should not be impaired, with an hourly output on the average of 30 ml/hour. Following fluid administration or blood replacement, the patient should be assessed for fluid overload, which may occur in the elderly and those with chronic left ventricular disease. The patient should have no further evidence of continued bleeding as demonstrated by an absence of active bleeding in emesis or stool and negative stool for guaiac.

Community/Home Care

Patients treated for GI bleeding should have normal fluid status restored and an absence of active bleeding prior to discharge home. The patient needs to be educated on how to prevent bleeding in those instances where the cause is preventable. Patients who take aspirin, NSAIDs, or steroids should discuss alternatives to these medications with the health care provider. Substituting acetaminophen for aspirin or NSAIDs if possible is a good solution. If eliminating these substances is not an option, taking them with food may decrease the risk of bleeding. In addition, the patient who has bleeding due to peptic ulcers will need to control those factors that aggravate the disorder and that predispose them to bleeding. This includes managing stress and limiting foods that cause irritation, such as acidic, fried, and spicy foods. Even though most people find the act repulsive, patients at home will need to observe their stool for blood, and in some instances may need to perform testing for occult blood. Patients who experienced bleeding due to perforated ulcers or cancers of the GI tract will need to undergo surgery to alleviate the cause of the bleeding, and post-operative care at home will involve caring for the incisional wound, modification of activities until healed, and follow-up care. Fatigue at home is caused by the loss of RBCs, which results in the loss of oxygen carrying capacity of the blood. This problem can be handled simply by informing the patient to perform activities as tolerated until stamina/endurance is re-established. This may take a number of days or weeks depending upon the extent of the bleeding. The patient can cluster activities around rest periods and seek the assistance of a family member for household chores or cooking. The patient typically has more energy during the early part of the day and may want to perform necessary tasks during this time. Planning by placing needed items within easy reach will help; for instance, the patient can place remote controls, books, liquids, snacks, and medications in the room where he or she will spend most of his or her time in order to limit numerous trips to other parts of the home. Eating iron-rich foods such as meat and leafy green vegetables should be encouraged. The health care provider may want the patient to return for a follow-up appointment to ensure that parameters such as RBCs, Hgb, and Hct have returned to normal.

Documentation

In this situation, document initial assessment findings such as blood pressure, pulse, respirations, temperature, skin status, and mental status. If there is an obvious bleeding source, document an estimate of blood loss, and measures implemented to stop bleeding. Chart results of stool and emesis for guaiac in keeping with agency guidelines. Document all interventions, such as IV catheter insertion, fluids initiated (type, rate), nasogastric tube insertion with description of the gastric contents returned (amount, color), and patient preparation for procedures or surgery. Be specific when charting patient responses to treatment so that other health care providers can clearly determine improvement or deterioration.

NURSING DIAGNOSIS 2

DECREASED CARDIAC OUTPUT

Related to:

Inadequate intravascular volume

Defining Characteristics:

Tachycardia

Decreased oxygen saturation

Skin cool to touch

Peripheral cyanosis

Diminished peripheral pulses

Delayed capillary refill > 2 seconds

Urinary output < 30 ml/hour

Narrowing pulse pressure

Goal:

Adequate cardiac output is restored.

Outcome Criteria

✔ The patient has pulse rate between 60 and 100.

✔ The patient's skin is warm and dry.

✔ Perfusion is restored as evidenced by absence of peripheral cyanosis and capillary refill is < 2 seconds.

✔ Urinary output is > 30 ml/hour average.

✔ The patient's blood pressure returns to patient's baseline.

NOC *Circulatory status*
Tissue perfusion: Cardiac
Tissue perfusion: Peripheral
Tissue perfusion: Cerebral
Cardiac pump effectiveness
Vital signs

INTERVENTIONS	RATIONALES
Assess vital signs, particularly blood pressure and pulse, as ordered but at least every 4 hours.	Changes in blood pressure and pulse give indicators to patient status. In severe fluid loss, a decreased blood pressure with narrowing pulse pressure may be noted; the pulse may be rapid, weak, and thready.
Assess neck veins.	Absence of visible neck veins when the patient is supine indicates decreased circulating volume.
Assess urinary output.	Decreased urinary output (< 30 ml/hour) indicates decreased perfusion to kidneys secondary to blood loss.
Assess skin temperature and color.	If bleeding is unchecked, perfusion to skin and periphery is inadequate to maintain warmth or normal color.
Assess peripheral pulses.	If cardiac output starts to decrease due to loss of blood, peripheral pulses become weak, diminished, or absent, as the heart is unable to maintain perfusion to extremities.
Assess mental status: level of consciousness, confusion, and agitation.	Changes in mental status indicate a decrease in cerebral tissue perfusion and indicates an inability of the body's compensatory mechanism to provide adequate oxygenation to cerebral tissue.
Assess respiratory status noting adventitious breath sounds and oxygen saturation.	Decreased cardiac output leads to decreased perfusion to lungs, causing crackles and dyspnea; loss of blood can create a decreased ability to perfuse tissues, resulting in lowered oxygen saturation.

(continues)

(continued)

INTERVENTIONS	RATIONALES
Implement strategies to control bleeding and restore intravascular volume as ordered (see nursing diagnosis "Deficient Fluid Volume").	Replacing intravascular volume is necessary to improve cardiac output.
Maintain bedrest during acute bleeding.	Helps to decrease the workload of the heart.

NIC *Cardiac care*
   Fluid management
   Fluid monitoring
   Vital signs monitoring

Evaluation

Note the degree to which outcome criteria have been achieved. The patient should demonstrate adequate cardiac output or improvement in abnormalities. Peripheral pulses should be present, and skin, when touched, should be warm. If cardiac output is improved, perfusion to the kidneys should be adequate, with the patient producing at least 30 ml of urine per hour on average. Blood pressure returns to the patient's normal range, and the pulse is strong, regular, and within 60 to 100 beats per minute. Oxygen saturation should be > 90 percent.

Community/Home Care

For most patients, once the bleeding source has been identified and fluid status is re-established, cardiac output is restored, and no further interventions are required in the home. However, there may be some residual effects on other systems that affect ability to perform usual activities. The patient who has experienced GI bleeding will need to know how to increase activities gradually when at home with a balance of rest and activity. The patient will need to monitor his or her response to activity, noting any shortness of breath, increased respiratory rate, or increased pulse rate. Home care follow-up may be required for some patients, especially if they verbalize feelings of anxiety or lack of knowledge about the emergency that necessitated in-hospital care. For those patients with disease processes such as cancer or cirrhosis, more aggressive treatments are required, and follow-up may center on treating the disease to prevent a recurrence. A follow-up appointment is necessary to be sure that the patient has returned to his or her normal level of functioning.

Documentation

Chart the results of a thorough assessment of the cardiac/respiratory system, including skin temperature, peripheral pulses, tolerance for activity, capillary refill, breath sounds, and vital signs. Document blood pressure and pulse according to agency protocol. Output should be recorded according to agency guidelines. Include in the record any patient complaint made relevant to the cardiac system or bleeding exactly as the patient states it. All interventions should be documented in a timely fashion with the patient's specific response to the intervention. Always include in the patient's record his or her psychological status: whether the patient appears anxious, restless, or fearful, and whether family members or significant others are present.

NURSING DIAGNOSIS 3

 ANXIETY

Related to:
   Active bleeding
   Emergency health problem
   Unknown health status

Defining Characteristics:
   Tachycardia
   Restlessness
   Verbalization of anxiety, concern, fear

Goal:
   Anxiety is relieved.

Outcome Criteria

✔ The patient exhibits no overt signs of anxiety such as restlessness or agitation.

✔ The patient verbalizes that anxiety has been reduced or alleviated.

✔ The patient asks appropriate questions regarding bleeding or any aspect of treatment.

NOC *Anxiety self-control*
   Symptom control

INTERVENTIONS	RATIONALES
Assess for verbal and nonverbal signs of anxiety and fear, including increased heart rate.	Helps to detect the presence of anxiety and for early intervention to prevent physiological alterations.
Monitor the intensity of anxiety/fear by having patient rate on a numerical scale.	Allows for a more objective measure of anxiety and fear levels.
Encourage patient to verbalize fears and anxiety regarding health status (bleeding).	Recognition of fear and anxiety is the first step to coping with issues and to avoid of negative feelings.
Teach the patient relaxation techniques (such as slow, purposeful breathing and guided imagery) and encourage their use.	Reduces anxiety and creates a feeling of comfort.
Reassure the patient by explaining procedures, such as EGD and colonoscopy; treatments; and hospital environment.	Fear of the unknown contributes to anxiety; knowing what to expect helps the patient maintain a sense of control.
Administer anti-anxiety agents as ordered.	Helps to decrease anxiety if unrelieved by non-pharmacological measures.
Stay with patient during critical times and during periods when fear and anxiety are evident.	Allows the nurse to offer comfort, care, and assurances to reduce anxiety and fear.
Keep significant others/family informed of patient's status.	The presence of significant others often has a calming effect on critically ill patients.
Teach the patient new methods of relaxing and coping.	The patient may require assistance in identifying and learning new coping techniques.

NIC   *Anxiety reduction*
Calming technique
Presence

Evaluation

Assess the patient for the degree that fear and anxiety have been controlled. The patient should verbalize feelings and indicate whether interventions have produced a tolerable state of anxiety and fear. Determine if the patient understands what has happened (GI bleeding) and interventions required for treatment by the health care provider and by the patient. During evaluation, be sure to inquire about the use of coping strategies and relaxation techniques.

Community/Home Care

The patient will need to develop coping strategies and relaxation techniques to utilize in the home setting. The nurse must adequately equip the patient with the knowledge necessary to make him or her feel in control. An understanding of what to expect following a diagnosis of GI bleeding and how to prevent it if possible will assist the patient to feel in control. In the home, the patient may be able to reduce anxiety more quickly through use of common everyday activities, such as taking a walk, reading, meditating, listening to music, and enjoying the emotional support of family and friends.

Documentation

Using a numerical scale, document the degree of fear or anxiety the patient is experiencing. Also, include any verbal, nonverbal, or physiological clues that could be indicators of anxiety or fear, such as restlessness, tachycardia, or diaphoresis. Document interventions implemented to treat anxiety or fear, along with the patient's responses, as well as instruction about relaxation techniques and the disease process.

CHAPTER 6.87

HEPATITIS (A, B, C, D, & E)

GENERAL INFORMATION

Hepatitis is an inflammation of the liver that may be caused by bacteria, viruses, toxic chemicals, or trauma. However, viral hepatitis is the most common form of hepatitis. **Hepatitis A** (infectious hepatitis, HA) is an infectious process caused by the hepatitis A virus. The range of symptomatology and disability may range from very mild to severe, and complete recovery usually occurs. It is transmitted by the fecal-oral route, most often through contaminated water and food. It is most commonly seen in children and young adults. A vaccine is available for prevention for those persons traveling to countries where it is endemic, but for those who have been exposed it must be given within 2 weeks of exposure. **Hepatitis B** (viral hepatitis, serum hepatitis, HB) is an inflammation of the liver caused by the hepatitis B virus. It is transmitted via blood, saliva, semen, and vaginal fluids. Frequently contamination occurs parenterally through contact with infected syringes, needles, blood products, or even instruments used for tattoos or body piercing. Complications can include cirrhosis, coma, and death. A preventative vaccine is available for Hepatitis B and is recommended for all health care workers, sanitary workers, and others who are at high risk for the disease. A small percentage of persons with Hepatitis B become chronic carriers of the virus and approximately 10 percent of patients eventually have chronic infection. Hepatitis B is also more likely to result in fulminant hepatitis than the other types of hepatitis. **Hepatitis C** (non-A/non-B hepatitis, HC) is an inflammation of the liver caused by the hepatitis C virus. It is transmitted via blood or high-risk sexual contact. Hepatitis C represents 20 percent of all cases of hepatitis officially reported to the CDC. The most common groups of people to contract Hepatitis C are intravenous drug users (most common mode of transmission in the U.S.),

hemophiliacs, renal dialysis patients, and health care workers. It is usually insidious and death rarely occurs but it is estimated that 50–80 percent of patients who acquire Hepatitis C will have chronic hepatitis and approximately 20 percent of patients with Hepatitis C will progress to cirrhosis. **Hepatitis D** (delta hepatitis, viral hepatitis D, HD) is an inflammation caused by the hepatitis D (Delta) virus. It is always accompanied by Hepatitis B and is transmitted via blood, serous body fluids, or sexual intercourse. Hepatitis D can be acute or it may also prove to be chronic and increases the severity of Hepatitis B. **Hepatitis E** (viral hepatitis E, enterically transmitted non-A/non-B, HE) is very similar to Hepatitis A. It is most commonly transmitted via feces-contaminated water and is caused by the hepatitis E virus. Although Hepatitis E is rare in the U.S. and is self-limiting, there appears to be a high mortality rate in pregnant women. It is a common form of hepatitis in third-world countries. **Toxic Hepatitis** (chemical hepatitis) is caused by exposure to a toxic chemical agent through ingestion, inhalation, or parenteral administration. Some causes of toxic hepatitis include acetaminophen, aspirin, INH, Thorazine, muscarine found in some mushrooms, carbon tetra-chloride found in dry cleaning fluids, glue containing toluene, and pesticides. Prognosis is based on the toxin and the amount of exposure. Clinical manifestations of hepatitis can be mild or severe and occur in three phases. In the pre-icteric phase, the patient may have fatigue, headaches, anorexia, abdominal discomfort, sore throat, and a fever. The icteric phase is characterized by the onset of jaundice, right upper quadrant pain, clay-colored stools, darkened urine, and pruritus. The post-icteric phase is characterized by fatigue, a return of stools and urine to a more normal color, and an improvement or resolution in jaundice. Most patients with hepatitis are treated as outpatients.

NURSING DIAGNOSIS 1

 ## IMBALANCED NUTRITION: LESS THAN BODY REQUIREMENTS

Related to:

Anorexia

Nausea and vomiting

Malabsorption of nutrients from foods

Increased metabolic needs causing increased caloric needs

Abdominal pain

No interest in eating

Defining Characteristics:

Weight loss

Decreased total protein and albumin levels

Decreased intake of food

Reports lack of energy

Lack of interest in eating

Complaint of abdominal pain

Goal:

The patient's normal nutritional status will be restored.

The patient's daily caloric requirements are met.

Outcome Criteria

✔ The patient will not lose weight.

✔ Electrolytes will be within normal limits.

✔ Albumin will return to normal limits.

✔ The patient verbalizes an understanding of the importance of adequate nutrition.

NOC *Nutritional status:*
Food and fluid intake
Nutritional status: Energy

INTERVENTIONS	RATIONALES
Complete a fluid and nutritional assessment, including assessing for nausea; vomiting; poor skin turgor; dry, pale mucous membranes; fatty stools; change in stool color/context: clay-colored or melena;	Patients who experience hepatitis often have a decreased nutritional status due to malabsorption of nutrients in the gastrointestinal (GI) tract due to the diseased state of the liver and a feeling of malaise
concentrated, dark, foul-smelling urine; dietary intake; fluid intake and output; weight loss; loss of appetite; decreased muscle tone; albumin levels; hemoglobin (Hgb); iron; and electrolytes.	that decreases appetite. Anorexia and nausea are common in hepatitis and add to the problem by preventing the patient from taking in enough nutrients to meet metabolic demands. The stool becomes clay-colored due to the lack of bilirubin from the liver; fat content in the stool increases because of an inability of the liver to metabolize it; and the urine is dark because of increased amounts of bilirubin now excreted via the kidneys. These laboratory results give clues to nutritional status and the effect of hepatitis on liver function.
Assess laboratory results: viral antigens, liver function studies—alanine aminotransferase (ALT), alkaline phosphatase (ALP), aspartate aminotransferase (AST), and gamma-glutamyltransferase (GGTP)—bilirubin, albumin, total protein, iron, electrolytes, folic acid, and thiamine level.	Viral antibodies specific to the type of causative virus can be found in the blood (anti-HAV, HBV surface antigen, anti-HBV antibodies, anti-HCV antibodies, positive delta antigen, anti-HDV antibodies, anti-HEV antibodies); liver enzymes will be elevated in hepatitis and give an indication that the liver's ability to function may be impaired; bilirubin will be increased; other lab values will be decreased due to the inability of the patient to eat and absorb adequate amounts of nutrients. Iron, folic acid, and electrolytes decrease as nutritional intake decreases.
Weigh patient and monitor weight daily or weekly.	Helps to establish baseline for comparison and to evaluate responses to interventions.
Collaborate with the dietician to develop an acceptable diet that considers usual habits, food intake, and any cultural or religious restrictions.	The dietician can discuss with the patient which foods may be digested better with the fewest untoward effects but the best nutritional results.
Encourage the patient to take increased nutrients through high-calorie and high-carbohydrate diets, as ordered, and suggest small meals with between-meal snacks.	Helps to promote adequate intake of nutrients; for patients with decreased appetite, a small meal is easier to ingest and more likely to be seen as desirable; the patient with hepatitis is often fatigued and may become tired before completing a large meal.

(continues)

(continued)

INTERVENTIONS	RATIONALES
Give the patient most of his or her calorie requirements early in the day.	Patients with hepatitis are more likely to be anorexic and nauseated in the evening and afternoon.
Give nutritional supplements as ordered: folic acid, thiamine, B_{12}, multivitamins.	Helps to supplement nutrient intake.
Provide between-meal snacks that taste good and contain supplemental calories.	These can include such things as pudding, ice cream, candy, fruit, juice, milk, soft drinks, and cookies, and may prove to be more appealing than the food served in normal meals.
Administer antivirals (interferon alpha for both chronic hepatitis B and C, combination therapy of interferon alpha with ribavirin for chronic hepatitis C, lamivudine for chronic hepatitis B), as ordered, and monitor for adverse effects.	Interferon alpha interferes with viral replication and reduces the viral load; lamivudine also decreases inflammation and subsequent scarring. Flu-like symptoms are a side effect.
Administer anti-emetics, as ordered.	Helps to decrease nausea and vomiting.
Administer antacids, as ordered.	Helps to reduce heartburn, stomach acids, and risk of ulcer formation.
Administer IV fluids with electrolytes and multivitamins, as ordered.	Hepatitis patients admitted to the hospital for acute care often have poor nutritional states and require IV fluids for hydration, as well as electrolytes and multivitamins; these are usually given until the patient can take adequate nutrients by mouth.
Assist with administration of total parenteral nutrition (TPN), as ordered.	Short-term TPN may be necessary if the patient is unable to meet daily caloric and vitamin requirements via oral intake, especially during times of acute illness.
Monitor and record intake and output according to agency protocol, being sure to include liquid stools as part of the fluid output.	Helps to detect dehydration and initiate early treatment.
Teach the patient and family about nutritional requirements and the role of the liver in maintenance of nutritional status.	Helps to enhance compliance with diet.

NIC   *Nutritional monitoring*
Nutritional management
Nausea management

Evaluation

The patient's nutritional status is stable as demonstrated by the laboratory values (albumin, total protein, iron, electrolytes, folate, etc.). The patient verbalizes an interest in eating and understands the need for increased nutrients due to the malnourished state. No further weight loss occurs, and the patient consumes regular meals. Liver enzymes and bilirubin are decreased and returning to normal.

Community/Home Care

The patient must continue to give attention to nutrition and the role of the liver in nutrition maintenance. A dietary consultation is crucial in assisting the patient in planning for nutritional needs. The patient and family require formal instruction regarding the restrictions that may be imposed due to dysfunction of the liver. Crucial areas include the need for increased calories, carbohydrates, and specifically, glucose. Glucose levels can drop due to poor intake of adequate amounts and because the diseased liver may not be able to adequately break down glycogen from its stores or manufacture new glucose. Giving the patient a list of foods that can provide good sources of the required nutrients will be helpful. With this in mind, the patient and family will need to remember the signs and symptoms of a hypoglycemic episode. Even though a diet rich in protein is not advised, the patient will need to have sufficient amounts to provide a source of energy, as fatigue will be a persistent problem throughout recovery. Significant others play a role in implementing strategies to improve nutrition by preparing meals and encouraging the patient to ingest them. Frequent small meals at home should be encouraged for the patient during the early convalescence period in order to increase the likelihood that the patient can ingest enough nutrients. Because the dietary recommendations may be easily forgotten, a handy, laminated reference guide can be created to give to the patient or family. This guide could include a list of foods that provide protein, foods that provide glucose, foods that provide iron, foods to avoid, foods that are acceptable, how much of any group to consume, and a schedule for small meals. Supplemental drinks can improve nutritional status during periods when the patient is unable to ingest adequate amounts of nutrition through normal meals due to anorexia, abdominal pain, or malaise. There are numerous products on the market (Boost, Ensure) but the patient may need to experiment with which ones are satisfying or appealing after consultation with the dietician. The patient may need to remain on multivitamins, folic acid, thiamine, electrolyte supplements, and other nutritional supplements for an extended period of time. Teach the patient to monitor nutrition/intake by keeping a log of what he or she eats, when he or she eats, and how he or she tolerates eating. If at any time a particular meal or food product causes pain or subsequent nausea/vomiting, the patient should note this in the log and eliminate this food from the diet. Weights should also be included in the log. Even though the patient may not want to weigh every day, weighing at least every other day is a good way to keep track of weight loss or stabilization. This information can be shared with the health care provider at each follow-up visit to provide data for revision in prescribed therapeutic interventions. The patient is more likely to have proper nutrition when supported by family and friends. Follow-up providers should assess the patient for weight loss and monitor laboratory results (liver enzymes, bilirubin, etc.) for improvement in the disease.

Documentation

Chart the results of a nutritional assessment that includes a history of usual intake. Document vital signs, weights, and intake and output according to agency protocol at least every shift or every 8 hours. Include in the chart the amount of food the patient consumes at each meal and what, if any, supplements are taken by the patient. For patients who are taking nutritional supplements (vitamins, liquid supplements, etc.) chart this in the patient's medication record. In most agencies there are specific guidelines for charting regarding total parenteral nutrition (TPN) that includes specific nutritional parameters, so the nurse should document accordingly. If the patient has complaints of any type, document these in the record with accompanying documentation indicating response to interventions. Always include in the record any referrals made, especially to the dietician.

 IMPAIRED SKIN INTEGRITY

Related to:

Increased bilirubin in the bloodstream and deposits of bile salts under the skin

Defining Characteristics:

Jaundice (skin and sclera)

Pruritus

Dry skin

Goal:

The patient's skin will remain intact and return to normal status.

Outcome Criteria

✔ Itching will be relieved.

✔ Skin will be moist.

✔ The patient's skin will have no areas of breakdown.

✔ Jaundice will resolve.

NOC *Comfort level*

Tissue integrity:
Skin and mucous membranes

INTERVENTIONS	RATIONALES
Perform a thorough skin assessment, noting jaundice, open areas, any bruising, petechiae, and color changes; monitor laboratory results of bilirubin, coagulation studies, and vitamin K.	Jaundice occurs as a result of the inability of the diseased liver to conjugate bilirubin and excrete it through urine and stool. As the bilirubin levels increase, the bile salts are deposited in the skin, giving it a yellow appearance and causing irritation. The abnormal itchy skin becomes a high-risk area for breakdown and frequent skin assessments are critical, especially given the compromised nutritional state of the patient. Due to the inability of the liver to exert its normal role in the absorption and storage of vitamin K and other clotting factors, patients bruise easily.

(continues)

(continued)

INTERVENTIONS	RATIONALES
Assess patient for itching and ask to describe.	Most patients with hepatitis experience itching, especially in the icteric phase, which can be attributed to increased levels of bilirubin and the deposition of bile salts in the skin. The itching may be described as intense and deep.
Administer antihistamines (Benadryl), as ordered.	Helps alleviate itching due to jaundice.
Ensure that the room is cool and humidified, and that bed clothing is light cotton and loose fitting.	These provide for maximum comfort.
Apply cool, moist compresses to areas that itch.	This will reduce itching, frustration level, and annoyance.
Discourage the patient from vigorous scratching and encourage to keep nails short.	Scratching can cause disruption to the skin that can lead to lesions that are difficult to heal.
Apply moisturizing products to the skin: oil-based shower gels or lotions, petroleum jelly, or oatmeal-based shower gels or lotions. Avoid products containing alcohol and deodorant soaps.	These products add moisture back to the skin and ease the itching. Alcohol-based products and most deodorant soaps cause further drying of the skin.
Instruct the patient to bathe in tepid rather than hot water.	Hot water increases pruritus.
Instruct the patient to pat dry and apply lotions or ointments before completely drying the skin following a shower or bath.	Vigorous rubbing or drying of the skin following a bath closes skin pores, rendering emollients ineffective.
Lower room temperature, especially at night.	Excessive warmth increases itching.
Encourage the use of distraction or relaxation therapy.	These will help change the perception of the itching and discomfort.

NIC　*Pruritus management*
　　　　Skin care: Topical treatments
　　　　Skin surveillance

Evaluation

Determine whether the stated outcome criteria have been achieved. The patient should report decreased itching, and the skin should be intact. Even though jaundice may still be present, the patient's comfort should improve. Skin is moist without scaliness. Bruising or petechiae should be minimal.

Community/Home Care

In the home setting, the patient will continue implementation of the interventions initiated by the nursing staff. The intensity of the pruritus will vary from time to time, often depending upon the amount of bilirubin present in the blood and being deposited onto the skin as well as environmental factors. The patient will need to experiment with a number of measures or products to relieve the itching. It is important that the patient pay attention to environmental factors at home that may contribute to itching, such as temperature in the home, types of linens used (coarse cotton sheets may increase itching, whereas flannel sheets may feel better), and common household items such as dishwashing detergent, household cleaning products, and hand soaps, all of which can worsen the condition. Clothes made of fabrics known to be irritating, such as wool, linen, and synthetics, should be avoided. If the patient cannot resist touching the skin when itching, he or she can place a thin layer of clothing or a thin towel over the area and rub it gently using wide circular motions. Remembering to reduce the temperature of bath water to lukewarm or tepid can make a difference in comfort, as can application of cool moist compresses when itching occurs. The patient may find that inexpensive home remedies will often work as well as commercial products and medications. The patient or significant other should inspect the skin for open areas or bruising on a regular basis so that early treatment can be instituted. The patient should understand when to take medications for itching and be aware that medicines such as Benadryl may cause drowsiness that limits the ability to engage in activities requiring alertness. As the patient moves into the post-icteric phase, itching should resolve.

Documentation

Chart any complaints of itching and interventions employed to treat it. If medications are given, document them on the medication record according to agency protocol with follow-up documentation regarding the patient's responses. Document skin assessments, specifically noting any abnormalities in the skin, including discoloration, bruising, or breakdown. Indicate education provided regarding skin impairment and suggested treatments.

NURSING DIAGNOSIS 3

 ### FATIGUE

Related to:

Decreased nutritional state

Decreased synthesis of tissue protein and utilization of nutrients

Defining Characteristics:

Lethargy

Verbalization of being tired

States a lack of energy

Inability to carry out normal activities without becoming exhausted

Goal:

Fatigue will be relieved.

Outcome Criteria

✔ The patient is able to perform activities of daily living (ADLs).

✔ The patient verbalizes that fatigue has improved or been eliminated.

NOC *Activity tolerance*
Endurance
Energy conservation
Nutritional status: Energy

INTERVENTIONS	RATIONALES
Obtain subjective data regarding normal activities, limitations, and nighttime sleep patterns.	Helps to determine the effect fatigue has on normal functioning. Adequate sleep is required for restoration of the body.
Monitor patient for signs of excessive physical and emotional fatigue (irritability, agitation, easily falls asleep during normal waking hours, inability to complete normal tasks).	Use as a guideline for adjusting activity and increasing rest periods.
Encourage periods of rest and activity.	Hepatitis interferes with synthesis of tissue proteins and utilization of nutrients required for energy; rest is required to decrease metabolic demands and allow for recovery of the liver. Conserves oxygen and prevents undue fatigue. Hepatitis patients often require extended periods of rest or sleep in order to feel rested.
Schedule activities so that excessive demands for oxygen and energy are avoided; for example, space planned activities away from mealtimes.	Digestion requires energy and oxygen; participation in activities close to meals will cause increased fatigue because of insufficient energy reserves.
Gradually increase activity, as tolerated.	In the post-icteric period, fatigue improves, but the patient may still require activity restrictions; monitoring tolerance to activity can provide information to indicate when activity may be increased or decreased. If any particular activity causes undue fatigue, it should not be attempted again until later in the recovery period.
Limit visitors during any periods of acute illness.	Socialization for long periods may cause fatigue.
Increase intake of high-energy foods such as poultry, dried beans and peas, whole grains, and foods high in vitamin C, within restrictions of the recommended diet.	These foods enhance energy metabolism, increase oxygen-carrying capacity, and provide ready sources of energy needed in hypermetabolic states such as acute inflammation and fever.
Encourage the patient to plan activities for times when he or she has the most energy, usually early in the day.	Helps to prevent fatigue.
Explore diversional activities with the patient and encourage quiet activities such as reading, video games, computer games, card games, television/movies, crossword puzzles, etc.	Because the recovery period may be extensive, the patient needs methods to alleviate boredom.
If family or significant others are not available, assist the patient to identify community resources that can be of assistance with daily activities such as housekeeping, laundry, and meal preparation.	The patient may need assistance with daily normal tasks due to fatigue, and a number of community resources are available to the chronically ill and/or disabled.
Assist the patient in developing a home schedule to minimize energy expenditure.	This will help the patient retain some independence while being cognizant of limitations and need for energy conservation.

NIC   *Energy management*

Evaluation

Obtain subjective information from the patient regarding the presence of fatigue. The patient should gradually report the ability to participate in ADLs and other normal activities with no fatigue.

Community/Home Care

Patients with hepatitis should understand that fatigue will persist for an extended period of time from diagnosis through the post-icteric phase. Appropriate education on ways to adapt self-care and household activities when fatigued is paramount. A history should be obtained from the patient regarding the usual routine for work, school, ADLs, and household chores, so that individualized interventions can be implemented. Attention to what the patient normally does and how the patient wants to make adaptations can only enhance compliance. The nurse must remain aware of cultural backgrounds that may influence a patient's perception of and adaptation to perceived dependency on others. During the period when the liver is attempting to heal from the inflammation but is still unable to carry out its detoxification function, fatigue will be more pronounced. The patient must understand how to adjust activity in response to feelings of fatigue, possibly even arranging for rest or nap periods in the afternoon. This may not be a realistic recommendation for some people who may try to continue to work and whose occupations preclude them from napping or even resting during the day. Strategies to enhance nighttime sleep should be implemented so that the patient can get adequate rest. Of particular concern is controlling itching that occurs with jaundice (see nursing diagnosis "Impaired Skin Integrity"). Attention to good nutrition should continue with intake of foods that are good sources of iron, vitamin C, and protein, within dietary restrictions (see nursing diagnosis "Imbalanced Nutrition: Less than Body Requirements"). The patient will need to return to the health care provider for evaluation of liver enzymes and bilirubin. If these parameters have not decreased or returned to normal, the patient may require further restrictions in activity.

Documentation

Chart the specific complaint of fatigue, including what activities the patient has been performing.

Document interventions implemented to address fatigue, being sure to document food intake as well as rest periods and the patient's response to activity. Include in the record the patient's particular verbalization of the degree of fatigue and response to treatment. An assessment of the patient's sleep patterns should also be documented. Be sure to document teaching implemented with the family.

NURSING DIAGNOSIS 4

DEFICIENT KNOWLEDGE

Related to:

New diagnosis of hepatitis

Lack of information about the disease and its treatment and prevention

Misinformation

Defining Characteristics:

Asks many questions

Asks no questions

Verbalizes misunderstanding

Goal:

The patient is compliant with disease treatment and preventive measures.

The patient is able to identify symptoms that would encourage him or her to seek early medical intervention.

Outcome Criteria

✔ The patient verbalizes a willingness and desire to learn the necessary information.

✔ The patient verbalizes an understanding of the disease process of hepatitis.

✔ The patient verbalizes an understanding of all treatment recommendations.

✔ The patient verbalizes an understanding of activity restrictions required during convalescence.

✔ The patient will be able to identify signs and symptoms of deteriorating liver function.

NOC   *Knowledge: Disease process*
          Knowledge: Health behavior
          Treatment behavior:
              Illness or injury

INTERVENTIONS	RATIONALES
Assess readiness of the patient to learn (motivation, cognitive level, and physiological status).	The patient must be motivated to learn, have the capability to learn the content, and be free of distractions from learning such as pain, fatigue, and emotional distress.
Assess the patient's knowledge of hepatitis.	The patient may have some knowledge about the disease, and teaching should begin with what the patient already knows.
Create a quiet environment conducive to learning.	Environmental noise can prevent the learner from focusing on what is being taught.
Teach incrementally, beginning with simple concepts.	The patient will learn and retain knowledge better when information is presented in small segments. Starting with simple information first allows for better understanding.
Collaborate with the physician to teach the patient and family members about the disease process of hepatitis and required interventions: — Normal function of the liver — Pathophysiology of hepatitis, including clinical manifestations — Prognosis for hepatitis patients — Transmission and prevention of hepatitis — Diagnostic and laboratory tests: liver enzymes, bilirubin — Treatment of the disease (rest, nutrition, skin care, medications) — Indications of a relapse or deteriorating liver function (urine returns to a dark color, stools lighten, fatigue worsens)	Understanding of normal function and pathophysiology helps the patient to understand the rationale for therapeutic interventions. Knowledge of diagnostic tests, treatments required, and prevention of complications empowers the patient to take control and be compliant.
Teach the patient regarding diet required: small meals; nutritious snacks; high-calorie, high-carbohydrate, and high-energy foods (see nursing diagnosis "Imbalanced Nutrition: Less than Body Requirements").	The patient will need to understand the role of nutrition in healing and implement strategies to provide for adequate nutrition.
Teach the patient how to conserve energy (see nursing diagnosis "Fatigue").	Fatigue continues to be a problem through all phases of the disease; the patient needs to implement strategies to ensure enough rest to allow for liver healing.
Assess the patient's and family's understanding of all teaching by encouraging them to repeat information and ask questions as needed.	This allows the nurse to hear in the patient's own words what was taught, makes it easier to know what information may need to be reinforced, and ensures that the patient has enough information to be compliant.
Establish that the patient has the resources required to be compliant, such as transportation to follow-up appointments for laboratory work or in-home assistance for household chores.	If needed resources such as finances and transportation to follow-up appointments are not available, the patient cannot be compliant; the nurse will need to make necessary referrals. This may be a real problem for patients from remote and rural areas, especially if family support is not available.
Give the patient written information.	Provides reference at a later time, and for review.

NIC *Teaching: Disease process*
Teaching: Individual

Evaluation

The patient is able to repeat all information for the nurse and asks questions about hepatitis, diagnostic tests, prevention of transmission, treatment modalities (rest, skin care, nutrition, medications), and possible outcomes. Prior to discharge, the patient verbalizes an understanding of the activity restrictions and agrees to be compliant. The patient is able to discuss signs that would indicate a relapse and how to address it. In addition, the patient agrees to return for follow-up appointments.

Community/Home Care

The possibility for the knowledge deficit to persist following hospitalization is very real due to the large volume of information the patient needs. In-home care focuses on the three most significant problems of nutrition, fatigue, and skin (jaundice, pruritus). The most difficult part of this will be compliance with the need for rest to allow healing of the diseased liver. Teaching must be structured and thorough to allow for adequate understanding by the patient. Written literature and instructions should be given to the patient and possibly placed in a colorful folder or envelope that is easily identified. Telephone numbers to be used to contact health care providers regarding any problems at home should be in the folder as well. The information should be written in simple terms that are easily read. This document should be kept in a handy place for quick reference. Evaluate the patient's knowledge level prior to discharge. The nurse should ensure that the patient understands exactly what having a diagnosis of hepatitis means and what to expect in the future. Follow-up with a health care provider focuses on assurance that no complications have occurred, energy levels are improving, jaundice has dissipated, and liver function studies are normal.

Documentation

Document all content taught and the patient's verbalization of understanding. Specific attention should be given to documentation of any specific concerns that the patient expresses. Include in the documentation the patient's willingness to comply with all recommendations made regarding diet, rest, medications, and follow-up care. Any area that requires further teaching should be clearly indicated in the record. Include in the record appointments that have been made for outpatient laboratory tests or check-ups. Chart any questions or concerns that the patient has verbalized. Always include the titles of any printed literature given to the patient for reinforcement.

CHAPTER 6.88

INFLAMMATORY BOWEL DISEASE

GENERAL INFORMATION

Inflammatory bowel disease (IBD) is the term used to classify or group the disorders of ulcerative colitis and Crohn's disease. The etiologies of these diseases have not been absolutely confirmed, but several theories have been suggested. These include an autoimmune response, allergies, heredity, and infections of the gastrointestinal (GI) system. Both ulcerative colitis and Crohn's disease have patterns of remission and exacerbation. IBD is most frequently seen among 15- to 30-year-olds, and is more common in whites, particularly those of Jewish descent or Middle European origin. Ulcerative colitis is isolated to the colon and involves the mucosal and sub-mucosal layers of bowel. The process is chronic and intermittent, usually starting in the rectum and sigmoid colon and then progressing upward. Clinical manifestations include diarrhea that contains mucous and is bloody, and abdominal pain that can be described as cramping to severe. The more severe the disease, the greater the number of stools and the more severe the bleeding. Crohn's disease (regional enteritis) is also a chronic inflammatory disorder, and most frequently involves the ileum and the ascending colon, but may occur anywhere along the GI tract. Pathophysiologically, it is characterized by discontinuous involvement with areas of normal bowel between areas of diseased bowel. It involves all four layers of bowel tissue. Clinical manifestations depend on the location of the disease but in general include pain that can be described as severe, intermittent, or constant usually in the right lower quadrant, which is relieved by defecation, diarrhea that is not bloody and not as severe as colitis, and abdominal distention. Most commonly, these two diseases are controlled by dietary restrictions and medical therapeutic interventions. If ulcerative colitis does not respond to medical management, a cure can be achieved by removing the colon and leaving the patient with a fecal diversion. Surgery is usually not recommended for Crohn's disease as it recurs in almost all instances; however, in some instances it is performed to relieve symptoms temporarily, provide bowel rest, and improve quality of life. Common complications of IBD include hemorrhage, perforation, obstruction, and toxic megacolon. This care plan addresses the medical management of uncomplicated IBD.

NURSING DIAGNOSIS 1

 CHRONIC PAIN

Related to:

Inflammatory change in the bowel

Skin irritation from frequent stool (diarrhea)

Defining Characteristics:

Complains of pain

Cramping in abdomen

Goal:

The patient states that pain is reduced.

Outcome Criteria

✔ The patient states that painful episodes occur less frequently.

✔ The patient states that pain is < 4 on a 10-point scale.

✔ The patient will verbalize that pain has been relieved 30 minutes after interventions.

✔ The patient will verbalize an understanding of what causes pain.

NOC *Pain level*

Pain control

Comfort level

INTERVENTIONS	RATIONALES
Assess for location, intensity, quality, and nonverbal signs of pain: grimacing, facial expressions, guarding of painful abdomen.	Identifying these will assist in accurate diagnosis and treatment.
Have the patient rate pain intensity using a pain rating scale.	Provides a more objective description of level of pain.
Administer anti-inflammatory agents as ordered (Azulfidine®) and monitor for side effects.	Azulfidine is a first-choice drug given to decrease inflammation by inhibiting prostaglandin synthesis in the colon. As inflammation decreases, pain subsides. Side effects include nausea, vomiting, and anorexia.
Administer steroidal preparations as ordered (prednisone PO, Solu-Medrol IV) and monitor for side effects.	Helps to decrease intestinal inflammation especially, during acute episodes. Pain subsides as the inflammation decreases. Common side effects include edema, GI upset (nausea, vomiting), and, with long-term therapy, a moon appearance to the face.
Administer anticholinergics, as ordered.	Helps to decrease cramping and intestinal spasms.
Administer immunosuppressants (such as 6-Mercaptopurine® Imuran®), as ordered, and monitor for side effects.	These medications are used in severe cases if the patient does not respond to more traditional medical management. They prolong remissions but have a slow onset requiring approximately 3 to 4 months before effects are seen in the patient.
Arrange for dietary consult to determine proper foods and intervals for eating.	Certain foods should not be eaten when the patient has IBD, as they may contribute to the pain and cause further inflammation. A dietician can prepare a menu using the patient's preferred foods while following dietary requirements.
Apply protective/healing skin ointment in anal region.	The tissue around the anus may be reddened and cracked due to frequent diarrhea episodes.

Implement non-pharmacological strategies to reduce pain and anxiety, such as staying with the patient, meditation, guided imagery, relaxation techniques, and playing soft music.	Anxiety often intensifies the pain experience.
Investigate the use of diversional activities.	Helps to decrease the attention or focus on the pain.
Encourage patient to find a position of best comfort and utilize it.	Helps to enhance medications and promote comfort.
Assess effectiveness of interventions to relieve pain.	Helps to determine if interventions have been effective in relieving pain or if new strategies need to be employed.

NIC   *Pain management*
Analgesic administration
Anxiety reduction

Evaluation

The patient reports that the abdominal pain or cramping has been reduced or alleviated following interventions. Pain in the anal area is relieved. The patient should have no observable signs of discomfort and report that relaxation techniques have been useful in helping to relieve discomfort.

Community/Home Care

The patient will need to learn how to manage chronic pain at home. The pain will improve as the inflammation improves, but some degree of mild pain or cramping may persist. Pain at home is usually managed with mild analgesics and anti-inflammatory agents. The patient will need to understand the schedule for these medications and how to control side effects. For both Azulfidine and steroidal preparations, the patient should take the medication after meals (Azulfidine) and with food (prednisone) to decrease the GI side effects. Health care providers often forget to inform the patient of side effects that may be less common, such as interference of Azulfidine with effectiveness of oral contraceptives or increased sensitivity to the sun. In addition, the patient should report any sore throat, difficulty swallowing, or mouth lesions to the health care provider at once. The patient will need to use sunscreen and shield him or herself from long exposure to the sun. For steroidal preparations, the patient at home needs to be able to monitor for fluid retention by weighing regularly and paying attention to the fit of shoes and of clothes in the waist. The patient needs to monitor response to pain medications and be able to identify those factors or positions that increase pain and those that relieve pain. Because IBD is a chronic disorder, the patient needs to understand methods to cope with persistent pain, possibly through diversional activities such as reading, meditating, using guided imagery, or engaging in hobbies. If anal discomfort occurs due to diarrhea, the patient can use a warm tub bath to help provide comfort. However, if the pain intensifies rather than improves, the patient should seek follow-up care with the health care provider.

Documentation

Document in the patient's own words the description and location of the pain, and the rating of the level of pain. Include in the documentation any other assessments made relevant to the pain. Chart all interventions employed for pain relief and the patient's responses. Medications are charted according to agency protocol.

NURSING DIAGNOSIS 2

 DIARRHEA

Related to:

Inflammation of the bowel

Defining Characteristics:

Frequent stools

Liquid stools

Bloody stools

Mucous in stools

Reddened cracked tissue around anus

Goal:

Diarrhea episodes occur less frequently.

Outcome Criteria

✔ The patient will have a decreased number of stools per day.

✔ The patient's stool is semi-formed to formed.

✔ Tissue breakdown does not occur.

✔ The patient will have decreased amounts of blood in stool.

✔ The patient will have no mucous in stool.

NOC *Bowel elimination*
Fluid balance
Hydration

INTERVENTIONS	RATIONALES
Assess the patient's bowel history for diarrhea frequency, episodes of uncontrolled diarrhea, bowel sounds, urine output, hyperactive bowel sounds, heme-positive stools, and inability to venture far from toilet facilities.	Helps to determine effect of the disease, establish a baseline to guide planning, and to evaluate response to therapy.
Monitor results of laboratory and diagnostic tests: electrolytes, blood urea nitrogen (BUN), albumin, complete blood count (CBC), hemoglobin (Hgb), hematocrit (Hct), colonoscopy, rectal biopsy, computed tomography (CT) scan, and magnetic resonance imaging (MRI).	Helps to confirm the disease, note extent of disease, monitor for systemic effects, and rule out other causes for the symptoms.
Monitor stools for frequency, amount, color, and consistency; record according to agency guidelines.	The number of stools is correlated with severity of disease and this can provide information about disease and response to treatment.
Weigh patient daily.	Weights are an accurate measurement of fluid lost. If diarrhea is severe, the patient may lose weight overnight.
Monitor for dehydration: poor skin turgor, decreased blood pressure with orthostatic hypotension, tachycardia, dry warm skin, and dry mucous membranes.	Dehydration occurs due to the high volume of liquid stools; early detection of dehydration leads to prompt treatment prior to complications.
Administer anti-diarrheal medication (such as Kaopectate®, Imodium®, Lomotil®), as ordered.	Antidiarrheal agents slow peristalsis and provide for fluid reabsorption and stool formation.
Administer IV fluids and electrolyte replacements, as ordered.	Helps to prevent dehydration or volume depletion due to frequency of diarrhea and to replace lost fluids and electrolytes.

(continues)

(continued)

INTERVENTIONS	RATIONALES
Administer anti-inflammatory medications, as ordered (see nursing diagnosis "Chronic Pain").	Helps to decrease inflammation of intestinal tissue.
Cleanse and apply protective/ antibacterial ointment to perianal area; assess each shift.	Frequent diarrhea stools will cause tissue irritation and fissures in the perianal area.
Consult with a dietician to revise the diet to eliminate roughage, fatty foods, and flatus-producing foods (see nursing diagnosis "Imbalanced Nutrition: Less than Body Requirements").	Fatty foods and roughage cause intestinal distention/abdominal bloating, as do flatus-producing foods, and worsen the problems of inflammation, pain, and diarrhea.
Maintain nothing-by-mouth (NPO) status, as ordered.	Helps to promote bowel rest, slow diarrhea, and decrease inflammation; peristalsis required for food transit through the lower GI system prevents healing.

NIC *Diarrhea management*
Fluid management
Fluid monitoring
Perineal care

Evaluation

The patient's stools become fewer in number. Consistency of the stools becomes more formed, and blood and mucous is decreased or absent. There are no signs of dehydration such as dry skin, poor skin turgor, or dry mucous membranes. Vital signs are normal and electrolytes return to normal range.

Community/Home Care

IBD is a chronic disease with periods of remission and exacerbation throughout its course. The patient needs to learn how to control the diarrhea and promote comfort. At home the patient will need to implement strategies to prevent dehydration from the loss of water in stools. Prescribed antidiarrheals become a part of life until the stools are controlled, which can take days to weeks. During periods of disease flare-up, the patient should avoid foods that are known to be great GI stimulants that increase peristalsis. A dietician can prepare a list of foods to avoid for the patient to keep in the kitchen as a handy reference guide. In addition, the patient will need to keep hydrated, as the stools are frequently liquid in nature, adding to dehydration. Keeping a bottle or large glass filled with their favorite drink (nonstimulant) close by at all times can serve as a reminder to drink fluids during relapses when diarrhea is present. The patient who is having numerous stools may become weak and require some assistance with activities such as household chores, ambulation, and driving until his or her usual energy level returns. At home, the patient may want to stay close to the bathroom during acute episodes during which diarrhea is frequent. The patient needs to monitor the number of stools each day by recording each episode in a journal or log, along with a description of the stool (particularly the presence of blood). The ability to work or go to school (college or high school) may be hampered due to the number of stools, weakness, and the embarrassment of needing to go to the bathroom frequently. This issue needs to be addressed with the patient by the health care provider, with some discussion about solutions to the problem such as getting a tutor, obtaining notes from others, or having assignments picked up by a friend. The patient should be instructed to return to the health care provider if the number of stools increases, if blood in the stool increases, or if the patient has worsening malaise.

Documentation

Document the number of stools, a description of the stools, and the consistency of stools. Include an assessment of the patient's hydration status with attention to skin turgor, mucous membranes, and vital signs (blood pressure and pulse). Intake and output is recorded according to agency protocol at least once a shift if the patient is hospitalized, remembering to record liquid diarrhea stools as part of the fluid output. Document all interventions carried out to resolve the problem of diarrhea with appropriate patient responses. Chart any prescribed medications on the medication administration record, and always chart the number of stools the patient has following antidiarrheal medications.

NURSING DIAGNOSIS 3

IMBALANCED NUTRITION: LESS THAN BODY REQUIREMENTS

Related to:

Malabsorption of nutrients

Diarrhea

Anorexia

Defining Characteristics:

Weight loss

Decreased albumin

Electrolyte abnormalities

Reports of lack of energy

Goal:

The patient's normal nutritional status will be restored.

Outcome Criteria

✔ The patient will not lose weight.

✔ Electrolytes will be within normal limits.

✔ Albumin will return to normal limits.

✔ The patient verbalizes an understanding of the required dietary recommendations and the importance of adequate nutrition.

NOC *Nutritional status:*
Food and fluid intake
Nutritional status: Energy

INTERVENTIONS	RATIONALES
Complete a fluid and nutritional assessment, including assessing for nausea; vomiting; poor skin turgor; dry, pale mucous membranes; diarrhea; dietary intake; fluid intake and output; weight loss; loss of appetite; decreased muscle tone; albumin levels; hemoglobin; iron; and electrolytes.	Patients who experience IBD often have a decreased nutritional status due to malabsorption of nutrients in the GI tract, the loss of electrolytes and fluids through diarrhea, and a feeling of malaise that decreases appetite. Anorexia and nausea add to the problem by preventing the patient from taking in enough nutrients to meet metabolic demands.
Assess laboratory results: albumin, iron, electrolytes, folic acid, and thiamine level.	All of these values will probably be decreased due to the inability of the patient to eat adequate amounts or control the loss of nutrients through malabsorption secondary to diarrhea. Iron, folic acid, and electrolytes decrease as nutritional intake decreases.
Weigh patient and monitor weight daily or weekly.	Helps to establish baseline for comparison and to detect significant weight loss early to allow for prompt treatment.
Monitor and record intake and output according to agency protocol, being sure to include liquid stools as part of the fluid output.	Helps to detect dehydration and initiate early treatment.
Encourage the patient to take increased nutrients through high-calorie, high-protein, and low-roughage diets as ordered (small meals with between-meal snacks).	Helps to promote adequate intake of nutrients; for patients with decreased appetite, a small meal is more likely to be ingested and to be seen as desirable.
Restrict the intake of raw fruit and vegetables.	Raw fruit and vegetables increase peristalsis and contribute to diarrhea.
Assess for lactose intolerance and restrict dairy products in diet if present.	Most patients with IBD are lactose intolerant and must eliminate dairy products from their diet.
During periods of acute exacerbation with diarrhea, limit intake of foods.	Particularly in Crohn's disease, limiting of foods is needed to allow for bowel rest and to slow the diarrhea.
Give nutritional supplements as ordered: folic acid, thiamine, multivitamins.	Helps to supplement nutrient intake; patients with IBD are likely candidates for malnutrition and need these supplements to improve nutritional status.
Collaborate with the dietician to develop an acceptable diet that considers usual habits, food intake, and any cultural or religious restrictions.	The dietician can discuss with the patient which foods may be digested better with the fewest untoward effects but the best nutritional results.
Administer total parenteral nutrition (TPN) as ordered.	TPN may be needed to restore the patient's nutritional state, especially during acute exacerbations and to allow for bowel rest.
Implement strategies to decrease or alleviate diarrhea (see nursing diagnosis "Diarrhea").	Diarrhea is the contributing factor for nutrient loss.

NIC *Nutritional monitoring*
Nutritional management

Evaluation

The patient's nutritional status is stable as evidenced by the laboratory values (iron, electrolytes, folate, etc.) and no weight loss. The patient verbalizes an interest in eating and understands the need for increased nutrients due to the loss that accompanies diarrhea. Weight loss is minimized and the patient consumes regular meals.

Community/Home Care

Once acute symptoms of IBD are alleviated, the patient must begin to develop plans to address the impact that IBD has on nutrition. Many patients suffer from some degree of malnutrition that needs attention due to the loss of nutrients and fluids through diarrhea. Family members and significant others play a role in implementing strategies to improve nutrition by preparing meals and encouraging the patient to ingest them. Frequent small meals at home should be encouraged for the patient in order to increase the likelihood that the patient can ingest enough nutrients. Foods should be bland, and avoidance of spicy foods or raw fruits and vegetables is crucial as these stimulate peristalsis and thus add to the problem of diarrhea. Many patients with IBD are also lactose intolerant and must remove dairy products from their diet. Supplemental drinks can improve nutritional status during periods when the patient is unable to ingest adequate amounts of nutrition through normal meals due to anorexia or malaise. A dietician should assist the patient with locating those products that are free of lactose, but the patient may need to experiment with which ones are tolerated. The patient may need to remain on multivitamins, folic acid, thiamine, electrolyte supplements, and other nutritional supplements for an extended period of time. Teach the patient to monitor nutrition/intake by keeping a log of food eaten, when eaten, and how tolerated, as well as episodes of diarrhea. If at any time a particular meal or food product causes pain or subsequent diarrhea, the patient should note this in the log and eliminate this food from the diet. In addition, include in the log frequency of diarrhea stools, medications taken for diarrhea, and weights. Even though the patient may not want to weigh every day, weighing at least every other day is a good way to keep track of weight loss or stabilization. This information can be shared with the health care provider at each follow-up visit to provide data for revision in prescribed therapeutic interventions. Despite aggressive measures by the family and nurse to develop an acceptable plan for nutrition, some patients will not be able to meet nutritional needs, and parenteral nutrition in the

home may be required. In this instance, referrals are made to appropriate home care agencies or infusion companies that can supply the patient with the resources (staff and supplies) needed for infusion therapy. The family and patient will need to be taught how to care for the central line or peripherally inserted catheter (PIC) line used for infusion when it is not in use. Priority care involves prevention of infection through strict hand hygiene and protection of the site from injury. Dressing changes can be performed by the infusion specialist in the home. Follow-up providers should assess the patient for weight loss and monitor laboratory results for improvement.

Documentation

Chart the results of a nutritional assessment, including a history of usual intake. Document vital signs, weights, and intake and output according to agency protocol at least every shift or every 8 hours. Include in the chart the amount of food the patient consumes at each meal and what, if any, supplements are taken by the patient. For patients who are taking nutritional supplements (vitamins, liquid supplements, etc.), chart this in the patient record. In most agencies, there are specific guidelines for charting about total parenteral nutrition that include specific nutritional parameters, so the nurse should document accordingly. Document any complaints and the number of stools that occur in the record with accompanying documentation indicating response to interventions. Always include in the record all therapeutic interventions implemented for the patient.

NURSING DIAGNOSIS 4

 ANXIETY

Related to:

Difficulty coping with new disease

Chronic diarrhea

Expressed fear

Disruption of lifestyle

Anticipation of fecal diversion surgery

Defining Characteristics:

States that he or she knows very little about the disease

Anger

Introversion

Avoidance of social interactions

Restlessness

Insomnia

Goal:

Anxiety is relieved.

Outcome Criteria

✔ The patient verbalizes that anxiety is reduced.

✔ The patient has no physiological signs of anxiety.

✔ The patient verbalizes an understanding of IBD, its treatment, and anticipated outcomes.

✔ The patient is able to develop coping techniques.

✔ The patient identifies one successful coping strategy.

NOC   *Anxiety control*

Acceptance: Health status

Knowledge: Disease process

Coping

Psychosocial adjustment: Life change

Anxiety self-control

INTERVENTIONS	RATIONALES
Assess level of anxiety using a numerical rating scale.	Helps to obtain an objective measure of the extent of the anxiety.
Encourage expressions of anxieties/fears.	Verbal expressions of anxiety can assist the patient in identifying sources of anxiety.
Provide safe, private environment for expressions of anxiety.	Assure the patient that expressions of feelings are okay and that they are confidential.
Teach patient about the disease of IBD, etiologic theories, therapeutic interventions (medications, diet, possible surgery), and possible long-term outcomes. Evaluate the patient's understanding and reinforce teaching as needed.	Patient understanding of the disease and the therapeutic interventions will facilitate mobilization of coping strategies and can diminish the patient's feelings of helplessness and anxiety, thus increasing coping skills. The patient and family can begin to plan (realistically) for
	discharge and home care with an understanding of why symptoms are occurring.
Identify misconceptions and provide correct information.	Misunderstandings can decrease the patient's ability to cope.
Have the patient identify coping strategies that have worked in the past and encourage their use.	Strategies that have worked in the past may work again and provide a starting place for dealing with anxiety.
Teach the patient new methods of relaxation and coping.	The patient may require assistance in identifying and learning new coping techniques.
Administer anti-anxiety medication, as ordered.	Helps to produce a calming effect and permit the patient rest periods.
Provide encouragement and feedback.	This will assist the patient to explore new coping skills and focuses patient away from negative attitudes.
Arrange for community support group involvement from agencies such as the Crohn's and Colitis Foundation of America.	The patient will be able to share experiences with others with the same disease. This agency may also be able to provide information about local support groups where the patient may meet someone who has gone through a similar situation and who is now able to function normally, is able to undertake all activities of daily living (ADLs), and may provide significant psychological support.

NIC   *Anxiety reduction*

Coping enhancement

Emotional support

Teaching: Diet

Teaching: Disease process

Teaching: Medications

Evaluation

Assess the patient to determine that anxiety has been reduced or eliminated. The patient should verbalize an understanding of IBD and ability to cope with the diagnosis. Treatment options are understood as well as the possible outcomes of the chronic condition. The patient has no physiological symptoms of anxiety, such as tachycardia and diaphoresis. In addition, the patient is able to identify at least one coping strategy that can be used in this situation.

Community/Home Care

The patient will need to know how to control anxiety in the home. IBD is a chronic disease that has periods of remissions and exacerbations with acute symptoms. If the patient is taught how to relax and call upon successful coping strategies, he or she will be better equipped to deal with the disease and its demands. A patient with a strong knowledge base about the disease and treatment will probably have fewer episodes of anxiety. The presence of profound diarrhea in some instances may increase anxiety and the sense of loss of control; however, if the patient is expecting it and knows how to control the diarrhea, he or she will not panic when it occurs but rather be proactive in its treatment. The patient has

to identify what options are available for coping and reducing anxiety. Non-pharmacological measures that can be used include meditating, deep breathing, using guided imagery, taking short walks, gardening, or having consultations with spiritual leaders. If the patient practices an organized religion visits at home with clergy can provide an avenue for expression of concerns and fears.

Documentation

Document the degree of anxiety experienced by the patient as the patient verbalizes it. Chart any physiological indicators of anxiety such as diaphoresis or tachycardia. Document verbalizations by the patient about ability to cope with the diagnosis of IBD. Chart all teaching done relevant to diagnosis and treatment with reference to the patient's understanding or the need for further education. Document all interventions employed to treat the patient's anxiety with the patient's responses clearly indicated.

CHAPTER 6.89

INTESTINAL OBSTRUCTION

GENERAL INFORMATION

Intestinal obstruction is the complete or partial stoppage of function of the intestines that inhibits the passage of intestinal contents through the intestines. This disorder can be categorized as mechanical or functional (also known as non-mechanical). Mechanical obstructions, which account for approximately 85 to 90 percent of all obstructions, are caused by occlusion of the lumen of the intestine, usually the small intestine. The most common causes of mechanical obstruction are adhesions (50 percent), hernias (15 percent), and neoplasms (15 percent). Neoplasms are the most common cause for large bowel obstruction. Other causes of mechanical obstructions are fecal impactions, volvulus, foreign bodies, inflammatory bowel disease, and intussusception. Functional obstructions are caused by neuromuscular or vascular disorders that prevent the action of peristalsis. The most common type of functional obstruction is paralytic ileus, which occurs frequently following gastrointestinal (GI) surgery. Other disorders that can cause functional obstruction are spinal cord injuries, peritonitis, hypokalemia, and decreased gastrointestinal tissue perfusion. The patient with bowel obstruction suffers from a fluid deficit as gas (from bacterial metabolism) and fluid collect in the bowel proximal to the obstruction, causing distention of the lumen, reducing absorption of fluids, and increasing capillary permeability. As a result, as much as 2 to 6 liters of fluid along with electrolytes escape into the peritoneal cavity, reducing the circulating volume. Clinical manifestations of bowel obstruction vary depending upon the location, the extent of the obstruction, and onset. Symptoms of small bowel obstruction typically have a rapid onset and include cramping or colicky pain, intermittent vomiting of large amounts, and in cases of low or distal obstruction of the small bowel, emesis that may be feculent. Early in mechanical obstruction, bowel sounds are characterized by a high-pitched sound and borborygmi with observable peristaltic waves, but later on the bowel sounds become silent. Clinical manifestations of large bowel obstruction have a gradual onset and include a crampy, deep pain; distended abdomen; high-pitched bowel sounds; and the absence of bowel movements. Vomiting occurs as a late sign, and severe pain is an indicator of perforation.

NURSING DIAGNOSIS 1

IMPAIRED BOWEL ELIMINATION*

Related to:

Obstruction of flow of fecal contents

Paralytic ileus

Defining Characteristics:

Obstipation

High-pitched bowel sounds

Absent bowel sounds

Deep, crampy, intermittent pain

Vomiting

Feculent appearance and odor to emesis

Goal:

Bowel function will return to normal.

Outcome Criteria

✔ Bowel sounds will be present in all quadrants.

✔ The patient will have one formed stool.

✔ Vomiting will be relieved.

✔ The patient will report an absence of abdominal pain.

NOC *Bowel elimination*

INTERVENTIONS	RATIONALES
Conduct a complete assessment of GI function every shift, noting abnormalities: bowel sounds that are high-pitched, absent, or borborygmi; obstipation; feculent vomitus (fecal smelling); peristaltic waves; oozing of stool; history of elimination patterns; tenderness in abdomen; palpable masses; nausea and vomiting; anorexia; abdominal distention; or abdominal tenderness/guarding.	Bowel obstructions cause a variety of symptoms that give clues to location. Oozing of stool may occur early as the feces left in the bowel try to exit the bowel; high-pitched sounds occur and peristaltic waves may be seen as peristalsis becomes stronger, trying to relieve the obstruction; feculent vomitus occurs in small bowel obstruction due to action of bacteria on contents; abdominal distention occurs due to accumulation of fluid in the peritoneal cavity.
Monitor results of laboratory and diagnostic tests: complete blood count (CBC), arterial blood gases (ABGs), serum electrolytes, abdominal x-rays, and lower GI series.	The CBC may reveal elevations in white blood cell (WBC) count due to an inflammatory response; ABGs reveal metabolic alkalosis due to loss of acidic contents of the GI tract; serum electrolyte measurements demonstrate a decrease in potassium and chloride; abdominal x-rays show dilated loops of intestine as well as the presence of gas and fluid; x-rays of the lower GI tract show the extent of the obstruction.
Monitor the color, amount, odor, and consistency of any vomitus.	Helps to detect changes that indicate worsening of the condition; feculent smelling vomitus indicates a small bowel obstruction.
Administer anti-emetics as ordered.	Anti-emetics relieve the discomfort of vomiting.
Monitor intake and output.	Helps to assess the extent of the fluid deficits (see nursing diagnosis "Deficient Fluid Volume").
For small bowel obstruction or paralytic ileus, insert a nasogastric tube and connect to low suction as ordered and monitor output; for large bowel obstructions, insert intestinal tube as ordered.	Helps to decompress the bowel and to rest the bowel. For approximately 90 percent of all small bowel obstructions, decompression with the nasogastric problem corrects the problem.
Secure the nasogastric tube to nose, and provide nose and mouth care 4 times a day, or as ordered.	Helps to promote comfort.

Irrigate nasogastric tube as ordered.	Helps to maintain patency.
Establish intravenous access and initiate intravenous fluids, as ordered.	Helps to restore circulating volume; large amounts of fluid escape into the peritoneal space with obstructions.
Maintain nothing-by-mouth (NPO) status for the patient.	Food is withheld until peristalsis and bowel function return.
Administer antibiotics intravenously (IV) as ordered.	Bacteria may leak into the peritoneal cavity due to changes in capillary permeability; antibiotics are needed to prevent peritonitis.
Measure abdominal girth and report increasing girth to physician	Helps to detect resolution or worsening of abdominal distention. Increased girth may indicate a perforation or increased leakage of fluid into the peritoneal cavity that requires aggressive intervention, possibly surgery.
Encourage the patient to ambulate if allowed.	Walking stimulates peristalsis.
Prepare the patient for surgery, as ordered.	If the bowel obstruction does not correct itself, surgery may be required, especially for obstructions caused by a volvulus, hernias, or foreign objects.

NIC *Bowel management*
Gastrointestinal intubation
Tube care: Gastrointestinal

Evaluation

Determine if the patient has a return of normal bowel function. Assessments should reveal bowel sounds returning to all quadrants. The patient has a normal bowel movement and there is no colicky pain. The output from the GI tube has diminished, and the nasogastric tube has been removed.

Community/Home Care

Bowel obstruction is an acute situation that has to be resolved prior to discharge. There should be no long-lasting effects requiring in-home visits, as the cause of the obstruction has been corrected. For those patients requiring surgery, the patient will need to understand post-operative wound care, activity restrictions, and dietary needs for healing.

Wound care most often will only involve keeping the wound clean, and no dressing may be required except to protect it from clothing. If a fecal diversion has been performed, the patient and a family member will need to learn how to care for the ostomy in the home (see nursing care plan "Fecal Diversions/Ostomies"). The patient may feel fatigued from being without nutrition for a period of time, and once at home will need to eat iron-rich and protein-rich foods such as spinach, meat, nuts, etc. Progressing activity gradually, as tolerated, will assist the patient to regain stamina over time. The patient will need to monitor bowel movements to ensure that normal bowel function has returned, making note of number, amount, consistency, and odor of stools. If the patient detects that bowel function has not returned to the usual pattern, the patient should report to the health care provider.

Documentation

Document the results of a thorough GI assessment, particularly of bowel sounds and abdominal girth. Include in the chart the insertion of nasogastric or intestinal tubes and information regarding drainage, including a description, any odor, and amount of drainage. All interventions carried out to treat the obstruction are documented with a specific reference to the patient's response. Be sure to document intake and output, and medications, according to agency protocol.

NURSING DIAGNOSIS 2

 DEFICIENT FLUID VOLUME

Related to:

Movement of fluid into the peritoneal cavity due to bowel obstruction

Anorexia

Nausea and vomiting

Defining Characteristics:

Tachycardia

Dry mucous membranes

Poor skin turgor

Hemoconcentration

Hypotension

Increased urine specific gravity

Electrolyte imbalance

Decreased urine output

Goal:

Normal fluid and electrolyte balance will be restored.

Outcome Criteria

✔ Vital signs (blood pressure and pulse) return to baseline.

✔ Mucous membranes become moist and pink.

✔ Skin turgor returns to normal (skin when pinched returns to normal position in < 3 seconds).

✔ Specific gravity, hematocrit (Hct), and hemoglobin (Hgb) return to normal levels.

NOC   *Hydration*
   Fluid balance
   Electrolyte and acid/base balance
   Vital signs

INTERVENTIONS	RATIONALES
Assess for signs of dehydration/ volume deficit: decreased blood pressure, increased pulse, dry mucous membranes, poor skin turgor, decreased urinary output, and elevated specific gravity.	These findings support the diagnosis of fluid deficit and determine the seriousness of the problem; helps to guide treatment and to assess effectiveness of treatments.
Establish IV access and initiate IV fluids, as ordered.	Helps to rehydrate patient and correct fluid and electrolyte imbalance.
Monitor intake and output.	Helps to assess fluid balance and monitor for improvement in fluid deficit.
Monitor serum electrolytes, especially serum potassium and chloride, and serum osmolality.	Helps to determine fluid and electrolyte replacement needs.
Administer electrolyte replacements (potassium and chloride) IV, as ordered.	Potassium and chloride are rich in the GI tract; a combination of fluid losses from the bowel, vomiting, and nasogastric suction causes decreases in serum levels, necessitating replacement.

(continues)

(continued)

INTERVENTIONS	RATIONALES
Monitor cardiac status: blood pressure, pulse (quality and rate), pulse pressure, and capillary refill. Take vital signs at least every 4 hours, or more often, as ordered.	For early detection of complications; decreases in circulating volume occurs due to loss of fluid from the bowel into the peritoneal cavity; changes in blood pressure and pulse give information relevant to changes in cardiac status; blood pressure decreases and the pulse increases; capillary refill will be an indicator of perfusion.
Insert indwelling urinary catheter and monitor output every hour.	Helps to monitor for renal function, decreased output indicates decreased renal perfusion secondary to decreased circulating volume.
Monitor skin temperature and color for baseline and during treatment for improvement.	Pale, cool, clammy skin indicates decreased perfusion. As treatment progresses, skin should be warm and return to normal color.
Monitor oxygen saturation using pulse oximetry.	Oxygen saturation is a way to assess ability to perfuse tissues.
Monitor results of laboratory studies: Hgb and Hct, ABG, blood urea nitrogen (BUN), and electrolytes.	Hct fluctuates in response to fluid status; severe absolute loss from volume would produce a decrease in Hct, with further drops during aggressive fluid resuscitation due to hemodilution; Hgb may be decreased. If volume loss is due to third spacing, Hct may be high initially and decrease as fluid is restored to the intravascular space. ABGs often reveal metabolic alkalosis as potassium and chloride are lost in the fluid exiting the bowel into the peritoneal cavity or through suctioning. BUN and electrolytes indicate renal function. BUN may be elevated initially but decrease due to hemodilution of fluid replacement.
Administer antibiotics, as ordered.	Helps to prevent an infection (peritonitis) due to bacteria in intestinal fluids, which have leaked into the peritoneal space.
Administer anti-emetic medications.	Helps to relieve nausea and vomiting that accompany bowel obstruction.

NIC *Hypovolemia management*
Intravenous therapy
Fluid monitoring
Electrolyte monitoring
Fluid/electrolyte management

Evaluation

Assess the patient for return of normal fluid volume. The patient's blood pressure and pulse should return to baseline. The pulse should be strong and regular and at the patient's baseline or only slightly increased. Skin should be warm, and color should return to the patient's normal appearance. Renal function should not be impaired, with an hourly output on the average of 30 ml/hour. Serum electrolytes, specific gravity, Hgb, and Hct should be within normal range. The patient's intake and output are balanced.

Community/Home Care

Patients treated for deficient fluid volume due to bowel obstruction should have normal fluid status restored within a short period of time. Attention to methods of replacing electrolytes is important because the patient almost always loses potassium and chloride. Once bowel function has returned, encourage the intake of frequent small amounts of clear liquid electrolyte solutions, such as Gatorade or other clear liquids. Plain water should be avoided because it makes nausea worse for some, but more importantly it contains no electrolytes. At home, the patient may not require any follow-up as this is an acute situation that for the most part has no long-term complications. Fatigue may be an issue; the patient should be instructed to perform activities as tolerated until stamina/endurance is re-established. The health care provider may want the patient to return for a follow-up appointment to ensure that parameters such as electrolytes, Hgb, Hct, and renal function studies have returned to normal.

Documentation

Document initial assessment findings relevant to hydration status such as intake and output, status of skin and mucous membranes, blood pressure, pulse, respirations, temperature, breath sounds, and mental status. Document all interventions, such as IV catheter insertion, fluids initiated (type, rate), and indwelling catheter insertion with description of urine returned (amount, color). Be specific when charting patient responses to treatment so that other health care providers can clearly determine improvement or deterioration.

NURSING DIAGNOSIS 3

 ### ACUTE PAIN

Related to:

Obstruction

Defining Characteristics:

Complains of abdominal pain

Nasogastric or intestinal tube in nares

Presence of colicky, intermittent pain

Abdominal tenderness

Goal:

The patient's level of comfort is improved.

Outcome Criteria

✔ The patient reports a decrease in level of pain.

✔ The patient reports that the discomfort caused by any tubes (rectal or nasogastric) is tolerable.

✔ The patient verbalizes relief of discomfort 30 minutes following interventions.

NOC *Pain level*

Pain control

Comfort level

INTERVENTIONS	RATIONALES
Assess for location, intensity, quality, duration, and precipitating factors.	Identifying these will assist in accurate diagnosis and treatment; most patients who have bowel obstructions have a colicky, deep abdominal pain that is intermittent. GI tubes also contribute to discomfort due to size and movement in the nares. If pain intensifies, this may signal a perforation or necrosis of the bowel.
Have patient rate pain or discomfort intensity using a pain rating scale.	Provides a more objective description of level of pain.
Assess for nausea and vomiting.	Nausea and vomiting are common with bowel obstruction and can add to a decreased comfort level and pain.
Administer anti-emetics as ordered.	Helps to increase comfort by relieving nausea and vomiting.
Assess respiratory status, including breath sounds, respiratory rate, depth, quality, and oxygen saturation.	For early signs of respiratory complications, patients who have bowel obstructions may have abdominal distention that places pressure on the diaphragm, adding to decreased ventilatory effort.
Administer mild analgesics, as ordered, and avoid opioid derivatives.	Strong analgesics may mask symptoms of complications; opioids decrease peristalsis.
Assist to position of comfort.	Patients will often be more comfortable in a side-lying position with the head of the bed elevated (to relieve pressure on the abdomen).
Provide nose and oral care every shift.	The tube in the nares adds to discomfort due to movement of the tube and the presence of a foreign object. The mouth can become dry due to mouth breathing, NPO status, and dehydration.
Implement non-pharmacological strategies to relieve pain and discomfort, such as relaxation techniques, playing soft music, distraction, and meditation.	Non-pharmacological interventions can assist in reducing pain by affecting the perception of the pain experience.
Assess effectiveness of all interventions.	Helps to determine if other interventions are required.
If the patient has had surgery, teach him or her to splint abdomen with a pillow or rolled bath blanket when moving or coughing.	Splinting provides support for the painful area, decreases stress on surgical site that may increase pain, and allows the patient to participate in coughing and deep breathing more comfortably.

NIC *Pain management*

Analgesic administration

Anxiety reduction

Evaluation

The patient is able to report that the pain has been reduced (is less than a 4 on a scale of 1–10) or alleviated following interventions. The patient reports that the pain is tolerable and verbalizes an understanding of why analgesic administration is limited. GI tubes are comfortable or tolerable without excessive movement. The patient should have no discomfort.

Community/Home Care

The patient's pain should be temporary and resolve once the bowel obstruction is resolved. If pain occurs at home, it can be managed with mild analgesics, and the duration of pain should be short. If the patient has had surgery for the obstruction, encourage him or her to use splinting when moving or coughing at home. The nurse should stress to the post-operative patient that weak respiratory efforts because of pain could cause respiratory problems such as pneumonia. If the pain worsens at home, the patient should contact the health care provider to determine other causes for the pain. If the recommended analgesics are not working, the patient should seek follow-up care with the health care provider.

Documentation

Document in the patient's own words the description of the pain and his or her rating of the level of pain. All assessments made relevant to the pain are documented. Chart all interventions employed and the patient's responses. Medications are charted on the medication administration record according to the agency guidelines. If pain is unrelieved, document this and indicate what revisions are made to the plan of care.

CHAPTER 6.90

OBESITY

GENERAL INFORMATION

Obesity is the presence of excess adipose tissue on the body as a result of consuming more nutrients than the body requires for energy expenditure. The extra calories that are not required for metabolism are stored by the body as fat. In some instances, obesity can be attributed to other causes such as genetic and hormonal disorders, but this constitutes a small percentage of all cases. Contributing factors include a sedentary lifestyle, a fast-paced lifestyle that relies on fast food meals, psychological problems such as low self-esteem, and a constant supply of ready-to-eat, high-fat foods for snacks. Obesity has reached epidemic proportions in the United States and is a growing health concern. Although there are several methods of identifying obesity or being overweight, most people use the simple weight calculation. However, a more accurate measure used by health care providers defines obesity in terms of body mass index (BMI) that is calculated by dividing the weight in kilograms by the height in meters squared. A BMI of 25 to 29.9 kg/m^2 is considered overweight, a BMI of > 30 kg/m^2 is considered obese, and morbidly obese is a BMI > 40 kg/m^2. Obesity is a significant health problem because of its role in worsening numerous disease processes including hypertension, diabetes, heart disease, osteoarthritis, stroke, and certain cancers (colon, breast). Treatment for obesity can be multifaceted and occurs as an outpatient unless the patient is undergoing surgical interventions. Gastric partitioning (gastroplasty, gastric stapling) and gastric bypass have gained popularity as surgical treatments of choice for morbid obesity. In gastric partitioning, the stomach is literally "stapled" so that just a small part of the stomach is available through which food can pass. This causes a feeling of "fullness," and the patient does not have cravings for large food supplies. Gastric bypass, although still occasionally performed, is risky due to the high incidence of liver failure. Obesity is seen more often in women and is more prevalent among African American and Hispanic populations.

NURSING DIAGNOSIS 1

IMBALANCED NUTRITION: MORE THAN BODY REQUIREMENTS

Related to:

Intake of more food than required for metabolic needs

Defining Characteristics:

Reports of binge eating

Excessive weight gain with BMI > 30

Verbalization of poor nutrition

Goal:

The patient verbalizes an understanding of dietary needs.

The patient demonstrates proper dietary intake.

Outcome Criteria

✔ The patient's weight is normal for height.
✔ The patient remains on target for projected weight loss.
✔ The patient verbalizes a need to refrain from binge eating.
✔ The patient will verbalize a desire to refrain from using food as a coping mechanism.
✔ The patient will verbalize an understanding of the dangers of being obese.

NOC *Nutritional status: Nutrient intake*

Weight: Body mass

Nutritional status: Food and fluid intake

INTERVENTIONS	RATIONALES
Gather a diet and weight history, including dietary habits and intake, methods of food preparation, meal schedule, favorite foods, 24-hour dietary recall, calorie count, weight gain, binge eating, history of episodes of weight gain/weight loss, history of previous diet regimens, and diets and weight loss plans attempted without long-term success.	These data provide evidence for the extent of the problem and a starting point for intervention. Health care providers need to know this baseline information in order to tailor a plan that is individualized to the patient. Many obese patients have a history of numerous efforts at weight loss, including fad diets.
Ascertain likes and dislikes, and assist patient in making healthy dietary choices based on the food pyramid.	It is important to help the patient retain a sense of control and confidence while feeling a sense of support; the patient needs to understand healthy diets.
Weigh patient on first encounter and monitor weekly.	The first weight establishes a baseline to use for evaluation of the success of interventions; weekly weights monitor progress.
Determine BMI.	The BMI considers weight and height, and is a better indicator of whether a person is overweight or obese.
Assess patient for usual activity level.	Many obese/overweight people have sedentary lifestyles with limited or no physical exercise, which is necessary to keep weight constant or to lose weight.
Have the patient keep a food log that records all food consumed, including often forgotten items such as a piece of hard candy or chewing gum.	This will allow the patient to examine intake more readily and to develop a thought process for change.
Encourage the patient to implement the following general strategies for better nutrition: — To the extent possible, plan all meals in advance to avoid last-minute, rushed meals that are likely to be high calorie and less nutritious. — Have set meal times and do not skip meals. — Learn to bake, broil, grill, or steam food.	These strategies help control unhealthy nutritional habits by changing eating behaviors. Having healthy snacks readily available assists the patient to make the right choice.

— Avoid snacking throughout the day, but have scheduled nutritious snacks.
— Cut up fresh fruit or raw vegetables and place in sealable plastic bags for easy access.
— Avoid highly concentrated sweets.
— When eating, take small bites and chew slowly to prevent early satiety, allowing 20 minutes minimum for meals.
— Stop eating as soon as you begin to feel full.
— Always eat at the same place.
— Drink 6 to 8 glasses of water each day.
— Avoid sweetened beverages.

Arrange a consultation with a dietician to assist the patient in planning a weight loss diet.	The dietician is best prepared to assess the patient's nutritional status and develop a plan of action for weight loss.
Discuss with the patient available community resources for weight loss, such as Weight Watchers®, Jenny Craig®, TOPS® (Take Pounds Off Sensibly), gyms, spas, health departments, etc.	A variety of weight loss programs exists in most communities. A formalized plan or a support group in the initial stages of the plan to lose weight may provide the emotional support needed.
Encourage the patient to undergo a complete physical examination before beginning a weight reduction plan.	Being obese or overweight has an effect on the patient's health, often without symptoms; before attempting to lose large amounts of weight, the patient should know his or her health status to prevent further health issues.
Have the patient set small realistic goals for weight loss, usually 1 to 2 pounds per week.	Setting realistic goals allows the individual to be motivated by success and prevents frustration.
Address the needs of patients who are morbidly obese and undergoing gastric bypass or stapling: **Pre-operative:** — Teach the patient about the operative procedure. — Provide professional pre-operative counseling about post-operative requirements for nutrition.	Gastric stapling severely reduces stomach size (to approximately 50 to 60 ml). Frequent nutritionally balanced small meals are a necessity.

INTERVENTIONS	RATIONALES

— Teach the patient post-operative care strategies (nasogastric [NG] tube, pain control, incision care, use of incentive spirometer [IS]).

— Teach turning, coughing, and deep breathing (TCDB) for post-operative use.

Post-operative:

— Perform routine post-operative assessments and care, as with any gastrointestinal (GI) surgical patient.

— Oral intake will begin with very small amounts of liquids and progress to allow for small, nutritionally balanced meals spread out over the day.

— Ensure that the patient knows the consequences of eating too much (feeling full, vomiting, rupture of staple line).

— Encourage patient to follow the post-operative dietary regimen carefully.

— Administer vitamins or other supplements as ordered to offset malabsorption.

— Instruct patient to avoid gas-forming foods that provide a feeling of fullness without adequate nutritional intake.

Carefully monitor and record weight loss (weigh at the same time of day for greater accuracy).	Weight loss should be in accordance with planned therapeutic goals.
Reinforce teaching by the dietician, teach patient and family members or significant other about the need for adequate nutrition for proper body functioning, and provide with sample menus.	Knowledge will enhance the patient's ability to implement suggested strategies to improve nutritional status.

NIC *Weight reduction assistance*
Nutritional counseling
Nutritional monitoring

Evaluation

Determine the degree to which the patient has achieved the stated outcome criteria. The patient should verbalize an understanding of the need for acceptable nutritional behaviors to avoid complications of chronic illness and should indicate a desire to stop overeating. The patient verbalizes an understanding of new behaviors required for healthy nutrition and verbalizes a willingness to comply. Following implementation of the stated strategies, the patient loses weight.

Community/Home Care

The patient seeking to lose weight needs to give attention to two areas: healthy eating and exercise. Education by a dietician is the best source of information about what is acceptable to eat and what to avoid. Even though calories are understandably limited for the obese patient, enough food needs to be consumed to meet nutrient requirements of the body. For many people, simple rules include making better food choices, avoiding overindulgent social eating habits, and incorporating exercise into the daily routine. At home, the patient will need to be sure that healthy snacks are readily available and that snack foods such as potato chips, cookies, sodas, and candy are not purchased. Fresh fruit and vegetables can be pre-sliced and placed in sandwich bags in the refrigerator, thus making a readily accessible snack. When buying groceries, the patient should make a list and stick to it rather than picking up tempting items that have no nutritional value. Early in the process of losing weight, the patient should keep a food diary of all food consumed, review it a few times a week, and revise intake accordingly if bad choices have been made. The patient needs information on how to determine portion sizes. Having the patient use common items to determine a serving size rather than weighing all food will enhance compliance. The dietician can provide the patient with this information and have the patient or other meal provider place it in a readily accessible place. An accurate scale should be obtained to allow the patient to weigh him or herself weekly and to enter weight into the food diary. Exercise is key to weight loss, and the patient needs to identify activities that are acceptable. Some recommendations include walking, riding a stationary bicycle, doing simple aerobics, and using simple handheld weights. Most experts recommend 20 to 30 minutes of exercise on most days of the week, but at least 3 to 4 times a week. If finances are not an issue, the patient may benefit from enrollment in a structured exercise program at a health club, spa, or YMCA. Continued monitoring of the patient's progress is necessary to be sure that eating behaviors have improved and weight reduction has begun. Health care providers should determine that the patient has learned new coping strategies to replace eating. Family members can play a vital role in the patient's achievement of goals by encouraging healthy eating habits, monitoring dietary intake, and making healthy eating a choice or activity for the total family. The patient will need to focus on retaining enough food to prevent malnutrition and electrolyte imbalance, and this is especially true for patients who have undergone surgical interventions. For these patients, aggressive follow-up with a health care provider is necessary to be sure that malabsorption syndromes do not occur and vomiting or diarrhea are not major problems. When the patient is discharged home, attention to wound care is important. The patient is at risk for wound dehiscence and infection due to poor circulation secondary to obesity. The patient or family should be aware of signs and symptoms of wound infection. Pain at home may be a problem simply because of the amount of adipose tissue that was incised to perform the procedure. Analgesics may be required for a period of several days to a week. Participation in groups such as Weight Watchers, Overeaters Anonymous®, and TOPS are often helpful and provide support from others experiencing the same problem. Treatment for obesity is usually time-intensive; treatment may last for a long period of time, and relapse is a possibility. Family or significant others will need to offer acceptance and support in the patient's effort to cope with obesity.

Documentation

Chart the patient's weight according to agency protocol. Include in the patient record the findings from a comprehensive dietary history and nutritional assessment. Of particular importance are the patient's 24-hour dietary recall and usual dietary habits. Document reports of binge eating, vomiting, or diarrhea. Include any reports of psychological problems that could be triggers for poor nutritional habits. All interventions are documented in the record along with whether the patient has achieved the stated outcomes. Chart all teaching done and referrals for follow-up.

NURSING DIAGNOSIS 2

DISTURBED BODY IMAGE

Related to:

Abnormal perception of self

Obesity

Morbid obesity

Failed efforts at weight loss

Defining Characteristics:

Reports personal loss of control

Has unkempt appearance

Verbalizes negative feelings about self

Indifferent toward caregivers/family

Uses denial frequently

States that he or she is embarrassed or feels shame

Goal:

The patient develops a positive body image and self-esteem.

Outcome Criteria

✔ The patient is able to establish realistic weight goals.

✔ The patient states one positive aspect of body and self.

✔ The patient verbalizes that self is liked.

✔ The patient verbalizes acceptance of body appearance.

✔ The patient makes no negative statements about self.

NOC *Body image*
Self-esteem

INTERVENTIONS	RATIONALES
Monitor for expressions such as referring to self as being fat or ugly, worry over others' acceptance, feelings about self/relationships, fear of loss of love of others due to weight; assess the patient's understanding of health risks with morbid obesity.	For many people, but especially for adolescents, acceptance by peers and others is important, and fears about appearance are common.
Monitor for expressions of self-value/interpersonal	The patient who is overweight often suffers from low self-esteem

INTERVENTIONS	RATIONALES
relationships: expressions of feelings about self, low self-esteem, inability to communicate well with family/friends, withdrawal from social contact, expressions of feeling overweight and unattractive or feelings that no one likes him or her.	and has feelings of having an unacceptable appearance. He or she may actually shun social contact because of fear of ridicule. Recognition of this helps the health care provider begin planning for intervention.
Talk to the patient about body appearances and how the body can be changed.	Open dialogue about body appearance helps the patient to start accepting his or her body.
Listen attentively to the patient and be aware of his or her fears and concerns. Also look for misinterpretations or misunderstandings.	Listening to the patient will help identify opportunities for teaching.
Help patient identify personal strengths and mobilize coping strategies.	Discussions like this will help the patient to cope with the situation.
Help client to set realistic goals, such as "I will lose 1 pound this week" or "I will exercise for 10 minutes on two consecutive days."	Setting small, achievable goals will help the patient to see rewards from his or her efforts; achieving small outcomes/goals instills hope in the patient at times when he or she may be experiencing frustration and negative thoughts about self.
Arrange for nutritional consultation.	Helps to provide strategies to resolve the overweight or obesity problem.
Implement strategies to change patient eating habits and assist with weight reduction (see nursing diagnosis "Imbalanced Nutrition: More than Body Requirements").	Success at weight reduction can improve body image.
Identify the effects of the patient's culture or religion on self-concept and body image.	A patient's culture and religion often help define reactions to changes in body image and self-worth.

 NIC   *Body image enhancement*
   Emotional support
   Self-esteem enhancement

Evaluation

The patient is able to express that a problem exists with nutritional practices. It is crucial that the nurse evaluates to what degree the patient is beginning to acknowledge that certain behaviors (overeating and poor diet choices) are detrimental to his or her health and well-being. Assess for verbalizations that would indicate that the patient is beginning to assimilate positive dietary habits into the daily routine and is asking appropriate questions related to nutrition or the recommended dietary requirements. Communication of feelings and concerns relevant to weight and the need to consume healthier foods and less food overall should be taken as a positive sign that progress is being made towards meeting outcome criteria. Determine whether the patient is able to openly discuss feelings with family or significant other.

Community/Home Care

At home, continued monitoring of the patient's perception of body image and self-esteem is necessary. Obesity, especially morbid obesity, may represent another psychological problem that needs to be addressed by a professional counselor. Frequently, depression or stress need to be treated in order for the patient to move forward with establishing healthy nutritional habits. Counselors assist the patient to create a feeling of acceptance of self and the body as it is by identifying positive attributes and strengths to build upon. Counselors will need to continue to work with the patient until he or she has garnered enough self-confidence and elevated self-esteem to the point of feeling good about him or herself. Finding the right counselor who can establish a good rapport with the patient may be a challenge, and choices for this type of service may be limited in rural areas. Family members, friends, and significant others must provide support to the patient who is obese, helping him or her to stick to the recommended diets in order to regain a healthier state and achieve an acceptable weight loss. Accomplishments, regardless of how small, should be recognized through positive statements to the patient. Because most obese patients are treated on an outpatient basis in the absence of medical complications, other psychosocial issues such as ineffective coping may not be evident to the health care provider unless they spend time taking a thorough psychological history. The nurse or other health care provider who sees the patient for follow-up will need to be alert to subtle hints indicating that the patient is not making progress towards changing unhealthy nutritional habits and losing weight. Open discussions about this disturbed body image and interventions to prevent social isolation and withdrawal should continue with the patient.

Documentation

Chart any specific behaviors or verbalizations that may indicate a lowered self-esteem or altered body image. In addition to a thorough assessment of the patient's psychological state, include all interventions employed to address this issue and the patient's responses. Note when and if the patient begins to verbalize positive statements about him or herself. Document the patient's stated goals for weight loss and feelings about the proposed changes in lifestyle. Referrals to counselors are included in the patient record. If printed materials are given, indicate them in the patient chart by title. Document all referrals made to counselors or nutritionists.

CHAPTER 6.91

PANCREATITIS: ACUTE

GENERAL INFORMATION

Pancreatitis is an acute inflammation of the pancreas caused by an autodigestion of the pancreatic tissue by its own enzymes. Several processes lead to the autodigestion: obstruction of the biliary system by gallstones or edema causes bile containing enzymes to back up into the pancreas rather than moving into the digestive tract; pancreatic juices in the duodenum back up into the pancreatic duct; obstruction of pancreatic outflow; and activation of the pancreatic enzymes while they remain in the pancreas. There are two major forms of pancreatitis, interstitial and acute hemorrhagic. Pathophysiological changes seen in interstitial pancreatitis include a swollen, inflamed gland. Changes in hemorrhagic pancreatitis are more severe and include acute inflammation, significant necrosis of glandular tissue, and hemorrhage. The most common contributing factors are alcoholism (leading cause in the United States) and biliary disease, combining for more than 80 percent of all cases. Clinical manifestations are sudden onset abdominal pain in the epigastric area or left upper quadrant (LUQ) that is steady with radiation to the back or flank area, nausea, vomiting (70–90 percent of patients), fever, and abdominal distention and tenderness. Other significant findings include Turner's sign (bruising in the flanks) and Cullen's sign (ecchymosis around the umbilicus). Pancreatitis occurs most often in middle-aged people, and is more common in men.

NURSING DIAGNOSIS 1

 ACUTE PAIN

Related to:

Inflammation of the pancreas

Necrosis of the pancreas

Defining Characteristics:

Sudden abdominal pain in LUQ

Epigastric pain

Pain after eating fatty foods

Pain radiating to flank and back

Grimacing

Goal:

The patient reports pain is reduced or relieved.

Outcome Criteria

✔ The patient will state pain is relieved 30 minutes after interventions.

✔ The patient will state that pain does not occur after eating.

NOC *Pain level*
Pain control
Comfort level

INTERVENTIONS	RATIONALES
Assess pain, character, location, severity, duration, and precipitating factors; use a pain rating scale.	The pain of pancreatitis is moderate to severe and occurs in the LUQ and around the umbilicus. It is worsened by food and alcohol. A thorough pain assessment can provide clues about the diagnosis and severity of the disease. Pain scales provide an objective way to measure pain.
Assist to position of comfort.	Patients will often be more comfortable in the fetal position (side-lying with knees drawn to chest) with the head of bed elevated.

(continues)

(continued)

INTERVENTIONS	RATIONALES
Administer narcotic analgesics as ordered (such as Demerol) and monitor for side effects.	Narcotics are usually required for pain relief; Demerol is often the drug of choice.
Administer anticholinergics.	Helps to reduce pancreatic secretions and bile duct spasms.
Keep the patient NPO (nothing by mouth), as ordered.	Food stimulates gastric secretions that cause the pancreas to secrete its enzymes, which further aggravates pain.
If oral intake is allowed, avoid fatty foods.	Fatty foods can precipitate pain by stimulating the pancreas to release pancreatic juices.
Encourage use of alternative methods of pain relief, such as relaxation techniques, music therapy, massage, distraction, and guided imagery.	These strategies can enhance the effectiveness of analgesics.
Avoid the ingestion of alcohol.	Alcohol stimulates the pancreas and produces pain.
Teach the patient causes of pain.	Understanding what precipitates the pain helps the patient to take control of pain and avoid precipitating factors.

Evaluation

The patient reports that the pain has been reduced or alleviated following interventions. The patient reports ability to eat without pain. There are no observable signs of discomfort.

Community/Home Care

The patient's pain should be temporary and resolve once medical treatment has been initiated. The patient should implement measures to decrease excessive stimulation of pancreatic activity such as eating fatty foods or drinking alcohol, both of which can contribute to subsequent episodes of acute pancreatitis (see nursing diagnosis "Imbalanced Nutrition: Less than Body Requirements"). Pain at home is usually managed with mild analgesics, and the duration of pain should be short for acute pancreatitis. Use of non-pharmacological measures such as guided imagery, relaxation techniques, and music should be encouraged. The nurse should stress to the patient that weak respiratory efforts because of pain could cause respiratory problems such as atelectasis and pneumonia. There is a need to practice deep-breathing exercises to prevent this. To decrease the discomfort, encourage the patient to support the LUQ with a pillow when moving if soreness or mild pain persists at home. If the pain worsens, this may signal pancreatic necrosis or incomplete healing, and the patient will need to contact the health care provider for assessment or to determine other causes for the pain. If the recommended analgesics are not working, the patient should seek follow-up care with the health care provider.

Documentation

Document in the patient's own words the description of the pain and rating of the level of pain. Chart all interventions employed and the patient's responses. Document administration of analgesics on the medication administration record, including a reassessment of the pain 30 minutes to 1 hour after medication. Include in the documentation assessments made relevant to the respiratory system (breath sounds and depth). Document any teaching in the patient record with an indication of the patient's level of understanding.

NURSING DIAGNOSIS 2

IMBALANCED NUTRITION: LESS THAN BODY REQUIREMENTS

Related to:

Pain with oral intake

Inflammation

Nausea and vomiting

Inability to utilize pancreatic enzymes

NPO status

Defining Characteristics:

Increased pancreatic enzymes

Decreased intake of food

Goal:

The patient's normal nutritional status will be restored.

Outcome Criteria

✔ The patient will not lose weight.

✔ Pancreatic pain will subside.

✔ Pancreatic enzyme levels will decrease and return to normal limits.

✔ Electrolytes will be within normal limits.

✔ Albumin will return to normal limits.

✔ The patient verbalizes an understanding of the importance of remaining NPO until pain subsides.

NOC *Nutritional status: Food and fluid intake*

INTERVENTIONS	RATIONALES
Complete a fluid and nutritional assessment, including assessing for nausea; vomiting; poor skin turgor; dry, pale mucous membranes; dietary intake before onset of pain; fluid intake and output; weight loss, and loss of appetite.	Patients who experience pancreatitis often have a decreased nutritional status due to pain with intake and lack of pancreatic enzymes in the digestive tract. Anorexia, nausea, and vomiting add to the problem by preventing the patient from taking in enough nutrients to meet metabolic demands.
Assess laboratory results: pancreatic enzymes (amylase, lipase), urine amylase, serum albumin, total protein, calcium, electrolytes, glucose, serum transferrin, iron, folic acid, and thiamine level.	Pancreatic enzymes will be elevated in pancreatitis. Lipase will increase within 2 to 12 hours of the onset of pancreatitis and remain elevated for 3 to 4 days; lipase is more specific than amylase and rises after 48 hours but remains elevated for 7 to 14 days; urine amylase is elevated; albumin and total protein are decreased due to malnutrition; calcium levels may be decreased due to calcium deposits into areas of necrosis in the pancreas; other electrolytes may be imbalanced due to loss through vomiting or poor intake; elevated glucose is seen due to the diseased pancreas' inability to produce/ release insulin; nutritional indicators (transferrin, iron, folic acid, thiamine) are decreased due to the patient's inability to eat and absorb adequate amounts of nutrients, particularly in alcoholic patients.
Weigh patient and monitor weight daily or weekly.	Helps to establish baseline for comparison.
Keep the patient NPO.	Helps to ensure that the pancreas rests and pancreatic enzymes are not released.
Insert nasogastric (NG) tube and connect to low suction as ordered.	Keeping the stomach decompressed decreases pancreatic secretion and vomiting.
Insert intravenous catheter and administer intravenous (IV) fluids and electrolytes, as ordered.	Helps to hydrate patient.
Monitor lipase and amylase levels.	Oral intake is resumed when the enzyme levels decrease and return to normal.
Assess for pain and treat as ordered (see nursing diagnosis "Acute Pain").	Food is withheld until pain resolves; persistent pain is an indicator of continuing inflammation.
Once food is allowed, collaborate with the dietician to develop an acceptable diet that considers usual habits, food intake, and any cultural or religious restrictions.	The dietician can discuss with the patient which foods may be digested better with the fewest untoward effects but the best nutritional results.
Offer clear liquid fluids first when oral intake is allowed and monitor for return or worsening of pain.	Helps to determine the patient's tolerance for intake.
Encourage the patient to take increased nutrients through high-calorie, moderate carbohydrate, and low-fat diets, as ordered, with small meals and between-meal snacks. Both alcohol and caffeine should be avoided.	Helps to promote adequate intake of nutrients; for patients with decreased appetite, a small meal is more likely to be ingested and to be seen as desirable. Fat is not generally tolerated by patients with pancreatitis and needs to be restricted. Snacks provide needed additional calories. Alcohol is a contributing factor to pancreatitis and can induce a repeat episode. Caffeine is a stimulant.
Give nutritional supplements as ordered: folic acid, thiamine, vitamins.	Helps to supplement nutrient intake; a majority of patients with pancreatitis are likely candidates for malnutrition and need these nutrients. This is especially true for those patients with pancreatitis caused by alcohol use.
Administer anti-emetics, as ordered.	Helps to decrease nausea and vomiting.
Administer antacids, as ordered.	Helps to reduce heartburn, stomach acids, and risk of ulcer formation.

(continues)

(continued)

INTERVENTIONS	RATIONALES
Assist with administration of total parenteral nutrition (TPN), as ordered.	TPN may be necessary if the patient is unable to meet daily caloric and vitamin requirements via oral intake, especially if the acute illness is prolonged.
Monitor and record intake and output according to agency protocol.	Helps to detect dehydration and initiate early treatment.
Teach the patient and family about nutritional restrictions, rationales for interventions, and the role of the pancreas in maintenance of nutritional status.	Helps to enhance compliance with nutritional interventions.

NIC *Nutritional monitoring*
Nutritional management
Nausea management

Evaluation

The acute pancreatitis is resolving as demonstrated by serum amylase and lipase returning to normal or improving. The patient's nutritional status is stable, as demonstrated by the laboratory values (albumin, total protein, iron, electrolytes, folate, etc.) returning to normal and no weight loss. The patient verbalizes an understanding of the interventions required (NPO, NG tube). When oral intake is allowed, the patient is interested in eating, understands the need for increased nutrients due to the malnourished state, and tolerates food and fluids without pain, eventually progressing to regular meals.

Community/Home Care

The patient must continue to give attention to nutrition and the role of the pancreas in nutrition maintenance. If the pancreatitis was caused by biliary disease, the problem will probably be completely resolved once at home following successful treatment of the biliary problem. However, if acute pancreatitis was caused by alcoholism, then interventions will need to continue, as it may recur. A dietary consultation is crucial in assisting the patient to identify those food items that should be restricted and those that are more suitable for the healing pancreas. Both the patient and family require formal instruction about the restrictions that may be imposed due to pancreatitis. The patient will need to eliminate fat or restrict it in the diet. Giving the patient a list of foods that are high in fat will be helpful, as fried foods are usually restricted until recovery is complete. A handy reference guide can be created to give to the patient or family that includes a list of foods that provide carbohydrates, foods that provide iron, foods to avoid, foods that are acceptable, how much of any group to consume, and a schedule for small meals. Nutritional snacks can be prepared in advance in ready-to-eat sizes and kept in the refrigerator, especially during the early periods of recovery when anorexia may be a problem. Family members and significant others play a role in implementing strategies to improve nutrition by preparing meals and encouraging the patient to ingest them. Frequent small meals at home should be encouraged to increase the likelihood that the patient can ingest enough nutrients. The patient may need to remain on multivitamins, folic acid, thiamine, electrolyte supplements, and other nutritional supplements for an extended period of time, especially if alcoholism is an issue. It should be clear to the patient and family that abstinence from alcohol is necessary to prevent future occurrences of acute pancreatitis. Providing the patient with information about how alcohol alters nutritional status and on self-help groups for alcohol cessation may lead to health-promoting behaviors. Teach the patient to monitor nutrition/intake by keeping a log of food eaten, when eaten, and whether eating causes pain or vomiting. If at any time a particular meal or food product causes pain or subsequent nausea/vomiting, the patient should note this in the log and eliminate this food from his or her diet. Weights should also be included in the log. Even though the patient may not want to weigh every day, weighing at least every other day is a good way to keep track of weight loss or stabilization. This information can be shared with the health care provider at each follow-up visit to provide data for revision in prescribed therapeutic interventions. The patient is more likely to have proper nutrition when supported by family and friends. Follow-up providers should assess the patient for weight loss and monitor laboratory results for improvement.

Documentation

Chart the results of a nutritional assessment that includes a history of usual intake. Document vital signs, weights, and intake and output according to agency protocol at least every shift or every 8 hours.

Include in the chart the amount of drainage from the NG tube suctioning (if present). Once oral intake is allowed, document the amount of food the patient consumes at each meal, tolerance for food, and what, if any, supplements are taken by the patient. If the patient experiences pain following a meal, document this along with the exact foods aggravating the pain and measures to relieve it. For patients who are taking nutritional supplements (vitamins, liquid supplements, etc.), chart this in the patient record. In most agencies there are specific guidelines for charting regarding TPN that include specific nutritional parameters, so the nurse should document accordingly. If the patient has complaints of any type, document this in the record with accompanying documentation indicating responses to interventions. Always include in the record any referrals made, especially to the dietician or alcohol cessation programs.

NURSING DIAGNOSIS 3

DEFICIENT FLUID VOLUME

Related to:

> Vomiting/nausea
>
> NPO restrictions
>
> NG tube to suction

Defining Characteristics:

> Hypotension
>
> Tachycardia
>
> Dry mucous membranes
>
> Decreased skin turgor
>
> Decreased urine output

Goal:

> Adequate fluid volume is restored.

Outcome Criteria

✔ Urinary output is > 30 ml per hour on average.

✔ Skin is moist.

✔ Mucous membranes are moist.

✔ Capillary refill is < 3 seconds.

✔ Vital signs return to baseline.

NOC   *Fluid balance*

INTERVENTIONS	RATIONALES
Assess the patient's fluid status: pulse, blood pressure, mucous membranes, skin turgor, and capillary refill.	These are all clues to hydration status; in states of dehydration, the blood pressure may decrease and the pulse increase, mucous membranes will be dry, and capillary refill time will be increased.
Monitor intake and output, noting color of urine.	Helps to assess fluid balance; urine output will decrease, and urine will be dark and concentrated in dehydration.
Measure abdominal girth.	A distended abdomen may occur in acute pancreatitis due to loss of fluids from the circulating volume and due to inflammation.
Establish IV access and administer IV fluids and electrolytes, as ordered.	Helps to maintain fluid and electrolyte balance while NPO.
Monitor output from NG tube suction and vomiting, and record every 8 hours, or as ordered.	Helps to detect excessive loss of fluid and provide information needed for treatment.
Resume intake of food and fluids by mouth, as ordered, when pain subsides and pancreatic enzymes return to normal.	Helps to return the patient back to a normal fluid status as soon as possible.

NIC   *Fluid management*
Fluid monitoring
Intravenous insertion
Intravenous therapy

Evaluation

Assess the patient for return of normal fluid volume. The patient's blood pressure and pulse should be at baseline. Mucous membranes should be moist and skin should be warm and dry. Renal output should not be impaired, with an hourly output on the average of 30 ml/hour. The patient has no nausea or vomiting. Output from the NG tube suction should be minimal.

Community/Home Care

Patients treated for fluid volume deficit secondary to pancreatitis have normal fluid status restored prior to discharge home. Patients experiencing the deficit secondary to vomiting or NG suction should receive education about prevention of fluid deficit through management of nausea/vomiting and the need to seek medical assistance in a timely manner. At home, the patient may not require any follow-up, as this is an acute situation that for the most part has no long-term complications. Once at home, the patient may have some initial anxiety or fear about the ability to take fluids and foods without vomiting or pain, and may be cautious about intake. For this reason, the patient should start the intake of oral substances with clear liquids and progress as tolerated. Fatigue secondary to fluid loss may need to be addressed; the fatigued patient should perform activities as tolerated until stamina/endurance is re-established. The health care provider may want the patient to return for a follow-up appointment to ensure that the fluid status has returned to normal.

Documentation

Findings from an assessment of the patient's fluid status are charted, including blood pressure, pulse, skin turgor, mucous membranes, and intake and output, with a description of the urine. Drainage from NG suction is charted on the patient's intake/output record according to agency guidelines. If the patient vomits, document this as well as strategies for relief. Chart insertion of IV catheters and the type and amount of IV fluid administered. Document all other interventions implemented to address the problem of fluid volume deficit. Be specific when charting patient responses to treatment so that other health care providers can clearly determine improvement or deterioration.

NURSING DIAGNOSIS 4

INEFFECTIVE BREATHING PATTERN

Related to:

    Pain in LUQ

    Vomiting

    Limited mobility due to pain

Defining Characteristics:

    Shallow breathing

    Decreased breath sounds

    Adventitious breath sounds

Goal:

    The patient will have effective breathing patterns.

Outcome Criteria

✔ Breath sounds will be equal and clear bilaterally.

✔ The patient will not develop atelectasis or pneumonia.

✔ The patient will demonstrate proper use of incentive spirometry (IS).

✔ The patient will demonstrate turn, cough, and deep breathe (TCDB) technique.

NOC   *Respiratory status: Gas exchange*
          Respiratory status: Ventilation
          Pain level

INTERVENTIONS	RATIONALES
Assess respiratory status, including rate, rhythm, effort, depth, and breath sounds.	Helps to obtain a baseline and to detect problems; because of the pain in the LUQ, the patient may take shallow breaths that predispose him or her to atelectasis and subsequently to pneumonia.
Assess for signs of pneumonia or atelectasis every shift.	Atelectasis is common in patients with pancreatitis and is characterized by diminished breath sounds in the bases; pneumonia occurs secondary to atelectasis, and the patient should be monitored for elevated temperature, shortness of breath, and expectoration of sputum.
Teach the patient how to turn, cough, and deep breathe, and encourage him or her to do so every 2 hours while awake.	Helps to stimulate deep breathing that can open distant airways and prevent atelectasis.
Have patient hold a pillow to LUQ when practicing TCDB exercises.	This provides support for the painful area.
Teach the patient how to use the IS, and encourage that it be used 10 times per hour.	Helps to open distant airways and prevent atelectasis.
Administer pain medications as needed.	If pain is relieved, the patient can breathe more effectively and is more willing to participate in breathing exercises.

INTERVENTIONS	RATIONALES
Assist with placement on mechanical ventilation, as ordered.	In cases of severe abdominal distention, breathing patterns may be ineffective in maintaining adequate oxygen, and ventilation assistance may be required.

NIC *Respiratory monitoring*
Positioning

Evaluation

Respirations should be easy with equal chest expansion bilaterally and a rate of 12 to 24 per minute. The patient's breath sounds are clear and equal bilaterally in all lobes. IS and TCDB exercises are understood and practiced as requested. The patient does not present with any symptoms of pneumonia. Diminished breath sounds, especially over left lung, should return to normal. Oxygen saturation results should provide evidence that breathing patterns are able to achieve adequate gas exchange.

Community/Home Care

At time of discharge, the patient's breathing patterns should be effective. There should be no long-term concerns that would necessitate special in-home care. Once at home, the patient may continue to have some tenderness in the area of the pancreas that may make him or her continue to breathe shallowly, but this should not pose a significant threat to respiratory status as the patient should be fully ambulatory, which will help prevent atelectasis. The patient should continue to utilize the IS as directed by the physician, and one should be sent home with the patient. The patient will need to be aware of respiratory symptoms of infection that warrant a return to the physician, such as fever, shortness of breath, large amounts of sputum, and a cough. Although a visiting nurse may not be required, the patient should be encouraged to return for a follow-up appointment with a health care provider.

Documentation

Chart the extent to which the outcome criteria have been achieved. Document the patient's breath sounds, respiratory rate, and extent of respiratory effort. If the patient practices TCDB and IS, document this in the chart. Always include all nursing interventions implemented to prevent or treat respiratory problems. Any signs of atelectasis or pneumonia are documented.

NURSING DIAGNOSIS 5

 DEFICIENT KNOWLEDGE

Related to:
Lack of information
Anxiety
No previous experience with pancreatitis

Defining Characteristics:
Has many questions
Has no questions
Verbalizes misunderstanding

Goal:
The patient verbalizes an understanding of pancreatitis and its treatment.

Outcome Criteria

✔ The patient verbalizes a willingness and desire to learn the necessary information.
✔ The patient verbalizes an understanding of pancreatitis.
✔ The patient verbalizes a willingness to be compliant with treatment recommendations.
✔ The patient verbalizes an understanding of dietary restrictions required.

NOC *Knowledge: Disease process*
Knowledge: Health behavior
Treatment behavior: Illness
or injury

INTERVENTIONS	RATIONALES
Assess readiness of client to learn (motivation, cognitive level, and physiological status).	Patient must be motivated to learn, have the capability to learn, and be free of distractions from learning such as pain and emotional distress.
Assess what the patient already knows.	The patient may have some knowledge about pancreatitis, and teaching should begin with what the patient already knows.

(continues)

(continued)

INTERVENTIONS	RATIONALES
Create a quiet environment conducive to learning.	Environmental noise can prevent the learner from focusing on what is being taught.
Teach the learners about the normal function of the pancreas (role of pancreas in digestion, insulin release) and the pathophysiology of pancreatitis.	Understanding of normal function and pathophysiology assists the patient to understand the rationale for therapeutic interventions.
Teach the patient deep breathing and coughing exercises.	Helps to maximize ventilatory excursion and reduce the likelihood of atelectasis and pneumonia.
If alcohol abuse is the causative factor, provide the patient with information about alcohol cessation programs.	Continued use of alcohol can predispose the patient to repeated episodes of pancreatitis and possible chronic pancreatitis.
Teach the patient about diet required: low fat, adequate proteins, no alcohol, and limited caffeine.	The patient needs to understand the dietary requirements for healing. Adequate calories and protein are needed for healing and energy. Diets that are high in fat are generally not well tolerated by patients with pancreatitis during the early convalescence, alcohol is toxic to the pancreas, and caffeine acts as both a stimulant and an irritant to the GI system.
Evaluate the patient's understanding of all content covered by asking questions.	Helps to identify areas that require more teaching and to ensure that the patient has enough information to ensure compliance.
Give the patient written information.	Provides reference at a later time, and for review.

NIC *Teaching: Disease process*
   Teaching: Individual
   Teaching: Diet

Evaluation

The patient is able to repeat all information for the nurse and asks questions about the pancreatitis and possible outcomes (positive and negative). Prior to discharge, the patient verbalizes an understanding of the diet restrictions and agrees to be compliant. The patient is able to state what pancreatitis is and what causes it. In cases of alcoholism, the patient verbalizes a willingness to seek professional help. The patient should be able to inform the nurse when health care assistance should be sought.

Community/Home Care

With the exception of elderly patients follow-up care in the home is rarely required unless complications have occurred. For patients who have had acute pancreatitis, the hospital stay may be short, which dictates that knowledge deficits be identified early in order to improve the likelihood that the patient will be prepared for self-care and self-monitoring. One of the most crucial parts of teaching should focus on the dietary restrictions and abstinence from alcohol. Specific information on availability of alcohol cessation programs should be given. Consultation with a social worker who can locate a program that is accessible to the patient (geographically and financially) is recommended. Initially, the patient should refrain from ingesting foods with high fat content as the pancreas continues to heal. Even though the dietician or nurse provides the patient with information about foods to avoid, items not on the list may cause problems as well. Therefore, some period of trial and error of diet may be required to rule out particular foods. The patient may find it helpful to try fatty foods in small amounts to be sure he or she can ingest them without nausea, vomiting, or pain. Teaching needs to be thorough, so that the patient will be able to monitor him or herself for improvement of symptoms, or onset of respiratory complications such as pneumonia. Follow-up with a health care provider focuses on assurance that no complications have occurred and that the patient has a clear understanding of what a diagnosis of pancreatitis entails.

Documentation

Document all content taught and the patient's verbalization of understanding. Specific attention should be given to documentation of any specific concerns that the patient expresses. Include in the documentation the patient's willingness to comply with all recommendations made about the diet and abstinence of alcohol. Any area that requires further teaching should be clearly indicated in the record. Include in the record all appointments that have been made for follow-up. Chart any questions or concerns that the patient has verbalized. Always include the titles of any printed literature given to the patient for reinforcement.

CHAPTER 6.92

PANCREATITIS: CHRONIC

GENERAL INFORMATION

Chronic pancreatitis is a recurring inflammation of the pancreas resulting in scarring and destruction of the pancreatic tissue that most often occurs due to long-term alcohol use. In alcoholic pancreatitis, this inflammation is caused in large part by an increased concentration of proteins that calcify and subsequently form plugs that block the normal outflow of pancreatic secretions. It is characterized by remissions and exacerbations with complaints of severe upper abdominal pain that may be continuous or a dull, nagging constant pain. Chronic pancreatitis is also demonstrated by significant weight loss, dark urine, and, late in the disease, signs of malabsorption. A common distinctive finding is stools that are frothy and foul-smelling due to the inability of the pancreas to exert its function in fat digestion. If beta cells have been destroyed or damaged, the patient also has elevated glucose levels due to lack of insulin release from the beta cells. The incidence among drinkers is 50 times greater than that seen in nondrinkers. It is estimated that 75 percent of all clients with chronic pancreatitis are alcoholics.

NURSING DIAGNOSIS 1

ACUTE AND CHRONIC PAIN

Related to:

Inflammation of the pancreas

Necrosis of the pancreas

Defining Characteristics:

Severe pain in left upper quadrant (LUQ)

Epigastric pain

Pain after eating fatty foods

Complaints of a constant, dull pain

Pain that is recurring

Grimacing

Goal:

The patient reports pain is reduced or relieved.

Outcome Criteria

✔ The patient will state pain is relieved 30 minutes after interventions.
✔ The patient will state that pain does not occur after eating.
✔ The patient states that pain is tolerable.

NOC *Pain level*
Pain control
Comfort level

INTERVENTIONS	RATIONALES
Assess pain, character, location, severity, duration, and precipitating factors; use a pain rating scale.	The pain of chronic pancreatitis is moderate to severe, occurs in the LUQ, and may be described as severe, constant, nagging, or dull. It is worsened by food and alcohol. A thorough pain assessment can provide clues about the diagnosis and how the disease impacts function. Pain scales provide an objective measure of the pain.
Assist to a position of comfort.	Patients will often be more comfortable in the fetal position (side-lying with knees drawn to chest), with the head of bed elevated.
Administer non-narcotic analgesics, as ordered.	Narcotics may be required for relief of acute pain or pain that has worsened; Demerol is often the drug of choice; however, the pain of chronic pancreatitis can be treated with less potent medications at other times.

(continues)

(continued)

INTERVENTIONS	RATIONALES
Administer proton pump inhibitors, such as Protonix or Prilosec, as ordered.	These medications suppress gastric secretions that lead to decreased pancreatic secretions; prevents ulcers.
Administer H$_2$ receptor antagonists, as ordered.	Suppresses gastric acid secretion.
Keep the patient NPO (nothing by mouth) as ordered if pain worsens.	Food stimulates gastric secretions that causes pancreas to secrete or attempt to secrete its enzymes, which further aggravates pain.
Avoid fatty foods during episodes of acute pain.	Fatty foods can precipitate pain by stimulating the pancreas to release pancreatic juices.
Encourage use of alternative methods of pain relief, such as relaxation techniques, music therapy, massage, distraction, and guided imagery.	These strategies can enhance the effectiveness of analgesics.
Administer synthetic hormone (Octreotide®) as ordered.	This medication is used if the patient has poor response to other interventions to control pain. It is a synthetic version of somatostatin that suppresses pancreatic secretion.
Evaluate the effectiveness of interventions to manage pain.	Helps to determine whether interventions have been successful or whether new interventions need to be added to the plan.

Evaluation

The patient is able to report that the pain has been reduced or alleviated following interventions. The patient verbalizes ability to tolerate pain without feeling anxious and is able to assist in the management of the pain through anxiety reduction and relaxation techniques. The patient should have no observable signs of discomfort.

Community/Home Care

The patient's pain is chronic and the patient will need to learn how to control or minimize the effect the pain has on quality of life. The pain at home is managed with mild analgesics and other medications that control the secretion of gastric juices, minimizing stimulation of the pancreas. It is of crucial importance that the patient implement measures to

eliminate fatty foods from the diet and abstain from alcohol; both fatty foods and alcohol can contribute to subsequent episodes of acute intensified pain and cause further damage to the pancreas. It may be necessary for the patient to seek professional help for alcohol cessation, and a dietician can help to prepare a tolerable diet. Use of non-pharmacological measures such as guided imagery, relaxation techniques, and music should be encouraged. Encourage the patient to support the LUQ with a pillow when moving if soreness or mild pain persists at home to decrease the discomfort. When the patient with chronic pancreatitis experiences severe abdominal or epigastric pain similar to that of acute pancreatitis, he or she should seek health care for possible pain management in an acute care setting. This may signal pancreatic necrosis or incomplete healing. If the recommended analgesics are not working, the patient should seek follow-up care with the health care provider.

Documentation

Document in the patient's own words the description of the pain and rating of the level of pain. Chart the administration of analgesics and all other interventions employed to treat the pain and the patient's responses. Include in the documentation any nonverbal signs of pain. Instruction about relaxation techniques and management of pain at home should be indicated in the patient record, along with the patient's level of understanding. Document all referrals made for assistance.

 NURSING DIAGNOSIS 2

IMBALANCED NUTRITION: LESS THAN BODY REQUIREMENTS

Related to:

Chronic pain

Inflammation

Inability to utilize pancreatic enzymes

Defining Characteristics:

Elevated pancreatic enzymes

Decreased intake of food

Weight loss

Steatorrhea

Nausea/vomiting

Anorexia

Goal:

> The patient's normal nutritional status will be restored.

Outcome Criteria

✔ The patient will not lose weight.

✔ Pancreatic pain will subside.

✔ Serum levels of pancreatic enzymes decrease.

✔ Fat content in stools will decrease or be eliminated.

✔ Electrolytes will be within normal limits.

✔ Albumin will return to normal limits.

✔ The patient verbalizes an understanding of the importance of remaining NPO until pain subsides.

✔ The patient verbalizes an understanding of and willingness to comply with medication regimen (pancreatic enzymes), nutritional restrictions, and abstinence from alcohol.

NOC *Nutritional status: Food and fluid intake*

INTERVENTIONS	RATIONALES
Complete a fluid and nutritional assessment, including assessing for nausea; vomiting; poor skin turgor; dry, pale mucous membranes; dietary intake before onset of pain; fluid intake and output; weight loss; and loss of appetite.	Patients who have chronic pancreatitis often have a decreased nutritional status due to pain with intake and lack of pancreatic enzymes in the digestive tract. Anorexia, nausea, and vomiting add to the problem by preventing the patient from taking in enough nutrients to meet metabolic demands.
Assess laboratory results: pancreatic enzymes (amylase, lipase), urine amylase, 24-hour stool for fat, serum albumin, total protein, calcium, electrolytes, glucose, serum transferrin, iron, folic acid, and thiamine.	Pancreatic enzymes will be elevated in pancreatitis. Lipase will increase within 2 to 12 hours of the onset of pancreatitis and remain elevated for 3 to 4 days; lipase is more specific than amylase and rises after 48 hours but remains elevated for 7 to 14 days; urine amylase is elevated; stools of patients with chronic pancreatitis are frothy and foul-smelling due to the presence of increased fat (steatorrhea); albumin and total protein are decreased due to malnutrition; calcium levels may be decreased due to calcium deposits into areas of necrosis in
	the pancreas; other electrolytes may be imbalanced due to loss through vomiting or poor intake; elevated glucose is seen due to the diseased pancreas' inability to produce/release insulin and gives an indication that the pancreas' ability to function may be impaired; nutritional indicators (transferrin, iron, folic acid, thiamine) are decreased due to the inability of the patient to eat and absorb adequate amounts of nutrients, particularly in alcoholic patients.
Weigh patient and monitor weight daily or weekly.	Helps to establish baseline for comparison and to monitor nutritional status.
Keep the patient NPO during recurrent episodes of acute pain.	Helps to ensure that the pancreas rests and is not stimulated by the presence of food in the gastrointestinal (GI) tract.
Insert nasogastric (NG) tube and connect to low suction as ordered during acute pain episodes.	Keeping the stomach decompressed decreases pancreatic secretion and vomiting.
Insert intravenous (IV) catheter and administer IV fluids and electrolytes, as ordered.	Helps to hydrate patient and prevent electrolyte imbalance.
Monitor lipase and amylase levels.	These levels guide treatment, and oral intake is resumed only when the enzyme levels return to the patient's baseline.
Assess for pain and treat as ordered (see nursing diagnosis "Acute and Chronic Pain").	Food is withheld until pain resolves; persistent pain is an indicator of continuing acute inflammation.
Once food is allowed, collaborate with the dietician to develop an acceptable diet that considers usual habits, food intake, and any cultural or religious restrictions.	The dietician can discuss with the patient which foods may be digested better with the fewest untoward effects but the best nutritional results.
Administer pancreatic enzymes (such as Pancrelipase®), as ordered, and monitor for response.	This is a supplemental enzyme given to patients with chronic pancreatitis who are unable to secrete enough enzymes for digestion, especially for the synthesis of fats. It also improves *(continues)*

(continued)

INTERVENTIONS	RATIONALES
	absorption. It must be given with meals or within one hour of meals. If the medication is effective, the number of stools should decrease, and stools should become less fatty (absence of frothy appearance, less foul-smelling).
Offer clear liquid fluids first when oral intake is allowed, and monitor for return or worsening of pain.	Helps to determine the patient's tolerance for intake.
Encourage the patient to take increased nutrients through high-calorie, high-protein, moderate carbohydrate, and low-fat diets, as ordered, with small meals and between-meal snacks. Both alcohol and caffeine should be avoided.	Helps to promote adequate intake of nutrients; fat is not generally tolerated by patients with chronic pancreatitis and needs to be avoided during episodes of acute pain; however, once acute episodes of pain have resolved, some fat can be ingested if the patient is taking supplemental pancreatic enzymes. The small meals may be easier to digest and will not give a sensation of fullness; a small meal is more likely to be consumed by patients with decreased appetites. Snacks provide needed additional calories. Alcohol is a contributing factor to pancreatitis, can induce a repeat acute episode, and should be avoided. Caffeine is a stimulant.
Give nutritional supplements as ordered: folic acid, thiamine, vitamins.	Helps to supplement nutrient intake; a majority of patients with chronic pancreatitis are likely candidates for malnutrition due to alcoholism, and need these nutrients. This is especially true for patients with chronic pancreatitis caused by alcohol use.
Administer anti-emetics, as ordered.	Helps to decrease nausea and vomiting.
Administer antacids, as ordered.	Helps to reduce heartburn, stomach acids, bloating, and risk of ulcer formation.
Check blood glucose using finger-stick method before each meal and administer insulin as ordered.	In patients with chronic pancreatitis, the pancreas is unable to perform its normal role in the release of insulin from

	the beta cells. Blood glucose levels are needed to determine the body's need for insulin.
Assist with administration of total parenteral nutrition (TPN), as ordered.	TPN may be necessary if the patient is unable to meet daily caloric and vitamin requirements via oral intake, especially if the acute episode is prolonged.
Monitor and record intake and output according to agency protocol.	Helps to detect dehydration and initiate early treatment.
Teach the patient and family about nutritional restrictions, rationales for interventions, and the role of the pancreas in maintenance of nutritional status.	Helps to enhance compliance with nutritional interventions.
Teach patient and family needed information for disease management (see nursing diagnosis "Deficient Knowledge").	Helps to ensure positive outcomes and prevent hospitalizations.

NIC   *Nutritional monitoring*
Nutritional management
Nausea management

Evaluation

The acute episode of pain with chronic pancreatitis is resolving. The patient's nutritional status is improved, as evidenced by the laboratory values (albumin, total protein, iron, electrolytes, folate, etc.) returning to normal or decreasing (pancreatic enzymes). Stools are no longer frothy or foul-smelling. The patient verbalizes an understanding of the interventions required for home maintenance (pancreatic enzymes, abstinence from alcohol). When oral intake is allowed, the patient is interested in eating, understands the need for increased nutrients due to the malnourished state, and tolerates food and fluids without pain. No further weight loss occurs, and the patient consumes regular meals.

Community/Home Care

The patient with chronic pancreatitis will need to implement a complex regimen in the home, giving much attention to nutrition and the role of the pancreas in nutrition maintenance. A dietary consultation is crucial in assisting the patient to identify those food items that should be restricted and those that are more suitable for the diseased pancreas. Both the patient and family require formal instruction about the restrictions that may be imposed due to chronic pancreatitis. The patient will need to eliminate fat or restrict it in the diet. Giving the patient a list of foods that are high in fat—usually including all fried foods—will be helpful. Because the dietary recommendations may be easily forgotten, a handy, laminated reference guide can be created for the patient or family. This guide could include a list of foods that provide carbohydrates, foods that provide iron, foods to avoid, foods that are acceptable, how much of any group to consume, and a schedule for frequent small meals to increase the likelihood that the patient can ingest enough nutrients. It is important that the patient understand the need to take the pancreatic enzymes at the scheduled time (with or before meals) to achieve the desired therapeutic effect. Skipping doses or taking them at odd hours if they have forgotten them will not provide satisfactory results in terms of being available to assist with absorption/digestion. Keeping written instructions with the medications and placing the medications in the kitchen in plain view may serve as a reminder, especially when the regimen is first initiated, when the patient is learning and adapting to the regimen. Supplemental drinks can improve nutritional status during periods when the patient is unable to ingest adequate amounts of nutrition through normal meals due to anorexia or abdominal pain. There are numerous products on the market, but the patient may need to experiment with which ones are tolerated after consultation with the dietician to determine which ones are allowed. The patient may need to remain on multivitamins, folic acid, thiamine, electrolyte supplements, and other nutritional supplements for an extended period of time, especially if alcoholism is an issue. Significant others play a role in implementing strategies to improve nutrition by preparing meals and encouraging the patient to ingest them. In the home, self-monitoring of blood glucose by the patient will need to be done prior to meals to determine insulin needs, as the diseased pancreas is unable to respond to meals with insulin release. The patient records the results of the glucose check as well as any insulin administration. The nurse needs to assist the patient to set up a log/journal for recording this information as well as other data relevant to nutritional status. Other important data to be recorded include food eaten, when eaten, and whether eating causes pain or vomiting. If at any time a particular meal or food product causes pain or subsequent nausea/vomiting, the patient should note this in the log and eliminate this food from the diet. Weight should also be included in the log. Even though the patient may not want to weigh every day, weighing at least every other day is a good way to keep track of weight loss or stabilization. A final piece of data that is part of the patient's in-home assessment includes observation of the stool to determine if the fat content is decreasing. The odor of the stool should become less foul, and the frothy appearance should decrease as the patient's therapy with pancreatic enzymes becomes effective. All of this information recorded in the log can be shared with the health care provider at each follow-up visit to provide data for revision in prescribed therapeutic interventions. The patient is more likely to have proper nutrition when supported by family and friends. Follow-up providers should assess the patient for weight loss and monitor laboratory results for improvement.

Documentation

Chart the results of a nutritional assessment that includes a history of usual intake (amount and type of food and liquid, including alcohol). Document vital signs, weights, and intake and output according to agency protocol at least every shift or every 8 hours. Include in the chart the amount of drainage from any NG tube suctioning. Once oral intake is allowed, document the amount of food the patient consumes at each meal, as well as tolerance for food. If the patient experiences pain following a meal, document this along with the exact foods aggravating the pain and measures to relieve it. For patients who are taking pancreatic enzymes or other nutritional supplements (vitamins, liquid supplements, etc.) chart this in the patient record according to protocol for medication administration. Chart results of glucose monitoring and coverage with insulin as required. In most agencies there are specific guidelines for charting regarding TPN that include specific nutritional parameters, so the nurse should document accordingly. If the patient has complaints of any type, record this along with accompanying documentation indicating response to interventions. Always include in the record any referrals made, especially to the dietician.

NURSING DIAGNOSIS 3

DEFICIENT KNOWLEDGE

Related to:

Lack of information

Anxiety

Chronic pancreatitis

Defining Characteristics:

Asks many questions

Has no questions

Verbalizes that do not understand the disease

Goal:

The patient verbalizes an understanding of chronic pancreatitis and its treatment.

Outcome Criteria

✔ The patient verbalizes a willingness and desire to learn the necessary information.

✔ The patient verbalizes an understanding of chronic pancreatitis.

✔ The patient verbalizes a willingness to be compliant with treatment recommendations relevant to fat and alcohol intake.

✔ The patient verbalizes an understanding of dietary restrictions required.

NOC *Knowledge: Disease process*
Knowledge: Health behavior
Treatment behavior: Illness or injury

INTERVENTIONS	RATIONALES
Assess readiness of client to learn (motivation, cognitive level, and physiological status).	The patient must be motivated to learn, have the capability to learn the content, and be free of distractions from learning such as pain and emotional distress.
Assess what the patient already knows.	The patient may have some knowledge about chronic pancreatitis, and instruction should begin with what the patient already knows.
Create a quiet environment conducive to learning.	Environmental noise can prevent the learner from focusing on what is being taught.
Teach the learners about the normal function of the pancreas and the pathophysiology of chronic pancreatitis (role of pancreas in digestion, insulin production).	Understanding of normal function and pathophysiology assists the patient to understand the rationale for therapeutic interventions.
If alcohol abuse is the causative factor, provide the patient with information about alcohol cessation programs.	Continued use of alcohol can predispose the patient to repeated episodes of acute exacerbations of pain and further destruction of pancreatitis tissue.
Teach the patient about pancreatic enzymes: — Action: assist with digestion of fats — Scheduling: given with meals, or within 1 hour of meals — Side effects: rare, but in large doses can cause GI upset	If the patient understands actions and why the medication is needed, he or she will be more likely to comply.
Teach the patient and one other person about aspects of self-monitoring of glucose and insulin administration, and have him or her demonstrate the skills: — Self-monitoring of blood glucose: how to perform finger-stick, how to operate the monitor, storage, recording results — Insulin administration: when to perform blood glucose checks, how to administer insulin, acceptable sites, and disposal of used syringes/needles — Signs of complications: hyperglycemia and hypoglycemia, treatment of hypoglycemia, recording administration, storage	The patient with chronic pancreatitis will need to monitor blood glucose in order to prevent episodes of hyperglycemia due to lack of insulin. The patient needs to know how to perform glucose checks as well as insulin administration. The nurse needs to have all parties demonstrate the skill to ensure its correct performance at home.
Teach the patient about diet required: low-fat, no alcohol, high-calorie, high-protein, moderate carbohydrates, and limited caffeine.	Adequate calories and protein are needed for proper nutrition and energy. Diets that are high in fat are generally not well tolerated by patients with chronic pancreatitis. Alcohol is toxic to the pancreas, and caffeine is a GI irritant.
Evaluate the patient's understanding of all content covered by asking questions.	Helps to identify areas that require more instruction and to ensure that the patient has enough information to ensure compliance.

INTERVENTIONS	RATIONALES
Give the patient written information on diet, medications, use of equipment for self-monitoring of blood glucose, and insulin administration.	Provides reference at a later time, and for review.

NIC *Teaching: Disease process*
Teaching: Individual
Teaching: Diet
Teaching: Psychomotor skill

Evaluation

The patient is able to repeat all information for the nurse and asks questions about chronic pancreatitis and possible outcomes (positive and negative). Prior to discharge, the patient verbalizes an understanding of pancreatic enzymes, self-monitoring of blood glucose, insulin administration, and diet restrictions, and agrees to be compliant. In addition, the patient is able to demonstrate the correct procedures for testing blood glucose and administering insulin. The patient is able to state what chronic pancreatitis is and what causes it. In addition, in cases of alcoholism the patient verbalizes a willingness to seek professional help. The patient should be able to inform the nurse when health care assistance should be sought.

Community/Home Care

For patients who have chronic pancreatitis, the therapeutic regimen will need to be continued in the home. Instruction by the health care team should be thorough, with opportunities for discussions. Knowledge needs are identified early in order to improve the likelihood that the patient will be prepared for self-care and self-monitoring once at home. Some follow-up care in the home should be made to ensure that the patient is progressing with treatments and responding. The major components of the regimen are dietary, medications, self-monitoring of blood glucose, pain control, and abstinence from alcohol (for detailed interventions see nursing diagnoses "Acute and Chronic Pain" and "Imbalanced Nutrition: Less than Body Requirements"). The nurse visiting the home should visit at a time when he or she can observe the patient performing the blood glucose check and administering insulin. This ensures that the patient is performing the skill correctly. Proper disposal of needles in the home is important, and they should be labeled if placed in household trash. Insulin is typically stored in the refrigerator, even though insulin is stable at room temperature for 30 days. Some adaptations in procedure may be required for the elderly patient who may have visual disturbances, such as obtaining insulin syringes with larger numbers or obtaining a magnifying glass for use in measuring. Be sure that the patient records information in the log correctly, as this will serve as a reference for health care providers at follow-up appointments. During visits in the home, the nurse needs to evaluate once more the patient's understanding of all content taught and ability and willingness to follow through. Follow-up with a health care provider focuses on assurance that no complications have occurred and that the patient has a clear understanding of how to manage all aspects of chronic pancreatitis.

Documentation

Document all content taught and the patient's verbalization of understanding. Specific attention should be given to documentation of any specific concerns that the patient expresses. Include in the documentation the patient's willingness to comply with all recommendations made about the diet, administration of pancreatic enzymes, pain control, checking glucose levels, and abstinence from alcohol. Include the patient's demonstration of how to perform self-monitoring of glucose and how to administer insulin. Any area that requires further instruction should be clearly indicated in the record. Include in the record appointments that have been made for outpatient procedures as well. Chart any questions or concerns that the patient has verbalized. Always include the titles of any printed literature given to the patient for reinforcement.

CHAPTER 6.93

PERITONITIS

GENERAL INFORMATION

Peritonitis is an inflammation of the peritoneum (the lining of the peritoneal cavity of the abdomen) caused by bacterial or chemical contamination/irritation. Primary peritonitis is caused by entry of bacterial organisms into the peritoneal cavity secondary to such disorders as ruptured appendix or diverticula, urinary tract infections (UTIs), pelvic inflammatory disease (PID), infection of peritoneal dialysis catheter sites, and bowel obstruction. Secondary peritonitis is caused by perforation of hollow abdominal viscus such as occurs in a ruptured appendix, perforated ulcer (release of gastric juices in the peritoneum), volvulus, trauma, or surgical injury. Regardless of the initiating event, (primary or secondary) inflammation and bacterial peritonitis is the result. The most common causative organism in a majority of the cases is *E. coli.* Other organisms are *Klebsiella, proteus, streptococci, gonococci,* or *pseudomonas.* With the entry of foreign substances into the sterile peritoneal cavity, the body's immune system activates the inflammatory response, leading to vasodilation and the release of histamine. In addition to the body's normal reaction of sending extra blood to the area of the inflammation, massive amounts of electrolyte-rich fluid (up to 500 ml/hour) can diffuse into the abdominal cavity from the circulating volume in response. If treatment is not prompt, septicemia and hypovolemic shock may result. The most common clinical manifestations include abrupt onset of severe abdominal pain and rigidity of the abdomen with guarding of the area. Other manifestations are nausea, vomiting, distention, and fever. As the disorder progresses untreated, the patient may demonstrate signs of early shock, such as tachycardia, increased respirations, diaphoresis, and decreased urine output. Elderly patients frequently present with less severe clinical symptoms but may be more critically ill.

NURSING DIAGNOSIS 1

INFECTION*

Related to:

Recent trauma (blunt or penetrating)

History of peptic ulcers

History of appendicitis

Recent history of abortion

History of PID

Infected foreign substance or object in abdominal wall (peritoneal dialysis catheter)

Bacterial invasion of peritoneal cavity

Defining Characteristics:

Fever

Chills

Positive cultures of peritoneal washings

Positive cultures of wounds

Elevated white blood cell (WBC) count

Abdominal rigidity

Abdominal pain and rebound tenderness

Abdominal distention

Redness/discoloration of surgical wounds or abdominal catheter insertion sites

Goal:

The patient's infection is resolved.

There are no further complications from infection.

Outcome Criteria

✔ The patient will be afebrile and have no chills.

✔ The patient will have negative cultures.

✔ WBCs will decrease and return to normal by discharge.

✔ The patient's abdomen will be soft and non-tender.

✔ Any surgical incisions or wounds will show signs of healing (no redness/discoloration, absence of warmth, and absence of drainage).

NOC *Infection severity*
Knowledge: Infection control

INTERVENTIONS	RATIONALES
Monitor results of diagnostic studies: WBC count, blood culture, culture and gram stain of any surgical incisions, peritoneal washings obtained during surgery, abdominal x-rays, diagnostic laparoscopic surgery, and abdominal computed tomography (CT) scan.	Positive cultures provide evidence for the specific organism that caused peritonitis; WBC count will reveal elevated WBCs; abdominal x-rays and CT scans provide evidence for causes of peritonitis and may demonstrate air- and fluid-filled spaces; laparoscopic surgery can visualize the pelvic and abdominal structures, and obtain specimens for analyses.
Assess for decreased or absent bowel sounds, abdominal rigidity, and distention by measuring abdominal girth.	Distention is a symptom of peritonitis or gas due to decreased peristalsis; decreased or absent bowel sounds may signal paralytic ileus post-operatively.
Monitor temperature every 4 hours and assess for chills.	Helps to establish baseline and monitor response to treatment; elevated temperature and chills are common in peritonitis.
Institute measures to reduce temperature: administer antipyretics (such as Tylenol) as ordered, apply cooling blanket, give a tepid sponge bath.	Helps to reduce temperature and decrease metabolic demands of the body.
Establish intravenous (IV) access and administer IV fluids as ordered; if the patient is allowed oral fluids, encourage their intake.	IV access is required for administration of antibiotics, and fluids are needed to prevent dehydration from fevers and decreased intake of fluids.
Administer antibiotics as ordered; monitor for and teach patient to monitor for side effects, and instruct patient on need to complete entire regimen. Broad-spectrum antibiotics are given until culture results are obtained.	These medications will resolve the infection through bacteriocidal or bacteriostatic activities.
If oral intake is allowed, provide a diet high in calories, and rich in iron, protein, and vitamin C.	Fatigue is common, and these measures will give the patient needed nutrients for energy and healing; iron-rich foods increase oxygen-carrying capacity of the blood.
Have patient remain resting in semi-Fowler's position.	This assists with comfort.
Practice good hand hygiene.	Good handwashing is the first line of defense against infection.
Change dressings on any incision or wound as ordered and clean area using sterile technique as ordered; if incision has been left open due to a contaminated surgical site, such as a gunshot wound or rupture of the appendix, pack the wound as ordered and cover with sterile dressing.	Maintenance of a clean wound or incisional site decreases the number of organisms and reduces the chance of infection; contaminated wounds are left unsutured/open and packed; healing by secondary intention and wound infection is often inevitable.
Irrigate wounds/incisions and change dressings over wounds/incisions or drainage devices using sterile technique.	Sterile technique is required to minimize bacteria count and prevent further infection.
If necessary, prepare patient for abdominal surgery as ordered and in accordance with agency protocol, and post-operatively implement any prescribed interventions.	In many cases of peritonitis, surgical interventions are required to repair the causative factor (such as appendicitis, ruptured peptic ulcer or diverticular, etc.), and the patient requires basic post-operative care with attention to gastrointestinal suction, wound care (usually left open), and fluid status.

NIC *Infection control*
Infection protection

Evaluation

Determine the extent to which the patient has achieved the expected outcomes. The patient should become afebrile, and there should be no signs or symptoms of infection. Specifically, the patient should have no abdominal rigidity, tenderness, or pain, and any drainage from wounds should decrease or be absent. WBCs are decreasing or within normal limits. The patient should verbalize an understanding of the infectious process of peritonitis and treatment measures being implemented with attention to prevention.

Community/Home Care

The causative factor for the peritonitis should be resolved by time of discharge home. However, peritonitis can be a serious illness that could lead to sepsis. For many patients, a feeling of malaise may linger for an extended period after hospital discharge. The patient will need to understand the importance of good nutrition in complete healing, recovery, and return to previous energy levels. The patient will need to increase activity gradually until stamina returns. Eating foods high in iron and protein, such as spinach, other green vegetables, and meat, can help with fatigue. If the patient has had surgery, incisional care will need to be taught to the patient, especially if the wound was left open due to the presence of an infection that caused the peritonitis. This will include packing the wound at least daily, and in some instances a visiting nurse may be employed to perform this task. Wearing loose-fitting clothes over incision lines may be needed for a period of time to prevent irritation to the site. Regardless of the type of incisional wound, the patient at home must practice good hand hygiene at all times and be aware that even normal bacteria can cause re-infection in open wounds and incision lines. It is crucial that the patient understand that the best intervention to prevent future infection is proper handwashing before touching any incisional site, catheter insertion sites, or other wounds. Antibiotics may be continued after the patient is at home, and monitoring for side effects will be necessary. The importance of completing the entire course of ordered antibiotics should be stressed. If any evidence of poor wound healing or infection should occur, the patient should be instructed to contact the health care provider. Follow-up care is required to ensure that the infection has been successfully treated.

Documentation

Document the findings from a comprehensive assessment with special attention to the gastrointestinal (GI) system. Chart the skin color on the abdomen or around any wounds, amount, color, and odor of any discharge from wounds, drainage devices, or catheters/tubes in the patient record, as well as vital signs and patient-specific complaints, such as pain at the site, fatigue, malaise, anorexia, or chills. Always chart therapeutic interventions implemented and the patient's specific responses to those interventions. Document all teaching and referrals.

 ACUTE PAIN

Related to:

Peritonitis (irritation of peritoneal cavity)
Abdominal ascites causing abdominal distention
Trauma to abdominal wall, organs, viscus
Surgical incision

Defining Characteristics:

Complaints of severe pain
Guarding
Tenderness on palpation
Grimace
Diaphoresis

Goal:

Pain control is achieved.

Outcome Criteria

✔ The patient will verbalize that pain is reduced or relieved.

✔ The patient will verbalize that the abdomen is not tender, and there is no guarding.

✔ The patient will have no grimacing.

NOC *Pain level*
Pain control
Comfort level
Medication response

INTERVENTIONS	RATIONALES
Monitor for complaints of severe abdominal pain, abdominal tenderness on palpation, guarding of abdomen, and abdominal rigidity. Have patient identify exact location of pain.	Helps to establish a baseline and give indicators of severity of disease.
Have patient rate pain for intensity using a pain rating scale.	Gives a more objective assessment of the pain intensity.

INTERVENTIONS	RATIONALES
Administer analgesics, as ordered, or encourage use of patient-controlled analgesia (PCA).	Helps to provide pain relief and decrease anxiety.
Position patient in semi-Fowler's position with knees and legs raised.	Improves circulation to the area and reduces stress on abdomen.
Teach appropriate relaxation techniques and other distraction techniques such as guided imagery and music.	Helps to enhance effects of pharmacological interventions.
Assess effectiveness of interventions to relieve pain.	Helps to determine whether interventions have been effective in relieving pain or whether new strategies need to be employed.
Establish a quiet environment.	Helps to enhance effects of analgesics.

NIC   *Pain management*
Analgesic administration
Anxiety reduction

Evaluation

The patient is able to report that the pain has been relieved or alleviated following interventions. Based on pain rating scales, the patient's pain has decreased. The absence of abdominal pain or tenderness should be noted. The patient should be able to ambulate without pelvic or abdominal pain.

Community/Home Care

Home care required for the management of pain is typically minimal. Once the infection has been controlled with antibiotics, the pain should start to subside and require only mild analgesics. If pain persists, the patient should return to a health care provider to determine if the inflammatory/infectious process has worsened, possibly with the development of abscesses. Teaching the patient how to utilize non-pharmacological measures to enhance the effects of analgesics will be crucial to obtaining satisfactory outcomes. Assessing pain control is an important facet of follow-up care.

Documentation

Document in the patient's own words the location of the pain, the description of the pain, and rating of the level of pain. Include factors that contribute to pain, such as ambulation and the degree to which pain limits tolerance for performing activities of daily living (ADLs). Chart the patient's responses to all interventions that have been employed. If pain control has not been achieved, indicate necessary revisions in the planned interventions.

NURSING DIAGNOSIS 3

DEFICIENT FLUID VOLUME

Related to:

Movement of fluid into the peritoneal cavity due to the inflammatory process

Possible NPO (nothing-by-mouth) status

Nasogastric (NG) suctioning

Vasodilation

Vomiting

Defining Characteristics:

Tachycardia

Dry mucous membranes

Poor skin turgor

Hemoconcentration

Hypotension

Increased urine specific gravity

Electrolyte imbalance

Decreased urine output

Dark colored urine

Goal:

Normal fluid and electrolyte balance will be restored.

Outcome Criteria

✔ Vital signs (blood pressure and pulse) return to baseline.

✔ Mucous membranes become moist and pink.

✔ Skin turgor returns to normal (skin when pinched returns to normal position in < 3 seconds).

✔ Hematocrit (Hct) and hemoglobin (Hgb) return to normal levels.

NOC *Hydration*
Fluid balance
Electrolyte and acid/base balance
Vital signs

INTERVENTIONS	RATIONALES
Assess for signs of dehydration/volume deficit: decreased blood pressure, increased pulse, dry mucous membranes, poor skin turgor, and decreased urinary output.	Helps to determine the seriousness of the problem, to guide treatment, and to assess effectiveness of treatments.
Establish IV access and initiate IV fluids (such as colloids), as ordered.	Helps to rehydrate patient and correct fluid and electrolyte imbalance; colloids provide osmotic "pull" for water from extravascular spaces to intravascular spaces.
Monitor and record intake and output and daily weights; report output < 30 ml/hour.	Helps to assess fluid balance.
Monitor serum electrolytes, especially serum potassium and chloride.	Helps to determine fluid and electrolyte replacement needs.
Administer electrolyte replacements (potassium and chloride) IV, as ordered.	Potassium and chloride are rich in the GI tract; a combination of fluid losses from the bowel, circulating volume, and NG suction causes decreases in serum levels necessitating replacement.
Monitor cardiac status: blood pressure, pulse (quality and rate), pulse pressure, and capillary refill. Take vital signs at least every 4 hours or more often, as ordered.	Cardiac output may decrease as fluids are lost from the circulating volume and from the bowel into the peritoneal cavity as a result of the inflammatory response; changes in blood pressure and pulse give information relevant to changes in cardiac status; blood pressure decreases and the pulse increases; capillary refill provides a way to assess perfusion.
Monitor skin temperature and color for baseline, and during treatment for improvement.	Pale, cool, clammy skin indicates decreased perfusion. As treatment progresses, skin should be warm and return to normal color.
Monitor oxygen saturation using pulse oximetry.	Oxygen saturation is a way to assess ability to perfuse tissues.
Monitor results of laboratory studies: Hgb and Hct, arterial blood gases (ABGs), blood urea nitrogen (BUN), and electrolytes.	Hct fluctuates in response to fluid status; severe absolute loss from volume would produce a decrease in Hct, with further drops during aggressive fluid resuscitation due to hemodilution; the Hgb may be decreased. If volume loss is due to third spacing, Hct may be high initially and decrease as fluid is restored to the intravascular space. ABGs often reveal metabolic alkalosis as potassium and chloride are lost in the fluid entering the peritoneal cavity. BUN and electrolytes indicate renal function; BUN may be elevated initially, but decrease due to hemodilution of fluid replacement.
Administer antibiotics as ordered after cultures have been obtained.	Helps to treat bacterial infection.

NIC *Hypovolemia management*
Intravenous therapy
Fluid monitoring
Electrolyte monitoring
Fluid/electrolyte management

Evaluation

Assess the patient for return of normal fluid volume. The patient's blood pressure and pulse should return to baseline. The pulse should be strong and regular and at the patient baseline or only slightly increased. Skin should be warm, and color should return to the patient's normal appearance. Mucous membranes are moist. Renal function should not be impaired, with an hourly output on average of 30 ml/hour. Serum electrolytes, Hgb, and Hct should be within normal range. The patient's intake and output are balanced.

Community/Home Care

Patients treated for deficient fluid volume due to peritonitis should have normal fluid status restored within a short period. Attention to methods of replacing electrolytes is important because the patient almost always loses them through fluid shifts. Once at home, encourage the frequent intake of clear liquid electrolyte solutions, such as Gatorade. Plain water should be avoided, as it contains no electrolytes. At home, the patient may not require any follow-up as this is an acute situation that for the most part has no long-term complications. Fatigue may need to be addressed at home, but usually it resolves in a short period. Until it does, the patient will need to perform activities as tolerated until stamina/endurance is re-established. The health care provider may want the patient to return for a follow-up appointment to ensure that parameters such as electrolytes, Hbg, Hct, and renal function studies have returned to normal.

Documentation

For the patient with peritonitis, document initial assessment findings relevant to hydration status such as mucous membranes, blood pressure, pulse, respirations, oxygen saturation, temperature, skin status, and mental status. Document all interventions such as intravenous catheter insertion, fluids initiated (type, rate), and urinary output with a description of urine (consistency, color). Chart intake and output in accordance with agency protocol, but at least every 8 hours. Be specific when charting patient responses to treatment so that other health care providers can clearly determine improvement or deterioration.

CHAPTER 6.94

TOTAL PARENTERAL NUTRITION (TPN)

GENERAL INFORMATION

Total parenteral nutrition (TPN) is a process of delivering enough essential nutrients to meet the body's metabolic demands when nutrition via normal routes through the gastrointestinal (GI) system cannot be accomplished or when the nutritional needs increase significantly due to disease states. TPN, formerly referred to as hyperalimentation, is usually administered through a multilumen central venous catheter, a large bore catheter inserted into a large central vein (referred to as a "central line"), such as the superior vena cava. In cases of short-term therapy, the solution can be adapted for infusion into a large peripheral vein, and this adaptation usually involves decreasing the glucose content of the solution to make it less hypertonic and thus less irritating to the peripheral veins. The TPN solution usually consists of concentrated glucose (25 to 30 percent), amino acids, electrolytes, minerals, and vitamins; in most instances, insulin is also added. Other additives are included based on the nutritional needs and specific organ involvement of the patient. The patient receiving TPN will also receive fat emulsions at least three times a week, possibly daily, to provide calories for energy, to prevent further tissue breakdown, and to prevent fatty acid deficiency. Patients who are candidates for TPN include those with increased nutritional needs due to trauma, burns, malabsorption disorders, inflammatory bowel disease, pancreatitis, inability to resume oral intake after 5 to 7 days of being NPO, cancer, eating disorders, and any other disorder that demands adequate or increased nutrient intake that cannot be met via normal routes. Complications of TPN to be prevented include infection at the catheter insertion site, hyperglycemia, and a fluid deficit due to osmotic diuresis secondary to the increased glucose.

NURSING DIAGNOSIS 1

IMBALANCED NUTRITION: LESS THAN BODY REQUIREMENTS

Related to:

Severe nausea, vomiting, and/or diarrhea

Esophageal dysfunction

Dysphagia

Other GI disorders

Need for excessive nutrition due to severe body stress conditions (sepsis, major burns, and antineoplastic therapy)

Anorexia/bulimia

Malabsorption of nutrients

Defining Characteristics:

Inability to consume enough nutrients for current metabolic demands

Weight loss

Decreased albumin

Decreased total protein

Electrolyte abnormalities

Reports of lack of energy

Poor wound healing

Goal:

The patient's normal nutritional status will be restored.

Outcome Criteria

✔ The patient will gain weight or not lose weight.

✔ Electrolytes will be within normal limits.

✔ Total protein and albumin will return to normal limits.

✔ The patient verbalizes an understanding of the importance of adequate nutrition.

NOC *Nutritional status: Food and fluid intake*

Nutritional status: Energy

Nutritional status: Biochemical measures

INTERVENTIONS	RATIONALES
Complete a fluid and nutritional assessment prior to initiation of TPN and daily during therapy, including assessing for nausea, vomiting, skin turgor, status of mucous membranes, any diarrhea, dietary intake, fluid intake and output, weight loss, loss of appetite, decreased muscle tone, albumin levels, hemoglobin, iron, electrolytes, and glucose.	Patients who require TPN have a decreased nutritional status for a variety of reasons, with accompanying loss of weight, malabsorption of nutrients in the GI tract, decreased or loss of electrolytes and fluids, and a feeling of malaise that decreases appetite. Persistent anorexia and nausea in some patients add to the nutrition problem by preventing the patient from taking in enough nutrients to meet metabolic demands.
Assist with placement of large bore central venous cannula.	The cannula is the tube via which the TPN is administered. Placing the TPN solution into a central vein will ensure adequate dilution of nutritional IV material.
Obtain subsequent chest x-ray, as ordered.	Validates proper placement.
Tape all TPN connections securely according to agency guidelines.	Helps to prevent accidental disconnection and prevent air entry into the system.
Use Luer-locks or other special locks, caps, or valves on all tubing connections, according to agency guidelines.	Helps to prevent accidental disconnection and prevent air entry into the system.
Administer prescribed TPN via an infusion pump, as ordered, according to agency guidelines/protocols but general guidelines include — Use a filter on all infusions. — Maintain the ordered infusion rate. — If solution runs out, hang dextrose 10 percent until the prescribed TPN solution is available.	TPN is used to ensure that adequate amounts of nutrients are provided given the patient's special needs; however, many precautions are required to protect the compromised patient from complications such as fluid overload, fluid deficiency, and infection. Filters are used to trap any crystals or microorganisms, or to vent air.

— If infusion is behind schedule, do not try to make up amount behind.
— Do not infuse or inject any other solution or medications through the central catheter lumen used for TPN.
— Use port of IV tubing closest to the patient for infusion of lipids/fat emulsions.

Infuse fat emulsion or lipids, as ordered.	Fat is required for body energy and to reserve protein for healing and nutritional requirements; fat is also needed for proper synthesis of some vitamins.
Assess laboratory results: albumin, iron, electrolytes, folic acid, and thiamine level.	All of these values will probably be decreased prior to therapy with TPN due to the inability of the patient to eat adequate amounts to meet metabolic demands. Iron, folic acid, and electrolytes decrease as nutritional intake decreases. Monitor for improvement as TPN becomes effective.
Monitor serum glucose levels via finger-stick method as ordered, administer insulin accordingly, and assess for signs and symptoms of hyperglycemia (thirst, increased urine output, increased hunger).	The TPN solution has high glucose content; the patient must be monitored for symptoms of hyperglycemia; an elevated serum glucose level can cause osmotic diuresis resulting in fluid volume deficit (see nursing diagnosis "Risk for Deficient Fluid Volume").
Weigh patient prior to initiation of TPN, and monitor weight daily or as ordered.	Helps to establish baseline for comparison and monitor for stabilization in weight or weight gain.
Monitor and record intake and output according to agency protocol, being sure to include any liquid stools as part of the fluid output.	Helps to detect dehydration and initiate early treatment.
If allowed and if patient is able, encourage him or her to take increased nutrients through high-calorie, high-protein, and low-roughage diets as ordered, trying small meals with between-meal snacks.	Helps to promote adequate intake of nutrients; for patients with decreased appetite, a small meal is more likely to be ingested and to be seen as desirable. Some patients on TPN may also be allowed to eat.

(continues)

(continued)

INTERVENTIONS	RATIONALES
When oral intake is allowed, collaborate with the dietician to develop an acceptable diet that considers usual habits, food intake, and any cultural or religious restrictions.	The dietician can discuss with the patient which foods may be digested better with the fewest untoward effects but the best nutritional results.
If the patient or family is to perform TPN at home, teach him or her how to perform the following skills: — Connecting the tubing to the central catheter — Disconnecting the tubing from the catheter — Connecting the solution to the tubing — Applying a filter — Setting the flow rate of the infusion — Dressing changes — Assessment of the site — Signs and symptoms of infection	If the patient or family is to perform the skill in the home, detailed instruction is required to ensure proper performance, to prevent infection or other complications, and to decrease anxiety.
Monitor BUN and creatinine levels as ordered (in some instances every third day), and urinary output.	Kidney function may become compromised due to the large concentration of amino acids administered in the TPN fluid. The nurse needs to monitor for changes in renal function as a result.

NIC   ***Total parenteral nutrition (TPN) administration***

Nutritional monitoring

Nutritional management

Teaching: Procedure/treatment

Teaching: Psychomotor skill

Evaluation

The patient's nutritional status is stable as demonstrated by the laboratory values (albumin, total protein, iron, electrolytes, folate, etc.). Weight is maintained, or the patient gains weight. The patient verbalizes an interest in eating and understands the need for increased nutrients due to the pathophysiological process. TPN is administered without complications. The patient is able to verbalize an understanding of how TPN works and the importance of adequate nutrition.

Community/Home Care

For some patients, TPN therapy may need to be continued in the home. The family and patient will need instruction on how to care for the access site and catheter as well as administer the solution. In some instances, the family or patient may be unable to carry out the procedures, and an in-home infusion service may be needed. The patient needs to locate a place to keep all supplies such as tubing, filters, and dressing. An airtight durable plastic box may be used for this purpose and can be found at almost any household retail or discount store. The TPN solution must be kept refrigerated in a specially identified place when not used; one solution might be to purchase a small compact refrigerator to be used for this exclusive purpose. For many patients, the infusion can be done during the evening or night hours so that they can remain active during the day. If the infusion is performed during the day, the patient may want to position him or herself in an easy chair or recliner and watch television or read during the time of the infusion. A small table containing items that may be needed, such as the telephone, remote controls, tissues, water, etc., can be placed nearby. It is important that the actual performance of the skill be taught by the nurse prior to discharge home, including how to perform all aspects of the skill, proper storage of supplies and solution, signs and symptoms of complications, and dressing changes. Likewise, it is crucial that the patient and family demonstrate all aspects of care including proper handwashing, setting up the infusion tubing with the solution, discontinuing the infusion, changing the dressing, and assessment of the site. The family and patient will need to be taught how to care for the central line or PIC (peripherally inserted catheter) line used for infusion when it is not in use. Priority care involves prevention of infection through strict hand hygiene and protection of the site from injury. Written detailed instructions relevant to care of the site and administration of the fluids should be given to the patient in duplicate, ideally laminated to prevent tearing or destruction by ordinary means such as spills. An in-home follow-up is required to reinforce teaching and assure proper performance at home. The family will need to know what to do in case of an emergency if the solution runs out without delivery of the next solution, which could happen in the event of a snowstorm or other natural disaster. A reliable scale is needed in the home to do weekly weights or weights as recommended. Even though the patient may not want to weigh every day, weighing at least every other day is a good way to keep track of weight loss or stabilization. A journal or log is needed for this purpose, and the patient should document in the journal temperatures, assessment of the site, results of glucose checks, and coverage with regular insulin. This information can be shared with the health care provider at each follow-up visit to provide data for revision in prescribed therapeutic interventions. If the patient is allowed oral intake, a caregiver, family member, or significant other will play a role in implementing strategies to improve nutrition by preparing meals and encouraging the patient to ingest them. Frequent small meals or nutritional snacks at home are encouraged for the patient in order to increase the likelihood that he or she can ingest the nutrients. Supplemental drinks can improve nutritional status during periods when the patient is unable to ingest adequate amounts of nutrition through normal meals due to anorexia or malaise. There are numerous products on the market (Boost, Ensure) but the patient may need to experiment with which ones are tolerated after consultation with the dietician. The patient may need to remain on multivitamins, folic acid, thiamine, electrolyte supplements, and other nutritional supplements for an extended period following the end of TPN. The patient is more likely to have proper nutrition when supported by family and friends. Follow-up providers should assess the patient for improved nutritional status as demonstrated by weight stabilization or gain and improvement in laboratory results.

Documentation

Chart the results of a nutritional assessment that includes a history of usual intake. Document vital signs, weights, and intake and output according to agency protocol at least every shift or every 8 hours. Include in the chart the insertion of the central line or PIC, initiation of TPN, infusion rate, and an assessment of the location of dressings. Results of glucose checks, with the administration of insulin for coverage, are documented according to agency protocol. If the patient is allowed oral foods, document the amount of food and fluid the patient consumes. Chart an assessment of the central line insertion site as well as dressing changes. In most agencies, there are specific guidelines for charting regarding TPN that includes specific nutritional parameters, so the nurse should

document accordingly. If the patient has complaints of any type, document this in the record with accompanying documentation indicating responses to interventions. Always include in the record all therapeutic interventions implemented for the patient.

NURSING DIAGNOSIS 2

RISK FOR INFECTION

Related to:

> High glucose concentration of TPN solution (excellent growth medium for microbials)
>
> Direct access to central circulation via central line
>
> Depressed immune response due to insufficient nutritional status

Defining Characteristics:

> None

Goal:

> Infection does not occur.

Outcome Criteria

✔ The patient remains afebrile.

✔ Central line insertion site has no redness/discoloration, drainage, or edema.

✔ The patient verbalizes no complaints of pain at central line insertion site.

✔ White blood cell (WBC) count remains within normal limits.

NOC *Infection severity*

> *Tissue integrity: Skin and mucous membranes*

INTERVENTIONS	RATIONALES
Always use sterile technique when dealing with the central line for tubing change, solution change, and dressing change.	Helps to reduce possibility of bacterial introduction into central line.
Change TPN filter, tubing, and bag based on institutional procedure (usually every 24 hours) using strict sterile technique.	Helps to prevent bacterial growth on filter, bag, and tubing walls.

(continues)

(continued)

INTERVENTIONS	RATIONALES
Use TPN line for TPN only: no blood draws, no medication administration. Do not use central line that has been used for things other than TPN.	Helps to reduce possibility of bacterial introduction into line.
Keep TPN solution refrigerated until ready for use; ensure currency of solution.	TPN has a high glucose concentration, which is a perfect medium for bacteria growth. Refrigeration inhibits bacterial growth.
Monitor central line insertion site for signs and symptoms of infection: redness/discoloration, swelling, purulent drainage, heat, increased pain.	Early identification of infection can expedite treatment.
Use strict sterile technique and wear a mask to change dressings and connect solution to administration tubing according to agency protocol. Dressings are typically changed at least every 72 hours and administration sets are changed every 24 hours.	Helps to decrease bacteria count on the skin and protect the insertion site from microorganism invasion; because of the glucose concentration the insertion site is a prime area for infection.
Monitor laboratory results for elevation of WBCs and for increased immature white blood cells (bands, known as shift to left).	Infection causes increased WBCs and increased immature WBCs to be released from the bone marrow into the blood.
Take temperature every 4 hours.	Temperature elevations may be indicative of infection.
Administer antipyretics (acetaminophen [Tylenol]), as ordered.	Helps to reduce fever.
Administer antibiotics, as ordered IV (intravenously) or PO (by mouth) if signs of infection are noted.	Helps to reduce the number of infective organisms and eliminate infection.
Teach the patient and family: — Proper handwashing — Dressing changes — Care of supplies and solutions used for TPN at home — Signs and symptoms of infection	The patient may need to administer TPN in the home and will need to monitor for signs of infection; handwashing is the number one defense against infection. This knowledge can prevent infection in the patient.

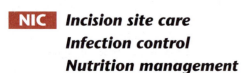

NIC   *Incision site care*
   Infection control
   Nutrition management

Evaluation

Evaluate the degree to which the outcome criteria have been met. The central line insertion site should be free of redness/discoloration, swelling, purulent drainage, pain, and heat. Any drainage from the insertion site should be minimal and serosanguineous in color. The patient should be afebrile, and WBC counts should be normal.

Community/Home Care

The patient receiving TPN is at high risk for infection due to the glucose concentration in the solution as well as the compromised nutritional state of the patient. In the home, the risk for infection remains and the family will need to know what symptoms may signal the onset of infection. For this reason, the patient and family will need to be taught to assess the site for redness/discoloration, heat, swelling, or pain. It is crucial that the patient understand that the best intervention to prevent infection is proper handwashing before touching the catheter insertion site; the patient should realize that even normal bacteria can cause infection. Dressing changes will need to be implemented with attention to strict aseptic technique as taught by the nurse. Inspection of the insertion site may be difficult due to its location on the chest; however, the patient can use a handheld mirror to get a better view daily. Proper storage of all equipment and solutions as recommended is also important. As previously stated, keeping solutions refrigerated and supplies properly stored reduces the likelihood of contamination and a visiting nurse should ascertain that this is being carried out. In addition, the patient's aseptic technique for dressing changes and handwashing technique should be evaluated. The importance of completing any ordered medications, such as antibiotics, should be stressed. The patient needs to learn how to take his or her temperature and monitor it daily keeping a written record. If the patient or family is unable to complete the necessary care, referrals are made to social workers for assistance. The patient should be instructed to contact the health care provider immediately if any evidence of infection should occur.

Documentation

Document assessment findings from the central line insertion site, including the presence of dressings, dressing type, skin color, and amount and color of any drainage. Be sure to note any sign of infection. Document vital signs according to agency protocol or as ordered. Chart medications given, such as antipyretics, in the medication administration record. Dressing changes are documented according to agency guidelines. Document in the patient record all interventions implemented for the prevention of infection, including any teaching implemented.

NURSING DIAGNOSIS 3

 ### RISK FOR DEFICIENT FLUID VOLUME

Related to:

Osmotic diuresis caused by hyperglycemia

Defining Characteristics:

None

Goal:

Adequate fluid volume is maintained.

Outcome Criteria

✔ Urinary output is > 30 ml per hour on average.
✔ Skin is moist.
✔ Mucous membranes are moist.
✔ Capillary refill is < 3 seconds.
✔ Vital signs return to baseline.
✔ Intake and output are balanced.

NOC *Fluid balance*

INTERVENTIONS	RATIONALES
Assess for signs of deficient volume, such as increased pulse, decreased blood pressure, dry mucous membranes, poor skin turgor, dry skin, increased capillary refill time, increased specific gravity, and decreased urine output.	These are all clues to hydration status and indicate a deficient circulating volume.
Monitor intake and output, noting color of urine.	Helps to assess fluid balance; dark, concentrated urine is a sign of dehydration.
Maintain TPN as ordered, keeping on schedule.	TPN provides fluid and electrolytes. Maintaining the correct rate of infusion prevents complications.
Administer any ordered supplemental IV fluids and electrolytes, as ordered.	Helps to maintain fluid and electrolyte balance; because of TPN-induced diuresis, the patient may require supplemental fluids while receiving TPN.
Offer fluids by mouth if not NPO.	Helps to supplement TPN .
Monitor glucose levels as ordered.	High levels of glucose in the TPN causes osmotic diuresis, which leads to volume deficit through increased urinary output.
Administer insulin, as ordered.	Helps to correct hyperglycemia and prevent osmotic diuresis.
Monitor serum albumin levels.	Low albumin levels due to compromised nutritional status can lead to the additional loss of fluids from the circulating volume.

NIC *Fluid management*
Fluid monitoring
Intravenous insertion
Intravenous therapy

Evaluation

Assess the patient for return of normal fluid volume with a balanced intake and output. The patient's blood pressure and pulse should be at baseline, skin turgor should be good, and capillary refill is < 3 seconds. Mucous membranes should be moist, and skin should be warm and dry. Renal output should not be impaired, with an hourly output on the average of 30 ml/hour. The patient has no complaints of excess thirst.

Community/Home Care

Patients receiving TPN will always be at risk for fluid volume deficit due to the glucose concentration in the solution. However, if any signs of hyperglycemia are detected and treated early, a deficiency should not occur. The patient and family will need to be cognizant of the signs and symptoms of dehydration to note such as dry skin, dark, concentrated urine, and decreased amounts of urine. The nurse should teach the patient how to measure output using a "hat" device, and if the patient is taking oral fluids, how to measure intake in common containers such as coffee cups or soda cans, or a favorite drinking glass. The patient can keep track of intake and output in a log or journal and note any imbalances that may indicate a volume deficit. The health care provider can evaluate the patient's fluid status at return appointments to ensure that parameters such as albumin, electrolytes, hematocrit (Hct), specific gravity, and renal function studies are normal.

Documentation

Findings from an assessment of the patient's fluid status are charted, including blood pressure, pulse, skin turgor, mucous membranes, and intake and output, with a description of the urine. If the patient complains of thirst, chart this along with the nursing interventions employed to relieve the problem. Type and amount of TPN and supplemental IV fluid administered are charted according to agency guidelines. When oral substances are resumed, document the type and the patient's tolerance. Document all interventions implemented to address the problem of fluid volume deficit. Be specific when charting patient responses to treatment so that other health care providers can clearly determine improvement or deterioration.

UNIT 7

HEMATOLOGICAL/ ONCOLOGICAL SYSTEMS

CHAPTER 7.95

ANEMIA

GENERAL INFORMATION

Anemia is the generic name for a number of diseases/conditions where, for whatever reason, red blood cell (RBC) counts drop below the normal range and the blood loses its ability to carry oxygen. Anemias are usually classified according to their pathogenesis or their RBC indices. The causes of anemia are nutritional deficiency, blood loss, hemolysis, decreased RBC production, and chronic disease or inflammation. Nutritional deficiency anemias include iron deficiency anemia, which results from chronic blood loss and insufficient intake of iron and megoblastic anemia caused by insufficient Vitamin B_{12} or folic acid resulting in large immature misshapen cells with decreased hemoglobin (Hgb) and hence an inability to carry enough oxygen as well as decreased numbers of RBCs produced. Blood loss is a contributing factor to anemia with common contributing disorders being gastrointestinal (GI) bleeding, post-operative status, menstruation, and coagulation deficits. Hemolysis (destruction of RBCs) is the cause of anemia in sickle cell anemia, thalassemia, enzyme deficiency anemia, drug-induced anemia, or anemia of transfusion reactions. Hemolysis can also occur through mechanical means in patients with prosthetic heart valves, or in patients on hemodialysis. Anemias attributed to decreased RBC production result from bone marrow suppression from chemotherapy, drugs, and radiation. Aplastic anemia, a type of anemia with decreased RBC production, is characterized by the suppression of all blood cell types (white blood cells, platelets, and RBCs). Chronic disease or inflammation anemia is thought to occur due to decreased resources to make RBCs due to the increased metabolic toll that occurs in chronic disease (such as renal failure) or infection. Clinical manifestations of anemia vary dependent upon the type, but common findings are fatigue, pallor of skin, tachycardia, and exertional dyspnea. Common laboratory findings include decreased RBCs, decreased iron and total iron-binding capacity (TIBC), decreased Hgb and hematocrit (Hct), decreased Vitamin B_{12}, decreased folic acid levels, and low serum ferritin.

NURSING DIAGNOSIS 1

ACTIVITY INTOLERANCE

Related to:

Imbalance between oxygen supply and demand

Decreased count of healthy RBCs

Defining Characteristics:

Fatigue

Weakness

Exertional discomfort

Dyspnea

Abnormal heart rate or blood pressure in response to activity

Goal:

The patient's activity level increases.

Outcome Criteria

✔ The patient will report the absence of fatigue or weakness.

✔ The patient will perform activities without shortness of breath.

✔ Heart rate and blood pressure will return to baseline within 5 minutes of ceasing activity.

NOC *Activity helps tolerance*
Energy conservation
Endurance

INTERVENTIONS	RATIONALES
Assess heart rate, blood pressure, and respiratory rate before and after activity.	Activity intolerance can result in vital sign changes as the heart attempts to meet oxygen demands.
Assist with activities as needed and encourage the patient to prioritize activities.	Helps to conserve energy and reduce oxygen demand; patient lacks enough oxygen-carrying capacity to supply oxygen to tissues during activities.
Encourage the patient to alternate periods of activity with periods of rest.	Helps to conserve energy.
Monitor response to activity (pulse, respiratory rate, oxygen saturation, and dyspnea).	Increased pulse and respirations, along with dyspnea, indicate an intolerance to the activity.
Instruct the patient to stop any activity that causes shortness of breath, chest pain, or dizziness.	These indicate intolerance to activity, and the level of activity being performed should be evaluated.
If shortness of breath occurs, administer oxygen as ordered.	Improves oxygenation and thus allows an increased activity level.
Encourage the patient to sleep 8 to 10 hours a night.	Sleep decreases oxygen requirements.
Collaborate with other disciplines such as physical therapy and respiratory therapy as ordered to assist with ambulation.	Respiratory therapy may need to provide oxygen when the patient first starts an activity program, and physical therapy can assist with monitoring activity progression.
Administer iron, folate, and vitamin B_{12}, as ordered.	These supplements are required for hematopoiesis.
Encourage foods rich in iron and folate.	Helps to improve oxygen-carrying capacity.
Prepare for transfusion of packed RBCs (as ordered).	Helps to increase oxygen-carrying capacity of the blood.

NIC *Activity therapy*
Energy management
Sleep enhancement

Evaluation

The patient is able to tolerate performance of self-care activities. The patient is able to walk short distances without fatigue or shortness of breath. The patient verbalizes an understanding of the need to progress activities gradually, restrict activity as needed, conserve energy, and monitor response to activity.

Community/Home Care

The patient may continue to experience some fatigue and intolerance to activity after discharge. At home, the patient must understand how to continue progression of activities and how to adjust activity in response to feelings of fatigue or shortness of breath. Instructions should include specific activity goals, monitoring response to activity, and energy conservation. Home maintenance will require the patient to evaluate which usual activities or routines can be continued. The home environment is assessed for factors such as stairs and distance to the bathroom from patient's usual resting place. In the early stages of treatment for anemia, the patient may need to alter the environment and shorten the distance to favorite places in the home by rearranging furniture and placing needed items (eyeglasses, tissues, remote control, medicines, etc.) close to the place of rest. In order to increase stamina and energy, the patient needs to increase foods that are good sources of iron, vitamin C, and protein in the diet. If the patient is unable to increase activity gradually, he or she should notify a health care provider.

Documentation

Document the specific activity goals prescribed for the patient. When the patient attempts activity, document the exact activity and the patient's response. Chart vital signs and record pulse and respirations before and after activity. If the patient verbalizes any complaints of fatigue or shortness of breath, document these in the patient's own words and document interventions carried out to obtain relief.

NURSING DIAGNOSIS 2

 IMBALANCED NUTRITION: LESS THAN BODY REQUIREMENTS

Related to:

Insufficient intake of foods that are necessary for RBC manufacture (foods that contain folate and iron)

Inability to absorb food products containing vitamin B_{12}

Defining Characteristics:

Weight loss

Fatigue, weakness

Dry, pale mucous membranes

Decreased activity level

Beefy red tongue

Spoon-shaped nails

Brittle nails

Goal:

The patient's nutritional status will improve.

Outcome Criteria

✔ The patient has dietary intake that contains sufficient folate, vitamin B_{12}, and iron.

✔ The patient's weight returns to normal.

✔ The patient's nails return to normal appearance.

✔ The patients tongue is no longer red or beefy.

NOC *Nutritional status*
Nutritional status: Energy
Nutritional status: Food and
     fluid intake

INTERVENTIONS	RATIONALES
Monitor intake and output of food and fluid carefully.	Enables caregiver to properly assess dietary intake.
Conduct a nutritional assessment: 24-hour recall, analysis of types of foods eaten, condition of skin and hair, mucous membranes, abnormalities such as beefy red tongue, brittle nails, spoon-shaped nails, cheilosis, pallor, cracks or fissures in corners of mouth, and pain in mouth.	A nutritional assessment will give the dietician clues to deficits in diet and areas for improvement to correct deficits that could improve anemia. It also gives clues to extent of the problem. Cheilosis, fissures, red tongue, and cracks in lips are all signs of nutritional deficiency anemia (decreased iron, folate, vitamin B_{12}).
Encourage intake of small meals with frequent snacks in between, including liquid dietary supplements.	The patient with anemia is fatigued, and it takes less energy to eat a small meal. Meals can be high in calories, proteins, iron, and folate.
Encourage meticulous mouth care: mouth washes every 2 hours and after meals.	Decreases the likelihood of infections and sores, promotes healing, and enhances the taste of food.
Apply ointments, such as petroleum jelly, to lips and corners of mouth.	Helps to promote comfort and enhance intake.
Encourage foods needed to improve nutritional anemia: folic acid: green vegetables, broccoli, organ meats, eggs, asparagus, and liver; vitamin B_{12}: liver, shrimp and oysters, dairy products, eggs, and most other meats; iron: beef, chicken, egg yolk, clams, oysters, turkey, veal, green vegetables, and whole grain breads.	These foods can help treat the causative factor in the nutritional deficiency.
Administer medications as ordered: iron, folic acid, or vitamin B_{12}.	These medications are given to improve the deficiency. Folic acid stimulates production of RBCs; iron corrects erythropoietic abnormalities but does not increase the production of RBCs, vitamin B_{12} helps with RBC maturation. Folic acid is especially needed by alcoholics who may be malnourished with anemia, as alcohol suppresses folate metabolism.
Monitor laboratory results: Schilling's test, hemoglobin, RBCs, bone marrow aspiration, iron, TIBC, ferritin, and hemoglobin (Hgb) electrophoresis.	Schilling's test is used to measure vitamin B_{12} absorption; Hgb determines the oxygen-carrying capacity of cells; the number of RBCs establishes the ability of the blood to transport Hgb; Hgb electrophoresis evaluates the status of hemolytic anemias and is useful in diagnosing thalassemia; bone marrow aspiration examines the elements of marrow production to determine ability of marrow to produce healthy RBCs; iron, TIBC, and ferritin provide data for iron-deficiency anemia.
Consult with dietician for patient teaching.	The dietician can teach the patient about proper food choices and assist the patient with menu preparation with preferable foods.

NIC *Skin care: Topical treatments*
Teaching: Prescribed diet
Nutrition therapy
Nutritional monitoring

Evaluation

The patient reports that the tongue and mouth are no longer sore. The beefy red appearance and cracks in mouth and lips have resolved. Dietary intake includes foods rich in folic acid, vitamin B_{12}, and iron. No weight loss has occurred due to the inability to eat due to alterations in mouth and mucous membranes. Laboratory indicators of nutritional anemia have improved.

Community/Home Care

Most patients with nutritional deficiency are treated at home unless diagnostic indicators show worsening of disease or the patient has difficulty maintaining nutrition. Home management focuses on the intake of a diet rich in the needed substances: folic acid, iron, or vitamin B_{12}. Most patients will need assistance in identifying the proper foods, and a dietician, physician, or nurse can assist with this. Foods included in the diet for folic acid deficiency include green leafy vegetables, broccoli, organ meats, eggs, asparagus, and liver. For vitamin B_{12} deficiency, the diet required is made up mostly of meats along with dairy products. Iron deficiency anemia requires foods such as beef, chicken, whole grain breads, oysters, clams, veal, and green vegetables. Vegetarian diets are a concern, as many of the foods that supply vitamin B_{12} come from meats. In this instance Vitamin B_{12} supplements may need to be offered. The health care provider should discuss what the patient normally eats, his or her likes and dislikes, and any cultural or religious restrictions. Based on this information, a list of foods that meet the nutritional needs and that are acceptable to the patient should be identified and provided to the patient. Keeping this list handy in the kitchen or when shopping for food can enhance compliance. Mouth care to relieve the discomfort of the red tongue, fissures/cracks, soreness, and dryness are needed to increase the likelihood that the patient will consume the necessary nutrients. Simple homemade mouthwashes can be made with salt and warm water, or a commercial product can be used. Follow-up with a health care provider is needed to monitor the progress of the anemia and resolution of symptoms.

Documentation

Document the results of a nutritional assessment, including the status of the oral mucous membranes and tongues. Chart the patient's weight on each visit for follow-up care and question the patient about the ability to take food. Include in the record the patient's understanding of dietary requirements for anemia. Document the patient's response to activity. All medications are charted according to agency protocols for charting medication administration. Any referrals are documented.

NURSING DIAGNOSIS 3

INEFFECTIVE PROTECTION

Related to:

Impaired RBC production

Destruction of RBCs

Poor absorption of iron and vitamin B_{12} from the GI tract

Bone marrow suppression

Defining Characteristics:

Fatigue

Decreased Hgb and Hct

Easy bruising

Prolonged bleeding

Blood in stool or emesis

Decreased RBC count

Outcome Criteria

✔ The patient will not experience bleeding or bruising.

✔ The patient will have no signs or symptoms of infections (urinary, respiratory, central access sites, skin areas).

✔ The patient will verbalize an understanding of the necessary precautions needed to prevent bleeding and prevent infection.

NOC *Blood coagulation*

Immune status

Knowledge: Infection control

Risk Control

INTERVENTIONS	RATIONALES
Monitor RBC, Hgb, Hct, iron, platelets, white blood cells (WBCs), vitamin B$_{12}$, and folic acid levels, as ordered.	Helps to detect abnormalities that place the patient at risk for bleeding and infection. Measures of RBC, Hgb, Hct, Vitamin B$_{12}$, iron, TIBC, and folic acid are used to evaluate the severity of some anemias. In some types of anemia, all blood cell components are decreased, including platelets and WBCs, due to bone marrow suppression.
Assess for evidence of bleeding: hematemesis, guaiac positive stool, hematuria, increased bleeding with menses, bruising, easy bleeding, petechiae, bleeding gums, nose bleed, or purpura.	Assessing for these may give clues to cause of anemia (chronic blood loss), or they may be a result of the anemia due to decreased RBCs and platelets; in addition, they may indicate that the body is unable to clot effectively. Monitoring these indices are needed for early detection of complications, which would allow for early treatment.
Perform a cardiovascular history and assessment monitoring for hypotension, tachycardia, pale skin and mucous membranes, flat neck veins, dry warm skin, capillary refill > 2 seconds, thin, dry hair, brittle nails, palpitations, history of GI bleed, and heavy menses.	These are indicators of decreased circulating volume.
Have patient use electric razors for shaving.	Helps to decrease risk for bleeding due to nicks; even small breaks in the skin can cause bleeding.
Teach the patient necessary precautions to prevent bleeding.	The patient will need to institute these precautions at home.
Monitor for signs of infection: elevated WBCs, redness or other discoloration, drainage or heat at any wound or intravenous (IV) access insertion site, fever, and chills.	With bone marrow suppression, there are decreased numbers of WBCs, placing the patient at higher risk for infection.
Administer IV fluid or blood products, as ordered.	Helps to replenish fluid volume or loss from excessive bleeding and to increase oxygen-carrying capacity.
Encourage patient and family members to practice good hand hygiene.	Handwashing is one of the best ways to stop the transmission of infection.
Encourage mouth care every 2 hours.	A sore mouth and tongue, open lesions, cracks and fissures at corners of mouth, etc., predispose the patient to infection in these areas, particularly if food particles are left in the mouth. Frequent mouth care cleanses the mouth and reduces risk of invasion by microorganisms.
Have the patient avoid crowds and people with upper respiratory infections.	Due to compromised immune status, being in crowds and exposure to persons with upper respiratory infections increases the risk of acquiring respiratory infections.

NIC *Bleeding precautions*
Risk identification
Surveillance

Evaluation

Evaluate whether outcome criteria have been met. The patient should have no bleeding; if bleeding occurs, it is detected and treated early. Infections have been prevented as evidenced by the absence of signs and symptoms. The patient ambulates with assistance without injury or complaints of dizziness. At time of discharge from the health care agency, the patient is able to verbalize precautions required to prevent bleeding and infection.

Community/Home Care

The patient with anemia will remain at risk for ineffective protection until the anemia has been resolved. In the home environment, the patient will need to practice safety-enhancing behaviors to prevent bleeding, physical injury, and infections. The patient must be vigilant in preventing or controlling bleeding promptly if it occurs as well as preventing falls due to fatigue. Implementing strategies to protect self from injuries, such as bruising or disruption of skin caused by bumping into objects, is important. This may include rearranging furniture or small objects around the house to make walking areas clear. Because the patient is prone to dizziness and fatigued until treatment has been effective, assistance with activities around the home may be required. Dietary interventions that can assist the patient with energy levels can prevent some of the fatigue and dizziness caused by decreased RBCs and subsequent impaired oxygen transport. Foods rich in iron should be encouraged; diet should take into consideration the patient's likes/dislikes, culture, religion, and any dietary restrictions. The patient with anemia may want to avoid large crowds or other activities that may increase risk for infection. Handshaking is a common expression of greeting but can also be the source of transmission of organisms. Practicing good handwashing techniques can minimize the risk of infection. Patients who have young children or grandchildren should avoid them, if possible, when they are sick with colds or the flu. Patients with anemia should be encouraged to take appropriate vaccines for influenza and pneumonia. At the first sign of infection, the patient should return to a health care provider for further assistance.

Documentation

Include in the patient chart findings from a thorough assessment of the patient for evidence of bleeding, such as bruises, bleeding gums, bleeding from access sites, etc. In addition, document the patient's activity level and response to activity (fatigue, dizzy). If the patient has any signs of infection, however minor, document this in the patient record with a clear indication of what actions were carried out in response. Chart all interventions implemented to address safety, bleeding, and prevention of infections. If teaching is implemented, include information about who the learners were and their level of understanding.

NURSING DIAGNOSIS 4

DEFICIENT KNOWLEDGE

Related to:

Lack of information about anemia and its treatment

Misinformation

Defining Characteristics:

Asks no questions

Has many questions/concerns

Noncompliant

Incorrect information

Poor dietary habits

Goal:

The patient will understand anemia and its treatment.

Outcome Criteria

✔ The patient verbalizes a willingness and desire to learn the necessary information.

✔ The patient verbalizes an understanding of anemia.

✔ The patient verbalizes a willingness to comply with treatment recommendations.

✔ The patient verbalizes an understanding of dietary recommendations.

NOC *Knowledge: Disease process*
Knowledge: Health behavior
Treatment behavior:
Illness or injury

INTERVENTIONS	RATIONALES
Assess readiness of client to learn (motivation, cognitive level, physiological status).	The patient must be motivated to learn, have the capability to learn the content, and be free of distractions from learning, such as pain and emotional distress.
Assess what the patient already knows.	The patient may have some knowledge about anemia, and teaching should begin with what the patient already knows.
Create a quiet environment conducive to learning.	Environmental noise can prevent the learner from focusing on what is being taught.
Teach incrementally, starting with simple concepts first and progressing to more complex concepts.	The patient will learn and retain knowledge better when information is presented in small segments.
Teach the learners about the normal function of the RBCs, WBCs, platelets, vitamin B_{12}, folic acid, iron, and bone marrow.	Understanding of normal function helps the patient to understand the disease process.
Teach the patient about the disease process (pathophysiology) of the specific anemia for which he or she is treated.	Understanding the pathophysiology of anemia will assist the patient to understand the rationale for therapeutic interventions.

(continues)

(continued)

INTERVENTIONS	RATIONALES
Teach the patient about nutritional deficiency anemias (see nursing diagnosis "Imbalanced Nutrition"): — Dietary needs: foods that are rich in iron, vitamin B_{12} or folic acid — Medications: supplements of iron, vitamin B_{12}, or folic acid, as required; side effects to recognize and prevent; scheduling	Patients who understand the necessary interventions related to diet and medications are more likely to be compliant.
Teach the patient with aplastic anemia about — Bone marrow transplant: matching, procedure, prognosis for success, preventing infection, avoidance of receiving transfusions from possible donors, possible rejection, signs of rejection (see nursing care plan "Organ and Tissue Transplantation") — Immunosuppressive therapy: medications used, side effects, prognosis for success, preventing infection	Bone marrow transplant from a matched donor with identical human leukocyte antigen is the treatment of choice for persons younger than 40, but the procedure carries some risk. The patient needs to be aware of these in order to make an informed decision. Immunosuppressant therapy is the treatment often prescribed for persons over 40.
Evaluate the patient's understanding of all content covered by asking questions.	Helps to identify areas that require more teaching and to ensure that the patient has enough information to comply.
Give the patient written information on diet and medications.	Provides reference at a later time, and for review.

NIC *Teaching: Disease process*
Teaching: Individual
Teaching: Diet
Teaching: Procedure/treatment
Teaching: Prescribed medication

Evaluation

The patient is able to state what anemia is and what causes it. The patient is able to repeat all information for the nurse and asks questions about anemia, prognosis, and possible outcomes (positive and negative). The patient verbalizes an understanding of prescribed medications and dietary recommendations,

and agrees to be compliant. In addition, in cases of patients requiring more invasive treatments, such as bone marrow transplant or immunosuppressant therapy, the patient verbalizes an understanding of the procedures and the risks prior to consenting for treatment. The patient knows and can inform the nurse when health care assistance should be sought.

Community/Home Care

For patients who have anemia, the therapeutic regimen is implemented in the home, with the exception of immunosuppressant therapy and bone marrow transplant. Teaching by the health care team should be thorough, with opportunities for discussions. Knowledge needs are identified early in order to improve the likelihood that the patient will be prepared for self-monitoring and prevention of complications from anemia, such as bleeding and injury due to undue fatigue. A follow-up telephone call from the health care provider can assess whether the patient has understood the teaching. It is helpful to provide the patient with a sample diet and list of foods that improve anemia that are in keeping with his or her preferences. A written schedule for medications can also be given, as many patients may be prone to forget but are more likely to check a schedule if one is available. This information can be condensed to fit on one sheet of paper, placed on a colorful sheet, and laminated for long-term use. Written instructions for pre-procedure care and post-procedure care should be given to the patient who will return for a bone marrow transplant or immunosuppression therapy. Follow-up with a health care provider focuses on assurance that no complications have occurred and that the patient has a clear understanding of how to manage all aspects of anemia.

Documentation

Document all content taught and the patient's verbalization of understanding. Specific attention should be given to documentation of any specific concerns that the patient expresses. Document the patient's willingness to comply with all recommendations made about the diet, medication administration, and follow-up care. Any area that requires further teaching should be clearly indicated in the record. Include in the record appointments that have been made for return visits for treatment procedures such as bone marrow transplant or immunosuppression therapy. Always include the titles of any printed literature given to the patient for reinforcement.

CHAPTER 7.96

CHEMOTHERAPY FOR CANCER

GENERAL INFORMATION

Chemotherapy is the administration of medications for cure, control, or palliation of cancer. It can be given orally (PO), topically, intravenously (IV), or intrathecally, and is usually given in spaced cycles. However, it may be given in individual, separate doses, spaced in a certain sequence or as a continuous dosage. Chemotherapy targets cancerous/malignant cells and can be the sole therapeutic modality for treatment of the cancer cells or in conjunction with radiation therapy and/or surgery. Cancer chemotherapy affects actively reproducing cells such as tumor cells. Healthy tissue cells that are actively reproducing are also vulnerable to the effects of chemotherapy. Cells of the skin and mucous membranes, bone marrow, reproductive system, and hair can be altered by the effects of chemotherapy. Side effects of chemotherapy include but are not limited to hair loss, nausea and vomiting, anorexia, fatigue, mucositis, pancytopenia, and sterility.

NURSING DIAGNOSIS 1

DEFICIENT KNOWLEDGE

Related to:

Lack of information about chemotherapy

Misinformation

Defining Characteristics:

Asks no questions

Has many questions/concerns

Shows no interest in learning about chemotherapy

Goal:

The patient verbalizes an understanding of chemotherapy.

Outcome Criteria

✔ The patient verbalizes a desire to learn the necessary information.

✔ The patient verbalizes an understanding of chemotherapy, including untoward effects of treatment.

✔ The patient verbalizes an understanding of the method of administration for chemotherapy.

✔ The patient agrees to comply with recommendations for treatment.

✔ The patient verbalizes an understanding of follow-up care required and expresses a willingness to comply.

NOC *Knowledge: Disease process*
Knowledge: Treatment regimen
Compliance Behavior

INTERVENTIONS	RATIONALES
Assess the patient's current knowledge, ability to learn, and readiness to learn.	The nurse needs to ascertain what the patient already knows and build on this; if the patient is not capable of learning or is not ready to learn, teaching will not be effective due to disinterest or inability to understand. The patient may not be ready to learn if in a state of denial or if extremely angry because of the diagnosis of cancer.
Teach incrementally, starting with the simplest information and moving to complex information.	The patient will learn and retain knowledge better when information is presented in small segments; patients can understand simple concepts easily and then can build on those to understand concepts that are more complex.

(continues)

(continued)

INTERVENTIONS	RATIONALES
Teach patient and family about chemotherapy and its effects: — Specific agents used for treatment — Method of action — Alopecia: assist the patient to plan for hair loss by investigating the purchase of wigs or having hair cut short and using hair for a specially made wig before alopecia; have men shave head prior to the loss of hair; find a resource that could teach women how to prepare fashionable head wraps — Nausea/vomiting: teach to use anti-emetics before meals prophylactically; avoid foods with strong odors, and in the hospital setting have lids removed from trays outside the room (when lids are removed from food trays the smell is often overwhelming to the gastrointestinal [GI] system and causes nausea); attempt frequent small meals, avoiding spicy foods — Care of access sites: prevention of infection by use of aseptic techniques and procedures according to agency protocol, how to protect site from injury — Control of fatigue: balance of rest and activity; on chemotherapy days a designated naptime may be needed — Prevention of infection: chemotherapy causes a depression of white blood cells (WBCs), predisposing the patient to infection; avoid people with infections and large crowds; practice good hand hygiene; know WBC counts — Signs and symptoms that would indicate a need to seek health care	Knowledge of all aspects of the chemotherapy process empowers the patient to take control, make informed decisions, and enhance compliance. Knowledge of what to expect helps the patient cope with untoward side effects and better equips him or her to take responsibility for managing the illness and engaging in self-care.
Provide the patient and family with information on hospice and other community service agencies, such as the American Cancer Society, as warranted.	These agencies can provide psychological support as well as resources to the patient and family.
Assess the patient's and family's understanding of all teaching by encouraging them to repeat information and ask questions as needed.	This allows the nurse to hear in the patient's own words what was taught and makes it easier to know what information may need to be reinforced.
Establish that the patient has the resources required to be compliant.	If needed resources such as finances and transportation to follow-up appointments are not available, the patient cannot be compliant; the nurse will need to make necessary referrals.
Provide written information or brochures to review.	The patient can review these for clarification of information.

NIC   *Chemotherapy management*
Learning readiness enhancement
Learning facilitation
Teaching: Prescribed medication

Evaluation

Evaluate the degree to which the patient has achieved the outcome criteria relevant to the teaching sessions. The patient asks questions and discusses the content with the nurse. The patient should verbalize an understanding of the content presented by repeating the information, particularly chemotherapy and medications for chemotherapy-induced nausea and vomiting. The nurse must determine whether the patient is capable of being compliant with the recommended chemotherapy regimen. If further teaching is required at time of discharge, the appropriate referrals should be made to continue education.

Community/Home Care

The patient receiving chemotherapy may travel to outpatient centers for treatment or spend time in a hospital setting and then go home. In either event, the patient is required to manage the effects of the chemotherapy. Common effects to control include hair loss, nausea, vomiting, and fatigue. The patient will need to understand all teaching relevant to chemotherapy in order to know what to expect. At times the nausea and vomiting can be unrelenting, making the patient quite uncomfortable; it is crucial that the patient understand how to minimize or alleviate these. Make handy resource sheets for the patient that are easy to read with large print on colorful paper; a sheet for each topic covered during teaching will make it easy for the patient to locate the necessary information when it is needed. The resource sheets can be kept in a colorful folder similar to ones used for school reports. Other information to be placed on information sheets includes the name of chemotherapy agent, its side effects, and how it works. A separate page should be used to record the schedule for chemotherapy appointments. Another aspect of the teaching for the patient receiving chemotherapy is to have the dietician assist the patient to prepare a diet that is both nutritional and easy to digest but that decreases the likelihood of nausea and vomiting. The nurse needs to be sure that the patient has understood teaching related to any care required of the access site being used for chemotherapy administration. In addition, the patient should have a clear understanding of the schedule of treatments at an outpatient facility. At home, the patient will likely experience fatigue following any of the treatments, but especially with chemotherapy treatments. Because the patient is seen on a regular basis for general follow-up for chemotherapy, health care providers can determine how the patient is managing the regimen and side effects and whether further teaching or reinforcement is required.

Documentation

Document the specific content taught and the titles of any printed documents given to the patient. Include in the chart the patient's degree of understanding of the content and the methods used to evaluate learning. An assessment of the patient's ability to be compliant with the regimen for chemotherapy or follow-up should be made in the chart with indicators of referrals made. Any areas that need to be reinforced should be documented to ensure appropriate follow-up. If family members are present for the teaching sessions, document this in the chart.

NURSING DIAGNOSIS 2

 NAUSEA

Related to:
Chemotherapy

Defining Characteristics:
Reports of nausea
Vomiting
Decreased intake of nutrients
Reports of anorexia
Weight loss

Goal:
Nausea will be reduced or eliminated.

Outcome Criteria

✔ The patient will not experience nausea; if nausea is present, the patient states that it is tolerable.
✔ The patient will not vomit.
✔ The patient will be able to eat at least 50 percent of meals.

NOC *Nausea and vomiting severity*
Nausea and vomiting control
Nutritional status: Food and fluid intake

INTERVENTIONS	RATIONALES
Assess for nausea and encourage patient to verbalize its presence.	Nausea and vomiting are common side effects of chemotherapy. Assessing for nausea and controlling it prevents the loss of nutrition through subsequent vomiting.
Administer anti-emetics prior to administration of chemotherapy, according to chemotherapy protocol.	Helps to prevent nausea before it occurs; nausea and vomiting are common with most types of chemotherapy.
Administer anti-emetics at other times as needed and 30 minutes before meals.	Helps to increase comfort and decrease the risk of vomiting.
Collaborate with the physician and consider "round the clock" anti-emetic administration rather than an "as needed" schedule.	Helps to be proactive in nausea prevention and control; decreases incidence and severity of episodes of nausea.
Provide oral/mouth care before meals.	Chemotherapy often alters taste buds, and a fresh mouth can enhance taste and makes food taste better.

(continues)

(continued)

INTERVENTIONS	RATIONALES
Open food containers away from the patient or outside door.	Removing lids from food containers at the bedside releases a strong aroma that can cause nausea, which would prevent the patient from eating.
Collaborate with the dietician to determine patient's likes, dislikes, and preferences, taking into consideration cultural and religious restrictions.	This information is needed to plan a diet for the patient to meet nutritional needs, to decrease nausea, and to increase the likelihood that the patient will eat.
Modify diet, including bland chilled foods with liquids served separately; avoid spicy foods, greasy foods, or foods that tend to cause gas (such as beans, cabbage, etc.), thick gravies or sauces, and highly concentrated sweets.	Helps to decrease bloating and nausea; spicy, greasy foods and foods that cause gas will increase the likelihood of nausea and vomiting.
Based on patient likes, dislikes, and preferences, offer bland foods or drinks that have a decreased likelihood of causing nausea such as toast, crackers, ginger ale, and gelatin.	These foods are usually well tolerated by patients on chemotherapy.
Encourage the patient to eat the most nutritious foods (such as meats) early in the day.	The patient becomes more fatigued as the day progresses and is less likely to eat. In addition, nausea may increase later in the day.
If nausea is present, offer cold rather than hot foods on the meal tray.	Cold foods tend to decrease nausea.
Have the patient keep hard candy available.	Sucking on hard candy can decrease the feeling of mild nausea.
Give nutritional supplemental drinks.	Helps to improve overall intake.
Assess amount of food consumed at each meal.	Helps to detect inability to consume adequate nutrients and intervene early.
Avoid excessive movement or reclining within 30 minutes of eating.	Frequent or rapid movements soon after meals and the recumbent position increase motility of food upwards.
Arrange for a cool, well-ventilated environment with low light and noise levels, free of noxious sights and smells.	Helps to decrease stimulation that may cause nausea.
Encourage relaxation and distraction.	Helps to enhance effects of anti-emetics and decrease episodes of nausea.
Teach positioning techniques if vomiting occurs: height of bed elevated, head turned to side.	Helps to reduce risk of aspiration.
Weigh the patient prior to initiation of chemotherapy.	Helps to establish a baseline for assessing nutritional status and for early detection of decreasing nutritional status during and after treatment.

NIC *Nutritional monitoring*
Nutritional management
Nausea and vomiting control
Nausea and vomiting disruptive
effects

Evaluation

The patient's nausea and vomiting are controlled and nutritional state is stable; the patient has a satisfactory nutrient intake. Assess the patient's weight and determine that the patient is not losing weight. The patient should be ingesting at least 50 percent of food served and should be tolerating it without nausea or vomiting. The patient should be able to eat and drink without nausea/vomiting and be able to verbalize methods to maintain nutrition in the home.

Community/Home Care

Difficulties with eating and drinking may continue at home for the patient receiving chemotherapy. The patient will need to continue efforts to ingest enough food and nutrients to meet the metabolic demands of a disease state. The patient needs encouragement to eat and at home may lose interest in eating due to depression or because of fatigue. A home nurse or other health care provider needs to monitor the patient's nutritional status on a regular basis to detect excessive weight loss and to note reports of increased nausea/vomiting. A strategy to address nausea at home is crucial for maintenance of nutrition. The physician will need to prescribe anti-emetics for the patient during chemotherapy, and there is a variety of medications available including Reglan, Zofran®, and Compazine®. These should be taken prophylactically before meals. A regimen that includes medications, diet, and relaxation methods in the home is more likely to be successful. Instruct the patient to maintain a supply of foods, recommended by the dietician or nurse, that can decrease the likelihood of nausea/vomiting, such as crackers, hard candy, gelatin, etc. Giving the patient a list of foods that can provide good sources of the required nutrients and minimize nausea will be helpful. A diet rich in protein is advised, and the patient will need to have sufficient amounts to provide a source of energy, as fatigue will be a persistent problem. Family members and significant others play a role in implementing strategies to improve nutrition by preparing meals and encouraging the patient to ingest them. Frequent small meals at home should be encouraged for the patient in order to increase the likelihood that the patient can ingest enough nutrients. Because the dietary recommendations may be easily forgotten, a handy, laminated reference guide can be created to give to the patient or family. This guide could include a list of foods that provide protein, foods that minimize nausea or bloating, foods that provide iron, foods to avoid because of risk for nausea/vomiting, foods that are acceptable, and a schedule for small meals. Supplemental drinks can improve nutritional status during periods when the patient is unable to ingest adequate amounts of nutrition through normal meals due to anorexia, vomiting, or malaise. There are numerous products on the market (Boost, Ensure), but the patient may need to experiment with which ones are satisfying or appealing after consultation with the dietician. The patient may need to take multivitamins or electrolyte supplements until the nutritional status stabilizes and chemotherapy treatment is complete. Teach the patient to monitor nutrition intake by keeping a log of nausea or vomiting episodes, anti-emetics taken, food eaten, mealtimes or snack times, and toleration of food. If at any time a particular meal or food product causes nausea or vomiting, the patient should note this in the log and eliminate this food from the diet. Weights should also be included in the log. Even though the patient may not want to weigh every day, weighing at least every other day is a good way to keep track of weight loss or stabilization. This information can be shared with the health care provider at each follow-up visit to provide data for revision in prescribed therapeutic interventions. Follow-up providers should assess the patient for weight loss and decrease in number of nausea and vomiting episodes.

Documentation

Chart the patient's weight daily. Document any difficulties that the patient experiences during meals, particularly nausea or vomiting, and any interventions (anti-emetics or other) implemented to address them. Record intake and output according to agency protocol, being sure to document the percentage of food consumed. The patient's tolerance to food and fluid intake is documented as part of an overall assessment. If the patient verbalizes concerns, include this in the chart, as well as strategies to address these concerns. Always document any referrals made to other disciplines, particularly the dietician. Document teaching done to address nutritional needs and whether the patient has understood.

NURSING DIAGNOSIS 3

 INEFFECTIVE PROTECTION

Related to:

Chemotherapy

Immunosuppression

Bone marrow suppression

Inadequate secondary defenses: leukopenia, neutropenia

Invasive procedures: central venous catheter

Thrombocytopenia

Defining Characteristics:

Neutropenia

Decreased platelet count

Decreased hemoglobin (Hgb) and hematocrit (Hct)

Leukocytosis

Immature WBCs

Easy bruising

Prolonged bleeding

Blood in stool or emesis

Fatigue

Goal:

The patient will have no infection or bleeding.

Outcome Criteria

✔ The patient will not experience bleeding or bruising.

✔ The patient will be afebrile.

✔ The patient will have no signs or symptoms of infections (urinary, respiratory, central access sites, skin areas).

✔ The patient will verbalize an understanding of the necessary precautions needed to prevent bleeding, infection, and injury.

NOC   *Blood coagulation*
Immune status
Knowledge: Infection control
Risk control

INTERVENTIONS	RATIONALES
Monitor WBCs, RBCs, Hgb, Hct, and platelets, as ordered.	Helps to detect abnormalities that place the patient at risk for injury and infection. Due to bone marrow suppression caused by most chemotherapeutic agents, the number and type of WBCs required to fight infection may be decreased. Anemia is common in chemotherapy patients and measures of RBC, Hgb, and Hct are indicators of severity. Fewer RBCs are produced due to bone marrow suppression secondary to chemotherapy. Platelets are decreased, placing the patient at high risk for bleeding.
Assess for fatigue, weakness, shortness of breath, and any alteration in mental status.	These symptoms occur due to the body's inability to transport enough oxygen to tissues secondary to decreased RBC and iron.
Monitor for indicators of bleeding abnormalities: bruising, easy bleeding, petechiae, bleeding gums, nosebleed, and purpura.	These indicate that the body is unable to clot effectively, and further examination and interventions may be warranted to prevent complications.
Assess all stools and emesis for blood by hemoccult, urine for blood using dipstick, sputum for blood by examination, and vaginal bleeding by counting pads or tampons during menses.	The lungs and gastrointestinal and genitourinary systems are highly vascular and prone to bleed; menses may be extremely heavy if the patient has thrombocytopenia.
Avoid the use of aspirin or aspirin-containing products.	These products increase the risk of bleeding.
Avoid excessive venipuncture or injections to the extent possible, and apply pressure to all puncture sites for 5 minutes.	Due to thrombocytopenia, the patient bleeds easily and pressure is required to stop bleeding effectively. At least 5 minutes may be required.
Brush teeth with a soft-bristle toothbrush.	Gums tend to bleed easily due to altered clotting factors and decreased platelets; soft toothbrushes prevent trauma to gums that can cause bleeding.
Have patient use an electric razor when shaving.	Helps to decrease the risk of bleeding due to nicks to the skin which often occur with use of a straight razor.
Encourage a soft diet.	Helps to avoid trauma to the mucous membranes of the mouth.
Avoid hot foods/liquids.	Heat causes vasodilation that may increase bleeding.
When in the hospital, place in protective isolation or on neutropenic precautions when cell counts decrease according to agency protocol: wear mask when in room, avoid raw fruit and vegetables, do not allow fresh flowers, make sure all visitors wash hands before entering room.	Helps to protect the patient from sources of infection.
Consider neutropenic diet.	Restriction of uncooked fruits and vegetables may decrease microorganisms entering the body.
Monitor for signs of infection: fever, redness or other discoloration, drainage or heat at any wound or IV access insertion site; urine for malodor, mucous; oral cavity for white coating; respiratory system for cough, sputum production, crackles in lungs; notify physician if any are noted.	With bone marrow suppression and decreased numbers of neutrophils, the patient is at higher risk for infection. A fever may be the only sign of infection, as the patient is unable to produce the normal inflammatory response due to immunosuppression.
Assess temperature frequently, at least every 4 hours.	Fever is an indicator of infection. When present, obtain a culture to identify the microorganism causing the fever, as ordered.
Practice good hand hygiene.	Handwashing is one of the best ways to stop the transmission of infection.
Have the patient avoid crowds.	Being in crowds increases the risk of acquiring respiratory infections.

INTERVENTIONS	RATIONALES
Increase iron-rich foods in diet.	Helps to increase oxygen-carrying capacity of RBCs.
Change any dressings over central line access sites in accordance with agency protocol, using strict sterile technique.	Central lines are easy portals for entry of organisms. Strict sterile technique is required to reduce risk for infection.
Administer antibiotics, as ordered.	Helps to prevent or treat infection.
Ensure adequate rest and hydration.	Rest and hydration are essential for infection prevention and control.
Teach the patient all safety precautions required related to bleeding and infection.	The patient needs to be informed in order to practice health promotion and disease prevention behaviors.

NIC *Bleeding precautions*
Infection protection
Risk identification
Surveillance

Evaluation

Evaluate whether outcome criteria have been met. The patient should have no bleeding; if bleeding does occur, it should be detected and treated early. Infections have been prevented as demonstrated by the absence of signs and symptoms. The patient ambulates as tolerated or with assistance without injury. At time of discharge from the health care agency, the patient is able to verbalize safety precautions required.

Community/Home Care

The patient receiving chemotherapy will remain at risk for ineffective protection throughout the course of treatment. Once at home, the patient will need to continue to practice safety-enhancing behaviors to prevent bleeding, physical injury, and infections. The patient must be vigilant in preventing or controlling bleeding promptly if it occurs, as well as preventing falls that could cause injury. Implementing strategies to protect self from injury such as bruising or disruption of skin resulting from bumping into objects is important. These strategies may include rearranging furniture or removing rugs to make walking areas clear. Because the patient is prone to be fatigued, assistance with ambulation or activities

requiring mental alertness may need to be restricted at times. Dietary interventions that can assist the patient with energy levels can prevent some fatigue caused by decreased RBCs and subsequent impaired oxygen transport. Iron-rich foods should be encouraged, taking into consideration the patient's likes/dislikes, culture, religion, and dietary restrictions. In cases of neutropenia, the diet may restrict raw fruits and vegetables (good sources of iron and electrolytes); therefore, it is crucial that the dietician make dietary recommendations only after a thorough consult with the patient and, if possible, a significant other. Discussion should include how to prepare favorite vegetables previously eaten raw or how to substitute fruit juices for their favorite raw fruit. At home, the patient should use electric razors for shaving, as even a small nick from a disposable straight razor can cause significant free bleeding. Dental floss, if used, should be waxed for easier sliding and prevention of trauma to gums, and a soft-bristle toothbrush is always required. Women should note changes in their menstrual cycle that would indicate more profuse bleeding, such as a significant increase in numbers of pads or tampons used and the passage of clots. If bleeding is noted in stools, emesis, or from any orifice or wound, the health care provider should be notified for prompt treatment. The patient receiving chemotherapy will need to avoid large crowds or other activities that may increase risk for infection. Handshaking can also be the source of transmission of organisms. The patient as well as any primary caregiver, such as a spouse or significant other, should remove him or herself from the vicinity of any person coughing or presenting with symptoms of respiratory infection. In addition, the patient may have to limit visitors to the hospital and to the home following discharge. Practicing frequent good handwashing techniques can minimize the risk of infection. Patients who have young children or grandchildren should avoid them if possible when they are sick with colds or the flu. Teach the patient to take his or her temperature and to record it daily. Central line access sites or other ports used for chemotherapy should be assessed daily for early detection of infection. At the first sign of infection, the patient should return to a health care provider for further assistance.

Documentation

Include in the documentation findings from a thorough assessment of the patient for evidence of bleeding such as bruises, bleeding gums, bleeding from access sites, etc. If bleeding occurs, document what interventions were carried out to control or stop the bleeding. In addition, document the patient's activity level and response to activity (fatigue, dizziness). If the patient has any signs of infection, even minor ones, document this in the patient record with a clear indication of what actions were carried out in response. Temperatures should be taken at least every 4 hours and recorded according to agency protocol. Chart all interventions implemented to address safety, bleeding, and prevention of infections. If teaching is implemented, include who the learners were and their level of understanding.

NURSING DIAGNOSIS 4

ACTIVITY INTOLERANCE

Related to:

Effects of chemotherapy

Increased metabolic demand from cancer

Imbalance between oxygen supply and demand

Decreased number of healthy RBCs

Anxiety

Defining Characteristics:

Fatigue

Lethargy

Exertional discomfort

Dyspnea

Abnormal heart rate or blood pressure in response to activity

Goal:

Fatigue is decreased and the patient's activity level increases.

Outcome Criteria

✔ The patient will report the absence of fatigue or weakness.

✔ The patient will perform activities without shortness of breath.

✔ The patient will be able to perform activities of daily living.

✔ Heart rate and blood pressure will return to baseline within 5 minutes of ceasing activity.

NOC *Activity tolerance*
Energy conservation
Endurance

INTERVENTIONS	RATIONALES
Assess heart rate, blood pressure, and respiratory rate before and after activity.	Activity intolerance can result in vital sign changes as the heart attempts to meet oxygen demands.
Assess level of energy and ability to perform activities of daily living (ADLs).	Helps to ascertain baseline energy and performance level.
Assist with activities as needed and encourage patient to prioritize activities.	Helps to conserve energy and reduce oxygen demand; patient lacks enough oxygen-carrying capacity to supply oxygen to tissues during activities.
Pace activities and encourage the patient to alternate periods of activity with periods of rest.	Helps to conserve energy and decrease demand for oxygen.
Monitor response to activity (pulse, respiratory rate, oxygen saturation, and dyspnea).	Increased pulse and respirations along with dyspnea that does not resolve when activity is stopped indicate an intolerance to the activity.
Instruct the patient to stop any activity that causes shortness of breath, chest pain, or dizziness.	These indicate intolerance to activity and the level of activity being performed should be evaluated.
If shortness of breath occurs, administer oxygen, as ordered.	Improves oxygenation and thus allows an increased activity level.
Encourage the patient to sleep 8 to 10 hours a night.	Sleep decreases oxygen requirements.
Collaborate with other disciplines such as physical therapy and respiratory therapy, as ordered, to assist with ambulation.	Respiratory therapy may be necessary to provide oxygen when patient first starts an activity program, and physical therapy can assist with monitoring activity progression.
Administer iron, folate, and vitamin B_{12} as ordered.	These supplements are required for hematopoiesis.
Encourage foods rich in iron and folate.	Helps to improve oxygen-carrying capacity.
Administer erythropoietin or other similar medications, as ordered.	Helps to stimulate hematopoiesis, increasing RBC production, and subsequently increases ability to deliver oxygen to tissues.

INTERVENTIONS	RATIONALES
Prepare for transfusion of packed RBCs, as ordered.	Helps to increase oxygen-carrying capacity of the blood.

NIC *Energy management*
        Sleep enhancement

Evaluation

The patient is able to tolerate performance of self-care activities. The patient is able to walk short distances without fatigue or shortness of breath. The patient verbalizes an understanding of the need to progress activities gradually, restrict activity as needed, conserve energy, and monitor response to activity.

Community/Home Care

The patient will continue to experience some fatigue and intolerance to activity for the duration of the chemotherapy treatments. At home, the patient must understand how to continue progression of activities and how to adjust activity in response to feelings of fatigue or shortness of breath. Instructions should include specific activity goals, monitoring response to activity, and energy conservation. Home maintenance will require the patient to evaluate which activities or routines can be continued. The home environment is assessed for factors such as stairs and distance to the bathroom from the patient's usual resting place. In the early stages of chemotherapy, the patient may need to alter the environment and shorten the distance between where he or she usually rests in the house and other places such as the bathroom or kitchen by rearranging furniture and placing frequently used items (eyeglasses, tissues, remote control, medicines, etc.) close to the patient's resting place. In order to increase stamina and energy, the patient needs to increase foods that are good sources of iron, vitamin C, and protein in the diet. On the day that the patient receives chemotherapy, he or she may require long naps or rest periods in a quiet comfortable place. It may also be helpful for the patient to discourage visitors immediately following chemotherapy and postpone social activities until after a rest period. If the patient is unable to gradually increase activity, he or she should notify a health care provider.

Documentation

Document the specific activity goals prescribed for the patient. When the patient attempts activity, document the exact activity and the patient's response. Document whether the patient requires assistance with ADLs and specify exactly how much assistance is required. Chart vital signs and record pulse and respirations before and after activity. If the patient verbalizes any complaints of fatigue or shortness of breath, document these in the patient's own words as well as interventions carried out to obtain relief.

NURSING DIAGNOSIS 5

IMPAIRED ORAL MUCOUS MEMBRANES

Related to:
   Chemotherapy
   Immunosuppression
   Lack of or decreased salivation
   Infection
   Decreased nutrition
   Decreased oral intake

Defining Characteristics:
   Oral lesions
   Oral pain or discomfort
   Dry mouth
   White patches, plaques

Goal:
   Oral mucous membranes will be intact.

Outcome Criteria

✔ The patient will report no pain in mucous membranes.

✔ Mucous membranes will be moist.

✔ The patient will not have an infection of the oral mucosa.

✔ Oral cavity will be free of ulcers, lesions, and white patches.

NOC *Tissue integrity: Skin and mucous*
        membranes
        Oral hygiene

INTERVENTIONS	RATIONALES
Assess oral mucosa daily.	Detects signs of mucositis.
Encourage a systematic oral care regimen consisting of cleansing, lubricating, and coating of the oral mucosa with prescribed agents.	Systematic oral hygiene is an important factor in decreasing mucositis incidence.
Encourage fluid intake of > 3000 ml/day.	Helps to promote moisture of oral mucosa.
Encourage intake of bland, soft, high-calorie, high-protein foods and liquids; avoid spicy and/or acidic foods.	Promotes nutrition but decreases the risk of irritating the oral mucosa; high-acid foods irritate the oral mucosa.
Use normal saline rinses and antimicrobial solutions after eating or drinking.	Particles may stick to the mouth; rinsing after eating cleans the mouth.
Assess for pain in mouth.	Excoriation of oral mucosa or infections can cause the oral cavity and specifically the tongue to become sore and in some instances painful.
Administer mild analgesics or analgesic mouthwashes.	Helps to promote comfort and enhance intake.

 NIC *Oral health restoration*
Oral health promotion

Evaluation

The mucous membranes are intact. The patient reports that discomfort has been relieved and no lesions or ulcers are noted in the mouth. An understanding of how to prevent oral impairment is verbalized by the patient.

Community/Home Care

The patient remains at risk for impairment of oral mucous membranes for a variety of reasons. The patient will need to develop a routine of inspection of the oral mucous membranes using a small dental mirror that can be inserted into the mouth. Any area that is painful should be noted, and the patient should apply prescribed agents to the site. Simple measures in the home that can assist with improvement or prevention of impairments include brushing the teeth, using an antiseptic mouthwash daily, and using a saline rinse after

each meal. This removes food particles that under normal circumstances may not be problematic but for the chemotherapy patient could be a source of infection. Mouthwashes that have a high percentage of alcohol should be avoided since this will cause more drying of the mucous membranes that can lead to easy excoriation. The patient needs to be sure to drink adequate fluids and maintain nutrition to ensure healthy skin and enhance the immune function. The patient needs to know which foods may cause irritation to the mouth and eliminate these from the diet. If the mouth becomes sore and prevents intake, the patient needs to seek health care, as any decrease in intake could further compromise a nutritional status that may already be poor due to nausea.

Documentation

Document the findings from a physical assessment of the oral cavity. Indicate any complaints from the patient of pain or discomfort. Chart all interventions implemented to address the problem of impaired oral mucous membranes, along with the patient's responses. Be sure to note the patient's ability to consume adequate food and fluids.

NURSING DIAGNOSIS 6

 DISTURBED BODY IMAGE

Related to:
Loss of hair (alopecia)

Defining Characteristics:
Withdrawal
Social isolation
Depression
Negative statements about physical appearance
Nonverbal response to change in appearance

Goal:
The patient accepts the change in physical appearance and continues social activities and interpersonal relationships.

Outcome Criteria

✔ The patient will verbalize acceptance of alopecia as temporary.

✔ The patient does not verbalize negative feelings toward self.

NOC *Body image*

INTERVENTIONS	RATIONALES
Encourage the patient to discuss feelings about changes in physical appearance openly, and assure the patient that his or her feelings are normal.	Talking about the changes may sometimes be the beginning of acceptance; the patient should understand that his or her emotions are real and should be expected.
Assess for and monitor patient for feelings about self, interpersonal relationships with family members and friends, withdrawal, social isolation, fear, anxiety, embarrassment by appearance, and desire to be alone.	Helps to detect early alterations in social functioning, to prevent unhealthy behaviors, and to intervene early through referral to counseling.
Provide information regarding progression of hair loss.	Helps to educate the patient about hair loss and new growth.
Encourage the patient to obtain scarves, turbans, hats, or wigs before hair loss. For women, an expert in wrapping scarves can teach methods for creating stylish wraps.	Helps to help the patient be prepared for change in appearance. Many men will shave their heads prior to hair loss.
Have the patient wash hair less frequently and use mild shampoo or other solutions.	Helps to minimize hair loss.
Avoid using dyes, relaxers, permanents, blow dryers, curling irons, and straightening combs or other hot objects on the head.	All of these can increase hair loss, and some may damage the tender scalp.
Encourage the patient to participate in at least one outside/public activity each week once health status permits.	Prevents patient from isolating self from others.
Identify the effects of the patient's culture or religion on body image.	A patient's culture and religion often help define reactions to changes in body image and self-worth.
Assist the patient in identifying coping strategies/diversionary activities that can be used to deal with the changed	Helps to provide diversionary activities so that not all thoughts are on the cancer and changed appearance.

appearance, chemotherapy, and the diagnosis of cancer.	
Encourage family and significant other support.	Support and acceptance from those close to the patient enhance the patient's acceptance of the change in physical appearance.

NIC *Body image enhancement*
Emotional support
Socialization enhancement

Evaluation

The patient is able and willing to learn about the strategies to improve psychosocial health. Determine whether the patient is able to verbalize feelings regarding hair loss. Time is required for the patient to completely assimilate the change in body appearance into their self-perception. It is crucial that the nurse evaluate the degree to which the patient is beginning to do this. Communication of feelings and concerns relevant to the change in appearance should be taken as a positive sign of progress towards meeting outcome criteria.

Community/Home Care

At home, continued monitoring of the patient's perception of body image is needed. The health care provider will need to be alert to subtle hints that may indicate that the patient has not completely adapted to the loss of hair and change in body appearance. Open discussions regarding physical changes and interventions to prevent social isolation and withdrawal should continue with patient and family. As the chemotherapy is completed and hair begins to return, the patient may feel better about his or her appearance; however, he or she may still be hesitant to allow family members, especially spouses or significant others, to see his or her balding head or sparse hair. This is especially true of women. Encouraging the patient to look at him or herself, and to identify other positive qualities, may improve the patient's ability to deal with body changes. Family members should encourage the patient to go out for short periods once allowed, starting with environments where the patient feels comfortable and where people are more likely to refrain from staring. Once hair returns, the body image issues may be resolved. However, the patient should be aware that frequently the new hair is not always the same hair type as prior to chemotherapy. Some support groups offer scarves to women with alopecia to wear following chemotherapy-induced alopecia. In addition, these groups often have people available who can demonstrate wrapping of the scarf to wear as a fashionable head wrap. Hats can also be purchased in a variety of styles and colors to wear outside the home. Some disturbed body image may persist, and the patient will need continued assessments and attention to the problem.

Documentation

Chart any specific behaviors or verbalizations that may indicate an altered body image. Include all interventions that have been employed to address this issue and the patient's responses. Note when and if the patient begins to verbalize feelings regarding the loss of hair and to demonstrate behaviors indicative of positive body image. Document the content of all teaching done and the patient's understanding of content. Any referrals made are documented in the patient record.

CHAPTER 7.97

HEMOPHILIA

GENERAL INFORMATION

Hemophilia, a deficiency or abnormal synthesis of coagulation factors A, B, or C, is a hereditary disease characterized by abnormal coagulation. Each factor in the clotting mechanism is a protein or glycoprotein that free-floats in plasma in an inactive form until activated by the previous factor. The clotting mechanism is activated when a laceration or bruising occurs. Factor XII is the first to activate, causing factor XI to activate. Factor XI activation causes factor X to activate, and so on, in domino-like fashion until prothrombin is activated. This activates fibrinogen, which releases fibrin and causes a clot to form. If any of the factors are missing, the entire clotting factor sequence will not be completed, and a clot will not form. An X-linked recessive disease, hemophilia (A and B) is carried by females and occurs in males. Hemophilia A, the most common form of the disease, is divided into three categories: severe, moderate, and mild. Severe hemophilia is evidenced by a concentration of factor VIII of < 1 percent of normal. Moderate hemophilia is evidenced by a factor VIII assay of 1 to 5 percent of normal. Mild hemophilia is evidenced by a factor VIII assay of > 5 percent, but < 35 percent. Hemophilia B disease (Christmas disease) accounts for approximately 15 percent of cases and is characterized by a deficiency in factor IX. Even though different points in the clotting mechanism are impaired, the two types (A and B) are identical in terms of clinical manifestation. The extent of the bleeding is directly proportional to the amount of factor present in the blood. The disease may be evidenced by blood collecting in the joints of the elbows, knees, ankles, spinal canal, gastrointestinal (GI) tract, or the urinary tract. Patients may also bleed from the nose and the mouth. It may first be detected at circumcision, when bleeding continues for prolonged periods.

NURSING DIAGNOSIS 1

INEFFECTIVE PROTECTION

Related to:

    Factor VIII deficiency or inadequacy

    Factor IX deficiency or inadequacy

Defining Characteristics:

    Difficulty clotting or inability of blood to clot

    Bleeding: epistaxis, oral, GI, urinary

    Bleeding easily from trauma

    Bruises

    Petechiae

Goal:

    Clotting occurs.

Outcome Criteria

✔ The patient has no bleeding or bruising.

✔ The patient's vital signs remain at baseline.

✔ Any bleeding will stop 10 minutes after interventions are implemented.

NOC *Blood coagulation*
      Risk control

INTERVENTIONS	RATIONALES
Monitor results of laboratory tests: factor VIII assay, factor IX assay, APTT (activated partial thromboplastin time), PT (prothrombin time).	Screening tests for factor VIII and IX deficiency demonstrate decreased amounts of these factors; increased activated partial thromboplastin time is present, and the prothrombin time is normal but is used to exclude other disorders.

(continues)

(continued)

INTERVENTIONS	RATIONALES
Monitor for indicators of bleeding abnormalities: skin for bruising, petechiae, easy bleeding, blood in emesis or stool, bleeding gums, nosebleeds, hematuria, and purpura.	Allows for early detection; these symptoms indicate that the body is unable to clot effectively and further examination and interventions may be warranted to prevent hemorrhage.
Test any emesis or stool for blood.	Helps to detect bleeding not recognizable through observation.
Assess for hemarthrosis by questioning patient about joint discomfort or any abnormal feelings in joints, and by reviewing x-rays of joints.	Bleeding into the joints is a common occurrence in hemophilia. Early detection can prevent long-term complications.
Administer fresh frozen plasma, fresh plasma, cryoprecipitate, factor VIII or concentrate, or factor IX, as ordered.	Helps to provide factor VIII and IX to continue the clotting cascade; fresh frozen plasma replaces all clotting factors. These should be administered prophylactically before any type of invasive procedure, surgery, or dental care.
Administer desmopressin (DDAVP), as ordered.	Helps to assist in clotting process in mild hemophilia; increases factor VIII activity.
Encourage the patient to ambulate carefully and refrain from high-risk activities, such as contact sports.	The patient is at high risk for bleeding; contact sports or simply bumping into objects places the patient at risk for bruising or frank bleeding from simple injuries.
Avoid injections or any other interventions that cause trauma to skin or mucous membrane if possible, but if puncture sites are necessary, apply pressure for 5 minutes.	Lack of sufficient clotting factors predisposes the patient to bleeding, even from simple procedures, and pressure is required to stop bleeding effectively.
If bleeding occurs from an injury or trauma, apply prolonged direct pressure; apply ice or topical hemostat agents.	Extensive pressure is required to enhance clotting, ice is a vasoconstrictor, and topical hemostat agents such as a gelatin sponge help control bleeding.
Brush teeth with soft-bristle toothbrush and use an electric razor for shaving.	Helps to prevent bleeding from minor abrasions. Gums tend to bleed easily due to altered clotting factors.
If nosebleeds occur, implement measures for cessation (see nursing care plan "Epistaxis").	The patient with hemophilia may have spontaneous nosebleeds and can lose a significant amount of blood if

	treatment is not implemented swiftly.
Teach the patient and family about safety precautions and all interventions employed to prevent hemorrhage and control any bleeding.	Providing information can decrease anxiety; the patient needs to be informed in order to comply with recommendations for care.
If bleeding occurs, monitor for signs of fluid volume deficit: tachycardia, decreased blood pressure, change in mental status, and decreased hemoglobin (Hgb) and hematocrit (Hct) (see nursing care plan "Hypovolemic Shock"), and report to physician.	If bleeding is profuse, the patient may show signs of cardiac compensation to maintain perfusion to vital organs by increasing heart rate; blood pressure drops as a result of decreased circulating volume; changes in mental status indicate decreased perfusion to cerebral tissue.
Have the patient obtain and wear a Medic-Alert bracelet.	In the event of injury or illness, this would alert others that there is a bleeding tendency, thus preventing hemorrhage or treating bleeding promptly.
Teach the patient and evaluate his or her understanding of the following: — Pathophysiology of hemophilia (hereditary transmission) — Treatments (clotting factors) — Complications: hemarthrosis — To observe for bleeding in stool, gums, urine, nose, bruising — How to protect self in home — Importance of wearing Medic-Alert bracelet — Not to take aspirin products	Knowledge enhances anxiety reduction and allows the patient to understand health status and implement health-promoting behaviors.

NIC *Bleeding precautions*
Blood products administration
Risk identification
Surveillance

Evaluation

Evaluate whether outcome criteria have been met. The patient should have no bleeding and if so, it is detected and treated early. Vital signs have returned to the patient's baseline. Any bleeding ceases spontaneously or after interventions. Any signs of abnormal bleeding such as petechiae resolve, no injuries occur, and bruising is avoided. At time of discharge from the health care agency, the patient is able to verbalize safety precautions required.

Community/Home Care

The patient with hemophilia will always be at risk for ineffective protection. Once at home, the patient will need to continue to practice safety-enhancing behaviors for bleeding and physical injury. The patient must be vigilant in preventing or controlling bleeding promptly if it occurs, as well as preventing injuries that could cause hemorrhaging. This may include rearranging furniture or removing rugs to make walking areas clear. Adequate lighting is essential, especially at night, so that the patient can see how to move about. The patient should be encouraged to place a light by the bedside so that it can be turned on prior to getting out of the bed. The patient will need to avoid any type of strenuous activities or rough sports such as football, soccer, or hockey, as directed by the physician. For younger patients especially, acceptable activities with a low risk for injury should be identified; these may include golf, swimming, or tennis. Those treating the patient for hemophilia should review the patient's medications to ascertain if any could potentiate the risk for bleeding, such as steroidal inhalers, aspirin, or aspirin-containing products, which many people take for cardiovascular prophylaxis or arthritis. Simple instructions about hygienic practices include reminding all hemophilia patients to shave with electric razors, to brush teeth with a soft-bristled toothbrush, and to floss using waxed dental floss. The patient is taught to apply pressure or a bandage to any injury site regardless of how minor it may appear. If spontaneous bleeding should occur, if bleeding is noted in stools, or if the patient starts to vomit blood, health care assistance should be sought for prompt treatment. The patient with hemophilia should also inform health care providers such as dentists and podiatrists that he or she has hemophilia so that precautions against bleeding can be taken during any procedures. Support groups can be located through the National Hemophilia Foundation but may not be available in rural or remote areas.

Documentation

Include in the documentation findings from a thorough assessment of the patient for evidence of bleeding such as bruises, petechiae, bleeding gums, bleeding from access sites, etc. In addition, chart the presence or absence of bleeding with an estimation of amount. If medical interventions, such as administration of clotting factors or frozen plasma, are implemented, document these according to agency protocol; document as well all nursing assessments and interventions employed during their administration. Document the results of tests for blood done on emesis or stool. Include all other interventions and patient responses in the patient record, recording them as specifically as possible. Document blood pressure and pulse readings indicating cardiac response to bleeding. If teaching is implemented, include who the learners were, what was taught, and their level of understanding.

NURSING DIAGNOSIS 2

 ACUTE PAIN

Related to:

Hemarthrosis

Defining Characteristics:

Complaints of pain in joint

Grimacing

Goal:

Pain is controlled.

Outcome Criteria

✔ The patient states that pain is < 4 on a 10-point scale.

✔ The patient will verbalize that pain has been relieved 30 minutes after interventions.

✔ The patient will verbalize an understanding of what causes pain.

NOC *Pain level*

Pain control

Comfort level

INTERVENTIONS	RATIONALES
Assess for location, intensity, quality, and other signs of pain: inability to move joint, grimacing, facial expressions, audible expressions of pain, and guarding of painful area.	Identifying these will assist in accurate diagnosis and treatment; hemophiliac patients bleed into joints, which cause a local inflammatory response and painful joints, especially with movement.

(continues)

(continued)

INTERVENTIONS	RATIONALES
Have the patient rate pain intensity using a pain rating scale.	Provides a more objective description of level of pain.
Assess status of affected joint, including pain at site, tenderness to touch, temperature, and edema.	For early signs of neurovascular dysfunction, patients with hemarthrosis are at risk for neurovascular compromise.
Administer analgesics as ordered on a regular schedule, not allowing pain to get intense.	Helps to provide comfort for patient; in addition, decreased pain will improve patient's ability to tolerate mobility.
Encourage the patient to elevate affected joint.	Helps to improve circulation, provide comfort, and reduce pressure points.
Apply ice packs: 20 minutes on.	Ice reduces swelling and bleeding through vasoconstriction, and reduces pain.
Move patient's extremity gently and cautiously.	Movement of affected joint causes pain, and careful movement provides support for the painful area.
Implement strategies to reduce anxiety such as relaxation techniques, guided imagery, and soft music.	Anxiety often intensifies the pain experience.
Investigate the use of diversional activities.	Helps to decrease the attention or focus on the pain.
Assess effectiveness of interventions to relieve pain.	Helps to determine whether interventions have been effective in relieving pain or whether new strategies need to be employed.

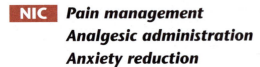 **Pain management**
  Analgesic administration
  Anxiety reduction

Evaluation

The patient is able to report that the pain has been reduced or alleviated following interventions. Joints should not be swollen, and tenderness is decreased. The patient should have no observable signs of discomfort. If the pain is controlled, the patient is able to use the affected joint with minimal discomfort.

Community/Home Care

The patient's pain should decrease once swelling due to bleeding into the joint has been eliminated. Teaching is done to give the patient the information needed to manage painful joints at home. Pain is usually managed with mild analgesics that do not contain aspirin. Ice can be used to promote comfort, and homemade ice packs can be created using a bag of frozen vegetables, such as peas, that molds to the joint. The bag can be wrapped in a towel and applied directly to the joint. For most patients, the duration of pain should be short; however, for some patients, repeated episodes of bleeding into a joint could cause permanent damage, especially in the elbow, hip, knee, and ankle. In this case, long-term management of chronic pain is required. The patient needs to monitor response to pain medications and be able to identify those activities or positions that increase or decrease the pain. Encourage the patient to use assistive devices such as canes and crutches to ambulate if necessary to reduce the risk of injury. If the recommended analgesics are not working, the patient should seek follow-up care with the health care provider.

Documentation

Document in the patient's own words the description of the pain and his rating of the level of pain. Chart all interventions employed and the patient's responses. Include in the documentation assessments made relevant to the pain, including an assessment of the affected joint. Document specifically the appearance of the joint in terms of swelling, tenderness to touch, deformities, heat, or discoloration. All teaching about pain management should be indicated in the patient record with an indication of the patient's level of understanding.

NURSING DIAGNOSIS 3

 IMPAIRED PHYSICAL MOBILITY

Related to:

Deformities of the joint: shoulder, hip, knee, elbow, ankle

Pain at joint area

Defining Characteristics:

Physical restriction

Inability to move with ease

Decreased range of motion

Decreased movement of extremity

Unable and unwilling to move affected joint

Goal:

The patient obtains physical mobility to the highest permissible level.

Outcome Criteria

✔ The patient demonstrates gradual improvement in movement in shoulder, elbow, knee, ankle, and hip.

✔ The patient can use adjunctive devices to assist mobility.

✔ The patient does not sustain injury.

INTERVENTIONS	RATIONALES
Assess affected joint for range of motion or notable deformities.	Helps to determine the extent of disability.
Assess for neurovascular complications by checking peripheral pulses, capillary refill, blanching, skin temperature, and color.	Neurovascular compromise may occur due to constriction of the extremity by hemorrhage into the joint, by edema, or by compression of nerves and blood vessels due to hemarthrosis.
Check results of diagnostic tests: x-rays of joints.	These exams confirm the diagnosis (hemarthrosis).
Support and immobilize the joint by elevating the joint.	Immobilization will prevent further damage to soft tissue of the joints.
Maintain proper alignment.	Proper alignment promotes maximum neurological and vascular function and minimizes pain.
Apply ice to the site.	Helps to decrease swelling and pain through numbing of the site and vasoconstriction.
Implement measures to decrease or prevent bleeding (see nursing diagnosis "Ineffective Protection").	Deformities, pain, and immobility are caused by bleeding into joints; controlling the bleeding prevents further damage to joints.
Encourage range of motion and ambulation as tolerated or ordered.	Activity and range of motion will prevent complications of immobility in joints and help resolve swelling.
Instruct on proper use of assistive devices such as slings, canes, and	Slings provide immobilization to the affected arm, elbow, or
crutches, etc., and encourage their use.	shoulder, and canes and crutches provide added support to the affected extremity for ambulation to prevent injury. This maintains some independence with movement if joint deformity is present or until the hemarthrosis resolves, and the patient needs to know how to use them properly when at home.
Administer pain medications, as ordered.	Mobility is easier if pain is resolved.

NIC *Positioning*

Exercise therapy: Ambulation

Exercise therapy: Joint mobility

Evaluation

Evaluate the degree to which the patient has achieved the stated outcome criteria. The patient should verbalize an understanding of interventions utilized to maintain mobility of the affected joints. Mobility is maximized through use of assistive devices, such as a cane or crutches for lower extremities, and the patient is able to ambulate. No deformities occur, and no symptoms of neurovascular compromise are noted secondary to the hemarthrosis.

Community/Home Care

The patient who has hemarthrosis and/or joint deformity may require some adaptations in performance of activities at home. Safety at home may be an issue for the patient, as the use of canes or crutches can create difficulty with ambulation. Crutches tend to create a feeling of imbalance and use of them will require some trial and error, during which time the patient is at higher risk for falling and subsequent traumatic injury that could lead to bleeding. The environment will need to be assessed to determine how the patient can maneuver safely. Look for hazards such as stairs and excessive furniture or clutter that poses a risk. Early in the convalescence period, the patient may need assistance with household tasks that require long periods of standing, such as cleaning, vacuuming, or cooking. Assistance might need to be sought through a social services agency if family or friends are not available to assist. For younger patients who will need to return to school or college, the challenges are great because the school or college environment is not always conducive to accommodating those with mobility issues. Investigation into how the person can manipulate the environment should be undertaken to determine whether someone will be needed to carry books or take notes, or in the case of joints in the lower extremities, how to get from one point to another on campus. The patient should be encouraged to implement strategies to alleviate pain, such as taking analgesics or using ice packs at home to enhance the level of mobility. Follow-up care is needed to determine whether permanent deformities are present and to check for resolution of hemarthrosis.

Documentation

Chart the findings from an assessment of affected joints, including movement, complaints of pain, tenderness, swelling, color, and neurovascular status. Include in the chart a note that describes ambulation and whether assistance is required. Chart the patient's ability to use upper extremities for self-care activities. If assistive devices such as slings, canes, or crutches are used, chart these. Document all interventions employed to address the problems with the affected joint and the patient's responses to them. Any complaints that the patient verbalizes should be documented in his or her own words.

CHAPTER 7.98

LEUKEMIA

GENERAL INFORMATION

Leukemia is a disorder involving malignant transformation of the white blood cells (WBCs) and their precursors in the bone marrow. Malignant transformation of WBCs results in abundant production of abnormal immature malignant cells and subsequent decreased production of other cell types, such as red blood cells (RBCs). Persons who have leukemia commonly develop other types of cell disorders, such as thrombocytopenia, anemia, and functional leukopenia. The cause of leukemia is not known; however, certain chromosomal aberrations, such as Down syndrome, have been linked with an increased incidence of leukemia. Exposures to certain chemicals, such as benzene or cancer chemotherapy, also increase the incidence. Leukemia can be classified as acute or chronic and by the cell type. If lymphocytes or their precursors in the bone marrow are the malignant cell type, the term *lymphocytic* or *lymphoblastic* is used. For abnormalities of myeloid stem cells in the bone marrow, the term *myelocytic* or *myeloblastic* is used. Acute leukemia has an acute onset with rapid progression that involves proliferation of poorly differentiated malignant cells called *blast cells*. The blast cells relentlessly proliferate as other blood-cell types decrease. Hepatosplenomegaly commonly develops as the blast cells accumulate in the lymphatic tissues of these organs (liver and spleen). Without treatment, patients with acute leukemia are likely to die from infection and/or bleeding within weeks to months. Chronic leukemia involves proliferation of more highly differentiated malignant blood cells. These malignant cells proliferate as other blood cell types decrease, but the process tends to be slower and more insidious. Patients with chronic leukemia often have problems with easy bruising, chronic infections, and fatigue. Patients with chronic leukemia often live for years with the disease. Ultimate transformation of chronic leukemia into acute leukemia is common. The four types of leukemia are acute lymphocytic (lymphoblastic), chronic lymphocytic (lymphoblastic), acute myelocytic (myeloblastic), and chronic myelocytic (myeloblastic). The disease is seen most often in adults, with the most common types being acute myeloblastic leukemia and chronic lymphocytic leukemia in adults.

NURSING DIAGNOSIS 1

DEFICIENT KNOWLEDGE

Related to:

No previous history of the disease/new onset of disease

Lack of information about the disease and its treatment and prevention

Misinformation

Patient/family denial

Defining Characteristics:

Asks no questions

Has many questions/concerns

No interest in learning about the disease

Goal:

The patient verbalizes an understanding of the disease and the required treatment.

Outcome Criteria

✔ The patient verbalizes a desire to learn necessary information.

✔ The patient verbalizes an understanding of the pathophysiology of leukemia.

✔ The patient understands possible treatment options (chemotherapy, stem cell, and bone marrow transplant), including untoward effects of treatment, disease prognosis, and possible complications of leukemia.

✔ The patient agrees to comply with recommendations for treatment.

✔ The patient verbalizes an understanding of diagnostic tests (bone marrow examination, complete blood count [CBC], platelets).

✔ The patient verbalizes an understanding of follow-up care required and expresses a willingness to comply.

NOC *Knowledge: Disease process*
Knowledge: Treatment regimen
Compliance behavior

INTERVENTIONS	RATIONALES
Assess the patient's current knowledge, as well as ability and readiness to learn.	The nurse needs to ascertain and build on what the patient already knows; if the patient is not capable of learning or is not ready to learn, teaching will not be effective due to disinterest or inability to understand. The patient may not be ready to learn if in a state of denial or if extremely angry.
Teach incrementally, starting with the simplest information and moving to complex information.	The patient will learn and retain knowledge better when information is presented in small segments; patients can understand simple concepts easily and then can build on those to understand concepts that are more complex.
Teach patient and significant others: — Disease process of leukemia (too many abnormal immature malignant WBCs, not enough of functional WBCs, decreased RBC and platelet production, particular classification of disease—acute or chronic, lymphocytic or myelocytic) — Prognosis (cure, remission, or control) — Available treatment options (chemotherapy, bone marrow transplant, stem cell transplant) and prognosis, based on type of disease	Knowledge of disease process, diagnostic procedures, identification of complications, and other information empowers the patient to take control and make informed decisions, and enhances compliance.
— Diagnostic studies: CBC, bone marrow examination, and platelets — Signs and symptoms that indicate a need to seek health care (bleeding, signs of infection, extreme fatigue, side effects of medications, persistent nausea, and vomiting)	
Teach patient and family about chemotherapy and its effects: — Method of action — Specific agents used for treatment — Stages of chemotherapy — Alopecia: plan for hair loss by investigating the purchase of wigs or having hair cut short and using hair for a specially made wig before alopecia; find a resource that could teach women how to prepare fashionable head wraps; for men, shave head before alopecia — Nausea/vomiting: use anti-emetics before meals prophylactically; avoid foods with strong odors, and in the hospital setting have lids removed from trays outside the room (when lids are removed from food trays the smell is often overwhelming to the gastrointestinal [GI] system and causes nausea); attempt frequent small meals, avoiding spicy foods — Care of access sites: prevention of infection by use of aseptic techniques and procedures according to agency protocol — Control of fatigue: balance of rest and activity, and on chemotherapy days a designated naptime should be scheduled — Prevention of infection: chemotherapy causes a further depression of WBCs, predisposing the patient to infection; avoid large crowds and people with infections; practice good hand hygiene; know WBC counts	Knowledge of what to expect helps the patient cope with untoward side effects and better equips him or her to take responsibility for managing the illness and to engage in self-care.

INTERVENTIONS	RATIONALES
Teach the patient and family about bone marrow and stem cell transplant therapy: — Mechanism of action — Process of transplant — Potential complications (nausea, infection) — No fresh plants or flowers, no gardening, no fresh Christmas trees — Special dietary precautions — Inspect oral cavity daily for breakdown and infection — Autologous (transplant of patient's own marrow or cells) — Allogenic (transplant of a donor's marrow or cells)	Stem cell and bone marrow transplant therapy is indicated as part of a regimen for patients who have received extensive chemotherapy and radiation, for patients not responsive to more traditional treatments, or as a treatment of choice for some types of leukemia. Knowing what to expect allays anxiety.
Teach patient and family about external radiation: — Method of action — Course/duration of treatment — Skin changes to note include redness, sloughing, and tenderness — Skin care: do not apply soap, ointments, lotions, creams, or powder to area; do not rub, scrub, or scratch the area; do not try to wash off markings; avoid exposing the treated area to the sun during the treatment and for 1 year following treatments — Wear loose-fitting clothes due to risk of irritation — Control of fatigue: energy conservation; intake of high energy foods rich in vitamin C, protein, and iron; taking a nap each day especially after treatment	Radiation is used to destroy abnormal cells in leukemia and is usually used in combination with other treatments, and the patient needs to be informed of what to expect. The radiated skin is sensitive and lotions, creams, ultraviolet rays, rubbing, etc., may cause burning and skin sloughing and interfere with radiation. The patient must know how to protect the skin from impairment; knowing what to expect in terms of radiation helps the patient to be more compliant and feel more in control.
Provide the patient and family with information on hospice and other community service agencies, such as American Cancer Society, as warranted.	These agencies can provide psychological support as well as resources to the patient and family.
Assess the patient's and family's understanding of all teaching by encouraging them to repeat information and ask questions as needed.	This allows the nurse to hear in the patient's own words what was taught and makes it easier to know what information may need to be reinforced.
Give the patient written information of all content taught.	Helps to serve as a handy reference tool for the patient; the volume of information

	needed by the patient is great, and the patient is not likely to remember everything.
Establish that the patient has the resources required to be compliant.	If needed resources such as finances and transportation to follow-up appointments are not available, the patient cannot be compliant; the nurse will need to make necessary referrals.

NIC *Learning readiness enhancement*
Learning facilitation
Teaching: Disease process
Teaching: Prescribed medication
Teaching: Procedure/treatment

Evaluation

Evaluate the degree to which the patient has achieved the outcome criteria relevant to the teaching sessions. The patient should verbalize an understanding of the content presented by repeating the information, particularly the disease process of leukemia, radiation treatment process, chemotherapy, bone marrow, and stem cell transplant procedures. The patient should be able to repeat the signs and symptoms of problems such as infection, anemia, or bleeding. The nurse must determine whether the patient is capable of being compliant with the recommended regimen. If further teaching is required at time of discharge, the appropriate referrals should be made to continue education.

Community/Home Care

The patient will need to implement the prescribed regimen in the home setting, and the amount of time that the patient will require visitation or follow-up will depend on the type of treatment employed. The success of this implementation will depend upon the degree to which the patient has received adequate teaching, has subsequently understood it, and has the resources to implement the recommendations. At home, the patient will need to understand how to manage fatigue following any of the treatments, but especially after radiation or chemotherapy treatments. Knowledge of chemotherapy and its side effects, such as hair loss, nausea, and vomiting, is needed to ensure that the patient can manage them successfully. The nurse needs to be sure that the patient has understood teaching related to radiation therapy to prevent complications and minimize untoward effects. In addition, the patient should have a clear understanding of the schedule of treatments at an outpatient facility. External radiation therapy patients will need to be monitored for ability to care for the skin properly in order to prevent further tissue destruction including avoidance of ultraviolet rays. The nurse should provide the patient with the content taught in an easy-to-read written format. Colorful paper can be used, and the documents can be placed in a folder or small three-ring notebook with dividers by subject matter. A schedule of appointments can be written on a calendar and kept in the binder as well. Because the patient is seen on a regular basis for general follow-up for chemotherapy or for radiation therapy, health care providers can determine whether further teaching or reinforcement is required.

Documentation

Document the specific content taught and the titles of any printed documents given to the patient. Include in the chart the patient's degree of understanding of the content and the methods used to evaluate learning. An assessment of the patient's ability to comply with the regimen in terms of preparation for transplants, radiation, chemotherapy, or follow-up should be made in the chart with indicators of referrals made. Any areas that need to be reinforced should be documented to ensure appropriate follow-up. If family members are present for the teaching sessions, document this in the chart.

NURSING DIAGNOSIS 2

 INEFFECTIVE COPING

Related to:

Fear related to prognosis

Diagnosis of leukemia

Uncertain stage of disease at time of diagnosis

Treatments required

Defining Characteristics:

Expressions of fear

Restlessness

Verbalizes anxiety

Crying

Withdrawn

Goal:

The patient expresses grief and identifies coping strategies.

Outcome Criteria

✔ The patient identifies and uses one coping mechanism.

✔ The patient verbalizes fears and concerns.

✔ The patient reports being less anxious.

✔ The patient demonstrates no outward signs of anxiety such as restlessness or agitation.

NOC   *Anxiety control*
   Comfort level
   Grief resolution
   Coping

INTERVENTIONS	RATIONALES
Assess level of anxiety (mild, moderate, severe); have patient rate on a scale of 1 to 10, with 10 being the greatest.	Gives the nurse an objective measure of the extent of the anxiety.
Assess the patient for the presence of the following feelings about self/disease: sadness, anger, tearfulness, withdrawal, and fear of dying, as well as anxiety about inability to carry out family responsibilities, finances, cost of hospitalization, cost of therapy.	The patient may experience all of these feelings as he or she tries to cope with the diagnosis and treatment. Knowing where the patient is in terms of coping helps to identify needed interventions.
Collaborate with physician to engage patient and family in open dialogue about options for treatment and care as well as the prognosis for the particular type of leukemia. Keep the patient informed of all that is going on, including information about diagnostic tests and planned therapeutic interventions.	Communication of information in a straightforward manner may help to relieve anxiety and fear. Discussion of care options allows the patient to be more in control, providing a sense of empowerment that may assist with coping with the diagnosis.
Give the patient brochures to read about treatment options.	Allows the patient to learn more about the disease and treatment independently.

INTERVENTIONS	RATIONALES
Encourage the patient to verbalize fears and concerns while listening attentively and assuring him or her that it is acceptable to be afraid or angry, or to cry.	Verbalization of fears contributes to dealing with concerns; being attentive relays empathy to the patient. Knowing that his or her feelings are normal gives the patient permission to accept these feelings and move forward.
Provide quiet time for the patient and be available for communication, if needed.	The patient may want or need quiet periods of time to think and adjust to the diagnosis, and to reflect on current situation and options.
Allow family or significant others to visit liberally.	Helps to provide emotional support and promote a sense of comfort.
Assist the patient to identify at least one coping mechanism that has worked in the past; encourage the use of relaxation, guided imagery, deep breathing, or meditation, or assist to develop new coping strategies.	Coping mechanisms that have worked in the past may work again; other relaxation techniques can decrease anxiety and give the patient a sense of calm; new strategies may be required to deal with serious illness.
Seek spiritual consult as needed or requested by the patient and/ or family.	Meeting the patient's spiritual needs helps him or her to deal with fears through the use of spiritual or religious rituals.
Recognize the role of culture in a patient's method of coping with illness and the acceptability of verbalizing fears and concerns.	Culture often dictates how a person copes, and the nurse must recognize this in order to support the patient in identifying successful coping strategies.
If the patient has the energy, time, and motivation, encourage him or her to document feelings in a diary.	This strategy can assist the patient to express self in an acceptable manner when he or she may feel uncomfortable talking to others.
Determine the availability of resources needed to comply with treatment requirements (money, transportation, emotional support).	Treatments for leukemia can be extensive, spanning months or even years. Transportation is needed for travel to appointments. These requirements may add to fear and anxiety. Social services can assist in location of needed resources.

NIC *Coping enhancement*
Emotional support
Grief work facilitation
Spiritual support

Evaluation

Evaluate the extent to which the outcome criteria have been achieved. The patient should be assessed for behaviors that would indicate adjustment to the diagnosis of leukemia. He or she should begin to accept the diagnosis, and should be able to identify and use acceptable coping, anxiety-reducing, and grieving strategies. The patient may still experience heightened anxiety and anticipatory grieving shortly after diagnosis as he or she attempts to deal with the unknown and the possibility of death. The patient should verbalize fears and concerns and be able to identify one way to cope with the diagnosis of leukemia. If the patient is unable to talk about the diagnosis and communicate concerns, the nurse should explore further interventions to assist the patient.

Community/Home Care

Nurses should assess which coping mechanisms work for the patient and encourage their use by the patient at home. Even among patients who have types of leukemia with high survival rates or who were treated successfully, problems with anxiety and fear of death may continue for a long period of time. At least one follow-up visit by a health care provider should be initiated to assess for ineffective coping. The patient should be encouraged to identify coping strategies that have been successful in the past and prompted to use those regularly. Anxiety about prognosis usually continues throughout treatment and recovery until a remission is achieved and the patient is able to resume normal activities. However, for those patients whose disease was detected in later stages with a poor prognosis, anxiety can be more pronounced. For this group, coping through use of support from outside sources such as hospice or nurse therapists may be required. Monitor for extreme withdrawal, self-isolation, and depression, reporting any symptoms to the physician. At home, the patient and family may benefit from visits from religious or spiritual leaders to assist with coping. For many patients and families, spiritual or religious rituals provide a means of coping with difficult, stressful situations. The patient's culture may dictate how he or she copes and/or grieves, and with whom. It is crucial that the nurse and family support the patient as needed to foster a healthy psychological state, recognizing that anger and denial are common. Even though friends and family intend well with their presence, the patient may benefit from quiet periods of meditation and solitude during the day. If questions should arise at home about the patient's health status or prescribed regimen, the patient should have a means of contact with a health care provider for answers.

Documentation

The degree to which the patient has demonstrated effective coping and decreased anxiety should be documented in the patient record. A rating system provides an objective way to relay to others the extent of the anxiety or expressions of fear. Include in the patient record findings from an assessment of the patient's psychological state, indicating whether there is depression, anger, crying sadness, etc. Document whether the patient is able to discuss feelings about a diagnosis of leukemia. Chart the patient's verbalizations as the patient states them, and include in the record coping mechanisms utilized by the patient. Document all referrals to hospice or religious leaders.

NURSING DIAGNOSIS 3

INEFFECTIVE PROTECTION

Related to:

> Chemotherapy
>
> Radiation therapy
>
> Immunosuppression
>
> Bone marrow suppression

Defining Characteristics:

> Fatigue
>
> Decreased hemoglobin (Hgb) and hematocrit (Hct)
>
> Leukocytosis
>
> Immature WBCs
>
> Decreased platelets
>
> Easy bruising
>
> Prolonged bleeding
>
> Blood in stool or emesis

Goal:

> The patient will have no infection or bleeding.

Outcome Criteria

✔ The patient will not experience bleeding or bruising.

✔ The patient will have no signs or symptoms of infections (urinary, respiratory, central access sites, skin areas).

✔ The patient will verbalize an understanding of the necessary precautions needed to prevent bleeding, infection, and injury.

NOC *Blood coagulation*
Immune status
Knowledge: Infection control
Risk control

INTERVENTIONS	RATIONALES
Monitor WBCs, RBCs, Hgb, Hct, and platelets.	Helps to detect abnormalities that place the patient at risk for injury and infection. The number and type of WBCs required to fight infection are decreased in leukemia and further decreases occur during treatment with chemotherapy. Anemia is common in chemotherapy patients and leukemia patients, and measures of RBC, Hgb, and Hct are indicators of severity. Fewer RBCs are produced due to bone marrow suppression secondary to chemotherapy. Platelets are decreased, placing the patient at high risk for bleeding.
Assess for fatigue, weakness, shortness of breath, and any alteration in mental status.	These symptoms occur due to the body's inability to transport enough oxygen to tissues secondary to decreased RBCs and iron.
Monitor for indicators of bleeding abnormalities: bruising, easy bleeding, petechiae, bleeding gums, nose bleed, and purpura.	These indicate that the body is unable to clot effectively, and further examination and interventions may be warranted to prevent complications.

INTERVENTIONS	RATIONALES
Assess all stools and emesis for blood by hemoccult, urine for blood using dipstick, and sputum for blood by examination.	The lungs, GI, and genitourinary (GU) systems are highly vascular and prone to bleeding; the nurse needs to monitor for bleeding to allow for early intervention if bleeding is noted.
Avoid the use of aspirin or aspirin-containing products.	These products increase the risk of bleeding.
Avoid venipuncture or injections to the extent possible, and apply pressure to all puncture sites.	Due to thrombocytopenia, the patient bleeds easily, and pressure is required to effectively stop bleeding. At least 5 minutes may be required.
Brush teeth with soft-bristle toothbrush.	Gums tend to bleed easily due to altered clotting factors and decreased platelets; use of a soft toothbrush is needed to decrease bleeding from gums.
When the patient is hospitalized, place him or her in protective isolation or on neutropenic precautions when cell counts decrease, according to agency protocol. All visitors should wear a mask when in the room and wash their hands before entering the room; no raw fruit and vegetables or fresh flowers should be brought into the room.	Helps to protect the patient from sources of infection.
Consider a neutropenic diet.	Restriction of uncooked fruits and vegetables may decrease microorganisms entering the body.
Monitor for signs of infection: fever; redness or other discoloration, drainage, or heat at any wound or intravenous (IV) access insertion site; urine for malodor, mucous; oral cavity for white coating; respiratory system for cough, sputum production, crackles in lungs; notify physician if any are noted.	With bone marrow suppression and decreased numbers of neutrophils, the patient is at higher risk for infection. A fever may be the only sign of infection, as the patient is unable to produce the normal inflammatory response due to immunosuppression.
Assess temperature frequently, at least every 4 hours.	Fever is an indicator of infection.
Practice good hand hygiene and have family members wash hands frequently.	Handwashing is one of the best ways to stop the transmission of infection.
Have the patient avoid crowds.	Being in crowds increases the risk of acquiring respiratory infections.
Increase iron-rich foods in diet.	Helps to increase oxygen-carrying capacity of RBCs.
Change any dressings over central line access sites in accordance with agency protocol using strict sterile technique.	Leukemia patients may have central line sites or other ports for chemotherapy administration. These sites are an easy portal for entry of organisms. Strict sterile technique is required to reduce risk for infection.
Administer antibiotics, as ordered.	Helps to prevent or treat infection.
Teach patient all safety precautions related to bleeding and infection.	The patient needs to be informed in order to practice health promotion and disease prevention behaviors.

NIC *Bleeding precautions*
Infection protection
Risk identification
Surveillance

Evaluation

Evaluate whether outcome criteria have been met. The patient should have no bleeding; if bleeding is present, it should be detected and treated early. Infections have been prevented as demonstrated by the absence of signs and symptoms. The patient ambulates with assistance and sustains no injury. At time of discharge from the health care agency, the patient is able to verbalize safety precautions required.

Community/Home Care

The patient with leukemia will remain at risk for ineffective protection throughout treatment. Once at home, the patient will need to continue to practice safety-enhancing behaviors for bleeding, physical injury, and infections. The patient must be vigilant in preventing or controlling bleeding promptly if it occurs as well as preventing falls. It is suggested that the patient have gauze pads or sponges available in a first aid kit at home and understand the concept of "applying pressure" to a bleeding site. The patient should understand the importance of avoiding aspirin or aspirin-containing products. Prior to taking any over-the-counter pain medicines, the patient should read the label or ask the pharmacist, as many products contain aspirin. Implementing strategies to protect self from injury, such as bumping into objects that may cause bruising or disruption of skin, is important. This may include rearranging furniture or removing rugs to make walking areas clear. Because the patient is prone to fatigue, he or she may need assistance with ambulation or restriction of activities requiring mental alertness at times. Dietary interventions that can assist the patient with energy levels can prevent some of the fatigue caused by decreased RBCs and subsequent impaired oxygen transport. Foods rich in iron should be encouraged, taking into consideration the patient's likes/dislikes, culture, religion, and dietary restrictions. In cases of neutropenia, the diet at home may need to restrict raw fruits and vegetables, making it crucial that the dietician provide dietary recommendations only after a thorough consult with the patient and, if possible, a family member or significant other. At home, the patient should use electric razors for shaving since even a small nick from a disposable straight razor can cause significant free bleeding. Dental floss, if used, should be waxed for easier sliding and prevention of trauma to gums, and a soft-bristle toothbrush is always required. Women should note changes in menstrual cycle that would indicate more profuse bleeding, such as a significant increase in numbers of pads used and the passage of clots. If bleeding is noted in stools, emesis, or from any orifice or wound, the health care provider should be notified for prompt treatment. The patient with leukemia receiving chemotherapy or bone marrow or stem cell transplant will need to avoid large crowds or other environments that may increase risk for infection. Handshaking is a common expression of greeting but can be the source of transmission of organisms from well-intending persons, and the patient will need to limit this activity and wash their hands thoroughly after shaking hands. The patient, as well as any primary caregiver such as a family member or significant other, should remove him or herself from the vicinity of any person coughing or presenting symptoms of respiratory infection. Practicing frequent good handwashing techniques can minimize the risk of infection. Patients with young children or grandchildren should avoid them if possible when they are sick with colds or the flu. Teach the patient to take his or her temperature three times a day and to record it. Any elevations are to be reported to the health care provider in accordance with recommended guidelines. For those patients receiving bone marrow transplant or stem cell transplant, more aggressive measures are required to prevent infection (see nursing care plan

"Organ and Tissue Transplantation"). At the first sign of infection, the patient should return to a health care provider for further assistance.

Documentation

Include in the documentation findings from a thorough assessment of the patient for evidence of bleeding, such as bruises, bleeding gums, bleeding from access sites, etc. Also, document the patient's activity level and response to activity (fatigue, dizziness). If the patient has any signs of infection, even minor ones, document this in the patient record with a clear indication of what actions were carried out in response. Temperature should be taken at least every 4 hours and recorded according to agency protocol. Chart all interventions implemented to address safety, bleeding, and prevention of infections. If teaching is implemented, include who the learners were and their level of understanding.

NURSING DIAGNOSIS 5

 ## ACTIVITY INTOLERANCE

Related to:

Effects of treatment

Imbalance between oxygen supply and demand secondary to leukemia and anemia

Defining Characteristics:

Lethargy/fatigue

Verbalization of tiredness

States a lack of energy

Inability to carry out normal activities without becoming exhausted

Goal:

The patient tolerates activity without fatigue.

Outcome Criteria

✔ The patient is able to perform activities of daily living (ADLs).

✔ The patient verbalizes that fatigue has improved or been eliminated.

✔ No exertional dyspnea occurs.

✔ Heart rate and blood pressure return to baseline 5 minutes following cessation of activity.

NOC *Activity tolerance*
Endurance
Energy conservation
Nutritional status: Energy

INTERVENTIONS	RATIONALES
Obtain subjective data about normal activities, limitations, and nighttime sleep patterns.	Helps to determine the effect fatigue has on normal functioning. Adequate sleep is required for restoration of the body.
Monitor patient for signs of excessive physical and emotional fatigue.	Provides a guideline for adjusting activity.
Alternate periods of rest and activity.	Helps to decrease the demand for energy and oxygen reserves; fatigue is a side effect of all types of chemotherapy and radiation, and periods of rest are required to restore body.
Encourage the patient to plan activities during times of greater energy, usually early in the day.	Helps to prevent fatigue.
Space planned activities away from mealtimes.	Digestion requires energy and oxygen. Participation in activities close to meals will cause increased fatigue because of insufficient energy reserves.
Gradually increase activity as tolerated, and take blood pressure and pulse before and after activity.	When treatment is complete, fatigue improves, but the patient may still require activity restrictions; monitoring tolerance to activity can provide information to indicate when activity may be increased or decreased. If any particular activity causes undue fatigue, it should not be attempted again until later in the recovery period.
Limit visitors during any periods of acute illness.	Socialization for long periods may cause fatigue.
Increase intake of high-energy foods such as poultry, dried beans and peas, whole grains, foods high in vitamin C, and adequate to liberal amounts of fluids within restrictions of the recommended diet.	These foods enhance energy metabolism, increase oxygen-carrying capacity, and provide ready sources of energy. High-carbohydrate foods help maintain glycogen stores required for energy, and increased fluids enhance

	excretion of metabolic wastes that can cause the patient to feel tired.
Administer iron, folate, vitamin B$_{12}$, or erythropoietin, as ordered.	All of these agents stimulate hematopoiesis.
Encourage the patient to sleep 8 to 10 hours each night.	Sleep decreases oxygen demand and adds to the feeling of restfulness.
Explore diversional activities with the patient, and encourage quiet activities such as reading, video games, computer games, card games or television/movies, crossword puzzles, etc.	Resolution of acute symptoms may take an extended period, and because the recovery period from treatment may be extended, the patient needs methods to alleviate boredom.
Assist the patient in identifying community resources that can be of assistance with daily activities such as housekeeping, laundry, and preparing meals.	A number of community resources may be available to the chronically ill and/or disabled for household assistance.
Assist the patient in developing a home schedule to minimize energy expenditure.	This will help the patient retain some independence while being cognizant of limitations and need for energy conservation.

NIC *Energy management*

Evaluation

Obtain subjective information from the patient about the presence of fatigue. The patient should gradually report the ability to participate in ADLs and other normal activities with no fatigue or exertional dyspnea. Blood pressure and pulse return to baseline range within 5 minutes of when activity is stopped.

Community/Home Care

Patients with leukemia should understand that fatigue might persist for an extended period from diagnosis through the treatment period. Appropriate education on ways to adapt self-care and household activities when the patient is fatigued is paramount. A history should be obtained from the patient about his or her usual routine for work, school, ADLs, and household chores, so that individualized interventions can be implemented. Attention to what the patient normally does and how the patient wants to make adaptations can only enhance compliance. The patient should make a list of all chores that need to be done during a week and make a schedule for them, with a balance of light duties and heavier duties. In addition, the patient, in consultation with family members (if available), can delegate chores to others. On days that the patient receives chemotherapy or radiation, the performance of even light activities will be limited due to fatigue. The nurse must remain aware of cultural backgrounds that may influence a patient's perception of and adaptation to perceived dependency on others. The patient must understand how to adjust activity in response to feelings of fatigue, possibly even arranging for rest or nap periods in the afternoon. This may not be a realistic recommendation for people who continue to work and whose occupations preclude napping or even resting during the day. Strategies to enhance nighttime sleep should be implemented so that the patient can get adequate rest. Attention to good nutrition that can improve energy levels should continue with intake of foods that are good sources of iron, vitamin C, and protein, within any dietary restrictions. The patient will need to return to the health care provider for evaluation of overall health status and progression.

Documentation

Chart the specific complaint of fatigue, including activities the patient has been performing. If the patient requires assistance with ADLs, document this with a description of the exact type of assistance required and response to treatment. Chart the patient's pulse and blood pressure before and after activity, and if the patient has exertional dyspnea, document this as well. An assessment of the patient's sleep patterns is also included. Document all interventions implemented to address activity intolerance and fatigue, being sure to document food intake.

CHAPTER 7.99

LYMPHOMA

GENERAL INFORMATION

Lymphoma is cancer of the lymph nodes that is diagnosed with lymph node biopsy. Primary lymphomas are classified as Hodgkin's or non-Hodgkin's. Hodgkin's disease occurs in a single lymph node or in a chain of nodes and easily spreads to nearby nodes. Diagnosis is confirmed through a biopsy of the lymph node that reveals the presence of Reed-Sternberg cells. The disease has four subtypes: lymphocyte predominant, nodular sclerosing, mixed cellularity, and lymphocyte depleted. Hodgkin's disease found in mixed cells and Hodgkin's disease that causes nodular sclerosis have a poor prognosis. The disease progression is divided into four phases/stages. Stage I is isolation of the disease to a single lymph node region (without disease spread). By Stage IV, the disease has spread to numerous body areas/systems. Nodular sclerosis is the most common form of the disease, and lymphocyte depleted is the least common form. The initial and most common symptom of the disease is the presence of a painless enlarged lymph node in the cervical or subclavicular region. Systemic clinical manifestations include fatigue, persistent fever of unexplained origin, night sweats, anorexia, weight loss, and severe pruritus. The spleen may be enlarged. Treatment for Hodgkin's disease ranges from chemotherapy to radiation therapy to bone marrow transplant, and combinations of two or all three. Hodgkin's disease is most often a disease of people between the ages of 15 and 35, and a second peak in incidence occurs in people over 50 years of age. The incidence is slightly higher in men.

Non-Hodgkin's disease is cancer arising from three specific lymphocyte cell systems (B-lymphocyte, T-lymphocyte, and histocytes) that occurs in the lymph nodes in the periphery and metastasizes early in the disease. Non-Hodgkin's disease can be divided into two general categories: nodular and diffuse. Each of these is graded from I to III, or low, moderate, or

high. Low-grade tumors have a better prognosis for cure, and higher-grade tumors have a poor prognosis and may have widely spread by the time of discovery. Clinical manifestations of non-Hodgkin's lymphoma are painless peripheral lymph nodes; if other organs are involved, the patient may demonstrate abdominal pain, nausea, and vomiting. The presence of headaches or other neurological symptoms implicate involvement of the central nervous system. The patient may have systemic manifestations of fever, sweats, fatigue, and weight loss similar to those of Hodgkin's disease, but these are not common findings. Treatment for non-Hodgkin's disease is a combination of chemotherapy, radiation therapy, and in some cases stem cell transplants. Non-Hodgkin's lymphoma occurs more frequently than Hodgkin's disease, occurring most often in older adults and men.

NURSING DIAGNOSIS 1

 DEFICIENT KNOWLEDGE

Related to:

No previous history of the disease/new onset of disease

Lack of information about the disease and its treatment and prevention

Misinformation

Patient/family denial

Defining Characteristics:

Asks no questions

Has many questions/concerns

Shows no interest in learning about the disease

Goal:

The patient verbalizes an understanding of the disease and the required treatment.

Outcome Criteria

✔ The patient verbalizes a desire to learn necessary information.

✔ The patient verbalizes an understanding of the pathophysiology of lymphoma.

✔ The patient understands possible treatment options (chemotherapy, radiation therapy, stem cell transplant), including untoward effects of treatment, disease prognosis, and possible complications of lymphoma.

✔ The patient agrees to comply with recommendations for treatment.

✔ The patient verbalizes an understanding of diagnostic procedures (biopsy, chest x-ray, abdominal computed tomography (CT) scan, and lymphangiography).

✔ The patient verbalizes an understanding of follow-up care required and expresses a willingness to comply.

NOC *Knowledge: Disease process*
Knowledge: Treatment regimen
Compliance behavior

INTERVENTIONS	RATIONALES
Assess the patient's current knowledge, ability to learn, and readiness to learn.	The nurse needs to ascertain what the patient already knows and build on this; if the patient is not capable of learning or is not ready to learn, teaching will not be effective due to disinterest or inability to understand. The patient may not be ready to learn if in a state of denial or if extremely angry about his or her diagnosis.
Teach incrementally, starting with the simplest information and moving to complex information.	The patient will learn and retain knowledge better when information is presented in small segments; patients can understand simple concepts easily and then can build on those to understand concepts that are more complex.
Teach patient and significant others: — Disease process of lymphoma (pathophysiology and staging of the disease)	Knowledge of disease process, diagnostic procedures, identification of complications, and other information empowers the patient to take
— Available treatment options (chemotherapy, radiation, stem cell transplant); the stage of disease guides treatment — Diagnostic studies: CT scan, biopsy, lymphangiography, chest x-ray, complete blood cell counts (CBCs) — Signs and symptoms that would indicate a need to seek health care	control and make informed decisions, and enhances compliance. CBC gives preliminary data in making the diagnosis; CT scans can demonstrate the presence of the enlarged lymph nodes; chest x-rays identify lymph nodes in the mediastinal area and also help to rule out metastasis to the lung; a biopsy will confirm the diagnosis and stage of disease; lymphangiography outlines the lymph nodes and can detect abnormalities.
Teach patient and family about external radiation: — Method of action — Course/duration of treatment — Skin changes to note include redness, sloughing, and tenderness — Skin care: do not apply soap, ointments, lotions, creams, or powder to area. Do not rub, scrub, or scratch the area; do not try to wash off markings; avoid exposing the treated area to the sun during the treatment and for 1 year following treatments — Wear loose-fitting clothes due to risk of irritation — Control of fatigue: importance of energy conservation, intake of high-energy foods rich in vitamin C, protein, and iron; taking a nap each day especially after treatment	Radiation is used with early stage Hodgkin's disease and in combination with chemotherapy for non-Hodgkin's disease; the patient needs to be informed of what to expect. The radiated skin is sensitive and lotions, creams, ultraviolet rays, rubbing, etc., may cause burning and skin sloughing, and interfere with radiation. The patient must know how to protect the skin from impairment; knowing what to expect in terms of radiation helps the patient to be more compliant and feel more in control.
Teach patient and family about chemotherapy and its effects: — Method of action — Specific agents used for treatment — Alopecia: assist the patient to plan for hair loss by investigating the purchase of wigs or having hair cut short and using hair for a specially made wig before alopecia; find a resource that could teach women how to prepare fashionable head wraps; men may want to shave head before the onset of alopecia	Knowledge of what to expect helps the patient cope with untoward side effects and better equips him or her to take responsibility for managing the illness and to engage in self-care.

INTERVENTIONS	RATIONALES

— Nausea/vomiting: teach to use anti-emetics before meals prophylactically; avoid foods with strong odors, and in the hospital setting, have lids removed from trays outside the room (when lids are removed from food trays the smell is often overwhelming to the gastrointestinal [GI] system and causes nausea); attempt frequent small meals, avoiding spicy foods

— Care of access sites: prevention of infection by use of aseptic techniques and procedures according to agency protocol

— Control of fatigue: balance of rest and activity; on chemotherapy days a designated naptime should be scheduled

— Prevention of infection: chemotherapy causes a depression of white blood cells (WBCs), predisposing the patient to infection; avoid people with infections and large crowds; practice good hand hygiene by washing hands often and thoroughly, and limiting handshaking; know WBC counts

Teach the patient and family about stem cell transplant therapy: — Mechanism of action — Procedure for transplant — Potential complications (nausea, infection, stomatitis) — Autologous (transplant of patient's cells) — Allogenic (transplant of donor cells) — Post-transplant care requirements — Extended length of stay in hospital before and after transplant	Stem cell therapy is indicated for patients not responsive to treatments that are more traditional or with advanced disease. Autologous transplant restores blood and immune cell function after bone marrow depression following radiation and high-dose chemotherapy. Knowing what to expect allays anxiety.
Provide the patient and family with information on hospice and other community service agencies, such as the American Cancer Society and the Leukemia and Lymphoma Society, as warranted.	These agencies can provide psychological support as well as resources to the patient and family.

Assess the patient's and family's understanding of all teaching by encouraging them to repeat information and ask questions, as needed.	This allows the nurse to hear in the patient's own words what was taught and makes it easier to know what information may need to be reinforced.
Establish that the patient has the resources required to be compliant.	If needed resources such as finances and transportation to follow-up appointments are not available, the patient cannot be compliant; the nurse will need to make necessary referrals.

NIC *Learning readiness enhancement*
Learning facilitation
Teaching: Disease process
Teaching: Prescribed medication
Teaching: Procedure/treatment

Evaluation

Evaluate the degree to which the patient has achieved the outcome criteria relevant to the teaching sessions. The patient should verbalize an understanding of the content presented by repeating the information, particularly the disease process, radiation treatment process, chemotherapy, and medications for pain or nausea. The nurse must determine whether the patient is capable of being compliant with the recommended regimen. If further teaching is required at time of discharge, the appropriate referrals should be made to continue education.

Community/Home Care

The patient will need to implement the prescribed regimen in the home setting, and the amount of time that the patient will require visitation or follow-up will depend on the type of treatment employed. The success of this implementation will depend upon the degree to which the patient has received adequate teaching and has subsequently understood and internalized it. At home, the patient will likely experience fatigue following any of the treatments, but especially with radiation or chemotherapy treatments. Thorough education on how to pace activities and conserve energy is crucial to the patient successfully managing energy and minimizing feelings of fatigue. Knowledge of chemotherapy and its side effects such as hair loss, nausea, and vomiting are needed to ensure that the patient can manage them successfully. The nurse needs to be sure that the patient has understood teaching related to radiation therapy to prevent complications and minimize untoward effects. In addition, the patient should have a clear understanding of the schedule of all treatments at an outpatient facility. External radiation therapy patients will need to be monitored for ability to care for the skin properly in order to prevent further tissue destruction including avoidance of ultraviolet rays. The nurse should provide the patient with the content taught in an easy-to-read format. Colorful paper can be used, and the documents placed in a folder or small three-ring notebook with dividers by subject matter. A schedule of appointments can be written down on a calendar and kept in the binder as well. If the patient is to receive a stem cell transplant, be sure he or she understands what is required before and after the procedure. Stem cell transplant patients are required to stay in close proximity to the hospital following the transplant, and for some this means staying at a hotel room or a hospital-run housing facility. Knowing this can help the patient prepare for being away from home. The patient may need emotional support from a variety of sources, but particularly from family or significant others. Because the patient is seen on a regular basis for general follow-up and for treatments, health care providers can determine whether further teaching or reinforcement is required.

Documentation

Document the specific content taught and the titles of any printed documents given to the patient. Include in the chart the patient's degree of understanding of the content and the methods used to evaluate learning. An assessment of the patient's ability to be compliant with the regimen in terms of radiation, chemotherapy, transplant, or follow-up should be made in the chart with indicators of referrals made. Document any concerns expressed by the patient and any areas that need to reinforcement to ensure appropriate follow-up. If family members are present for the teaching sessions, document this in the chart.

NURSING DIAGNOSIS 2

INEFFECTIVE COPING

Related to:

Fear

Diagnosis of lymphoma

Uncertain stage of disease at time of diagnosis

Defining Characteristics:

Expressions of fear

Restlessness

Verbalizes anxiety

Crying

Goal:

The patient expresses grief and identifies coping strategies.

Outcome Criteria

✔ The patient identifies and uses one coping mechanism.

✔ The patient verbalizes fears and concerns.

✔ The patient reports being less anxious.

✔ The patient demonstrates no outward signs of anxiety, such as restlessness or agitation.

NOC *Anxiety control*
         Comfort level
         Coping

INTERVENTIONS	RATIONALES
Assess level of anxiety (mild, moderate, severe); have the patient rate on a scale of 1 to 10, with 10 being the greatest.	Gives the nurse a better perception of extent of the anxiety.
Assess the patient about feelings related to the diagnosis: sadness, anger, tearfulness, withdrawal, and fear of dying, as well as anxiety about inability to carry out family responsibilities, finances, cost of hospitalization, and cost of therapy.	The patient may experience all of these feelings as he or she tries to cope with the diagnosis and treatment. Knowing where the patient is in terms of coping helps to identify interventions.
Keep the patient informed of all that is going on, including information about diagnostic tests and planned therapeutic interventions.	Communication of information in a straightforward manner may help to relieve anxiety and fear.
Use a calm, reassuring manner with the patient.	Gives the patient a sense of well-being.
Allow family to visit liberally.	Helps to provide emotional support and promote a sense of comfort.

INTERVENTIONS	RATIONALES
Encourage the patient to verbalize any fears or concerns and listen attentively.	Verbalization of fears contributes to dealing with concerns; being attentive relays empathy to the patient.
Assist the patient to identify at least one coping mechanism that has worked in the past; encourage the use of relaxation, guided imagery, deep breathing, or meditation, or assist to develop new coping strategies.	Coping mechanisms that have worked in the past may work again; other relaxation techniques can decrease anxiety and give the patient a sense of calm; new strategies may be required to cope with serious illness.
Seek spiritual consult as needed or requested by the patient and or family.	Meeting spiritual needs of the patient helps the patient to deal with fears through use of spiritual or religious rituals.
Recognize the role of culture in a patient's method of coping with illness and perception of the acceptability of verbalizing fears and concerns.	Culture often dictates how a person copes, and the nurse must recognize this in order to support the patient in identifying successful coping strategies.
Collaborate with physician to engage patient and family in open dialogue about options for treatments and care.	Discussion of care options allows the patient to be more in control and provides a sense of empowerment that may assist with coping with the diagnosis.
If the patient has the energy, time, or motivation, encourage him or her to document feelings in a diary.	These strategies assist the patient to express him or herself in an acceptable manner when he or she may feel uncomfortable talking to others.

NIC *Coping enhancement*
Emotional support
Spiritual support

Evaluation

Evaluate the extent to which the outcome criteria have been achieved. The patient should be assessed for behaviors that would indicate adjustment to the diagnosis of lymphoma. Even though most cases of lymphoma have a good prognosis, the patient may still experience heightened anxiety and anticipatory grieving shortly after diagnosis while attempting to deal with the unknown and the possibility of death. The patient should verbalize fears and concerns and be able to identify one way to cope with the diagnosis of cancer. The extent to which the

patient displays appropriate coping behaviors should be noted. If the patient is unable to talk about the diagnosis and communicate concerns, the nurse should explore further interventions to assist the patient.

Community/Home Care

Nurses should assess which coping mechanisms work for the patient and encourage their use by the patient at home. Even for those patients whose disease was detected early and treated successfully, problems with anxiety and ineffective coping may continue for a long period of time. At least one follow-up visit by a health care provider should be initiated to assess for ineffective coping. The patient should be encouraged to identify coping strategies that have been successful in the past and prompted to use those regularly. Anxiety about prognosis usually continues throughout treatment and recovery until the patient achieves remission and is able to resume normal activities. However, for those patients whose disease was detected in later stages with a poor prognosis, anxiety can be more pronounced. For this group, coping through use of support from outside sources such as hospice or nurse therapists may be required. Monitor for extreme withdrawal, self-isolation, and depression, and report any symptoms to the primary care provider. For many patients and families, spiritual or religious rituals provide a means of coping with difficult stressful situations. If this is true for the patient, suggest visits in the home from the religious or spiritual leader. The patient's culture may dictate how he or she copes and/or grieves and with whom. It is crucial that the nurse and family support the patient as needed to foster a healthy psychological state and recognize that anger and denial are common. Even though friends and family intend well with their presence in the home, the patient may benefit from quiet periods of meditation and solitude during the day. If questions should arise at home about the patient's health status or prescribed regimen, the patient should have a means of contact with a health care provider for answers.

Documentation

Document the degree to which the patient has demonstrated effective coping and decreased anxiety in the patient record. A rating system provides an objective way to relay to others the extent of the anxiety or expressions of fear. Document whether the patient is able to discuss feelings about a diagnosis of lymphoma. Chart the patient's verbalizations as stated and include in the record coping mechanisms utilized by the patient. Document findings from an assessment of the patient's psychological state, indicating whether there is depression, anger, crying, sadness, etc. Include in the patient record referrals to support groups, hospice, or religious leaders.

NURSING DIAGNOSIS 3

 ### IMBALANCED NUTRITION: LESS THAN BODY REQUIREMENTS

Related to:

> Nausea
>
> Anorexia
>
> Effects of chemotherapy

Defining Characteristics:

> Reports of decreased appetite
>
> Nausea
>
> Loss of weight
>
> Eats little of food served

Goal:

> Adequate dietary and fluid intake is maintained.

Outcome Criteria

✔ The patient does not lose weight.

✔ The patient consumes 50 percent of food served.

✔ The patient tolerates meals without nausea or vomiting.

NOC   *Nutritional status: Food and fluid intake*

        Nutritional status: Nutrient intake

        Oral hygiene

INTERVENTIONS	RATIONALES
Assess laboratory results: albumin, electrolytes, glucose, protein (total), and iron.	These indicate nutritional status.
Assess the patient's ability to eat and drink, and ability to retain intake.	Helps to identify specific problems such as nausea, vomiting, or indigestion the patient is experiencing and to intervene accordingly.
Weigh patient and monitor weight daily or weekly when at home.	Helps to establish a baseline for comparison and, as the patient progresses, to allow for early intervention for nutritional deficits.
Monitor intake and output, and assess for dehydration (oral mucous membranes, skin turgor).	Helps to assure adequate hydration and implement appropriate action promptly.
Consider a dietician consult to ascertain the patient's ability to take in enough food to meet caloric demand and to determine the patient's likes, dislikes, and preferences within the prescribed diet with consideration to cultural or religious preferences.	For patients who have cancer, weight loss is common for a variety of reasons, especially during chemotherapy or in later stages; sufficient caloric intake is necessary to prevent wasting, if possible, and the patient will be more likely to consume foods that he or she likes; the dietician will be useful in determining what the patient needs.
Encourage the patient to eat small, frequent meals.	Food may be more tolerable in small portions, and smaller portions require less energy for consumption. The patient undergoing treatment for lymphoma is frequently fatigued, and smaller meals may prevent this discomfort.
Allow adequate time for meals.	The patient may take longer to eat due to lack of energy and interest in foods.
In consultation with the dietician, offer meals that are high in calories and rich in protein, vitamin C, and iron.	These foods promote healing and are energy-rich.
Create a pleasant environment for meals.	The environment can enhance the patient's willingness to eat.
Provide oral/mouth care before meals.	Chemotherapy and stem cell transplant often alter taste buds, and a fresh mouth can enhance taste and makes food taste better.
Open containers away from the patient or outside door.	Especially for the patient receiving chemotherapy, removing lids from containers at the bedside releases a strong aroma that can cause nausea, which would prevent patient from eating.

INTERVENTIONS	RATIONALES
Give anti-emetics, as ordered, prior to chemotherapy and prn 30 minutes before meals.	Helps to prevent nausea and vomiting.
Avoid spicy foods, greasy foods, and foods that tend to cause gas (such as beans, cabbage, etc.), as well as thick gravies or sauces and highly concentrated sweets.	These foods will increase the likelihood of nausea and vomiting and are more difficult to digest.
Based on patient likes, dislikes, and preferences, offer bland foods or drinks that have a decreased likelihood of causing nausea, such as toast, crackers, ginger ale, and gelatin.	These foods are usually well tolerated by patients on chemotherapy.
Encourage patient to take the most nutritious foods (such as meats) early in the day.	The patient becomes more fatigued as the day progresses and is less likely to eat; in addition, nausea may increase later in the day.
If nausea is present, offer foods on the meal tray that are cold rather than hot.	Cold foods tend to decrease nausea.
Have the patient keep hard candy available.	Sucking on hard candy can decrease the feeling of mild nausea.
Give nutritional supplemental drinks such as Boost, Ensure, and milkshakes.	These high-calorie drinks also contain vitamins and minerals, and are used to improve overall nutritional intake.

NIC *Nutritional monitoring*
Nutritional management

Evaluation

The patient's nutritional state is stable, and the patient has a satisfactory method for nutrient intake. Assess the patient's weight and determine that the patient is not losing weight. The patient should be ingesting at least 50 percent of foods served and tolerating them without nausea or vomiting. Laboratory results should reveal a normal albumin level as well as total protein and electrolytes. Prior to discharge, the patient should be able to eat and drink without nausea/vomiting and be able to verbalize methods to maintain nutrition in the home.

Community/Home Care

Difficulties eating and drinking may continue at home for the patient who has lymphoma during the period of chemotherapy and radiation therapy as well as following stem cell transplant. The patient will need to continue efforts to ingest enough food and nutrients to meet the metabolic demands of a disease state. The patient needs encouragement to eat and at home may lose interest in eating due to depression or because of fatigue. In addition, the prescribed medications and stem cell transplants may alter taste buds. A home nurse or other health care provider needs to monitor the patient's nutritional status on a regular basis to detect poor eating patterns and excessive weight loss, and to note reports of increased nausea/vomiting. The patient can keep the mouth fresh by sucking on hard candy or chewing gum. If a mouthwash is used, the patient should avoid alcohol-based products as they cause drying of the oral mucosa that can lead to soreness, in turn altering ability to take in nutrients. A strategy to address nausea at home is crucial for maintenance of nutrition. The physician will need to prescribe anti-emetics for the patient during chemotherapy, and there are a variety of medications available, including Reglan, Zofran, and Compazine. These should be taken prophylactically before meals, and a regimen that includes medications, diet, and relaxation methods in the home is more likely to be successful. Instruct the patient to maintain a supply of foods recommended by the nutritionist or nurse that can decrease the likelihood of nausea/vomiting, such as crackers, hard candy, gelatin, etc. Provide the patient with a list of foods that can provide good sources of the required nutrients and minimize nausea. A diet rich in protein is advised, and the patient will need to have sufficient amounts to provide a source of energy, as fatigue will be a persistent problem. Significant others and family members play a role in implementing strategies to improve nutrition by preparing meals and encouraging the patient to ingest them. Frequent small meals at home should be encouraged for the patient in order to increase the likelihood that the patient can ingest enough nutrients. Because the dietary recommendations may be easily forgotten, a handy, laminated reference guide can be created to give to the patient or family. This guide could include a list of foods that provide protein, foods that minimize nausea or bloating, foods that provide iron, foods to avoid because of risk for nausea/vomiting, foods that are acceptable, and a schedule for small meals. Supplemental drinks can improve nutritional status during periods when the patient is unable to ingest adequate amounts of nutrition through normal meals due to anorexia, vomiting, abdominal pain, or malaise. There are numerous products on the market (Boost, Ensure, and Resource®) but the patient may need to experiment with which ones are satisfying or appealing after consultation with the dietician. A less expensive, nutritious milkshake can be made with a kitchen blender using low-fat ice cream and skim milk. The patient may need to take multivitamins or electrolyte supplements until the nutritional status stabilizes and treatment is complete. Teach the patient to monitor nutrition/intake by keeping a log of food eaten, when eaten, and how tolerated, noting any nausea or vomiting. If at any time a particular meal or food product causes nausea or vomiting, the patient should note this in the log and eliminate this food from the diet. Weights should also be included in the log. Even though the patient may not want to weigh every day, weighing at least every other day is a good way to keep track of weight loss or stabilization. This information can be shared with the health care provider at each follow-up visit to provide data for revision in prescribed therapeutic interventions. Follow-up providers should assess the patient for weight loss and monitor laboratory results for improvement in nutritional status.

Documentation

Chart the patient's weight daily. Document any difficulty that the patient experiences during meals, particularly nausea or vomiting, and any interventions (anti-emetics or other) implemented to address them. If the patient verbalizes complaints or concerns, such as inability to taste foods, document this in the chart. Record intake and output according to agency protocol, being sure to document the percentage of food consumed. Always document any referrals made to other disciplines, particularly the dietician. Document teaching done to address nutritional needs and whether the patient has understood.

NURSING DIAGNOSIS 4

INEFFECTIVE PROTECTION

Related to:
  Chemotherapy
  Stem cell transplant
  Immunosuppression
  Bone marrow suppression

Defining Characteristics:
  Fatigue
  Decreased hemoglobin (Hgb) and hematocrit (Hct)
  Leukocytosis
  Decreased platelets
  Easy bruising
  Prolonged bleeding
  Blood in stool or emesis

Goal:
  The patient will have no infection or bleeding.

Outcome Criteria

✔ The patient will not experience bleeding or bruising.

✔ The patient will have no signs or symptoms of infections (urinary, respiratory, central access sites, skin areas).

✔ The patient will verbalize an understanding of the necessary precautions needed to prevent bleeding, infection, and injury.

NOC *Blood coagulation*
       Immune status
       Knowledge: Infection control
       Risk control

INTERVENTIONS	RATIONALES
Monitor WBCs, RBCs, Hgb, Hct, and platelets, as ordered.	Helps to detect abnormalities that place the patient at risk for injury and infection. The number and type of WBCs required to fight infection are decreased in lymphoma and further decreases occur during treatment with chemotherapy. Anemia is common in chemotherapy patients, and measures of RBC, Hgb, and Hct indicate severity. Fewer RBCs are produced due to bone marrow suppression secondary to chemotherapy. Platelets are decreased, placing the patient at high risk for bleeding.

INTERVENTIONS	RATIONALES
Assess for fatigue, weakness, shortness of breath, and any alteration in mental status.	These symptoms occur due to the body's inability to transport enough oxygen to tissues secondary to decreased RBC and iron.
Monitor for indicators of bleeding abnormalities: bruising, easy bleeding, blood in emesis or stool, petechiae, bleeding gums, nosebleed, and purpura.	These indicate that the body is unable to clot effectively, and further examination and interventions may be warranted to prevent complications.
Test any emesis or stool for blood.	Helps to detect bleeding not recognizable through observation.
Avoid the use of aspirin or aspirin-containing products.	These products increase the risk of bleeding.
Avoid excessive venipuncture or injections to the extent possible, and apply pressure to all puncture sites.	Due to thrombocytopenia, the patient bleeds easily, and pressure is required to effectively stop bleeding. At least 5 minutes may be required.
Brush teeth with a soft-bristle toothbrush.	Gums tend to bleed easily due to altered clotting factors and decreased platelets; a soft brush is needed to decrease the risk of bleeding from the gums.
Monitor for signs of infection: fever; redness or other discoloration; drainage or heat at any wound or intravenous (IV) access insertion site; urine for malodor, mucous; oral cavity for white coating; respiratory system for cough, sputum production, or crackles in lungs; notify physician if any are noted.	With bone marrow suppression and decreased numbers of neutrophils, the patient is at higher risk for infection. A fever may be the only sign of infection, as the patient is unable to produce the normal inflammatory response due to immunosuppression.
Administer platelets.	When platelet counts decrease below set parameters, platelet administration is required.
Practice good hand hygiene.	Handwashing is one of the best ways to stop the transmission of infection.
Have the patient avoid crowds.	Being in crowds increases the patient's risk of acquiring respiratory infections.
The hospitalized patient should be placed in protective isolation or on neutropenic precautions when cell counts decrease, according to agency protocol: no raw fruit and vegetables, no fresh	Helps to protect the patient from infection.

flowers, all visitors wash hands before entering room, both visitors and health care providers wear a mask in the room.	
Increase iron-rich foods in diet.	Helps to increase oxygen-carrying capacity of RBCs.
Change any dressings over central line access sites in accordance with agency protocol using strict sterile technique.	Central lines are an easy portal for entry of organisms. Strict sterile technique is required to reduce risk for infection.
Administer antibiotics, as ordered.	Helps to prevent or treat infection.
Teach the patient safety precautions required to prevent falls, bleeding, and infection.	The patient needs to be informed in order to practice health promotion and disease prevention behaviors.

NIC *Bleeding precautions*
Risk identification
Self-care assistance
Surveillance

Evaluation

Evaluate whether outcome criteria have been met. The patient should have no bleeding; any bleeding that does occur should be detected and treated early. Infections have been prevented as demonstrated by the absence of signs and symptoms. The patient ambulates with assistance and sustains no injury. At time of discharge from the health care agency, the patient is able to verbalize safety precautions required.

Community/Home Care

The patient being treated for lymphoma will remain at risk for ineffective protection throughout treatment. Once at home, the patient will need to continue to practice safety-enhancing behaviors for bleeding, physical injury, and infections. The patient must be vigilant in preventing or controlling bleeding promptly if it occurs, preventing falls, and implementing strategies to protect self from injuries resulting from bumping into objects, such as bruising or disruption of skin. Strategies may include rearranging furniture or removing rugs to make walking areas clear. Because the patient is prone to fatigue, assistance with ambulation or activities requiring mental alertness, such as operating machinery or driving, may need to be restricted. Dietary interventions that can assist the patient with energy levels can prevent some of the fatigue caused by decreased RBCs and subsequent impaired oxygen transport. Foods rich in iron should be encouraged, taking into consideration the patient's likes/dislikes, culture, religion, and dietary restrictions. In cases of neutropenia, the diet should restrict raw fruits and vegetables (good sources of iron and electrolytes); the dietician should make dietary recommendations only after a thorough consult with the patient and, if possible, a significant other or family member. At home, the patient should use electric razors for shaving, as even a small nick from a disposable straight razor can cause significant free bleeding. Dental floss should be waxed for easier sliding and prevention of trauma to gums, and a soft-bristle toothbrush is always required. Women should note changes in menstrual cycle that would indicate more profuse bleeding, such as a significant increase in numbers of pads or tampons used and the passage of clots. If bleeding is noted in stools, emesis, or from any orifice or wound, the health care provider should be notified for prompt treatment. The patient with lymphoma will need to avoid large crowds or activities that may increase risk for infection. Handshaking can be the source of transmission of organisms; if possible, the patient should refrain from handshaking, and if it does occur, the patient should wash his or her hands as soon as possible. The patient and primary caregivers should avoid being near any person coughing or presenting symptoms of respiratory infection. Thorough and frequent handwashing by the patient and caregiver can minimize the risk of infection. Visitors should also wash their hands when they enter the home prior to contact with the patient. Patients with young children or grandchildren should avoid them if possible when they are sick with colds or the flu. Teach the patient to take his or her temperature and to record it daily. At the first sign of infection, the patient should return to a health care provider for further assistance.

Documentation

Include in the documentation findings from a thorough assessment of the patient for evidence of bleeding such as bruises, bleeding gums, bleeding from access sites, etc. In addition, document the patient's activity level and response to activity

(fatigue, dizziness). If the patient has any signs of infection, even minor ones, document this in the patient record with a clear indication of what actions were carried out in response. Temperatures should be taken at least every 4 hours and recorded according to agency protocol. Chart all interventions implemented to address safety, bleeding, and prevention of infections. If teaching is implemented, include who the learners were and their level of understanding.

NURSING DIAGNOSIS 5

 FATIGUE

Related to:

Disease process

Defining Characteristics:

Lethargy

Verbalization of being tired

States a lack of energy

Inability to carry out normal activities without becoming exhausted

Goal:

Fatigue will be relieved.

Outcome Criteria

✔ The patient is able to perform activities of daily living (ADLs).

✔ The patient verbalizes that fatigue has improved or been eliminated.

NOC *Activity tolerance*
Endurance
Energy conservation
Nutritional status: Energy

INTERVENTIONS	RATIONALES
Obtain subjective data about normal activities, limitations, and nighttime sleep patterns.	Helps to determine the effect fatigue has on normal functioning. Adequate sleep is required for restoration of the body.

INTERVENTIONS	RATIONALES
Monitor the patient for signs of excessive physical and emotional fatigue.	Use as a guideline for adjusting activity.
Encourage periods of rest and activity.	Helps to maintain oxygen reserves and limit energy expenditure; fatigue is a side effect of all types of chemotherapy and radiation.
Space planned activities away from mealtimes.	Digestion requires energy and oxygen. Participation in activities close to meals will cause increased fatigue because of insufficient energy reserves.
Encourage the patient to plan activities at times of greatest energy, usually early in the day.	Helps to prevent fatigue.
Gradually increase activity, as tolerated.	When treatment is complete, fatigue improves, but the patient may still require activity restrictions; monitoring tolerance to activity can provide information to indicate when activity may be increased or decreased. If any particular activity causes undue fatigue, it should not be attempted again until later in the recovery period.
Limit visitors during any periods of acute illness.	Socialization for long periods may cause fatigue.
Increase intake of high-energy foods such as poultry, dried beans and peas, whole grains, and foods high in vitamin C, as well as adequate to liberal amounts of fluids within restrictions of the recommended diet.	These foods enhance energy metabolism, increase oxygen-carrying capacity, and provide ready sources of energy. High-carbohydrate foods help maintain glycogen stores required for energy, and increased fluids enhance excretion of metabolic wastes that can cause the patient to feel tired.
Explore diversional activities with the patient and encourage quiet activities, such as reading, playing games, watching television/movies, doing crossword puzzles, etc.	Lymphoma goes into remission for 75 percent of patients, but resolution may take an extended period of time, and because the recovery period from chemotherapy or radiation may be extended, the patient needs methods to alleviate boredom.
Assist the patient in identifying community resources that can be of assistance with daily activities such as housekeeping, laundry, and preparing meals.	A number of community resources are available to the chronically ill and/or disabled.
Assist the patient in developing a home schedule to minimize energy expenditure.	This will help the patient retain some independence while being cognizant of limitations and need for energy conservation.

NIC *Energy management*

Evaluation

Obtain subjective information from the patient about the presence of fatigue. The patient should gradually report the ability to participate in ADLs and other normal activities with no fatigue.

Community/Home Care

Patients with lymphoma should understand that fatigue might persist for an extended period of time from diagnosis through the treatment period. Appropriate education on ways to adapt self-care and household activities when the patient is fatigued is paramount. A history should be obtained from the patient about his or her usual routine for work, school, ADLs, and household chores so that individualized interventions can be implemented. Attention to what the patient normally does and how the patient wants to make adaptations can only enhance compliance. On days that the patient receives chemotherapy or radiation, the performance of even light activities will be limited due to fatigue. The nurse must remain aware of cultural backgrounds that may influence a patient's perception of and adaptation to perceived dependency on others. The patient must understand how to adjust activity in response to feelings of fatigue, possibly even arranging for rest or nap periods in the afternoon. This may not be a realistic recommendation for people who continue to work and whose occupations preclude them from napping or even resting during the day. Strategies to enhance nighttime sleep should be implemented so that the patient can get adequate rest. Attention to good nutrition that can improve energy levels should continue with intake of foods that are good sources of iron, vitamin C, and protein within any dietary restrictions. The patient will need to return to the health care provider for evaluation of overall health status and resolution of symptoms.

Documentation

Chart the specific complaint of fatigue, including activities the patient has been performing. Record the patient's response to activity, including pulse, blood pressure, and any exertional dyspnea. Describe the type of assistance the patient requires when performing ADLs. Document interventions implemented to address fatigue, being sure to document food intake. Include in the record the patient's particular verbalization of the degree of fatigue and response to treatment. An assessment of the patient's sleep patterns should also be documented. Be sure to document teaching implemented with the family.

NURSING DIAGNOSIS 6

 ## RISK FOR IMPAIRED SKIN INTEGRITY

Related to:

Effect of Hodgkin's lymphoma: Pruritus

Defining Characteristics:

None

Goal:

The patient's skin will remain intact.

Outcome Criteria

✔ The patient will report that itching has been relieved.

✔ Skin will be moist.

✔ No breakdown will occur.

NOC *Tissue integrity: Skin and mucous membranes*

INTERVENTIONS	RATIONALES
Assess the patient for itching and ask to describe.	Patients with Hodgkin's lymphoma experience itching that is described as severe.
Discourage the patient from vigorous scratching and encourage to keep nails short.	Scratching can cause disruption to the skin that can lead to lesions difficult to heal.

INTERVENTIONS	RATIONALES
Apply moisturizing products to the skin: oil-based lotions, petroleum jelly, and oatmeal or oil-based shower gels or lotions. Avoid products containing alcohol or perfume and deodorant soaps.	These products add moisture back to the skin and ease the itching. Alcohol-based products and most deodorant soaps cause further drying of the skin.
Instruct the patient to bathe in tepid rather than hot water.	Hot water increases pruritus.
Instruct the patient to apply lotions before completely drying the skin following a shower or bath.	Vigorous rubbing or drying of the skin following a bath closes skin pores yielding emollients ineffective.
Lower room temperature, especially at night.	Excessive warmth increases itching.
Administer Benadryl or Atarax, as ordered.	Both medications relieve itching.
Encourage the use of distraction or relaxation therapy.	These will help change the perception of the itching and discomfort.

NIC *Skin care: Topical treatments*
Skin surveillance

Evaluation

Determine whether the stated outcome criteria have been achieved. The patient should report decreased itching, and the skin should be intact. Skin is moist without scaliness.

Community/Home Care

In the home setting, the patient will continue implementation of the interventions initiated by the nursing staff. The intensity of the pruritus will vary from time to time. Any personal care items such as soap, shower gels, lotions, or deodorants that contain alcohol or perfume should be avoided, as they cause excessive dryness of the skin. The patient will need to experiment with a number of measures or products to relieve the itching. If the patient does not want to cut nails short, he or she should sleep in gloves to prevent scratching during sleep. Placing a thin cloth over the itchy spot and rubbing gently or rubbing with gloves on can also relieve mild itching. It is important that the patient pay attention to environmental factors at home that may contribute to itching, such as room temperature, types of linens used (coarse cotton sheets may increase itching, whereas flannel sheets may feel better), household cleaning products, and hand soaps, which all can worsen the condition. The patient or family members should inspect the skin for open areas, edema, or bruising on a regular basis so that early treatment to prevent disruption of the skin can be instituted. Bruised skin (due to decreased platelets) that also itches is a prime area for breakdown and needs to be protected from further injury at home. The patient should be clear on when to take medications for itching and be aware that medicines such as Benadryl may cause drowsiness that limits the ability to engage in activities requiring alertness.

Documentation

Chart any complaints of itching and interventions employed to treat it. If medications are given, document them on the medication record according to agency protocol, with follow-up documentation about the patient's response. Any abnormalities in the skin, including evidence of abnormal bleeding or breakdown, should be included in the documented assessment findings. Document education provided about skin impairment and suggested treatments.

CHAPTER 7.100

SICKLE CELL ANEMIA

GENERAL INFORMATION

Sickle cell anemia is a genetically determined anemia caused by an autosomal recessive disorder. Red blood cells (RBCs) contain > 50 percent of their hemoglobin (Hgb) in the form of hemoglobin S. The name "sickle cell" is derived from the shape of the red blood cells, which is "sickled." These cells carry normal amounts of Hgb but have a tendency to clump together because of their shape. Sickle cell anemia is classified as a hemolytic anemia because the process of sickling causes RBCs to be viewed as abnormal by macrophages in the spleen, liver, and circulatory system. Consequently, the RBC lifespan is decreased because of early hemolysis (destruction) by macrophages. Under conditions of decreased oxygen, tension in the blood, such as hypoxia, dehydration, and acidosis the Hgb S causes the RBCs to lose their ability to squeeze flexibly through capillary beds, resulting in clumping, vascular occlusion, ischemia, inflammation, intense pain, and potential infarction of affected tissues. When this happens it manifests itself in severe pain, often in joints and the abdomen and is classified as a sickle cell crisis. Common sites of obstruction in adults are the large joints of the shoulder, hip and knee, the long bones, and the lumbar spine. Clinical manifestations of sickle cell anemia include symptoms of anemia such as fatigue, pallor, dyspnea, tachycardia, and rapid respirations with exertion. The disease is not curable, and long-term complications due to repeated infarctions and obstructions are possible including destruction of hip and knee joints that may require surgical replacement. The disease occurs most often in African Americans or people of African descent, with a rate of 1 in 600 births. Most children are screened as newborns as part of well-child checks, with 40 states requiring the screening.

NURSING DIAGNOSIS 1

 INEFFECTIVE TISSUE PERFUSION: PERIPHERAL AND GASTROINTESTINAL

Related to:

Clumping of RBCs

Sickled cells

Obstruction of blood flow

Defining Characteristics:

Joint pain

Pallor

Prolonged capillary refill

Edema

Warmth over joints

Reddened, tender joints

Abdominal pain

Difficulty walking

Goal:

The patient will have effective tissue perfusion.

Outcome Criteria

✔ Peripheral pulses are strong.

✔ Capillary refill will be < 2 seconds.

✔ Skin will be warm and dry.

✔ The patient will verbalize that mobility has improved.

NOC *Tissue perfusion: Peripheral*

Tissue perfusion: Abdominal organs

INTERVENTIONS	RATIONALES
Assess for ineffective tissue perfusion: capillary refill, skin color, temperature, peripheral pulses, edema in extremities, abdominal pain, extremity joint pain, and ulcers on lower extremities.	Clumped sickled red cells are difficult to move through blood vessels, resulting in decreased circulation to the periphery and abdomen, with a subsequent decrease in oxygen to tissues. Ulcers on lower extremities are common due to ischemia.
Monitor laboratory tests: Hgb electrophoresis, serum bilirubin, arterial blood gases (ABGs), oxygen saturation, and complete blood cell counts (CBCs).	Hemoglobin electrophoresis is used to diagnose sickle cell anemia and determines the type of Hgb present and how much of each is present. In sickle cell anemia, 70 percent of the Hgb is Hgb S; serum bilirubin is elevated due to the removal/degradation of old, damaged, and abnormal RBCs by the liver and bone marrow; the heme part of the RBC is oxidized to bilirubin; ABG test assesses the patient's respiratory status and need for oxygen; oxygen saturation provides clues to the ability to perfuse tissues and often shows decreased oxygen; CBC provides information about the number of RBCs circulating and also white blood cell (WBC) counts, which can monitor for infection.
Administer humidified oxygen at a high flow, as ordered.	Oxygen administered at a high flow maximizes oxygen delivery to the cells.
Initiate intravenous (IV) fluid therapy, as ordered.	Hydration makes it easier for blood to move through vessels and can improve circulation in areas of vascular occlusion and diminish clumping of sickled cells.
Encourage fluid intake.	Fluids prevent increased blood viscosity.
Apply moist heat to affected joints in hands or legs.	Heat causes vasodilation that can improve circulation around areas of occlusion.
Administer RBC transfusions, as ordered.	Transfusing normally round cells that do not sickle decreases likelihood of clumping; increased numbers of normal cells improves oxygen-carrying ability.
If the patient smokes, encourage discontinuance or at least no smoking during symptomatic state.	Smoking causes vasoconstriction that worsens tissue perfusion, making it more difficult for cells to move through the circulation.
Monitor the patient for embolus: sudden pain, decreased color, and absent or diminished peripheral pulses.	Because of the viscosity of the blood due to sickling, emboli may occur.
Keep patient warm at all times, especially during cold months.	Cold causes vasoconstriction, which can precipitate a crisis.

NIC *Surveillance*
       Circulatory care
       Embolus precautions

Evaluation

Evaluate whether the outcome criteria have been met. The patient should have evidence of adequate tissue perfusion such as strong peripheral pulses, normal skin color, and normal capillary refill (< 2 seconds). There should be no evidence of inflammation of the joints of the hands or lower extremities. The patient is able to ambulate without complaints of pain in joints.

Community/Home Care

The patient with sickle cell anemia is treated as an outpatient unless experiencing an acute crisis. In-home considerations for peripheral tissue perfusion are focused on preventing increased blood viscosity. It is quite important that the patient implement strategies to increase fluid intake to at least 4 to 6 quarts each day. Although this may be challenging, the patient must be vigilant about its implementation. A schedule for intake can be developed that has the patient drinking every 2 hours unless sleeping. Favorite fluids can be placed in a water bottle, or small bottles of acceptable liquids can be purchased. Keeping these fluids handy can enhance the likelihood of reaching the fluid intake goal. Caffeinated beverages should only be taken occasionally because they tend to cause some degree of vasoconstriction. The patient will need to implement strategies to maintain warmth of extremities to promote vasodilation. In winter months, the patient can wear wool socks or tights, and inside the house wear slippers that keep the feet warm. The patient should monitor for signs of decreased peripheral perfusion, such as change in skin color, coolness of extremities, ulcers on lower extremities, and pain in joints. When symptoms are noted, the health care provider should be notified.

Documentation

Chart the findings from an assessment of peripheral tissue perfusion, including peripheral pulses, capillary refill, skin temperature, and color. Document any complaints of pain or discomfort, noting specific locations and intensity. All interventions implemented (IV fluids or transfusions) to treat or prevent ineffective peripheral tissue perfusion are documented.

NURSING DIAGNOSIS 2

ACUTE PAIN

Related to:

> Sickled, clumped RBCs
>
> Vascular occlusion
>
> Ischemia
>
> Infarction
>
> Necrosis

Defining Characteristics:

> Complaint of severe, sharp pain in head, lumbar spine, joints, abdomen
>
> Difficulty walking
>
> Tachycardia
>
> Hypertension
>
> Diaphoresis
>
> Facial grimace
>
> Guarding
>
> Pain upon movement

Goal:

> Pain will be alleviated.

Outcome Criteria

✔ The patient states that pain is resolved.

✔ Pain is rated < 5 on a 10-point scale

✔ The patient will verbalize that pain has been relieved 30 minutes after interventions.

✔ The patient will verbalize an understanding of what causes pain.

NOC *Pain level*
Pain control
Comfort level

INTERVENTIONS	RATIONALES
Assess for location, intensity, quality, duration, other signs of pain: inability to move joint, grimacing, facial expressions, audible expressions of pain, and guarding of affected area.	Pain is one of the characteristic findings in sickle cell anemia. Accurate assessments will assist in identifying areas of occlusion and can guide analgesic treatment.
Have the patient rate pain intensity using a pain rating scale.	Provides a more objective description of level of pain.
Assess status of affected area, including pain at site, tenderness to touch, temperature, and edema.	For validating signs of ineffective perfusion, which is the causative factor for pain (see nursing diagnosis "Ineffective Tissue Perfusion: Peripheral and Gastrointestinal").
Encourage bedrest but perform range of motion exercises on extremities.	Helps to decrease oxygen demand by tissues, which may decrease anaerobic metabolism and subsequent pain.
Elevate affected limbs above heart level.	Helps to decrease edema, promote circulation, and reduce pressure and pain.
Administer narcotic analgesics and anti-inflammatory agents as ordered for joint, back, and abdominal pain.	Narcotic analgesics produce vasodilation as well as narcotic/pain relief effects; anti-inflammatory agents decrease inflammation that can add to pain.
Apply moist, warm packs to abdomen and joints.	Warmth will cause vasodilation, which may reduce the obstruction and induce cellular oxygenation.
Administer hydroxyurea, as ordered.	This medication is thought to interfere with the sickling process by increasing the levels of fetal Hgb.
Administer non-narcotic/ non-aspirin analgesics, as ordered, for headache.	Aspirin products are not recommended in sickle cell disease because an acidotic pH (caused by aspirin) will increase sickling.
Encourage the use of non-pharmacological methods of pain relief, such as relaxation techniques, massage, music, distraction, and meditation.	These techniques enhance the effects of medications.

INTERVENTIONS	RATIONALES
During a crisis, initiate patient-controlled analgesia (PCA).	Helps to provide the patient with control over pain.
Consider administration of packed red cells, as ordered.	Packed red cells will increase the ratio of normal cells to sickled cells, which may reduce sickling and obstruction, resulting in relief of pain.
Implement strategies to increase fluid volume (see nursing diagnosis "Ineffective Tissue Perfusion").	Helps to decrease the viscosity of the blood to prevent occlusion that contributes to pain in joints.
Implement strategies to reduce anxiety such as staying with the patient, using relaxation techniques, and playing soft music.	Anxiety often intensifies the pain experience.
Assess effectiveness of interventions to relieve pain.	Helps to determine if interventions have been effective in relieving pain or if new strategies need to be employed.

NIC *Pain management*
Analgesic administration
Anxiety reduction

Evaluation

The patient is able to report that the pain has been reduced or alleviated following interventions. The patient should have no facial grimacing or other observable signs of discomfort. If the pain is controlled, the patient is able to participate in self-care activities and ambulate unassisted. The patient verbalizes that he or she can understand what is causing the pain in the joints.

Community/Home Care

The patient's pain should decrease once the ischemia of the vessels has been resolved; it does, however, remain as a constant threat to those with sickle cell anemia. Pain at home is usually managed with analgesics, fluid therapy, non-pharmacological agents, and in some cases hydroxyurea. Attempting to prevent a crisis is a keystone to pain management. The patient needs to be aware of intake and be sure to remain hydrated by drinking liberal amounts of water throughout the day. When engaging in activities that cause dehydration, such as exercising or working outside in the heat, the patient needs to take fluid breaks. It is important that water

or other liquids be readily available. If away from home, the patient should carry a water bottle. The patient needs to monitor response to pain medications and be able to identify those factors or positions that increase pain. In the home, the patient may find comfort in elevating the affected extremity when sitting and using a heating pad to promote comfort. The patient should deal with stressors by developing coping strategies that are effective in reducing stress and anxiety, as stress contributes to a sickle cell crisis. If the recommended interventions for pain relief are not working, the patient should seek follow-up care with the health care provider.

Documentation

Document in the patient's own words the description of the pain and rating of the level of pain. Include in the documentation assessments made relevant to the pain. Chart all interventions employed and the patient's responses. Document any medications given or IV fluids administered on the medication administration record or according to agency protocol.

NURSING DIAGNOSIS 3

ACTIVITY INTOLERANCE

Related to:
 Imbalance between oxygen supply and demand
 Decreased count of healthy RBCs

Defining Characteristics:
 Fatigue
 Weakness
 Pain with activity
 Exertional discomfort
 Dyspnea
 Abnormal heart rate or blood pressure in response to activity

Goal:
 The patient's activity level increases.

Outcome Criteria

✔ The patient will report the absence of fatigue, weakness, or pain with activity.

✔ The patient will perform activities without shortness of breath.

✔ Heart rate and blood pressure will return to base-line within 10 minutes of ceasing activity.

NOC *Activity tolerance*
Energy conservation
Endurance

INTERVENTIONS	RATIONALES
Assess heart rate, blood pressure, and respiratory rate before and after activity.	Activity intolerance can result in vital sign changes as the heart attempts to meet oxygen demands.
Assist with activities as needed and encourage patient to prioritize activities.	Helps to conserve energy and reduce oxygen demand; patient lacks enough oxygen-carrying capacity to supply oxygen to tissues during activities.
Pace activities, alternating periods of activity with periods of rest.	Helps to reduce oxygen demand by conserving energy.
Monitor response to activity (pulse, respiratory rate, oxygen saturation, and dyspnea).	Increased pulse and respirations along with dyspnea indicate an intolerance to the activity.
Instruct the patient to stop any activity that causes shortness of breath, chest pain, or dizziness.	These indicate intolerance to activity, and the level of activity being performed should be evaluated. If the heart rate does not slow after 4 minutes, this indicates cardiac decompensation.
If shortness of breath occurs, administer oxygen, as ordered.	Improves oxygenation and thus allows an increased activity level.
Encourage the patient to sleep 8 to 10 hours a night.	Sleep decreases oxygen requirements and restores the body.
Collaborate with other disciplines, such as physical therapy and respiratory therapy, as ordered, to assist with ambulation.	Respiratory therapy may need to provide oxygen when patient first starts an activity program, and physical therapy can assist with monitoring activity progression.
Administer iron, folate, and vitamin B_{12}, as ordered.	These supplements are required for hematopoiesis.
Administer erythropoietin, as ordered.	Helps to stimulate hematopoiesis.
Encourage foods rich in iron and folate.	Helps to improve oxygen-carrying capacity.
Prepare for transfusion of packed RBCs (as ordered).	Helps to increase oxygen-carrying capacity.

NIC *Activity therapy*
Energy management
Sleep enhancement

Evaluation

The patient is able to tolerate performance of self-care activities. The patient is able to walk short distances without fatigue, pain, or shortness of breath. The patient verbalizes an understanding of the need to progress activities gradually, restrict activity as needed, conserve energy, and monitor response to activity.

Community/Home Care

The patient may continue to experience some fatigue and intolerance to activity at home. The patient must understand how to continue progression of activities and how to adjust activity in response to pain, feelings of fatigue, or shortness of breath. Instructions should include specific activity goals, how to monitor response to activity, and how to conserve energy. Alternating periods of rest and activity will be needed at home to prevent fatigue and decrease oxygen demands. Home maintenance will require the patient to evaluate which activities or routines can be continued. The feasibility of returning to work should be explored with the patient. Immediately following a crisis, recovery at home prior to return to work is needed. The home environment is assessed for factors such as stairs and distance to the bathroom from the patient's usual place of rest. In the periods following a crisis, the patient may need to alter the environment and shorten the distance that he or she must walk by rearranging furniture and placing more frequently used or needed items (liquids, eyeglasses, tissues, remote control, medicines, etc.) close to his or her usual place of rest. In order to increase stamina and energy, the patient needs to increase foods that are good sources of iron, vitamin C, and protein. If the patient is unable to gradually increase activity, he or she should notify a health care provider.

Documentation

Document the specific recommendations made for the patient. When the patient attempts activity, document the exact activity and the patient's response to the activity. Chart vital signs and record pulse and respirations before and after activity. If the patient verbalizes any complaints of pain, fatigue, or shortness of breath, document these in the patient's own words and interventions carried out to obtain relief. Include in the record teaching provided to the patient on how to manage fatigue.

NURSING DIAGNOSIS 4

 ## DEFICIENT KNOWLEDGE

Related to:

Lack of information about sickle cell anemia and its treatment

Misinformation

Defining Characteristics:

Asks no questions

Has many questions/concerns

Has incorrect information

Anxiety about diagnosis

Goal:

The patient will understand sickle cell anemia and its treatment.

Outcome Criteria

✔ The patient verbalizes a willingness and desire to learn the necessary information.

✔ The patient verbalizes an understanding of sickle cell anemia.

✔ The patient verbalizes a willingness to be compliant with treatment recommendations.

✔ The patient verbalizes an understanding of recommendations for hydration and pain control.

NOC *Knowledge: Disease process*
Knowledge: Health behavior
Treatment behavior: Illness
or injury

INTERVENTIONS	RATIONALES
Assess the patient's readiness to learn (motivation, cognitive level, and physiological status).	The patient must be motivated to learn, have the capability to learn the content, and be free of distractions from learning such as pain, fatigue, shortness of breath, and emotional distress.
Assess what the patient already knows.	The patient may have some knowledge about sickle cell anemia, and teaching should begin with what the patient already knows.
Create a quiet environment conducive to learning.	Environmental noise can prevent the learner from focusing on what is being taught.
Teach incrementally starting with simple concepts first and progressing to more complex concepts.	The patient will learn and retain knowledge better when information is presented in small segments.
Teach the learners about the normal function of the RBCs, vitamin B_{12}, folic acid, iron, and bone marrow.	Understanding of normal function helps the patient to understand the disease process.
Teach the patient about the disease process (pathophysiology) of sickle cell anemia and long-term complications.	Understanding the pathophysiology of sickle cell anemia will assist the patient to understand the rationale for therapeutic interventions.
Teach the patient about the pain of crisis (see nursing diagnosis "Acute Pain"): — Cause: sickling of cells that clump and are unable to move through vessels to perfuse tissues resulting in hypoxia leading to ischemia (lack of oxygen) of tissues, joints, and abdomen — Precipitating factors that cause hypoxia and crisis: dehydration, infection, emotional stress, fatigue, exposure to cold, strenuous exercise — Encourage the patient to avoid dehydration, infection, emotional stress, fatigue, cold, and strenuous exercise — Treatment: analgesics and hydroxyurea, supplements of iron, Vitamin B_{12} or folic acid, fluid therapy	If the patient understands the cause of a crisis/pain, he or she is more likely to comply. Medications attempt to decrease the number and severity of crisis episodes. Folic acid helps restore folic acid levels that improve RBC production in the marrow.
Teach the patient the importance of adequate fluid intake: drink liberally, 4 to 6 quarts daily.	Adequate amounts of fluid are needed to decrease viscosity of blood and reduce pain.
Instruct the patient on the risks of pregnancy and need for possible genetic counseling.	Patients with sickle cell anemia are at high risk for complications during pregnancy as oxygen demands of the body increase. In addition, the patient needs to

(continues)

(continued)

INTERVENTIONS	RATIONALES
	understand the genetic basis for sickle cell anemia prior to conceiving.
Provide the patient with information on the Sickle Cell Anemia Association or a local support group.	These entities can provide useful information about the disease and how to cope.
Evaluate the patient's understanding of all content covered by asking questions.	Helps to identify areas that require more teaching and to ensure that the patient has enough information to comply.
Give the patient written information on sickle cell anemia.	Provides reference at a later time, and for review.

NIC *Teaching: Disease process*
Teaching: Individual
Teaching: Prescribed medication

Evaluation

The patient is able to state what sickle cell anemia is and what causes it. The patient is able to repeat all information for the nurse and asks questions about sickle cell anemia, prognosis, and possible outcomes (positive and negative). The patient verbalizes an understanding of prescribed medications and fluid recommendations, and agrees to be compliant. The patient reports how to prevent or control the pain of crisis. The patient knows and can tell the nurse when health care assistance should be sought.

Community/Home Care

For patients who have sickle cell anemia, the therapeutic regimen is implemented in the home. Teaching by the health care team should be thorough, with opportunities for discussions. Knowledge needs are identified early in the disease process in order to improve the likelihood that the patient will be prepared for self-monitoring and prevention of complications from sickle cell anemia, such as limited mobility and repeated sickle cell crises. Successful education will allow the patient to address the issues of pain, tissue perfusion, and activity at home (see home care in nursing diagnoses "Ineffective Tissue Perfusion," "Acute Pain," and "Activity Intolerance"). Education focuses on creating a sense of control for the patient that will allow for continued quality of life and ability to participate in a relatively normal lifestyle. Further education may be needed; this should be ascertained in follow-up visits with the health care provider. A follow-up telephone call from the health care provider can assess whether the patient has understood the teaching. It is helpful to provide the patient with written information about sickle cell anemia that the patient can keep as a reference. Follow-up with a health care provider focuses on assurance that no complications have occurred and that the patient has a clear understanding of how to manage all aspects of sickle cell anemia, particularly pain.

Documentation

Document all content taught and the patient's verbalization of understanding. Specific attention should be given to documentation of any specific concerns that the patient expresses. Included in the documentation is the patient's willingness to comply with all recommendations made about hydration, pain control, prevention of crises, medication administration, and follow-up care. Any area that requires further teaching should be clearly indicated in the record. If family or significant others are present for teaching, document this in the patient chart. Include in the record appointments that have been made for outpatient visits, laboratory tests, or other procedures. Always include the titles of any printed literature given to the patient for reinforcement. If the patient is unable to comply with recommendations due to lack of resources, document this and any referrals made to social services for assistance.

CHAPTER 7.101

THROMBOCYTOPENIA

GENERAL INFORMATION

Thrombocytopenia is a disorder in which the platelet count is > 100,000 per cubic mm, placing an individual at high risk for abnormal bleeding. The causes for the decrease in platelet numbers can be categorized into several major groups: decreased platelet production, increased platelet destruction (most common), sequestration of platelets in the spleen, or increased platelet consumption. Acute idiopathic thrombocytopenia (ITP), caused by platelet destruction, is the most common type and occurs because of a viral illness. Chronic ITP is caused by an autoantibody reaction against a platelet antigen and is referred to as autoimmune thrombocytopenia purpura. Other causes of thrombocytopenia include medications, bone marrow suppression (as seen in chemotherapy), aplastic anemia, leukemia, cirrhosis, splenomegaly, hemorrhage, and disseminated intravascular coagulation (DIC). The decreased number of platelets leads to abnormal bleeding, which results in bleeding into the skin or other tissues. Bleeding risk escalates as the platelet count drops below 50,000 cubic mm, and the likelihood of spontaneous bleeding increases if the platelet count drops below 20,000 per cubic mm. Clinical manifestations include bruising, purpura, bleeding from the gums, increased bleeding with menses, and nosebleeds. Chronic ITP occurs more often in women in their 20s and 30s, and acute ITP occurs more often in children.

NURSING DIAGNOSIS 1

 INEFFECTIVE PROTECTION

Related to:

Destruction of platelets

Consumption of platelets

Sequestration of platelets in the spleen

Loss of platelets from hemorrhage

Defining Characteristics:

Decreased platelet count

Ecchymosis

Purpura

Nosebleeds

Menorrhagia

Hematuria

Blood in stool

Hematemesis

Petechiae

Goal:

The patient will not hemorrhage.

Outcome Criteria

✔ Platelet count will return to normal.

✔ Any patient bleeding will stop 10 minutes after interventions are implemented.

✔ The patient's vitals signs (blood pressure and pulse) will be within patient's baseline.

✔ The patient will not experience bleeding or bruising.

✔ The patient will verbalize an understanding of the necessary precautions needed to prevent bleeding and injury.

NOC *Blood coagulation*

Immune status

Risk control

INTERVENTIONS	RATIONALES
Monitor results of laboratory and diagnostic tests: platelets, APTT,	Platelets are monitored to assess the patient's risk for bleeding

(continues)

(continued)

INTERVENTIONS	RATIONALES
PT, vitamin K, and bone marrow aspiration.	and monitor response to therapy—the lower the platelet count, the higher the risk for bleeding; APTT and PT results provide additional evidence to assess the bleeding risk. Results of bone marrow examination give clues to exact cause (may demonstrate presence of the precursors to platelets, which means the problem is probably platelet destruction; the absence or decreased numbers of the precursors implies lack of production in the marrow).
Monitor for indicators of bleeding abnormalities: skin for bruising, petechiae, easy bleeding, menorrhagia, blood in emesis or stool, bleeding gums, nosebleed, and purpura.	These indicate that the body is unable to clot effectively, and further examination and interventions may be warranted to prevent complications. Due to decreases in platelets, vascular sites bleed easily.
Assess for intracranial bleeding by evaluating level of consciousness, changes in mental status such as restlessness or agitation, pupillary equality and reaction to light, presence of headaches, and Cushing's triad (slowed respirations, bradycardia, rising systolic blood pressure).	The brain is very vascular and vulnerable to bleeding, especially when the platelet count is < 20,000.
During menses, assess for excess vaginal bleeding by counting pads or tampons.	Menses may be heavy in patients with thrombocytopenia.
Take vital signs at least every 4 hours; if bleeding occurs, monitor for signs of fluid volume deficit: tachycardia, decreased blood pressure, change in mental status, decreased hemoglobin (Hgb) and hematocrit (Hct), and report to physician.	The patient may exhibit signs of hemorrhagic shock: decreased blood pressure and increased pulse due to loss of volume are compensatory mechanisms. If bleeding is profuse, the patient may show signs of cardiac compensation in an effort to maintain perfusion to vital organs by increasing heart rate; blood pressure drops because of decreased circulating volume; changes in mental status indicate decreased perfusion to cerebral tissue.
Test any emesis or stool for blood by guaiac test.	Helps to detect bleeding not recognizable through observation.
Administer corticosteroids, as ordered.	Helps to decrease antibody production by suppressing the autoimmune response.
Prepare the patient for platelet transfusion in patients who are bleeding acutely.	Based on platelet counts, the patient may require platelets to help control active bleeding. Platelets are used frequently in secondary thrombocytopenia but may not be as useful in disorders caused by destruction of platelets as the infused platelets will also be destroyed.
Encourage intake of soft diet.	Helps to avoid trauma to the mucous membranes of the mouth.
Avoid hot foods and liquids.	Heat causes vasodilation that may increase bleeding.
Administer stool softeners.	Helps to prevent constipation and straining to pass hard stools that increases the risk of rectal bleeding.
Encourage the use of electric razors to shave.	Helps to decrease bleeding from shaving nicks.
Avoid injections if possible, but if puncture sites are necessary, apply pressure for 5 minutes.	Lack of sufficient platelets for clotting predisposes the patient to bleeding even from simple procedures, and pressure is required to effectively stop bleeding; pressure also provides time for coagulation factors to accumulate and stop the hemorrhage.
Apply ice to bleeding sites.	Ice causes vasoconstriction and decreases hemorrhage.
Brush teeth with soft-bristle toothbrush.	Gums tend to bleed easily due to altered clotting factors; a soft toothbrush prevents trauma to gums that could cause bleeding.
Assist patient with careful ambulation and other activities.	Due to weakness and fatigue, the patient is at higher risk for falls and bumping into objects, which may cause bruising.
If interventions are not successful, prepare patient for splenectomy as directed or in accordance with agency policies.	One of the spleen's normal functions is to destroy platelets. Platelets that are antibody-coated (ITP) function normally, but the spleen reacts to the antibody as if it were a foreign substance and destroys the platelet prematurely. Removal of the spleen cures the disease.

INTERVENTIONS	RATIONALES
Teach the patient and family about all interventions needed to prevent or control bleeding, and also about safety precautions.	Providing information can decrease anxiety; the patient needs to be informed in order to comply with regimen.
Educate the patient on the disease of thrombocytopenia, treatments, and complications.	Knowledge enhances reduction of anxiety and allows the patient to understand health status.

NIC *Bleeding precautions*
Risk identification
Surveillance

Evaluation

Evaluate whether outcome criteria have been met. The patient should have no bleeding; if bleeding does occur, it is detected and treated early. Vital signs have returned to the patient's baseline. Platelet counts improve, petechiae resolve, no injuries occur, and bruising is avoided. The patient ambulates and performs usual activities without injury. At time of discharge from the health care agency, the patient is able to verbalize safety precautions required.

Community/Home Care

The patient with thrombocytopenia will always be at risk for ineffective protection unless the disease progression is halted. Once at home, the patient will need to continue to practice safety-enhancing behaviors for bleeding and physical injury. The patient must be vigilant in preventing or controlling bleeding promptly if it occurs, as well as preventing falls. Implementing strategies to protect self from injury, such as bumping into objects that may cause bruising or disruption of skin, is important. This may include rearranging furniture or removing rugs to make walking areas clear. The patient will need to avoid strenuous activities, as directed by the physician, due to risk for injury. Those treating the patient for thrombocytopenia should review the patient's medications to ascertain if any could be increasing the risk for bleeding, such as steroidal inhalers, aspirin, or aspirin-containing products, which many people take for cardiovascular prophylaxis or arthritis.

Simple instructions regarding hygienic practices include reminding all patients (male and female) to shave with electric razors, to brush teeth using a soft-bristle toothbrush, and to floss using the waxed type of dental floss. Women should take note of increased bleeding at time of menses each month, which can occur due to the absence of adequate amounts of platelets. The patient is taught to apply pressure or a bandage to any injury site regardless of how minor it may appear. If spontaneous bleeding should occur, if bleeding is noted in stools, or if the patient starts to vomit blood, health care assistance should be sought for prompt treatment. The patient with thrombocytopenia should also inform health care providers such as dentists and podiatrists of the disorder so that precautions against bleeding can be taken during any procedures.

Documentation

Include in the documentation findings from a thorough assessment of the patient for evidence of bleeding, such as bruises, petechiae, bleeding gums, bleeding from access sites, etc. In addition, chart the presence or absence of bleeding, with an estimation of amount. If medical interventions such as platelet transfusion are implemented, document this according to agency protocol, as well as all nursing assessments and interventions employed. Document the results of tests for blood done on emesis, urine, or stool. All other interventions and patient responses should be included in the patient record as specifically as possible. Blood pressure and pulse readings that indicate cardiac response to bleeding should be documented. In addition, document the patient's activity level and response to activity (fatigue, dizziness). If teaching is implemented, include who the learners were, what was taught, and their level of understanding.

NURSING DIAGNOSIS 2

 DEFICIENT FLUID VOLUME

Related to:

Hemorrhage

Insufficient platelets for clotting

Defining Characteristics:

Hypotension with tachycardia

Postural hypotension

Pale, cool, clammy skin

Delayed capillary refill

Dry mucous membranes

Urine output < 30 ml/hour

Bleeding manifestations

Goal:

The patient will have fluid volume restored.

Outcome Criteria

✔ The patient will have blood pressure at baseline.

✔ Pulse will be < 100.

✔ The patient will have no evidence of bleeding.

✔ Skin will be warm and dry with good turgor.

NOC *Hydration*
Fluid balance
Vital signs

INTERVENTIONS	RATIONALES
Assess for signs of volume deficit: decreased blood pressure, narrowing pulse pressure, restlessness, increased pulse, dry mucous membranes, and decreased urinary output.	Helps to determine the seriousness of the problem, to guide treatment, and to assess effectiveness of treatments.
Establish intravenous (IV) access and initiate IV fluids, as ordered.	Helps to replenish fluid volume lost due to hemorrhage.
Monitor cardiac status: blood pressure, pulse (quality and rate), pulse pressure, and capillary refill; take vital signs at least every 4 hours or more often, as ordered.	Cardiac output may decrease, as fluids are lost from the circulating volume and changes in blood pressure and pulse give information relevant to changes in cardiac status; blood pressure decreases and the pulse increases; capillary refill will be an indicator of perfusion, and in the presence of bleeding, refill time will be prolonged.
Monitor skin temperature and color for baseline and during treatment for improvement.	Pale, cool, clammy skin indicates decreased perfusion. As treatment progresses, skin should be warm and return to normal color.

Monitor oxygen saturation using pulse oximetry.	Oxygen saturation is a way to assess ability to perfuse tissues.
Monitor and record intake and output.	Monitors fluid balance. Output < 30 ml/hour may suggest impaired renal perfusion and should be reported to the physician.
Establish IV access and administer platelets, as ordered.	Platelets are needed to correct the underlying problem (bleeding due to inadequate platelet aggregation for clotting) that is causing the volume deficit.

NIC *Hypovolemia management*
Intravenous therapy
Blood products administration
Fluid monitoring

Evaluation

Assess the patient for return of normal fluid volume. The patient's blood pressure and pulse should return to baseline. The pulse should be strong and regular and at the patient's baseline or only slightly increased. Skin should be warm, and color should return to the patient's normal appearance. Mucous membranes are moist. Renal function should not be impaired, with an hourly output on the average of 30 ml/hour. Bleeding is controlled, and platelet count has improved.

Community/Home Care

Patients treated for deficient fluid volume due to hemorrhage should have normal fluid status restored within a short period. At home, the patient may not require any follow-up as this is an acute situation that is corrected before exiting the health care institution. Rather, attention is given to educating the patient about how to prevent or control bleeding (see nursing diagnosis "Ineffective Protection"). The patient will need to carry out assessments for bleeding by examining stool and urine as well as inspecting oral mucous membranes for blood. Women should take note of increases in pad or tampon use during menses that can be easily overlooked until signs of volume depletion occur. The patient will need to drink adequate amounts of fluid so that sufficient volume is available for tissues. Fatigue may need to be addressed at home, and can be handled by informing the patient to perform activities as tolerated until stamina/endurance is re-established. The health care provider may want the patient to return for a follow-up appointment to ensure that parameters such as platelets and Hct have returned to normal.

Documentation

Document initial assessment findings relevant to hydration status, such as mucous membranes, blood pressure, pulse, respirations, temperature, breath sounds, skin status, and mental status. Document all interventions, such as intravenous catheter insertion, fluids initiated (type, rate), and urinary output, with a description of urine (amount, color). Always include in the patient record specific information regarding any bleeding and methods used to control it. Chart intake and output in accordance with agency protocol but at least every 8 hours. Be specific when charting patient responses to treatment so that other health care providers can clearly determine improvement or deterioration.

CHAPTER 7.102

TRANSFUSION

GENERAL INFORMATION

Transfusion of whole blood or packed red blood cells (RBCs) may be ordered for a variety of reasons. Whole blood is usually transfused in patients who require replacement of volume to maintain cardiac output. These patients frequently have lost blood due to hemorrhage and need to receive a large amount of blood. If the patient receives more than 50 percent of his or her total estimated blood volume over a three-hour period or less, it is considered a massive transfusion. RBCs are infused in patients who are not necessarily volume-depleted but rather require cell replacement for oxygen transport. In some instances, the patient has minimal blood loss as is seen post-surgery or with monthly menses. For other patients, RBCs are needed due to impairments of RBC production, low hemoglobin (Hgb) levels, or destruction such as occurs in patients with certain cancers, anemias, and renal disease. Other blood components that can be infused include fresh frozen plasma, platelets, and salt-poor albumin. Transfusions require that the recipient is typed to determine blood type and Rh factor in order to ensure that the blood received matches the patient's own. There are three types of transfusions: autologous, in which the patient donates his or her own blood for future use; homologous, in which the patient receives blood from another person; and directed, in which the donor donates blood for a specific person at a specific time. Blood that is banked may present the caregiver with a host of problems/complications added to the original condition for which the patient received blood. These problems/complications may include hypothermia, hyperkalemia, hypocalcemia, fluid overload, acidosis, and alkalosis.

NURSING DIAGNOSIS 1

 DEFICIENT KNOWLEDGE

Related to:

Transfusion

Defining Characteristics:

Has no prior experience with transfusion

Asks many questions

Asks no questions

Has misconceptions

Goal:

The patient will understand all aspects of blood transfusion.

Outcome Criteria

✔ The patient will verbalize an understanding of the blood donor process and transfusion process.

✔ The patient will verbalize an understanding of measures taken to decrease likelihood of transmission of diseases (hepatitis, HIV/AIDS) in blood supply.

✔ The patient verbalizes an understanding of signs and symptoms of a transfusion reaction.

NOC *Knowledge: Treatment procedure*

INTERVENTIONS	RATIONALES
Assess the patient's readiness and ability to learn (motivation, cognitive level, and physiological status).	The patient must be motivated to learn, have the capability to learn the content, be physiologically stable enough to learn, and be free from distractions such as pain or shortness of breath.
Assess what the patient already knows about blood transfusions.	Many people have some notion of transfusions but also have misconceptions. Teaching must begin with what the patient knows in order to dispel myths or misinformation.

INTERVENTIONS	RATIONALES
Determine whether the patient desires the transfusion of blood or blood products.	Even though the health care provider has recommended or prescribed blood, the patient may not want to receive it. Some religions (such as Jehovah's Witnesses) and cultures may forbid transfusions, and the patient may choose to forego the transfusion.
Inform the patient of why the transfusion is needed in his or her particular situation and how the type of solution to be administered will correct the problem.	An informed patient is better equipped in decisions regarding care and treatment; this also allays anxiety.
Explain how blood is screened for diseases prior to administration.	Many people are unclear as to how blood banks test blood for diseases such as HIV/AIDS, syphilis, and hepatitis, and perceive the risks to be higher than they are. The patient should know that all blood is tested for a variety of diseases when donated, but blood banks cannot ensure with 100 percent accuracy that the blood is disease-free. Providing information helps to reduce anxiety.
Teach the patient how the blood transfusion is actually carried out: — Blood is drawn for typing and crossmatching; correct match is located and the blood prepped — Establishment of intravenous (IV) access with normal saline started before the blood — Vital signs are taken before transfusion — Transfusion starts very slowly; nurse remains at the bedside for the first 15 minutes, and vital signs taken every 15 minutes for the first hour. — Monitoring during the transfusion for any reaction — Nurse should be notified in case of itching, rash, abdominal/back pain, flushing, or shortness of breath	Providing this step-by-step procedure will help the patient to understand exactly what will happen and allay anxiety about the process.
Inform the patient of blood type.	This is good information for the patient to have for future reference.
Instruct the patient to inform the nurse or health care provider if any signs or symptoms of a reaction (flushing, headache, backache, abdominal pain, shortness of breath, itching) occur, regardless of how minor the symptoms.	The patient will need to know what signs indicate a transfusion reaction or allergic reaction, which should be reported to a health care provider. The patient's prompt reporting allows rapid response to prevent serious complications.
Evaluate the patient's understanding of all information presented.	Helps to allow the patient to ask questions, and to determine that the patient understood the teaching.

NIC *Teaching: Procedure/treatment*

Evaluation

The patient verbalizes an understanding of the blood donation and screening process. The patient is able to repeat how the transfusion is carried out and why it is needed, as well as to state correctly the signs and symptoms of a transfusion reaction.

Community/Home Care

There are no specific community or home care knowledge needs specific to the transfusion. Any needs of the patient are likely related to the underlying disease process. Patients who have received transfusions should be given written information relevant to their blood type and what type of product they received. The patient can then file this information with other important papers or medical records for future reference. Instruct the patient to contact a health care provider if feeling faint or weak after returning home. Follow-up care is needed to determine that the problem that necessitated the transfusion has resolved or improved.

Documentation

Document the specific information on blood transfusions taught by the nurse, and the patient's verbalization of understanding. Include in the chart any patient questions or misunderstandings. Always document concerns, particularly any related to the receipt of blood and religious beliefs, and interventions employed to address them. If further teaching is required, document the specific information that needs reinforcement.

NURSING DIAGNOSIS 2

INEFFECTIVE PROTECTION

Related to:

Administration of blood or blood products

Defining Characteristics:

Elevated temperature and chills

Rash, hives, and itching

Shortness of breath

Crackles

Pain

Flushing

Goal:

The patient will be protected and treated promptly if transfusion reaction occurs.

Outcome Criteria

✔ The patient's temperature will remain in normal range.

✔ Blood pressure and pulse will be at patient's baseline.

✔ The patient does not experience fluid overload (no crackles or shortness of breath).

✔ The patient has no wheezing, flushing, or shortness of breath.

✔ The patient's skin will remain in its usual state, and any rashes, hives, or itching are relieved.

✔ Any reactions will be treated promptly with no long-term complications.

NOC *Blood transfusion reaction*

INTERVENTIONS	RATIONALES
Perform a history and physical prior to starting blood transfusion; inquire about previous receipt of blood or blood products and any reactions (minor or serious); assess respiratory rate, rhythm, and depth, as well as cardiac rate and rhythm, blood pressure, and capillary refill.	A history is needed to alert the nurse to the risk for reactions; if a patient has had a reaction in the past, especially febrile or allergic, he or she is likely to have another; the physical assessment establishes a baseline for comparison if a reaction occurs.
Check the patient's chart for the prescribed amount of blood and results of type and cross-matching.	The nurse needs to be sure of the number of units of blood and the type of blood.
Establish intravenous (IV) access with a large bore catheter, at least a #18 gauge.	Blood and blood products are viscous and require a large bore catheter to ensure proper flow rate; a smaller gauge catheter may cause significant hemolysis of RBC, which can cause the release of potassium and lead to hyperkalemia.
Administer any ordered medications, such as antihistamines or antipyretics.	If the patient has a history of febrile or allergic reactions, these medications are given prophylactically before the transfusion.
Obtain blood or RBCs, as ordered, and initiate transfusion: — Take vital signs before starting transfusion. — Check blood label for blood type and Rh compatibility, as well as expiration date, and compare to patient data. — Check recipient number, patient identification number, and compare to information on blood product; in most states, the nurse practice acts require two registered nurses for this activity. — Connect normal saline to blood administration set/tubing; connect to IV catheter and prime. — Connect blood to administration tubing and start infusion slowly, approximately 25 to 30 ml per hour for the first 15 minutes. — Take vital signs every 15 minutes for the first hour and every 30 minutes thereafter. — Stay with the patient for the first 15 minutes of the transfusion, or as agency requires. — Instruct the patient to notify the nurse if any abnormal symptoms occur.	Double-checking labels for correct type and patient is a safety measure to prevent errors; normal saline is the standard solution to be used for priming as it has no reaction with blood products, and if a reaction occurs, it will be needed to keep the IV line open; many reactions occur in the early part of the transfusion, and a change in vital signs may take place; staying with the patient allows for early detection and prompt treatment.
After the first 15 minutes, set the prescribed administration rate and check the infusion frequently to ensure that it is flowing properly.	In most instances, one unit of blood or packed RBCs should hang no longer than 4 hours. Hanging longer increases the risk of bacterial contamination.
Administer a diuretic such as Lasix, as ordered, following transfusion.	For elderly patients or those with a history of congestive heart failure, Lasix is given to prevent

INTERVENTIONS	RATIONALES
	fluid overload, the patient does not require volume but rather blood components, such as RBCs. Administration of Lasix is especially needed if multiple units are ordered.
Monitor the patient for a febrile reaction: abrupt onset of fever, chills, headache; if these symptoms occur, stop the infusion, begin normal saline IV, notify physician, implement orders (antipyretics and antihistamines), and follow agency protocol.	Febrile reactions are caused by a reaction to the donor's white blood cells (WBCs). If the patient has a history of febrile reactions, antipyretics and Demerol can be given before the transfusion to prevent the symptoms. Leukocyte-reduced blood components can be used in the future along with a special leukocyte filter.
Monitor the patient for an allergic reaction: rash, hives, itching, and flushing; if these symptoms occur, stop the infusion, begin normal saline, notify the physician, implement orders (antihistamines, epinephrine, and steroids), and follow agency protocol.	This type of reaction occurs due to sensitivity of the recipient to the donor's plasma protein. Some physicians may order Benadryl and continue the infusion at a slower rate in the absence of respiratory symptoms.
Monitor for the life-threatening hemolytic reaction: chills, fever, back pain, hypotension, tachycardia, blood in the urine, dyspnea, and facial flushing. If these symptoms occur, stop transfusion immediately, remove tubing from IV catheter, start normal saline at rapid rate, administer oxygen, notify physician, and implement orders such as insertion of urinary catheter; administer medications to raise blood pressure, assess vital signs every 15 minutes, and follow agency protocol. Obtain blood sample and save the unit of blood or RBCs; in many places tubing may be sent to the lab.	This type of reaction occurs due to the administration of incompatible blood and can be fatal. The reaction occurs almost immediately, which is why the nurse should stay with patients during the first 15 minutes of a transfusion.
Monitor the patient for signs of fluid overload: crackles in lungs and shortness of breath. If these symptoms occur, slow the infusion, dangle feet (place in dependent position), notify the physician, administer diuretics as ordered, and monitor response.	Fluid overload occurs if the amount of solution placed in the circulating volume cannot be handled by the cardiac system due to impaired left ventricular function, especially in patients with a history of congestive heart failure.
Inform patient and family of what is occurring if reactions occur.	Helps to decrease anxiety.
Monitor laboratory results for response to treatment: RBCs, Hgb, and Hct.	These laboratory indices should show improvement with administration of blood products.

NIC *Blood products administration*

Evaluation

The patient shows improvement in laboratory results such as Hgb, Hct, and RBCs. No reactions should occur, but if they do, they are treated promptly and no long-lasting effects are noted. The patient's vital signs are within baseline, with temperature at normal level or only slightly elevated. The patient offers no complaints of headache, chills, itching, or pain, etc.

Community/Home Care

There are no considerations for home care for the patient who has a transfusion. If problems are present, they can usually be attributed to the underlying disorder that dictated the transfusion. The one area that the patient needs to be attuned to is the effect of hospitalization on energy levels and ability to resume usual activities. Low energy is easily remedied by encouraging the patient to perform activities as tolerated and to rest as needed, maybe getting short periods of rest throughout the day. If reactions have occurred, the patient should remember what type of reaction he or she experienced so that this information can be shared with subsequent health care providers, especially in the event of future transfusions. The patient can write this on a note card to laminate and keep with insurance cards so that it is easily accessible.

Documentation

Include in the patient record all assessments made before, during, and after the transfusion, particularly vital signs. Document other information relevant to the transfusion as required by agency protocol; usually this includes charting the time the transfusion was started, the identification or unit number of the blood, the type of solution, the amount of solution, the time the transfusion was ended, and the patient's tolerance. If the patient has any type of reaction or any complaint, document a description of the reaction along with what measures were taken to resolve the symptoms, and the patient's status following treatment. If the transfusion is completed without incident, document this as well as the patient's vital signs.

UNIT 8

IMMUNOLOGICAL SYSTEM

CHAPTER 8.103

ACQUIRED IMMUNODEFICIENCY SYNDROME (AIDS)/HIV-POSITIVE

GENERAL INFORMATION

Acquired immunodeficiency syndrome (AIDS) is a disease caused by the human immunodeficiency virus (HIV) that produces profound immunosuppression. Not all HIV-positive patients have AIDS, but most progress to that syndrome. The human immunodeficiency virus is a retrovirus that affects T4 (T-helper) lymphocytes, macrophages, B-cells, and cells of vital body organs such as the brain, spleen, and lungs. HIV also affects the cells of the lymphatic system. AIDS is diagnosed by a CD_4 cell count < 200, whether symptomatic or asymptomatic. Because of the profound immunosuppressive effect, the patient is susceptible to a host of opportunistic infections such as pneumocystis carinii pneumonia, tuberculosis, cancers such as Kaposi's sarcoma, nutritional deficits (wasting syndrome), and neurological disorders such as AIDS encephalopathy. Transmission of the HIV virus occurs through contact with infected body fluids parenterally (injecting intravenous [IV] drugs with contaminated needles, incidental contact with contaminated needles), sexual contact, and contaminated transfused blood. HIV can also be transmitted to fetuses via the maternal-fetal blood barrier and to neonates via breastfeeding from an HIV-positive mother. It can also be contracted via contaminated blood or fluid exposure to a highly vascular mucosal area or disrupted skin. The high-risk population includes IV drug users, those who practice unprotected sex with HIV carriers or multiple sexual partners, those who receive blood transfusions (although this risk has been greatly reduced due to careful screening of donor blood), and health care workers who are accidentally exposed to the blood or fluid from an HIV-positive patient. Flu-like symptoms (malaise, fatigue, fever, sore throat) occur several weeks up to 6 months after infection, and last for approximately 1 to 2 weeks. Following this stage, the patient becomes HIV-positive and may have no symptoms of disease except persistent lymphadenopathy for as long as 10 to 15 years. Eventually the immune system becomes compromised due to attack by the virus, and a variety of clinical manifestations occur, including fever, night sweats, dyspnea, lethargy, anorexia, nausea, diarrhea, and candida. Numerous other disease entities and syndromes occur in the HIV/AIDS patient that complicate treatment regimens and affect patient outcomes. The largest-growing group of HIV-positive persons includes heterosexual women. In most recent statistics, African Americans and Hispanics account for over 54 percent of all cases of AIDS and more than 75 percent of all cases in women. More than half of all new HIV infections occur among African Americans. The care plan presented here represents only a few of the numerous nursing diagnoses, which are applicable to the patient with HIV/AIDS.

NURSING DIAGNOSIS 1

INFECTION*

Related to:

Invasion of body with human immunodeficiency virus (HIV)

Defining Characteristics:

Early disease:

Fever

Sore throat

Arthralgias

Enlarged lymph nodes

Headache

Nausea and vomiting

Night sweats

Later disease:

General malaise

Weight loss

Memory loss

Difficulty concentrating

Diarrhea

Decreased CD_4 cell count

Increased viral load

Goal:

The disease of AIDS stabilizes, and complications are minimized.

Outcome Criteria

✔ The patient is afebrile.

✔ The viral load decreases.

✔ The patient has no symptoms of opportunistic infections.

✔ Night sweats, arthralgias, headaches, nausea, vomiting, and diarrhea are controlled.

✔ There are no further decreases in CD_4 cell count.

NOC *Infection severity*

   Immune status

   Community risk control: Communicable disease

INTERVENTIONS	RATIONALES
Monitor diagnostic studies: ELISA (enzyme linked immunosorbent assay), Western immunoblot test, CD_4 levels, and HIV-RNA levels (viral loads).	The ELISA test is the most often used initial test for diagnosing AIDS/HIV and is very specific for detecting HIV antibodies. The antibody occurs approximately 6 to 12 weeks after exposure. Western immunoblot test is done to confirm the findings of a positive ELISA. CD_4 cell count will be decreased indicating the extent of the immunodeficiency, with CD_4 counts $< 200/mm^3$ indicating immunodeficiency. HIV RNA or viral load will be elevated and measures how much viral activity or replication of the virus is occurring; a viral load of > 5000 to $10,000$ is

used by many as an indicator for treatment; loads $> 100,000$ indicate an extremely high likelihood that AIDS will occur.

Monitor for the presence of symptoms of HIV infection: fever, arthralgias, headache, sore throat, enlarged lymph nodes, night sweats, or any other abnormal report.	These represent complaints experienced by the patient during early infection and disease. Later symptoms include those of opportunistic infections and alterations in a variety of body systems.
Monitor vital signs, especially temperature, every 4 hours.	HIV infection affects all body systems; a baseline of vital signs is needed for future evaluation purposes. Fever is common in early disease.
Monitor the patient's response to the report of being positive for HIV and provide emotional support or arrange for counseling, as needed.	The confirmation of the diagnosis is usually met with a variety of significant emotional responses due to the overwhelming physical and psychological challenges that come with the diagnosis.
Instruct the patient about the medication regimen required and administer as ordered: — Nucleoside reverse transcriptase inhibitors: these medications act by suppressing synthesis of viral DNA by reverse transcriptase, inhibiting the viral copying. Commonly used medications include zidovudine (AZT), didanosine (Videx®), zalcitabine (Hivid®), and lamivudine (Epivir™). Side effects of this class depend upon the particular medication but include peripheral neuropathy, gastrointestinal (GI) intolerance, bone marrow suppression, anemia, stomatitis, and headache. — Nonnucleoside reverse transcriptase inhibitors: these medications act by blocking HIV replication through binding with the active center of reverse transcriptase, suppressing the enzyme's activity. Medications in this group include nevirapine (Viramune®),	These medications are given in an attempt to halt the progression of the disease interfering with the multiplication. Side effects occur frequently, and compliance with the regimen is problematic. Extensive teaching from the health care provider or specialist in a specialized HIV/AIDS clinic or other practice is recommended.

(continues)

(continued)

INTERVENTIONS	RATIONALES
delavirdine (Rescriptor®), and efavirenz (Sustiva®). Side effects include rash, impaired liver function, headaches, and fatigue. — Protease inhibitors: This is said to be the most effective class of medications and exert their action by interfering with HIV replication at the stage when the virus is attempting to make long protein chains necessary to reproduce. Protease is the enzyme required for the process to make the cells infectious. Medications in this group include indinavir (Crixivan), ritonavir (Norvir), saquinavir (Invirase), and nelfinavir (Viracept). Side effects include blurred vision, headache, dizziness, rash, metallic taste in mouth, and thrombocytopenia, and GI intolerance.	
Administer the prescribed medications or encourage the patient to take the prescribed medications exactly as ordered, and monitor for side effects	The aim of medications is to halt viral reproduction by being aggressive with drug therapy. The HAART (highly active antiretroviral therapy) approach to treating HIV/AIDS consists of at least three medications, such as two nucleoside analogues and a protease inhibitor. The patient needs to be aware of side effects to allow for early treatment; in some instances, the patient must learn to live with and attempt to manage the side effects, as discontinuance of the drug may not be recommended depending on the severity of the side effect.
Monitor the response to antiretroviral medications by reviewing CD$_4$ cell counts and viral loads.	Laboratory results should show an improvement in CD$_4$ cell counts and a decrease in measures of viral activity.
Instruct patient, family, and friends of infection protection measures required (see nursing diagnosis "Deficient Knowledge").	Preventing the transmission of the disease to others is an issue. Due to confidentiality regulations, it may be difficult to warn others of the possibility of infection.

Give a diet high in calories and rich in iron, protein, and vitamin C.	Good nutrition enhances immune system function; in addition, fatigue is common in infectious states, and these measures will give the patient needed nutrients for energy; iron-rich foods increase oxygen-carrying capacity of the blood, which is needed due to anemia that is common in HIV/AIDS.
Monitor the patient for signs of Kaposi's sarcoma: dark blue, red, or purple papules on the skin that may be painful and itch.	Kaposi's sarcoma is the most common type of cancer found in HIV/AIDS infected patients. The nurse needs to monitor for its presence so that prompt treatment with chemotherapy or radiation can be initiated.
Monitor the patient for signs of AIDS dementia complex or encephalopathy.	The patient has signs of altered cognitive function and thought processes due to the effects of the virus on the nervous system; in some instances, these symptoms can be caused by opportunistic infections. Note memory loss, confusion, inability to concentrate, inability to complete usual tasks at work, and eventual loss of some motor function due to spasticity and tremors.
Conduct extensive teaching to patient and family prior to discharge from hospital, or if in the community setting, on repeated visits to an outpatient facility (see nursing diagnosis "Deficient Knowledge").	Noncompliance is a serious threat with the regimen because of the complexity and the number of medications required, the need for some to be taken with food, and the fact that some cannot be taken together. Teaching is crucial to ensure compliance with medication regimen exactly as prescribed.
Collaborate with physician to make necessary referrals to the community health department for follow-up and assistance with carrying out the medication regimen.	HIV/AIDS is a public health concern, and follow-up with a health care provider or public health entity is required.

NIC   *Infection control*
        Health screening
        Communicable disease
           management

Infection protection
Medication management

Evaluation

Determine the extent to which the patient has achieved the expected outcomes. The viral load decreases and CD$_4$ cell counts should increase. Signs of early infections, such as fever, night sweats, arthralgias, headache, and diarrhea will abate (temporarily). The patient should verbalize an understanding of the diagnostic tests and treatment measures being implemented.

Community/Home Care

All patients with a diagnosis of HIV/AIDS will require follow-up and management by a health care provider or public health program for prevention of communicable disease in keeping with the Centers for Disease Control and Prevention guidelines. The patient, when discharged home, needs to be assessed for the ability to manage the disease and may require in-home visitation for further assessment and teaching reinforcement. The nurse should establish that the patient understands how to take the prescribed medication regimen, is taking all medications as prescribed by the physician, and knows the importance of staying on the regimen. Noncompliance is a danger as the patient may need to take 8 to 16 pills per day just for the HIV/AIDS. Encouragement and support are crucial for the patient, but in reality, many may not have the required social support that enhances compliance. A written schedule for medications can also be given to the patient, as many patients may be prone to forget but are more likely to check a schedule if one is available. Some medications need to be given with food others on an empty stomach, so include on the schedule information about suggested meal times. This information can be condensed to one sheet of paper, placed on a colorful sheet, and laminated for long-term use. A separate sheet on a different color of paper should list the common side effects of each medication taken and which ones need to be reported to the physician. Assist the patient to create a medication diary in which to chart medication administration and record other information such as side effects and temperature. This information can then be shared with the health care provider on subsequent visits. A follow-up telephone call from the

health care provider can assess whether the patient has understood the teaching. The patient will require frequent follow-up, and prior to discharge the social worker or nurse should ascertain whether the patient has the means to be compliant financially, as the medication regimen may cost as much as $15,000 per year. Family members in the household may experience some anxiety about the possibility of transmission of the virus and need to be taught measures to reduce the chance of infection. In-home strategies to prevent transmission include avoiding sharing of personal hygiene objects such as razors. Any body fluid spill, such as blood or urine, should be cleaned with soap and water using gloves and then disinfected by wiping with a 1:10 bleach solution. Bathrooms should also be cleansed with bleach if people other than the patient are using it. If the patient is injured in any way that causes bleeding, it is crucial that the family members protect themselves before rendering aid to the patient; keeping clean gloves in the home at all times is recommended. The patient needs to be protected from others with infections. Discourage visits from people with any type of upper respiratory infection and limit handshaking due to the spread of organisms through this common greeting. Teach the patient how to take a temperature without a thermometer, using products available at drugstores, and record the finding. With special populations such as the homeless or those at high risk for noncompliance, the health care provider, social worker, and local health department will need to be creative or innovative in developing strategies for effective treatment of the infection and to prevention of transmission of the virus to others (see nursing diagnosis "Deficient Knowledge").

Documentation

Document a thorough physical assessment of the patient, specifically noting any complaints or signs of early infection such as arthralgias, headaches, night sweats, nausea/vomiting, lymphadenopathy, or diarrhea. Specific attention should be given to documentation of any specific concerns, especially those of a psychosocial nature that the patient expresses and how they are addressed. Chart interventions carried out to address the infection in the patient's record, including a notation on all content taught and the patient's verbalization of understanding. Included in the documentation is the patient's expression of ability and willingness to comply with all recommendations made about medication regimen and follow-up care. Document appointments made for laboratory tests such as CD_4 counts and viral loads. Always include the titles of any printed literature given to the patient for reinforcement.

NURSING DIAGNOSIS 2

INEFFECTIVE MANAGEMENT OF THERAPEUTIC REGIMEN

Related to:

New diagnosis of HIV/AIDS

Insufficient knowledge of HIV/AIDS

Noncompliance with therapeutic regimen due to deficient knowledge and understanding

Complexity of prescribed regimen

Defining Characteristics:

Asks many questions

Asks no questions about health status

Verbalizes a lack of knowledge/understanding

Misinformed about HIV/AIDS

Goal:

The patient verbalizes an understanding of HIV/AIDS and the required treatment regimen.

Outcome Criteria

✔ The patient demonstrates knowledge of HIV/AIDS and how to prevent transmission.

✔ The patient demonstrates knowledge of medications, including dosage, scheduling, and side effects.

✔ The patient verbalizes a desire to learn necessary information.

✔ The patient verbalizes a willingness to keep appointments and to follow prescribed regimen.

NOC *Knowledge: Disease process*

Knowledge: Treatment regimen

Compliance behavior

INTERVENTIONS	RATIONALES
Assess the patient's current knowledge, ability and readiness to learn, and risk for noncompliance.	Teachings need to be tailored to the patient's ability and willingness to learn for maximum effectiveness; assessment of the patient for likelihood of noncompliance will allow the nurse to intervene early.
Identify a family member or significant other who will also learn the content and assist the patient with compliance.	This person can reinforce the teaching and assist with implementation if the patient becomes incapable of follow-through.
Create a quiet environment conducive to learning.	Environmental noise and distractions can prevent the learner from focusing on what is being taught.
Teach the learners the following information about HIV/AIDS: — Disease process of HIV/AIDS — Prevention of transmission to others (not sharing needles, safe sex, standard precautions, proper disposal of personal use items, good handwashing) — In-home care required — Medications: (nucleoside reverse transcriptase inhibitors, non-nucleoside reverse transcriptase inhibitors, protease inhibitors), including action, side effects, dosing schedule, importance of adhering to the regimen exactly as prescribed — Importance of good nutrition — Signs and symptoms of complications to be reported	Knowledge empowers the patient to take control and be compliant; stressing adherence to the regimen as prescribed will help to prevent drug resistance; identification of side effects will minimize anxiety if these untoward effects should occur.
Teach patient about high-risk behaviors that predispose the patient to infect others: sharing needles, unprotected sex, multiple sex partners.	The most common route for transmission is through unprotected sexual intercourse in both homosexual and heterosexual populations and sharing of IV drug paraphernalia.
Teach patient about opportunistic infections that are often a part of HIV/AIDS: — Pneumocystis carinii — Mycobacterium avium — Herpes simplex — Candidiasis — Cytomegalovirus	Opportunistic infections seem to be a part of the progression of the disease. The patient needs to understand the possibilities in order to identify them if they occur and seek medical attention.

INTERVENTIONS	RATIONALES
Teach patient about cancers that are often part of HIV/AIDS: — Kaposi's sarcoma — Cervical cancer — Non-Hodgkin's lymphoma — Primary lymphoma of the brain	When the immune system becomes compromised, the risk of certain cancers increases. The most current definition of AIDS by the Centers for Disease Control and Prevention (CDC) includes these cancers. Kaposi's sarcoma is the most frequently seen cancer in AIDS patients, and may be present at time of diagnosis of AIDS. When lymphomas and cervical cancers occur in AIDS patients, they are extremely aggressive.
Teach the patient about other disorders that occur with HIV/AIDS: — HIV/AIDS encephalopathy — Wasting syndrome	AIDS encephalopathy or dementia complex is the most frequently occurring cause of changes in mental status. The patient may demonstrate near normal mental capacity but very quickly revert to memory loss, confusion, and profound changes in ability to function. Eventually the complex causes severe dementia and impaired motor function that resembles the later stages of Alzheimer's. The wasting syndrome occurs in approximately 90 percent of all patients with AIDS and is defined as the unintentional loss of > 10 percent of total baseline weight, accompanied by chronic diarrhea.
Teach patient and caregiver how to improve nutritional status.	The wasting syndrome is a common occurrence, and the patient will need to develop strategies to enhance intake of nutrients (see nursing diagnosis "Imbalanced Nutrition: Less than Body Requirements").
Stress to the patient and family the need for vaccines: influenza, pneumonia, hepatitis B.	Due to the impaired immune system, the patient will be prone to develop infections. Vaccines will help protect the patient.
Encourage the patient to discuss HIV status with any sexual partners.	Helps to prevent further transmission.
Provide the patient with information about drug rehabilitation programs or clean needle programs, if needed. If the patient reports reusing needles, provide information on how to	A realistic approach is one that attends to the patient's reported lifestyle. If the patient is not willing or ready to stop drug use, teaching alternative practices to decrease likelihood

INTERVENTIONS	RATIONALES
cleanse with bleach solution (1:10 bleach to water).	of infecting others is suggested. Washing with a hypochlorite solution reduces HIV on equipment.
Provide the patient with information on services available to HIV/AIDS patients, or refer to a social worker.	The patient may need assistance from community organizations for purchase of medications or location of housing, etc. The social worker can be a vital key to locating these for the patient.
Discourage pregnancy and discuss with female patients the dangers of pregnancy when HIV-positive or when they have AIDS (transmission to child and medical complications to the mother).	A significant number of children born to HIV-positive mothers also have the virus and will require treatment.
Ask the patient to repeat information, and ask questions as needed.	This allows the nurse to hear in the patient's own words what was taught, making it easier to know what information may need to be reinforced.
Establish that the patient has the resources required to be compliant.	If needed resources such as finances, transportation, and psychosocial support are not available, the patient cannot comply.
Refer to appropriate disciplines, as needed (social worker, public health agency, etc.).	These disciplines can provide additional services to help the patient be compliant with prescribed regimen.
Give printed material to the patient of information covered in teaching session.	The patient may be more comfortable at home knowing that there is printed material for future reference.

NIC ***Teaching: Disease process***
Teaching: Prescribed medication
Teaching: Safe sex
Learning readiness enhancement
Learning facilitation

Evaluation

The patient verbalizes an understanding of the complex therapeutic regimen, particularly the prescribed HIV/AIDS medications. The patient should be able to identify all medications by name, state when they should be taken, and report the common side effects. It is important that the patient understand how to prevent the transmission of the virus and how to protect him or herself from infections. The patient is able to repeat the information for the nurse and asks questions about the information that has been taught. The patient should be able to inform the nurse about signs and symptoms that would necessitate contact with a health care provider. The nurse must determine that the patient is capable of being compliant, and it should also be ascertained whether the patient expresses a willingness to comply with the somewhat complex regimen.

Community/Home Care

For patients with HIV/AIDS, community and home care is crucial. Because of the complexity of the regimen with a variety of medications that have significant, annoying side effects, the risk for noncompliance is high. At home, the patient may be unsure about the ability to comply with the medical regimen. Successful management will depend on the patient's understanding of the information provided in teaching sessions and the internal motivation to implement health-promoting behaviors. The patient will need to implement strategies to prevent the transmission of the HIV virus to other members of the household, as well as to sexual partners. A solution made of 1:10 bleach to water can be used to cleanse surfaces such as commodes. The patient should practice good hand hygiene for protection of him or herself from infection. Items contaminated with blood or other body fluids should be properly disposed of by placing them in a plastic bag and sealing. Personal care items such as razors or toothbrushes should not be shared at any time. Condom use is stressed for all sexual encounters, and condoms are available free at many public health clinics. Teaching will need to be reinforced periodically due to the large volume of information required, especially the medications. The nurse should make the patient some type of educational packet that has information summarized succinctly. A medication schedule should be written out for the patient showing all the medications to be taken for the entire day. Follow-up by a community health nurse is required once the patient is at home to check on medication administration and check for signs and symptoms of side effects of medications. Medications should be kept in a place that is highly visible for the patient, such as a bedroom dresser, but out of sight of visitors to the home. This will enhance the possibility that the patient will remember to take it at the designated times. If it is determined that the patient is noncompliant, the health care provider needs to attempt to determine the reason. It is crucial that the patient be assessed for the ability to be compliant (availability of resources) or desire to be compliant. The teaching may be extensive, but because of the patient's lifestyle, attitudes about the diagnosis, denial, and inability to cope with the diagnosis, changes in behavior may not occur.

Documentation

Document the specific content taught and the titles of printed materials given to the patient or family. Chart the patient's and family's understanding of the content and the methods used to evaluate learning. The nurse must clearly indicate areas that need to be reinforced. After the teaching session is complete, the nurse should document whether the patient indicates a willingness to comply with health care recommendations. If the teaching included a significant other, indicate this in the documentation. In addition, any referrals made should be documented.

NURSING DIAGNOSIS 3

INEFFECTIVE COPING

Related to:

New diagnosis of HIV/AIDS

Social stigma associated with the disease

Lack of needed resources for management of the disease

Defining Characteristics:

Anger

Denial

Crying

Anxiety

Fear

Expressed loneliness

Goal:

The patient will express an ability to cope.

Outcome Criteria

✔ The patient will verbalize fears and concerns.

✔ The patient identifies one way to cope with serious illness.

✔ The patient will express a willingness to learn new ways to cope.

✔ The patient reports coping with the disease, and anxiety is reduced.

✔ The patient will identify one community resource to assist with disease management.

NOC *Coping*
Social support
Fear level

INTERVENTIONS	RATIONALES
Assess level of anxiety (mild, moderate, severe); have patient rate on a scale of 1 to 10, with 10 being the greatest.	Gives the nurse a better perception of extent of the anxiety.
Assess the patient's psychological state for feelings about self/disease: sadness, anger, anxiety, tearfulness, withdrawal, fear of dying, and worry about inability to carry out family responsibilities, finances, cost of medications, and possible loss of employment.	The patient may experience all of these feelings while trying to cope with the diagnosis and treatment. Knowing where the patient is in terms of coping helps to identify interventions.
Keep the patient informed of all that is going on, including information about diagnostic tests and planned therapeutic interventions.	Communication of factual information in a straightforward manner may help to relieve some of the anxiety and fear.
Assess whether the patient has a social support network of friends or family.	As the patient learns to adapt to the diagnosis and move forward with treatment, a social support will be needed to enhance coping and for emotional support. Oftentimes family members may turn away from the patient with HIV/AIDS.
In collaboration with the physician and other health care providers, be realistic with the patient about prognosis.	The patient needs to hear realistic information and not be given false assurances about health status.
Allow family and friends to visit liberally, if desired by the patient.	Provides emotional support and promotes a sense of comfort.
Assist the patient to identify at least one coping mechanism that has worked in the past; encourage the use of relaxation, guided imagery, deep breathing, writing,	Coping mechanisms that have worked in the past may work again; other relaxation techniques can decrease anxiety and give the patient a sense of
or meditation, or assist to develop new coping strategies.	calm. Because of the overwhelming nature of HIV/AIDS, new coping strategies may be needed.
Seek spiritual or religious consult as needed or requested by the patient.	Meeting spiritual needs of the patient helps the patient to deal with fears through use of spiritual or religious rituals; if the patient practices an organized religion, this may serve as a source of support and a method of coping; the visit may bring peace to the patient.
Recognize the role of culture in a patient's method of coping with an illness such as HIV/AIDS and the acceptability of verbalizing fears and concerns.	Culture often dictates how a person copes, and the nurse must recognize this in order to support the patient in identifying successful coping strategies. In addition, some cultures may frown upon the patient with HIV/AIDS.
Engage patient and family in open dialogues about the complex nature of the medication regimen and the numerous other syndromes and complications that can occur with AIDS and what will be required of them.	Discussion of the possible sequence of events with HIV/AIDS and the needed care will allow the patient to be more in control and provide a sense of empowerment that may assist with coping with the diagnosis.
If the patient has the energy, time, and motivation, encourage him or her to write feelings down.	This will assist the patient to express him or herself in an acceptable manner at a time when he or she may feel uncomfortable talking to others.
Refer to HIV/AIDS support groups and encourage participation.	People from support groups can provide assistance and emotional support to the patient by providing advice on how to cope with aspects of the disease.

NIC *Coping enhancement*
Emotional support
Spiritual support

Evaluation

Evaluate the extent to which the outcome criteria have been achieved. The patient should be assessed for behaviors that would indicate adjustment to the diagnosis of HIV/AIDS. Most patients experience heightened anxiety and anticipatory grieving shortly after receiving word of the diagnosis of HIV/AIDS. As he or she attempts to deal with the unknown and the possibility of death, the patient should be able to verbalize fears and concerns and be able to identify one way to cope. The extent to which the patient displays appropriate coping behaviors should be noted. If the patient is unable to talk about the diagnosis and communicate concerns, the nurse should explore further new interventions to assist the patient.

Community/Home Care

Nurses should assess which coping mechanisms work for the patient and encourage their use by the patient at home. At least one follow-up visit by a health care provider should be initiated to assess for ineffective coping. The patient should be encouraged to identify coping strategies that have been successful in the past and prompted to use those regularly. For some patients, ineffective coping is displayed through inappropriate behaviors such as drinking, excessive drug use, and inappropriate unsafe sexual activity. The patient needs to identify other acceptable means of coping that will assist in alleviating anger and frustrations, activities may include hitting baseballs or golf balls, screaming, hitting a punching bag, meditation, etc. Anxiety about prognosis usually continues throughout the disease, especially as the patient may stabilize or improve but is never cured and must take the medication for the duration of his or her life. The impact that HIV/AIDS has on lifestyle can be overwhelming, and coping through use of support from sources such as support groups, family, friends, and significant others can help the patient maintain a healthy outlook. At follow-up visits, the health care provider should continue to monitor the patient for extreme withdrawal, isolation, and depression, reporting any symptoms to the physician. For many patients and families, spiritual/religious rituals may provide a means of coping with difficult, stressful situations. The patient's culture may dictate how he or she copes and/or grieves and with whom. It is crucial that the nurse and family support the patient as needed to foster a healthy psychological state, recognizing that anger and denial are common. If questions should arise at home about the patient's health status or prescribed regimen, the patient should have a means of contact with a health care provider for answers.

Documentation

Document the degree to which the patient has demonstrated effective coping and decreased anxiety in the patient record. A rating system provides an objective way to relay to others the extent of the anxiety or expressions of fear. Document whether the patient is able to discuss feelings about the diagnosis of HIV/AIDS. Chart the patient's verbalizations as stated and include in the record coping mechanisms utilized by the patient. Document findings from an assessment of the patient's psychological state, indicating whether there is depression, anger, crying, sadness, etc. Document referrals to support groups, social workers, counselors, or religious leaders. Make a note in the patient record about visits from family or friends during hospitalization.

NURSING DIAGNOSIS 4

INEFFECTIVE BREATHING PATTERN

Related to:

    Respiratory opportunistic infections: Pneumocystis carinii pneumonia, mycobacterium tuberculosis, bacterial pneumonia

Defining Characteristics:

    Chest x-ray demonstrates disease

    Positive cultures

    Fever

    Night sweats

    Cough with expectoration

    Fatigue

Goal:

    Infection will be resolved.

Outcome Criteria

✔ The patient will be afebrile.

✔ Breath sounds will be clear.

✔ The patient will have no cyanosis, and arterial blood gases (ABGs) will return to normal.

✔ The patient will verbalize an understanding of treatment required.

NOC   *Infection severity*

    Respiratory status: Ventilation

    Knowledge: Infection control

INTERVENTIONS	RATIONALES
Monitor diagnostic studies: PPD (purified protein derivative), skin test for tuberculosis (TB) (also called Mantoux), pulmonary function studies, sputum culture/smear, bronchial washings culture/smear, and chest x-ray.	PPD is the initial screening for TB but may not always be positive in the immuno-compromised patient, in HIV/AIDS patients an induration of > 5 mm is considered positive because of a delayed type hypersensitivity response and in some cases no reaction to the PPD (anergy) occurs at all; sputum cultures are done to detect infectious agents; sputum smear for acid fast bacilli is a quicker way to identify the tubercle bacillus; bronchial washings for culture and smears are obtained via bronchoscopy if the patient is unable to produce a sputum specimen; chest x-ray will demonstrate active disease.
Monitor temperature every 4 hours.	Helps to establish a baseline and monitor response to treatment.
Perform a complete respiratory assessment, including breath sounds, respiratory rate, presence of cough and expectoration (note color, amount, consistency, presence of blood), shortness of breath, or exertional dyspnea.	Helps to detect symptoms of disease and their resolution, and to monitor patient's response to treatment.
Monitor results of oxygen saturation or ABGs, if ordered.	Helps to note any alterations in the respiratory system's ability to maintain oxygenation and gas exchange.
If the patient is hospitalized due to positive cultures, place in respiratory isolation and follow agency isolation procedures by wearing a mask when entering the room and a gown and gloves if soiling is expected.	A special well-ventilated negative pressure room with scheduled air exchange is required for a diagnosis of tuberculosis, and use of isolation protocols is needed to protect others.
Give oxygen as ordered and in accordance with ABGs and oxygen saturation.	Respiratory infections cause impaired gas exchange and increase the work of breathing; oxygen will enhance oxygenation to tissues and decrease the work of breathing.
Increase fluids if not contraindicated.	Helps to thin secretions.
Place patient in semi- or high Fowler's position	Increases chest excursion and ability to breathe adequately.
Have patient cough and deep breathe.	Helps to maximize airway space and enhance expectoration of mucous.
In the hospital setting, implement strategies to prevent the spread of organisms: — Teach patient correct handling of secretions: to cover mouth and nose when coughing or sneezing. — Keep tissues at bedside, tape plastic bag to bedrail for disposal, or place wastebasket directly beside bed. — Teach and encourage use of frequent proper handwashing after handling secretions. — If patient leaves room, have him or her wear a mask (if on respiratory isolation). — Educate visitors about proper isolation procedures to be employed when visiting infectious patients. — Be sure that any isolation requirements are posted at doorway. — Keep door closed at all times (if on respiratory isolation).	Proper disposal of infectious items and minimizing droplet contact from person to person is standard to the prevention of the spread of organisms and is crucial to protect the public health.
Give a diet high in calories and rich in iron, protein, and vitamin C.	Fatigue is common in HIV/AIDS, and foods rich in these nutrients will give the patient needed nutrients for energy and healing; iron-rich foods increase oxygen-carrying capacity of the blood.
Administer medications as ordered and monitor for side effects: — For pneumoncysti carinii pneumonia, administer Bactrim/Septra® (TMP-SMX), pentamidine, or others as required. Side effects are rashes, GI upset, anorexia, and weakness (Bactrim); and hyperkalemia, cough, bronchospasm, and local reactions at site of injection (pentamidine). — For mycobacterium tuberculosis, administer the standard drug therapy of isoniazid/isonicotinic acid hydraide (INH), rifampin,	These medications will resolve the infection by killing or halting the growth of organisms, and protect the health of the larger community by stopping transmission. The regimen is prescribed by the physician and is intended to treat the infection aggressively in the immunosuppressed patient. Anti-tuberculosis regimens always contain two or more drugs to decrease the risk for development of drug-resistant organisms. Monitoring for side effects allows for dosage adjustment and prevention of complications.

(continues)

(continued)

INTERVENTIONS	RATIONALES
and pyrazinamide, and either ethambutol or streptomycin. (See nursing care plan "Tuberculosis"). — For bacterial pneumonia, administer antibiotics according to culture results, or give a broad-spectrum antibiotic. — For any other opportunistic infections administer antibiotics, antifungals, or antivirals, as ordered.	
If the patient has tuberculosis or other transmissible infections, collaborate with other disciplines to protect the community. For patients with tuberculosis, make necessary referrals to the community health department for follow-up and assistance with carrying out the medication regimen.	Prevention of transmission of infection to others is important to the health of the community. Tuberculosis is a public health concern, and follow-up with a public health entity is required.
Conduct extensive teaching to patient and family prior to discharge from hospital, or if being cared for in the home, teach at office visits.	Noncompliance is a serious danger for the HIV/AIDS patient. Because the patient already takes numerous drugs for HIV/AIDS, adding more only complicates the regimen further. Education is crucial to teach the patient and others the importance of compliance with medication regimen exactly as prescribed.

NIC   *Infection control*
          Health screening
          Communicable disease
              management
          Infection protection
          Medication management
          Respiratory monitoring

Evaluation

Determine the extent to which the patient has achieved the expected outcomes. The patient should become afebrile and have no signs of respiratory infection. Breath sounds should be clear, and any cough should diminish with little or no expectoration. Arterial blood gases (ABGs) should return to normal or improve, and oxygen saturation is > 90 percent. The patient should verbalize an understanding of the treatment measures being implemented, particularly medication administration and any isolation precautions required.

Community/Home Care

All patients who experience ineffective breathing pattern due to opportunistic infections, especially tuberculosis, will require some degree of follow-up and management by a visiting nurse. The patient, when discharged home, needs to be assessed for the ability to manage respiratory infections. The nurse should establish that the patient is taking all medications as prescribed by the physician and knows the importance of staying on the regimen for its duration. Follow-up sputum specimens and a thorough assessment of the patient's physical status will be needed to ascertain effectiveness of treatment. For patients with tuberculosis, there is no need for airborne precautions at home, as family members have already been exposed to the disease. Protecting the patient from future infections is required because the patient is immunocompromised and likely to be a prime host for respiratory infections. Avoidance of crowds, those with upper respiratory infections, and frequent handshaking are suggested because of the high risk of cross-contamination. Stress to the patient the importance of consuming nutritious foods and liquids; monitor general feelings and evaluate whether symptoms are abating. Proper disposal of infectious items such as tissues should be implemented in the home by using paper bags placed inside plastic garbage bags or by placing a small trashcan lined with a plastic bag in an easily accessible place. Throughout the treatment for respiratory opportunistic infections, the patient should be monitored for side effects of the medications and referred appropriately for medical assistance. Effective teaching is crucial for the patient and family, and reinforcement is vital to ensure that the patient is managing the regimen as prescribed.

Documentation

Document the findings from a comprehensive respiratory assessment with special attention to the presence or absence of cough and a description of the sputum. Include patient-specific complaints such as fatigue, malaise, or anorexia. Chart oxygen saturation results with the vital signs according to agency guidelines. Always chart therapeutic interventions implemented and the patient's specific response to those interventions. Document medication administration and results of any skin testing according to agency protocol. Indicate all teaching and referrals in the patient's record.

NURSING DIAGNOSIS 5

IMBALANCED NUTRITION: LESS THAN BODY REQUIREMENTS

Related to:

Nausea

Anorexia

Diarrhea

Stomatitis

Effects of medications

Defining Characteristics:

Reports of decreased appetite

Loss of weight/wasting

Eats little of food served

Goal:

Adequate dietary/fluid intake is maintained.

Outcome Criteria

✔ The patient does not lose weight.

✔ The patient consumes 50 percent of food served.

✔ The patient tolerates meals without nausea or vomiting.

✔ Stomatitis resolves.

NOC *Nutritional status: Food and fluid intake*

Nutritional status: Nutrient intake

Oral hygiene

INTERVENTIONS	RATIONALES
Assess laboratory results: albumin, electrolytes, glucose, protein (total), and iron.	These give indications of nutritional status.
Assess the patient's ability to eat or drink and to retain intake without nausea, vomiting, mouth pain, or abdominal pain.	Helps to identify specific problems the patient is experiencing in order to intervene accordingly.
Weigh patient and monitor weight daily (in hospital) or weekly (at home).	Helps to establish a baseline for comparison and as patient progresses to allow for early intervention for nutritional deficits.
Monitor intake and output; assess for dehydration by checking for moisture of oral mucous membranes and skin turgor (skin should be elastic).	Helps to assure adequate hydration and implement appropriate action promptly if problems are noted.
Consider a dietician consult to ascertain the patient's ability to take in enough food to meet caloric demand and to determine the patient likes, dislikes, and preferences within the prescribed diet, with consideration given to cultural or religious preferences.	For patients who have HIV/AIDS, especially in later stages, weight loss and even wasting (loss of > 10 percent of baseline weight) may occur; sufficient caloric intake is necessary to prevent wasting, if possible, and the patient will be more likely to consume foods that he or she likes; utilization of the dietician will be useful in determining what the patient needs and can tolerate.
Create a pleasant environment for meals.	The environment can enhance the patient's willingness to eat.
Plan for small frequent (six) meals that are high in calories and protein.	Food may be more tolerable in small portions and require less energy for consumption. Frequently, the patient undergoing treatment for HIV/AIDS is fatigued, and smaller meals are more likely to be consumed.
Provide oral/mouth care before meals.	Taste buds may be altered due to a variety of medications, and a fresh mouth can enhance taste.
Give anti-emetics as ordered or 30 minutes before meals.	Helps to prevent nausea and vomiting.
Administer appetite-stimulating medications such as Megace®, as ordered.	This is an appetite stimulant given to increase chances that the patient will consume food.
Based on patient likes, dislikes, and preferences, offer bland foods or drinks that have a decreased likelihood of causing nausea, such as toast, crackers, ginger ale, or gelatin.	These foods are usually well tolerated by nauseated patients.

(continues)

(continued)

INTERVENTIONS	RATIONALES
Open containers away from the patient or outside the door.	Especially for the patient who is experiencing nausea and vomiting, removing lids from containers at the bedside releases a strong aroma that can cause nausea, which would prevent the patient from eating.
Encourage the patient to take most nutritious foods (such as meats) early in the day.	The patient becomes more fatigued as the day progresses and is less likely to eat; in addition, nausea may increase later in the day.
If nausea is present, offer cold rather than hot foods on the meal tray.	Cold foods tend to decrease nausea.
For candida infections that irritate the mouth, have the patient rinse mouth well after meals using oral antifungal agents such as Mycostatin® (nystatin) as ordered.	This improves comfort and corrects candida that can cause mouth pain and ulceration.
Monitor the number of diarrhea stools and administer antidiarrheal medications after each stool, as ordered.	The HIV/AIDS patient frequently suffers from diarrhea that can cause nutritional deficits, electrolyte imbalances, and subsequent weight loss.

NIC *Nutritional monitoring*
Oral health maintenance
Oral health restoration
Nausea management
Nutritional management

Evaluation

The patient's nutritional state is stable and the patient has a satisfactory method for nutrient intake. Assess the patient's weight and determine that the patient is not losing weight. The patient should be ingesting at least 50 percent of food served and should be tolerating meals without nausea or vomiting. The patient's mouth is free of any lesions or candida. Laboratory results should reveal a normal albumin level as well as total protein and electrolytes. The patient should be able to eat and drink without nausea or pain in the mouth and be able to verbalize methods to maintain nutrition in the home.

Community/Home Care

Difficulties with eating and drinking may continue at home for the patient who has HIV/AIDS due to the effects of the disease process, opportunistic infections, and altered thought processes due to AIDS dementia complex/AIDS encephalopathy. The patient will need to continue efforts to ingest enough food and nutrients to meet the metabolic demands of a disease state. The patient needs encouragement to eat and at home may lose interest in eating due to pain in the mouth due to stomatitis or candida, depression, nausea, or fatigue that may be caused by frequent diarrhea. A home nurse or other health care provider needs to monitor the patient's nutritional status on a regular basis to detect excessive weight loss (wasting syndrome) and to note reports of increased nausea/vomiting. A strategy to address nausea at home is crucial for maintenance of nutrition. The physician may prescribe anti-emetics for the patient, and these should be taken prophylactically before meals; a regimen that includes medications, diet, and relaxation methods in the home is the most likely to be successful. Strategies that promote oral comfort, such as rinsing the mouth before and after meals and the use of agents such as Mycostatin, will enhance the ability to eat. Instruct the patient to maintain a supply of foods recommended by the dietician or nurse that can decrease the likelihood of nausea/vomiting and diarrhea, such as bland foods, crackers, hard candy, gelatin, etc. It is helpful to provide the patient with a list of foods that can provide good sources of the required nutrients and minimize GI distress. A diet high in calories and rich in protein is advised, and the patient will need to have sufficient amounts to provide a source of energy, as fatigue will be a persistent problem. Family members and significant others play a role in implementing strategies to improve nutrition by preparing meals, encouraging the patient to ingest them, and assisting the patient as needed. Frequent small meals at home should be continued for the patient in order to increase the likelihood that the patient can ingest enough nutrients. Supplemental drinks or even ice cream can improve the number of calories and nutrients that the patient can consume during periods when the patient is unable to ingest adequate amounts of nutrition through normal meals due to pain in the mouth, anorexia, vomiting, diarrhea, or malaise. The patient should use caution with commercial products such as Boost or Ensure as some popular products cause diarrhea as a side effect in some people. The patient may need to experiment with which products are tolerated, satisfying, or appealing after consultation with the dietician. The patient may need to continue to take appetite stimulants as well as multivitamins or electrolyte supplements until the nutritional status stabilizes. Diarrhea should be treated with prescribed anti-diarrheal agents to prevent electrolyte and nutrient loss through stools. Teach the patient to monitor his or her nutrition/intake by keeping a log of food eaten, when eaten, and how well tolerated (whether any nausea, vomiting, or diarrhea occurs). If at any time a particular meal or food product causes nausea or vomiting, the patient should note this in the log and eliminate this food from the diet. Weights should also be included in the log. Even though the patient may not want to weigh every day, weighing at least every other day is a good way to keep track of weight loss or stabilization. This information can be shared with the health care provider at each follow-up visit to provide data for revision in prescribed therapeutic interventions for nutrition. Follow-up providers should assess the patient for weight loss and condition of mouth, and monitor laboratory results for improvement in nutritional status. Despite the best nutritional plan, the HIV/AIDS patient may still suffer from wasting syndrome.

Documentation

Document an assessment of the condition of the patient's mouth along with any complaints of pain in the oral cavity. Chart the patient's weight daily. Document any difficulty that the patient experiences during meals, particularly nausea or vomiting, and any interventions (anti-emetics or other) implemented to address them. Record intake and output according to agency protocol, being sure to document the percentage of food consumed, any appetite stimulants administered, and amount of any diarrhea stools. If the patient verbalizes concerns, include these in the chart. Document all interventions implemented to address the issue of nutrition in the patient record. Always document any referrals made to other disciplines, particularly the dietician. Document teaching done to address nutritional needs and whether the patient has understood.

CHAPTER 8.104

LATEX SENSITIVITY

GENERAL INFORMATION

Latex sensitivity is a cumulative sensitivity that may begin with a skin rash or wheezing and result in full-blown anaphylaxis and/or respiratory arrest. Response to exposure to latex products is classified into three categories: irritant reaction, type IV reaction, and type I reaction. Irritant reactions are caused by direct contact with latex resulting in dryness, redness, or skin chapping, and are not true allergic responses. Although irritant reactions are not in and of themselves immunologic responses, they may be the primary cause of the latex allergen entering the body system circulation. Type IV reactions are a cell-mediated response to the substances in the latex affecting the area of the body that was exposed. There is no antibody formation, and evidence of the reaction (tissue inflammation: erythema, rash, and vesicle formation) may be delayed from 6 to 48 hours after exposure. Type I reactions are systemic and occur due to a massive antibody response to the latex allergen, usually because of repeated exposures to latex allergens. Immunoglobulin E (IgE) antibodies are formed by the body in response to the allergen so that subsequent exposures result in a massive allergic response that occurs quickly, with symptoms ranging from rashes/hives or mild respiratory symptoms to hypotension and frank anaphylaxis. This response can occur with skin contact, inhalation, or ingestion of the latex protein. Those at risk for latex sensitivity are health care workers/dental workers who are in a high-latex-glove-use environment; environmental workers, bakery workers, and food service workers who use latex gloves; patients who have had three or more major surgeries where there has been high exposure to latex gloves on mucous membranes; and patients who have had repeated exposure/contact with latex products, such as urinary catheters. Significant emphasis must be placed on prevention of sensitivity reactions and decreasing the amount of latex in the environment. Health care workers should make every attempt to ensure a latex-safe environment for all patients, including being alert at all times to the possibility of latex-based components in any items with which the patient may come into contact. Cornstarch powder containing latex proteins will be in the air if latex gloves are used in any unit or department, and latex is contained in medical devices, such as stethoscope tubing, blood pressure cuffs, endotracheal tubes, urinary catheters, intravenous fluid tubing, stoppers in medication vials, and other medical equipment.

NURSING DIAGNOSIS 1

 LATEX ALLERGY RESPONSE

Related to:

Hypersensitivity

Exposure to latex or protein in latex rubber

Defining Characteristics:

Dermatitis

Hives

Wheezing

Sneezing

Shortness of breath

Severe hypotension

Tachycardia

Feeling of uneasiness

Diaphoresis

Weakness

Mental status changes (restless, agitated, or anxious)

Goal:

The patient will not experience anaphylactic shock.

The patient's cardiac output is maintained.

Outcome Criteria

✔ The patient has no wheezing or shortness of breath.

✔ Skin reactions are resolved.

✔ The patient and/or family verbalize an understanding of latex allergies and interventions required.

✔ The patient has a pulse rate between 60 and 100.

✔ The patient is not agitated or restless and reports decreased anxiety.

✔ Urinary output is > 30 ml/hour average.

✔ The patient's blood pressure returns to patient's baseline.

NOC *Allergic response: Localized*

Immune hypersensitivity response

Tissue integrity: Skin and mucous membranes

Circulatory status

Tissue perfusion: Cardiac

Tissue perfusion: Cerebral

Vital signs

INTERVENTIONS	RATIONALES
Assist in identification of the specific item containing latex that the patient was exposed to and initiate interventions to treat the cause, as ordered.	Identification of the specific item will assist in correct treatment and prevention of future episodes. In a hospital setting or at home, numerous items may cause a reaction.
Assess respiratory status, noting adventitious breath sounds: for patients experiencing a latex allergy response/anaphylaxis, assess for wheezing, stridor, and other signs of respiratory distress.	Histamine, released in response to the exposure, causes a leak of fluid into alveoli, also causing pulmonary congestion, which manifests itself as crackles; histamine also causes smooth muscle constriction in the lungs, resulting in bronchospasms and laryngospasms that manifest as wheezing and stridor.
Assess blood pressure and pulse every 15 minutes.	Changes in blood pressure and pulse give indicators to patient status. A decreased blood pressure with narrowing pulse pressure may be noted, and the pulse may be rapid, weak, and
	thready, both of which are signs of shock.
Complete a thorough cardiovascular assessment: cardiac rate, rhythm, and vital signs (blood pressure and pulse); the patient should be assessed for hypotension, tachycardia, dysrhythmias, and warm skin.	Helps to evaluate for decreased cardiac output and establish baseline for evaluation of response to interventions. All of the above manifestations occur because of massive vasodilation with subsequent changes in cardiac effectiveness that would indicate progression to anaphylactic shock.
Give oxygen, as ordered.	Due to hypoperfusion, tissues may be hypoxic; oxygen is needed to increase the amount of oxygen available for gas exchange and to maintain pO_2 at > 90 percent.
If symptoms of cardiac compromise occur, place patient with trunk flat, head not higher than 10 degrees, and legs elevated 20 degrees.	This position increases venous return to the heart from the periphery and is needed if the patient progresses to anaphylaxis; prevents decrease in cardiac output.
Assess for other signs of shock: skin temperature and color, peripheral pulses, and mental status, including level of consciousness, confusion, and agitation.	If shock occurs, perfusion to skin and periphery is inadequate to maintain warmth or normal color. Peripheral pulses may become weak, diminished, or absent, as the heart is unable to maintain perfusion to extremities. Changes in mental status indicate a decrease in cerebral tissue perfusion and an inability of the body's compensatory mechanism to provide adequate oxygenation to cerebral tissue.
Establish intravenous (IV) access and initiate fluid, as ordered.	Helps to have access for administration of emergency medications and to maintain a route for fluid replacement if the patient progresses to anaphylaxis.
Administer medications, as ordered (epinephrine IV; Benadryl PO or IV; bronchodilators, metaproterenol/beta agonists, steroids).	Antihistamines decrease the amount of circulating histamines that caused the vasodilation; epinephrine acts directly on alpha and beta receptors, strengthens myocardial contraction, and increases cardiac output. In addition, epinephrine inhibits histamine release and as a result decreases

(continues)

(continued)

INTERVENTIONS	RATIONALES
	respiratory symptoms, particularly bronchospasm.
Assess the patient for a quick resolution of symptoms of latex allergy response. Note respiratory status, particularly breath sounds, effort, and rate; pulse, blood pressure, output, mental status—especially anxiety—and presence of any other symptoms of allergic reaction such as hives or itching.	Helps to evaluate the effectiveness of interventions and determine the need for further action.
Have patients avoid latex if they have food allergies for bananas, kiwi, avocados, tropical fruits, or chestnuts.	Patients with these allergies frequently have a cross-reaction between the latex and these foods.
If the patient progresses to anaphylactic shock, assist with hemodynamic monitoring and other interventions, as ordered.	If the initial allergic response to latex is not treated or the patient does not respond, more aggressive measures are required to maintain cardiac output.
Post a sign at bedside indicating the latex allergy.	Helps to notify others of the allergy and to prevent accidental contact with latex.
Assess the patient's current knowledge about latex allergy and use of latex products.	An assessment is required prior to implementing instruction about latex allergy and instruction needs to start with what the patient already knows.
Teach the patient and family the following: — Definition of latex allergy — Signs and symptoms of an allergic response — Emergency interventions required for treatment (Benadryl, epinephrine) — How to use an EpiPen — Importance of wearing a Medic-Alert bracelet identifying the allergy — Prevention of exposure to latex (acceptable gloves, avoidance of certain foods) — Creation of a latex-free environment — Common health care items and household items that contain latex — Avoid use of condoms containing latex — Objects or products that contain latex	Education is a key to preventing future episodes of latex allergy response.

Refer patient to an allergist.	Helps to assist with management of the latex allergy.
Assist the patient in identifying an appropriate support group. Provide information about latex allergy/latex sensitivity support on the Internet, such as ELASTIC, a latex allergy support newsletter.	A support group or other resources can assist the patient in coping with this allergy and may provide useful information on items containing latex.

NIC *Latex precautions*
Allergy management
Anaphylaxis management
Fluid monitoring
Vital signs monitoring

Evaluation

Note the degree to which the outcome criteria have been achieved. Respiratory status has stabilized with no wheezing or distress. The patient should demonstrate adequate cardiac output or improvement in abnormalities. Peripheral pulses should be present and skin, when touched, should be warm. If cardiac output is improved, perfusion to the kidneys should be adequate, with the patient producing at least 30 ml of urine per hour on average. The pulse should be within the patient's baseline and should be strong and regular. The patient and family can verbalize an understanding of the information taught about latex allergy and are willing to comply with recommendations. No signs of impaired cerebral perfusion such as restlessness are present.

Community/Home Care

Patients who have experienced a reaction to latex require structured education about latex allergy responses and how to prevent future episodes. This involves identifying common items that may contain latex, which is a daunting task. Health care workers have a role in assisting the patient with this activity, and an allergist may be best equipped to assist. As items are identified, the patient should write them down in a notebook or other place for reference. The patient also needs to eliminate from their diet foods that are likely to have a cross-reaction with latex, including most tropical or exotic fruits such as kiwi and mangoes. It is important that the patient understand the signs and symptoms of a reaction, realizing that respiratory distress is an emergency to be treated promptly. Most patients are told to keep Benadryl available in the home to be taken if exposure occurs. If an EpiPen is prescribed, be sure that the patient knows how to use and store it. In the weeks immediately following identification of the allergy, the patient should carry the EpiPen when leaving the home, as many patients are still not quite sure when a reaction may occur due to the widespread use of latex in ordinary products. Wearing of a Medic-Alert bracelet is crucial so that others, including family members, know about the allergy. Teaching about strategies required to prevent shock when exposed to latex needs to be done with the patient, family members, and/or significant other. Home care follow-up may be required for some patients, especially if they verbalize feelings of anxiety or lack of knowledge about the emergency that necessitated immediate care. A follow-up appointment is needed to be sure that the patient understands the requirements for preventing subsequent responses or anaphylaxis.

Documentation

Chart the results of all assessments made, particularly respiratory and cardiac. Note particularly the presence of any wheezing, stridor, or shortness of breath. For patients who have experienced a latex allergy response, document an assessment of the skin for rashes, redness/discoloration, and edema, especially of the lips, eyes, and tongue. Document the administration of antihistamines and epinephrine or other medications in the medication administration record as required, with a follow-up note about the patient outcome in response to treatment. Chart vital signs and intake and output according to agency protocol, including presence of IV infusions. All other interventions should be documented in a timely fashion with the patient's specific response to the intervention. Always include the patient's psychological status: whether he or she appears anxious, restless, fearful, and whether family members or significant others are present.

NURSING DIAGNOSIS 2

INEFFECTIVE BREATHING PATTERN

Related to:

Type I latex reaction

Bronchospasm

Laryngeal edema

Allergic reaction

Facial edema

Defining Characteristics:

Wheezing

Stridor

Decreased oxygen saturation

Dyspnea

Tachypnea

Abnormal blood gases (ABGs) (decreased pO_2 and increased pCO_2)

Restlessness and anxiety

Goal:

The patient's respiratory status is normal.

Outcome Criteria:

✔ The patient will have no wheezing or stridor.

✔ The patient will have no cyanosis.

✔ Oxygen saturation will be > 90 percent.

✔ ABGs are normal or improved.

NOC *Respiratory status: Airway patency*
Respiratory status: Ventilation
Allergic response: Systemic

INTERVENTIONS	RATIONALES
Assess respiratory status: breath sounds, respiratory rate, oxygen saturation; note abnormalities, such as wheezing, stridor, dyspnea, presence of cyanosis, retractions, use of accessory muscles, flaring of nostrils, and angioedema.	Abnormal breathing patterns may signal worsening of condition; stridor, retractions, and flaring of nostrils indicate a significant decline in respiratory status; angioedema of the facial area or mouth contributes to the inability to breathe; initial assessments establish a baseline and subsequent assessments allow for monitoring response to interventions.
Monitor the patient for signs of occluded airway: cyanosis, cessation of wheezing, absence of breath sounds over lungs, or continuous coughing.	If bronchospasm is severe, there may be no air movement, and therefore no wheezing. Be very careful when auscultating the chest to pay particular attention to the sound of any air movement, as focusing on picking up adventitious sounds may cause one to miss the fact

(continues)

(continued)

INTERVENTIONS	RATIONALES
	that there is no air movement; the patient may cough almost continuously in an attempt to open the airway.
Monitor ABGs, as ordered.	Initially, ABG analysis will reveal respiratory alkalosis as the tachypnea blows off more carbon dioxide, but as the airway narrows, the lungs are unable to blow off carbon dioxide, and acidosis is noted.
Assess for anxiety and reassure patient with presence.	The patient experiencing anaphylaxis is already anxious because of the allergic response; inability to breathe causes more anxiety and fear; the patient needs a calming presence; anxiety increases the demand for oxygen.
Provide humidified oxygen, as ordered, to maintain oxygen saturation at > 90 percent.	Helps to improve oxygenation to cells.
Establish IV access.	Helps to ensure a route for rapid-acting medications.
Administer epinephrine, as ordered.	Inhibits histamine release, reduces pulmonary congestion, and decreases laryngospasm as well as bronchospasm by its effect on alpha and beta receptors.
Place the patient in a high Fowler's position, if possible, and support with an overbed table, as needed.	Maximizes chest excursion and subsequent movement of air.
Assist respiratory therapist with administration of beta-adrenergic agonists (such as albuterol, metaproterenol) via nebulizer or metered dose inhaler, as ordered, and monitor for side effects.	Stimulates beta$_2$-adrenergic receptor sites in the pulmonary system to increase levels of cyclic adenosine monophosphate (cAMP), which relaxes smooth muscles causing bronchodilation, thereby reducing bronchospasm; common side effects include tremors, tachycardia, and anxiety.
Administer corticosteroids (such as Solu-Medrol IV, Prednisone PO, Flovent inhaled) or antihistamines (Benadryl), as ordered, and monitor for side effects.	Corticosteroids suppress the inflammatory response and decrease mucosal edema; systemic side effects from oral or IV administration include acne, bruising, increased appetite, muscle weakness, and, with oral

intake, GI upset; effects from inhaled corticosteroids include candidiasis, hoarseness, and dry cough; antihistamines block the release of histamine, the substance that causes bronchiole constriction; side effects of antihistamines include drowsiness and dry mouth.

Teach the patient and family about latex allergy, prevention, treatment, and home care (see nursing diagnosis "Latex Allergy Response").	Knowledge increases the chance that the patient can engage in health-promoting behaviors to prevent future allergic reactions.
If the patient's respiratory status does not improve, transfer to a critical care environment and assist with implementation of mechanical ventilation.	If stridor occurs, the patient is unable to maintain effective respiratory efforts for oxygenation and will need the assistance of intubation.
Inform family members or significant other about patient's condition.	Emergencies such as anaphylaxis often cause anxiety and fear in family members and significant others. Holistic nursing care recognizes the importance of family members and seeks to allay their anxiety, as well as the patient's.

NIC *Presence*
Respiratory monitoring
Oxygen therapy
Ventilation assistance

Evaluation

Assess the patient to determine the extent to which the outcome criteria have been met. Assessments of the respiratory system should reveal that acute respiratory symptoms of anaphylaxis, such as wheezing, have been resolved. Breathing should be unlabored, and even though some mild wheezing may be noted, this should be improved. ABGs and oxygen saturation should indicate adequate oxygenation, and there should be no cyanosis.

Community/Home Care

The patient who has experienced respiratory distress due to a latex allergy reaction may not need any monitoring when discharged home. The patient and family will be able to implement strategies to manage future allergic reactions themselves with the use of EpiPens or Benadryl. The patient and a family member should demonstrate how to use the EpiPen so that if it is needed in an emergency, they are comfortable with the procedure. Prior to discharge from the acute setting, the patient should attempt to identify known products in the environment that contain latex. If possible, these should be minimized or alleviated altogether before entering the home. The patient and family will need to know the signs of allergic reactions that indicate a possible progression to respiratory distress, what interventions could be implemented prior to seeking emergency care, and thorough information on medications. All patients who have a latex allergy should carry medical information at all times and wear a Medic-Alert bracelet to alert others.

Documentation

Document a comprehensive respiratory assessment. Include in the patient record all interventions carried out for the patient and the patient's responses. Note specifically changes in breath sounds in response to interventions, along with vital signs and oxygen saturation. Document the introduction of new medication regimens and the patient's responses, or lack thereof. Chart an assessment of the patient's emotional state. Teaching initiated relevant to the latex allergy and prevention of respiratory symptoms should be charted with a clear indication of what was taught and to whom.

NURSING DIAGNOSIS 3

 ## ANXIETY

Related to:

Emergency health problem

Unknown health status

Defining Characteristics:

Tachycardia

Restlessness

Verbalization of anxiety, concern, fear

Goal:

Anxiety is relieved.

Outcome Criteria

✔ The patient reports feeling calm and relaxed.

✔ The patient verbalizes that anxiety has been reduced or alleviated.

✔ The patient asks appropriate questions about latex allergy response or any aspect of treatment.

NOC *Anxiety self-control*
Symptom control

INTERVENTIONS	RATIONALES
Assess for verbal and nonverbal signs of anxiety and fear, including increased heart rate. Have the patient rate the level of anxiety using a numerical rating scale.	Helps to detect the presence of anxiety and allows for early intervention to prevent physiological alterations. A rating scale provides an objective measure of the anxiety.
Encourage the patient to verbalize fears and anxiety about health status.	Recognition of fear and anxiety is the first step to understanding and coping.
Teach the patient relaxation techniques (such as slow, purposeful breathing) and encourage their use.	Reduces anxiety and creates a feeling of comfort.
Explain what is happening, including procedures, treatments, and critical care or emergency room environment.	Reassures the patient; fear of the unknown contributes to anxiety; knowing what to expect helps the patient maintain a sense of control. Patients with sudden onset of symptoms such as difficulty breathing or the sensation of feeling their lips and face swelling most often feel panicky and fearful.
Stay with patient during critical times and during periods when fear and anxiety are evident.	Helps to offer comfort, care, and assurances to reduce anxiety and fear.
Keep significant other or family members informed of the patient's status and allow them to stay with the patient, if possible.	The presence of family members and significant others often has a calming effect on seriously ill patients.

NIC *Anxiety reduction*
Calming technique
Presence

Evaluation

Assess the patient for the degree that fear/anxiety has been controlled. The patient should verbalize feelings and indicate whether interventions have produced a comfortable psychological state, and whether anxiety and fear are improved. Determine whether the patient understands latex allergies and interventions required for treatment. During evaluation, be sure to inquire about the use of coping strategies and relaxation techniques.

Community/Home Care

The patient will need to develop coping strategies and relaxation techniques to utilize in the home setting. The nurse must adequately equip the patient with knowledge about latex allergy necessary to make him or her feel in control. Anxiety may persist for a while due to the fear that another exposure to the offending substance may produce the same consequences. Adequate instruction is needed about prevention and emergency treatment that can be implemented prior to seeking health care. In the home, the patient may be able to reduce anxiety more quickly through use of common everyday activities such as walking, reading, meditating, listening to the radio, and spending time with emotionally supportive family and friends.

Documentation

Using a numerical scale, document the degree of fear or anxiety the patient is experiencing. In addition, include any verbal, nonverbal, or physiological clues that could indicate anxiety or fear, such as restlessness, tachycardia, or diaphoresis. Record interventions implemented to treat anxiety or fear, along with the patient's responses. Document instruction about relaxation techniques and the disease process.

NURSING DIAGNOSIS 4

 ## IMPAIRED SKIN INTEGRITY

Related to:

　Allergic reaction

Defining Characteristics:

　Itching

　Hives

　Edema of lips, eyelids

　Urticaria

　Redness/discoloration

Goal:

　The patient's skin will return to a normal state.

Outcome Criteria

✔ The patient's skin will not be red or discolored.

✔ The patient will have no rashes or hives.

✔ Edema of lips, tongue, face, or eyelids will be alleviated.

NOC *Allergic response: Localized*
Tissue integrity: Skin and
mucous membranes

INTERVENTIONS	RATIONALES
Assess for urticaria/hives/rashes; pruritus; edema of lips, eyelids, and tongue; and redness/discoloration. Inquire about ingestion of recent foods and drugs or exposure to other possible allergens such as animals, hay, mold, etc.	For patients experiencing latex allergy response, exposure to an offending substance causes a hypersensitivity reaction that often produces skin changes such as hives, redness, rash, and edema of the facial area. Questioning the patient about other allergies rules them out as the cause of the current reaction.
Administer medications as ordered (Benadryl, epinephrine).	Benadryl or other antihistamines will block histamine release, decreasing symptoms; epinephrine will relieve sympathetic system responses and ultimately decrease swelling in facial area as well as the amount of circulating histamine.
Apply ice pack to area of itching.	Helps to decrease discomfort caused by pruritus.
Apply anti-itch lotions or ointments, as ordered (Caladryl, hydrocortisone).	Helps to increase comfort.
Encourage the patient to avoid scratching areas of rash or redness.	Scratching can lead to excoriation and further alterations in skin integrity.
Avoid putting substances containing alcohol or perfume or harsh deodorant soaps on affected areas.	The skin is sensitive, and harsh products and alcohol can further dry the area, making itching worse and contributing to excoriation.

INTERVENTIONS	RATIONALES
If the patient has difficulty not scratching, especially during sleep, encourage him or her to wear soft gloves.	The discomfort from itching may be so severe that scratching is inevitable. During sleep, the patient is not aware that he or she is scratching. Having the patient wear soft gloves minimizes trauma to the skin.
Wear an eye patch at night if edema is present in eye area.	If swelling of the eye is extensive and prevents complete closure of the eye, a patch will protect the eye from dryness or damage.
Assess skin, eyes, face, tongue, and other areas following interventions.	Helps to detect improvement, resolution, or need for revision of therapeutic interventions.

 NIC *Skin surveillance*

Eye care

Allergy management

Evaluation

The patient's skin has returned to a normal state. The patient verbalizes no complaints of itching, and areas of redness/discoloration, hives, or rash resolve. In addition, edema of the eyes, face, or other areas has been eliminated. The patient experienced no further alterations in skin, and no areas of excoriation are noted.

Community/Home Care

The patient who has impaired skin integrity due to an allergic reaction may possibly go home with some symptoms still present. Continued care of skin at home may include applying substances for itching and monitoring for complete resolution of edema of eyes or other areas. The patient requires education about how to care for the skin, especially rashes, hives, and itching. Simple measures to employ at home include taking cool baths rather than hot ones, as hot water tends to make pruritus worse, and avoidance of everyday household products that can worsen symptoms, such as perfumed body lotions, soaps, and common cleansing agents such as Clorox® or Pine Sol®. Placing a thin cloth or piece of clothing over the itching area and rubbing it gently can help provide some relief from itching. If the causative agent for the reaction is known, the patient should avoid it at all times, and if contact occurs, institute measures quickly to prevent problems. This may include taking a dose of Benadryl or possibly use of an EpiPen in accordance with discharge instructions from the physician. The patient should always have these items nearby and be encouraged to carry them when traveling away from home. This is especially true for latex allergies, as often times it is not known whether an item contains latex.

Documentation

Document findings from the assessment of all skin, especially on the back, as well as the tongue, mucous membranes, and eyes. Describe specifically what types of skin changes are seen, including their specific locations. Inspect for edema over entire body but especially around the eyes and on feet, hands, and tongue. Document all therapeutic interventions employed. After interventions, always document the patient's responses and improvement, or changes required.

CHAPTER 8.105

ORGAN TRANSPLANT

GENERAL INFORMATION

Organ transplantation is a treatment modality that harvests organs from one source and transplants them into persons in need of them for a variety of diseases. Transplant types include heart, heart-lung, liver, kidney, and pancreas. A variety of tissues can also be transplanted, the most common being corneas, but heart valve, bones, cartilage, and parts of the ear can also be transplanted. Sources of organs include living donors, cadaver donors, and xenografting (use of animal organs that for the most part remains experimental). Chronic kidney disease is the leading cause of organ transplant followed by liver failure. Following transplantation, patients must strictly adhere to a therapeutic regimen of daily medications to suppress their immune system in order to avoid organ rejection. Patients are instructed to take anti-rejection medications without fail and to monitor for side effects, signs of infection, or organ rejection. The major reasons that transplant patients are readmitted to the hospital after transplant are organ rejection and infection, but hypertension is also a common occurrence thought to occur as a side effect of the prescribed medications. Those in need of transplants are placed on a national registry or waiting list from which recipients are selected when organs become available. There is a dearth of organs in the United States, and the waiting list is extensive, with additions estimated to occur every 20 minutes. The following care plan focuses on care of the patient in the post-operative period.

NURSING DIAGNOSIS 1

DEFICIENT KNOWLEDGE

Related to:

Lack of information about organ transplant and post-transplant care

Defining Characteristics:

Asks no questions

Asks many questions

No prior knowledge about transplantation

Goal:

The patient will understand principles of transplantation.

Outcome Criteria

✔ The patient verbalizes a willingness and desire to learn the necessary information.

✔ The patient verbalizes an understanding of transplantation.

✔ The patient verbalizes a willingness to be compliant with treatment recommendations.

✔ The patient is able to state correctly the required medications and the schedule for administration.

✔ The patient verbalizes an understanding of the signs of infection and rejection.

NOC *Knowledge: Health behavior*
Treatment behavior: Illness or injury

INTERVENTIONS	RATIONALES
Assess readiness of the patient to learn (motivation, cognitive level, and physiological status).	The patient must be motivated to learn, have the capability to learn the content, and be free of distractions from learning, such as pain and emotional distress.
Assess what the patient already knows.	The patient may have some knowledge about transplantation, and teaching should begin with what the patient already knows.

INTERVENTIONS	RATIONALES
Create a quiet environment conducive to learning.	Environmental noise can prevent the learner from focusing on what is being taught.
Teach incrementally, starting with simple concepts first and progressing to more complex concepts.	The patient will learn and retain knowledge better when information is presented in small segments.
Teach the learners about organ or tissue transplant and care required post-transplant.	If the patient understands the procedures and post-operative care the patient is more likely to avoid complications and hospital visits decrease.
Teach the patient to maintain a strict medication regimen as prescribed with anti-rejection medications and others as ordered: — Calcineurin inhibitors: cyclosporine (inhibits T-cell interleukin-2 production), Prograf® (prevents production and release of interleukin-2), and sirolimus (suppresses lymphocyte proliferation) — Steroids: suppress the inflammatory response — CellCept®: inhibits T- and B-lymphocyte proliferation responses, inhibiting antibody formation (used in allogenic transplants of kidney or heart) — Azathioprine (Imuran) suppresses T-cell effects to prevent rejection of kidney allografts and is given in conjunction with other immunosuppressants — Instruct on dosage, schedule, purpose, side effects of medications, and how to reduce occurrence of side effects	Adherence to the medication regimen is required to decrease likelihood of rejection. Medications are needed daily for the remainder of the patient's life. Compliance improves when patients understand all aspects of the regimen.
Teach the patient signs and symptoms of infection: feeling of malaise, low-grade fever, drainage from any open area, and increased pulse rate.	Infections are the most common cause of illness and death in the transplant patient, and the patient should be able to detect signs early. Immunosuppression therapy may prevent the normal signs of infection from occurring, and the earliest sign may be tachycardia and malaise.
Teach the patient about signs and symptoms of rejection: fever, fatigue, shortness of breath,	Rejection can be of three types: hyperacute rejection occurs immediately within minutes to
tenderness over site of graft, and decreased urine output.	hours of transplant, usually attributed to a bad match; acute rejection usually occurs within the first three months; chronic rejection has a more insidious onset, occurring after 3 months, and often results in loss of the graft. The patient needs to be aware of the signs of rejection in order to get immediate care to save the transplant.
Teach the patient about any dietary restrictions specific to the type of transplant received.	Although the transplant may lift some of the dietary restrictions previously required, some caution must still be taken, especially for heart transplants (low fat, low sodium) and renal transplants (low sodium). Other restrictions may be required, and the patient will need to understand and agree to comply with recommendations.
Inform the patient and family of appropriate phone numbers for health care providers.	The patient needs a way to contact health care providers in case of emergency or complications that require prompt treatment.
Evaluate the patient's understanding of all content covered by asking questions.	Helps to identify areas that require more teaching and to ensure that the patient has enough information to ensure compliance.
Give the patient written information on medications, signs of infection, diet recommendations, and any other information covered.	Provides reference at a later time, and for review.

NIC *Discharge planning*
Teaching: Individual
Teaching: Diet
Teaching: Prescribed medication

Evaluation

The patient is able to discuss the process of transplantation and the post-operative requirements for care. It is crucial that the patient verbalize accurate information about the anti-rejection medication regimen. The patient is able to repeat all other information for the nurse and asks questions about what to anticipate following transplant, including possible outcomes (positive and negative). Signs and symptoms of infection and rejection are stated correctly. The patient agrees to be compliant with all recommendations. The patient should know and be able to inform the nurse when health care assistance should be sought.

Community/Home Care

For patients who have had a transplant the hospital, stay may be lengthy, but continued care is required in the home. Teaching by the health care team should be thorough, with opportunities for discussions. The most crucial information is the regimen for anti-rejection medications and preventing infection. A written schedule for medications can also be given to the patient, as many patients may be prone to forget but are more likely to check a schedule if one is available. This information can be condensed to one sheet of paper, placed on a colorful sheet, and laminated for long-term use. Assist the patient to create a medication diary in which to chart medication administration but also record temperature, pulse rates, intake/output, or any other information the patient desires. This information can then be shared with the health care provider on subsequent visits. The signs and symptoms of infection and rejection should also be printed on one sheet of paper and given to the patient. Strategies that the patient must implement, especially in the early days following discharge home, are reviewed with the patient (see nursing diagnosis "Risk for Infection"). A follow-up telephone call from the transplant team or other health care provider can assess whether the patient has understood the teaching. The patient will require frequent follow-up, and prior to discharge the social worker or nurse should ascertain that the patient has transportation and the means to be compliant financially. In some instances, the patient may be required to remain in close proximity to the hospital for follow-up, and it is crucial that acceptable, affordable living arrangements are available. Follow-up with a health care provider focuses on assurance that no complications have occurred and that the patient has a clear understanding of how to manage all aspects of the post-transplant care.

Documentation

Document all content taught and the patient's verbalization of understanding. Specific attention should be given to documentation of any specific concerns that the patient expresses and how they are addressed. Include in the documentation the patient's expression of ability and willingness to comply with all recommendations made about medication administration and follow-up care. Any area that requires further teaching should be clearly indicated in the record, along with appointments for follow-up and referrals made. Always include the titles of any printed literature given to the patient for reinforcement.

NURSING DIAGNOSIS 2

RISK FOR INFECTION

Related to:

Immunosuppressant medication regimen

Defining Characteristics:

None

Goal:

The patient will not develop an infection.

Outcome Criteria

✔ The patient will be afebrile.
✔ The patient will report the absence of malaise and fatigue.
✔ The patient will have no edema at or drainage from surgical sites.

NOC *Immune status*
Knowledge: Infection control
Risk control

INTERVENTIONS	RATIONALES
Monitor for signs of infection: fever (take temperature every 4 hours); drainage or heat at any wound or intravenous (IV) access insertion site; urine for malodor or mucous; oral cavity for white coating; respiratory system for cough, sputum production, or crackles in lungs; notify physician if any are noted.	With immunosuppression, the patient is at higher risk for infection. A fever or systemic signs such as malaise may be the only sign of infection, as the patient is unable to produce the normal inflammatory response due to immunosuppression.

INTERVENTIONS	RATIONALES
Institute compromised host precautions: private room, good handwashing, restriction of visitors with symptoms of infections, requirement that all visitors wash hands before entering room; restriction of cut flowers and potted plants.	Helps to protect the patient from sources of infection.
If signs of infection occur, obtain blood cultures or cultures from other sites.	When the immunosuppressed person has a fever, a culture is needed in order to identify the causative organism to allow for specific treatment.
Practice good hand hygiene.	Handwashing is one of the best ways to prevent or stop the transmission of infection.
Have the patient avoid crowds.	Being in crowds increases the risk of acquiring respiratory infections.
Administer antibiotics, as ordered.	Helps to prevent or treat infection.
Assess surgical site and central line access sites for signs of infection, and change any dressings using strict sterile technique.	Skin that is broken by surgery or central line insertion is an easy portal for entry of organisms. Strict sterile technique is required to reduce risk of infection.
Ensure adequate rest, nutrition, and hydration.	Rest and hydration are both needed for restoration of the body and to prevent infection; good nutrition is needed for healing.

NIC   *Infection control*
        Infection protection
        Risk identification
        Self-care assistance
        Surveillance

Evaluation

Evaluate whether outcome criteria have been met. Infections have been prevented, as demonstrated by the absence of signs and symptoms. The patient verbalizes strategies needed to prevent infection and agrees to comply with them. At time of discharge from the health care agency, the patient has no malaise, fatigue, or fever.

Community/Home Care

The patient who has had a transplant will remain at risk for infection for his or her lifetime due to immunosuppression therapy. Once at home, the patient will need to continue to be vigilant in the practice of safety-enhancing behaviors for the prevention of infections. The diet may restrict raw fruits and vegetables early in treatment because of the risk of contamination; however, cooked fresh vegetables are allowed. Some care providers recommend that the patient avoid food buffets since these may also be a source of infection for an immunsuppressed patient. Specific dietary recommendations based on type of transplant and calorie requirements are made only after a thorough consult with the patient, and if possible, a significant other or family member. The patient will need to avoid crowds and activities that may increase risk for acquiring respiratory infection. Handshaking is a common expression of greeting but can also be the source of transmission of organisms from well-intending persons. This activity can transport organisms easily, so the patient should wash his or her hands afterwards or avoid the activity. Practicing good handwashing techniques can minimize the risk of infection. Visitors to the home and all caregivers should wash their hands prior to visiting with the patient in the early convalescent period. All persons in the home should practice meticulous handwashing, and children should be supervised washing their hands to ensure that it has been done properly before interacting with the patient. The patient, as well as any primary caregiver such as a family member or significant other, should avoid any person coughing or presenting with symptoms of respiratory infection. Patients who have young children or grandchildren should avoid them if possible when they are sick with colds or the flu. Teach the patient to take his or her temperature three times a day and to record it daily. At the first sign of infection, the patient should return to a health care provider for further assistance.

Documentation

Include in the documentation findings from a thorough assessment of the patient for evidence of infection. If the patient has any signs of infection, even minor ones, document this in the patient record with a clear indication of what actions were carried out in response. Temperatures should be taken at least every 4 hours and recorded according to agency protocol. Chart all interventions implemented to address infection prevention or treatment, including placing the patient on protective isolation. If teaching is implemented, include who the learners were and their levels of understanding.

NURSING DIAGNOSIS 3

 ## IMPAIRED SKIN INTEGRITY

Related to:

Surgical interventions

Defining Characteristics:

Incision on body

Staples or sutures present

Drainage device insertion sites

IV sites

Central line access sites

Goal:

Wounds will heal by primary intention.

Outcome Criteria

✔ Incision will be well approximated.

✔ Incisions will have no signs of infection (discoloration, purulent drainage, heat, or edema) at site.

✔ The patient will remain afebrile.

NOC *Wound healing: Primary intention*

INTERVENTIONS	RATIONALES
Monitor surgical sites, central line insertion sites, and any drainage device insertion sites for signs and symptoms of infection (discoloration, swelling, purulent drainage, heat, or edema).	Early identification of infection can expedite treatment.
Assess the surgical incision for approximation and signs of healing.	The site should be closed, with no open areas.
Take temperature every 4 hours.	Helps to detect elevations that may signal infection.
Change dressings as ordered and clean area using sterile technique, cleansing site of drainage devices last.	Maintenance of a clean incisional site decreases number of organisms and reduces chance of infection.
Practice good hand hygiene.	Effective handwashing is the first-line prevention measure. Most hospital-acquired infections can be prevented by adequate handwashing.
Administer antipyretics (acetaminophen [Tylenol]), as ordered.	Helps to reduce fever.
Administer antibiotics, as ordered, IV or PO (by mouth).	Helps to reduce number of infective organisms and eliminate or prevent infection.
Assess for increasing pain in surgical site and administer analgesics, as ordered.	Increasing pain at surgical site may signal infection; analgesics are needed to decrease post-operative pain.
Restrict visitors with colds or other upper respiratory infections.	Helps to reduce likelihood of patient exposure to infective agents.
Encourage adequate nutritional intake orally, parenterally, or enterally, especially intake of protein, vitamin C, and iron.	Adequate nutrient intake, especially of vitamin C, protein, zinc, and iron, is required for healing and tissue repair.
Monitor white blood cell (WBC) count.	WBCs may not always increase significantly due to immunosuppressive therapy, but should be monitored.

NIC *Incision site care*
Infection control
Nutrition management
Wound care
Wound care: Closed drainage

Evaluation

Evaluate the degree to which the outcome criteria have been met. The surgical site, drainage device insertion sites, chest tube insertion sites (heart or lung transplants), and any central line sites are intact healing by primary intention, with incision well approximated with staples or sutures intact. Discoloration, swelling, purulent drainage, and heat should be absent from the site. Drainage from the drainage devices should be serosanguineous and decreasing in amount. The patient should be afebrile.

Community/Home Care

The status of the surgical site may remain a problem after the patient has been discharged home;

however, for most patients the incision site has healed prior to discharge, as the length of stay is 7 days or longer for most transplants. For those patients whose incisions are not healed, the risk for infection remains once discharged, and the family will need to know proper incision care. Care of the incision may include dressing changes, but in many instances, the incision will be left open to air with staples intact. It is crucial that the patient or family realize the importance of refraining from touching the surgical wounds unless hands have been thoroughly washed. Irritation of the incision by clothing and bedcovers needs to be prevented, possibly by applying a light, clean dressing. The patient will need to understand the importance of good nutrition in complete wound healing and include foods rich in vitamin C, protein, iron, and zinc in the diet, unless contraindicated. The nurse completing discharge teaching should provide the patient with a list of foods that meet this requirement. The patient should understand the importance of completing any ordered antibiotics once at home. The patient should be instructed to contact the health care provider if he or she has a fever or if the wound opens or there is any evidence of infection or injury.

Documentation

Document dressing changes along with assessment findings from the wound, including color, approximation, and drainage, being sure to note any sign of infection. Chart the status of drainage devices or tubes indicating the color, amount, and consistency of drainage. Document vital signs according to agency protocol, as ordered for post-operative patients. Indicate any medications administered in the medication administration record according to agency protocol.

NURSING DIAGNOSIS 4

ANXIETY

Related to:

Lack of knowledge about organ transplantation
Complexity of treatment regimen
Fear of death
Serious illness

Defining Characteristics:

Expressions of fear
Verbalization of concern about medications
Restlessness
Tachycardia

Goal:

Anxiety is decreased or alleviated.

Outcome Criteria

✔ The patient will express feelings about organ transplantation, medication regimen, and side effects.

✔ The patient reports being less anxious.

✔ The patient demonstrates no outward signs of anxiety, such as restlessness or agitation.

NOC *Anxiety control*
        Comfort level
        Coping

INTERVENTIONS	RATIONALES
Assess level of anxiety (mild, moderate, severe); have patient rate on a scale of 1 to 10, with 10 being the greatest.	Gives the nurse a more objective measure of extent of the anxiety and how the patient is coping.
Provide accurate information about all aspects of the transplantation, particularly the post-operative therapeutic regimen for anti-rejection medications (see nursing diagnosis "Deficient Knowledge").	Communication about interventions in a reassuring, calm, and straightforward manner may help to relieve anxiety.
Encourage the patient to verbalize questions, fears, and concerns about the transplant.	Verbalization of fears contributes to dealing with concerns and moves the patient forward in terms of acceptance and successful health maintenance.
Control multiple sources of stimuli that could cause sensory overload.	Overstimulation can worsen anxiety.
Help the patient to identify successful coping mechanisms.	The patient needs to cope with a change in health status that has an impact on lifestyle and may need new coping strategies.

(continues)

(continued)

INTERVENTIONS	RATIONALES
Seek spiritual consult, as needed or requested by the patient and/or family.	Meeting the patient's spiritual needs helps him or her to deal with fears through the use of spiritual or religious rituals.
Teach the patient how to reduce anxiety with relaxation techniques, such as music, reading, meditation, distraction, writing, deep breathing, and guided imagery, and encourage their use.	These strategies can reduce anxiety and make the patient feel calm and in control.
Arrange for consultation with social worker to explore resources available for assistance with care needs.	Transplantation may require significant resources from the patient in terms of keeping appointments and obtaining medications. A social worker should be able to provide information about programs available to the patient.

NIC *Anxiety reduction*
Coping enhancement
Emotional support

Evaluation

The patient is able to identify ways to cope with anxiety and the changes in health status. Physiological signs of anxiety such as tachycardia will be absent. The patient will verbalize a decrease in anxiety and fear. Restlessness and agitation will be absent.

Community/Home Care

Anxiety is common during the post-operative period for patients following transplantation surgery. At home, the patient will need to practice relaxation techniques that can reduce anxiety and promote a sense of calm or peace. Nurses should discuss coping mechanisms with the patient and encourage the patient to use them at home. Methods of controlling the anxiety include reading, listening to music, having backrubs, watching television, and using guided imagery. The patient will need to experiment with several to determine what works. If the patient practices an organized religion, in-home visits by the religious/spiritual leader should be planned. This provides an avenue for expression of concerns and fears. Having printed materials for reference about medication schedule and side effects will also help relieve anxiety, as the patient will not have to memorize the information. If questions should arise at home about the patient's health status or prescribed regimen, the patient should have a means of contact with a health care provider for answers to further decrease anxiety.

Documentation

Document whether the patient is able to verbalize a feeling of decreased anxiety and whether there are outward signs of anxiety. A rating system provides an objective way to relay to others the extent of the anxiety. Blood pressure and pulse rates should be documented, as anxiety often causes an increase in both vital signs. Document coping methods the patient uses to decrease anxiety. Include in the chart all interventions that have been implemented to reduce anxiety, including teaching.

UNIT 9

INTEGUMENTARY SYSTEM

CHAPTER 9.106

BURNS: THERMAL/CHEMICAL

GENERAL INFORMATION

Burns (thermal and chemical) occur as a result of exposure to harmful chemicals, flames, hot liquids or superheated steam, or hot objects. Thermal burns are the result of contact with flames or moist heat, such as steam or hot liquids. Thermal burns are the most common type of burn in the United States, with an estimated one million people suffering a thermal injury. Most burns are caused by unsafe cooking practices or careless smoking habits, both of which can cause clothes to ignite. Chemical burns are caused when the skin comes in contact with caustic substances that erode or burn the skin. Acid or alkaline agents can cause these burns, but alkaline agents tend to produce a more severe burn. Common agents that cause chemical burns include lye, or products containing lye, ammonia, bleach, oven cleaners, and drain cleaners. Burns are commonly categorized based on the thickness of the burned skin and the percentage (extent) of the body surface area (BSA) burned, with consideration given to the age of the patient. Skin thickness categories of burns include superficial, partial thickness, and full thickness. The percentage or extent of BSA burn is determined using guides such as the rule of nines and the Lund and Browder charts. The rule of nines is a quick and easy assessment method that can be used in the field, while the Lund and Browder chart is more complex and accurate, taking into consideration the patient's age. Burns are classified as minor, moderate, or major using American Burn Association guidelines regarding percentage of body surface area burned, depth of the burn, and the particular part of the body burned. The severity of a burn injury is also based on the age of the patient, the presence of concomitant smoke inhalation, or other trauma, and the presence of a co-morbid factor, such as chronic illnesses. It is recommended that all patients with moderate and major burns be treated in specialized burn units. A severe burn injury is one of the most significant insults that can happen to a human body, both in physiologic terms and in psychological terms. If the patient survives a critical burn injury, the recovery and rehabilitation period may span years, and the psychological and financial toll to both the patient and the patient's family may be great. It is estimated that 75 percent of all burn injuries result from accidents, usually unsafe practices such as leaving cooking substances unattended, handling pans or grease that are on fire, rigging up unsafe electrical wiring, smoking in bed, using highly volatile substances inappropriately, etc. Estimates are that there are as many as two million burn injuries each year, with 45,000 patients requiring hospital admissions and 4500 people succumbing to burn injuries each year in the United States. There are a vast number of nursing diagnoses appropriate for the patient who has been burned, but the diagnoses for this plan are only a few of the most significant.

NURSING DIAGNOSIS 1

 INEFFECTIVE BREATHING PATTERN/INEFFECTIVE AIRWAY CLEARANCE

Related to:

Smoke inhalation

Edema of the airway

Burns to face, neck or chest

Defining Characteristics:

Severe dypsnea

Poor SaO$_2$ and arterial blood gas (ABG) values

Coughing

Soot in nose, around face and mouth, and in mouth and pharynx

Respiratory stridor

Decreased level of consciousness

Goal:

Breathing pattern is effective in maintaining oxygenation.

Outcome Criteria

✔ Oxygen saturation improves to 90 percent.

✔ Blood gas values return to normal.

✔ No dyspnea is present.

✔ Respirations are supported with mechanical ventilation.

NOC *Respiratory status: Airway patency*
Respiratory status: Ventilation
Respiratory status: Gas exchange
Anxiety level

INTERVENTIONS	RATIONALES
Assess for the presence of burns on face, neck, and chest, and determine their extent.	Burns to the neck and face are accompanied by edema that constricts the airway, making breathing difficult; chest burns restrict chest movement so that breathing is ineffective.
Perform a respiratory assessment and monitor for open airway, oxygen saturation, ABGs, carboxyhemoglobin level, struggling to breathe, use of accessory muscles of respiration, carbon particles in oropharynx and vocal cords, tachypnea, rales/rhonchi in chest auscultation, and ineffective chest wall excursion.	A detailed assessment of respiratory function is crucial to determine the ability to maintain airway patency and adequate gas exchange. Damage to the respiratory system may occur secondary to inhalation of smoke or burns to neck and face that cause edema that occludes the airway, or due to the body's systemic response. If carbon dioxide is present, it will displace oxygen on the hemoglobin molecule to form carboxyhemoglobin with the resultant decrease in oxygen available for tissues (hypoxia), and the level will be elevated. ABGs will reveal a decreased percentage of oxygen in the arterial blood.
Administer 100 percent humidified oxygen.	Helps to maximize oxygen saturation and decrease carbon monoxide levels (carbon monoxide toxicity is the most common cause of deaths in fires).
Elevate head of bed at least 30 degrees.	Helps to maximize chest expansion.
If burns are on face, neck, or chest, assist with placement on mechanical ventilation.	Mechanical ventilation is required due to the high risk for airway obstruction.
Suction frequently as ordered; if the patient is alert, encourage the use of incentive spirometry (IS) and turn, cough, deep-breathe (TCDB) exercises.	Suctioning is required to remove secretions and debris; IS and TCDB serve to open the distal airways and prevent atelectasis.
Provide airway adjuncts (early on), as ordered: oropharyngeal airway, endotracheal tube.	Helps to maintain open airway.
Prepare patient for creation of surgical airway: cricothyrotomy, tracheostomy.	Because of laryngeal edema, a surgical airway may be necessary. Cricothyrotomy is an emergent airway, and tracheostomy is an "elective" airway. Tracheostomy is usually performed if the patient is to be on mechanical ventilation longer than 3 weeks.
Provide positive pressure and mechanical ventilation, as ordered.	Helps to provide the required percentage of oxygen under pressure sufficient to deliver oxygen to the alveolar-capillary cellular membrane level through chemically damaged lungs.
If circumferential chest wall burns are present, prepare for surgical escharotomy.	Circumferential chest wall burns may limit chest wall excursion, prohibiting adequate gas exchange. In this life-threatening situation, surgical incisions are made along the lateral borders of the chest to release the scarred tissue and permit excursion of the chest wall.
Assess the patient for and implement strategies to reduce anxiety and fear, such as providing soft music, touching the patient, and informing the patient of all that is happening.	The patient is usually anxious due to the injury, difficulties breathing, and fear of what is happening. Anxiety increases the need for oxygen, which may worsen the respiratory status.
Inform family members or significant others about health status and treatments being implemented.	Keeping the family informed prevents undue anxiety and allows them to cope better.

NIC *Respiratory monitoring*
Oxygen therapy

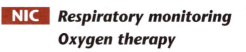

Airway management
Airway suctioning
Anxiety reduction
Mechanical ventilation

Evaluation

Assess the client to determine the extent to which the outcome criteria have been met. Assessments of the respiratory system should reveal that any acute symptoms of ineffective breathing pattern and airway obstruction have been resolved. The patient's airway should be clear, and the patient should be breathing easy. Breath sounds should be present, and even though some mild wheezing may be noted as the respiratory system attempts to re-establish adequate respirations, this should be improved. ABGs and oxygen saturation should indicate adequate oxygenation, and there should be no cyanosis. The patient should be alert and back at a normal level of consciousness. Patients requiring mechanical ventilation or with serious burn injury may remain comatose or semi-comatose, but respiratory status should have stabilized.

Community/Home Care

For the burn patient who has experienced ineffective breathing pattern or airway obstruction, time in the hospital may be prolonged due to the burn injury itself. By the time the patient is able to return home, respiratory complications have been resolved and the patient probably will not require in-home follow-up for breathing difficulties. The prevention of pneumonia is of great concern as it can develop as a late event. The patient should continue to practice TCDB exercises and IS. Health care providers should instruct the patients about signs of infection, such as increased sputum production, cough, fever, and fatigue. Little home care is required for the patient who has experienced airway obstruction except as it applies to other complications of the burn. If the patient is going home with a tracheostomy, teaching and some assistance may be needed (see nursing care plan "Tracheostomy").

Documentation

Document a comprehensive respiratory assessment, including respiratory status during the early phase of burn treatment and treatment of ineffective breathing pattern. Of particular note should be breath sounds, color, oxygenation status, respiratory rate, depth, and any nonverbal signs from the patient of difficulty breathing. Documentation about the mechanically ventilated patient is done in accordance with agency guidelines. Include in the patient record interventions carried out to treat the ineffective breathing pattern and ineffective airway clearance, and the patient's responses. Include an assessment of the patient's respiratory status once the problem has been resolved. Document vital signs according to agency protocol. Always include in the documentation the patient's progress towards achievement of the stated outcome criteria.

NURSING DIAGNOSIS 2

 IMPAIRED SKIN INTEGRITY

Related to:

　　Burns

　　Damage to the protective skin

　　Scarring of the skin causing a tourniquet effect

Defining Characteristics:

　　Loss of skin layers

　　Redness of skin

　　Blisters at site of burn

　　Dark, thick-burned skin

　　Severe tissue edema

　　Loss of circulation distal to burn injury

Goal:

　　Wound healing occurs.

Outcome Criteria

✔ The burns heal without signs of infection.

✔ Edema at the site of burns decreases.

✔ No signs of loss of circulation occur: severe pain in area, cyanosis, necrosis.

NIC *Medication administration: Skin*
Skin care: Topical treatments
Skin surveillance
Bathing
Infection protection
Circulatory precautions

Skin care: Donor site
Skin care: Graft site

INTERVENTIONS	RATIONALES
Identify the location of all burns and assess the amount of area burned using the Lund and Browder chart or rule of nines, according to agency protocol.	The Lund and Browder chart considers the patient age when determining the total BSA burned and is used to guide treatment of the skin as well as fluid replacement; this method is more accurate.
Assess the depth of all burns: — Superficial burns are dry, red, and painful, with no edema. — Partial-thickness superficial burns have blisters and are pink and very painful. — Partial-thickness deep burns have blisters, are pale or mottled, and very painful. — Full-thickness burns are dry with eschar that has a leathery appearance, have a charred, dark appearance or white, and are not painful.	This assessment is needed to determine skin care and to have data to determine the severity of the burn.
Assess all patient skin, especially areas in close proximity to the burn area.	The patient will most likely spend time in bedrest; breakdown must be prevented to all intact skin, as skin grafting may be needed.
Assess amount of pain experienced by the patient.	Superficial and partial-thickness burns are painful, especially deep partial-thickness burns. Full-thickness burns are not painful due to the destruction of nerve endings.
If the wound has not been cleansed prior to arrival in the burn unit, cleanse as directed by physician: — For chemical burns: Flush away/rinse chemicals using aseptic technique; irrigate wounds thoroughly, and remove jewelry and clothing that may contain the chemical. — For thermal burns: Remove clothing and jewelry, and initiate tub hydrotherapy and debridement, as ordered. — All hair in and close to the burned skin is shaved or clipped.	Debris and hair need to be removed to prevent the introduction of bacteria; use sterile gloves, mask, gown, and a hair covering. All invasive procedures should be done using sterile technique.
Following cleansing and debridement, administer topical antibiotics, such as mafenide acetate cream (Sulfamylon®), sulfadiazine cream (Silvadene®), and silver nitrate soaks, as ordered, and monitor for side effects.	These are broad-spectrum topical antibiotics that can prevent infection in the burn area. The choice of agent is physician-dependent, with consideration for extent of burn, type of dressing to be used, other treatments to be employed, etc. Sulfadiazine is the most commonly used agent.
Using sterile technique, apply loose bulky dressings, and change at intervals, as ordered.	Dressings are used to provide protection to the burned area.
Take temperature frequently, as ordered.	Due to the loss of skin, the body loses heat and the patient experiences hypothermia.
Administer pain medications as ordered, at least 30 minutes before scheduled dressing changes.	Dressing changes can be painful, especially in superficial and partial thickness burns.
Keep blisters intact, if possible.	Blisters provide protection from bacteria.
Prepare the patient for and assist with escharotomy, as ordered.	Escharotomy is done when the burned eschar restricts circulation to an area. It is often done at the bedside, and involves making lateral and horizontal incisions to loosen the eschar. It is usually required for full-thickness burns that restrict extremities or the chest, impairing adequate chest expansion for respiration. Some bleeding may occur from the tissue beneath the eschar.
Monitor patient for signs of infection: elevated white blood cells (WBCs), purulent drainage from burns, increased redness/discoloration, fever, positive blood cultures, and swelling at the burn site or the area close to the burn.	One of the most common complications of burns is infection; if infection occurs, mortality rate increases. It is crucial that care providers utilize strict sterile technique when working with the burn area. Cultures are obtained at regular intervals to monitor for the presence of organisms as well as the effectiveness of topical anti-microbial agents.
Administer antibiotics intravenously (IV) as ordered.	Patients receive antibiotics prophylactically due to the high risk of infection, especially if burns are extensive or the

(continues)

(continued)

INTERVENTIONS	RATIONALES
	patient is elderly or has other chronic illnesses that predispose him or her to infections such as diabetes mellitus.
Cleanse the patient's perineal and rectal area following elimination, especially if burns are in these areas.	Helps to minimize the entry of organisms into the burns through contamination from urine and feces.
Assist with application of temporary biological/biosynthetic grafts such as a homograft (allograft) and heterograft (xenograft), as ordered.	Helps to promote wound coverage until a more permanent graft can be performed, and reduces loss of fluid and heat from the site. Homografts are taken from cadavers and have been kept in skin banks. Heterografts are taken from other animals, such as pigs, and are usually kept frozen until time of use.
Prepare the patient for surgery for deep wound debridement and permanent graft placement: autograft (taken from the patient).	Debridement is required to remove devitalized tissue; the graft promotes wound coverage with permanent skin. Special care is required for both the donor site and the graft site, and most burn units have established protocols for their care.
Provide care to the graft and donor site according to agency protocol using aseptic technique.	A variety of types of grafts can be used, and each has specific care requirements.
Determine if the patient needs a tetanus toxoid immunization and administer as ordered.	Helps to prevent infection in the contaminated wound by clostridium tetani. The area beneath eschar tissue is an anaerobic environment that is perfect for growth of the tetanus organism.
Collaborate with physical therapist or occupational therapist.	Physical therapy is required to maintain range of motion in affected extremities as well as unaffected extremities. The occupational therapist provides assistance with development of special devices to be used in self-care when the hands have been burned or in providing diversional activities.
Teach the patient or family necessary wound care for in-home	Most patients will go home still requiring care for the burn area;

treatment, as ordered: infection prevention, care of burned area, application of topical ointments, and dressing changes.

there is a need for adequate teaching to ensure compliance with recommendations.

NIC *Infection protection*
Medication administration: Skin
Skin care: Donor site
Skin care: Graft site
Skin care: Topical treatments
Skin surveillance
Wound care

Evaluation

Evaluate the degree to which the outcome criteria have been met, which may be a prolonged period of time depending upon the extent of the burn. The burn site should show evidence of healing without signs of infection, such as redness, swelling, purulent drainage, and heat. There is no eschar tissue at the burn site or graft donor site. The patient should be afebrile, and WBC counts should be within normal ranges.

Community/Home Care

The status of the burns may remain a problem after the patient has been discharged home. The risk for infection remains, and the family will need to know what symptoms may signal the onset of infection. A family member, the patient, or a home nurse may perform wound care in the home environment. Adequate and extensive education by the nurse regarding wound care is necessary if the patient or family will be performing care of the burn site. The patient at home must practice good hand hygiene at all times, keeping in mind that even normal bacteria can cause infection in burn wounds. Dressing changes are usually done once a day when the patient is at home. Continued application of creams such as silver sulfadiazine may be required until healing is evident. The patient or family should demonstrate how to perform the skill (cleansing, applying cream, and applying dressing) correctly prior to discharge. Use of silver sulfadiazine can predispose the patient to sulfa crystals in the urine, and so even at home, the patient should be encouraged to drink liberal amounts of liquids. A list of the supplies the patient needs for wound care are given to the patient and a determination is made as to how the patient will obtain them. All supplies used in the care of the burn wounds should be kept in an easily accessible place in the patient's bedroom. These items can be stored in a covered heavy plastic box or crate with a lid like those used to store sweaters or shoes. Healing wounds can also cause a feeling of tightening, especially in the extremities, and the patient will need to continue exercises to preserve mobility and function. The physical therapist and occupational therapist play a key role in teaching exercises and assuring that those charged with their performance can carry them out correctly and understand their importance. Exercise also stimulates circulation to the area that can improve healing. Special support garments that apply pressure to the burn area are used to reduce scarring and may be ordered for the patient to wear for an extended period following discharge. The patient and family members are given instructions on the care of these garments and the correct way to wear them. If no special garments are required, the patient should wear loose-fitting clothes over the burns to prevent irritation to the site. The patient should be aware not only of signs of infection but also of indications of development of eschar tissue either on the burn itself or on any graft donor sites. The patient can use a hand-held mirror to get a better view of difficult-to-see areas and will need to assess those areas daily. If any evidence of poor wound healing or infection should occur, the patient should contact the health care provider. The patient will need to understand the importance of good nutrition in complete wound healing and recovery. A nutritious diet rich in proteins, vitamin C, and zinc promotes healing of impaired tissue. In addition, avoidance of people with respiratory infections is necessary due to the likelihood of transmission of organisms to the burn patient. The importance of completing any ordered medications such as antibiotics once at home should be stressed. It is also important to review safety practices and teach the patient fire-safety behaviors if the burn injury was preventable, as in the case of burns resulting from cooking, dangerous burning, inappropriate use of chemical agents, etc. In addition, be sure that the patient has a smoke detector and a fire extinguisher in the home, and that he or she understands how to use the extinguisher. Health care providers should inform the patient about follow-up care needed for burns, such as additional grafts or plastic surgery.

Documentation

Document assessment findings from the burned areas, including the location, depth, extent, and a description of the area. Record the exact type of skin care provided, including the names of antimicrobial topical agents used on the burn. Following grafts, document an assessment of the donor sites. During the entire period of hospitalization, document any signs of infection at either the site of the burn or the donor site. Chart vital signs according to the unit protocol, as ordered for burn patients or post-operative patients. Include in the patient record all interventions implemented for wound care.

NURSING DIAGNOSIS 3

 DEFICIENT FLUID VOLUME

Related to:

Loss of fluid through loss of skin

Fluid shifting from intravascular and intracellular spaces

Burn injuries > 20 percent BSA

Defining Characteristics:

Tachycardia

Hypotension

Delayed capillary refill (> 2 seconds)

Cool, clammy skin

Decreased urinary output

Hypotension

Hemoconcentration

Urine output < 30 ml/hr

Restlessness, agitation

Edema

Goal:

The patient will have adequate fluid volume restored.

Outcome Criteria

✔ The patient's skin will be warm and dry, and mucous membranes will be moist.

✔ The patient will have blood pressure at baseline.

✔ Pulse will be < 100.

✔ Electrolytes are within normal limits.

✔ Urinary output will be ≥ 30 ml/hour.
✔ Hematocrit (Hct) and hemoglobin (Hgb) are within normal range.

NOC *Fluid balance*
        Electrolyte and acid/base balance

INTERVENTIONS	RATIONALES
Assess fluid status: skin turgor, skin temperature, urine output, tachycardia, restlessness, lethargy, decreased blood pressure, and thirst.	Helps to determine the extent of the fluid loss. The first 48 hours are crucial for the burn patient. Capillary membranes become permeable, causing a shift of fluids from the vascular and cellular spaces, and some fluid is lost with the burning of the skin.
Obtain weight in kilograms and estimate total BSA burned.	Formulas used to determine fluid resuscitation are based on weight in kilograms and percent of body burned.
Monitor results of laboratory studies: Hgb and Hct, ABGs, BUN, electrolytes.	Hct fluctuates in response to fluid status; severe absolute loss from volume would produce a decrease in Hct, with further drops during aggressive fluid resuscitation due to hemodilution; the Hgb may be decreased. If volume loss is due to third spacing, Hct may be high initially and decrease as fluid is restored to the intravascular space. ABGs are done to determine oxygen and carbon dioxide levels; if the patient is progressing to shock, metabolic acidosis may occur due to anaerobic metabolism, as the respiratory and cardiac systems are unable to sustain adequate oxygenation to tissues. BUN and electrolytes indicate renal function. BUN may be elevated initially, but decreases due to hemodilution of fluid replacement. Potassium levels will be high initially as potassium exits from destroyed tissue, but as adequate fluid volume is restored, potassium level will decrease.
Monitor cardiac status: blood pressure, pulse (quality and rate), pulse pressure, and capillary refill.	Changes in blood pressure and pulse give information relevant to effectiveness of fluid resuscitation and are used to monitor for impending burn shock. A pulse rate above 120 is an indication of continued decreased cardiac output due to decreased volume. Capillary refill is an indicator of perfusion, and in the early stages of burn treatment it is > 2 seconds.
Monitor skin temperature and color for baseline and during treatment for improvement.	Pale, cool, clammy skin indicates decreased perfusion. As treatment progresses, skin should be warm and return to normal color.
Monitor oxygen saturation using pulse oximetry. It may be necessary to use the ear or nose.	Oxygen saturation indicates ability to perfuse tissues; in the presence of decreased cardiac output, perfusion to the fingers or toes may not be sufficient to obtain readings in these sites, and these areas may be burned.
Establish IV access with 2 large bore catheters (16 gauge or larger).	IV access is crucial to treatment; large gauge catheters allow for fluids to be given quickly.
Collaborate with physician to use Parkland formula or other formula to determine fluid replacement needs and infuse, as ordered (e.g., IV Ringer's lactate at 4 ml per kilogram of weight times percentage of BSA burned).	When skin is burned, histamine is released, causing increased capillary permeability and capillary leaking, with intravascular volume leaking into the interstitial spaces. This causes generalized edema, hemoconcentration, and hypotension. In addition, some fluid is lost from the skin due to the burn process. General rules of replacement suggest giving Ringer's lactate initially, half of the total volume required in the first 8 hours post-burn and half of total over next 16 hours post-burn. In the second 24 hours, 5 percent dextrose in water may be used to maintain urine output at 30 ml/hour in patients with large burns, but protocols for solutions vary based on provider and particular burn unit. Supplemental potassium and plasma or plasma volume expanders to maintain normal blood pressure and pulse may accompany fluid replacement.

INTERVENTIONS	RATIONALES
Strictly monitor intake and output every hour, or as ordered.	Helps to monitor fluid balance. Because of the massive fluid deficit, the kidneys may be hypoperfused as a compensatory mechanism and output decreases. In some burn units, fluids are titrated to maintain urine output at either 30 to 50 ml/hour or 0.5 ml/kg/hour. As fluid status is corrected, urine output should increase.
Insert indwelling urinary catheter.	The indwelling catheter is used to accurately measure urinary output.
Assess effectiveness of interventions to restore circulating volume.	Helps to determine whether revisions are required.
If urine output is inadequate and renal function studies decline, assist with institution of hemodialysis, usually continuous veno-venous hemodialysis (CVVHD). Monitor for side effects of the procedure.	CVVHD may be required due to acute renal failure. Renal failure can occur for several reasons, such as decreased perfusion secondary to decreased cardiac output and often due to acute tubular necrosis caused by myoglobin and Hgb release from damaged tissue that can precipitate in the renal tubules. CVVHD allows for slow removal of fluids, as the rapid removal can disrupt cardiac output in critically ill and unstable burn patients due to decreases in blood pressure. Side effects for CVVHD include hypothermia.
Assess the patient for fluid overload by noting adventitious breath sounds and distended neck veins.	Crackles in the lung may indicate fluid overload and the beginning of pulmonary edema; distended neck veins indicate increased volume.

NIC *Fluid resuscitation*

Fluid/electrolyte management

Fluid monitoring

Electrolyte management:
   Hyperkalemia

Hypovolemia management

Intravenous insertion

Intravenous therapy

Evaluation

Assess the patient for return of normal fluid volume. The patient's blood pressure should return to baseline or be > 70 systolic. The pulse should be strong, regular, and < 100, as higher rates may indicate continued decreased circulating volume. Skin should be warm, and color should return to the patient's normal appearance. Renal function should not be impaired, with an average hourly output of 30 to 50 ml/hour. Following fluid replacement, the patient should also be assessed for fluid overload that may occur in the elderly and those with chronic left ventricular disease. Oxygen saturation should demonstrate adequate oxygenation, and ABGs reveal a normal acid/base balance.

Community/Home Care

Patients treated for deficient fluid volume have normal fluid status restored prior to discharge home. At home, the patient does not require any follow-up for fluid status specifically, as this is an emergency acute situation that is corrected quickly long before the patient is ready for discharge and for the most part has no long-term complications. Fatigue may need to be addressed at home by having the patient perform activities as tolerated until stamina/endurance is re-established. The health care provider may want the patient to return for a follow-up appointment to ensure that parameters such as Hgb, Hct, electrolytes, and renal function studies have returned to normal.

Documentation

In this emergency situation, document initial assessment findings such as blood pressure, pulse, respirations, temperature, breath sounds, oxygen saturation, skin status, and mental status. Include in the chart any flow sheets used to document the calculation of fluid replacement for the first 48 hours. Document the specific solutions used and the rate of administration. Other interventions to be documented include IV catheter insertion and indwelling catheter insertion, with description of urine returned (amount, color). Intake and output are generally recorded every hour. Be specific when charting patient responses to treatment so that other health care providers can clearly determine improvement or deterioration. If hemodynamic monitoring is initiated, document readings as required by agency/unit-specific protocols.

NURSING DIAGNOSIS 4

ACUTE PAIN

Related to:

    Burn injuries

    Destruction of tissue

Defining Characteristics:

    Restlessness

    Tachycardia

    Tachypnea

    Grimacing and moaning

    Complaints of pain

Goal:

    The patient's pain is relieved.

Outcome Criteria

✔ The patient will verbalize that pain has been relieved 30 minutes after interventions.

✔ The patient has no grimacing or moaning.

NOC *Pain level*

      Pain control

      Comfort level

INTERVENTIONS	RATIONALES
Assess for location, intensity, quality, and precipitating factors.	Identifying these will assist in accurate diagnosis and treatment; most patients who experience burns experience some pain, especially with wound care procedures and movement. Third degree burns are not painful initially due to loss of nerve endings.
If possible, have patient rate pain intensity using a pain rating scale.	Provides a more objective description of level of pain.
Monitor for nonverbal cues to pain: grimacing/other facial expressions of pain, tachycardia, audible moans, and uncontrolled shivering. If the patient is alert but unable to speak due to intubation, use head nods or blinks to assess degree of pain.	All of these could indicate discomfort or pain. For patients unable to speak, alternative methods of evaluating pain are required.
Administer morphine or other narcotic analgesic (IV) in small doses, as ordered on a regular schedule, not allowing pain to get intense; narcotics may be required for a period of time. If able, use patient-controlled analgesia (PCA).	Decreased pain will improve patient's ability to tolerate dressing changes, participate in any prescribed physical therapy activities, and will also decrease oxygen demand.
Administer anti-anxiety medications (such as diazepam [Valium]), as ordered.	Helps to relieve severe agitation and provide sedative actions, which enhance effects of analgesics.
Move patient gently and cautiously when repositioning.	Movement of the patient causes pain in the burn areas, and careful movement provides support for the painful area.
Administer pain medication prior to morning care.	Morning care for patients with burns can take an extensive period of time, especially if dressing changes are done at the same time. Such a long period of activity is painful for the patient.
Implement non-pharmacological strategies to reduce anxiety, such as staying with the patient, using relaxation techniques, playing soft music, and keeping informed about interventions.	Anxiety often intensifies the pain experience, and reducing anxiety enhances effect of pain reduction measures.
Assess effectiveness of interventions to relieve pain.	Helps to determine if interventions have been effective in relieving pain or if new strategies need to be employed.
Teach the patient how to manage pain at home.	Pain will need to be controlled in the home, as healing may require a period of time beyond the time the patient is hospitalized.

NIC *Pain management*

     Analgesic administration

     Anxiety reduction

Evaluation

The patient is able to report that the pain has been reduced or alleviated following interventions. The degree to which the patient is able to assist in the management of the pain through anxiety reduction and relaxation techniques is assessed. The patient should have no observable signs of being uncomfortable, and the pulse rate remains at baseline. If the pain is controlled, the patient is able to tolerate dressing changes and movement without significant increases in pain.

Community/Home Care

The patient's pain should decrease once the burn areas begin to heal, but depending upon the length of hospitalization, may still be an issue at time of discharge to home. Teaching should be done to give the patient the information he or she needs to manage pain. Pain at home is usually managed with moderate analgesics, and the duration of pain is variable. For a short time, the patient will probably benefit from taking the pain medicine on a regular schedule rather than prn. The patient needs to monitor his or her response to activities that he or she participates in around the house and be able to identify those activities or even positions that increase pain. Encourage the patient to use any special devices such as slings or special garments that support the burned areas to relieve pressure on the affected site. Once at home, the patient should keep a pain diary that documents pain occurrence, rating of pain, and interventions used to treat the pain. Relaxation techniques such as meditation, reading, playing quiet music, and using guided imagery can assist with pain management in the home. The patient should be informed to notify a health care provider if pain worsens, as this may indicate infection. If the recommended analgesics are not working, the patient should also seek follow-up care with the health care provider.

Documentation

Include in the documentation a thorough pain assessment that includes nonverbal indicators of pain. Document in the patient's own words the description of the pain and rating of the level of pain. Chart all interventions (pharmacological and non-pharmacological) employed and the patient's responses. All teaching done relevant to pain control at home should be indicated in the patient record with an indication of the patient's level of understanding.

NURSING DIAGNOSIS 5

IMBALANCED NUTRITION: LESS THAN BODY REQUIREMENTS

Related to:

    Inability to eat

    Loss of protein and fluids from the burn area

    Increased metabolic demands

Defining Characteristics:

    No oral intake

    Decreased albumin levels

    Decreased iron and hemoglobin

    Loss of skin tissue

Goal:

    Nutritional status is maintained.

Outcome Criteria

✔ The patient does not lose weight.

✔ Albumin, iron, and Hgb are within normal limits.

✔ The family verbalizes an understanding of the patient's nutritional needs, including artificial means of delivering nutrition.

NOC *Nutritional status: Food and fluid intake*

    Weight: Body mass

INTERVENTIONS	RATIONALES
Assess indicators of nutrition: iron, Hgb, albumin, total protein, and BUN.	These are assessed to establish a baseline for evaluation of nutritional status following interventions. Iron, Hgb, and Hct provide evidence for the detection of anemia. Albumin and total protein give an indication of current nutrition status, especially the availability of proteins for healing. BUN gives clues to nitrogen balance, and a negative nitrogen balance indicates a lack of adequate proteins.
Weigh patient on admission and daily using bed scales.	Helps to determine baseline weight and for future comparisons to determine if nutritional status stabilizes and weight loss is prevented.
Collaborate with physician to obtain consultation with dietician to determine nutritional requirements.	The dietician is best qualified to develop a plan to meet nutritional needs. In most cases, the Curreri formula is used to determine the calorie requirements. This formula is (25 kcal/kg body weight) + (40 kcal × percent TBSA burn) = total kcal required.

(continues)

(continued)

INTERVENTIONS	RATIONALES
If the patient is able to take oral foods and liquids, encourage the intake of a high-calorie, high-protein diet, and enough carbohydrates and fats to provide energy.	Proteins are needed for wound healing; more carbohydrates and fats are needed to ensure enough nutrients for energy needs for the patient. The patient may need as much as 1.5 to 3 g/kg of body weight.
Assist with ordered alternative means of providing nutrition according to agency protocol such as enteral tube feedings via nasogastric (NG) or gastrostomy tubes.	Because of the increased metabolic demand, initiation of a means to provide nutrition is started quickly (within 24 hours of admission) to prevent protein depletion that could cause a negative nitrogen balance and delayed skin healing.
If tube feedings are initiated, offer water with each bolus feeding or every 4 hours for continuous feedings, or as ordered by the physician.	Many tube-feeding solutions are metabolized easily but leave very little free water, causing the patient to experience dehydration. Because many solutions are also high in protein, water is needed to protect the kidneys.
Follow agency protocol for administration of tube feedings, in general: — Check placement of tube (aspirate stomach contents and test for ph). — Keep patient elevated at least 30 degrees during feedings. — Flush the tube at least every 4 hours. — Check residual prior to each bolus feed, or every 8 hours for continuous feedings. — Hold tube feedings for specified amount of residuals as ordered (~150 cc). — For patients on continuous feeds, discard administration bag every 24 hours or according to agency protocol. — Refill feeding bag every 4 hours with only enough formula for a 4-hour time period for patients on continuous feedings.	These are all accepted standards of care for patients receiving tube feedings. Tube placement is assured by aspirating stomach contents, not auscultating for injected air; if mercury weighted tubes are used, placement is confirmed by x-ray; keeping the patient elevated prevents aspiration; flushing the tube maintains patency, especially if the tube is being used for medication administration; large amounts of residual indicate a lack of absorption or digestion of feedings; administration bags that hang longer than 24 hours become a medium for bacteria growth; placing only enough tube feed solution in the bag for 4 hours decreases chance for proliferation of bacteria.
Provide oral care to the patient using commercial preparations or gauze pads saturated with warm water.	Helps to minimize drying of oral mucous membranes and promote comfort.
Administer total parenteral nutrition, as ordered.	This is another means of supplying nutrients needed for healing (see nursing care plan "Total Patenteral Nutrition").
Provide information to family members or significant other on recommended strategies for providing nutrition and support them in decisions regarding implementation.	The family will need sufficient information in order to make an informed decision regarding the need and desire for artificial nutrition.

NIC *Nutritional monitoring*
Enteral tube feeding
Nutrition therapy

Evaluation

Determine whether the patient has met the stated outcome criteria. The patient should have a means of providing nutritional intake and fluids. Weight loss is prevented and laboratory results indicate a stable nutritional status. The family indicates an understanding of the nutritional needs of the patient and is supported in decisions regarding artificial means of delivering nutrition. The family will understand what is required to maintain an adequate nutritional status and has learned how to implement tube feedings in the home if necessary. Burn wounds show evidence of healing.

Community/Home Care

The burn patient will have continued nutritional needs when discharged home due to the continued need for increased nutrients for healing. If the patient is able to consume a diet through normal means, he or she will need education on what type of foods are needed. The patient may need to eat several meals a day with supplements and nutritional snacks that are high in calories. Milkshakes and fruit smoothies provide calories, but the patient may also need increased protein for healing, and can be encouraged to eat meat, eggs, beans, etc. It might be helpful to have the patient or caregiver make sample menus before discharge for the dietician to review. In addition, a schedule for meals and in-between snacks might make it easier for the patient to be more mindful of nutrient intake. Consideration should be given to the patient's usual dietary habits, food preferences, and cultural or religious requirements. The dietician should provide the patient with a list of foods and their corresponding calorie counts as well as how much protein they provide. This information can be kept in the kitchen for easy reference when planning meals. The patient will need to obtain a scale and weigh him or herself daily. Any weight loss should be met with increased intake. Encourage the patient to keep a log of intake and weights to be shared with the health care provider at return visits. If the burn patient goes home with tube feedings, the family members must learn how to administer tube feedings, most likely via a gastrostomy tube, as NG tubes usually are not used for long-term feedings. Family members or caregivers will need to have a realistic view of what administering tube feedings in the home will entail. Included in the teaching should be equipment to be used (syringe for bolus feedings, pumps, and bags for continuous feedings, as well as syringes for checking for residual), type of solution used, complications to anticipate (occlusion, diarrhea, constipation, excess residual), and how to correct them. Of utmost importance is positioning of the patient at home to prevent aspiration. A hospital bed is desirable if one can be obtained and afforded because it is easily elevated to a Fowler's or semi-Fowler's position. A nurse should be in the home the first time the family does the procedure, even if the family has demonstrated the procedure in the hospital. There is a certain level of comfort in performing tasks with nursing staff standing by at the bedside for support or assistance. It is a totally different experience to be at home with no health care personnel and possibly having a different set of equipment that makes the task more threatening. Someone should be on call to answer questions and troubleshoot for the family in case problems occur. The family will need to understand how to clean equipment and store it when not in use, particularly syringes used in the feeding procedure. Cleansing them in hot soapy water, rinsing well, and storing in the refrigerator should decrease bacteria count, but syringes should be replaced on a regular basis as both bulb and plunger types lose their ability to suction or operate smoothly with repeated use. It is important that the family understand the need for water as well as the feeding solution and be given specific instructions for the amount to be given and how often. In case of emergency such as running out of feeding solution, teach the family types of substances that can be substituted on a temporary basis—juices, sugar water, whole milk (unless contraindicated)—but first verify with the physician. A backup source of nutrition needs to be available in case the main caregiver becomes ill or for some other reason is unable to render the service. The family should be given written instructions that outline the procedure, give pointers for common trouble areas, and state clearly the solution, amount to be given, frequency, and amount of water to be given and how often. It is suggested that this document be made in duplicate and laminated so that it does not tear or soil resulting in an unreadable document.

Documentation

Document all strategies implemented for nutritional support. Include in the patient record assessments of nutritional status such as weight, condition of burned skin, and hydration status. Document referrals to the dietician. For patients taking nutrition orally document the percentage of meals and snacks taken, and in some instances assist with calorie counts. Document the patient's understanding of the diet required for proper healing and the rationale for increased calories and protein. For enteral feedings, chart feedings given according to agency protocol including amount of residual. Also record any untoward effects of tube feedings such as diarrhea or vomiting and the interventions used to correct them. Document all teaching and the family's verbalization of understanding. If the patient is going home with tube feedings, have the family demonstrate correct technique for performing the feedings prior to discharge.

NURSING DIAGNOSIS 6

 ## DISTURBED BODY IMAGE

Related to:

Changes in skin secondary to burns

Visible scar tissue

Defining Characteristics:

Withdrawal

Social isolation

Depression

Negative statements about physical appearance

Attempts to cover burn areas when visitors are present

Fear that no one will ever want to look at him or
her again

Fear/anxiety over image/loss of function

Expresses desire to die

Goal:

The patient accepts the change in physical
appearance and continues social activities and
interpersonal relationships.

Outcome Criteria

✔ The patient states a willingness to look at and
touch burn areas.

✔ The patient looks at self or areas of burn in the
mirror.

✔ The patient verbalizes an understanding of recommended skin grafting or plastic surgery required.

✔ The patient verbalizes an understanding of how
to perform wound care and exercises for the
skin that can reduce development of further skin
abnormalities.

✔ The patient verbalizes one positive statement regarding self or body image.

NOC *Body image*

INTERVENTIONS	RATIONALES
Provide assurance that feelings are very normal following burn injury.	Helps to stop the patient from thinking that his or her feelings are abnormal.
Encourage patient to look at him or herself in mirror while hospitalized.	Helps to allow patient time to adjust to appearance without concern for how others react.
Encourage the patient to communicate feelings about changes in physical appearance.	Talking about the changes may sometimes be the beginning of acceptance.
Teach patient and family how to care for any burn wounds or graft sites.	If the patient is comfortable with self-care, that comfort level may translate into acceptance for the change in appearance and incorporation of body appearance change into a positive self-image.
Monitor for feelings about self, interpersonal relationships with family members and friends, withdrawal, isolation, anxiety, embarrassment by appearance, fear that appearance will frighten	Helps to detect early alterations in social functioning, prevent unhealthy behaviors, and intervene early through referral to counseling.

loved ones, or expressions of desire to be alone.	
Encourage the patient to participate in at least one outside/public activity each week once health status permits.	Prevents patient from isolating self from others.
Identify the effects of the patient's culture or religion on perceived body image.	A patient's culture and religion often help define reactions to changes in body image and self-worth.
Assist the patient in identifying coping strategies/diversionary activities.	Helps to provide diversionary activities so that not all thoughts are on disfigurement.
Provide reassurance.	Explain that the burned area appears worse closer to the injury event due to swelling and discoloration. As time progresses, the burned area may appear better as edema subsides, and skin begins to heal.
Arrange for psychological counseling, if required.	Helps to provide psychological assistance to the patient and psychosocial evaluation.
Collaborate with the physician to arrange consultation with a plastic surgeon.	A plastic surgeon can explain procedures that can be done in the near or distant future to reduce scarring and restore the skin. It is often helpful for the patient to see "before" and "after" photos of other burn patients with similar appearances who have had plastic surgery intervention.

NIC *Body image enhancement*
Emotional support
Socialization enhancement

Evaluation

The patient is able and willing to learn about care
required following burn injury and adaptations required for self-care. Time is required for the patient
to assimilate the change in body image into his or
her self-perception. It is crucial that the nurse evaluates to what degree the patient is beginning to do
this. Look for behaviors such as touching the site,
looking at the disfigurement in the mirror, or asking
appropriate questions. Communication of feelings
and concerns relevant to the change in appearance
should be taken as a positive sign that progress towards meeting outcome criteria is being made.

Community/Home Care

At home, continued monitoring of the patient's body image is needed. Patients with facial disfigurement or disfigurement to areas that are visible to others may be self-conscious about their physical appearance. The nurse will need to be alert to subtle hints that may indicate that the patient has not completely adapted to the change in appearance. Open discussions regarding this change and interventions to prevent social isolation and withdrawal should continue with the patient and family. The patient may benefit from talking to others who have experienced changes in physical appearance. Gradual resumption of outside activities should be undertaken with visits to areas where the patient has felt comfortable in the past, such as church or social groups, community organizations, or volunteer activities.

Having the patient visit the hospital cafeteria when returning for follow-up visits may be helpful as well. This is an environment where there may be a variety of people with different medical devices attached and skin impairments, but also visitors who may stare. The combination may be a more comfortable environment for starting public appearances. Discussions with health care providers regarding future reconstructive/plastic surgery should be encouraged.

Documentation

Chart any specific behaviors or verbalizations that may indicate an altered body image. Include all interventions that have been employed to address this issue and the patient's responses. Note when and if the patient begins to ask questions and participate in care. Document all referrals made.

CHAPTER 9.107

BURNS: ELECTRICAL

GENERAL INFORMATION

Electrical burns are caused by the entrance of a high-voltage current into the body, either through a manmade electrical source (such as power lines or electrical wiring) or naturally occurring lightning. The current will pass through the body along the path of least resistance, usually traveling along nerves, blood vessels, and muscles (especially the heart), and exiting through another part of the body. Electrical burns are usually very different from thermal or chemical burns because there may be very little visible damage to superficial tissue except at the entrance and exit sites of the current. The problem, however, is that there may be massive muscle and tissue injury that cannot be visualized, and severe cardiac dysrhythmias, especially ventricular tachycardia and ventricular fibrillation. The full extent of damage caused by an electrical burn may not be evident for 7 to 10 days. Factors that affect the extent of the damage include duration of contact with the body, intensity of the current, the type of current, the pathway it takes through the body, and the resistance of the tissues it encounters. It is important to check the patient carefully for concurrent trauma in addition to electrical burn injuries.

NURSING DIAGNOSIS 1

 DECREASED CARDIAC OUTPUT

Related to:

Passage of electrical current through heart

Dysfunctional electrical conductivity of cardiac cells

Ineffective/decreased myocardial function

Defining Characteristics:

Cardiac dysrhythmias: Ventricular tachycardia and/or ventricular fibrillation

Asystole

Hypotension

Decreased capillary refill

Pale, cool skin

Decreased urine output

Altered mental status

Decreased, thready peripheral pulses

Pale extremities

Abnormal heart sounds

EKG changes

Goal:

The patient exhibits improved cardiac output, and dysrhythmias will be alleviated.

Outcome Criteria

✔ Pulse rate is < 100 but > 60.

✔ Blood pressure is at patient's baseline.

✔ Heart sounds are normal.

✔ The patient will have a normal sinus rhythm.

✔ Peripheral pulses return.

✔ Skin is warm and is patient's normal color.

✔ The patient is alert and oriented.

✔ Urine output will be > 30 ml/hour.

NOC *Cardiac pump effectiveness*
Circulation status
Tissue perfusion:
    Cerebral
Tissue perfusion:
    Peripheral
Vital signs
Medication response

INTERVENTIONS	RATIONALES
Monitor for tachycardia, dysrhythmias (ventricular tachycardia, ventricular fibrillation), abnormal heart sounds (murmur, S_3, S_4) and changes in blood pressure; take both apical and radial pulse, noting rate, rhythm, quality, and any pulse deficit.	Assessment of cardiac status gives early clues to cardiac damage and response to interventions and establishes a baseline; hypotension and pulse deficits may result from decreased cardiac output.
Assess peripheral perfusion: skin color, temperature, peripheral pulses, and capillary refill.	Helps to monitor for decreased perfusion secondary to decreased cardiac output: decreased peripheral pulses and increased capillary refill > 2 seconds are indicators of poor perfusion.
Monitor for changes in mental status (confusion, restlessness, agitation).	These indicate decreased cerebral tissue perfusion.
Conduct a respiratory assessment: monitor for respiratory rate, rhythm, depth, tachypnea, difficulty breathing, and signs of ineffective airway.	Helps to determine the effect cardiac alterations have on ability to exchange gases, for early identification of ineffective airway clearance.
Monitor arterial blood gases (ABGs) and oxygen saturation level.	These are measures of the ability of the heart to perfuse tissues with oxygenated blood.
Assist with obtaining 12-lead EKG and any other ordered diagnostic tests such as chest x-ray, and monitor results.	These tests reveal definitive diagnosis of the effect the electric current had on the cardiac system and aids in monitoring the response to interventions. Twelve-lead EKGs are ordered and will show any dysrhythmias; the chest x-ray will give information regarding any other internal damage caused by the electric current.
Place the patient on continuous cardiac monitoring, monitor cardiac monitor strips, and document rhythm according to agency protocol.	The nurse is responsible for monitoring for dysrhythmia and intervening according to protocol or notifying physician for prompt treatment.
Insert urinary indwelling catheter; monitor urine output and results of urinalysis.	Decreased urine output of less than 30 ml/hour may indicate decreased tissue perfusion to the kidneys because of decreased cardiac output. Following electrical burns, acute renal failure is a significant problem due to release of myoglobin and

INTERVENTIONS	RATIONALES
	hemoglobin (Hgb) from deep muscle injury that may precipitate and clog the renal tubules, resulting in myoglobinuria.
Administer supplemental oxygen as ordered based on results of ABGs and oxygen saturation.	Helps to maximize the amount of oxygen available for gas exchange, which assists in alleviating signs of hypoxia; hypoxia can be a cause of dysrhythmia.
Administer antidysrhythmic medications as ordered based on type of dysrhythmia (examples: lidocaine, amiodarone, epinephrine, procainamide, atropine).	Helps to correct the abnormality before complications occur.
Establish intravenous (IV) access.	Provides a means to give medications as ordered and to have access available in case of emergency.
Prepare for electrical intervention according to agency protocols.	Some patients require synchronized cardioversion, defibrillation, or a pacemaker to correct dysrhythmia. These medical interventions performed by qualified cardiologists restore normal electrical activity and conduction in the heart tissue.
For patients who are tachycardic, encourage the Valsalva maneuver as directed.	This maneuver (vagal nerve stimulation) stimulate the parasympathetic nervous system and decrease heart rate.
Encourage the patient to rest; provide assistance with activities, and monitor for fatigue.	Patients who experience dysrhythmias secondary to electrical burns are often fatigued easily, and rest and assistance will promote conservation of energy.
For life-threatening dysrhythmias or asystole, prepare to initiate advanced cardiac life support (ACLS), as needed.	Advanced cardiac life support (ACLS) implementation is the definitive treatment for certain dysrhythmias.

NIC *Dysrhythmia management*
Cardiac care: Acute
Oxygen therapy
Vital signs monitoring

Medication management
Code management

Evaluation

The patient has no signs of decreased cardiac output. Dysrhythmias have been alleviated, with a return to normal sinus rhythm as demonstrated by the cardiac monitor readings. Urinary output has been maintained at or above 30 ml/hour. The patient's pulse and blood pressure have returned to baseline/normal, and skin is warm and color is at patient's baseline.

Community/Home Care

The patient with decreased cardiac output following electrical burns may not require any in-home care for the problem once discharged. The cardiac dysrhythmias will be resolved quickly with either medication or invasive procedures due to their ability to be life-threatening. The patient may have problems such as fatigue due to the impact of serious illness on stamina. It is anticipated that the patient will need to incorporate rest periods into the daily routine to ensure that the demands for oxygen can be met by the myocardium that has been traumatized. Encourage the patient to increase activities slowly by monitoring the response at home and keeping a log to monitor progress. There should be no need for continued cardiac medications or treatment. However, the patient will require a follow-up visit with a health care provider for an EKG to assure that the normal sinus rhythm has remained. Psychomotor skills required for management of the regimen include knowing how to monitor pulse for rate and rhythm and what constitutes a finding that should be reported to the health care provider.

Documentation

Chart the status of achievement of outcomes with specific patient behaviors. Include pulse, blood pressure, oxygenation saturation, heart sounds, and type of rhythm noted on the cardiac monitor. Document all indicators of cardiac output and tissue perfusion. Document all interventions, EKG, medications, or cardioversion according to agency protocol, with corresponding documentation of the patient's responses. Include in the chart the patient's understanding of what has occurred.

NURSING DIAGNOSIS 2

 IMPAIRED SKIN INTEGRITY

Related to:
    Electrical current
    Damage to the protective skin

Defining Characteristics:
    Entry wound for electricity
    Exit wound for electricity
    Hard, tight limbs
    Shiny, stretched skin
    Redness of skin
    Blisters at site of burn

Goal:
    Wound healing occurs.

Outcome Criteria

✔ Exit and entry wounds heal without infection.
✔ Redness or excoriation at sites will dissipate.
✔ Edema at the site of burns decreases.
✔ No signs of loss of circulation occur: severe pain in area, cyanosis, or necrosis.

NIC *Medication administration: Skin*
    Skin care: Topical treatments
    Skin surveillance
    Infection protection
    Circulatory precautions

INTERVENTIONS	RATIONALES
Perform an extensive examination of the body to locate all burns, exit and injury sites of electricity, the amount of area burned, and any other signs of trauma, especially broken bones.	Electrical burns do not usually result in significant body surface burns, but rather, internal damages. Electrical jolts usually cause the patient to fall with resultant traumatic injuries, such as compression fractures.
Assess the extent of injury especially areas of burn at the entry or exit points of the electrical current; these burns are usually superficial burns	This assessment is needed to determine skin care and to have data to determine the severity of the burn.

INTERVENTIONS	RATIONALES
that are red, dry, with no edema, and painful or partial thickness superficial burns that are pink, very painful, and have blisters.	
Assess all patient skin, especially areas in close proximity to the burn area.	The patient will most likely spend time on bedrest; breakdown must be prevented to all intact skin.
Assess amount of pain experienced by the patient.	Superficial and partial thickness burns are painful and require pain medication.
If the wound has not been cleansed prior to arrival in the burn unit, cleanse as directed by physician.	Debris and hair need to be removed to prevent the introduction of bacteria; use sterile gloves, mask, gown, and hair covering. All invasive procedures should be done using sterile technique.
Following cleansing, administer topical antibiotics such as mafenide acetate cream (Sulfamylon®) or sulfadiazine cream (Silvadene) as ordered, and monitor for side effects.	These are broad-spectrum topical antibiotics that can prevent infection in the burn area. The choice of agent is physician-dependent, with consideration for extent of burn, type of dressing to be used, other treatments to be employed, etc. Sulfadiazine is the most commonly used agent.
Using sterile technique, apply dressings to entry or exit wounds and change at intervals, as ordered.	Dressings are used to provide protection to the burned area.
Take temperature frequently as ordered.	The patient who has sustained any type of burn is at risk for infection with accompanying fever and hypothermia.
Administer pain medications as ordered at least 30 minutes before scheduled dressing changes.	Dressing changes can be painful, especially in cases of superficial and partial thickness burns.
Keep blisters intact if possible.	Blisters provide protection from bacteria.
Monitor patient for signs of infection: elevated white blood cells (WBCs), purulent drainage from burns, increased redness, fever, positive blood cultures, and swelling at the burn site or the area close to the burn.	Even though burn wounds from electrical burns are smaller, infection may still occur. It is crucial that care providers utilize strict sterile technique when working with the burn area. Cultures are obtained at regular intervals to monitor for the presence of organisms and also

	the effectiveness of topical antimicrobial agents.
Determine if the patient needs a tetanus toxoid immunization, and administer as ordered.	Helps to prevent infection in the contaminated wound by *Clostridium tetani*.
If the patient is unable to move or if fractures have occurred, collaborate with physical therapist for appropriate activity.	Physical therapy is required to maintain range of motion in extremities until the patient is mobile or ambulatory.
Prepare for exploratory fasciotomies.	If internal damage to muscles is suspected, the surgeon will explore subcutaneous tissue to evaluate damage, repair damage, and debride devitalized tissue.
If the entry or exit wounds require wound care, teach the patient necessary wound care for in-home treatment as ordered: infection prevention, care of burned area, application of topical ointments, and dressing changes.	If the patient is to go home still requiring care for the burn area, there is a need for adequate teaching to ensure compliance with recommendations.

NIC *Infection protection*
Medication administration: Skin
Skin care: Topical treatments
Skin surveillance
Wound care

Evaluation

Evaluate the degree to which the outcome criteria have been met. The burn site should show evidence of healing without signs of infection such as redness/discoloration, swelling, purulent drainage, and heat. There is no edema or continued excoriation at the electric current entry or exit point. The patient should be afebrile, and white blood cell (WBC) counts should be within normal ranges.

Community/Home Care

In general, the patient who has sustained an electrical burn does not have substantial wound care needs at home. The status of the burns may not be a problem after the patient has been discharged home because the wounds from electrical burns tend to be smaller and may heal quickly. However, the risk for infection may remain, even with a small wound, and the family will need to know what symptoms may signal the onset of infection. Wound care is performed by the family, patient, or in-home nurse. The patient at home must practice good hand hygiene at all times and realize that even normal bacteria can cause infection in burn wounds. Dressing changes are usually done once a day when the patient is at home. Simple cleansing with normal saline and the application of antibiotic ointments are usually sufficient, but that is determined by the physician. Prior to discharge, the patient or family should demonstrate how to perform dressing changes correctly. A list of the supplies needed are given to the patient and a determination is made as to how the patient will obtain them. All supplies used in the care of the burn area should be kept in an easily accessible place in the patient's bedroom. These items can be stored in a covered heavy plastic box or crate with a lid, like those used to store sweaters or shoes. Continued application of creams or ointments may be required until healing is evident. The patient needs to assess the wounds daily and can use a handheld mirror to get a better view of difficult-to-see areas. The patient will need to understand the importance of good nutrition in complete wound healing, energy, and recovery. The importance of completing any ordered medications such as antibiotics once at home should be stressed. It is important to review safety practices and teach the patient safety behaviors related to electric current, such as rigging up electric devices and repairing electrical problems, and behaviors to avoid, such as touching live electric wires and using frayed electric wiring, etc. Health care providers should provide information to the patient regarding follow-up needed for further care, such as EKGs or x-rays of extremities, etc.

Documentation

Document assessment findings from the burned areas including the location, depth, extent, and a description of the area. Record the exact type of skin care provided, including the names of antimicrobial topical agents used on the burn. If evidence of other injury is present, document this with notation of any treatments performed. For the entire period of hospitalization, document any signs of infection at either the entry site or the exit site. Document vital signs according to the unit protocol, as ordered for burn patients. Include in the patient record all interventions implemented for wound care.

NURSING DIAGNOSIS 3

ACUTE PAIN

Related to:
Electrical burn
Destruction of internal muscle
Possible fractures
Impairment of skin

Defining Characteristics:
Verbalization of pain
Painful extremities
Paresthesias
Facial expressions
Grimacing
Moaning
Pain with movement

Goal:
Patient pain is decreased or relieved.

Outcome Criteria

✔ The patient will verbalize that pain has been relieved 30 minutes after interventions.

✔ The patient does not grimace or moan.

NOC *Pain level*
Pain control
Comfort level

INTERVENTIONS	RATIONALES
Assess for location, intensity, quality, and precipitating factors.	Identifying these will assist in accurate diagnosis and treatment; most patients who experience burns experience some pain, and the internal damage to muscles that occurs with electrical burns may cause pain, especially with movement.
If possible, have the patient rate pain intensity using a pain rating scale.	Provides a more objective description of level of pain.
Monitor for nonverbal cues to pain: grimacing/other facial expressions of pain, tachycardia,	All of these could be indicators of discomfort or pain. For patients unable to speak,

INTERVENTIONS	RATIONALES
audible moans, uncontrolled shivering, grimacing with movement, and increased pulse when extremities are moved. If the patient is alert but unable to speak due to intubation, use head nods or blinks to assess degree of pain.	alternative methods of evaluating pain are required.
Administer morphine or other narcotic analgesic (IV [intravenously], patient-controlled analgesia [PCA], or PO [by mouth]) as ordered on a regular schedule, not allowing pain to get intense.	Decreased pain will improve the patient's ability to tolerate dressing changes and participate in any prescribed physical therapy activities, and will also decrease oxygen demand. Patients with electrical burns may also have traumatic injuries that cause pain.
Move patient gently and cautiously when repositioning.	Movement of affected areas, especially limbs, causes pain, and careful movement provides support for the painful area.
Administer pain medication prior to morning care.	Morning care can increase pain due to movement and manipulation of injured areas.
Administer anti-anxiety medications (such as Valium), as ordered.	Helps to relieve severe anxiety or agitation.
Implement non-pharmacological strategies to reduce anxiety, such as staying with the patient, relaxation techniques, soft music, diversional activities, and keeping informed about interventions.	Anxiety often intensifies the pain experience; these activities may decrease the attention or focus on the pain and enhance effects of analgesics.
Assess effectiveness of interventions to relieve pain.	Helps to determine if interventions have been effective in relieving pain or if new strategies need to be employed.
Teach the patient how to manage pain at home.	Pain will need to be controlled in the home as healing may require a period of time beyond hospitalization.

NIC *Pain management*
      Analgesic administration
      Anxiety reduction

Evaluation

The patient is able to report that the pain has been reduced or alleviated following interventions. The degree to which the patient is able to assist in the management of the pain through anxiety reduction and relaxation techniques is assessed. There should be no observable signs of discomfort, and the pulse rate remains at baseline. If the pain is controlled, the patient is able to tolerate any dressing changes, physical therapy, activities of daily living (ADLs), and movement without significant increases in pain.

Community/Home Care

The patient's pain should decrease once the burn areas or traumatic injuries begin to heal, but depending upon the extent of the injuries and the length of hospitalization, may still be an issue at time of discharge to home. Pain at home is usually managed with moderate to mild analgesics, and the duration of pain is variable. For a short time, the patient will probably benefit from taking the pain medicine on a regular schedule rather than prn. The patient needs to monitor response to activities around the house and be able to identify those activities or even positions that increase pain. Encourage the patient to use any special devices such as slings, canes, or crutches that assist the burned or injured areas to relieve pressure on the affected site. Once at home, the patient should keep a pain diary that documents pain occurrence, rating of pain, and interventions used to treat the pain. Relaxation techniques, such as meditation, reading, playing quiet music, and using guided imagery can assist with pain management in the home. Teaching about pain management should be done, and the patient should be informed to notify a health care provider if pain worsens, as this may indicate infection. If the recommended analgesics are not working, the patient should seek follow-up care with the health care provider.

Documentation

Include in the documentation a thorough pain assessment that includes nonverbal indicators of pain. Document in the patient's own words the description of the pain and rating of the level of pain. Chart all interventions (pharmacological and non-pharmacological) employed and the patient's responses. Document all teaching done relevant to pain control at home in the patient record with an indication of the patient's level of understanding.

CHAPTER 9.108

PRESSURE ULCERS (DECUBITUS ULCERS)

GENERAL INFORMATION

Pressure ulcers, also known as decubitus ulcers, are wounds or lesions caused by pressure on an area for extended periods of time. The unrelieved pressure causes compression of blood vessels that supply the underlying tissue, which leads to tissue hypoxia due to decreased or lack of tissue perfusion. Eventually, tissue breakdown and death occur. There are several other causes of pressure ulcers. Movement of patients in a manner that creates friction and a shearing force also cause ulcers; as the patient is pulled up in bed, the tissue moves in a counter-direction against the bed. Urinary incontinence can cause an ulcer by emaciating the skin with constant wetness and irritating effects of ammonia byproducts in the urine. Other contributing factors leading to pressure ulcer development include immobility, poor nutritional status, and existing co-morbidities. Pressure ulcers typically occur on bony prominences or any other areas exposed to prolonged pressure. Common sites include the sacrum/coccyx area, hips, buttocks, heels, ankles, and inner aspect of knees. Pressure ulcers are classified into four stages: stage I ulcers are characterized by redness that is not relieved when pressure is removed; stage II is a partial thickness loss of skin that is characterized by loss of epidermis, dermis, or both, and that appears as a superficial lesion often described as excoriated; stage III is a loss of the full thickness of skin with impairment of the subcutaneous tissue but with no involvement of the fascia. The lesion is described as a crater. Stage IV is the most serious stage of pressure ulcers and is a loss of the full thickness of skin with extensive damage and loss of tissue with involvement of the muscle, bone, or other structures. This stage of pressure ulcer often has necrotic tissue and drainage, and undermining or tracking is common.

NURSING DIAGNOSIS 1

 IMPAIRED SKIN INTEGRITY

Related to:
Prolonged pressure
Immobility
Incontinence
Imbalanced nutrition
Shearing force
Chronic disease

Defining Characteristics:
Open ulcers
Draining wound
Necrotic tissue
Redness/discoloration and excoriation to skin
Stage I, II, III, or IV ulcer

Goal:
Pressure ulcers will heal.

Outcome Criteria

✔ The ulcer will have granulation tissue.
✔ The ulcer will be pink.
✔ The ulcer will decrease in size.
✔ Pressure ulcers will heal without infection.
✔ Pressure will be relieved.

NOC *Tissue integrity: Skin and mucous membranes*
Immobility consequences: Physiological
Wound healing: Secondary intention

INTERVENTIONS	RATIONALES
Assess pressure ulcers for color, drainage (amount, color, consistency, odor), size, heat, and stage using a standard staging method or agency guidelines.	It is important that pressure ulcers are assessed each shift to detect improvement or worsening, and to revise the plan of care as needed. Staging gives other care providers information on the seriousness of the ulcer. A description of drainage is needed to differentiate normal drainage due to healing from drainage that might indicate infection. The size is a way of assessing improvement; easy-to-use measuring tools exist, and if these are not available, a tape measure can be used.
Complete a thorough skin assessment of all other skin with particular attention to high-risk areas over bony prominences every shift, noting areas of redness, pallor, edema, and any denuded or open areas, with particular attention to sacrum/coccyx, heels, ears, hips, inner aspects of knees, and elbows.	A thorough assessment establishes a baseline; areas subject to pressure are higher risk for breakdown, and these include most bony prominences.
Use the Braden Risk Assessment Scale.	This is an objective method of assessing the patient's risk for skin breakdown, and includes parameters such as sensory perception, moisture, activity, mobility, nutrition, friction, and shear. Information from this assessment adds to the general assessment and allows for planning to resolve causative factors and predict new areas of breakdown.
Identify other disease processes that impact skin integrity, such as diabetes, renal insufficiency, liver disease, and AIDS.	Many other diseases place the patient at risk for pressure ulcers due to alterations in homeostasis and elasticity of skin.
Monitor laboratory tests: albumin, blood urea nitrogen (BUN), and creatinine.	Decreased levels of albumin, BUN, and creatinine indicate a state of protein depletion that prevents the patient from having adequate protein stores for healing; this is also a sign of malnutrition indicating a lack of nutrients for tissue health.
Turn the patient every 2 hours using turn sheets and acceptable patient handling techniques, avoiding friction and shearing force.	Most patients prone to breakdown are unable to sense the pressure on prone areas, and immobility prevents self-repositioning; pressure causes vasculature to be compressed and unable to provide nutrients to the high-risk areas; friction and shearing damages the skin and underlying vasculature.
Post a turning schedule at the patient's bedside.	Helps to ensure that all health care workers are aware of the need for turning; the schedule prevents the patient from being repositioned in a particular position too often.
Keep the patient's head in the lowest tolerable position and avoid positioning with head and feet both elevated.	When the head is elevated above 30 degrees the patient tends to slide down in bed, creating shearing; if head and feet are both elevated, pressure is increased on the sacrum.
Provide wound care using sterile technique as ordered. In general, wounds require cleansing, dressings, and medicated preparations to promote healing.	In order for a wound to heal, it must be kept clean, and cleansing is usually done with normal saline if infections are not present. Saline is preferred because it will not harm other tissue and is effective in cleansing. Numerous types of dressings and healing preparations are available, and the type used depends on the stage of ulcer and physician preference. Dressings may include wet-to-moist for debridement, hydrocolloid dressings such as Tegaderm® to prevent friction and shear, and packing of deep wounds with dressings impregnated with special ointments, to name a few.
For deep wounds requiring irrigation, use a 35 ml syringe.	Irrigation is needed for wounds that have debris, necrotic tissue, and pus. To be effective, the irrigation should be injected at a pressure of 4 to 15 pounds of pressure per square inch.
If the wound has eschar tissue, prepare the patient for	Pressure ulcers cannot heal in the presence of eschar, which

(continues)

(continued)

INTERVENTIONS	RATIONALES
debridement and assist as required.	prevents new granulation in the wound bed and is a source of infection.
Apply heel and elbow protectors bilaterally; be sure heels are kept off the surface of the bed by suspending the feet off a pillow.	Helps to prevent excoriation to bony areas.
Place thin pillows between knees.	Helps to prevent bony areas of knees from rubbing against one another, causing breakdown.
Keep patient clean and dry by washing well (avoiding friction) with warm water after each incontinent episode of urine or stool; changing sheets if patient is diaphoretic; apply protective ointment after cleansing.	Enzymes and chemicals found in urine and feces can irritate tissues, as can the moisture from urine. Hot water should be avoided because it causes dryness of the skin. Friction causes trauma to sensitive at risk skin. Cleansing is required after each episode to clean the irritants away from skin.
Avoid use of incontinent pads or briefs with plastic liners.	The plastic holds moisture next to the skin and promotes the production of heat next to the skin, which predisposes the patient to further breakdown.
Institute use of special mattresses, such as air or water mattress, as ordered.	Special mattresses are intended to relieve pressure on high-risk areas, especially the sacrum and coccyx.
Avoid massaging over bony prominences.	Pressure from massage increases the risk for ulcer formation due to excessive friction on areas already at risk.
Provide topical moisturizing agents, as ordered.	Skin that is dry and flaky is more likely to experience breakdown.
Assess the patient's hydration and nutritional status, and give a diet rich in protein and vitamin C; use supplements such as Boost and Ensure, if not contraindicated.	An adequate diet and hydration are necessary for healthy skin and healing.
Teach family members or other caregivers techniques for preventing skin breakdown.	If family members plan to care for the patient with pressure ulcers at home, they will need to know how to prevent new areas of skin breakdown.

NIC *Pressure ulcer care*
Pressure ulcer prevention

Skin surveillance
Positioning

Evaluation

Determine that the patient has met the outcome criteria. Pressure ulcers show signs of healing, and no eschar tissue is present. The patient's remaining skin will be intact; no areas of redness or excoriation and no signs of infection are present. The skin will be warm with no edema. In addition, the patient's risk for future breakdown will be minimized.

Community/Home Care

The type of care required of the pressure ulcer is prescribed by the physician, and a determination is made as to whether the family can perform the necessary care in the home. In some instances, the ulcer may be too extensive for the family to care for, and the services of a home health nurse will be utilized until the wound decreases in size or severity. Because of possible alterations in sensory perception, nutritional status, elimination patterns, and mobility, the patient remains at high risk for additional breakdown and persistence of current pressure ulcers. The family that cares for a patient with pressure ulcers in the home will need to have detailed teaching on strategies to treat and prevent skin breakdown. Teaching must also include instruction on the signs and symptoms of infection, deterioration in the condition of the wound, and measuring the wound. All supplies used in the care of the ulcer should be kept in an easily accessible place in the patient's bedroom. These items can be stored in a covered heavy plastic box or crate with a lid. The family will need to implement other strategies identified in the interventions section, with emphasis placed on turning, positioning, and cleanliness of the skin. Oftentimes, families caring for totally dependent patients in the home do not have a realistic perception of what total patient care involves. The nurse needs to enlist the family members to participate in the care while the patient is still in long-term care facilities or hospitalized so that they may perform pressure ulcer care under the nurse's supervision. This would also allow for any questions to be answered. The most critical aspects of care in the home will be turning the patient regularly on some type of schedule to relieve pressure on high-risk areas. A schedule that outlines which position the patient should be in at specific times will be helpful, particularly if there will be multiple caregivers. A sign with this information on it can be posted in the patient's bedroom above the bed for all to see. It is also crucial that the family learn how to use bed pillows or possibly a small rolled throw/cover to support the patient in the side-lying position, and smaller, semi-flat pillows between the knees to prevent rubbing of the bony inner aspects against each other. The family can also use a pillow or a smooth texture blanket to place beneath the feet to keep heels off the bed. The second area of emphasis in the home is handling incontinence. Many patients who have been in bed long enough to obtain a pressure ulcer also experience incontinence. All too often, when patients experience urinary incontinence caregivers remove the soiled pad and replace it with a clean one without cleaning the skin. The harsh components of urine can continue to irritate the skin contributing to further breakdown. Family caregivers must be diligent in cleansing the skin well after each episode of incontinence (urine and stool) with mild soap and warm water. There are many commercial barrier products on the market, but these can be expensive to use for totally incontinent patients. Good inexpensive substitutes that act as barriers, especially to urine, include petroleum jelly and zinc oxide paste. Even though the patient has on incontinent briefs, he or she should still be checked at least every 2 hours for wetness, and caregivers can check for wetness or stool at the same time they reposition the patient. Trashcans with plastic liners that are removable for washing should be used in the home for disposing of incontinent pads, and the family can place the pad or brief inside a plastic bag, tie it, and then put in the trashcan. These two strategies can drastically reduce or eliminate any odor from the soiled pads or briefs. In addition, the family will need to learn how to learn the signs of beginning skin breakdown, such as redness, pallor, warmth, or any open area. Attention to nutritional needs is important to promote healing of the ulcer. If the patient is able to consume an oral diet, the family should be sure that the patient receives adequate amounts of protein and vitamin C. Offering the patient nutritional snacks between meals is a good way to increase calories and nutrients. Caregivers may need some assistance in determining what types of snacks are appropriate for the patient, and should also be provided with written instructions. For those patients unable to eat, nutrients are generally prescribed via tube feedings of some sort, and the family will need to maintain the prescribed feedings to ensure adequate nutrients needed for tissue maintenance. If the family detects any change in the skin, a health care provider must be notified and a visit from a visiting nurse may be warranted.

Documentation

Chart the results of a thorough assessment of the patient's skin, including the results of the Braden Scale assessment. If any signs of new skin breakdown are noted, chart a thorough description of the area. Always include in the patient record all nursing interventions implemented to treat the pressure ulcer, with particular attention to a description of the wound, dressing changes completed, and the size of the wound. If the patient is incontinent, immobile, or has poor nutrition, document this as well. All actions employed to prevent skin impairment are also documented, including teaching to caregivers. If special mattresses or beds are used, document according to agency policy. Referrals to wound care specialists are included in the nurse's notes.

NURSING DIAGNOSIS 2

 RISK FOR INFECTION

Related to:

Open ulcer

Necrotic tissue on ulcer

Compromised nutritional state of patient

Defining Characteristics:

None

Goal:

The patient's skin will be free of infection.

Outcome Criteria

✔ The pressure ulcer will have no odor.

✔ The pressure ulcer will have no eschar tissue.

✔ The pressure ulcer will have no purulent drainage.

✔ The pressure ulcer bed will have healthy pink granulation tissue.

✔ The patient will be afebrile.

✔ No new areas of breakdown or new infections will occur.

NOC　*Infection severity*
Tissue integrity: Skin and mucous membranes

INTERVENTIONS	RATIONALES
Assess skin and pressure ulcers every shift or according to agency guidelines (see nursing diagnosis "Impaired Skin Integrity"), noting the presence of any new lesions.	Assessment of ulcers and skin in general establishes a baseline and allows for early detection of complications and infection.
Assess pressure ulcers for signs of infection: purulent drainage, odor, extreme redness, and warmth to surrounding skin; increasing size.	Infected ulcers may have large amounts of purulent drainage, a strong odor, exudates, increased pain at the site, and evidence of tissue necrosis.
Obtain culture of ulcers and monitor results.	Ulcers should be cultured to detect the presence of organisms that cause infection. Organism growth $> 10^3$ (100,000 organisms/ mm^3) indicates infection, and the causative organism is identified. In some cases, ulcers may be infected without some of the classic signs.
Monitor vital signs every 4 hours.	Temperature elevation is a classic sign of infection. The pulse rate also increases in the presence of infection.
Monitor white blood cell (WBC) count.	WBC count will be elevated in infectious states, but it should be noted that the elderly, the immunosuppressed, and those who take NSAIDs may not have elevations due to an inability to produce a normal inflammatory response to invasion by organisms.
Administer antibiotics (intravenously [IV] or by mouth [PO]) or topical antibiotic preparations, as ordered.	Helps to treat or prevent infections. Often, physicians may order topical antibiotics to go directly into the wound of uninfected ulcers to prevent infection.
Perform wound care as ordered (see nursing diagnosis "Impaired Skin Integrity").	Proper wound care is needed to promote healing.
Ensure that patient has an adequate diet rich in protein.	Nutrition is vital to skin healing and treatment/prevention of infection.

Cleanse patient with warm, soapy water after each incontinent episode.

For ulcers in the vicinity of the perineal area (sacrum, femur, coccyx), the risk for infection and recontamination is high due to the presence of organisms in feces and in the perineal area that easily invade the ulcer.

NIC　*Infection control*
Nutrition management
Wound care

Evaluation

Evaluate the degree to which the outcome criteria have been met. The pressure ulcers should be healing without signs of infection. Redness/ discoloration, swelling, purulent drainage, and heat should be absent from the site, and pink granulation tissue is evident. Drainage from the pressure ulcer, if present, should be serosanquinous and decreasing in amount. The patient should be afebrile, and WBC counts should return to normal. No new areas of breakdown develop, and ulcers should not become infected.

Community/Home Care

The risk for infection and actual infection remain as an active problem after the patient has been discharged home. Prevention and treatment of infection in the pressure ulcer are accomplished by good wound care, and the prevention of subsequent ulcers (see nursing diagnosis "Impaired Skin Integrity"). As long as the ulcer is present, the risk for infection remains, and the family will need to know what symptoms may signal a new onset of infection (redness/discoloration, purulent drainage, heat, increased pain). When teaching the family, the nurse should stress the importance of handwashing as the single most effective way to decrease infection risk. Although most people believe that they understand how to wash their hands, most do it ineffectively. Teaching how to wash, when to wash, and how long to wash is a good approach. Pressure ulcer care will need to be taught to the family, including proper cleansing, dressing, and application of topical agents. The caregiver should be aware not only of signs of infection, but also of signs that would indicate that the wound is not healing. The patient and caregiver will need to understand the importance of good nutrition in complete wound healing and recovery, and implement strategies to provide a nutritious diet. Completing any ordered medications such as antibiotics once at home should be stressed. If any evidence of poor wound healing or infection should occur, the patient should be instructed to contact the health care provider.

Documentation

Document general assessment findings from the wound, with particular attention to a general description of the ulcer, color, and odor of any drainage, and the presence of necrotic tissue. Vital signs and medications are documented according to agency protocol as ordered. Document all interventions that were implemented to address an actual infection or to prevent an infection.

NURSING DIAGNOSIS 3

DEFICIENT KNOWLEDGE

Related to:

No prior experience with pressure ulcers

Lack of knowledge about therapeutic interventions and prevention of ulcers

Limited knowledge regarding pressure ulcers

Defining Characteristics:

Asks many questions

Has misconceptions regarding disease

Has no questions

Goal:

The patient verbalizes an understanding of pressure ulcers and required treatment.

Outcome Criteria

✔ The patient and family verbalize a willingness and desire to learn the necessary information.

✔ The patient verbalizes an understanding of pressure ulcers.

✔ The patient verbalizes an understanding of the prescribed therapeutic interventions to treat pressure ulcers, the prevention of pressure ulcers, and the prevention and control of infection.

✔ The caregiver demonstrates proper technique for performing wound care.

NOC *Knowledge: Disease process*
Knowledge: Health behavior
Treatment behavior: Illness or injury

INTERVENTIONS	RATIONALES
Assess the patient's readiness to learn (motivation, cognitive level, physiological status).	The patient must be motivated to learn, have the capability to learn the content, and be free of distractions from learning, such as pain and emotional distress.
Assess what the patient already knows.	The patient may have some knowledge about pressure ulcers and their sequelae, and teaching should begin with what the patient already knows.
Create a quiet environment conducive to learning.	Environmental noise can prevent the learner from focusing on what is being taught.
Teach the patient and family about pressure ulcers: — Causes of pressure ulcers (unrelieved pressure on bony prominences, immobility) — Prevention of pressure ulcers (turning, good nutrition) — Early detection of skin impairment (redness of prone areas) — Treatment required (cleansing and dressings) — Prevention of infection (cleansing after incontinence, handwashing) — Assessments needed (for signs of infection and/or healing) — Role of good nutrition in healing (need for protein and calories, vitamin C) — Importance of turning every 2 hours and use of a turn schedule — Good hygiene with attention to cleansing following incontinent episodes	The caregiver needs to understand information relevant to the development, treatment, and prevention of pressure ulcers with understanding of rationale for therapeutic interventions, such as wound care, turning, good nutrition, and relief of pressure through use of pillows, rolls, special mattresses, and pads. When the patient and family understand the interventions that prevent and treat pressure ulcers and their complications, they are better able to make decisions regarding ability to care for the patient. Education also empowers them to be good caregivers.
Teach the family how to perform cleansing of ulcer and dressing changes, as ordered.	The family needs to understand the importance of wound care. Cleansing the wound is crucial to healing, and dressings protect the ulcer from organisms and injury.

(continues)

(continued)

INTERVENTIONS	RATIONALES
Teach incrementally.	The patient will learn and retain knowledge better when information is presented in small segments.
Offer printed materials and other audiovisual aides.	Printed and audiovisual aides enhance learning; printed materials can serve as reference materials later.
Evaluate the patient's understanding of all content covered by asking questions.	Helps to identify areas that require further teaching and to ensure that the patient has enough information to ensure compliance.
Investigate the need for a visiting nurse.	A nurse may be needed to perform wound care initially and to monitor healing.

NIC   *Teaching: Disease process*

Teaching: Psychomotor skill

Teaching: Individual

Evaluation

The patient and caregiver are able to repeat the information taught and ask appropriate questions about pressure ulcers, their treatment and prevention, and possible complications. The caregiver is able to demonstrate how to cleanse the ulcer and apply the prescribed dressing. The patient and/or caregiver verbalize a willingness to comply with prescribed therapies and follow-up. The patient knows the signs and symptoms of infection and reasons to return to the physician.

Community/Home Care

Knowledge deficits need to be identified early so that the family is better prepared to care for the pressure ulcer and to prevent future ones in the home. Home visits by a nurse may be required to ensure that the family is correctly performing procedures for wound care. In addition, the nurse can evaluate whether the family and patient have understood the teaching, whether the patient has completed any medications (i.e., antibiotics), and whether the pressure ulcer is healing. The family will need to implement a detailed treatment plan that includes turning, pressure relief measures, nutrition, assessment of ulcers, and hygienic practices, to name a few. At times this may prove overwhelming, but if the teaching has been thorough and detailed, the patient and family may have a sense of control. It may be helpful for the caregiver to develop a schedule for implementing the interventions and keep a record to show to health care providers. This would include assessments of the wound as well as nutritional intake. Providing the caregiver with telephone numbers to use if assistance is needed will be helpful in case of a crisis.

Documentation

Include documentation of the teaching session in the patient record, including the specific content taught and methodologies used. Document the patient's verbalization of understanding of the content, particularly the information relevant to treating and preventing pressure ulcers. If the patient and/or family verbalize concerns or indicate an inability to be compliant with the recommendations for pressure ulcer treatment in the home, document this in the record. Specify what areas need reinforcement or further teaching. Always include the titles of any printed literature given to the patient and family and any referrals made.

CHAPTER 9.109

HYPOTHERMIA (ACCIDENTAL)

GENERAL INFORMATION

Hypothermia is defined as the state of decreased temperature caused by decreased heat production or loss of the body's ability to regulate temperature. When the core temperature of the body drops below 95 degrees F (35 degrees C) for any reason, the condition is hypothermia. Severe or profound hypothermia is known as a core body temperature of 90 degrees F (32.2 degrees C) or less. When profound hypothermia is present, physiologic responses occur that are detrimental to cell survival, and death will usually occur if the core body temperature falls below 78 degrees F (25.6 degrees C). Hypothermia causes cellular metabolism to slow down. When hypothermia is present, renal blood flow slows, resulting in a reduced glomerular filtration rate. When this occurs, water is not reabsorbed, resulting in dehydration. At the same time, respiratory rate and depth decrease, causing carbon dioxide retention and resultant metabolic acidosis as well as hypoxia. In addition, glucose supply drops exponentially, resulting in severe hypoglycemia. Hypothermia causes myocardial cells to increase in sensitivity, causing dysrhythmias to become evident quickly. Hypothermia is classified as mild, 89.6 to 95 degrees F (32 to 35 degrees C), moderate, 82.4 to 89.6 degrees F (28 to 32 degrees C), or severe, temperature below 82.4 degrees F (temperature below 28 degrees C). Hypothermia can be caused by a variety of factors, such as submersion in water, exposure during cold weather, anesthesia, systemic infection, overdose, alcohol intoxication, rapid fluid resuscitation, and certain types of trauma. Clinical manifestations of hypothermia vary depending on the temperature, but typically include shivering (that worsens as the temperature is lowered), increased muscle rigidity, peripheral and central cyanosis, poor judgment, decreased heart rate, dysrhythmias, decreased urinary output, and change in level of consciousness. Older adults are at higher risk due to ineffective thermoregulation.

NURSING DIAGNOSIS 1

 HYPOTHERMIA

Related to:

Prolonged exposure to cold weather

Immersion in cold water

Anesthesia

Fluid replacement

Overdose or alcohol intoxication, or other situations that could cause body temperature drop

Defining Characteristics:

Decreased core temperature to < 90 degrees F

Shivering

Loss of manual coordination

Slurred speech

Amnesia

Muscular rigidity

Cyanosis

Dysrhythmias

Hemoconcentration

Stupor leading to coma

Decreased respirations

Cold diuresis

Goal:

The patient's temperature returns to normal.

Outcome Criteria

✔ The patient's temperature rises and gradually returns to normal.

✔ The patient's level of consciousness improves.

✔ Cardiac dysrhythmias diminish.

✔ Cardiac output is improved (blood pressure and pulse return to normal).

✔ Urine output is normal (30 ml per hour).

NOC _Thermoregulation_
Vital signs

INTERVENTIONS	RATIONALES
Determine causes of hypothermia and consider patient's age.	Knowing the cause can aid in determining appropriate treatment; the elderly and very young are at higher risk for hypothermia. There are numerous causes, including exposure, water submersion, drugs, alcohol intoxication, etc.
Assess vital signs, with particular attention to temperature.	Helps to know what level of hypothermia exists; after treatment has begun, allows monitoring of response. In patients with moderate to severe hypothermia, special thermometers that register below 35 degrees are needed; blood pressure and pulse may decrease as metabolic rate decreases.
Assess peripheral perfusion by noting peripheral pulses, capillary refills, color, and skin temperature.	Helps to determine effects of and severity of hypothermia. In the initial stages, there is vasoconstriction due to the coldness, but as hypothermia progresses, vasodilation occurs, predisposing the patient to further heat loss. Cyanosis and capillary refill > 2 seconds may be present, and peripheral pulses are decreased.
Monitor urinary output for increased amount (diuresis) followed by decreased output.	Cold diuresis occurs because of peripheral vasoconstriction that causes a smaller vascular compartment; this in turn causes greater volume pressure in the vascular system, which is detected by the kidneys, resulting in increased excretion of fluids in an effort to decrease pressure. Eventually, the excessive output will lead to decreased renal perfusion secondary to volume depletion, and decreased output then occurs.
Monitor respiratory status: respiratory rate, rhythm, depth; skin color and temperature.	Allows for early detection and treatment of respiratory complications. Note abnormalities of decreased

SaO_2, cyanotic skin, and arterial blood gases (ABGs), which validate metabolic acidosis and hypoxia.

Monitor electrocardiogram (EKG) changes.	Patients who are hypothermic are prone to development of dysrhythmias and conduction disturbances. Note abnormalities of bradycardia and any variety of dysrhythmias; however, ventricular fibrillation is common.
Monitor neurological status: level of consciousness, motor activity, reflexes, shivering, irrational behavior, decreased manual coordination, slurred speech, amnesia, muscular rigidity, and decreased deep tendon reflexes.	Helps to detect and treat early changes in neurological function.
Monitor laboratory and diagnostic tests: ABGs, oxygen saturation (O_2Sat), serum glucose, urinalysis.	Hypothermia can cause a number of alterations in physiological function. Metabolic acidosis will be noted in ABGs; oxygen saturation will be decreased, serum electrolytes will vary, glucose will be decreased, and following cold diuresis, specific gravity of urine will be decreased (concentrated urine).
Perform a complete health examination of the patient.	Helps to gather information regarding effects of hypothermia on all body systems.
Place patient in a warm bath: 104 to 110 degrees F (40 to 43.3 degrees C).	Helps to remove chill and rewarm patient.
Increase the environmental heat.	A warm environment adds to the heat of the patient.
Be sure the patient is warmly dressed, including a hat or other head covering.	Helps to provide warmth; a large amount of heat is lost from the body via the head.
Apply warming blankets as ordered.	Helps to warm the patient; this will not, however, warm the inner core.
Administer warm fluids by mouth (PO) that contain glucose (calories/sugar).	Helps to re-hydrate patient and provide glucose and calories that will assist the body to produce heat.
In cases of severe hypothermia, re-warm the core before peripheral extremities.	For patients in severe/profound hypothermic states, it is essential to re-warm the core of the body prior to the peripheral extremities. This will prevent re-warming

INTERVENTIONS	RATIONALES
	shock, which occurs when the extremities are re-warmed faster than the core, causing lactic acid that was being pooled in the peripheral extremities to be rapidly shunted to the core and the heart, and resulting in ventricular fibrillation. Severe hypothermia also results in hypotension caused by peripheral vasodilation that produces relative hypovolemia.
In cases of severe hypothermia, administer warm, humidified oxygen with positive pressure.	Warm, humidified oxygen will prevent pulmonary heat loss.
In cases of severe hypothermia, administer warm, peritoneal, and/or gastric lavage, as ordered.	Helps to effect core re-warming.
Administer warmed intravenous (IV) solutions, as ordered, for severe hypothermia.	Helps to prevent the heat loss that would occur if patient were given room temperature fluids.
Assist in preparing patient for cardiopulmonary bypass or hemodialysis (severe hypothermia).	Helps to provide rapid core re-warming via blood.
Continuously monitor the patient for the return of normal physiological functioning, complications, and re-warming.	Helps to evaluate effectiveness of interventions.

NIC *Hypothermia treatment*
Vital signs monitoring
Oxygen therapy
Temperature regulation

Evaluation

The patient has a temperature that is compatible with cellular metabolism. The temperature gradually rises and returns to normal. Cardiac output is restored, with a blood pressure and pulse at the patient's baseline, without dysrhythmias. Urine output is normal, and the patient's level of consciousness and behavior is normal.

Community/Home Care

Prior to discharge, the patient has a return to normal temperature, and temperature regulation is not an issue. Attention needs to be given to the patient who suffered hypothermia due to preventable causes such as exposure or water submersion. These patients need education on safety precautions against accidents that subsequently lead to lowering of temperature. If the patient is homeless, the health care worker should utilize social workers to assist the patient in finding shelter, especially on extremely cold nights. Encourage the patient to wrap in blankets over layers and wear coverings on his or her head at all times. Those patients who experienced hypothermia due to drug abuse, overdose, or alcohol intoxication need education on causes of hypothermia as well as assistance with cessation of substance abuse habits. For all patients, a return visit to a health care provider is needed to ensure that all body systems have returned to normal.

Documentation

Chart the patient's temperature. Findings from a complete physical assessment are included in the patient's record, and any abnormalities, particularly cardiac and neurological deficits, are noted. Document all therapeutic interventions implemented (IV fluids, warming blankets, wraps, gastric lavage, hats, etc.) to raise the patient's temperature and to treat abnormalities. Chart the patient's responses to interventions, specifically body temperature, mental status, and skin temperature. All medications and vital signs are charted according to agency guidelines.

NURSING DIAGNOSIS 2

 DECREASED CARDIAC OUTPUT

Related to:

Decreased temperature

Increased sensitivity of cardiac cells

Decreased renal perfusion leading to decreased fluid reabsorption leading to fluid volume deficit

Defining Characteristics:

Increased, then decreased, urinary output

Atrial fibrillation leading to ventricular fibrillation

Hypotension

Tachycardia

Hemoconcentration

Goal:

Cardiac output is restored.

Outcome Criteria

✔ The patient's core temperature returns to normal.

✔ Cardiac dysrhythmias are resolved.

✔ The patient has a pulse rate between 60 and 100.

✔ The patient's skin is warm and dry.

✔ Perfusion is restored, as demonstrated by absence of peripheral cyanosis, and capillary refill is < 2 seconds.

✔ Urinary output is > 30 ml/hour average.

✔ The patient's blood pressure returns to patient's baseline.

NOC *Circulatory status*
Tissue perfusion: Cardiac
Tissue perfusion: Peripheral
Tissue perfusion: Cerebral
Vital signs

INTERVENTIONS	RATIONALES
Assess blood pressure and pulse every 4 hours, or as ordered.	Changes in blood pressure and pulse give indicators of patient status.
Assess neck veins.	Absence of visible neck veins when the patient is supine indicates decreased circulating volume.
Assess urinary output.	Decreased urinary output (< 30 ml/hour) indicates decreased perfusion to kidneys secondary to decreased cardiac output.
Assess skin temperature and color.	Changes in skin and temperature occur as perfusion to skin and periphery is inadequate to maintain warmth or normal color.
Assess peripheral pulses.	Peripheral pulses become weak, diminished, or absent, as the heart is unable to maintain perfusion to extremities.
Assess mental status: level of consciousness, confusion, and agitation.	Changes in mental status indicate a decrease in cerebral tissue perfusion and an inability of the body's compensatory

	mechanism to provide adequate oxygenation to cerebral tissue; acidotic states and hypoglycemia seen in hypothermia also contribute to changes in neurological function.
Monitor for cardiac dysrhythmias via EKG or bedside cardiac monitor.	Dysrhythmias are common in hypothermia and need to be corrected in order to restore cardiac output.
In cases of severe hypothermia, assist with hemodynamic monitoring according to agency/unit protocol (pulmonary artery pressure, central venous pressures, arterial pressures).	Helps to assess the effects of severe hypothermia and to evaluate patient response to treatment; these measures can give information to evaluate left ventricular function (cardiac output).
Give oxygen, as ordered.	Helps to maintain pO_2 at > 90 percent; due to hypoperfusion, tissues may be hypoxic; oxygen increases amount of oxygen available for gas exchange.
Proceed with core re-warming (see nursing diagnosis "Hypothermia").	Cardiac dysrhythmias resulting from hypothermia will not usually respond to traditional antidysrhythmic medications and/or electrical interventions. Dysrhythmias will usually be resolved when core temperature returns to normal or close to normal.
Administer warmed IV fluids, as ordered.	Helps to prevent heat loss and to replace volume lost due to cold diuresis; replacing intravascular volume is necessary to improve cardiac output.

NIC *Hypothermia treatment*
Temperature regulation
Invasive hemodynamic monitoring
Cardiac care
Vital signs monitoring

Evaluation

Note the degree to which outcome criteria have been achieved. The patient should demonstrate adequate cardiac output or improvement in abnormalities. Peripheral pulses should be present, and skin, when touched, should be warm. If cardiac output is improved, perfusion to the kidneys should be adequate, with the patient producing at least 30 ml of urine per hour on average. The pulse should be within the patient's baseline and should be strong and regular. The parameters from invasive hemodynamic monitoring should show improvement and a gradual return to normal. ABGs should return to normal or show compensation, and oxygen saturation should be > 90 percent. There should be no dysrhythmias, and the patient's temperature returns to normal. The patient is alert, and mental status is at patient's baseline.

Community/Home Care

Patients who have experienced decreased cardiac output due to hypothermia have been seriously ill and will need to know how to increase activities gradually at home with a balance of rest and activity. The patient will need to monitor the response to activity, noting any shortness of breath, increased respiratory rate, and increased pulse rate. Home care follow-up may be required for some patients, especially if they verbalize feelings of anxiety or lack of knowledge about the emergency situation that

necessitated in-hospital care. The patient needs to understand the causative factors for development of hypothermia and the effect on the cardiac system, with a focus on prevention once out of the hospital environment. For most patients, once the temperature is returned to normal, cardiac output is restored and no further interventions are required in the home. However, a follow-up appointment is needed to be sure that the patient has returned to a normal level of functioning.

Documentation

Chart the results of all assessments made, particularly respiratory and cardiac, including respiratory effort, capillary refill, blood pressure, pulse, skin temperature, and urinary output. All interventions should be documented in a timely fashion, with the patient's specific response to the intervention. Chart readings from hemodynamic monitoring according to agency/unit protocol. Always include the patient's psychological status: whether he or she appears anxious, restless, or fearful, and whether family members or significant others are present. Document all vital signs in accordance with agency protocol.

CHAPTER 9.110

MELANOMA/SKIN CANCER

GENERAL INFORMATION

Melanoma is a malignant cancer of the melanocytes of the skin, epidermal cells that synthesize melanin (the dark pigment of the skin). Approximately a third of all melanomas originate in existing nevi (common moles), while the remainder originate in melanocytes. Melanoma is classified into sub-categories: melanoma in situ, superficial spreading melanoma (most common type), lentigo maligna melanoma, nodular melanoma (worst prognosis), and acral lentiginous melanoma. The lesions are typically slow-growing in the early stages, with growth taking place over a number of years while confined to the epidermis. In this early period, the lesions are most often flat, asymmetrical, and > 6 mm in diameter, but in the later stages the lesions become more nodular in appearance, with smaller nodules in close proximity. Common sites of metastasis include regional lymph nodes, lungs, liver, and brain. Although the appearance of the lesions may vary, in general the clinical manifestations include lesions with irregular borders; lesions that appear to have color that "leaks out" from the mole's edges; a variety of colors, including a freckled appearance to some lesions; and an existing mole or nevus that has changed in size, shape, or color. In the later stages of the disease, the lesion may bleed or ooze and feel lumpy, hard, swollen, tender, or itchy. The lesions occur most often on the neck, hands, head, and lower extremities. Melanoma is the most commonly occurring cancer and is thought to arise in over 50,000 people each year, occurring more frequently in fair-skinned people with increased incidences among Caucasians as well as people who live in sunny climates, who work outdoors, and who visit suntanning parlors regularly.

NURSING DIAGNOSIS 1

 IMPAIRED SKIN INTEGRITY

Related to:

Changes in skin secondary to melanoma

Defining Characteristics:

Flat asymmetrical lesions

Nodular appearing lesions

Numerous moles

Drainage from lesions

Discoloration of skin

Bleeding from lesions

Ulceration of lesions

Goal:

Cancerous cells will be eliminated and/or cancer cell growth will be retarded.

Outcome Criteria

✔ Skin will heal without complications following surgery, radiation, or chemotherapy.

✔ There will be no drainage or bleeding from melanoma lesions.

NOC *Tissue integrity: Skin and mucous membranes*

Nausea and vomiting control

INTERVENTIONS	RATIONALES
Assess skin changes noting location of lesions, size of lesions, and a description of lesions, as well as presence and color of drainage. Pay close attention to the areas close to the eye.	Helps to establish a baseline to guide treatment and monitor response to treatments. The lesions vary in color, are usually > 6 mm in diameter, have irregular borders, and are asymmetrical; bleeding and drainage are signs of late disease.
Obtain a history from the patient about any mole that grows, changes color, develops hair, or changes shape.	This information will help validate the diagnosis.

INTERVENTIONS	RATIONALES
Prepare the patient for biopsy, excision of melanoma, and lymph node dissection, as ordered.	Helps to confirm diagnosis, determine depth of lesion's invasion, and remove cancerous tissue.
Prepare the patient for surgical removal of the lesion (resection of the lesion, any involved lymph nodes, and marginal tissue surrounding the lesion), as ordered or according to agency protocols for pre-operative preparation.	Surgery is the first choice treatment. This method removes the lesion and surrounding tissue to reduce chance of recurrence; any involved lymph nodes are removed to reduce metastasis.
Assess excisional site for drainage, increasing redness, and bleeding. Keep dressings on and cleanse as ordered; teach the patient post-operative care as directed by the physician: usually, the patient is directed to keep the area covered, to observe for infection, and to take no aspirin, aspirin-containing products, or anticoagulants for 1 week following surgery.	The excisional site of deep surgery must be assessed for delayed healing and signs of infection. The patient needs to know how to care for the site in the home.
Prepare the patient for cryosurgery, in which tissue is destroyed by rapid chemical freezing that destroys the cells of the melanoma.	This is another method of removing melanomas.
Assess the site of cryosurgery for tissue necrosis; a bulla may form; phases of healing of the site include a serous drainage in week 1, followed by scab formation and subsequent dropping off of the scab after 3 weeks. Teach the patient post-operative care: keep site dry, do not try to remove the crust, place a light dressing over area if desired, and observe for infection.	The site of cryosurgery must be assessed for complications, and the patient must understand how to care for the wound in the home.
Administer pain medications prn post-operatively.	The site of melanoma excision may be painful for a period of time after surgery.
Assist with or administer anti-neoplastic agents, such as DTIC (dacarbazine), tamoxifen citrate (Nolvadex®), or others, as ordered.	Helps to kill cancer cells that were not removed by other methods; DTIC is frequently the drug of choice.
Implement agency protocol for control of chemotherapy-induced	Most agencies have established protocols for controlling nausea
nausea and vomiting, including administering anti-emetics, as ordered.	and vomiting that include anti-emetics at set times prior to, during, and after chemotherapeutic infusions. This is required to prevent dehydration and electrolyte imbalance.
Prepare the patient for radiation therapy, as ordered.	Helps to destroy cancerous cells that were not destroyed by chemotherapy or to treat the malignancy as a palliative measure.
Assess for infection: purulent drainage, redness, or discoloration; heat at the site; elevated temperature; increased pulse; and malaise.	Early detection of infection allows for early treatment; open skin lesions of malignant melanoma are a prime target for infection.
Practice aseptic techniques when working with skin, and practice good hand hygiene.	Asepsis is required to prevent introduction of organisms into the melanoma site; the first line of defense against infection is good handwashing.
Teach the patient about the diagnostic procedure of biopsy, recommended surgical interventions, chemotherapy, radiation, and skin care.	Helps to enhance the patient's and family's ability to manage care at home; knowledge promotes compliance with regimen.

NIC *Chemotherapy management*
Skin surveillance
Nausea management
Radiation therapy management
Surgical preparation

Evaluation

The melanoma has been removed. There are no signs of infection at the site of treatment, and lesions are without drainage. Following cryosurgery, the lesions have scabbed over, or scabs have fallen off. Itching has been relieved, and the patient reports a sense of comfort.

Community/Home Care

In the home setting, the patient with malignant melanoma will need to implement strategies for skin care, as the lesions will be in a stage of scabbing following cryosurgery or healing by primary intention following excision. The patient who has had surgery will provide self-care for the lesions as instructed by the physician. For cryosurgery, it is important for the patient to refrain from scratching the scab and instead allow it to fall off on its own. If the site itches, the patient can use clean gloves and pat it gently or place a light towel over it and pat. The wound from surgery will need to be dressed with a light bandage, and cleansing is performed according to instructions given by the physician. The patient and family will need to be aware of the signs and symptoms of infection at the site of excision, such as purulent drainage, redness or discoloration, heat, and increased pain. Practicing meticulous handwashing is important to prevent infection at the site. For the patient receiving chemotherapy, caution should be taken to prevent contracting respiratory illnesses due to immunosuppression. Avoidance of crowds and other people with upper respiratory infections is needed. If the patient is receiving a course of chemotherapy, controlling nausea/vomiting is also required. Taking anti-emetics prior to meals and eating bland foods will be helpful. Avoiding foods with strong odors is suggested during chemotherapy, as odors often trigger nausea. The patient can still institute measures to prevent skin cancer, as there is a likelihood of new sites in the future or recurrence in the same site (see nursing diagnosis "Deficient Knowledge"). The patient will need to be aware of changes in the skin that would warrant a return visit to the health care provider. Follow-up appointments are crucial to assess the status of the lesions but also for continued treatments, such as radiation or chemotherapy.

Documentation

Document the results of a thorough assessment of the patient's skin, particularly the presence and description of the melanoma site and any other moles, rashes, or skin lesions. Chart all nursing interventions implemented to address the problem of impaired skin integrity, including radiation therapy, chemotherapy, preparation for surgery, and biopsy. Include all teaching implemented and the patient's understanding in the patient record. Document the patient's verbalization of any complaints or concerns. Document referrals to dermatologists.

NURSING DIAGNOSIS 2

DISTURBED BODY IMAGE

Related to:

Skin lesions on body

Disfigurement due to surgery

Defining Characteristics:

Withdrawal

Social isolation

Depression

Negative statements about physical appearance

Attempts to cover face or sites of other lesions in the presence of others

Goal:

The patient accepts the change in physical appearance and continues social activities and interpersonal relationships.

Outcome Criteria

✔ The patient states a willingness to look at lesions on the body.

✔ The patient does not verbalize negative feelings toward self.

✔ The patient verbalizes an acceptance of body appearance.

NOC *Body image*

INTERVENTIONS	RATIONALES
Encourage the patient to discuss his or her feelings about changes in physical appearance openly, and assure the patient that his or her feelings are normal.	Talking about the changes may sometimes be the beginning of acceptance; the patient should understand that his or her emotions are real and should be expected.
Allow the patient privacy when bathing, dressing, or toileting, unless assistance is requested.	Helps to allow patient time to adjust to appearance without concern for how others react.
Teach the patient methods to care for skin lesions (see nursing diagnosis "Impaired Skin Integrity").	Protecting the skin from secondary infections that worsen the melanoma lesions will improve appearance and prevent further problems.
Monitor the patient for feelings about self, interpersonal relationships with family members and friends, withdrawal, social isolation, fear, anxiety, embarrassment by appearance, and desire to be alone.	Helps to detect early alterations in social functioning, prevent unhealthy behaviors, and intervene early through referral to counseling.
Encourage the patient to participate in at least one outside/public activity each week.	Prevents patient from isolating self from others.

INTERVENTIONS	RATIONALES
Identify the effects of the patient's culture or religion on perception of body image.	A patient's culture and religion often help define reactions to changes in body image and self-worth.
Assist the patient in identifying coping strategies/diversionary activities that can be used to deal with the changed appearance and the diagnosis of skin cancer.	Helps to provide diversionary activities so that not all thoughts are on skin cancer and changed appearance.
Encourage family members and significant other to support the patient.	Support and acceptance from family and significant other enhance the patient's acceptance of the change in physical appearance.
Collaborate with the physician to provide patient with realistic and factual information about how the lesions may appear once healed.	The patient may cope better with the change if he or she understands how the lesion will appear and change in appearance following treatment.

NIC ***Body image enhancement***
Emotional support
Socialization enhancement

Evaluation

The patient is able and willing to learn about the strategies to improve psychological health. Determine if the patient is able to verbalize feelings about skin changes. The patient is able to look at the lesions and verbalizes an understanding of how the lesion may change appearance. Time is required for the patient to completely assimilate the change in body appearance into his or her self-perception. Communication of feelings and concerns relevant to the change in appearance should be taken as a positive sign that progress is being made towards meeting outcome criteria.

Community/Home Care

At home, continued monitoring of the patient's perception of body image is needed. The health care provider who sees the patient for follow-up will need to be alert to subtle hints that may indicate that the patient has not completely adapted to the change in body appearance. Open

discussions about physical changes and interventions to prevent social isolation and withdrawal should continue with the patient and family members. As the melanoma site heals following treatment, the patient may feel better about his or her body appearance; however, he or she may still hesitate to allow family members, especially a spouse or significant other, to see the healing lesions. This is especially true in lesions that have scabs following cryosurgery. Encouraging the patient to look at the lesions and assess them may improve the patient's ability to deal with body changes. If the lesions are hidden by clothes, going out in public may not be a major problem. However, if lesions are on the face, hands, or neck, the patient may impose self-isolation. Family members should encourage the patient to go out for short periods once allowed, starting with environments where the patient feels comfortable and where others are more likely to refrain from staring, such as religious services. Once lesions are completely healed and the scabs have fallen off, or the surgical site is healed, the body-image issues should be resolved. If, however, treatments were not effective in removing the lesions, some disturbed body image may persist, and the patient will need continued assessments and attention to the problem.

Documentation

Chart any specific behaviors or verbalizations that may indicate an altered body image. Include all interventions that have been employed to address this issue and the patient's responses. Note when and if the patient begins to verbalize feelings about the skin changes and demonstrates behaviors indicative of positive body image.

NURSING DIAGNOSIS 3

 DEFICIENT KNOWLEDGE

Related to:

New diagnosis of malignant melanoma

Lack of information about the disease and its treatment and prevention

Misinformation

Patient/family denial

Defining Characteristics:

Asks no questions

Has many questions/concerns

Shows no interest in learning about melanoma

Goal:

The patient verbalizes an understanding of the disease and the required treatment.

Outcome Criteria

✔ The patient verbalizes a desire to learn necessary information.

✔ The patient verbalizes an understanding of the pathophysiology of melanoma.

✔ The patient understands possible treatment options (surgery, chemotherapy, radiation therapy), including untoward effects of treatment, disease prognosis, and possible complications of melanoma.

✔ The patient agrees to comply with recommendations for treatment.

✔ The patient verbalizes an understanding of diagnostic procedures (excisional biopsy).

✔ The patient verbalizes an understanding of follow-up care required and expresses a willingness to comply.

NOC *Knowledge: Disease process*
Knowledge: Treatment regimen
Compliance behavior

INTERVENTIONS	RATIONALES
Assess patient's current knowledge, ability to learn, and readiness to learn.	The nurse needs to ascertain what the patient already knows and build on this; if the patient is not capable of learning or is not ready to learn, teaching will not be effective due to disinterest or inability to understand. The patient may not be ready to learn if in a state of denial or if angry about the diagnosis.
Teach incrementally, starting with the simplest information, and move to complex information.	The patient will learn and retain knowledge better when information is presented in small segments; patients can understand simple concepts easily and then can build on those to understand concepts that are more complex.
Teach patient and significant others: — Disease process of melanoma (pathophysiology and staging of the disease) — Available treatment options (surgery, chemotherapy, radiation) — Diagnostic studies: excisional biopsy — Signs and symptoms that would indicate a need to seek health care (severe pain, purulent drainage from site, excessive redness, or discoloration)	Knowledge of disease process, diagnostic procedures, identification of complications, and other information empowers the patient to take control, make informed decisions, and enhances compliance.
Collaborate with the physician to teach patient and family about surgical interventions: *Surgical excision* — Involves resection of the lesion, any involved lymph nodes, and marginal tissue surrounding the lesion; this method removes the surrounding tissue to reduce chance of recurrence; any involved lymph nodes are removed to reduce metastasis. — Assess excisional site for drainage, increasing redness, and bleeding. — Site care: cleanse as ordered; keep area covered; observe for infection. — Take no aspirin, aspirin-containing products, or anti-coagulants for 1 week following surgery. *Cryosurgery* — Involves destruction of tissue by rapid chemical freezing that destroys the cells of the melanoma; a bulla may form. — Phases of healing of the site include a serous drainage in week one, followed by scab formation, and subsequent dropping off of the scab after 3 weeks. — Site care: keep site dry, do not try to remove the crust, place a light dressing over area if desired, and observe for infection.	The excisional site of deep surgery must be assessed for delayed healing and signs of infection. The patient needs to know how to care for the site in the home; the site of cryosurgery must be assessed for complications, and the patient must understand how to care for the wound in the home.

INTERVENTIONS	RATIONALES

Teach patient and family about external radiation:
— Method of action
— Course/duration of treatment
— Skin changes to note include redness, sloughing, and tenderness
— Skin care: do not apply soap, ointments, lotions, creams, or powder to area. Do not rub, scrub, or scratch the area; do not try to wash off markings; avoid exposing the treated area to the sun during the treatment and for 1 year following treatments
— Wear loose-fitting clothes due to risk of irritation
— Control of fatigue: importance of energy conservation; intake of high-energy foods rich in vitamin C, protein, and iron; and taking a nap each day especially after treatment

Radiation is used with melanoma, especially with small tumors or in some cases where metastasis has occurred, and the patient needs to be informed of what to expect. The radiated skin is sensitive, and lotions, creams, ultraviolet rays, rubbing, etc., may cause burning and skin sloughing and interfere with radiation. The patient must know how to protect the skin from impairment; knowing what to expect in terms of radiation helps the patient to be more compliant and feel more in control.

Teach patient and family about chemotherapy and its effects:
— Method of action
— Specific agents used for treatment
— Alopecia: assist the patient to plan for hair loss by investigating the purchase of wigs or having hair cut short and using hair for a specially made wig before alopecia; men can have hair shaved prior to alopecia; find a resource that could teach women how to prepare fashionable head wraps
— Nausea/vomiting: teach to use anti-emetics before meals prophylactically; avoid foods with strong odors, and in the hospital setting have lids removed from trays outside the room (when lids are removed from food trays, the smell is often overwhelming to the gastrointestinal [GI] system and causes nausea); attempt frequent small meals avoiding spicy foods
— Care of access sites: prevention of infection by use of aseptic

Knowledge of what to expect helps the patient cope with untoward side effects and better equips him or her to take responsibility for managing the illness and engaging in self-care.

techniques and procedures according to agency protocol
— Control of fatigue: balance of rest and activity and on chemotherapy days a designated naptime
— Prevention of infection: chemotherapy causes a depression of white blood cells (WBCs), predisposing the patient to infection; avoid people with infections and large crowds; practice good hand hygiene; know WBC counts

Teach the patient and family about prevention of skin cancer:
— Avoid exposure to ultraviolet rays of the sun, especially during periods when the sun's rays are more pronounced, 11 a.m. to 4 p.m.
— Limit exposure in tanning salons.
— Wear sunscreen when in the sun with a sun protection (SPF) rating of at least 15.
— Wear a wide-brimmed hat or long-sleeved clothing if prolonged exposure is expected.

These precautions protect the skin from exposure to ultraviolet rays that can increase the risk of melanoma.

Teach the patient and family how to assess skin for signs of malignant melanoma:
— Be aware of changes in a mole or wart such as size, shape, color, especially if the mole spreads out or becomes raised.
— Examine birthmarks regularly for changes.
— Note any drainage or oozing from a mole.
— Note scaliness or ulceration of an area of skin.
— Use mirrors to examine areas that are difficult to see.

The patient needs to be able to identify changes that may indicate problems. In some cases, patients with melanoma experience new areas of malignant growth or a recurrence in the same site. Early detection allows for early treatment.

Assess the patient's and family's understanding of all teaching by encouraging them to repeat information and ask questions as needed.

This allows the nurse to hear in the patient's own words what was taught and makes it easier to know what information may need to be reinforced.

Establish that the patient has the resources required to be compliant.

If needed resources such as finances and transportation to follow-up appointments are not available, the patient cannot be compliant; the nurse will need to make necessary referrals.

NIC   *Learning readiness enhancement*
Learning facilitation
Teaching: Disease process
Teaching: Procedure/treatment

Evaluation

Evaluate the degree to which the patient has achieved the outcome criteria relevant to the teaching sessions. The patient should verbalize an understanding of the content presented by repeating the information, particularly the disease process and methods of treatment, including surgical interventions, radiation treatment process, and chemotherapy. In addition, the patient should understand how to control nausea and vomiting and how to care for any wounds. The nurse must determine if the patient is capable of being compliant with the recommended regimen. If further teaching is required at time of discharge, the appropriate referrals should be made to continue education.

Community/Home Care

The patient will need to implement the prescribed regimen in the home setting. The success of this implementation will depend upon the degree to which the patient has received adequate teaching and has subsequently understood and internalized it. For patients who have had surgery, care of surgical sites is generally undertaken in the home by the patient (see nursing diagnosis "Impaired Skin Integrity"). The patient will need to keep the site clean and dry while monitoring it for infection. Being mindful of scabs over the site will assist in preventing accidental dislodging due to trauma, especially sites on hands and feet, and the patient is allowed to cover the site lightly. If chemotherapy is employed, hair loss, nausea, and vomiting can also occur as a result of treatments. For the patient receiving chemotherapy, it is important to monitor the patient's weight at home if he or she is experiencing nausea and vomiting. Health care providers or dieticians can assist the patient to prepare a diet that is both nutritional and easy to digest. External radiation therapy patients will need to be monitored for ability to care for skin properly to prevent further tissue destruction. The patient will need to avoid exposure to the sun and refrain from rubbing or scratching the affected areas. In addition, no commercial products such as ointments or lotions should be applied to the areas being treated. At home, the patient will likely experience fatigue following any of the treatments, but especially after radiation or chemotherapy treatments. The patient will need to schedule rest periods during the day and space activities as tolerated. The patient should have a clear understanding of the schedule for any treatments as an outpatient. Providing written information covering all recommendations will help the patient comply with the regimen. Because the patient is seen on a regular basis for general follow-up, for chemotherapy, or for radiation therapy, health care providers can determine whether further teaching or reinforcement is required.

Documentation

Document the specific content taught and the titles of any printed documents given to the patient. Include in the chart the patient's degree of understanding of the content and the methods used to evaluate learning. Assess the patient's ability to comply with the regimen in terms of radiation, chemotherapy, care of wounds, or follow-up, and document the assessment in the chart indicating referrals made. Any areas that need to be reinforced should be documented to ensure appropriate follow-up. If family members are present for the teaching sessions, document this in the chart.

NURSING DIAGNOSIS 4

INEFFECTIVE COPING

Related to:

Fear

Diagnosis of malignant melanoma

Possible metastasis to other organs

Uncertain stage of disease at time of diagnosis

Surgery

Defining Characteristics:

Expressions of fear

Restlessness

Verbalizes anxiety

Crying

Goal:

The patient expresses grief and identifies coping strategies.

Outcome Criteria

✔ The patient identifies and uses one coping mechanism.

✔ The patient verbalizes fears and concerns.

✔ The patient reports being less anxious.

✔ The patient demonstrates no outward signs of anxiety, such as restlessness or agitation.

NOC *Anxiety control*
Comfort level
Coping

INTERVENTIONS	RATIONALES
Assess level of anxiety (mild, moderate, severe); have patient rate on a scale of 1 to 10, with 10 being the greatest.	Gives the nurse a better perception of extent of the anxiety.
Assess the patient for feelings about self/disease, sadness, anger, withdrawal, fear of dying, and anxieties about inability to carry out family responsibilities, finances, cost of hospitalization, and cost of therapy.	The patient may experience all of these feelings while trying to cope with the diagnosis and treatment. Knowing where the patient is in terms of acceptance and coping helps to identify interventions.
Keep the patient informed of all that is going on, including information about diagnostic tests and planned therapeutic interventions.	Communication of factual information in a straightforward manner may help to relieve anxiety and fear.
Use a calm, reassuring manner with the patient.	Gives the patient a sense of well-being.
Assist the patient to identify at least one coping mechanism that has worked in the past; encourage the use of relaxation, guided imagery, deep breathing, or meditation, or assist to develop new coping strategies.	Coping mechanisms that have worked in the past may work again; other relaxation techniques can decrease anxiety and give the patient a sense of calm.
Encourage the patient to verbalize any fears or concerns, and listen attentively.	Verbalization of fears contributes to dealing with concerns; being attentive relays empathy to the patient.
Seek spiritual consult as needed or requested by the patient and/or family.	Meeting the patient's spiritual needs helps him or her to deal with fears through use of spiritual or religious rituals.
Recognize the role of culture in a patient's method of coping	Culture often dictates how a person copes, and the nurse

with illness and perception of the acceptability of verbalizing fears and concerns.	must recognize this in order to support the patient in identifying successful coping strategies.
Review therapeutic interventions, and give the patient as much information as possible about what to expect; engage the patient and family in open dialogue about options for treatments and care.	Fear of the unknown produces anxiety; discussion of care options allows the patient to be more in control and gives him or her a sense of empowerment that may assist with coping with the diagnosis.
Arrange for a visit from a melanoma survivor or facilitate participation in a support group.	Meeting other patients who have been through similar experiences and survived helps to relieve anxiety.
If the patient has the energy, time, and motivation, encourage him or her to document feelings in a diary.	These strategies assist the patient to express him or herself in an acceptable manner when he or she may feel uncomfortable talking to others.

NIC *Coping enhancement*
Emotional support
Spiritual support

Evaluation

Evaluate the extent to which the outcome criteria have been achieved. The patient should be assessed for behaviors that would indicate adjustment to the diagnosis of melanoma. Even though most cases of melanoma have a good prognosis, especially if detected early, the patient may still experience heightened anxiety and anticipatory grieving shortly after diagnosis as he or she attempts to deal with the unknown and the possibility of death. The patient should verbalize fears and concerns and be able to identify one way to cope with the diagnosis of melanoma. The coping strategies utilized by the patient should be noted. If the patient is unable to talk about the diagnosis and communicate concerns, the nurse should explore new interventions to assist the patient.

Community/Home Care

Nurses should assess which coping mechanisms work for the patient and encourage their use by the patient at home. Even for those patients whose disease was detected early and treated successfully, problems with anxiety and ineffective coping may continue for a long period of time. The patient should be encouraged to identify coping strategies that have been successful in the past and prompted to use those regularly. Anxiety about prognosis usually continues throughout treatment and recovery until the patient is able to resume normal activities. However, for those patients whose disease was detected in later stages with a poor prognosis, anxiety can be more pronounced. For this group, coping through use of support from outside sources such as hospice or nurse therapists may be required. Monitor for extreme withdrawal, self-isolation, and depression, and report any symptoms to the physician. For many patients and families, spiritual and religious rituals provide a means of coping with difficult stressful situations. The patient's culture may dictate how he or she copes and/or grieves and with whom he or she shares this process. It is crucial that the nurse and family support the patient as needed to foster a healthy psychological state, recognizing that anger and denial are common. Even though friends and family intend well with their presence, the patient may benefit from quiet periods of meditation and solitude during the day. At least one follow-up visit with the health care provider should be initiated to assess how the patient is coping. If questions should arise at home about the patient's health status or prescribed regimen, the patient should have a means of contacting a health care provider for answers.

Documentation

Document findings from an assessment of the patient's psychological state, indicating whether there is depression, anger, crying, sadness, etc. The degree to which the patient has demonstrated effective coping and decreased anxiety should be documented in the patient record. A rating system provides an objective way to relay to others the extent of the anxiety or expressions of fear. Document whether the patient is able to discuss feelings about a diagnosis of melanoma. Chart the patient's verbalizations as the patient states them, and include in the record coping mechanisms utilized by the patient. Document referrals to hospice, religious leaders, support groups, or others.

CHAPTER 9.111

SCLERODERMA

GENERAL INFORMATION

Scleroderma is a relatively rare inflammatory autoimmune disease affecting blood vessels, connective tissue, and body organs. Scleroderma is characterized by thickening, tightening, and fibrosis of the skin, which is most frequently limited to the skin of the face and fingers. Even though its etiology is unknown, theorists suggest environmental, genetic, and immune factors as contributors to development of the disease. The disease is characterized by proliferation of fibrous connective tissue in a variety of organs. It can be limited to the skin only or it can affect both skin and visceral organs (generalized systemic sclerosis). Approximately 80 percent of diagnosed patients with the generalized type have what is called CREST syndrome: **C**alcinosis (calcium deposits in tissue), **R**aynaud's phenomenon (sequential color changes in fingers from pallor, cyanosis, extreme redness when exposed to cold), **E**sophageal dysfunction, **S**clerodactyly (scleroderma of the fingers), and **T**elangiectasia (dilated, superficial blood vessels). The patient experiences non-pitting edema of the hands and fingers; as the edema eases, gradual tightening and thickening of the skin develop. The skin may appear shiny and taut with loss of normal skin folds. Late in the course of the illness, the skin tends to soften and atrophy. A patient with scleroderma may exhibit rapidly progressive skin involvement or may have long intervals of stable or even improving skin thickening. Later in the disease, the patient may take on an expressionless or frozen face as the muscles become inelastic with limited ability to move, and lips become tightly pursed. Joint manifestations may progress to very limited movement of the wrist as the skin connecting the fingers and hands to the wrist become more tightened. Scleroderma occurs four times more frequently in women, is most common in middle-aged women, and has a higher incidence in African Americans.

NURSING DIAGNOSIS 1

IMPAIRED TISSUE INTEGRITY

Related to:

Inflammation

Fibrosis of tissue

Defining Characteristics:

Non-pitting edema

Thickening of skin

Smooth, taut, shiny skin

Hyperpigmentation of skin

Pain

Tightening of facial skin/Inelasticity of skin

Arthralgias

Raynaud's syndrome (when exposed to cold, fingers change colors from pallor, to cyanosis, and then reactive hyperemia/excess redness)

Difficulty swallowing

Goal:

Tissue integrity is restored or maintained.

Outcome Criteria

✔ The patient's skin will not lose elasticity.

✔ The patient's skin will remain intact.

✔ The patient will verbalize an understanding of the disease process and required skin care.

NOC *Tissue integrity: Skin and mucous membranes*

INTERVENTIONS	RATIONALES
Perform a thorough skin assessment, including special attention to fingertips.	Helps to determine the status of skin (integrity, elasticity, thickening) and tissue in order to establish a baseline and individualize plan for skin; fingertips may be sensitive due to calcinosis, and small ulcers may occur.
Monitor results of laboratory tests: scleroderma antibody (SCL-70); serum rheumatoid factor; complete blood count (CBC); erythrocyte sedimentation rate (ESR); and x-rays of joints, lungs, and gastrointestinal (GI) system.	SCL-70 will be present in approximately 35 percent of patients; rheumatoid factor is present in 30 percent of patients, CBC will reveal anemia, ESR will be elevated because of the chronic inflammatory nature of the disease. X-rays: joints, especially fingers, may show deposits of calcium; bilateral pulmonary fibrosis may be evident; esophageal motility is decreased. Examination of these results will help confirm the diagnosis.
Encourage the patient to perform therapeutic exercises such as range of motion of wrist and fingers and yawning with mouth open. Consult with physical therapist as required.	Helps to maintain flexibility of the skin and promote circulation; the mouth frequently tightens, and yawning maintains some degree of elasticity.
Apply moisturizing agents such as lanolin, Lubriderm®, or glycerin to the skin by rubbing for an extended period of time.	Helps to keep skin moisturized and to prevent dry, cracking skin; the thickened skin of systemic sclerosis requires rubbing for an extensive period of time to assure that the substances are penetrating the skin.
Protect the skin on feet and hands from cold by wearing warm socks or hose and gloves during cold or cool weather; provide warm blankets, socks, slippers, mittens in layers; instruct the patient to avoid restrictive clothing or shoes.	Helps to maximize vasodilation and avoid vasoconstriction. Cold weather will cause vasoconstriction in the hands and feet, creating a flare-up of Raynaud's phenomenon.
Use moist heat on skin and feet.	Helps to promote skin flexibility, thus preventing contractures.
Pad areas of bony prominence: elbows, heels, and sacrum.	Helps to avoid skin breakdown due to friction; skin with edema and thickening is more likely to break down.
Administer calcium channel blockers, as ordered, to patients with Raynaud's phenomenon.	Helps to produce vasodilation and improve circulation; maintains tissue integrity.
Consult with dietician for dietary instructions: no foods/drinks containing caffeine.	Caffeine causes vasoconstriction, which should be avoided.
Teach the patient all interventions to improve tissue integrity and prevent further tightening as well as the rationale for all recommendations.	The patient and family will need to implement the strategies at home; an understanding of why they are needed will enhance compliance. The patient and family need to know that once elasticity is lost, it cannot be regained.
Teach the patient and family about the pathophysiology of the disease process, including long-term complications and progression of the disease with major organ involvement (renal disease, hypertension, pulmonary fibrosis, pericarditis, right-sided heart failure, and GI disturbances) and the treatments required.	The patient needs to know about the disease in order to manage it effectively and comply with prescribed regimens.
Monitor patient for alterations in tissue integrity of the renal system by examining laboratory results: creatinine, urinalysis, and blood urea nitrogen (BUN), and assess the patient for elevated blood pressure.	Renal disease is a major cause of death in scleroderma. It usually manifests itself as hypertension and proteinuria. Elevated creatinine and BUN represent failure of the renal system that may require dialysis.
Assess the respiratory system for signs of respiratory complications (indications of impaired gas exchange and heart failure).	Pulmonary fibrosis that occurs with scleroderma occurs due to pleural thickening, leading to impaired function that often causes the patient to have shortness of breath, especially with activity, and to develop a cough. Assessments can assist with early intervention and prevention of infections.

NIC *Skin surveillance*
   Teaching: Prescribed
     activity/exercise
   Teaching: Disease process

Evaluation

Determine the degree to which the outcome criteria have been met. Skin should not be taut or inflexible. The patient should report an understanding of the importance of performing skin-stretching exercises. No ulcerations are noted on fingers or toes.

Community/Home Care

At home, the patient will need to implement strategies to maintain skin in an optimal state. In the early stages of the disease, home visits from nursing or other disciplines may not be required; however, follow-up with a health care provider is needed to monitor progress of the disease. The patient should focus attention on maintaining flexibility of skin, preventing ulcerations, and minimizing episodes of Raynaud's phenomenon. The nurse plays a vital role in the patient's ability to achieve these outcomes by educating the patient about methods to maintain skin flexibility. Interventions at home can include massaging skin on face, fingers, and feet and exercising the muscles of the face through yawning or other facial movements. If the patient smokes, cessation is needed to prevent vasoconstriction that could precipitate an episode of Raynaud's phenomenon. During winter months, it is crucial that the patient remain warm and dress in loose layers with special attention to the hands and feet, possibly requiring that the patient wear wool socks even when inside. Failure to provide the patient with this information precludes the patient from implementing necessary interventions to prevent loss of mobility of facial muscles and elasticity of skin over fingers and feet. When the tissue becomes tight and inelastic, home care providers will be faced with the issue of adequate nutrition and communication as movement of the mouth becomes difficult. As the distortion of the face progresses, the patient may withdraw from others. Follow-up care will require that the health care provider assess skin for ulcerations, mobility, and sensation and be sure that the patient recognizes signs and symptoms of organ involvement (renal and pulmonary) or disease progression. Attention should also be given to the patient's psychological well-being, including any verbalization of social isolation or negative talk about self.

Documentation

Chart the status of the patient's skin, including any ulcerations, edema, change in pigmentation, or inelasticity. Specifically note the status of facial muscles. Note any episodes of Raynaud's phenomenon that the patient reports. Include in the record any teaching done by the health care providers, along with documentation of the patient's understanding.

NURSING DIAGNOSIS 2

 ## IMBALANCED NUTRITION: LESS THAN BODY REQUIREMENTS

Related to:

Abdominal inflammation
Decreased intestinal motility
Esophageal strictures and/or scarring
Decreased esophageal motility
Diarrhea
Abdominal pain

Defining Characteristics:

Weight loss
Difficulty swallowing
Gastric reflux

Goal:

Nutritional status is maintained.

Outcome Criteria

✔ The patient is able to digest a normal diet.
✔ The patient does not lose weight.
✔ The patient reports no difficulty swallowing.

NOC *Swallowing status*
Swallowing status: Esophageal phase
Nutritional status: Food and fluid intake
Weight: Body mass

INTERVENTIONS	RATIONALES
Assess the patient's ability to swallow a variety of food types.	Helps to determine the extent of difficulty in swallowing and to make decisions about type of diet required; scleroderma causes strictures and scarring of the esophagus, making swallowing difficult.
Assess the patient's ability to open mouth wide enough to consume adequate foods and chew.	The face, especially the mouth, is often affected by scleroderma; the muscle surrounding the mouth tightens, and the patient may only be able to put small amounts of food into oral cavity at one time.

(continues)

(continued)

INTERVENTIONS	RATIONALES
Consult with a dietician, as ordered or as necessary.	The dietician can provide recommendations for adequate nutrient intake to prevent weight loss.
Weigh patient on first contact with health care system and monitor at follow-up visits.	It is important to establish a baseline weight and monitor weight over the progression of the disease to determine whether patient is able to take in enough food.
Administer proton pump linhibitors before meals as ordered; teach patient about the purpose of medications, side effects, and drug interactions.	Helps to prevent/relieve gastric reflux and heartburn by decreasing secretion of gastric acids; most proton pump inhibitors should be given before breakfast; food may decrease absorption.
Administer antacids 30 to 60 minutes after meals.	Helps to neutralize gastric acids.
Assist patient in assuming high Fowler's position for meals and have him or her remain upright for 1 hour after eating.	Helps to prevent gastric reflux.
Arrange for small meals, served frequently (6 times a day).	Helps to facilitate digestion; patients with scleroderma may have a narrowed oral opening and will tire before consuming a large meal; difficulty swallowing also makes it difficult for the patient to consume a large meal before tiring.
Elevate the patient in bed at night.	Helps to prevent gastric reflux when sleeping.
Give foods that are easy to chew, swallow, and digest, such as mashed potatoes, applesauce, pureed meats, or other soft-consistency foods.	If foods are easy to chew and swallow, the patient is more likely to have adequate intake of nutrients.
Teach the patient all strategies/ interventions to maintain or improve nutritional status, and encourage their use at home.	The patient needs to implement strategies to promote swallowing, digestion, and maintenance of nutrition to prevent weight loss.

Evaluation

The patient reports having the ability to swallow without difficulty. Weight remains stable, and patient states satisfaction with diet. The patient should report decreased episodes of gastric reflux and abdominal discomfort. In addition, the patient should verbalize an understanding of all required interventions and rationales for implementation.

Community/Home Care

At home, the patient should continue to implement strategies to maintain nutritional status. Even though a nurse or other health care provider may not be required for home visits, the patient's nutritional status will need to be monitored through some mechanism. Because of the difficulty with eating, chewing, and swallowing, it will be easy for the patient to lose interest in eating, leading to a gradual loss of weight, which over time may become pronounced. Teaching by the dietician or nurse should focus on providing information or lists of foods that are nutritional and easy to consume. The patient should be provided with printed information for later reference. The teaching should consider any cultural or religious practices or restrictions. At the conclusion of teaching, the patient should be able to identify those foods that have nutritional value and not just substances that are easy to consume. Some patients may be hesitant to eat in the presence of others because of difficulty eating and the extended time it may take to finish a meal. Family members should be encouraged to eat with the patient and discouraged from drawing attention to adaptations made to methods for chewing or promoting food intake. Liquid nutritional supplements may be beneficial to the patient to consume between meals or as snacks, as they contain multiple nutrients. However, the patient would need to use these cautiously if renal impairments are present, as many of these supplements are high in protein, which would further stress the renal system. In this case, the patient could use a supplement, such as Nepro®, that is especially formulated for renal disease patients. In the home, the patient may experiment with using a small baby spoon for eating if the mouth muscles are tight and the patient has difficulty opening the mouth. Strategies to control gastric reflux will be important for the patient at home, and adaptations to sleeping arrangements may be required. One suggestion is for patients to use pillows to elevate themselves in the bed at night. A schedule for administration of proton pump inhibitors and antacids should be written for the patient. Follow-up visits with a health care provider should include an assessment of the patient's ability to chew and swallow, along with obtaining a weight at each visit. A 24-hour recall of food intake with a calorie count can serve to identify the need for further intervention by a dietician.

Documentation

Chart the patient's weight and the findings from an assessment of the patient's ability to chew and swallow. Document specific verbalizations made by the patient about ability to eat and any complaints of abdominal pain or gastric reflux. Include in the patient record the percentage of food consumed. Chart all interventions implemented, the patient's responses, and all teaching including verbalization of understanding or the need for reinforcement. Document all referrals made in the patient record.

NURSING DIAGNOSIS 4

ACUTE PAIN

Related to:

> Inflamed joints
>
> Joint contractures
>
> Inelasticity of skin

Defining Characteristics:

> Complains of joint pain and/or pain upon movement of joint
>
> Joint(s) appear swollen, red, and warm to the touch

Goal:

> Pain is decreased.

Outcome Criteria

✔ The patient states pain has decreased 1 hour after intervention.
✔ The patient states mobility has improved.
✔ The patient verbalizes methods to reduce pain.

NOC *Pain: Disruptive effects*
Pain level
Pain control

INTERVENTIONS	RATIONALES
Assess the patient's pain using a pain rating scale.	Provides a more subjective assessment.
Assess or take a history about onset, location, precipitating factors, relieving factors, and effect on function.	These will assist in accurate diagnosis and treatment; knowing how pain affects function will provide information needed to assist patient with home care needs.
Administer nonsteroidal anti-inflammatory drugs (NSAIDs) or other analgesic agents, as ordered.	Helps to decrease inflammation and reduce pain.
Maintain joints in a position of function.	In the event that mobility and motion are limited, joints in position of function can be essential to future independence and use of assistive devices.
Arrange for physical/occupational therapy consultation.	Physical/occupational therapists can provide the patient with alternatives to foster mobility while decreasing the pain response.
Apply moist heat to affected joints.	Helps to aid muscle relaxation and decrease pain.
Assess effectiveness of all interventions implemented for pain, particularly medications.	Helps to determine whether revisions in the plan of care are required.

NIC *Heat/cold application*
Analgesic administration
Pain management

Evaluation

Assess the degree to which the patient expresses satisfaction with pain control. Determine the effectiveness of the individual interventions in order to decide which ones work best or least for the patient. If pain persists, the nurse should determine whether there are other causes of the pain and should investigate additional measures to relieve pain.

Community/Home Care

The patient with scleroderma is treated as an outpatient except at times when systemic complications occur. The pain that occurs with scleroderma is generally manageable with mild analgesics, and pain control is not the priority of home care. Maintenance of joint mobility and skin elasticity will help decrease episodes of pain in joints and tight skin. Therefore, strategies in the home to address skin and mobility will also enhance strategies to alleviate pain. Side effects of analgesics should be thoroughly explained to the patient with an explanation of what to do if they should occur. Generalized systemic scleroderma patients are at risk for kidney involvement that results in hypertension. For these patients, over-the-counter NSAIDs should be used cautiously, as some of these products can cause a significant increase in blood pressure. Follow-up care with a health care provider is crucial in order to monitor disease progression and to monitor for organ involvement that may require further evaluation and additional treatment.

Documentation

Document the results of the pain assessment, along with all interventions implemented to address the pain. It is important that the record reflect as much description about the pain as possible: location, intensity, precipitating factors, and a general description of the type of pain. Chart the achievement of outcome criteria with specific patient behaviors that validate achievement. Include in the patient record the patient's verbalization of satisfaction with pain control.

NURSING DIAGNOSIS 5

DISTURBED BODY IMAGE

Related to:

Physical deformities of hands (swelling, tightening of skin)

Limited movement of mouth

Difficulty communicating

Defining Characteristics:

Withdrawal

Social isolation

Depression

Negative statements about physical appearance

Attempts to cover hands and mouth in the presence of others

Goal:

The patient accepts the change in physical appearance and continues social activities and interpersonal relationships.

Outcome Criteria

✔ The patient states a willingness to look at and touch hands and face.

✔ The patient does not verbalize negative feelings toward self.

NOC *Body image*

INTERVENTIONS	RATIONALES
Encourage patient to communicate feelings about changes in physical appearance.	Talking about the changes may sometimes be the beginning of acceptance.
Teach the patient methods to care for hands and face to slow the process of tightening and edema (see nursing diagnosis "Impaired Tissue Integrity").	Exercising the face, hands, wrist, and fingers can slow the disease progression of tightening of face and skin around wrists and fingers.
Teach the patient and family how to maintain optimal self-care functioning.	If the patient is able to remain independent with self-care activities and common household tasks, that comfort level may translate into acceptance of the change in appearance and incorporation of body appearance change into a positive self-image.
Monitor the patient's feelings about self, interpersonal relationships with family members and friends, withdrawal, social isolation, anxiety, embarrassment by appearance, fear that appearance will frighten loved ones, and desire to be alone.	Helps to detect early alterations in social functioning, prevent unhealthy behaviors, and intervene early through referral to counseling.
Encourage the patient to participate in at least one outside/public activity each week once health status permits.	Prevents the patient from isolating self from others.
Identify the effects of the patient's culture or religion on body image.	A patient's culture and religion often help define reactions to changes in body image and self-worth.
Identify educational resources and community support groups through the Scleroderma Foundation.	Discussions with other patients with a similar situation is good for the patient who will be able to share thoughts with and hear thoughts from those who understand what the patient is going through; provides the patient with support and the courage to move forward in

INTERVENTIONS	RATIONALES
	terms of acceptance of the change. The Scleroderma Foundation also provides literature to patients and their families.
Assist the patient in identifying coping strategies or diversionary activities.	Helps to provide distraction from health status so that not all thoughts are on disfigurement.
Arrange for psychosocial counseling, as ordered.	Helps to provide psychological evaluation and assistance to the patient.

NIC *Body image enhancement*
Emotional support
Support group
Socialization enhancement

Evaluation

The patient is able to willingly learn about the strategies to improve functioning and manage own activities to the extent possible. Determine whether the patient is able to verbalize feelings about the deformities and the impact they will have on role performance. Time is required for the patient to completely assimilate the change in body appearance into his or her self-perception. It is crucial that the nurse evaluates to what degree the patient is beginning to do this. Communication of feelings and concerns relevant to the change in appearance should be taken as a positive sign that progress towards meeting the outcome criteria is being made.

Community/Home Care

At home, continued monitoring of the patient's perception of body image is needed. The nurse who visits will need to take the time to recognize any subtle hints that may indicate that the patient has not completely adapted to the change in body appearance. For the patient with scleroderma, the change in facial structure will be obvious to others as the mouth opening and face become tightened, making the patient's voice sound different and making eating difficult, both of which would be quite noticeable. Open discussions about this change and interventions to prevent social isolation and withdrawal should continue with patient and family. Discuss with the patient and family the types of activities that have previously enjoyed and the people with whom they are more comfortable. Use this information as a starting point for encouraging the patient to remain engaged in social relationships. The health care provider should inquire about participation in social activities. Community support groups should be explored as a way to provide support to the patient and family by talking to others who have had to deal with this issue.

Documentation

Chart any specific behaviors or verbalizations that may indicate an altered body image. Document a precise description of the physical change in appearance that is causing the disturbed body image. Include all interventions that have been employed to address this issue and the patient's responses. Note when and if the patient begins to verbalize feelings about the deformities of the face and fingers. All referrals should be documented in the patient record.

CHAPTER 9.112

HERPES ZOSTER/VARICELLA (SHINGLES)

GENERAL INFORMATION

Herpes zoster, also known as shingles, is a viral infection that occurs when there is reactivation of a latent varicella virus in persons who have had chickenpox. The disease is characterized by groupings of lesions along a dermatome that follow the path of peripheral sensory nerves. These lesions usually are vesicles that appear unilaterally without crossing the body's midline. Vesicles typically erupt 1 to 2 days after the development of pain and itching and clear in 2 to 3 weeks. If however, the period of time between appearance of pain and the appearance of lesions is > 2 days, the course of the disease is longer. The patient is contagious from the day before the appearance of the rash until all the lesions begin to have scab formation (usually 5 days). The incubation period for the varicella zoster virus is from 7 to 21 days, with the course of the disease ranging from 2 to 5 weeks. The lesions of herpes zoster consist of macules, papules, and vesicles that can be noted on the face, trunk, scalp, and thoracic regions of the body. In some cases the eyes are also involved, which may leave the patient with visual deficits. Other clinical manifestations include pain at the site, itching, malaise, and fever prior to eruption of the vesicles. The disease is seen most often in persons over the age of 50 and in people who are immunocompromised, such as those with HIV, lymphoma, and leukemia.

NURSING DIAGNOSIS 1

IMPAIRED SKIN INTEGRITY

Related to:

Invasion of skin with herpes zoster

Defining Characteristics:

Vesicles

Rash

Purulent drainage

Itching of skin

Goal:

Skin will heal without secondary infection.

Outcome Criteria

✔ Vesicles will scab and fall off.

✔ Itching will cease.

✔ No purulent drainage will be noted in vesicles.

NOC *Tissue integrity: Skin and mucous membranes*

Infection severity

Knowledge: Infection control

INTERVENTIONS	RATIONALES
Assess skin changes noting location of vesicles and a description of lesions, as well as presence and color of drainage. Pay close attention to the areas close to the eye.	Helps to establish a baseline to guide treatment and monitor response to treatments. The vesicles may have drainage initially but gradually dry up with scab formation. In the case of secondary infection, the drainage may become purulent; if the virus invades the eye, visual impairment, including blindness, may occur.
Obtain a history from the patient regarding itching and scratching.	This information will give clues to the extent of discomfort caused by the lesions.
Monitor results of laboratory tests: complete blood count (CBC), culture of vesicles, varicella virus antigen, Tzanck smear.	Helps to validate the diagnosis and extent of infection.
Assess for secondary infection in the vesicles: purulent drainage, increased white blood cell (WBC) count, lymphadenopathy	These are common findings in the infection, and identification allows for early intervention.

INTERVENTIONS	RATIONALES
(palpable lumps in neck, axilla, and groin), fever, and chills.	
Administer anti-virals such as acyclovir (Zovirax®), as ordered, and monitor for side effects	Helps to stop the proliferation of the virus. Anti-virals exerts their actions better if therapy is started within 1 to 2 days of the appearance of the vesicles. Side effects include nausea, vomiting, diarrhea, and headache.
Administer antipyretics, such as Tylenol, as ordered.	Helps to decrease fever.
Apply topical anti-pruritics (such as calamine lotion), as ordered.	Helps to reduce itching and need to scratch, which will erode the skin and introduce bacteria.
Administer antihistamines (such as Benadryl), as ordered.	Prevents histamine release, which causes reaction to varicella. An antihistamine will reduce the itching sensation and the need to scratch.
Use mild soaps for bathing or use commercial products, such as oatmeal bath lotion.	Helps to decrease itching.
Apply cool compresses.	Helps to provide relief from itching.
Cut fingernails short to avoid introduction of bacteria into vesicular skin eruptions when scratching.	Inevitably, the patient will scratch the vesicles. Keeping fingernails short will reduce the risk of bacterial introduction into the open vesicles.
Implement contact isolation and universal precautions.	Helps to prevent the spread of organisms during incubation period. Pregnant health care workers and those who have never had chickenpox should not work with the patient.
Assess the patient and family for: knowledge of disease, therapeutic interventions, mode of ransmission, and prognosis.	Helps to determine learning needs of the patient and family.
Teach the patient and family: disease process, treatments (skin care, medications), isolation precautions, mechanism of transmission, how to assess lesions, and ways to increase comfort.	Helps to enhance the patient's and family's ability to manage home care; knowledge promotes compliance with regimen.

 Medication administration: Skin
Skin care: Topical treatments

Skin surveillance
Infection control

Evaluation

The patient's skin returns to its normal state. There are no signs of secondary infection, and lesions are without drainage and have scabbed over or scabs have fallen off. Itching has been relieved, and the patient reports a sense of comfort.

Community/Home Care

In the home setting, the patient with herpes zoster will need to implement strategies for skin care, as the lesions will be in a stage of scabbing. Because of the potential for altered body image due to the possible scars that healed vesicles will create, especially in darker-skinned persons, it is important for the nurse to be sure that the patient has received adequate teaching about what is required. Topical ointments to prevent itching as the skin heals will be helpful to the patient. Daily baths with soothing preparations such as oatmeal can be continued at home using warm water rather than hot, as hot water increases itching. Cool compresses can be easily fashioned using a hand towel or washcloth dipped in cold water and applied to the itching or painful area. The patient needs to assess the skin for signs of secondary infection and notify a health care provider if vesicles start to drain purulent liquid. Practicing meticulous hand washing is important to prevent the spread of organisms, and the patient should refrain from contact with people who are at high risk for development of herpes zoster, such as the immunocompromised, pregnant women, and those who have never had chickenpox. At home, the patient should sleep alone and wash bed linens, towels, washcloth, and clothing items separately for at least 2 weeks. If the patient normally seeks hair care from a professional hairdresser, he or she will need to inform them of the possibility of healed scabs in the head so that gentle shampooing and mild products can be used. The patient should avoid using chemical products such as relaxers and dyes until complete healing has occurred. The patient will need to be aware of changes in the skin that would warrant a return visit to the health care provider.

Documentation

Document the results of a thorough assessment of the patient's skin, particularly the presence and description of any rashes, ulcers, or skin lesions. Chart all nursing interventions implemented to address the problem, including any attention given to psychosocial needs, such as disturbed body image. Complaints are documented and interventions to address them are charted, along with a follow-up note indicating whether the problem has been resolved. All medications administered are documented according to agency protocol. All teaching implemented and the patient's understanding should be included in the patient record. Referrals to dermatologists are also documented. Document whether the outcome criteria have been achieved.

NURSING DIAGNOSIS 2

 ### ACUTE PAIN

Related to:

> Purulent macular, papular, vesicular rash
> Fever

Defining Characteristics:

> Complaint of pain
> Grimacing

Goal:

> The patient's pain is resolved.

Outcome Criteria

✔ The patient states pain has decreased 1 hour after intervention.
✔ The patient verbalizes methods to reduce pain.
✔ The patient states that the pain/itching is reduced.

NOC *Pain: Disruptive effects*
Pain level
Pain control

INTERVENTIONS	RATIONALES
Obtain a history regarding onset of pain, including location.	In herpes zoster, a patient history is helpful in determining incubation period and length of time for vesicles; patient reports pain 1 to 2 days before appearance of vesicles/rash.
Assess the patient's pain using a pain rating scale.	Provides a more objective assessment.
Assess or take a history regarding onset, location, precipitating factors, relieving factors, and effect on function.	These will assist in accurate diagnosis and treatment; knowing how pain affects function will provide information needed to assist patient with home care needs.
Administer analgesics as ordered.	Helps to decrease pain. In some instances of severe pain, narcotic analgesics are required for relief.
Administer antihistamines (Benadryl), as ordered.	Reduces sensitivity reaction by blocking histamine release.
Apply topical anti-pruritic agents (calamine lotion), as ordered.	Helps to reduce itching and increase comfort.
Apply cool compresses.	Helps to reduce itching pain and provide soothing relief.
Encourage the patient to wear loose cotton bed clothing and supply light cotton bed linens.	Helps to reduce irritation and encourage air circulation.
Administer antivirals such as Acyclovir, as ordered.	Helps to decrease the severity of the disease and thus decrease pain.
Assess effectiveness of all interventions implemented for pain, particularly medications.	Helps to determine if revisions in the plan of care are required.
Teach the patient methods to control pain in preparation for home care.	Gives the patient a sense of control and allows for adequate pain control when in the home environment.

NIC *Analgesic administration*
Pain management

Evaluation

Assess the degree to which the patient expresses satisfaction with pain control. Determine the effectiveness of the individual interventions in order to decide which ones work best or least for the patient. If pain persists, the nurse should determine if there are other causes of the pain and should also investigate additional measures to relieve pain.

Community/Home Care

The pain that occurs with herpes zoster (shingles) is treated with mild analgesics and in the home environment, pain is usually a major concern, as it may persist for 4 weeks. At home, the patient should continue to take analgesics as needed throughout the day on a regular schedule. Strategies to relieve itching should continue and include warm water tub baths using commercial oatmeal bath solutions. If the patient takes Benadryl for itching, he or she should be cognizant of its potential to cause serious drowsiness and a feeling of tiredness that would make operation of machinery or driving hazardous. Clothing should be loose and made of material that is not scratchy (such as wool and crisp linen). Suggested fabrics are cotton or soft woven knits. If vesicles are present on the trunk, patients should avoid pants or skirts that fasten securely around the waist, but rather instead wear items that have elastic that is loose. During sleep, the patient can wear cotton gloves to decrease the chance of excoriating the skin lesions unknowingly by scratching during sleep. It is crucial that the patient understand strategies to be used for pain control. Side effects of analgesics and antivirals should be thoroughly explained to the patient, along with an explanation of what to do if they should occur. Follow-up care with a health care provider is crucial in order to monitor disease progression and to monitor for complications such as secondary infection, post-herpetic neuralgia, and visual changes.

Documentation

Document the results of the pain assessment. It is important that the record reflect as much description about the pain as possible: location, intensity, precipitating factors, and a general description of the type of pain. Document all interventions implemented, including special baths or topical preparations. Chart the achievement of outcome criteria with specific patient behaviors that validate achievement. Include in the patient record the patient's verbalization of satisfaction with pain control. Medications are charted according to the agency procedures, and temperatures are charted according to the agency's procedure for documenting vital signs.

NURSING DIAGNOSIS 3

DISTURBED BODY IMAGE

Related to:

Skin lesions on body

Defining Characteristics:

Withdrawal

Social isolation

Depression

Negative statements about physical appearance

Attempts to cover face in the presence of others

Goal:

The patient accepts the change in physical appearance and continues social activities and interpersonal relationships when no longer contagious.

Outcome Criteria

✔ The patient states a willingness to look at lesions on body.

✔ The patient does not verbalize negative feelings toward self.

✔ The patient verbalizes acceptance of body appearance.

NOC *Body image*

INTERVENTIONS	RATIONALES
Encourage the patient to get feelings out in the open and assure the patient that these feelings are normal.	The patient should understand that his or her emotions are real and should be expected.
Allow the patient privacy when bathing, dressing, or toileting, unless assistance is requested.	Helps to allow patient time to adjust to appearance without concern for how others react.
Encourage patient to communicate feelings about changes in physical appearance.	Talking about the changes may sometimes be the beginning of acceptance.
Teach the patient methods to care for skin lesions (see nursing diagnosis "Impaired Skin Integrity").	Protecting the skin from excoriation and secondary infections that worsen lesions will improve appearance and prevent further problems.
Monitor patient's feelings about self, interpersonal relationships with family members and friends, withdrawal, social isolation, fear, anxiety, embarrassment by appearance, and desire to be alone.	Helps to detect early alterations in social functioning, prevent unhealthy behaviors, and intervene early through referral to counseling.

(continues)

(continued)

INTERVENTIONS	RATIONALES
Encourage patient to participate in at least one outside/public activity each week once lesions are no longer contagious and health status permits.	Prevents patient from isolating self from others.
Identify the effects of the patient's culture or religion in terms of body image.	A patient's culture and religion often help define reactions to changes in body image and self-worth.
Assist the patient in identifying coping strategies/diversionary activities.	Helps to provide diversionary activities so that thoughts are not focused on current appearance.

NIC *Body image enhancement*

Emotional support

Socialization enhancement

Evaluation

The patient is able to look at lesions and verbalizes acceptance of changes in body appearance. Determine whether the patient is able to verbalize feelings regarding skin changes. The patient has no negative verbalizations about self. Communication of feelings and concerns relevant to the change in appearance should be taken as a positive sign that progress towards meeting outcome criteria is being made.

Community/Home Care

At home, continued monitoring of the patient's perception of body image is needed. Health care providers that see the patient for follow-up will need to be alert to subtle hints that may indicate that the patient has not completely adapted to the change in body appearance. Open discussions regarding physical changes and interventions to prevent social isolation and withdrawal should continue with patient and family. As the vesicles heal, the patient may feel better about his or her appearance; however, the person may still be hesitant to allow family members, especially a spouse or significant other, to see the healing lesions. Encouraging the patient to look at the lesions and assess them may improve the patient's ability to deal with body changes. Because the lesions are often hidden by clothes, going out in public may not be a major problem. However, if lesions are on the face, the patient may impose self-isolation. Family members should encourage the patient to go out for short periods once allowed, starting with environments where the patient feels comfortable and others are more likely to refrain from staring, such as religious services. Once lesions are completely healed and the scabs have fallen off, body image issues should be resolved.

Documentation

Chart any specific behaviors or verbalizations that may indicate an altered body image. Include all interventions that have been employed to address this issue and the patient's responses. Note when and if the patient begins to verbalize feelings regarding the skin changes and demonstrates behaviors indicative of positive body image.

UNIT 10

SENSORY/VISUAL SYSTEMS

CHAPTER 10.113

DETACHED RETINA

GENERAL INFORMATION

Detachment of the retina occurs when the inner sensory layers of the retina are separated from the outer pigmented epithelium (choroid) of the retina. This separation can occur because of inflammation or bleeding, or if the retina is torn and vitreous humor seeps between the retina and the choroid. When the separation occurs, there is a subsequent decrease in blood and oxygen supply to the retina, which renders the retina unable to perceive light. The loss of vision may occur quickly (in cases of trauma) or may progress over years. In cases of gradual loss, the patient may not have any noticeable symptoms. When present, symptoms include floating spots, flashes of light, and a gradual loss of vision in one area. Patients experiencing a rapid separation, usually due to trauma, often compare the effect to a curtain or veil being drawn over their eyes. The most common causes of retina detachment are myopic degeneration and trauma (usually from a blow to the head or globe of the eye). Aging is a risk factor for retinal detachment due to the shrinkage of vitreous humor that pulls the retina away from the choroid. Other risk factors include aphakia (absence of lens), which is seen following cataract surgery.

NURSING DIAGNOSIS 1

 DISTURBED SENSORY PERCEPTION: VISUAL

Related to:

Separation of sensory layers from choroids layer

Tear in retina

Defining Characteristics:

Gradual or sudden loss of vision

Pain in globe of eye following trauma

Inability to perceive light

Perceptions of flashes of light

"Veil" or "curtain" effect in the eye

Floating spots in eye

Goal:

The patient has no further deterioration of vision.

Outcome Criteria

✔ The patient reports an improvement in vision.

✔ The patient states that "veil" or "curtain" effect has resolved.

✔ The patient states that flashing lights and floaters are absent.

NOC *Sensory function: Vision*
Vision compensation behavior

INTERVENTIONS	RATIONALES
Assess for alterations in vision: decreased vision in one area, flashing lights, floaters, presence of "curtain" or "veil," blindness (with involvement of macula), and pain in globe of eye.	Helps to establish a baseline of visual functioning to serve as a basis for assistance to the patient.
Monitor results of diagnostic tests (B-scan ultrasonography, ophthalmoscopic exams, and slit lamp microscopy).	Ultrasonography provides an accurate assessment of the retina and allows for visualization of the detachment, and can detect fluid leakage within the eye behind the retina. Ophthalmoscopic exam identifies the area of detachment as well as the extent of the tear. Slit lamp microscopy allows for visualization of the far periphery of the retina. Early diagnosis is

INTERVENTIONS	RATIONALES
	critical so that early treatment is initiated to prevent blindness.
Enforce strict bedrest with head immobilized if retinal detachment/ tear is large or there is a possibility of damage to the macula.	The patient needs to avoid any excess movement that may cause further retinal detachment.
Assess the patient for signs of pain in the eye, such as keeping eyelids tightly closed and facial grimaces, and question the patient about headache and pain in globe of eye. Treat as ordered with mild analgesia.	Pain in the eye occasionally occurs with detachment due to trauma.
Orient the person to the environment, especially if hospitalized (see nursing diagnosis "Risk for Injury").	Disturbances in vision are present, and the person needs to know where objects are to prevent injury.
Apply bilateral eye patches, if ordered.	It is necessary to restrict movement of eyes to prevent further damage; if only the affected eye is patched, the good eye will continue to move to follow objects, causing the affected eye to move as well.
Administer medications, such as cycloplegics and corticosteroids, as ordered.	Cycloplegics paralyze and thus rest the eye; corticosteroids decrease inflammation.
Prepare the patient for surgery according to protocols or as ordered by surgeon.	Retinal detachments that create risk for vision compromise are corrected surgically, most with a 90 percent success rate. The goal of all interventions is to return the retina back to its normal position. Cryopexy is commonly used and involves using subfreezing nitrous oxide or carbon dioxide to the area of the tear to produce an inflammatory response with adhesions that hold the two layers together. Often the surgeon will combine this procedure with scleral buckling where an indention is created in the sclera and the choroids that bring the choroid in contact with the retina. An artificial band of substance is then placed around the eye in order to keep the choroids in contact with the tear or detachment and prevent

	traction on the tear. Pneumatic retinopexy is a procedure that injects an expandable gas or air into the vitreous area of the retina to apply pressure to the retina causing it to come back into contact with the choroids. The gas is absorbed.
Following retinopexy, position the patient in prone position (face down) or angled toward the unaffected side; use pillows to maintain position, and check patient often to be sure patient is compliant.	This position allows the gas bubble to rise in the eye and create pressure on the repair, it is a difficult position, and the patient may need assistance and reminders to remain in this position.
For other types of surgery, keep the patient positioned so that the area of detachment is dependent or inferior, and avoid bending or rapid head movements.	Maintains pressure on the area of the tear so that contact with the choroids is maintained; prevents pain and avoids increasing intraocular pressure, which could affect detachment or area of repair.
Keep lights in the patient's room turned down low.	Surgery to the eye and medications instilled in the eye make the eye more sensitive to light.
Post-operatively assess the affected eye for drainage, hemorrhage, or cloudy appearance to the cornea, and question the patient about sudden pain in the eye.	These are signs of complications that may indicate an emergency requiring prompt attention from a physician to safeguard sight.
Use books with large print and large numbers or letters on household items such as clocks.	Helps to enhance the environment to compensate for diminished vision.
Assist the patient with meals, particularly if he or she has bilateral eye patches, by helping with menu selection and preparing of foods on tray by describing the location of foods using positions on the clock (for example meat is at 12 o'clock); assure the patient that it is okay to get assistance.	The patient may not eat if he or she cannot readily find food, and may be embarrassed to ask for help.

NIC   *Eye care*
  Communication enhancement:
    Visual deficit
  Environmental management

Evaluation

Assess the degree to which outcomes have been achieved. The patient should have no further deterioration in visual ability. There is an absence of floaters, flashing lights, or sensation of a "curtain." The patient reports that there are no new variations in visual ability and is able to assist with activities of daily living.

Community/Home Care

For most patients with detached retinas, treatment is done on an outpatient basis through physician's offices, and if surgery is required, it is generally performed as a same-day procedure. However, some patients may remain overnight or the stay may be prolonged depending upon the individual patient's response to treatment and availability of resources after discharge. The patient should be encouraged to keep follow-up appointments as scheduled to ensure early detection and treatment of any further visual problems. Patients treated surgically need education on post-operative recommendations, including activity and position restrictions, instillation of eye drops, proper use of eye patches, signs and symptoms of infection, and use of sunglasses when outside in the sun (see nursing diagnosis "Deficient Knowledge"). Evaluations should be made to determine what assistance the patient may need in the home environment to compensate for altered visual ability. If no family member is available to assist, the patient may need the services of a home health aide until performance of activities of daily living (ADLs) and household chores can be performed independently. Signs and symptoms that necessitate immediate attention should be made clear to the patient and/or family members. Evaluate whether the patient has the resources to purchase medications and receive follow-up care, including the availability of transportation for appointments.

Documentation

Chart all assessments related to the status of the patient's vision. Include the patient's responses to interventions and understanding of all procedures. Document preparation for surgery, including pre-operative teaching, and post-operative assessments, according to agency protocol and guidelines. Any teaching should be documented with a clear indication of the patient's understanding of information. All referrals are included in the patient record.

NURSING DIAGNOSIS 2

 ### RISK FOR INFECTION

Related to:

    Enhanced opportunity for invasion by organisms

    Surgical intervention to repair detachment

Defining Characteristics:

    None

Goal:

    The patient will not acquire infection in eye.

Outcome Criteria

✔ The patient will have no redness or drainage from eye.

✔ The patient will have no pain in eye.

✔ The patient will remain afebrile.

NOC *Infection severity*

       Knowledge: Infection control

INTERVENTIONS	RATIONALES
Assess eye for drainage and redness, and question patient regarding increased pain.	These are signs of infection; pain in the eye is a common complaint when the eye becomes infected; identification allows for early intervention.
Monitor temperature every 4 hours.	An elevated temperature is indicative of infection.
Monitor white blood cell (WBC) count.	Elevations in WBC count indicate infection.
Administer antibiotic eye drops, as ordered.	Antibiotic eye drops are used prophylactically to prevent infection following surgical intervention.
Use sterile technique when changing eye dressings or patches.	Helps to reduce the opportunity for introduction of organisms into the eye.
Provide adequate diet rich in vitamin C and protein.	Good nutrition is required for enhanced immune status and wound healing.
Teach patient and significant other signs and symptoms of infection.	Infection may develop after the patient is discharged home, and the patient will need to be able to recognize the signs and symptoms to report to the health care provider.

NIC *Surveillance*
Infection protection

Evaluation

Evaluate the extent to which the projected outcome criteria have been met. The patient should be free of infection as demonstrated by the absence of drainage, increased pain in the eye, or redness. The patient is able to verbalize the signs and symptoms of infection prior to discharge.

Community/Home Care

Most patients treated for detached retina are not usually hospitalized for any extended period of time. For this reason, monitoring for infection becomes the responsibility of the patient or family members at home. It is crucial that health care providers teach the patient and family the signs and symptoms of infection and assure that they understand. The patient and family/significant others should understand that the patient should return for immediate follow-up if these symptoms occur. They should also be aware of the correct techniques for changing dressings or eye pads to avoid contamination or injury that could increase the risk of infection. The importance of good handwashing should be stressed, and the patient and family should be encouraged to wash hands prior to touching the affected eye.

Documentation

Document findings from an assessment of the eye, including gross visual acuity. Additionally, include subjective information from the patient, particularly regarding pain or other abnormal feelings in the eye. Document all nursing interventions performed, including antibiotic medications. Chart teaching performed and patient's understanding of the information presented.

NURSING DIAGNOSIS 3

RISK FOR INJURY

Related to:

Decreased vision

Loss of vision

Use of eye patches

Inability to see to the side

Inability to see items in environment clearly

Restrictions on movement of head

Defining Characteristics:

None

Goal:

The patient will be safe.

Outcome Criteria

✔ The patient will participate in ADLs without injury.

✔ The patient will verbalize an understanding of the need to adapt the home environment to prevent injury.

NOC *Safe home environment*
Fall prevention behavior

INTERVENTIONS	RATIONALES
Assess the patient's environment for hazards that could predispose him or her to falls.	Common items often place the patient at risk for injury when vision is impaired.
Orient the patient to the environment, especially if in the hospital setting, and do not rearrange items without telling the patient.	Patients will feel more comfortable if they are familiar with the environment; changes may create hazards, as the patient will not know where items are.
Instruct the patient to limit movement of the head when ambulating and to turn body to see objects around him or her.	Helps to decrease head movements, as gravity helps keep the retina in proper position following surgery; turning the entire body helps the patient scan the perimeter and identify obstacles to prevent falls.
Encourage the use of walls, rails, or other stable items when ambulating.	Helps to provide support and assistance with ambulation to prevent imbalance or falls.
Assist with ambulation as needed by walking ahead of the patient and having him or her hold your arm or elbow and warn the patient of any hazards/obstacles in his or her path.	Helps to guide the patient, provide a sense of safety, and maintain mobility; the first time the patient gets up, the sense of proprioception may be altered due to the presence of eye patches.
Following surgery, remain with patient for first ambulation.	Patients generally feel uncomfortable about walking, and visual acuity is not known immediately post-operatively.

(continues)

(continued)

INTERVENTIONS	RATIONALES
Have the patient avoid picking up heavy objects, avoid bending and lifting, and avoid straining for bowel movements.	These activities increase intraocular pressure and cause stress on the operative area of the retina.
Place the call light and other frequently used items within easy reach for the person at home or in the hospital.	Makes the environment more familiar and allows for independence.
In the home, remove clutter, such as scatter rugs or extra chairs, from rooms and hallways, and limit the use of electrical extension cords in open spaces.	Items that are in open spaces create obstacles that the patient may not be able to see; scatter rugs and other small pieces of furniture are frequently the cause of falls for the person with limited vision.
Use adequate lighting in the home or hospital, avoiding extremely bright lights.	Bright, direct light often causes glare, creating more of a hazard for falls.
Instruct the patient to wear an eye shield at night.	Helps to prevent accidental scratching or damage to the eye during sleep.

NIC *Environmental management: Safety*

  Fall prevention

  Surveillance: Safety

Evaluation

The proposed outcomes have been met, as evidenced by the fact that the patient sustains no injury. The patient is able to verbalize the need for adaptations to be made in the environment to ensure safety. In addition, the patient reports how to make changes in ambulation and daily living to prevent injury, and is willing to comply.

Community/Home Care

In the home setting, the patient that has been treated for retinal detachment will need to adapt the home to enhance vision and promote safety until the success of the surgery is known, usually several weeks later. The patient must be assessed for the ability to perform ADLs and household chores, keeping in mind the need to maintain independence if possible. Changes to the environment that would decrease the risk for falls must be undertaken in collaboration with the patient and family. Particular attention should be given to removal of scatter rugs, excess furniture, and small items sitting around in close proximity to frequently traveled paths (such as the way to the bathroom). Many patients with visual deficits limit social activities because of anxiety, fear of falling, and inability to maintain the same level of engagement in previous activities. Give the patient realistic expectations of what types of activities may be possible without risking injury.

Documentation

Documentation should include measures implemented to prevent injury in outpatient settings and whether the proposed outcomes were met. Chart the patient's understanding of the need for adaptations at home to promote safety. Include in the chart the patient's ability to participate in ADLs and ambulation. Content of teaching sessions should also be documented.

NURSING DIAGNOSIS 4

 ANXIETY

Related to:

  Vision loss

  Fear of blindness

Defining Characteristics:

  Restlessness and anxiety

  Expresses much concern about lifestyle change that will occur due to a loss of visual acuity

Goal:

  Anxiety is relieved.

Outcome Criteria

✔ The patient verbalizes that anxiety has been decreased.

✔ The patient is able to identify resources within his or her family/community.

✔ The patient asks appropriate questions about retinal detachment.

NOC *Anxiety control*

  Acceptance: Health status

INTERVENTIONS	RATIONALES
Have patient rate anxiety on a numerical scale.	Allows for a more objective measure of anxiety level.
Provide open, honest communication with the patient/family.	Fear of the unknown contributes to anxiety; the patient needs to know what to expect and have a realistic view of expectations and outcomes.
Teach the patient about the disease, therapeutic interventions, prevention of complications, adaptations in lifestyle, and success rates of interventions (90 percent with surgery).	The patient can focus on current therapeutic interventions and ways to adapt, and will understand importance of interventions to prevent further complications.
Encourage the patient to verbalize concerns about health status and the impact visual deficits will have on lifestyle.	Verbalizing concerns and getting accurate information may decrease anxiety and can help patient deal with health issues.
Assess for satisfactory coping mechanisms.	The patient and family may need coping mechanisms to deal with changes that a loss of vision can create; identifying them before they are needed enhances the ability to use them successfully.

NIC   *Anxiety reduction*
        Emotional support

Evaluation

Assess the patient for the degree that anxiety has been controlled or reduced. The patient should verbalize feelings regarding the alteration in vision and indicate whether the interventions or coping mechanisms have been successful. The health care provider should ascertain whether the patient has a clear understanding of retinal detachment and its effect on vision.

Community/Home Care

Retinal detachment is an acute condition that is most often resolved when treated surgically. However, because the recovery period requires the use of eye patches and limitations on activities using the eyes, the patient will still need to learn how to control anxiety. The patient must be equipped with knowledge to deal with daily nuances of decreased vision that will occur in the home. The patient who learns how to make adaptations and is willing to implement those changes will be more likely to

achieve a positive attitude towards visual loss. If visual impairment is not corrected, and blindness or other permanent visual impairments occur, support groups may prove beneficial for the patient and family through information sharing.

Documentation

Document the degree of anxiety experienced by the patient based on the numerical rating scale or the patient's own statements. Chart any observable indications of anxiety such as restlessness or physiological signs such as tachycardia or diaphoresis. Include any verbalization of concern, fear, and anxiety about visual deficits in the patient record, as well as any therapeutic interventions implemented. Include subsequent assessments made to determine the effectiveness of the therapeutic interventions and the patient's own coping strategies.

NURSING DIAGNOSIS 5

 DEFICIENT KNOWLEDGE

Related to:

No previous history of the disease/new onset of disease

Lack of information about retinal detachment and its treatment

Patient/family difficulty coping

Defining Characteristics:

Ask no questions

Has many questions/concerns

Shows an interest in learning about retinal detachment

Goal:

The patient verbalizes an understanding of retinal detachment and its treatment.

Outcome Criteria

✔ The patient verbalizes a desire to learn necessary information.

✔ The patient verbalizes a willingness to keep appointments and follow prescribed regimen.

✔ The patient demonstrates knowledge of disease (detached retina).

✔ The patient demonstrates knowledge of prescribed medications.

✔ The patient demonstrates correct method for instillation of eye drops.

NOC *Knowledge: Disease process*
Knowledge: Treatment regimen
Knowledge: Treatment procedure
Compliance behavior

INTERVENTIONS	RATIONALES
Assess readiness of patient to learn (motivation, cognitive level, and physiological status).	The patient must be motivated to learn, have the capability to learn the content, and be free of distractions to learning such as pain and noisy environments.
Assess the patient's current knowledge.	The nurse needs to ascertain what the patient already knows and build on this.
Start with the simplest information first.	Patients can understand simple concepts easily and then can build on those to understand concepts that are more complex.
Identify a family member or significant other who will also learn the content and assist the patient with compliance.	This person can reinforce the teaching and assist with implementation if the client becomes incapable of follow-through.
Create a quiet environment conducive to learning.	Environmental noise can prevent the learner from focusing on what is being taught.
Teach the learners about the pathophysiology of detached retina in the initial teaching session, including complications.	The patient must understand what retinal detachment is and how it affects vision before he or she can understand the rationale for treatments.
Explain the suggested procedures to be utilized to correct detached retina.	The patient needs to understand the surgical interventions to be employed; knowledge decreases anxiety.
Teach the learners about prescribed medications (see nursing diagnosis "Disturbed Sensory Perception: Visual"), including action, side effects,	Knowledge of why the medication is needed and how it works will focus the patient's attention on importance of the medication.
dosing schedule, and correct instillation of eye drops.	Identification of side effects will minimize anxiety if these untoward effects should occur.
Teach patient the correct technique for instilling eye drops, including anatomical structures instrumental in proper instillation of medications (orbit, lacrimal duct, conjunctiva sac, tear duct, inner canthus): — Slightly hyperextend head. — Look up at ceiling. — Pull downward against the bony orbit to expose the conjunctiva sac and apply slight pressure to the inner canthus. — Hold medication dispenser approximately $\frac{1}{2}$ to $\frac{3}{4}$ inch above the conjunctival sac and instill. — Close the eye, move around, and apply pressure over lacrimal duct for approximately 1 minute. — If medication lands on eyelid or cheek, repeat steps.	The patient must understand correct techniques for medication administration of eye drops to get the full benefit of the medication. (Minimizes drainage into tear duct.) (Reduces blink reflex.) (Exposes the lower conjunctiva sac; pressure blocks the tear duct to prevent medication from entering and being absorbed systemically.)
Instruct the patient to avoid coughing, sneezing, bending, or lifting.	These activities can increase intraocular pressure that would cause pressure on operative site.
Teach the patient which signs and symptoms to report to a health care provider.	Monitoring for signs and symptoms early can prevent a crisis.
Evaluate the patient's understanding of all content covered by asking questions.	Helps to identify areas that require more teaching and to ensure that the patient has enough information to ensure compliance; if the patient can demonstrate the correct procedure for administering medications, he or she will feel more comfortable using them.
Give the patient written information, especially a written procedure for instilling eye drops.	Provides material for reference later and for review.
Establish that the patient has the resources required to be compliant.	If needed resources such as finances, transportation, and psychosocial support are not available, the patient cannot be compliant.

INTERVENTIONS	RATIONALES
Teach how to prevent injury (see nursing diagnosis "Risk for Injury").	Decrease in visual acuity will persist for several weeks following repair of retinal detachment, and some loss of depth perception may occur with unilateral vision loss, predisposing the patient to injury, especially falls.

NIC *Learning readiness enhancement*
Learning facilitation
Teaching: Psychomotor skill
Teaching: Disease process
Teaching: Prescribed medication

Evaluation

Evaluate the degree to which the patient has achieved the outcome criteria relevant to the teaching sessions. The patient is able to repeat all information for the nurse and asks questions about all recommendations. The patient can identify any medications by name and report the common side effects, as well as the dosing schedule. Patients should demonstrate the ability to give their own eye drops. The patient knows and should be able to inform the nurse when health care assistance should be sought, as in the case of acute symptoms or a deterioration in vision.

Community/Home Care

The patient will need to implement the medical regimen in the home setting. Because the patient is sent home the same day as surgery, teaching is paramount if the patient is to recover without complications. A follow-up telephone call from a health care provider would allow an assessment of the patient's ability to function at home, incorporating all the interventions required for safety and protection of the eye. The patient with visual disturbances will need to know how to prevent injury in the home by constantly monitoring the environment for hazards and making adjustments (see nursing diagnosis "Risk for Injury"). Follow-up care should focus on assessing the return of the patient's normal vision or improvement in vision, ability to perform ADLs with some attention to role performance and prevention of social isolation. Adequate financial resources should be in place for purchase of medications and for follow-up care. Assistance with this should be made through social services prior to discharge from the acute care setting. During follow-up visits with healthcare providers, the patient should be asked to demonstrate correct technique for instillation of eye drops. Realistic assessments of the patient's ability to engage in all previous activities especially those requiring excellent visual acuity (i.e. driving, operating machinery) should be discussed with the family and the patient. The patient should understand what constitutes a need for seeking unscheduled medical attention.

Documentation

Document the specific content taught and the titles of printed materials given to the patient or family. Chart the patient's understanding of the content and the methods used to evaluate learning. The patient's successful demonstration of the proper use of eye drops should be documented. The nurse must clearly indicate areas that need to be reinforced. After the teaching session is complete, the nurse should note whether the patient indicates a willingness to comply with health care recommendations. If the teaching includes a family member or significant other, indicate this in the documentation. In addition, document any referrals made in the patient record.

CHAPTER 10.114

GLAUCOMA

GENERAL INFORMATION

Glaucoma is a disorder of the eye caused by an accumulation of aqueous humor in the anterior chamber of the globe of the eye as more fluid is produced than can drain out, which results in increased intraocular pressure. This causes decreased circulation to the retina, compression of the optic nerve, and eventual blindness. There is an absence of recognizable symptoms until the disease has progressed to its later stages. When they do occur, the most common one is a decrease in visual field. In open-angle glaucoma (known as chronic simple), the angle between the iris and the cornea is normal, but there is an obstruction to the outflow of aqueous humor through the trabecular meshwork and into the Canal of Schlemm (Lemone and Burke, 2004). As its evolution is very slow, the patient may not be aware of its presence, and sight is gradually lost. Late in the disease, common manifestations that the patient may experience include decreased or absence of peripheral vision, a need for frequent eyeglass change, halos around lights, and an inability to adapt to dark environments. This type of glaucoma accounts for 90 percent of all cases of glaucoma. Angle closure glaucoma (known as closed-angle or narrow angle) occurs suddenly due to closure of the anterior chamber angles. This is a medical emergency, as blindness will occur unless immediate therapeutic intervention takes place. Other types of glaucoma include secondary glaucoma due to trauma, tumors, surgery, hemorrhage, or inflammation, and congenital glaucoma seen in neonates and infants. Therapeutic intervention will depend on the etiology. Glaucoma is the third leading cause of blindness in the United States but is the number one cause of blindness among African Americans.

NURSING DIAGNOSIS 1

DISTURBED SENSORY PERCEPTION: VISUAL

Related to:

Optic nerve degeneration

Obstruction of outflow of aqueous humor

Increased intraocular pressure

Defining Characteristics:

Blurred vision

Decreased vision

Decreased peripheral vision

Halos around lights

Goal:

Vision loss is stabilized, and further visual loss is prevented.

Outcome Criteria

✔ The patient will maintain visual acuity at baseline and report an ability to participate in activities of daily living (ADLs).

✔ The patient will report an absence of headaches, pain in eyes, or halos around lights.

NOC *Sensory function: Vision*

Vision compensation behavior

INTERVENTIONS	RATIONALES
Assess for visual acuity: peripheral vision, decreased peripheral vision, pupil dilation, headache, poor night vision, and halos around lights.	Helps to establish a baseline of visual functioning to serve as a basis for assistance to the patient.

INTERVENTIONS	RATIONALES
Monitor results of diagnostic tests (tonometry, tonography, gonioscopy).	Tonometry measures intraocular pressure, reveals an increase between 22 and 32 mm of Hg in patients with glaucoma (normal is 10 to 21 mm), and is used for routine screening; tonography measures the outflow of aqueous humor from the eye; gonioscopy measures the depth of the anterior chamber of the eye and can differentiate between open-angle and closed-angle glaucoma. All tests provide clues to presence of disease and type of glaucoma, and assist in determining treatment.
Instill topical miotics/cholinergics, as ordered.	Used to cause pupillary constriction and iris sphincter contraction that opens the trabecular meshwork, allowing room for aqueous humor to leave the anterior chamber and decreasing intraocular pressure.
For open-angle (chronic) glaucoma: administer beta blockers such as timolol maleate (Timoptic®) and levobunolol (Betagan®), as ordered.	Helps to decrease the production of aqueous humor (if the patient has reactive airway disease or a cardiac condition where bradycardia is evident, use of beta blockers may be contraindicated).
For open-angle (chronic) glaucoma: administer carbonic anhydrase inhibitors, as ordered.	Slows down the rate of aqueous humor production, leading to decreased intraocular pressure.
For closed-angle (acute) glaucoma: administer carbonic anhydrase inhibitors, osmotic diuretics, or glycerin, as ordered.	Slows down the rate of aqueous humor production, leading to decreased intraocular pressure; produces osmotic diuresis and decreases overall body fluid volume (including aqueous humor).
For open-angle glaucoma: administer prostaglandin agonist (such as Xalatan®), as ordered.	This prostaglandin analog increases aqueous humor outflow, thereby decreasing intraocular pressure. This eye preparation has a long duration of action and is administered in the evening.
For all medications, teach patient and family correct technique for administering eye drops, side effects of medications, symptoms	Educating patients about medications enhances compliance and decreases anxiety.

to report, and expected outcomes following administration (see nursing diagnosis "Deficient Knowledge").	
Assess for signs of pain in eye, such as keeping eyelids tightly closed, facial grimace, headache, and severe pain in globe of eye.	Pain in the eye may indicate acute glaucoma and needs to be treated immediately.
For closed-angle (acute) glaucoma: administer narcotic analgesics (morphine sulfate)/sedatives, as ordered, for complaints of severe pain.	The analgesics will help control the pain and decrease intraocular pressure. The sedatives will help to reduce anxiety caused by pain and vision loss.
Teach patient to avoid activities that increase intraocular pressure (see nursing diagnosis "Deficient Knowledge").	The most important complication of medical and surgical therapy is increased intraocular pressure (IOP); patients can prevent further visual field loss if they avoid activities that increase IOP.
Orient the person to the environment, especially if hospitalized (see nursing diagnosis "Risk for Injury").	Peripheral vision is disturbed and the person needs to know where objects are in the environment.
Teach to turn head from side to side to see objects in close proximity.	Peripheral vision is often the first visual disturbance to occur in glaucoma.
Use bright lights, books with large print, and large numbers or letters on household items such as clocks.	Helps to enhance the environment to compensate for diminished vision.
Assist the patient with meals if vision is impaired by helping with menu selection and preparing of foods on tray and by describing position of foods on tray using positions on the clock (for example meat is at 12 o'clock); assure the client that it is okay to get assistance.	The patient may not eat if he or she cannot readily find food.
Prepare patient for surgical intervention (trabeculoplasty) as ordered or according to agency protocol.	Most often, this is the surgery of choice; following laser burning of areas around the trabecular meshwork, scars are formed during healing that cause tension and stretching that create an opening through the trabecula connecting the

(continues)

(continued)

INTERVENTIONS	RATIONALES
	anterior chamber to the conjunctiva; this allows for the drainage of aqueous humor.
Prepare patient for surgical intervention (trabeculectomy) and teach post-operative care.	A fistula is created to drain aqueous humor from anterior chamber of the eye into the conjunctival space where it is absorbed into systemic circulation.
In closed-angle (acute) glaucoma, prepare the patient for iridotomy or iridectomy and teach post-operative care.	In an iridectomy, a segment of the iris is removed to allow space through which aqueous humor can flow; in an iridotomy, several small lacerations are cut in the iris to allow aqueous humor to drain from the posterior chamber into the anterior chamber, out through the trabecular meshwork, and into the canal of Schlemm.

NIC *Eye care*

    Communication enhancement: Visual deficit

    Environmental management

Evaluation

Assess the degree to which outcomes have been achieved. The patient should have no further deterioration in visual ability. There is an absence of pain or headaches, and the patient reports having the ability to be self-sufficient in ADLs.

Community/Home Care

For most patients with glaucoma, treatment is done on an outpatient basis through physician's offices, and if surgery is required, this is generally performed as a same-day procedure. The patient treated medically should be encouraged to keep follow-up appointments as scheduled to ensure early detection and treatment of any further visual problems. Patients treated surgically need education on recommended post-operative activities and restrictions. Evaluations should be made to determine what assistance the patient may need in the home environment to compensate for altered visual ability. The patient and/or family will need to clear walking paths and give some attention to items that may be off to the side of the

normal path that the patient may not see (see nursing diagnosis "Risk for Injury"). It is crucial that the patient understand the need for proper instillation of eye drops in order to prevent increased intraocular pressure that further intensifies glaucoma. A health care provider should be sure that the patient is willing and able to undertake this task. Prior to leaving the doctor's office or outpatient clinic, the patient or significant other/family member should be required to demonstrate the proper way to instill eye drops. Evaluate whether the patient has the resources to purchase medications and receive follow-up care, including the availability of transportation for appointments.

Documentation

Chart all assessments related to the status of the patient's vision. Be specific about what the patient reports relevant to his or her vision. Include the patient's responses to interventions and understanding of all procedures. Any teaching should be documented with a clear indication of the patient's understanding of information. All referrals are included in the patient record.

NURSING DIAGNOSIS 2

RISK FOR INJURY

Related to:

    Decreased peripheral vision

    Loss of vision

    Inability to see to the side

    Inability to see items in environment clearly

Defining Characteristics:

    None

Goal:

    The patient will be safe.

Outcome Criteria

✔ The patient will participate in ADLs without injury.

✔ The patient will perform usual household activities or chores without injury.

✔ The patient will verbalize an understanding of the need to adapt the home environment to prevent injury.

NOC *Safe home environment*
Fall prevention behavior

INTERVENTIONS	RATIONALES
Assess the environment for hazards that could predispose the patient to falls.	Common items often place the patient at risk for injury when vision is impaired
Orient the patient to the environment, especially in the hospital setting, and do not rearrange items without telling the patient.	Patients will feel more comfortable if they are familiar with the environment; changes may create hazards, as the patient will not know where items are.
Instruct the patient to turn head from side to side before moving or when ambulating.	The patient should scan the entire perimeter and identify obstacles to prevent falls.
Encourage the use of wall, rails, or other stable items when ambulating.	Helps to provide support and assistance with ambulation to prevent imbalance or falls.
Assist with ambulation as needed by walking ahead of patient and having him or her hold your arm or elbow, and warn the patient of any hazards/obstacles in his or her path.	Helps to guide the patient and give him or her a sense of safety and maintain mobility.
Following surgery, remain with patient for first ambulation.	Patients generally feel uncomfortable about walking, and visual acuity is not known immediately post-operatively.
Have the patient avoid picking up heavy objects, avoid bending and lifting, and avoid straining for bowel movements.	These activities increase intraocular pressure.
Place the call light and other frequently used items within easy reach for the person at home or in the hospital.	Makes the environment more familiar and allows for independence.
In the home, remove clutter such as scatter rugs or extra chairs from rooms and halls, and limit the use of electrical extension cords in open spaces.	Items in open spaces create obstacles that the patient may not be able to see; scatter rugs and other small pieces of furniture are frequently the cause of falls in the person with limited vision.
Use adequate lighting in the home or hospital, avoiding extremely bright lights.	Bright direct light often causes glare, creating more of a hazard for falls.

NIC *Environmental management:*
Safety
Fall prevention
Surveillance: Safety

Evaluation

The proposed outcomes have been met as demonstrated by the fact that the patient sustains no injury. The patient is able to verbalize the need for adaptations to be made in the environment to ensure safety. In addition, the patient reports how to make changes in ambulation and daily living to prevent injury, and is willing to comply.

Community/Home Care

In the home setting, the patient with glaucoma, especially those being managed medically, will need to adapt the home to enhance vision and promote safety. The patient must be assessed for the ability to perform ADLs and household chores, keeping in mind the need to maintain independence if possible. Changes to the environment that would decrease the risk for falls must be undertaken in collaboration with the patient and family. Particular attention should be given to removal of scatter rugs, excess furniture, and small items in close proximity to frequently traveled paths (such as the way to the bathroom). Many patients with visual deficits limit social activities because of anxiety, fear of falling, and inability to maintain the same level of engagement in previous activities. Give the patient realistic expectations of what types of activities may be possible without risking injury.

Documentation

Documentation should include measures implemented to prevent injury in outpatient settings and whether the proposed outcomes were met. Chart the patient's understanding of the need for adaptations at home to promote safety. Include in the chart the patient's ability to participate in ADLs and ambulation. Document content of teaching sessions.

NURSING DIAGNOSIS 3

 ANXIETY

Related to:

Vision loss
Fear of blindness

Defining Characteristics:

> Restlessness
>
> Expresses much concern about lifestyle change that will occur due to a loss of visual acuity

Goal:

> Anxiety is relieved.

Outcome Criteria

✔ The patient verbalizes that anxiety has been decreased.

✔ The patient is able to identify resources within family/community.

✔ The patient asks appropriate questions about glaucoma.

NOC　*Anxiety control*
　　Acceptance: Health status

INTERVENTIONS	RATIONALES
Have patient rate anxiety on a numerical scale.	Allows for a more objective measure of anxiety level.
Encourage the patient to verbalize concerns about health status and the impact visual deficits will have on lifestyle.	Verbalizing concerns can help patient deal with issues, avoid negative feelings, and allow the health care provider to introduce alternative activities and methods of doing things.
Provide open, honest communication with the patient/family.	Fear of the unknown creates anxiety; the patient needs to know what to expect and have a realistic view of expectations and outcomes.
Teach the patient about the disease, therapeutic interventions, prevention of complications, and adaptations in lifestyle that are required.	The patient needs to understand what to expect from the disease, which will allow him or her to better understand the rationale for needed therapeutic interventions and adaptations to ensure safety and maintenance of optimal visual functioning.
Provide information to the family and patient regarding available support groups.	These groups often can provide emotional support and share real experiences on how to adapt to visual changes.
Assess for satisfactory coping mechanisms.	The patient and family may need coping mechanisms to deal with changes that a loss of vision can create; identifying them before they are needed enhances the ability to use them successfully.

NIC　*Anxiety reduction*
　　Emotional support

Evaluation

Assess the patient for the degree that anxiety has been controlled or reduced. The patient should verbalize feelings about the alteration in vision and indicate whether the interventions or coping mechanisms have been successful. The health care provider should ascertain whether the patient has a clear understanding of glaucoma and its effect on vision.

Community/Home Care

Because glaucoma is a chronic disorder, the patient will need to learn how to control anxiety. The patient must be equipped with knowledge to deal with daily nuances that will occur in the home with decreased vision. The patient who learns how to make adaptations and is willing to implement those changes will be more likely to achieve a positive attitude towards visual loss. Support groups for persons with visual loss may prove beneficial for the patient and family through information sharing. In addition, simple strategies to reduce anxiety and feelings of frustration include meditation, reading (large print books), listening to music, and any other activity that has had a calming effect on the patient in the past.

Documentation

Document the degree of anxiety experienced by the patient based on the numerical rating scale or in the patient's own words. Chart any observable or physiological signs of anxiety such as restlessness, tachycardia, or diaphoresis. Any verbalization of concern, fear, and anxiety regarding visual deficits should be included in the patient record, as well as any therapeutic interventions implemented. Include subsequent assessments made to determine the effectiveness of the therapeutic interventions and the patient's own coping strategies.

NURSING DIAGNOSIS 4

 ## DEFICIENT KNOWLEDGE

Related to:

> No previous history of the disease/new onset of disease

Lack of information about the disease and its treatment

Patient/family difficulty coping

Defining Characteristics:

Asks no questions

Has many questions/concerns

Shows an interest in learning about glaucoma

Goal:

The patient verbalizes an understanding of glaucoma and its treatment.

Outcome Criteria

✔ The patient verbalizes a desire to learn necessary information.

✔ The patient verbalizes a willingness to keep appointments and follow prescribed regimen.

✔ The patient verbalizes an understanding of glaucoma.

✔ The patient demonstrates knowledge of prescribed medications.

✔ The patient demonstrates correct method for instillation of eye drops.

NOC *Knowledge: Disease process*
Knowledge: Treatment regimen
Knowledge: Treatment procedure
Compliance behavior

INTERVENTIONS	RATIONALES
Assess readiness of patient to learn (motivation, cognitive level, and physiological status).	The patient must be motivated to learn, have the capability to learn the content, and be free of distractions from learning such as pain, anxiety, or a noisy environment.
Assess the patient's current knowledge.	The nurse needs to ascertain what the patient already knows and build on this.
Start with the simplest information first.	Patients can understand simple concepts easily and then can build on those to understand concepts that are more complex.
Identify a family member or significant other who will also learn the content and assist the patient with compliance.	This person can reinforce the teaching and assist with implementation if the patient becomes incapable of follow-through.
Create a quiet environment conducive to learning.	Environmental noise can prevent the learner from focusing on what is being taught.
Teach the learners about the pathophysiology of glaucoma in the initial teaching session, including complications.	The patient must understand what the disease is and how it affects vision before understanding the rationale for treatments.
Teach the learners about prescribed medications (see nursing diagnosis "Disturbed Sensory Perception: Visual"), including action, side effects, dosing schedule, and correct instillation of eye drops.	Knowledge of why the medication is needed and how it works will focus the importance of the medication. Identification of side effects will minimize anxiety if these untoward effects should occur. The patient needs to be clear about when and how to take medications to ensure therapeutic effect.
Teach the patient and family the correct technique for instilling eye drops, including anatomical structures instrumental in proper instillation of medications (orbit, lacrimal duct, conjunctiva sac, tear duct, inner canthus):	The patient must understand correct techniques for medication administration of eye drops to get the full benefit of the medication.
— Slightly hyperextend head.	(Minimizes drainage into tear duct.)
— Look up at ceiling.	(Reduces blink reflex.)
— Pull downward against the bony orbit to expose the conjunctiva sac and apply slight pressure to the inner canthus.	(Exposes the lower conjunctiva sac; pressure blocks the tear duct to prevent medication from entering and being absorbed systemically.)
— Hold medication dispenser approximately ½ to ¾ inch above the conjunctival sac and instill.	
— Close the eye, move the eye around and apply pressure over lacrimal duct for approximately 1 minute.	
— If medication lands on eyelid or cheek, repeat steps.	
Teach the patient to notify the physician or another health care provider if slow pulse, tiredness, or shortness of breath occurs.	These are symptoms of systemic effects of medications and indicate a need for further teaching.
Instruct patient to avoid bending, lifting, or taking steroids.	These activities can increase intraocular pressure.
Teach the patient to consult a physician before using over-the-counter cough preparations.	Many of these preparations block the effect of miotics.

(continues)

(continued)

INTERVENTIONS	RATIONALES
Teach the patient which signs and symptoms to report to a health care provider.	Monitoring for signs and symptoms early can prevent a crisis. It is important for patients to know when to seek health care assistance to avoid complications.
Evaluate the patient's understanding of all content covered by asking questions, and have patient demonstrate use of eye drops.	Helps to identify areas that require more teaching and to ensure that the patient has enough information to ensure compliance; if the patient can demonstrate the correct procedure for administering medications, he or she will feel more comfortable using them when needed, and anxiety should be decreased.
Give the patient written information.	Provides reference at a later time, and for review.
Establish that the patient has the resources required to be compliant.	If needed resources such as finances, transportation, and psychosocial support are not available, the patient cannot be compliant.
Teach how to prevent injury due to visual deficit (see nursing diagnosis "Risk for Injury").	Decrease in peripheral vision and/or loss of depth perception that occur with unilateral vision loss predispose the patient to injury, especially falls.

NIC   *Learning readiness enhancement*
Learning facilitation
Teaching: Psychomotor skill
Teaching: Disease process
Teaching: Prescribed medication

Evaluation

Evaluate the degree to which the patient has achieved the outcome criteria relevant to the teaching sessions. The patient is able to repeat all information related to the pathophysiology of glaucoma for the nurse and asks questions about the prescribed regimen. The patient can identify all medications by name and report the common side effects, as well as the dosing schedule. Glaucoma patients should demonstrate the ability to give their own eye drops. The patient knows when health care assistance should be sought for acute symptoms or continued deterioration of vision.

Community/Home Care

The patient will need to implement the medical regimen in the home setting. The success of treatment for glaucoma depends upon the degree to which the patient has received adequate teaching and has subsequently understood and internalized it. The patient with glaucoma will need to know how to prevent injury in the home by constantly monitoring the environment for hazards and making adjustments. Follow-up care should focus on assessing the patient's ability to perform ADLs with some attention to role performance and prevention of social isolation. Adequate financial resources should be in place for purchase of medications and for follow-up care. Assistance with this should be made through social services. During follow-up visits with health care providers, the patient should be asked to demonstrate correct technique for instillation of eye drops. Realistic assessments of the patient's ability to engage in all previous activities, especially those requiring excellent visual acuity (i.e. driving, operating machinery), should be discussed with family and patient. The patient should understand what constitutes a need for seeking unscheduled medical attention.

Documentation

Document the specific content taught and the titles of printed materials given to patient or family. Chart the patient's understanding of the content and the methods used to evaluate learning. The patient's successful demonstration of the proper use of eye drops should be documented. The nurse must clearly indicate areas that need to be reinforced. After the teaching session is complete, the nurse should note whether the patient indicates a willingness to comply with health care recommendations. If the teaching included a significant other or family member, indicate this in the documentation. In addition, if referrals are made, these should be documented in the patient record.

UNIT 11

REPRODUCTIVE SYSTEM

CHAPTER 11.115

BENIGN PROSTATIC HYPERTROPHY/ HYPERPLASIA (BPH)

GENERAL INFORMATION

Benign prostatic hypertrophy or hyperplasia (BPH) is a non-malignant enlargement of the prostate gland that occurs when the number of normal cells increases (hypertrophy) and the consistency of the prostatic tissue becomes nodular (hyperplasia). These changes are most often noted in the area of the prostate that surrounds the urethra. The changes are related to increased estrogen, increased androgen, and decreased free testosterone. The androgen that stimulates prostatic growth is dihydrotestosterone (DHT), the effects of which are enhanced by estrogen. During aging, the prostate gland becomes more sensitive to the effects of DHT, and with increasing levels of estrogen during aging, the effect of DHT is more pronounced, causing the enlargement and hyperplasia. Clinical manifestations include post-void dribbling, decreased force of the urinary stream, urinary frequency, inability to empty the bladder completely, and difficulty initiating the urinary stream. The most common complication is urinary tract/urethral obstruction due to the enlargement of the prostate putting pressure on the urethra, causing urinary retention. It usually occurs in men over age 50, and has a higher incidence in African American men and a lower incidence in native Japanese men.

NURSING DIAGNOSIS 1

URINARY RETENTION

Related to:

Enlarged prostate causing mechanical obstruction

Chronic bladder distention that leads to dystonic bladder

Defining Characteristics:

Urinary dribbling

Urinary incontinence

Difficulty starting urination

Stop-and-start urination

Incomplete bladder emptying

Distended bladder

Goal:

The patient is able to void without difficulty.

Outcome Criteria

✔ The patient will have no bladder distention/ urinary retention.

✔ The patient will implement strategies to reduce symptoms of impaired urinary elimination.

✔ The patient will void sufficient amounts with each voiding (200 cc).

NOC *Urinary elimination*
Symptom control

INTERVENTIONS	RATIONALES
Assess the patient for ability to void; firm, full bladder on palpation; history of urinary tract infections; urinating in dribbles, difficulty in starting to void, urinary frequency; urinary urgency, and nocturia. Utilize the American Urological Association (AUA) Symptom Score Tool to assess severity of symptoms.	These are symptoms of BPH and can be used to establish a baseline. They are caused by pressure on the bladder and around the urethra; the AUA Symptom Score Tool is used to determine how severe the symptoms are and provides subjective data.
Monitor results of diagnostic tests: prostate specific antigen (PSA) levels, blood urea nitrogen (BUN),	PSA is divided into bound and free levels. A high percentage of free PSA tends to imply BPH;

INTERVENTIONS	RATIONALES
creatinine, urinalysis, urine culture and sensitivity, complete blood count (CBC), ultrasound (transrectal), cystogram/ cystourethroscopy, intravenous pyelogram (IVP), and cystometry.	tests of renal function (BUN, creatinine) are done to determine if there is any alteration in kidney function due to obstruction or retention; CBC elevations, urine culture and sensitivity, as well as urinalysis are used to monitor for the presence of urinary tract infection which could occur due to retention; transrectal ultrasound is capable of determining the size of the prostate and to differentiate BPH from prostate cancer; cystourethroscopy is used to decide if there is outflow obstruction and to note any alterations in the bladder; IVP can be used to determine any effect on urinary structures, particularly to visualize distended ureters; cystometry is used to evaluate all aspects of bladder function and can diagnose prostatic obstruction.
Perform a sexuality assessment: monitor for concerns about sexual relations, worry about libido if disease progresses, concern about ability to have sex as disease progresses, concern about urinary incontinence during sex.	Patients frequently have some concerns about sexual function, especially following surgical interventions.
Instruct patient to attempt to void every 2–3 hours and have patient double void: void, sit on toilet for 3 to 5 minutes, and then void again.	This will assist to empty the bladder, avoiding urinary retention and bladder distention.
Teach patient to palpate bladder to check for distention.	The patient can detect bladder distention and intervene prior to bladder fully distending and becoming painful, which may result in incontinence and dribbling.
Monitor post-void residual.	Helps to determine the degree of retention with each voiding.
Administer antispasmodics (PO, PR), as ordered.	Helps to decrease bladder spasms, relax musculature.
Administer androgen inhibitor (PO): Finasteride (Proscar®), as ordered.	Proscar is a specific inhibitor of the steroid 5 Alpha-reductase, an enzyme that enhances the conversion of testosterone into

	androgen (DHT) leading to a reduction in the size of the prostate gland and improvement in urine flow.
Administer alpha adrenergic receptor blockers (such as Hytrin®) as ordered.	These drugs promote smooth muscle relaxation in the prostate gland where the receptors are abundant. Because of relaxation, urinary outflow improves, reducing retention. These agents are used in patients without serious symptoms.
Implement dietary strategies to control urinary retention and incontinence: avoid alcohol, give or increase zinc and vitamin E in diet, avoid over-the-counter decongestants or other anti-cholinergic or alpha agonist medications.	Alcohol exacerbates retention, Zinc and Vitamin E help reduce nocturnal urinary symptoms; over the counter decongestants increase smooth muscle tone of the prostate that increases the risk for urinary retention.
Limit intake of fluids after 6 pm and avoid consuming large amounts of fluid at one time.	Fluid intake after 6 pm increases the likelihood of nocturia; consuming large volumes of fluid at one time is more likely to cause retention.
Teach patient/family how to insert straight catheter to empty bladder of urine.	If urinary retention is persistent, the patient may require frequent catheterization. Patient/family will retain independence if they can learn how to safely and effectively do this.
Teach the patient the signs and symptoms of urinary tract infection: fever, cloudy urine, foul-smelling urine, hematuria, (see nursing diagnosis "Risk for infection").	Urinary tract infections can occur due to retention of the urine in the bladder and subsequent back-up or reflux into the ureters and kidney.
Teach patient and family about disease process and possible options for treatment of BPH: transurethral resection, open prostatectomy, medications.	Knowledge of the disease and its treatment allows the patient to make informed decisions.
Prepare for possible surgical or other invasive procedures according to orders or agency protocol.	Dependent upon the state of the disease and patient's symptoms, prostatectomy may be indicated (see nursing diagnosis "Deficient Knowledge ").

NIC   *Urinary elimination*
    management
Urinary retention care

Evaluation

Determine the degree to which the outcomes have been achieved. The patient should report an improvement in symptoms of impaired urinary elimination. Urinary output is sufficient and bladder distention is absent. The patient will verbalize an understanding of all strategies needed to improve urine output.

Community/Home Care

At home, the patient will need to implement strategies to improve urinary output. A health care provider will need to teach the patient and significant other how to handle symptoms that could be annoying. It is crucial that the patient understands the concepts of urinary retention and bladder distention and be able to relieve this if possible. Encourage the patient to keep a record of intake and to make a conscious effort to refrain from drinking after 6 p.m. to reduce nocturia. Both alcohol and over-the-counter cough preparations can cause urinary retention, and the nurse's instructions to the patient to avoid these items must be explicit. The patient at home needs to make a concerted effort to empty the bladder at regular intervals to avoid distention. Intake of fluids throughout the day is needed to maintain bladder tone, prevent bladder hypertrophy, and prevent urinary stasis. Keeping a diary that records intake and number of bathroom trips may be helpful for follow-up visits with the health care provider. This diary can also serve as a place to record any other urinary symptoms that the patient may experience. The patient should know how to perform a self-catheterization to relieve distention and how to measure the output. It is crucial that the patient understand the symptoms of urinary obstruction so that if they should occur, immediate medical attention can be sought in order to avoid effects to the kidney parenchyma. Follow-up care is needed to assess the progression of the disease and to determine what interventions might be needed.

Documentation

Chart an assessment of the urinary system, including the AUA symptom score and any current complaints of altered urinary function. Intake and output should be documented with attention to amount voided with each voiding. If the patient has been catheterized for residual, document this in the patient notes, including amount obtained. Always include in the documentation the interventions implemented and the patient's responses. If teaching has been done, document this along with the patient's understanding.

NURSING DIAGNOSIS 2

RISK FOR INFECTION

Related to:

> Surgical interventions
> Enhanced opportunity for invasion by organisms
> Urinary retention

Defining Characteristics:

> None

Goal:

> The patient does not acquire an infection.

Outcome Criteria

✔ The patient will have a negative urine culture.
✔ The patient will report no frequency, dysuria, hematuria, or flank tenderness.
✔ The patient's urine will be clear with no odor.
✔ Patient will be afebrile and have no chills.

NOC *Infection severity*
     Knowledge: Infection control

INTERVENTIONS	RATIONALES
Assess the patient for signs and symptoms of urinary infection: costovertebral angle tenderness, flank tenderness on palpation, hematuria, frequency, urgency, nocturia, and dysuria.	These are all symptoms of urinary tract infection (UTI) and give clues to severity of the infection; costovertebral angle tenderness and flank tenderness are symptoms of pyelonephritis, indicating invasion of the renal tissue. Many of the symptoms that the patient experiences with BPH are also indicators of urinary tract infection; knowing what symptoms the patient normally has can help distinguish the two. If the patient has had surgery, some hematuria may be present in the early post-operative period.

INTERVENTIONS	RATIONALES
Obtain urine specimen for routine urinalysis and culture and sensitivity, and send to lab immediately. Monitor results for positive culture of organisms.	Provides a definitive diagnosis and identifies the causative organism that is needed for appropriate antibiotic therapy. A colony count of 10^3 organisms per milliliter of urine constitutes a positive culture. Immediate transport to the lab is needed, for if urine is left at room temperature, bacterial count will double every 30 to 40 minutes; routine urinalysis will reveal the presence of casts, white blood cells (WBCs), and bacteria.
Observe urine, noting amount, color, and presence of any blood or odor.	Infected urine is usually cloudy and foul-smelling, and may contain small amounts of blood due to irritation; amounts at each voiding may be small; monitor for improvement in response to treatment.
Monitor results of other diagnostic tests: WBC, blood cultures, serum creatinine, BUN, IVP.	These tests give indications of any impaired renal function; blood cultures assist in determining if bacteremia is present; IVP can demonstrate obstructed urine flow.
Administer antibiotics specific to culture and sensitivity, as ordered. Often the first choice antibiotic is trimethoprim-sulfamethoxazole (Bactrim).	Helps to decrease bacteria through bacteriocidal or bacteriostatic action.
Teach patient to take medications until the prescribed regimen is complete (see nursing diagnosis "Deficient Knowledge").	Patients often discontinue taking medications when symptoms are relieved, increasing the risk of inadequate resolution of the infection.
Increase fluids to at least 3 to 4 liters per day by mouth if not contraindicated due to cardiac disease.	Helps to dilute urine and prevent irritation of the bladder.
Avoid liquids containing caffeine; include liquids such as cranberry or prune juice.	Caffeine is a bladder irritant and will aggravate symptoms; cranberry and prune juice will acidify urine, and bacteria generally do not flourish in acidic urine.
Have the patient void every 2 hours.	Helps to prevent stasis of urine and enhance emptying of bladder.
If an indwelling catheter is present, maintain aseptic technique when handling and perform perineal care every shift.	The indwelling catheter is a frequent source of infection, and maintaining aseptic technique in its care decreases the risk for infection.
Take temperature every 4 hours and administer antipyretics, as ordered.	Helps to monitor for elevations that may occur with UTI; give antipyretics to reduce fever and monitor response.
Implement strategies to address impaired urinary elimination (see nursing diagnosis "Urinary Retention").	Strategies to reduce bladder distention/retention can help prevent infection by preventing backflow of urine to ureters and decreasing the possibility of bacteria growth in stagnant urine in the bladder.

NIC   ***Urinary elimination management***
Infection control
Surveillance
Infection protection

Evaluation

Assess the patient's status overall with regard to the urinary system. Evaluate the degree to which the outcome criteria have been met. The patient should have no evidence of UTI, such as pain, frequency, urgency, fever, or chills. Laboratory results indicate decreased WBCs and a negative urine culture.

Community/Home Care

The patient with BPH remains at high risk for UTIs and will need to implement measures consistently to decrease that risk by preventing urinary retention (see nursing diagnosis "Urinary Retention"). Fluid intake is a key aspect of in-home self-care for the patient at risk for infection, and the role of fluids in maintaining an aseptic environment in the urinary system is stressed. The patient should drink fluids in adequate amounts throughout the day, but stop fluid intake by 6 p.m. if nocturia is a problem. Because most lay people cannot determine how much fluid they have consumed, this skill will need to be taught to the patient using common containers that the patient uses at home, such as a favorite drinking glass or cup. Making a planned schedule for intake and then keeping a record of intake will help the patient be more mindful of drinking at regular schedules. If infection does develop, health care providers may encounter problems regarding compliance with the antibiotic regimen. Because the risk for upper UTI is great for the patient with urinary retention, prevention of retention is important. In addition to drinking at scheduled intervals, the patient at risk for retention should void at least every 2 hours. If the patient has been treated surgically for BPH and has been discharged home with an indwelling catheter, the risk for infection is even greater. An in-home nurse should be sure that the patient or a family member knows how to care for the catheter properly, measures needed to prevent UTIs, and signs and symptoms of infection (see nursing diagnosis "Deficient Knowledge"). A follow-up visit with a health care provider should be recommended to ensure that no infection has occurred. Be sure that the patient has financial means to purchase antibiotics and return to the health care provider for follow-up.

Documentation

Chart the results of all assessments. Urinary elimination patterns should be documented, including any complaints of urgency, frequency, dysuria, and feelings of fullness or burning on urination. Also chart whether an indwelling urinary catheter is present, and give a description of the urine, noting color, amount, and whether there is hematuria. Patient complaints of pain are documented with follow-up assessment following interventions. Document all interventions that have been implemented to address the problem of risk for urinary infection, and the patient's response to treatment. Vital signs, especially temperature, are documented in accordance with agency standards. If specimens are sent to the laboratory, note this in the patient's record.

NURSING DIAGNOSIS 3

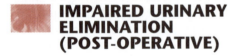

IMPAIRED URINARY ELIMINATION (POST-OPERATIVE)

Related to:

Surgical intervention for BPH

Defining Characteristics:

Incontinence

Bladder distention

Blood in urine

Bladder spasms

Presence of indwelling urinary catheter

Goal:

Urine output will be adequate.

Outcome Criteria

✔ Urine output will be ≥ 50 cc per hour postoperatively and return to normal color after 48 hours.

✔ There will be no bladder distention.

✔ The patient will have no symptoms of fluid overload due to bladder irrigation.

NOC   *Urinary elimination*
         Fluid balance

INTERVENTIONS	RATIONALES
Post-operatively assess for decreased urinary output, hemorrhage (decreased hemoglobin [Hgb] and hematocrit [Hct], tachycardia, hypotension), blood clots, and bladder spasms.	Bleeding and passage of clots are more common during the first 24 hours, and the patient should be assessed frequently for early identification; clots can obstruct the drainage device; bladder spasms need to be treated to prevent pain and decreased output.
Following transurethral resection of the prostate; maintain continuous bladder irrigation (CBI) with normal saline to keep the output light pink or very pale yellow (diluted urine); maintain patency of indwelling three-way catheter, noting the presence of any clots or frank bleeding; if present, increase irrigant in accordance with agency protocol or as ordered.	Following surgical interventions for BPH, clots may develop and cause a blockage to the outflow of urine; this is more likely during the first 24 to 48 hours. CBI maintains patency and flushes the bladder of any clots.
Accurately monitor intake and output every 1 to 2 hours, especially the amount of irrigant.	Careful calculation is required to determine that irrigant is not excessive and actual urine output is sufficient.
Teach patient to avoid trying to void around catheter.	The presence of a large ballooned catheter creates a sensation of pressure and the need to void, but if the patient tries to void around the catheter, bladder spasms will increase.

INTERVENTIONS	RATIONALES
Give patient medications for pain or bladder spasms, as ordered.	Spasms can increase pain, and the patient's comfort should be a priority.
Assess patient for signs of water intoxication (TURP syndrome) if on CBI: confusion, restlessness, and decreased serum sodium levels. If present, slow irrigant and notify physician.	These occur as the irrigant is absorbed; early identification allows for initiation of treatment before serious neurological or cardiovascular complications occur.
For the patient without CBI, irrigate catheter as ordered or according to agency protocol.	Helps to maintain patency of catheter by preventing obstruction from sediment or clots.
Encourage intake of 2 to 3 liters of fluid daily.	Helps to dilute urine and prevent bacteria growth.
Implement strategies to prevent infection (see nursing diagnosis "Risk for Infection").	Use of instrumentation such as indwelling catheters predisposes the patient to infection, and urinary retention prior to surgery may also predispose the patient to infection.
Remove catheter when ordered, and monitor output, color, and consistency of urine. Assess the patient for retention as well as dribbling following removal. Explain to the patient that he or she may perceive a sensation to void, and with initial voiding, may experience small amounts of blood in the urine, some dribbling, and some discomfort.	These symptoms occur as the bladder adapts to removal of the large ballooned catheter and attempts to recapture normal tone. The blood is most likely due to irritation, not frank bleeding.
Teach patient Kegel exercises: voluntary tightening and relaxing of the perineal and gluteal muscles that support the bladder and urethra.	Helps restore tone and minimize incontinence.

NIC *Pelvic muscle exercise*
Bladder irrigation
Fluid monitoring
Urinary elimination management

Evaluation

Examine the extent to which the patient has achieved the outcome criteria. Urine output should be > 50 cc per hour, have no frank bleeding or clots, and gradually return to a normal color. The patient should have no signs or symptoms of water intoxication and report an absence of bladder spasms. In addition, the patient should have no indications of hemorrhage.

Community/Home Care

The patient who has had surgery for BPH will need follow-up care to ensure that urinary output and bladder function return to normal. For some patients, discharge home is accomplished with the indwelling catheter still in place, and for this group the patient and a family member must be taught how to care for it, including emptying, proper positioning, measuring output, and appropriate perineal care. A return demonstration of the techniques for emptying, attaching leg bags, and care of ports should be required. If the patient goes home without a catheter, he will need to monitor output to be sure that retention is not an issue. Adequate fluid intake (2000 to 3000 ml/day) is necessary to prevent infection and retention, and to help restore bladder tone. The patient can keep fluids close at hand and sip on them throughout the day. Of concern for the patient following TURP and prostatectomy is the possibility of incontinence and altered sexual function. During follow-up visits, the health care provider should question the patient regarding these two areas and institute necessary measures to address them. The patient needs to know which signs and symptoms necessitate immediate return to the health care provider (see nursing diagnosis "Deficient Knowledge").

Documentation

Document the findings from a thorough assessment regarding the urinary system. Include the presence of catheters and a description of the output from the drainage device. Record the amount of urine and the amount of irrigant on the appropriate intake and output records according to agency protocol. The patient's subjective reports of any type are also charted. If the patient has pain or spasms, document specific complaints, interventions implemented to address them, and their effectiveness.

NURSING DIAGNOSIS 4

 DEFICIENT KNOWLEDGE

Related to:

No previous history of the disease/new onset of disease

Lack of information about the disease and its treatment

Misinformation

Concern about sexuality

Defining Characteristics:

Asks no questions

Has many questions

First experience with BPH

Outcome Criteria

✔ The patient and family members/significant other verbalize a desire to learn necessary information.

✔ The patient verbalizes an understanding of BPH treatment options (surgery, medications), including untoward effects of treatment and possible complications such as altered sexual function and urinary incontinence.

✔ The patient verbalizes an understanding of follow-up care required and expresses a willingness to comply.

NOC *Knowledge: Disease process*
Knowledge: Treatment regimen
Compliance behavior

INTERVENTIONS	RATIONALES
Assess the patient's current knowledge as well as his ability to learn and readiness to learn.	The nurse needs to ascertain what the patient already knows and build on this, if the patient is not capable of learning or is not ready to learn, teaching will not be effective due to disinterest or inability to understand. The patient may not be ready to learn if he has not accepted the diagnosis.
Start with the simplest information and move to more complex information.	Patients can understand simple concepts easily and then can build on those to understand concepts that are more complex.
Collaborate with physician to teach patient and significant others: — Disease process of BPH and possible treatments (surgery, medications) — Signs and symptoms that would indicate a need to seek health care (being unable to urinate, chills, and fever)	Knowledge of disease, treatments required, and prevention of complications empowers the patient to take control and be compliant; being unable to urinate indicates obstruction; fever and chills may indicate infection.
— Strategies to prevent infections (urinary and wound) as well as signs and symptoms of urinary tract infection and wound infection (see nursing diagnosis "Risk for Infection") — Complications following treatment: alterations in sexual function and incontinence, and ways to address them	
Teach the patient and family about medications used to treat BPH: — Specific agents used for treatment (such as Proscar, Hytrin) — Method of action — Side effects (Proscar: impotence, decreased libido; Hytrin: weakness, headache, dizziness, impotence) — Dosing schedule	Knowledge about medications and their effects will assist with compliance, and the patient can make informed decisions about therapy options. Knowing what to expect in terms of sexuality can help the patient cope or minimize frustrations with alterations in sexuality.
For patients who had prostatectomies, teach — Care of indwelling catheter: prevention of infection by use of aseptic techniques and procedures according to agency protocol; how to empty the drainage bag; signs and symptoms of UTI; proper use of leg bag if going home with indwelling catheter, including how to empty and cleanse and the need to empty the leg bag every 2 to 3 hours to prevent reflux of urine into bladder — Care of incision: keep perineal and abdominal incisions clean and dry; gently flush perineal incision with warm water daily when discharged home and after each bowel movement; wash hands thoroughly before touching surgical incision; how to change dressing if required — No sex for 6 weeks — No heavy lifting or strenuous activity for 4 to 8 weeks — Take showers, but not tub baths — Control of fatigue: balance of rest and activity, including a nap time	Knowledge of what to expect helps the patient cope with untoward side effects and better equips him to take responsibility for managing the illness and engaging in self-care. Sex, strenuous activity, or lifting all could disrupt incisional lines. Other interventions are aimed at preventing complications such as infections.

INTERVENTIONS	RATIONALES
Teach patient to implement dietary strategies to prevent constipation, and ensure adequate output and dilution of urine: — Intake of 2000 to 3000 ml of fluid — Increased fiber in diet; intake of prune juice or apple juice — Stool softeners or laxatives as needed or prescribed	Adequate fluid intake is necessary to keep urine diluted and prevent infection. Constipation can cause disruption of the surgical incision, and straining to defecate increases pain in patients who have had prostatectomies, especially perineal types.
For incontinence, teach Kegel exercises; instruct on use of pads with odor-control substances.	Kegel exercises improve perineal muscle tone and may reduce incontinence; pads keep the patient dry and promote hygiene.
Teach the patient and family the need for follow-up care.	Follow-up is required for post-operative assessments and removal of any indwelling catheters, and to monitor urinary system function.
Assess the patient's and family's understanding of all teaching by encouraging them to repeat information and ask questions as needed.	This allows the nurse to hear in the patient's own words what was taught and makes it easier to know what information may need to be reinforced.
Establish that the patient has the resources required to be compliant, such as transportation to follow-up appointments, finances to buy medications and supplies, and assistance with care.	The patient may need assistance in the home with care and household chores following surgery. If needed resources such as finances and transportation to follow-up appointments are not available, the patient cannot be compliant; the nurse will need to make necessary referrals. This may be a real problem for patients from remote and rural areas, especially if family support is not available.
Provide the patient with written materials that contain the information that was taught.	Provides material for review and as a reference later.

NIC *Learning readiness enhancement*

Learning facilitation

Teaching: Procedure/ treatment

Teaching: Psychomotor skill

Teaching: Disease process

Teaching: Prescribed medication

Evaluation

Evaluate the degree to which the patient has achieved the outcome criteria relevant to the teaching sessions. The patient should verbalize an understanding of content presented by repeating the information, particularly the disease process, treatments (surgery), and medications. The nurse must determine if the patient is capable of being compliant with the recommended regimen. If further teaching is required at time of discharge, the appropriate referrals should be made to continue education.

Community/Home Care

The patient and family will need to implement the medical regimen in the home setting over an extended period. The success of this implementation will be dependent upon the degree to which the patient has received adequate teaching and has subsequently understood and internalized it. In most instances, the patient will need to return to an outpatient facility or doctor's office for follow-up visits to assess urinary function. As indicated in the preceding teaching plan, there are many facets of care that the patient and family need to understand. The volume of information may prove overwhelming at first and in almost all instances, a visiting nurse should be employed to assist and determine that the patient is able to employ the strategies outlined. The ability to care for incisions, drainage devices, and indwelling catheters should be reassessed once the patient is at home. Questions that the patient or family may have include what to empty the urine or other drainage into, how to empty in the commode without soiling oneself, how to cleanse the bag, how to apply a leg bag, and how to store the urinary drainage bag at home. The nurse should watch the patient perform the psychomotor skills in the home. The nurse can assist the patient in the home by making note cards with instructions on them especially for information such as signs and symptoms of infections, symptoms to notify a health care worker about, and how to perform Kegel exercises. The cards can be color-coded and a ring placed through the upper corner to keep them together.

Documentation

Document the specific content taught and the titles of any printed documents given to the patient. Include in the chart the patient's degree of understanding of the content and the methods used to evaluate learning. The nurse should be sure to include specifically the patient's ability to perform psychomotor skills such as dressing changes and care of indwelling catheters. Any areas that need to be reinforced should be documented to ensure appropriate follow-up. If family members are present for the teaching sessions document this in the chart, and always document any referrals made.

CHAPTER 11.116

BREAST CANCER WITH MASTECTOMY/ LUMPECTOMY (POST-OPERATIVE)

GENERAL INFORMATION

Breast cancer is the most frequently diagnosed non-skin cancer in women and is the second leading cause of cancer deaths in the United States (lung cancer is first). Cancers of the breast are categorized as invasive or non-invasive, with most cancers being adenocarcinomas located in the upper outer quadrant of the breast and the tail of Spence. Infiltrating ductal carcinomas account for approximately 70–80 percent of all cases. Infiltrating lobular cancers account for 5 to 10 percent of all cases, and non-invasive ductal carcinoma accounts for 4 to 6 percent of all cases. Risk factors for the development of breast cancer include history of the disease in a first-degree relative, presence of BRCA-1 gene on chromosome 17, presence of BRCA-2 gene on chromosome 11, early menarche (earlier than 12 years of age), late menopause (after 50 years), nulliparity, first childbirth after age 30, and use of estrogen replacement therapy. The most common presenting finding for breast cancer is a lump or breast mass found on palpation by the patient or health care provider or through routine mammography. The mass is most often nontender, hard, non-movable, and irregularly shaped. Other clinical manifestations include dimpling, nipple retraction, nipple discharge or flaking, edema with peau d'orange (inflammatory breast cancer), and burning or stinging. There are significant unexplained cultural/ethnic differences in breast cancer incidence and mortality rates. Although Caucasian women have a higher incidence of breast cancer than other groups, African American women have a higher mortality rate even when diagnosed at an early stage. African American and Hispanic women are diagnosed at later stages of the disease. Hispanic women, especially Mexican Americans, have the lowest rate of participation in cancer screening of any ethnic group and tend to have larger tumors that are more advanced at time of diagnosis, which can account for their higher mortality rate. Mastectomy is done to help eliminate the spread of breast cancer, and may be undertaken in conjunction with chemotherapy, radiation therapy, and/or bone marrow transplant. It was estimated that there would be 212,930 new cases of breast cancer in 2005, and approximately 1690 new cases were projected in men. The death rate for breast cancer in 2005 was estimated to be 40,870 in women and 460 in men.

NURSING DIAGNOSIS 1

DEFICIENT KNOWLEDGE

Related to:

New onset of disease (breast cancer)

Treatments required

Possible complex treatment protocol

Misunderstanding of information

Defining Characteristics:

Many or no questions

Verbalizes a lack of knowledge/understanding

Goal:

The patient will understand breast cancer and its treatment.

Outcome Criteria

✔ The patient verbalizes a desire to learn necessary information.

✔ The patient verbalizes an understanding of diagnostic procedures (mammography, percutaneous needle biopsy, stereotactic needle biopsy, excisional biopsy, computed tomography [CT] scan, clinical breast exam).

✔ The patient verbalizes an understanding of treatment options (surgery, radiation, chemotherapy, hormonal therapy).

✔ The patient verbalizes an understanding of pain management.

✔ The patient verbalizes an understanding of follow-up care required and expresses a willingness to comply.

NOC *Knowledge: Disease process*
Knowledge: Treatment regimen
Knowledge: Treatment procedures
Compliance behavior

INTERVENTIONS	RATIONALES
Assess the patient's current knowledge and ability and readiness to learn.	The teacher needs to ascertain what the patient already knows and build on this; if the patient is not capable of learning or is not ready to learn, teaching will not be effective due to disinterest or inability to understand. The patient may not be ready to learn if in a state of denial or if extremely angry.
Start with the simplest information and move to more complex information.	Patients can understand simple concepts easily and then can build on those to understand concepts that are more complex.
Teach patient and significant others: — Disease process of breast cancer: pathophysiology (clinical manifestations), clinical staging of the disease, lymph node involvement, and metastasis — Available treatment options (chemotherapy, radiation therapy, surgery, hormonal therapy, bone marrow/stem cell transplant) and reconstructive surgery — Diagnostic studies: mammography, percutaneous needle biopsy, stereotactic needle biopsy, excisional biopsy, CT scan, clinical breast exam, carcinoembryonic antigen (CEA), and bone scans.	Knowledge of disease process and identification of complications empowers the patient to take control and be compliant; stages of breast cancer range from stage 0 (tissue in situ) to stage IV (distant metastasis); staging is based on size of tumor, involvement of regional lymph nodes, and distant metastasis; the stage of disease guides treatment, which also considers the woman's age; a combination of treatment modalities (chemotherapy, radiation, surgery) can be utilized, and the patient needs to be aware of these in order to make an informed decision regarding options; mammography is used most often for initial diagnosis;
	CT scans can demonstrate the presence of a mass; percutaneous and stereotactic needle biopsies aspirate cells and fluids for cytology examination and provide a definitive diagnosis through direct analysis of tissue; excisional biopsy removes the discovered lump for histological analysis; CEA is a tumor marker and elevates in the presence of cancerous growths; clinical breast exam is a screening method that identifies the location of any palpable mass; bone scans and x-rays of other structures are often done to detect possible sites of metastasis (common sites are bone, brain, lung, liver, and lymph nodes).
Teach patient and family regarding various types of surgical interventions and post-operative care required (see nursing diagnosis "Impaired Skin Integrity"): — Lumpectomy: removes the tumor and the surrounding margin of breast tissues — Simple mastectomy: removal of breast only — Modified radical mastectomy: removal of the breast tissue and lymph nodes under the arm — Radical mastectomy: removes the entire breast, lymph nodes under the arm, and underlying chest muscles — Post-operative interventions: drainage devices, pain control, incision, prevention of injury to affected side, and possibility of lymphedema (see nursing diagnosis "Impaired Physical Mobility") — Exercises: hand wall climbing, scissors, and elbow pull-in	Most patients with breast cancer undergo some type of surgical intervention and need to have information regarding the type of surgery recommended and post-operative expectations; exercises should be started 24 hours post-operatively to help develop collateral drainage and prevent lymphedema.
Teach or reinforce teaching regarding reconstructive surgery: breast implants/tissue expansion, transverse rectus abdominis musculocutaneous (TRAM) flap (the most commonly used flap operation), and nipple-areolar reconstruction.	Reconstruction should be discussed by the surgeon prior to the mastectomy so that the patient can make an informed decision regarding type of mastectomy. Breast implants and use of tissue expanders requires additional surgical

INTERVENTIONS	RATIONALES
	interventions following healing, and the TRAM flap requires reconstruction of the breast in a procedure that requires an additional incision with 2 to 8 hours of surgery followed by a recovery of 4 to 6 weeks. Nipple reconstruction gives the breast a normal appearance, which promotes better body image, and is performed a few months after initial reconstruction.
Teach patient and family about external radiation: — Method of action — Course/duration of treatment, usually five treatments each week for 4 to 6 weeks — Skin changes to note (redness/discoloration, sloughing, and tenderness) — Skin care: do not apply soap, ointments, lotions, creams, or powder to area. Refrain from using deodorant; do not rub, scrub, or scratch the area; do not try to wash off markings; avoid exposing the treated area to the sun during the treatment and for 1 year following treatments — Wear loose-fitting clothes; bras may need to be avoided due to risk of irritation — Control of fatigue: importance of energy conservation; intake of high-energy foods rich in vitamin C, protein, and iron; and taking a nap each day especially after treatments	Radiation for breast cancer is employed in combination with other types of treatment, and the decision to recommend radiation is based on staging of tumor and the other type of treatments to be used. It is almost always used in early disease (stage I and II) when a lumpectomy is the surgical option. The radiated skin is sensitive, and lotions, creams, ultraviolet rays, rubbing, etc., may cause burning and skin sloughing, and interfere with radiation. The patient must know how to protect the skin from impairment, and understanding what to expect in terms of radiation helps the patient to be more compliant and feel more in control.
Teach the patient and family about chemotherapy and its effects: — Specific agents used for treatment and method of action — Procedure for administration and duration of therapy — Alopecia: assist the patient to plan for hair loss by investigating the purchase of wigs or having hair cut short and using hair for a specially made wig before alopecia; find a resource that could teach women how to prepare fashionable head wraps	Knowledge of what to expect helps the patient cope with untoward side effects and better equips her or him to take responsibility for managing the illness and engaging in self-care.
— Nausea/vomiting: teach to use anti-emetics before meals prophylactically; avoid foods with strong odors, and in the hospital setting have lids removed from trays outside the room (when lids are removed from food trays the smell is often overwhelming to the gastrointestinal [GI] system and causes nausea); attempt frequent small meals, avoiding spicy foods — Care of access sites: prevent infection by use of aseptic techniques and procedures according to agency protocol — Control of fatigue: balance rest and activity, and on chemotherapy days, schedule a designated nap time — Prevention of infection: chemotherapy causes a depression of white blood cells (WBCs), predisposing the patient to infection; avoid people with infections and large crowds; practice good hand hygiene; know WBC counts	
Teach or reinforce teaching about hormonal therapy.	Some breast tumors are estrogen dependent (ER+) and to stop growth their estrogen supply needs to be suppressed. Estrogen and progesterone receptor assay are done to direct decisions; a value > 10 is positive and indicates that hormone therapy may be beneficial.
Reinforce information provided on bone marrow transplant and ensure that the patient has questions answered.	Bone marrow transplants are used for patients with metastatic disease in efforts to prolong survival; the patient's own bone marrow (autologous BMT) or the patient's circulating blood stem cells (referred to as peripheral blood stem cell transplant) can be used.
Provide patient and family with information on Reach to Recovery, and if disease is in the later stages provide information on hospice and other community service agencies such as American Cancer Society.	These agencies can provide psychological support as well as resources to the patient and family.

(continues)

(continued)

INTERVENTIONS	RATIONALES
Assess the patient's and family's understanding of all teaching by encouraging them to repeat information and ask questions as needed.	This allows the nurse to hear in the patient's own words what was taught and makes it easier to know what information may need to be reinforced.
Establish that the patient has the resources required to be compliant, including transportation to follow-up appointments and to radiation or chemotherapy treatments.	If needed resources such as finances and transportation to follow-up appointments are not available, the patient cannot be compliant; the nurse will need to make necessary referrals.
Monitor for understanding of treatments, operative and diagnostic procedures, recovery period, expected outcomes, prognosis, knowledge of any prosthetic devices, and reconstructive options.	Even though the patient may verbalize understanding following teaching, the patient's emotional state may distract and preclude her or him from retaining all information. The need for reinforcements is likely, and the nurse should monitor for this.
Provide the patient with written materials containing the information taught.	The patient may be distracted due to her or his emotional state at receiving the diagnosis of breast cancer and may not remember all the information given by the nurse. Written information can be used as a reference and reviewed later.

NIC *Learning readiness enhancement*
Learning facilitation
Teaching: Disease process
Teaching: Prescribed medication
Teaching: Procedure/treatment

Evaluation

Evaluate the degree to which the patient has achieved the outcome criteria relevant to the teaching sessions. The patient should verbalize an understanding of the content presented by repeating the information, particularly the disease process, treatment options (radiation, chemotherapy, surgery), and medications for pain or nausea. The nurse must determine if the patient is willing to comply with recommendations for treatment and if he or she is capable of being compliant with the recommended regimen. The patient should be able to discuss the possible diagnostic tests that may be performed and options for reconstruction. If further teaching is required at time of discharge, the appropriate referrals should be made to continue education.

Community/Home Care

The treatment of breast cancer can be complex and extend over a long period of time. The patient will need to implement aspects of the prescribed regimen in the home setting and the amount of time that the patient will require for visitation or follow-up will depend on the type of treatment employed. Teaching is crucial to enhance the patient's sense of being in control and to maintain some degree of independence. At home, the patient will likely experience fatigue following any of the treatments, but especially with surgery, radiation, or chemotherapy treatments. If chemotherapy is employed, hair loss, nausea, and vomiting may also occur because of treatments. For the patient receiving chemotherapy it is important to monitor the patient's weight if the patient is experiencing nausea and vomiting. Health care providers or dietitians can assist the patient to prepare a diet that is both nutritional and easy to digest. If the patient is receiving external radiation therapy, he or she will need to return to an outpatient facility. External radiation therapy patients will need to be monitored for ability to care for skin properly to prevent further tissue destruction. For the patient treated by surgical intervention alone, teaching regarding wound care and activity restrictions should be undertaken with reinforcement by a visiting nurse (see nursing diagnosis "Impaired Skin Integrity"). Attention to wound healing and the prevention of lymphedema if lymph nodes have been removed will be needed for patients who have had surgery. The patient should demonstrate the correct technique for performing arm exercises that prevent lymphedema, and the health care provider should follow up to be sure that the patient is actually practicing them at home. Because the patient is seen on a regular basis for general follow-up, for post-operative care, for chemotherapy, or for radiation therapy, health care providers can use these opportunities to determine if further teaching or reinforcement is required. Pain control following mastectomy is achieved with mild narcotics but will be a bigger part of home care in the later stages of the disease if a cure has not been effected by treatments and will require frequent follow-up to ensure patient satisfaction (see nursing diagnosis "Acute Pain"). The ability of the patient to implement the recommended regimen will be dependent upon the degree to which the patient has received adequate teaching and has subsequently understood and internalized it.

Documentation

Document the specific content taught and the titles of any printed documents given to the patient. Include in the chart the patient's degree of understanding of the content and the methods used to evaluate learning. An assessment of the patient's ability to be compliant with the regimen in terms of radiation, chemotherapy, and other prescribed follow-up should be made in the chart with indicators of referrals made. Any areas that need to be reinforced should be documented to ensure appropriate follow-up. If family members are present for the teaching session, document this in the chart.

NURSING DIAGNOSIS 2

 ## INEFFECTIVE COPING

Related to:

Fear of the unknown

Diagnosis of breast cancer

Uncertain stage of disease at time of diagnosis

Surgery

Defining Characteristics:

Expressions of fear

Restlessness

Verbalizes anxiety

Crying

Withdrawal

Verbalizations of anxiety

Goal:

The patient expresses grief and identifies coping strategies.

Outcome Criteria

✔ The patient identifies and uses one coping mechanism.

✔ The patient verbalizes feelings, fears, and concerns.

✔ The patient reports being less anxious.

✔ The patient demonstrates no outward signs of anxiety, such as restlessness or agitation.

NOC *Anxiety control*
Comfort level
Coping

INTERVENTIONS	RATIONALES
Assess level of anxiety (mild, moderate, severe); have patient rate on a scale of 1 to 10, with 10 being the greatest.	Gives the nurse a better perception of extent of the anxiety.
Assess the patient to determine feelings regarding the diagnosis of breast cancer, and support her or him as appropriate letting the patient know that these feelings are normal. Assess for expressions of — Fear of terminal disease diagnosis — Depression, crying — Anger, denial — Sorrow — Fearfulness — Worry about metastasis (real or unfounded) — Concern about what will happen to family — Worry about financial issues/ job security	The patient may experience a wide array of emotions and fears; the nurse needs to be mindful of the emotional toll that a diagnosis of breast cancer may have on the patient, especially if the diagnosis is made in the later stages or if metastasis is present. Assisting the family to deal with the diagnosis will enhance his or her ability to cope with serious illness.
Keep the patient informed of all that is going on, including information about diagnostic tests (mammogram, scans, and biopsy) and planned therapeutic interventions.	Providing factual information and communicating in a straightforward manner may help to relieve anxiety and fear.
Use a calm, reassuring manner with the patient.	Gives the patient a sense of well-being.
Encourage the patient to verbalize any fears or concerns, while listening attentively.	Verbalization of fears contributes to dealing with concerns; being attentive relays empathy to the patient.
Seek spiritual consult if requested by the patient and/or family.	Meeting spiritual needs of the patient helps the patient to deal with fears through use of spiritual or religious rituals.

(continues)

(continued)

INTERVENTIONS	RATIONALES
Recognize the role of culture in a patient's method of coping with illness and the acceptability of verbalizing fears and concerns.	Culture often dictates how a person copes and the nurse must recognize this in order to support the patient in identifying successful coping strategies.
Engage the patient and family in open dialogue regarding options for treatments and care with particular attention to reconstructive surgery.	Discussion of care options allows the patient to be more in control and gives her or him a sense of empowerment that may assist with coping with the disease and its prognosis.
Discuss with the family/patient and investigate the need for services of home health agencies or support services such as those provided by Reach to Recovery, Hospice, and the American Cancer Society if diagnosed in the later stages of the disease.	In late disease or recurrences that have not been adequately treated, as the disease progresses the patient and family may require services of these groups for nursing care, durable medical supplies, psychological support, and assistance with pain control. Having these discussions and planning ahead prevents any delays in obtaining services when needed and can reduce anxiety that accompanies decision making at a time of crisis. Reach to Recovery may be beneficial to women at any stage of the disease as it provides volunteers who have experienced breast cancer and provides valuable emotional support as the patient makes decisions regarding reconstruction or prosthesis.
If the patient has energy, time, and the desire, encourage her or him to document her or his feelings in a diary or journal; if the patient is in the later stages of disease or has metastasis and has young children, she or he can also record messages for them via a tape recording or written words.	These strategies assist the patient to express her or himself in an acceptable manner when she or he may feel uncomfortable talking to others; audio recordings or written messages for children leave a legacy and may provide comfort for the patient.
For the patient who has metastasis and a poor prognosis, give the patient printed literature for future reading, such as "I Still Buy Green Bananas: Living with Hope, Living with Breast Cancer."	This quick-read booklet offers some hope and provides insights from other people who have experienced breast cancer with a difficult prognosis. The nurse or patient can locate a copy through the local chapter of the American Cancer Society or at the local health department.

NIC *Coping enhancement*
Emotional support
Spiritual support

Evaluation

Evaluate the extent to which the outcome criteria have been achieved. The patient should be assessed for behaviors that would indicate adjustment to the diagnosis of breast cancer. The survival rate is good for breast cancer, but the patient may still experience anticipatory grieving and extreme anxiety shortly after diagnosis as he or she attempts to deal with the unknown and the possibility of death. The patient should verbalize fears and concerns and be able to identify one way that to cope with the diagnosis of cancer. The extent to which the patient displays appropriate coping behaviors should be noted. If the patient is unable to talk about the diagnosis and communicate concerns, the nurse should explore new interventions to assist the patient.

Community/Home Care

Nurses should assess which coping mechanisms work for the patient and encourage their use by the patient at home. Even for those patients whose disease was detected early and treated effectively (especially mastectomy patients), problems with anxiety may continue for a long period. At least one follow-up visit by a health care provider should be initiated to assess for ineffective coping. The patient should be encouraged to identify coping strategies that have been successful in the past and be prompted to use those regularly. For the patient undergoing reconstruction with either implants or TRAM, anxiety regarding upcoming surgeries may occur once at home, and the patient needs easy access to health care providers to have questions answered. Anxiety regarding prognosis usually continues regardless of stage of disease and is more pronounced for those patients for whom the disease was detected in the late stages. Coping through use of support from outside sources such as hospice, support groups, or nurse therapists may be required. Monitor the patient for extreme withdrawal, isolation, and depression, and report any symptoms to the physician. For many patients and families, spiritual/religious rituals provide a means of coping with difficult stressful situations. The patient's culture may dictate how she or he copes and/or grieves, and with whom she or he shares this process. It is crucial that the nurse and family support the patient as needed to foster a healthy psychological state, recognizing that anger and denial are common. As the disease progresses, the patient may require new strategies for coping with the disease and the anticipated loss of life. Even though friends and family intend well with their presence, the patient may benefit from quiet periods of meditation and solitude during the day. Support to long-term caregivers will be important, as they too need to be supported in a grief process. Hospice can play an important role in the home situation through provision of counselors, chaplains, and in-home care providers. If questions should arise at home regarding the patient's health status or prescribed regimen, the patient should have a means of contact with a health care provider for answers.

Documentation

The degree to which the patient has demonstrated effective coping and decreased anxiety should be documented in the patient record. A rating system provides an objective way to relay to others the extent of the anxiety or expressions of fear. Document whether the patient is able to discuss feelings regarding a diagnosis of breast cancer. Chart the patient's verbalizations as the patient states them and include in the record coping mechanisms utilized by the patient. Document findings from an assessment of the patient's psychological state: whether there is depression, anger, crying, sadness, etc. Document all referrals that are made to Reach to Recovery, hospice, religious leaders, or any other organization.

NURSING DIAGNOSIS 3

IMPAIRED SKIN INTEGRITY

Related to:

Surgical procedures (mastectomy, reconstructive surgery)

Defining Characteristics (if infection occurs):

Presence of surgical incisions

Drainage devices

Redness, swelling, drainage around wound

Goal:

Incision heals without complications.

Infection is prevented or eliminated.

Outcome Criteria

✔ The patient's surgical site has no redness/discoloration, purulent drainage, or heat.

✔ The patient remains afebrile.

✔ Incision is well approximated.

✔ WBC count remains within normal limits.

NOC *Wound healing: Primary intention*
Tissue integrity: Skin

INTERVENTIONS	RATIONALES
Monitor surgical site and any drainage tube insertion sites for signs and symptoms of infection: redness/discoloration, swelling, purulent drainage, poor approximation, heat, and increased pain.	Early identification of infection can expedite treatment and prevent irreparable damage to the site.
Maintain patency of any drainage devices (Jackson Pratt or Hemovac), and assess drainage for amount, color, and consistency.	The drainage device helps prevent accumulation of drainage in the surgical site; drainage may be bloody initially, but should become serosanguineous.
Assess surgical site dressing for bleeding according to unit protocol or as ordered.	Allows for early detection of post-operative hemorrhage.
Maintain drainage device (prevent kinking, secure to patient clothing) and empty drainage devices according to agency protocol or when one-third full.	Drainage is a source of infection; emptying when one-third full and attaching to clothing prevents unnecessary pull on skin.
Change dressings as ordered (first dressing change to be done by surgeon) and clean area using sterile technique; cleansing site of drainage devices last.	Maintenance of a clean incisional site decreases number of organisms and reduces chance of infection.
Administer antibiotics, as ordered IV (intravenously) or PO (by mouth).	Reduces number of infective organisms and eliminates or prevents infection.
Take temperature every 4 hours.	Temperature elevations may be indicative of infection.
Administer antipyretics (such as acetaminophen [Tylenol]), as ordered.	Helps to reduce fever.
Implement strategies to prevent lymphedema on affected side and	Lymphedema is a common complication following modified

(continues)

(continued)

INTERVENTIONS	RATIONALES
prevent injury (see nursing diagnosis "Impaired Physical Mobility").	and radical mastectomies. Injury to the site can cause lymphedema, as can improper positioning.
Encourage adequate nutritional intake with intake of protein, vitamin C, and iron.	Adequate nutrient intake and especially vitamin C, protein, and iron is required for healing and tissue repair but also enhances the immune system.
Teach patient to turn, cough, and deep breathe and proper use of incentive spirometry (IS), if ordered, and encourage their use.	Helps to open airways, improve oxygenation, and prevent atelectasis post-operatively.
Teach the patient and/or family how to care for drainage devices: emptying, compressing, and cleaning around area; ask patient to demonstrate emptying of the device.	Because of the short stay, the patient may go home with the drainage apparatus in place and will need to understand how to care for it.
Teach the patient how to care for incisional site as ordered or according to protocol and to notify physician if signs of infection occur (redness, warmth, purulent drainage, hardness, or increased pain).	The patient will need to assume care of incision at home and needs education on wound infection, expected care, and what should be reported to a health care provider.
If the patient has had radiation therapy, teach care of the skin following radiation (see nursing diagnosis "Deficient Knowledge").	The patient needs to understand how to care for the sensitive skin following radiation to prevent further damage to cells.

NIC *Incision site care*
Infection control
Nutrition management
Wound care
Wound care: Closed drainage

Evaluation

Evaluate the degree to which the outcome criteria have been met. The surgical site should be intact, healing by primary intention with incision well approximated. Redness, swelling, purulent drainage, and heat should be absent from the site. Drainage from the drainage devices (if present) should be serosanguineous and should be decreasing in amount. The patient should be afebrile, and WBC counts should return to normal.

Community/Home Care

The status of the surgical site remains as an active problem after the patient has been discharged home due to the short hospital stay for mastectomy patients. The risk for infection remains, and the family will need to know what symptoms may signal the onset of infection (redness/discoloration, purulent drainage, heat, and increased pain). Incisional care will need to be taught to the patient, including proper cleansing and maintenance of drainage devices, which are removed at the time of the postoperative follow-up visit. The nurse visiting in the home should assess the patient's ability to care for the drainage device by asking her to demonstrate emptying and compression. The patient should be aware of signs of infection and indications of wound dehiscence. At home, the patient should avoid any activity that would stretch the site or cause undue stress on the site, such as reaching for objects or lifting heavy objects. The patient will need to understand the importance of good nutrition in complete wound healing and recovery and consume a diet rich in protein and vitamin C. Completing any ordered medications such as antibiotics once at home should also be stressed. If any evidence of poor wound healing or infection should occur, the patient should be instructed to contact the health care provider.

Documentation

Document the assessment findings from the wound, including skin color and approximation of the incision. If any signs of infection such as redness, purulent drainage, hardness around site, or increased pain are detected, this should be noted. Chart the status of drainage devices or tubes, indicating the color, amount, and consistency of drainage or any odor. All interventions implemented in the care of the incision are documented. Vital signs are documented according to agency protocol as ordered for postoperative patients. Medications are charted according to agency protocol. All teaching is documented along with an indication of the patient's understanding.

NURSING DIAGNOSIS 4

 ### ACUTE PAIN

Related to:

Presence of breast cancer

Surgical interventions

Metastasis of cancer to other sites

Defining Characteristics

Facial grimace

Moaning

Complaints of pain in breast, bone, or surgical site

Goal:

Pain control is achieved.

Outcome Criteria

✔ The patient will verbalize that pain is reduced or relieved 30 minutes after interventions.

✔ The patient has no grimacing or moaning.

NOC *Pain level*

Pain control

Comfort level

Medication response

INTERVENTIONS	RATIONALES
Have patient rate pain for intensity using a pain rating scale.	Gives a more objective assessment of the pain intensity.
Encourage use of patient-controlled analgesic (PCA) narcotics post-operatively, or administer analgesics as ordered (varies with stage of disease); late in the disease narcotics such as morphine may be required.	Provides pain relief, promotes rest, and decreases anxiety.
Teach appropriate non-pharmacological measures for pain relief such as relaxation techniques, back massage, guided imagery, music, and positioning.	Enhances effects of pharmacological interventions; repositioning can reduce "pull" or tension on muscles and soft tissues.
Assess effectiveness of interventions to relieve pain.	Helps to determine interventions have been effective in relieving pain or if new strategies should be employed.
Establish a quiet environment.	Enhances effects of analgesics and promotes rest.

NIC *Pain management*

Analgesic administration

Anxiety reduction

Evaluation

The patient is able to report that the pain has been relieved or alleviated following interventions. Based on pain rating scales, the patient's pain has decreased. The degree to which the patient is able to assist in the management of the pain through anxiety reduction and relaxation techniques is assessed.

Community/Home Care

Home care required for the management of pain will depend on the type of treatments implemented and the stage of the cancer. For the patient who is being treated with chemotherapy and radiation, the problem will probably become more pronounced as the disease progresses, as these treatments only provide tumor shrinkage and slowing of growth. Initially, pain medications may be given by mouth to obtain satisfactory pain control. However, in the later stages pain control may require the services of hospice or a home nurse when more invasive means of administering narcotics may be needed for control. In some instances, ethical conflicts may arise as the family wants the patient to be alert but successful pain control creates a lethargic, drowsy state. Ineffective in-home management of pain may cause undue emotional stress for the patient and family, necessitating hospitalization. Teaching the patient how to utilize non-pharmacological measures to enhance the effects of analgesics will be crucial to obtaining satisfactory outcomes. Because the average length of stay for a mastectomy patient is 2 to 3 days, acute pain control is still a need for the patient at time of discharge. This need is greater if the patient is going home with drainage devices such as HemoVacs or bulb suction apparatuses (Jackson Pratts) in place. However, for the mastectomy patient the pain is typically temporary, subsiding as the wound heals. If pain becomes worse once at home, the patient should contact the health care provider for investigation of complications, particularly infection. Assessing pain control is an important facet of follow-up care by the home health nurse, hospice, or other health care worker, and should include the patient's ability to purchase prescribed analgesics.

Documentation

Document in the patient's own words the description of the pain and rating of the level of pain. Chart the patient's responses to all interventions, indicating what is effective for pain control and what is not. Those interventions that are ineffective should be removed from the plan of care. Include in the documentation all assessments made relevant to the status of the reproductive system and pain control. All teaching should be indicated in the patient record with an indication of the patient's level of understanding. Document in the chart the patient's and the family's indication of expectation for pain control.

NURSING DIAGNOSIS 5

 ### DISTURBED BODY IMAGE

Defining Characteristics:

> Verbalization of loss of affection from significant other
>
> Verbalization of concerns regarding body appearance
>
> Refusing to discuss health status
>
> Crying, anger (grieving process)
>
> Withdrawal
>
> Depression
>
> Inability to look at chest

Goal:

> The patient is able to verbalize feelings.
>
> The patient has accepted the current health status and has begun to cope.

Outcome Criteria

✔ The patient states willingness to discuss change in structure of body.

✔ The patient verbalizes a satisfaction with body appearance.

✔ The patient makes no negative statements regarding self.

✔ The patient accepts the change in body appearance and continues social activities and interpersonal relationships.

✔ The patient expresses a willingness to discuss changes with significant other or spouse.

✔ The patient verbalizes an understanding of possible reconstruction methods.

NOC   *Body image*
Psychosocial adjustment:
   Life change
Self-esteem

INTERVENTIONS	RATIONALES
Monitor for expressions such as worry over significant other's response or acceptance, grieving over "loss of breast," expressed feelings of "no longer sexually attractive," feelings about self/relationships, feelings about sexuality/sexual desirability/intimacy, fear of rejection and repulsion, fear of loss of significant other, withdrawal/social isolation, and desire to be alone.	These feelings are common following mastectomy and need to be noted and addressed to facilitate effective grieving and coping with loss of body part. Being attuned to these will help in early detection of alterations in social functioning, prevent unhealthy behaviors, and facilitate early intervention through referral to counseling.
Provide assurance that feelings are very normal following a mastectomy, the removal of a body part associated with sexuality.	Helps to prevent the patient from thinking that feelings are abnormal. It is very normal for the patient to run the gamut of emotions following mastectomy.
Identify the effects of the patient's culture or religion on self-concept and body image.	A patient's culture and religion often help define reactions to changes in body image and self-worth.
Provide quiet, private space where the patient can feel free to cry, grieve, or have privacy with family.	Newly diagnosed disease that may be terminal or may create problems with sexuality or role relationships can cause emotional disturbances. The patient needs private time and time alone with significant other or family to work through the grief process and begin to mobilize coping mechanisms.
Listen attentively to the patient and be aware of fears and concerns. In addition, look for misinterpretations or misunderstandings.	Listening to the patient will assist in coping and help identify opportunities for teaching.
Encourage the patient to communicate feelings about changes in physical appearance.	Talking about the changes may sometimes be the beginning of acceptance.
Assist the patient in identifying and mobilizing coping strategies and in recognizing personal strengths.	Discussions like this will help the patient to cope with the situation.

INTERVENTIONS	RATIONALES
Encourage the patient to look at the surgical site and participate in the care of the incision, but do not force the patient to do so.	Looking at the change in body appearance is the first step towards acceptance of the change; participating in the care of the incision also assists the patient to cope with the change. Forcing the patient to look at the site or participate in care may be emotionally traumatic if the patient is not ready.
Teach patient and family how to care for any wounds or surgical sites.	If the patient is comfortable with self-care, that comfort level may translate into acceptance for the change in appearance and incorporation of body appearance change into a positive self-image.
Allow the patient and significant other to express concerns about sexuality and sexual function.	Helps to confirm or refute misunderstanding, misconceptions.
Encourage the patient to participate in at least one outside/public activity each week once health status permits.	Prevents the patient from isolating self from others.
Arrange for psychosocial counseling if required.	Helps to provide psychological assistance to the patient and psychosocial evaluation.
Encourage a visit from Reach to Recovery to talk to the patient.	A volunteer from this agency can provide emotional support to the patient and provide suggestions on how to handle the emotional impact of breast cancer.
Review options for prosthetic devices or reconstruction and arrange for a specialist and/or previous mastectomy patient with prosthesis or reconstruction to visit.	Allows patient the opportunity to explore options, and seeing other patients may help the patient through this difficult time.
Provide the patient with literature regarding dealing with breast cancer such as "For Single Women with Breast Cancer" and "When the Woman You Love Has Breast Cancer."	These publications are easy-to-read materials that give suggestions on how to cope with breast cancer from the emotional perspective and are available from the Y-Me National Breast Cancer Organization.

NIC *Body image enhancement*
       Emotional support
       Self-esteem enhancement
       Role enhancement

Evaluation

The patient is able and willing to learn about care required following the mastectomy. Time is required for the patient to completely assimilate the change in body structure and appearance into self-concept. It is crucial that the nurse evaluates to what degree the patient is beginning to do this. Assess for verbalizations by the patient that would indicate beginning acceptance of the change, such as asking appropriate questions related to post-op care or the recommended therapeutic regimen (for example, radiation, chemotherapy, reconstruction). Communication of feelings and concerns relevant to the change in the body should be taken as a positive sign that progress towards meeting outcome criteria is being made. Determine if the patient is able to discuss her or his feelings with her or his significant other or spouse.

Community/Home Care

At home, continued monitoring of the patient's self-concept and body image is needed. For the patient who has had a mastectomy, the change in the body may cause mental grief and cause the patient to shut out significant others. Until the patient can work through the loss, he or she may be self-conscious about how the significant other or spouse perceives her or him in regards to sexuality or sexual desirability, or may express concerns regarding the impact the loss of the breast may have on future relationships. This threat to role performance may contribute to depression if not addressed by the patient and nurse. Because the length of stay for mastectomy is extremely short (1 to 2 days), psychosocial issues may not be evident until the patient is at home. The nurse or other health care provider who sees the patient for follow-up will need to be alert to subtle hints that may indicate that the patient has not completely adapted to the change in the body. For the patient who is undergoing reconstruction, the impact of the loss of a breast may not be as pronounced, as the person knows that the structural change will be corrected in the near future. Open discussions regarding this disturbed body image and interventions to prevent social isolation and withdrawal should continue with the patient. Encourage the patient to participate in support groups after discharge as an outlet for expressions of concern and as a coping mechanism.

Documentation

Chart any specific behaviors or verbalizations that may indicate a disturbed body image. In addition to a thorough assessment of the patient's psychological state, include all interventions that have been employed to address this issue and the patient's responses. Note when and if the patient looks at the operative site, participates in care, and begins to ask questions relevant to sexuality following mastectomy. If printed materials are given, indicate them in the patient chart by title. Document all referrals made, especially to agencies such as Reach to Recovery.

NURSING DIAGNOSIS 6

 ### IMPAIRED PHYSICAL MOBILITY (AFFECTED ARM)

Related to:

> Removal of lymph nodes under arm
>
> Tissue trauma secondary to surgery

Defining Characteristics:

> Hesitance to use arm on affected side
>
> Difficulty moving affected arm
>
> Pain in arm
>
> Heaviness in arm
>
> Lymphedema

Goal:

> The patient will have complete range of motion of affected side.

Outcome Criteria

✔ The patient will demonstrate appropriate exercises to prevent immobility of affected arm.

✔ The patient will maintain complete range of motion in affected arm and shoulder.

✔ There will be no injury to affected arm.

✔ The patient will have no lymphedema of arm or, if present, lymphedema will not restrict movement.

NOC *Mobility*
> *Knowledge: Prescribed*
> *activity*

INTERVENTIONS	RATIONALES
Assess the patient for limited movement of arm on affected side.	Due to surgical intervention on the affected side with removal of lymph nodes, soreness that inhibits movement may be noted.
Assess for the presence of lymphedema or complaints of numbness or tingling (described as pins and needles) on affected side.	Lymphedema occurs because of removal of lymph nodes or the radiation of nodes. Because of this, the nodes cannot return lymph drainage to the circulation. As a result, the drainage accumulates in the space created by surgery rather than going into the venous circulation; numbness and tingling are normal but may indicate possible nerve damage that may resolve in time but that needs to be monitored.
Avoid using the arm on the affected side for blood sticks, IV access, or measuring blood pressure, and post signs over the patient's bed during hospitalization to inform other health care providers.	Compression (applying tourniquets or blood pressure cuffs) of the arm on the affected side can cause lymphedema; the operative arm is subject to trauma and cellulitis even from minor insults and needs to be protected.
Keep affected arm immobile for the first 24 hours.	Helps to prevent strain on incisional line.
Elevate the affected arm with the hand and arm higher than the elbow and the elbow is higher than the shoulder; use pillows.	This position prevents accumulation of fluid in lymphatic and venous systems.
Measure the circumference of the arm above and below the elbow.	Measures the size of the arm objectively and subsequently the amount of fluid accumulation; used to evaluate the effectiveness of strategies to relieve or prevent fluid accumulation.
Implement hand or arm exercises as ordered such as — Range of motion — Ball squeezing — Hand wall climbing (face the wall and place palms on wall at shoulder level; slowly walk hands up the wall until they are fully extended; slowly walk down the wall) — Brushing or combing hair	These exercises promote mobility of the arm and help prevent accumulation of fluid in the arm and underneath the arm.

INTERVENTIONS	RATIONALES
Teach patient to implement strategies that protect the affected arm: — Wear gloves or long-sleeved shirts when working outside or gardening, especially if working in shrubs such as holly or roses that could cause pricks. — Wear rubber gloves when washing dishes and an oven mitt when cooking. — Do not shave underarms with straight razors. — Avoid tight-fitting clothes that may constrict the arm or operative site; bras may need to be avoided until wound healing has occurred or adaptations may need to be made to provide for comfort such as padding.	These strategies protect the surgical site and the affected arm from injury.

NIC *Positioning*

Teaching: Prescribed activity/exercise

Evaluation

The patient has experienced no injury to the affected arm. Lymphedema is absent or minimal and does not impair movement of the extremity. The patient demonstrates complete range of motion and implements exercises as prescribed. Following mastectomy, the patient demonstrates an understanding of the need to protect the affected arm and to monitor any edema that occurs.

Community/Home Care

The risk for injury to the affected arm continues for the patient after discharge from the hospital and may be a continuing problem for the patient. Strategies to prevent injury to the arm should continue, which necessitates that the patient be vigilant in protecting the arm when performing routine activities such as gardening and housework. The prevention of lymphedema through exercises and elevation of the extremity should be undertaken religiously by the patient. Family members can assist the patient by reminding her or him to perform the exercises or to elevate the extremity. It may be helpful if the patient measures the extremity once a week to detect small changes in size of the extremity. This early detection can prevent problems that are more serious because the patient can implement more aggressive strategies to alleviate the edema. Symptoms that necessitate notification of the health care provider include worsening symptoms of tingling and numbness, tightness in the extremity, increasing lymphedema, and signs of cellulitis (redness or other discoloration, heat, edema). Home visits by a home care nurse should incorporate an assessment of the affected arm for injury and lymphedema as well as reinforcement of any teaching.

Documentation

Chart the status of the affected arm, including an assessment of the skin, presence or absence of edema, and assessment of sensation. Include in the chart teaching of exercises to prevent limitations in mobility and the patient's performance of these activities. Range of motion when performed should be documented in the patient record and referrals to physical therapy for exercise teaching and implementation should be included in the documentation. When assessments reveal problems, document the nursing strategies implemented to address the problems.

CHAPTER 11.117

HYSTERECTOMY

GENERAL INFORMATION

The uterus may be removed for various reasons, such as chronic endometriosis, benign or malignant tumors and other malignancies, uterine rupture, or severe/chronic pelvic inflammatory disease (PID). Hysterectomies can be accomplished via two surgical approaches: abdominal or vaginal. Vaginal hysterectomy may be the surgical approach of choice when a cystocele or rectocele is present, when the patient is morbidly obese, when uterine prolapse is evident, or when there is a tumor at the distal third of the uterus. The abdominal surgical approach is chosen when there will be a partial (subtotal) removal of the uterus, when both the uterus and cervix will be resected, or when the fallopian tubes and ovaries are resected, along with the uterus and cervix. This is known as a total hysterectomy with bilateral salpingo-oophorectomy. This procedure is usually done when there is cervical or uterine cancer with a high likelihood of metastasis, when uterine hemorrhage is difficult to control, or when endometriosis is uncontrolled. More extensive procedures such as pelvic exoneration may be done when metastasis is widespread, but this procedure comprises only a small percentage of cases.

NURSING DIAGNOSIS 1

ACUTE PAIN

Related to:

Surgical interventions

Defining Characteristics:

Complaints of pain

Obvious signs of pain

Grimacing and moaning

Goal:

The patient's pain is relieved.

Outcome Criteria

✔ The patient will verbalize that pain has been relieved 30 minutes after interventions.

✔ The patient will verbalize satisfaction with pain control measures.

NOC *Pain level*

Pain control

Comfort level

INTERVENTIONS	RATIONALES
Assess for location, intensity, quality, and precipitating factors.	Identifying these will assist in accurate diagnosis and treatment; most patients who undergo surgical interventions experience some pain.
Have the patient rate pain intensity using a pain rating scale.	Provides a more objective description of level of pain.
Assess respiratory status, including breath sounds, respiratory rate, depth, quality, and oxygen saturation.	Patients who have had abdominal surgery tend to breathe shallowly due to the pain associated with inspiration; this compromises respiratory function and may lead to preventable complications such as atelectasis and pneumonia.
Administer analgesics, as ordered, on a regular schedule, not allowing pain to get intense.	The patient needs to be comfortable in order to participate in care; decreased pain will improve patient's respiratory efforts and makes it easier for the patient to participate in coughing and deep breathing.
Implement non-pharmacological strategies to enhance effects of pain medication, such as relaxation techniques, playing soft music, and distraction.	Non-pharmacological interventions can assist in reducing pain by affecting the perception of the pain experience.

INTERVENTIONS	RATIONALES
Teach the patient to splint abdomen when moving or coughing with a pillow or rolled bath blanket.	Splinting provides support for the painful area, decreases stress on surgical site that may increase pain, and allows the patient to participate in coughing and deep breathing more comfortably.
Assess effectiveness of interventions to relieve pain.	Helps to determine if interventions have been effective in relieving pain or if new strategies need to be employed.

NIC *Pain management*
Analgesic administration
Anxiety reduction

Evaluation

The patient is able to report that the pain has been reduced or alleviated following interventions. The degree to which the patient is able to assist in the management of the pain through anxiety reduction and relaxation techniques is assessed. The patient should appear calm and have no observable signs of being uncomfortable.

Community/Home Care

The patient's pain should be temporary and be re-solved once the surgical wounds heal. Pain at home is usually managed with mild analgesics, and the du-ration of pain should be short. The patient should take the medications as prescribed with decreasing frequency over time. The nurse should stress to the patient that weak respiratory efforts because of pain can cause respiratory problems such as pneumonia. Encourage the patient to use splinting when moving or coughing at home by placing a bed pillow or small decorative pillow against the surgical site. If the pain worsens at home, the patient should con-tact the health care provider to determine other causes for the pain; most often increased pain sig-nals a wound infection. If the recommended anal-gesics are not working, the patient should seek follow-up care with the health care provider.

Documentation

Document in the patient's own words the descrip-tion of the pain and rating of the level of pain.

Chart all interventions employed and the patient's responses. Include in the documentation assess-ments made relevant to the pain and to the respira-tory system. All teaching should be indicated in the patient record with an indication of the patient's level of understanding.

NURSING DIAGNOSIS 2

 IMPAIRED SKIN INTEGRITY

Related to:

Surgical procedures (abdominal or vaginal)

Defining Characteristics:

Incision with staples or sutures

Drainage tubes in place

Goal:

Incision heals by primary intention.

Infection is prevented or eliminated.

Outcome Criteria

✔ The patient's incision is well approximated.
✔ The patient's surgical site has no redness/discol-oration, purulent drainage, or heat.
✔ The patient remains afebrile.
✔ White blood cell (WBC) count remains within normal limits.

NOC *Wound healing: Primary intention*

INTERVENTIONS	RATIONALES
Monitor surgical site and any drainage tube insertion sites for signs and symptoms of infection: redness/discoloration, swelling, purulent drainage, poor approximation, heat, and increased pain.	Early identification of poor healing and infection will expedite treatment.
Maintain patency of any drainage devices, and assess drainage for amount, color, and consistency.	The drainage device helps prevent accumulation of drainage from surgical site; drainage may be bloody initially, but should become serosanguineous.

(continues)

(continued)

INTERVENTIONS	RATIONALES
Assess vaginal bleeding according to unit protocol or as ordered.	Following hysterectomy, some vaginal bleeding is expected, there should be less than one pad saturated in 4 hours.
Take temperature every 4 hours.	Temperature elevations may be indicative of infection.
Change dressings as ordered and clean area using sterile technique, cleansing site of drainage devices last; for vaginal hysterectomies, provide for sitz baths as ordered; give perineal care after each voiding or bowel movement, as ordered.	Maintenance of a clean incisional site decreases number of organisms and reduces chance of infection; wound infection is more common in vaginal hysterectomies due to close proximity of the surgical site to the rectum.
Administer antipyretics (acetaminophen [Tylenol]), as ordered.	Helps to reduce fever.
Administer antibiotics, as ordered IV (intravenously) or PO (by mouth).	Helps to reduce number of infective organisms and eliminate or prevent infection.
Encourage adequate nutritional intake, especially of protein, vitamin C, and iron.	Adequate nutrient intake, especially of vitamin C, protein, and iron, is required for healing and tissue repair.
Teach the patient to turn, cough, and deep breathe and proper use of incentive spirometry (IS), if ordered.	Helps to open airways, improve oxygenation, and prevent atelectasis.
Monitor for signs and symptoms of urinary tract infection (UTI) and retention.	Patients who have a hysterectomy have usually had an indwelling catheter, which places them at risk for UTI, and those with a vaginal hysterectomy are at high risk due to site of surgical intervention; burning or pain on urination, urine that is cloudy, and urine with an offensive odor may indicate infection; feeling of fullness in the pelvic area, distended abdomen, and decreased or absent voiding signal retention that increases the risk for infection. Distention puts stress on the incision that can disrupt the incisional line.

NIC   *Incision site care*
        Infection control

Nutrition management
Wound care
Wound care: Closed drainage

Evaluation

Evaluate the degree to which the outcome criteria have been met. The surgical site should be intact, healing by primary intention with incision well approximated. Redness, swelling, purulent drainage, and heat should be absent from the site. Drainage from the drainage devices (if present) should be serosanguineous and should be decreasing in amount. The patient should be afebrile, and WBC counts should return to normal. The patient should show no signs of UTI.

Community/Home Care

The status of the surgical site may remain a problem after the patient has been discharged home. The risk for infection remains, and the family will need to know what symptoms may signal the onset of infection. Infections of the abdominal surgical site or vaginal site or UTIs may occur once the patient is at home. Incisional care and perineal care will need to be taught to the patient (see nursing diagnosis "Deficient Knowledge"). For the patient with an abdominal hysterectomy, be sure the patient knows when to return for removal of sutures or staples. The patient may need to wear loose-fitting clothes over the abdomen to prevent irritation to the suture line. The patient should be aware of signs of infection as well as indications of wound dehiscence. The importance of completing any ordered medications such as antibiotics once at home should be stressed. The patient will need to understand the importance of good nutrition in complete wound healing and recovery. Meals should include foods that are rich in protein, vitamin C, and zinc, as well as adequate amounts of fluids. If any evidence of poor wound healing or infection should occur, the patient should be instructed to contact the health care provider.

Documentation

Document assessment findings of the wound including the presence of sutures or staples, drainage, approximation, and skin color. Be sure to note any signs of infection at the incision site such as redness/discoloration, purulent drainage, excessive pain, and heat. Chart the status of drainage devices or tubes, indicating the color, amount, and consistency of drainage.

Vital signs are documented according to agency protocol, as ordered, for post-operative patients.

NURSING DIAGNOSIS 3

 DISTURBED BODY IMAGE

Related to:

Loss of function of female reproductive organs

Inability to bear children

Fear of loss of sexuality

Defining Characteristics:

Verbalization of loss of affection from significant other

Verbalization of concern regarding role performance

Refusing to discuss health status

Crying, anger (grieving process)

Withdrawal

Depression

Goal:

The patient is able to verbalize feelings.

The patient has accepted the current health status and has begun to cope.

The patient accepts the change in function and continues social activities and interpersonal relationships.

Outcome Criteria

✔ The patient states a willingness to discuss change in female reproductive system.

✔ The patient verbalizes a satisfaction with body function.

✔ The patient verbalizes an understanding of the changes in function of the reproductive system.

✔ The patient makes no negative statements about herself.

NOC *Body image*
Psychosocial adjustment:
   Life change
Role performance
Self-esteem

INTERVENTIONS	RATIONALES
Monitor for expressions such as worry over acceptance by significant other, grieving over inability to reproduce, expressed feelings of "no longer a woman," expressed feelings of "no longer sexually attractive," withdrawal, social isolation, fear, anxiety, desire to be alone.	These feelings are common following hysterectomy and need to be noted and addressed to facilitate effective grieving and coping with loss of function; monitoring can detect alterations in social functioning, prevent unhealthy behaviors, and intervene early through referral to counseling.
Provide assurance that feelings are very normal following hysterectomy/removal of reproductive organs.	Helps to stop the patient from thinking that her feelings are abnormal. It is very normal for the patient to have an array of emotions following a hysterectomy. If the patient is aware that this may happen, it will provide reassurance that the emotion will pass; if the emotions do not pass, the patient will know that she or he needs to seek professional counseling.
Provide a quiet, private space where the patient can feel free to cry, grieve, and have privacy with her family.	Newly diagnosed diseases that may be terminal or may eliminate reproductive abilities can cause emotional disturbances. The patient needs private time and time alone with family to work through the grief process and begin to mobilize coping mechanisms.
Encourage the patient to communicate feelings about changes in body function, listen attentively to the patient, and be aware of her fears and concerns. Also look for misinterpretations or misunderstandings.	Talking about the changes may sometimes be the beginning of acceptance; listening to the patient will help the nurse to identify opportunities for teaching.
Help the patient identify personal strengths and mobilize coping strategies.	Discussions like this will help the patient to cope with her situation.
Teach the patient and family how to care for any wounds or surgical sites.	If the patient is comfortable with self-care, that comfort level may translate into acceptance for the change in body function and incorporation of change into a positive self-image.
Allow the patient and significant other to express concerns about sexuality and sexual function.	Helps to confirm or refute understanding, misconceptions.

(continues)

(continued)

INTERVENTIONS	RATIONALES
Encourage the patient to participate in at least one outside/public activity each week once health status permits.	Prevents the patient from isolating herself.
Identify the effects of the patient's culture or religion on self-concept and body image.	A patient's culture and religion often help define reactions to changes in body image and self-worth.
Assist the patient in identifying coping strategies/diversionary activities.	Helps to provide diversionary activities so that not all thoughts are on the loss.
Arrange for psychosocial counseling if required.	Helps to provide psychological assistance to the patient and psychosocial evaluation.

NIC   *Body image enhancement*

Emotional support

Self-esteem enhancement

Role enhancement

Evaluation

The patient is able and willing to learn about care required following the hysterectomy. Time is required for the patient to completely assimilate the perceived change in body function and reproductive ability into her self-perception. It is crucial that the nurse evaluate the degree to which the patient is beginning to do this. Assess for verbalizations that would indicate that the patient is beginning to assimilate changes into self-concept, such as asking appropriate questions related to post-op care or recommended therapeutic regimen. Communication of feelings and concerns relevant to the change in the female body should be taken as a positive sign that progress towards meeting outcome criteria is being made. Determine if the patient is able to discuss her feelings with her significant other or spouse.

Community/Home Care

At home, continued monitoring of the patient's body image is needed. For the patient who has had a hysterectomy, the changes may cause mental grief and cause the patient to shut out significant others. Until the patient can work through the loss, she may be concerned about how her significant other or spouse perceives her with respect to sexuality or sexual desirability. Teaching will need to include information about resumption of sexual activities, change in hormonal status, and expectations relevant to hormonal therapy (see nursing diagnosis "Deficient Knowledge"). The threat to role performance may contribute to depression if not addressed by the patient and nurse. Because the length of stay for hysterectomy is extremely short (1 to 2 days), psychological problems may not be evident until the patient is at home. The nurse or other health care provider who sees the patient for follow-up will need to be alert to subtle hints indicating that the patient has not completely adapted to the change in the body. Open discussions regarding this change and interventions to prevent social isolation and withdrawal should continue with the patient.

Documentation

Chart any specific behaviors or verbalizations that may indicate a low self-concept or altered body image. In addition to a thorough assessment of the patient's psychological state, include all interventions that have been employed to address this issue and the patient's responses. Note when and if the patient begins to ask questions relevant to sexuality following hysterectomy. Document all referrals made.

NURSING DIAGNOSIS 4

 DEFICIENT KNOWLEDGE

Related to:

> Post-operative care
>
> Lack of information
>
> Anxiety

Defining Characteristics:

> Has many questions
>
> Has no questions
>
> Verbalizes misunderstanding

Goal:

> The patient verbalizes an understanding of the operative procedure and prescribed post-operative regimens.

Outcome Criteria

✔ The patient verbalizes a willingness and desire to learn the necessary information.

✔ The patient verbalizes an understanding of the operative procedure and interventions required.

✔ The patient verbalizes an understanding of activity restrictions required during convalescence.

✔ The patient will be able to identify signs and symptoms of urinary and wound infection.

NOC *Knowledge: Disease process*
Knowledge: Health behavior
Treatment behavior: Illness
or injury

INTERVENTIONS	RATIONALES
Assess readiness of client to learn (motivation, cognitive level, and physiological status).	The patient must be motivated to learn, have the capability to learn the content, and be free of distraction from learning, such as pain and emotional distress.
Assess what the patient already knows.	The patient may have some knowledge about hysterectomy and its sequelae, and teaching should begin with what the patient already knows.
Create a quiet environment conducive to learning.	Environmental noise can prevent the learner from focusing on what is being taught.
Teach the learners about the pathophysiology of what happens when the uterus and/or other reproductive organs are removed (loss of menses, no menopausal symptoms unless oophorectomy also performed).	Understanding of pathophysiology assists with rationale for therapeutic interventions.
Teach the patient deep-breathing and coughing exercises.	Helps to maximize ventilatory excursion and reduce likelihood of atelectasis and pneumonia.
Teach the patient activity restrictions as ordered: — Do not lift any objects heavier than 5 pounds. — Refrain from strenuous activities such as aerobics, horseback riding, and jogging. — No driving for at least 4 to 6 weeks, or as prescribed by physician. — Limit stair climbing for 1 month or as prescribed by the physician.	Protects the surgical site; sitting for long periods causes pelvic congestion.

— Avoid sitting for long periods of time.
— Encourage pelvic rest.
— Ambulate as tolerated.
— Splint incision when ambulating.

Teach the patient wound care and infection control measures: — Keep incision clean and dry. — Rinse perineal area with warm water using a spray bottle as ordered following use of the bathroom. — Avoid tub baths, douches, or use of tampons. — If dressing is applied, change it using an aseptic technique. — Monitor for signs of wound infection: warmth, redness/discoloration, purulent drainage, and increased pain. — Monitor for signs of UTI: burning on urination, frequency, malodorous urine, or cloudy urine. — Monitor for urinary retention: inability to void, discomfort low in pelvic area, or distended abdomen. — Report signs and symptoms of infection to a health care provider.	Due to the short hospital stay following hysterectomy, the patient is likely to be at home when post-operative infections occur, so it is crucial that the patient know what to look for that would signal onset of infections.
Provide the patient with information related to sexuality: — No sexual activity for 4 to 6 weeks or as prescribed by physician — Use of water-soluble lubricants for initial sexual intercourse	The patient may express apprehension about the possibility of pain with intercourse, and information on what to expect can allay anxiety. It may take upwards of 4 to 6 weeks for proper healing to occur; the vaginal vault may be tight following hysterectomy and require lubrication during initial sexual intercourse.
Teach the patient signs and symptoms of thrombophlebitis to report to a health care provider: pain in calf, swollen calf or lower leg, warmth over calf, or pain with ambulation.	Positioning for hysterectomy predisposes the patient to pooling and stasis of blood in the pelvic vessels that place the patient at risk for development of thrombus; the patient needs to be aware of the indicators of thrombophlebitis to allow for early intervention.
Teach or reinforce teaching on hormone replacement therapy	If both uterus and ovaries are removed, the patient will

(continues)

(continued)

INTERVENTIONS	RATIONALES
as required if both ovaries are removed. — Benefits: controls symptoms of menopause such as hot flashes, dry vagina, mood swings — Risks: fluid retention, increased risk for blood clots in legs, increased risk of certain types of breast cancer — Types of dosing	experience menopause; hormonal replacement controls some of the symptoms of surgically induced menopause that can begin as early as 1 to 2 days following surgery.
Evaluate the patient's understanding of all content covered by asking questions.	Helps to identify areas that require more teaching and to ensure that the patient has enough information to comply.
Give the patient written information.	Provides reference at a later time, and for review.

NIC   *Teaching: Disease process*
Teaching: Individual
Positioning

Evaluation

The patient is able to repeat all information for the nurse and asks questions about the operative procedure (hysterectomy) and possible outcomes. Prior to discharge, the patient verbalizes an understanding of the activity restrictions required, including sexual activity, and agrees to be compliant. The patient is able to demonstrate to the nurse how to splint the incision when breathing and moving and how to perform deep-breathing exercises; the patient is also able to identify measures to relieve pain. Signs and symptoms of infection can be accurately stated, as well as signs and symptoms of thrombophlebitis. The patient knows when health care assistance should be sought, and is aware specifically of indicators of worsening respiratory status and signs and symptoms of respiratory infection.

Community/Home Care

For patients who have had a hysterectomy, the hospital stay is short, which dictates that knowledge deficits be identified early in order to improve the likelihood that the patient will be prepared for self-care and self-monitoring. With the exception of elderly patients, follow-up care in the home is rarely required. The patient will need to monitor herself for onset of wound infections, UTIs, respiratory complications such as pneumonia, and thrombophlebitis. Follow-up care with a health care provider focuses on assurance that no complications have occurred and any wounds are healing as expected. An additional priority of the health care provider is to assess the patient for psychological concerns such as sexuality, depression, and self-esteem. It is critical that the health care provider broach the topic rather than relying on the patient to express concerns. As the patient resumes more of her normal activity, she may discover that fatigue persists for up to 2 to 3 months but should resolve with time. Often when teaching is done shortly after a loss, such as loss of a body part, the learner may not comprehend or even hear the information, making it necessary for a thorough assessment of what the patient knows prior to discharge.

Documentation

Document all content taught and the patient's verbalization of understanding. Specific attention should be given to documentation of any specific concerns or questions that the patient or her significant other expresses. If a significant other was included in the teaching sessions, chart this information. Include in the documentation the patient's willingness to comply with all recommendations made regarding activity restrictions. Any area that requires further teaching should be clearly indicated in the record. Always include the names of any printed literature given to the patient for reinforcement.

CHAPTER 11.118

CERVICAL CANCER

GENERAL INFORMATION

Cervical cancer is a common neoplasm of the female reproductive system with an estimated 13,000 cases each year and 4800 deaths annually. Most cervical cancers are squamous cell and occur in the epidermal layer of the cervix. Dysplasia of the cervix, also known as preinvasive cancer or precursor lesions, are classified as cervical intraepithelial neoplasia (CIN) and divided into three stages. CIN I is mild to moderate dysplasia, CIN II is moderate to severe dysplasia, and CIN III is severe dysplasia to carcinoma in situ. Squamous cell cancer generally spreads locally in the pelvic region by direct extension, even though metastasis to distant sites can occur via the lymphatic system. Although there is no known cause for cervical cancer, one of the most important risk factors is human papillomavirus (HPV) infection. Other reported risk factors include sexual activity before age 16, multiple sex partners, low socioeconomic status, compromised immune status including HIV-positive status, and chlamydia infections of the reproductive organs. Pre-invasive cancer of the cervix rarely has obvious clinical manifestations, but is found on routine Papanicolaou smears (Pap tests). Early signs of invasive cancer of the cervix are a watery vaginal discharge, occasional spotting, especially after sexual intercourse, and painless bleeding. As the disease progresses, symptoms worsen and include dark, foul-smelling discharge, abdominal discomfort, pain in back and thighs, leg edema (due to obstruction of venous flow secondary to enlarged lymph nodes), anemia, and weight loss. With the widespread use of Pap test screening, the early identification of cancer of the cervix has resulted in a significant decrease in deaths due to the disease. Cancer of the cervix is more common in African Americans than in whites and the death rate for African Americans is twice that of whites (American Cancer Society, 2000).

NURSING DIAGNOSIS 1

DEFICIENT KNOWLEDGE

Related to:

New onset of disease

Treatments required

Possible complex treatment protocol

Misunderstanding of information

Defining Characteristics:

Has many or no questions

Verbalizes a lack of knowledge/understanding

Goal:

The patient will understand cervical cancer and its treatment.

Outcome Criteria

✔ The patient verbalizes a desire to learn necessary information.

✔ The patient verbalizes an understanding of diagnostic procedures (colposcopy, cervical biopsy, Pap smear, and computed tomography [CT] scan).

✔ The patient verbalizes an understanding of cervical cancer treatment options (surgery, radiation, chemotherapy), including untoward effects of treatment and possible complications of cervical cancer.

✔ The patient verbalizes an understanding of pain management.

✔ The patient verbalizes an understanding of follow-up care required and expresses a willingness to comply.

NOC *Knowledge: Disease process*
Knowledge: Treatment regimen
Compliance behavior

INTERVENTIONS	RATIONALES
Assess the patient's current knowledge as well as her ability and readiness to learn.	The nurse needs to ascertain what the patient already knows and use this as a starting point for teaching; if the patient is not capable of learning or is not ready to learn, teaching will not be effective due to disinterest or inability to understand. The patient may not be ready to learn if in a state of denial or if extremely angry.
Start with the simplest information and move to complex information.	Patients can understand simple concepts easily and then can build on those to understand concepts that are more complex.
Teach the patient and significant others: — Diagnostic studies: Pap smear, cervical biopsy, CT scan, colposcopy — Disease process of cervical cancer — Pain medications used to treat cancer pain, including dosage, frequency, side effects, scheduling, and interactions with other medications — Signs and symptoms that would indicate a need to seek health care (severe pain and poor pain control, moderate to severe vaginal bleeding, severe edema of the legs)	Knowledge of disease process, diagnostic tests, treatments, and identification of complications empowers the patient to take control and be compliant; a Pap smear is the first-line screening for cervical cancer and is a histological analysis of swabs of cells from the cervix; cervical biopsy is performed under local anesthesia following an abnormal Pap smear and involves excising a sample of tissue for pathological analysis; colposcopy is direct visualization of the vagina, cervix, and its canal with a lighted scope looking for abnormalities.
Instruct patient regarding internal radiation: — Internal radiation: implants will be placed and remain in place for 24 to 72 hours; — Remain flat in bed; no ambulation — Maintain urinary drainage device — Cleanse bowel prior to start of treatment — Gauze packing to keep implants in place — Possibility of uterine contractions — Radiation safety precautions for visitors/family — Monitor for symptoms of radiation syndrome: nausea, vomiting, anorexia, and malaise	If the patient knows what to expect, anxiety can be reduced, and the patient is better equipped to make decisions and is more likely to be compliant.
— Post-treatment: presence of foul-smelling vaginal discharge; douche at home to control odor; slight vaginal bleeding possible for several months	
Teach patient and family about external radiation: — Method of action — Course/duration of treatment, usually five treatments each week for 4 to 6 weeks — Skin changes to be noted, including redness/discoloration, sloughing, and tenderness — Skin care: do not apply soap, ointments, lotions, creams, or powder to area; do not rub, scrub or scratch the area; do not try to wash off markings; avoid exposing the treated area to the sun during the treatment and for 1 year following treatments — Wear loose-fitting clothes; panties may need to be avoided due to risk of irritation — Control fatigue: importance of energy conservation, intake of high-energy foods rich in vitamin C, protein, and iron; take a nap each day especially after treatment	Radiation is used with cervical cancer when surgery is not an option or in the presence of metastasis, and the patient needs to be informed of what to expect. The radiated skin is sensitive, and lotions, creams, ultraviolet rays, rubbing, etc., may cause burning and skin sloughing, and interfere with radiation. The patient must know how to protect the skin from impairment; knowing what to expect in terms of radiation helps the patient to be more compliant and feel more in control.
Teach the patient and family about chemotherapy and its effects: — Specific agents used for treatment — Method of action — Alopecia: assist the patient to plan for hair loss by investigating the purchase of wigs or having hair cut short and using hair for a specially made wig before alopecia; find a resource that could teach patient how to prepare fashionable head wraps — Nausea/vomiting: teach to use anti-emetics before meals prophylactically; avoid foods with strong odors, and in the hospital setting have lids removed from trays outside the room (when lids are removed from food trays the	Knowledge of what to expect helps the patient cope with untoward side effects and better equips him or her to take responsibility for managing the illness and engage in self-care.

INTERVENTIONS	RATIONALES
smell is often overwhelming to the gastrointestinal [GI] system and causes nausea); attempt frequent small meals, and avoid spicy foods — Care of access sites: prevent of infection by use of aseptic techniques and procedures according to agency protocol — Control of fatigue: balance rest and activity, and on chemotherapy days a designated nap time should be scheduled — Prevention of infection: chemotherapy causes a depression of white blood cells (WBCs), predisposing the patient to infection; avoid people with infections and large crowds; practice good hand hygiene; know WBC counts	
Teach the patient and family about post-operative hysterectomy care if this is the treatment option (see nursing care plan "Hysterectomy").	Hysterectomy is often the first treatment implemented, especially in the absence of metastasis; the patient will need to know post-operative care requirements.
Provide the patient and family with information on hospice and other community service agencies, such as the American Cancer Society.	These agencies can provide psychological support as well as resources to the patient and family.
Assess the patient's and family's understanding of all teaching by encouraging them to repeat information and ask questions as needed.	This allows the nurse to hear in the patient's own words what was taught, and makes it easier to know what information may need to be reinforced.
Establish that the patient has the resources required to be compliant.	If needed resources such as finances and transportation to follow-up appointments are not available, the patient cannot be compliant; the nurse will need collaborate with the physician to make necessary referrals.

NIC *Learning readiness enhancement*
Learning facilitation
Teaching: Disease process

Teaching: Prescribed medication
Teaching: Procedure/treatment

Evaluation

Evaluate the degree to which the patient has achieved the outcome criteria relevant to the teaching sessions. The patient should verbalize an understanding of the content presented by repeating the information, particularly the disease process, radiation treatment process, chemotherapy, and medications for pain or nausea. The nurse must determine if the patient is capable of being compliant with the recommended regimen. If further teaching is required at time of discharge, the appropriate referrals should be made to continue education.

Community/Home Care

The patient will need to implement the medical regimen in the home setting over an extended period of time. Without planned teaching by the nurse, implementation of the regimen may not be successful. At home, the patient will likely experience fatigue following radiation or chemotherapy treatments. If chemotherapy is employed, hair loss, nausea, and vomiting may also occur as a result of treatments. For the patient receiving chemotherapy, it is important to monitor weights if the patient is experiencing nausea and vomiting. Health care providers or dieticians can assist the patient to prepare a diet that is both nutritional and easy to digest. If the patient is receiving external radiation therapy, she will need to return to an outpatient facility for treatments. External radiation therapy patients will need to be monitored for ability to care for skin properly to prevent further tissue destruction. For the patient treated by surgical intervention alone, teaching regarding wound care and activity restrictions should be undertaken with reinforcement by a visiting nurse (see nursing care plan "Hysterectomy"). Because the patient is seen on a regular basis for general follow-up, for post-operative care, for chemotherapy, or for radiation therapy, health care providers can determine if further teaching or reinforcement is required. Pain control is a big part of home care especially in the later stages of the disease and will require frequent follow-up to ensure patient satisfaction. Those health care workers providing follow-up care need to ensure that the family and patient understand that dependence on medication should not be a concern for the cancer patient and that comfort is the ultimate goal.

Documentation

Document the specific content taught and the titles of any printed documents given to the patient. Include in the chart the patient's degree of understanding of the content and the methods used to evaluate learning. An assessment of the patient's ability to be compliant with the regimen in terms of radiation, chemotherapy, or follow-up should be made in the chart with indicators of referrals made. Any areas that need to be reinforced should be documented to ensure appropriate follow-up. If family members are present for the teaching session, document this in the chart, and always document any referrals made.

NURSING DIAGNOSIS 2

INEFFECTIVE COPING

Related to:

Diagnosis of cervical cancer

Fear of dying

Defining Characteristics:

Angry

Expressions of fear

Restlessness and anxiety

Crying

Expresses distress at potential loss

Goal:

The patient expresses grief.

Outcome Criteria

✔ The patient identifies one coping mechanism to be used.

✔ The patient verbalizes fears and concerns.

✔ The patient reports being less anxious.

✔ The patient demonstrates no outward signs of anxiety such as restlessness or agitation.

NOC *Grief resolution*

Anxiety control

Comfort level

Coping

INTERVENTIONS	RATIONALES
Assess level of anxiety (mild, moderate, severe); have patient rate on a scale of 1 to 10, with 10 being the greatest.	Gives the nurse a better perception of extent of the anxiety.
Assess the patient to determine her feelings regarding the diagnosis of cervical cancer and prognosis, and support her as appropriate by answering questions and making referrals.	Assisting the patient to deal with the diagnosis and prognosis will enhance her ability to cope with serious illness.
Use a calm, reassuring manner with the patient.	Communication in a reassuring, calm, and straightforward manner may help to relieve anxiety and give the patient a sense of well-being.
Engage the patient and family in open dialogue regarding options for treatment and care; keep the patient informed of all that is going on, including information about diagnostic tests and therapeutic nursing interventions.	Knowledge can allay anxiety and assist the patient to cope; during the final stages of disease, the patient and family may not be able to care for patient alone; discussion of care options early in the disease allows the patient to be more in control, giving her a sense of empowerment that may assist with coping with the disease.
Provide the patient with information required for informed decisions and self-care.	Being informed about the disease and its treatment will help allay anxiety and fear; assists the patient to be in control.
Allow the family to visit liberally.	Helps to provide emotional support.
Encourage the patient to verbalize fears, concerns, and expressions of grief, and listen attentively.	Verbalization of fears contributes to dealing with concerns; being attentive relays empathy to the patient.
Ask the patient to identify one method of coping with stressful situations that has been successful in the past.	Coping strategies that have been successful in the past can be tried again and used as a starting point for development of new strategies.
Seek spiritual consult as needed or requested by the patient and or family.	Meeting the patient's spiritual needs helps her to deal with fears through use of spiritual or religious rituals.
Recognize the role of culture in the patient's method of coping, grieving, and verbalization of fears and concerns.	Culture often dictates how a person grieves, and the nurse must recognize this in order to support the patient in a successful grief process.

NIC *Grief work facilitation*
      Coping enhancement
      Emotional support
      Spiritual support

Evaluation

Evaluate the extent to which the outcome criteria have been achieved. The patient should be assessed for behaviors that would indicate adjustment to the diagnosis of cervical cancer. The patient should verbalize fears and concerns and be able to identify one way to cope with the diagnosis of cancer, especially if metastasis is present. The extent to which the patient displays appropriate coping behaviors should be noted. If the patient is unable to talk about the diagnosis and communicate concerns, the nurse should explore further new interventions to assist the patient.

Community/Home Care

Nurses should assess which coping mechanisms work for the patient and encourage their use by the patient at home. Problems with grieving may continue for a long period of time, and follow-up by a health care provider can detect ineffective coping. Family should be taught what is appropriate grieving and coping and what is not. Extreme self-isolation and depression should be noted and reported to a health care provider. For many patients and families, spiritual/religious rituals provide a means of coping with difficult, stressful situations.

The patient's culture may dictate how she grieves and with whom she shares this process. It is crucial that the nurse and family support the patient as needed to foster a healthy psychological state, recognizing that anger and denial are common. If a cure was not effected with surgery, as the disease progresses the patient may require new strategies for coping with the disease and the anticipated loss of life. The patient may benefit from quiet periods of meditation during the day. Support to caregivers will be important, as they too need to be supported in a grief process. Hospice can play an important role in the home situation through provision of counselors, chaplains, and in-home care providers. If questions should arise at home regarding the patient's health status or prescribed regimen, the patient should have a means of contact with a health care provider for answers.

Documentation

The degree to which the patient has achieved the outcome criteria should be documented in the patient record. The extent of the patient's verbalization of fears, concerns, and grieving should be documented. Document whether the patient is able to discuss feelings regarding a diagnosis of cervical cancer. Chart the patient's verbalizations as the patient states them and include in the record coping mechanisms utilized by the patient. Document findings from an assessment of the patient's psychological state, whether there is depression, anger, crying, or sadness. Document referrals to hospice or religious leaders.

CHAPTER 11.119

OVARIAN CANCER

GENERAL INFORMATION

Ovarian cancer is a malignancy of the ovaries that is most often (90 percent of the time) epithelial carcinoma, the cause of which is unknown. Recent theories indicate an association with mutations of the BRAC genes that normally inhibit or suppress tumor growth. A familial history of ovarian cancer is the greatest risk factor for development of the disease. Other risk factors include nulliparity, early menarche, familial history of breast cancer, late menopause, and use of hormone replacement therapy. Ovarian cancer is the leading cause of death from reproductive malignancies, with an estimated 13,900 deaths each year and a five-year survival rate of < 50 percent (American Cancer Society, 2004). Even though ovarian cancer can occur at any age, the most common form of the disease affects women over age 50, while germ cell tumors (accounting for 10 percent of cases) affect younger women (frequently women under 20 years of age). White women are more likely to have ovarian cancer than other ethnic groups. Ovarian cancer has few symptoms in its early stages, which makes early diagnosis quite difficult and is a major reason for the high mortality rate. Late in the disease, clinical manifestations include abdominal or pelvic discomfort; vague gastrointestinal (GI) symptoms such as dyspepsia, indigestion, feelings of fullness, flatulence, and distention; dysfunctionsal bleeding; and a palpable abdominal mass upon examination. Ovarian cancers grow rapidly, spread fast, and are often bilateral so that at time of diagnosis or discovery the disease is usually at an advanced stage. Common sites for metastasis include the uterus, bladder, bowel, and omentum, with some spread through the lymphatic system. For most patients, treatment involves chemotherapy and/or radiation therapy as well as surgery. For patients whose cancer is diagnosed early, surgical intervention includes a hysterectomy with bilateral oophorectomy and salpingectomy (see nursing care plan "Hysterectomy" for care of the patient receiving surgical intervention).

NURSING DIAGNOSIS 1

 DEFICIENT KNOWLEDGE

Related to:

New onset of disease (ovarian cancer)

Treatments required

Possible complex treatment protocol

Misunderstanding of information

Defining Characteristics:

Asks many or no questions

Verbalizes a lack of knowledge/understanding

Goal:

The patient will understand ovarian cancer and its treatment.

Outcome Criteria

✔ The patient verbalizes a desire to learn necessary information.

✔ The patient verbalizes an understanding of diagnostic procedures (laparotomy exploration with biopsy, computed tomography [CT] scan, pelvic examination, CA-125).

✔ The patient verbalizes an understanding of treatment options (surgery, radiation, chemotherapy), including untoward effects of treatment and possible complications of ovarian cancer.

✔ The patient verbalizes an understanding of pain management.

✔ The patient verbalizes an understanding of follow-up care required and expresses a willingness to comply.

NOC *Knowledge: Disease process*
Knowledge: Treatment regimen
Compliance behavior

INTERVENTIONS	RATIONALES
Assess the patient's current knowledge, ability to learn, and readiness to learn.	The teacher needs to ascertain what the patient already knows and build on this; if the patient is not capable of learning or is not ready to learn, teaching will not be effective due to disinterest or inability to understand. The patient may not be ready to learn if in a state of denial or if extremely angry.
Start with the simplest information and move to complex information.	Patients can understand simple concepts easily and then can build on those to understand concepts that are more complex.
Teach patient and significant others: — Disease process of ovarian cancer (pathophysiology and staging of the disease) — Available treatment options — Diagnostic studies: laparotomy/biopsy, CT scan, CA-125, pelvic examination — Pain medications, including dosage, frequency, side effects, scheduling, and interactions with other medications — Signs and symptoms that would indicate a need to seek health care (severe pain and poor pain control, moderate to severe vaginal bleeding, and severe edema of the legs)	Knowledge of disease process and identification of complications empowers the patient to take control and be compliant; stage of disease guides treatment: stage I is usually treated with a total hysterectomy with bilateral oophorectomy and salpingectomy along with as much of the tumor as possible combined with chemotherapy or radiation therapy; stage II patients usually have some type of surgical debulking of the tumor but the primary treatment is either radiation therapy (internal or external) or chemotherapy and in some instances a combination of both may be used. Stage III and IV disease are generally treated with chemotherapy, even though in some instances surgical debulking may also be done in these advanced stages. A pelvic exam can identify an ovarian mass on palpation; laparoscopic exam is a direct visualization of the ovaries, and a biopsy can be obtained for histological analysis of cells from the ovarian tumor; CA-125 is a tumor marker specific to the ovaries, however it is not specific enough to be a primary diagnostic tool but can be used to monitor therapy; CT scans can demonstrate the presence of an ovarian mass; pain control is

INTERVENTIONS	RATIONALES
	a crucial component of care in the later stages of the disease (see nursing diagnosis "Acute Pain"); development of untoward side effects of therapies as well as indicators of advancing disease should be reported, including ascites, alterations in bowel and bladder function, and shortness of breath due to ascites.
Instruct the patient regarding internal radiation, and assist with implementation, as ordered: — Internal radiation: implants will be placed and remain in place for 24 to 72 hours. — Remain flat in bed on strict bedrest with head of bed elevated no more than 20 degrees. — Maintain urinary drainage device. — Cleanse bowel prior to start of treatment. — Use gauze packing to keep implants in place. — There is a possibility of uterine contractions, and analgesics may be needed. — Maintain fluid intake of 2500 ml. — Review radiation safety precautions for visitors/family. — Monitor for symptoms of radiation syndrome: nausea, vomiting, anorexia, and malaise. — Post-treatment: foul-smelling vaginal discharge is possible; douche at home to control odor; slight vaginal bleeding may continue for several months. — Possible need for vaginal dilation due to stenosis. — Long-handled forceps may be needed in case of dislodgement.	If the patient knows what to expect, anxiety can be reduced, and the patient will be better equipped to make decisions and is more likely to be compliant.
Teach patient and family about external radiation: — Method of action — Course/duration of treatment is usually five treatments each week for 4 to 6 weeks — Skin changes to note include redness, sloughing, and tenderness	Radiation is used with ovarian cancer when surgery is not an option or in the presence of metastasis, and the patient needs to be informed of what to expect. The radiated skin is sensitive, and ointments, creams, ultraviolet rays, and rubbing, etc., may cause

(continues)

(continued)

INTERVENTIONS	RATIONALES
— Skin care: do not apply soap, ointments, lotions, creams, or powder to area. Do not rub, scrub, or scratch the area; do not try to wash off markings; avoid exposing the treated area to the sun during the treatment and for 1 year following treatments — Wear loose-fitting clothes; panties may need to be avoided due to risk of irritation — Control fatigue through energy conservation and intake of high-energy foods rich in vitamin C, protein, and iron; take a nap each day, especially after treatment	burning, skin sloughing, and interfere with radiation. The patient must know how to protect the skin from impairment; knowing what to expect in terms of radiation helps the patient to be more compliant and feel more in control.
Teach patient and family about chemotherapy and its effects: — Method of action — Specific agents used for treatment — Alopecia: assist the patient to plan for hair loss by investigating the purchase of wigs or having hair cut short and using hair for a specially made wig before alopecia; find a resource that could teach patient how to prepare fashionable head wraps — Nausea/vomiting: teach to use anti-emetics before meals prophylactically; avoid foods with strong odors, and in the hospital setting have lids removed from trays outside the room (when lids are removed from food trays, the smell is often overwhelming to the GI system and causes nausea); attempt frequent small meals, avoiding spicy foods — Care of access sites: prevent infection by use of aseptic techniques and procedures according to agency protocol — Control of fatigue: balance rest and activity, and on chemotherapy days a designated nap time should be scheduled	Knowledge of what to expect helps the patient cope with untoward side effects and better equips her to take responsibility for managing the illness and engage in self-care.
— Prevention of infection: chemotherapy causes a depression of white blood cells (WBCs), predisposing the patient to infection; avoid people with infections and large crowds; practice good hand hygiene; know WBC counts	
Teach the patient and family regarding post-operative hysterectomy care if this is the treatment option (see nursing care plan "Hysterectomy").	Hysterectomy is often the first treatment implemented, especially in early stage I ovarian cancer in the absence of metastasis; the patient will need to know post-operative care requirements.
Provide the patient and family with information on hospice and other community service agencies, such as the American Cancer Society.	These agencies can provide psychological support as well as resources to the patient and family.
Assess the patient and family's understanding of all teaching by encouraging them to repeat information and ask questions as needed.	This allows the nurse to hear in the patient's own words what was taught and makes it easier to know what information may need to be reinforced.
Establish that the patient has the resources required to be compliant.	If needed resources such as finances and transportation to follow-up appointments are not available, the patient cannot be compliant; the nurse will need to make necessary referrals.

NIC　*Learning readiness enhancement*
Learning facilitation
Teaching: Disease process
Teaching: Prescribed medication
Teaching: Procedure/treatment

Evaluation

Evaluate the degree to which the patient has achieved the outcome criteria relevant to the teaching sessions. The patient should verbalize an understanding of the content presented by repeating the information, particularly the disease process, treatment options, and medications for pain or nausea. The nurse must determine if the patient is capable of being compliant with the recommended regimen. If further teaching is required at time of discharge, the appropriate referrals should be made to continue education.

Community/Home Care

The patient will need to implement the prescribed regimen in the home setting, and the amount of time that the patient will require visitation or follow-up will depend on the type of treatment employed. The success of this implementation will depend on the degree to which the patient has received detailed teaching and has subsequently understood and internalized it. At home, the patient will likely experience fatigue following any of the treatments, but especially with radiation or chemotherapy treatments. If chemotherapy is employed, hair loss, nausea, and vomiting may also occur because of treatments. For the patient receiving chemotherapy, it is important to monitor the patient's weight if the patient is experiencing nausea and vomiting. An inexpensive scale can be placed in the bathroom or bedroom so that the patient can weigh herself and report weight to the health care provider. Health care providers or dieticians can assist the patient to prepare a diet that is both nutritional and easy to digest. As the disease progresses, nutrition becomes more of a problem due to the increasing size of the tumor and presence of ascites that places pressure on abdominal contents. Alternate means of receiving nutrition may need to be employed with the help of in-home nurses (see nursing diagnosis "Imbalanced Nutrition: Less than Body Requirements"). If the patient is receiving external radiation therapy, she will need to return to an outpatient facility. External radiation therapy patients will need to be monitored for ability to care for skin properly to prevent further tissue destruction. The patient treated with internal radiation will need to continue perineal hygiene for several weeks at home, as the vaginal discharge may continue, requiring daily douches. Of critical importance at home for the woman who has had internal radiation is the likelihood of vaginal stenosis requiring dilation several times a week. If not performed, the vagina may become so stenosed that examination and sexual intercourse may become virtually impossible. Most sources recommend that if the woman has a sexual partner that dilation be achieved through regular sexual intercourse, however in the presence of advanced disease, fatigue, and pain, this may not be an option. For the patient treated by surgical intervention alone, teaching regarding wound care and activity restrictions should be undertaken with reinforcement by a visiting nurse (see nursing care plan "Hysterectomy"). Because the patient is seen on a regular basis for general follow-up for post-operative care, for chemotherapy, or for radiation therapy, health care providers can determine if further teaching or reinforcement is required. Pain control following hysterectomy is achieved with mild narcotics but will be a bigger part of home care in the later stages of the disease if a cure was not effected with surgery, and will require frequent follow-up to ensure patient satisfaction (see nursing diagnosis "Acute Pain"). Those health care workers providing follow-up care need to ensure that the family and patient understand that dependence on medication should not be a concern for the cancer patient and that comfort is the ultimate goal.

Documentation

Document the specific content taught and the titles of any printed documents given to the patient. Include in the chart the patient's degree of understanding of the content and the methods used to evaluate learning. An assessment of the patient's ability to be compliant with the regimen in terms of radiation, chemotherapy, or follow-up should be made in the chart, with indicators of referrals made. Any areas that need to be reinforced should be documented to ensure appropriate follow-up. If family members are present for the teaching sessions, document this in the chart.

NURSING DIAGNOSIS 2

ANTICIPATORY GRIEVING

Related to:

Fear

Diagnosis of ovarian cancer

Uncertain stage of disease at time of diagnosis

Poor prognosis

Surgery (hysterectomy)

Defining Characteristics:

Expressions of distress

Expressions of fear

Restlessness

Verbalizes anxiety

Crying

Goal:

The patient expresses grief and identifies coping strategies.

Outcome Criteria

✔ The patient identifies and uses one coping mechanism.

✔ The patient verbalizes feelings, fears, and concerns regarding the diagnosis of ovarian cancer.

✔ The patient reports being less anxious and demonstrates no outward signs of anxiety such as restlessness or agitation.

NOC *Grief resolution*
Anxiety control
Comfort level
Coping

INTERVENTIONS	RATIONALES
Assess level of anxiety (mild, moderate, severe); have patient rate on a scale of 1 to 10, with 10 being the greatest.	Gives the nurse a better perception of extent of the anxiety.
Assess the patient to determine her feelings regarding the diagnosis of ovarian cancer and the prognosis, and support her as appropriate.	Assisting the patient to deal with the diagnosis and prognosis will enhance her ability to cope with serious illness.
Encourage the patient to verbalize feelings, fears, or concerns, and listen attentively to any expressions of grief.	Verbalization of feelings and fears is a first step to healthy grieving and contributes to dealing with concerns; attentiveness relays empathy to the patient.
Keep the patient informed of all planned therapeutic interventions, including information about diagnostic tests, and answer any questions.	Keeping the patient informed assists her to make informed decisions and allays anxiety.
Engage the patient and family in open dialogue regarding options for treatments and care.	Discussion of care options allows the patient to be more in control, giving her a sense of empowerment that may assist with coping with the disease and its poor prognosis.
Use a calm, reassuring manner with the patient.	Communicating in a calm, straightforward manner may help to relieve anxiety and gives the patient a sense of well-being.
Provide privacy for the patient so that she can grieve privately as she adapts to the diagnosis.	Each person's response to a diagnosis of ovarian cancer is unique; privacy gives the patient the opportunity to grieve in her own way (crying, moaning, praying, expressions of anger, talking to loved ones, etc.) without fear of interruptions; this quiet alone time may promote a sense of comfort.
Seek spiritual consult as needed or requested by the patient and/or family.	Meeting the patient's spiritual needs helps her to deal with fears through use of spiritual or religious rituals.
Recognize the role of culture in a patient's grief process and method of coping with illness and the acceptability of verbalizing fears and concerns.	Culture often dictates how a person copes, and the nurse must recognize this in order to support the patient in identifying successful coping strategies.
Discuss with the family/patient and investigate the need for services of home health agencies or support services such as those provided by hospice and the American Cancer Society when at home later in the disease.	As the disease progresses, the patient and family may require services of these groups for nursing care, durable medical supplies, psychological support, and assistance with pain control. Having these discussions and planning ahead prevents any delays in obtaining services when needed and can reduce anxiety that accompanies decision making at a time of crisis.
If the patient has the energy, time, and desire, encourage her to document feelings in a diary; if the patient has young children, she can also leave messages for them via a tape recording or written words.	These strategies assist the patient to express herself in an acceptable manner when she may feel uncomfortable talking to others; audio recordings or written messages for children leave a legacy and may provide comfort for the patient.

NIC *Grief work facilitation*
Active listening
Coping enhancement
Emotional support
Spiritual support

Evaluation

Evaluate the extent to which the outcome criteria have been achieved. The patient should be assessed for behaviors that would indicate adjustment to the diagnosis of ovarian cancer. The prognosis for ovarian cancer is poor, so the patient may experience anticipatory grieving and extreme anxiety shortly after diagnosis as she attempts to deal with the unknown and the possibility of death. The patient should verbalize fears and concerns and be able to identify one way to cope with the diagnosis of cancer. The extent to which the patient displays appropriate coping behaviors should be noted. If the patient is unable to talk about the diagnosis and communicate concerns, the nurse should explore further new interventions to assist the patient.

Community/Home Care

Nurses should assess which coping mechanisms work for the patient and encourage their use by the patient at home. Even for those patients whose disease was detected early and treated surgically, problems with anticipatory grieving and anxiety may continue for a long period of time. At least one follow-up visit by a health care provider should be initiated to assess for ineffective coping. The patient should be encouraged to identify coping strategies that have been successful in the past and prompted to use those regularly. Anxiety regarding prognosis usually continues due to the poor prognosis with ovarian cancer and is more pronounced for those patients for whom the disease was detected in the late stages. Coping through use of support from an outside source such as a hospice or a nurse therapist may be required. Monitor for extreme withdrawal, isolation, and depression, and report any symptoms to the physician. For many patients and families, spiritual/religious rituals provide a means of coping with difficult, stressful situations, especially the anticipated loss of life. The patient's culture may dictate how she copes and/or grieves, and with whom she shares this process. It is crucial that the nurse and family support the patient as needed to foster a healthy psychological state, recognizing that anger and denial are common. As the disease progresses, the patient may require new strategies for coping with the disease and the anticipated loss of life. Even though friends and family intend well with their presence, the patient may benefit from quiet periods of meditation and solitude during the day. The patient should be encouraged to participate in activities that have brought her joy in the past for as long as health permits. These activities often can serve as a distraction and provide mental peace. Support to long-term caregivers will be important, remembering that they too need to be supported in a grief process. Hospice can play an important role in the home situation through provision of counselors, chaplains, and in-home care providers. If questions should arise at home regarding the patient's health status or prescribed regimen, the patient should have a means of contact with a health care provider for answers.

Documentation

The degree to which the patient has demonstrated effective coping and decreased anxiety should be documented in the patient record. A rating system provides an objective way to relay to others the extent of the anxiety or expressions of fear. Document whether the patient is able to discuss feelings regarding a diagnosis of ovarian cancer. Chart the patient's verbalizations as she states them and include in the record coping mechanisms utilized by the patient. Document findings from an assessment of the patient's psychological state, indicating whether there is depression, anger, crying, sadness, etc. Document referrals to hospice or religious leaders.

NURSING DIAGNOSIS 3

ACUTE PAIN

Related to:

Presence of ovarian tumor

Pressure on abdominal contents

Metastasis of cancer to other sites

Defining Characteristics:

Facial grimace

Complaints of pain in abdomen or pelvic area, lower back pain

Goal:

Pain control is achieved.

Outcome Criteria

✔ The patient will verbalize that pain is reduced or relieved 1 hour after interventions.

✔ The patient reports satisfaction with pain management measures.

 NOC *Pain level*

Pain control

Comfort level

Medication response

INTERVENTIONS	RATIONALES
Complete a pain assessment by noting location and quality of pain and have the patient rate pain for intensity using a pain rating scale.	Gives a more objective assessment of the pain intensity.
Administer analgesics, as ordered (varies with stage of disease); late in the disease narcotics such as morphine may be required.	Provides pain relief and decreases anxiety.
Teach appropriate non-pharmacological measures for pain relief such as relaxation techniques, back massage, guided imagery, and music, and encourage their use.	Helps to enhance effects of pharmacological interventions.
Assess effectiveness of interventions to relieve pain.	Helps to determine interventions have been effective in relieving pain or if new strategies need to be employed.
Establish a quiet environment.	Helps to enhance effects of analgesics.
If abdominal hysterectomy has been performed, implement strategies to reduce post-operative pain, including splinting abdomen when moving.	Supports incisional site and prevents stress on operative area.

 NIC *Pain management*
          Analgesic administration
          Anxiety reduction

Evaluation

The patient is able to report that the pain has been relieved or alleviated following interventions. Based on pain rating scales the patient's pain has decreased. The degree to which the patient is able to assist in the management of the pain through anxiety reduction and relaxation techniques is assessed. The patient reports being satisfied with pain control efforts.

Community/Home Care

Home care required for the management of pain will depend on the type of treatments implemented and the stage of the cancer. For the patient who is being treated with chemotherapy and radiation, the problem will probably become more pronounced as the disease progresses, as these treatments only provide

tumor shrinkage and slowing of growth. Initially, pain medications may be given by mouth to obtain satisfactory pain control. However, in the later stages, pain control may require the services of hospice or a home nurse when more invasive means of administering narcotics may be needed for control. If injectable medications are to be used, a family member or significant other who can learn the technique for administering the medication will need to be identified. In some instances, ethical conflicts may arise as the family wants the patient to be alert but successful pain control creates a lethargic, drowsy state. Ineffective in-home management of pain may cause undue emotional stress for the patient and family, necessitating hospitalization. Teaching the patient how to utilize non-pharmacological measures to enhance the effects of analgesics will be crucial to obtaining satisfactory outcomes. For the patient who has had surgery, the pain may be temporary, subsiding as the wound heals. Assessing pain control is an important facet of follow-up care by the home health nurse, hospice, or other health care worker, and should include the patient's ability to purchase prescribed analgesics.

Documentation

Document in the patient's own words the description of the pain and rating of the level of pain. Chart the patient's responses to all interventions, indicating what is effective for pain control and what is not. Those interventions that are ineffective should be removed from the plan of care. Include in the documentation all assessments made relevant to the reproductive system and pain control. All teaching should be indicated in the patient record with an indication of the patient's level of understanding. Also document in the chart the patient's and family's indication of expectations for pain control.

NURSING DIAGNOSIS 4

 IMBALANCED NUTRITION: LESS THAN BODY REQUIREMENTS

Related to:

Anorexia

Feeling of fullness due to ascites or pressure from tumor

Defining Characteristics:

Reports of decreased appetite

Abdominal distention

Reports feeling full

Loss of weight

Eats little of food served

Goal:

Adequate dietary/fluid intake is maintained.

Outcome Criteria

✔ The patient does not lose weight.

✔ The patient consumes 50 percent of food served.

✔ The patient tolerates meals without nausea, vomiting, diarrhea, and dyspepsia.

NOC *Nutritional status: Food and fluid intake*

Nutritional status: Nutrient intake

Oral hygiene

INTERVENTIONS	RATIONALES
Assess laboratory results: albumin, electrolytes, glucose, total protein, and iron.	These give indications of nutritional status.
Assess the patient for ability to eat/drink, ability to retain intake, feeling of fullness after limited intake, nausea, and indigestion.	Helps to identify specific problems the patient is experiencing and to intervene accordingly.
Weigh patient and monitor weight daily or weekly when at home.	Establishes a baseline for comparison and as patient progresses allows for early intervention for nutritional deficits.
Monitor intake and output; document according to agency protocol.	Helps to assure adequate hydration, which is needed for wound healing.
Consider dietician consult to ascertain the patient's ability to take in enough food to meet caloric demand and to determine the patient likes, dislikes, and preferences within the prescribed diet with consideration to cultural or religious preferences.	For patients who have cancer, especially in later stages, weight loss is common for a variety of reasons; sufficient caloric intake is necessary to prevent wasting if possible, and the patient will be more likely to consume foods that she likes; utilization of the dietician will be useful in determining what the patient needs.
Encourage the patient to take small frequent meals.	Food may be more tolerable in small portions, and smaller portions require less energy for consumption. Frequently the patient with ovarian cancer complains of feeling full, and smaller meals may prevent this discomfort.
Allow adequate time for meals.	The patient may take longer to eat due to lack of energy and interest in foods.
Give foods that are rich in protein, vitamin C, and iron.	These foods promote healing and are energy-rich foods.
Create a pleasant environment for meals.	The environment can enhance the patient's willingness to eat.
Provide oral/mouth care before meals.	A fresh mouth makes food taste better.
Open containers away from the patient or outside door.	Removing lids from containers at the bedside releases a strong aroma that can cause nausea, especially in patients receiving chemotherapy; nausea would prevent the patient from eating.
Give anti-emetics, as ordered, 30 minutes before meals.	Helps to prevent nausea and vomiting.
Monitor for ascites (measure abdominal girth) and implement strategies to relieve any ascites (give diuretics, assist with paracentesis if required, and assist to assume Fowler's position).	Ascites may occur in later stages of ovarian cancer and can cause pressure on abdominal cavity and thoracic cavity, which causes patient to have a sense of fullness before adequate intake is achieved.

NIC *Nutritional monitoring*

Nutritional management

Evaluation

The patient's nutritional state is stable, and the patient has a satisfactory method for nutrient intake. Assess the patient's weight and determine that the patient is not losing weight. The patient should be ingesting at least 50 percent of food served and should be tolerating food without nausea, vomiting, or diarrhea. Laboratory results should reveal a normal albumin level as well as total protein and electrolytes. Prior to discharge, the patient should be able to eat and drink without pain or difficulty and be able to verbalize methods to maintain nutrition in the home.

Community/Home Care

Difficulties eating and drinking may continue at home for the patient who has ovarian cancer. The patient will need to continue efforts to ingest enough food and nutrients to meet the metabolic demands of healing. A home nurse needs to monitor the patient's nutritional status on a regular basis to detect excessive weight loss and to note reports of decreased intake due to feelings of fullness, pain, anxiety, fatigue, or nausea/vomiting. The family can assist the patient by preparing foods that are easy to chew and swallow, that the patient likes, and that also have nutritional value. The patient needs encouragement to eat and at home may lose interest in eating due to depression or because of fatigue. The patient may never return to the pre-disease nutritional state, and as the disease progresses the patient may completely refrain from eating or simply become unable to eat. Because in most cultures food is considered a basic need for all people, family members may experience some frustration and emotional conflict, as they have no means to provide food to the patient. Placement of enteral feeding tubes or intravenous (IV) feeding via total parenteral nutrition (TPN) are usually seen as futile and are not usually employed. Support for the family and patient will be important at this time to assist in implementing coping strategies and dealing with impending death.

Documentation

The patient's tolerance to food and fluid intake is documented as part of an overall assessment. Document any difficulty that the patient experiences during meals, particularly pain, feeling full, nausea and/or vomiting, and any interventions implemented to address these difficulties. Record intake and output according to agency protocol, being sure to document the percentage of food consumed. If the patient verbalizes concerns, include this in the chart. Chart the patient's weight daily. Always document any referrals made to other disciplines, particularly the dietician.

CHAPTER 11.120

PELVIC INFLAMMATORY DISEASE (PID)

GENERAL INFORMATION

Pelvic inflammatory disease (PID) is an infection of one or more of the pelvic organs or structures, including the fallopian tubes, the ovaries, the cervix, the uterus, or the pelvic peritoneum, and is most commonly caused by chlamydia. Other common causative organisms are gonococci and streptococci. These bacteria migrate up the cervical canal to the fallopian tubes where they spread to other organs in the pelvis via the lymphatic system or through direct contact with mucosa. The invading organisms may enter during sexual intercourse, following surgery involving the reproductive organs, after abortions, and after giving birth. Clinical manifestations include the most common complaint of lower abdominal pain that may be described on a continuum from mild to severe. The other symptoms include pain with intercourse, pain when walking, fever, dysuria, and large amounts of a purulent, foul-smelling discharge. Risk factors for the development of PID include placement of intrauterine devices, multiple sex partners, frequent use of vaginal douches, and a history of sexually transmitted diseases (STDs).

NURSING DIAGNOSIS 1

INFECTION (ACTUAL)*

Related to:

Bacterial invasion of reproductive organs

Defining Characteristics:

Lower abdominal pain

Fever

Chills

Elevated white blood cell counts

Positive cultures of vaginal discharge

Purulent drainage

Goal:

The patient's infection is resolved.

There are no further complications from infection.

Outcome Criteria

✔ The patient will be afebrile.

✔ The patient experiences no chills.

✔ White blood cell (WBC) counts will return to normal.

✔ The patient will have negative cultures.

✔ The patient's vaginal discharge will be alleviated.

NOC *Infection severity*
Knowledge: Infection control

INTERVENTIONS	RATIONALES
Monitor diagnostic studies: complete blood count (CBC), blood culture, culture and gram stain of genital/vaginal/cervical tract, and diagnostic laparoscopic surgery.	Positive cultures provide evidence for the specific organism that caused PID; most cases of PID are caused by chlamydia or gonococci; CBC will reveal elevated WBCs; laparoscopic surgery can visualize the pelvic structures and obtain specimens from any abscesses.
Monitor temperature every 4 hours and assess for chills.	Establishes a baseline and monitors response to treatment.
Institute measures to reduce temperature: administer antipyretics as ordered, apply cooling blanket, and give a tepid sponge bath.	Reduce temperature and decrease metabolic demands of the body.
Administer antibiotics as ordered; monitor for and teach patient to monitor for side effects; and instruct patient on need to complete entire regimen. Broad-spectrum	These medications will resolve the infection through bacteriocidal and bacteriostatic activities. For the patient treated as an outpatient, oral antibiotic therapy usually lasts for 14 days.

(continues)

(continued)

INTERVENTIONS	RATIONALES
antibiotics are given until culture results are obtained (e.g., doxycycline, cefoxitin, clindamycin, erythromycin, ofloxacin, metronidazole, and Rocephin®).	Hospitalized patients remain on intravenous (IV) antibiotics until clinical improvement is demonstrated and there is no abdominal pain for 24 hours. Monitoring for side effects allows for dosage adjustment and prevention of complications.
Administer analgesics, as ordered.	Helps to reduce or alleviate pain (see nursing diagnosis "Acute Pain").
For hospitalized patients, establish IV access and administer fluids as ordered; for all patients, encourage oral intake of fluids.	IV access is required for administration of antibiotics, and fluids are needed to prevent dehydration from fevers.
Have patient remain on bedrest in a semi-Fowler's position.	This assists with drainage of pelvic area, which prevents abscess development.
Avoid tub or sitz baths, use of tampons, and sexual activity until infection is completely treated.	Helps to prevent re-infection.
Cleanse perineal area after each voiding or bowel movement.	Minimizes bacteria count.
Assist with removal of intrauterine devices (IUDs), if present.	IUDs can be the source of PID and should be removed during treatment.
Give a diet high in calories and rich in iron, protein, and vitamin C.	Fatigue is common, and these measures will give the patient needed nutrients for energy and healing; iron-rich foods increase oxygen-carrying capacity of the blood.
Complete a sexual history and monitor for sexual promiscuity and multiple/ frequent sexual partners.	Sexual promiscuity and multiple partners predisposes a patient to PID; information is required to provide counseling on disease prevention.
Be supportive of the patient and significant other.	Because PID is often caused by sexually transmitted diseases, the patient may be embarrassed about having the disease and will need emotional, nonjudgmental support from caregivers.
Teach the patient the signs and symptoms of PID: lower abdominal or pelvic pain; pain with sexual activity; purulent, foul-smelling vaginal discharge; elevated temperature; and malaise.	PID often reoccurs, and the patient needs to know what symptoms may signal re-infection.

NIC *Infection control*
Infection protection

Evaluation

Determine the extent to which the patient has achieved the expected outcomes. The patient should become afebrile and have no chills, and there should be no signs or symptoms of infection. In particular, the patient should have no abdominal tenderness or pain, and vaginal discharge should decrease or be absent. The patient should verbalize an understanding of the infectious process of PID and treatment measures being implemented with attention to prevention.

Community/Home Care

PID can be a serious illness that could lead to sepsis. Antibiotics are continued after the patient is at home, and monitoring for side effects will be necessary. Because many patients discontinue taking antibiotics when symptoms abate, it is crucial that the patient understand the need to take the medication for the full prescribed period. A chart that outlines the dosing schedule and has bright reminders attached that offer a reminder to continue taking medication may serve as motivation to adhere to the regimen. Recurrence is a concern, especially if the patient resumes sexual activity prematurely. Health care providers should provide the patient with information on prevention of PID in the future (see nursing diagnosis "Deficient Knowledge") and how to recognize the early signs of infection. Because a majority of patients who experience PID are infected with chlamydia or gonococci, sexual activity needs to be discussed with the patient. Notification of sexual partners should be undertaken, and for reportable cases of sexually transmitted diseases, assistance of the local health department may be needed. For many patients, whether treated at home or in a hospital, a feeling of malaise may linger for a period of time following completion of antibiotic therapy. Continued attention to nutrition is required so that the patient returns to a normal state of energy. Follow-up care is required to reinforce teachings regarding sexual activity and medications, and to ensure that the disease has been successfully treated.

Documentation

Document the findings from a comprehensive assessment with special attention to the reproductive system. Chart the amount, color, and odor of any vaginal discharge in the patient record as well as patient-specific complaints such as abdominal or pelvic pain, fatigue, malaise, anorexia, chills, and vital signs. Always chart therapeutic interventions implemented and the patient's specific responses to those interventions. All teaching and referrals are documented in the patient's record.

NURSING DIAGNOSIS 2

 ### ACUTE PAIN

Related to:

Inflammation and infection of reproductive organs

Defining Characteristics:

Complains of pelvic or abdominal pain

Holds abdomen

Complains of pain when walking

Dyspareunia

Grimacing when moving

Goal:

Pain control is achieved.

Outcome Criteria

✔ The patient will verbalize that pain is reduced or relieved 1 hour after interventions.

✔ The patient reports an ability to move and walk without pain.

NOC *Pain level*

Pain control

Comfort level

Medication response

INTERVENTIONS	RATIONALES
Have the patient identify location and quality of the pain, and aggravating factors, and rate pain for intensity using a pain rating scale.	Gives a more objective assessment of the pain intensity; pain is usually located in the lower abdominal area and usually occurs with movement.
Monitor for nonverbal indicators of pain, such as difficulty	Establishes a baseline and gives indicators of severity of disease.
ambulating, hunching over, small steps, hands on lower abdomen, and slow movement.	
Administer analgesics, as ordered.	Helps to provide pain relief and decrease anxiety.
Apply heat to abdomen.	Improves circulation and decreases pain.
Teach appropriate relaxation techniques and other distraction techniques, such as guided imagery and music.	Enhances effects of pharmacological interventions.
Encourage "pelvic rest."	The patient should refrain from sexual activity or pelvic exams until the infection/inflammation is resolved.
Assess effectiveness of interventions to relieve pain.	Helps to determine interventions have been effective in relieving pain or if new strategies need to be employed.
Establish a quiet environment.	Helps to enhance effects of analgesics.

NIC *Pain management*

Analgesic administration

Anxiety reduction

Evaluation

The patient is able to report that the pain has been relieved or alleviated following interventions. Based on pain rating scales, the patient's pain has decreased. The absence of abdominal pain or tenderness should be noted. The patient should be able to ambulate without pelvic or abdominal pain.

Community/Home Care

Home care required for the management of pain is typically minimal. Once the infection has been controlled with antibiotics, the pain should start to subside and require only mild analgesics. If pain persists, the patient should return to a health care provider to determine if the infectious process has worsened, possibly with the development of abscesses. Teaching the patient how to utilize non-pharmacological measures to enhance the effects of analgesics will be crucial to obtaining satisfactory outcomes. Assessing pain control is an important facet of follow-up care provided by the health care worker.

Documentation

Document in the patient's own words the location of the pain, the description of the pain, and rating of the level of pain. Include factors that contribute to pain, such as ambulation. Chart the patient's responses to all interventions that have been employed. Document analgesic medication on medication administration records according to agency guidelines. If pain control has not been achieved, indicate necessary revisions in the planned interventions.

NURSING DIAGNOSIS 3

 ### DEFICIENT KNOWLEDGE

Related to:

New onset of disease

Lack of knowledge about disease, therapeutic interventions, prevention

Limited knowledge regarding STDs

Defining Characteristics:

Asks many questions

Has misconceptions regarding disease

Has no questions

Goal:

The patient verbalizes an understanding of disease and required regimen.

Outcome Criteria

✔ The patient verbalizes willingness and desires to learn the necessary information.

✔ The patient verbalizes an understanding of the disease process of PID.

✔ The patient verbalizes an understanding of the prescribed therapeutic interventions, and the prevention and control of infection.

NOC *Knowledge: Disease process*
Knowledge: Health behavior
Treatment behavior:
Illness or injury

INTERVENTIONS	RATIONALES
Assess the patient's readiness to learn (motivation, cognitive level, and physiological status).	The patient must be motivated to learn, have the ability to learn, and be free of distractions from learning, such as pain and emotional distress.
Assess what the patient already knows.	The patient may have some knowledge about PID, and teaching should begin with what the patient already knows.
Create a quiet environment conducive to learning.	Environmental noise can prevent the learner from focusing on what is being taught.
Teach incrementally, starting with simple concepts first, and move to more complex concepts.	The patient will learn and retain knowledge better when information is presented in small segments.
Teach the patient and family about PID: — Pathophysiology — Complications: infertility, scarring of fallopian tubes, adhesions — Treatment with antibiotics: taking complete course of antibiotics; failure to do so will prevent complete resolution of infection and make re-infection likely — Signs of improvement — Importance of follow-up care	Understanding of pathophysiology, prescribed sexual restriction, and medication regime assists the patient with understanding the rationale for therapeutic interventions and helps prevent complications; the patient needs to understand the possible complications and the impact on reproduction; follow-up care is required to ensure that the infection is cured and to assess for complications.
Provide information regarding sexuality issues: — Avoid sexual intercourse until advised by physician that infection is eliminated. — Avoid use of tampons until infection is resolved. — Practice safe sex including use of condoms to protect against disease transmission. — Refrain from use of IUDs. — During menses, change pads or tampons frequently (every 2 to 3 hours). — Discuss infection with sexual partner.	Sexual intercourse and tampons can cause re-infection of the pelvic area; a large number of cases of PID are attributed to STDs, so the patient needs to discuss sexual health with partner to prevent re-infection; good hygiene practices, such as pad and tampon changes, minimize bacteria count; menstrual discharge can provide a means for entry of microorganisms into pelvic cavity.
Offer printed materials and other audiovisual aides.	Printed and audiovisual aides enhance learning; printed materials can serve as a reference later.

INTERVENTIONS	RATIONALES
Evaluate the patient's understanding of all content covered by asking questions.	Helps to identify areas that require further teaching and to ensure that the patient has enough information to ensure compliance.

NIC *Teaching: Safe sex*
Fertility preservation
Teaching: Individual

Evaluation

The patient is able to repeat the information taught and asks appropriate questions about PID, its treatment, and possible complications. Prior to exiting the health care system (inpatient or outpatient), the patient should verbalize a willingness to comply with prescribed therapies of antibiotics, pelvic rest, and return for follow-up. The patient knows the signs and symptoms of infection and reasons to return to the health care provider.

Community/Home Care

Knowledge deficits need to be identified early so that the patient can be better prepared for self-care. For many patients, treatment of PID does not require hospitalization, but for all patients the cornerstone of treatment is antibiotic therapy and prevention of transmission of infection. Oral antibiotics may be required for 14 days, increasing the likelihood of noncompliance with the entire prescribed regimen. It is important that the patient understand that this practice raises the risk of continued infection with the possibility of long-term complications due to scarring of the reproductive organs. Home visits by a nurse are not generally required, but some follow-up with a health care provider is warranted to ensure that the patient has understood the teaching and completed the medications, and that the symptoms have abated. Teaching and discussions centered on safe sex practices and prevention of future infections are important.

Documentation

Include documentation of the teaching session in the patient record, including the specific content taught and methodologies used. Document the patient's verbalization of understanding of the content, particularly the information relevant to antibiotic therapy and sexual activity. If the patient verbalizes concerns or indicates an inability to be compliant, document this in the record. Specify what areas need reinforcement or further teaching. Always include the titles of any printed literature given to the patient and family.

CHAPTER 11.121

PROSTATE CANCER

GENERAL INFORMATION

Cancer of the prostate gland is the most common cancer in American men and is the second leading cause of cancer deaths. Cancers of the prostate gland are usually adenocarcinoma and typically begin in outer peripheral tissue of the gland that has atrophied. Its exact etiology is unknown, but the development of prostate cancer has been linked to hormonal changes, particularly the change in androgen level that accompanies aging, and men that have been castrated do not get prostate cancer. In the early stages, the patient may be asymptomatic, but as the disease progresses, the patient experiences symptoms similar to those of benign prostatic hypertrophy (BPH), including decreased force of the urinary stream, frequency, nocturia, hematuria, and dysuria. The patient's initial symptom may be bone pain, particularly hip and back pain, which indicates early metastasis. Upon digital rectal exam of the prostate gland a hard, firm nodule or other abnormality of the prostate is felt. The most common complication is urinary tract/urethral obstruction due to the tumor exerting pressure on the urethra, causing urinary retention. Treatment for prostate cancer is based on the stage of the tumor and the symptoms of the patient. In many instances, treatment may be conservative because the tumor is slow-growing, and the patient may have a low life expectancy and be a high surgical risk. The three approaches to treatment are surgical intervention, drug therapy (hormonal, chemotherapy), and radiation therapy. African American men have a higher incidence of prostate cancer (3 times that of other groups), are more likely to be diagnosed later in the disease, and have a mortality rate twice that of men from other ethnic groups.

NURSING DIAGNOSIS 1

URINARY RETENTION

Related to:

Adenocarcinoma in the prostate gland causing mechanical obstruction

Defining Characteristics:

Hematuria

Dysuria

Stop-and-start urination

Incomplete bladder emptying

Distended bladder

Goal:

The patient is able to void without difficulty.

Outcome Criteria

✔ The patient will have no bladder distention/urinary retention.

✔ The patient will void sufficient amounts with each voiding (200 cc).

✔ The patient will implement strategies to reduce symptoms of impaired urinary elimination.

NOC *Urinary elimination*
Symptom control

INTERVENTIONS	RATIONALES
Assess the patient for ability to void, firm, full bladder on palpation, history of urinary tract infections (UTIs), urinating in dribbles, difficulty in starting	These are symptoms of obstruction and prostate cancer and can be used to establish a baseline. These symptoms are caused by pressure on the

INTERVENTIONS	RATIONALES
to void, urinary frequency, urinary urgency, and nocturia; utilize the American Urological Association (AUA) Symptom Score Tool to assess severity of symptoms.	bladder and around the urethra; this tool is used to determine how severe the symptoms are and provides subjective data.
Monitor results of diagnostic tests: prostate-specific antigen (PSA) levels, blood urea nitrogen (BUN), creatinine, urinalysis, urine culture and sensitivity, complete blood count (CBC), ultrasound (transrectal), cystogram/cystourethroscopy, intravenous pylegram (IVP), transrectal ultrasonography (TRUS), computed tomography (CT) scan and MRI, tissue biopsy, and cystometry.	Total PSA will be elevated; PSA can be divided into bound and free levels. A low percent of free PSA with a total PSA of 4 tends to imply prostate cancer; test of renal function (BUN, creatinine) are done to determine if there is any alteration in kidney function due to obstruction or retention; CBC elevations, urine culture and sensitivity, as well as urinalysis are used to monitor for the presence of UTI, which could occur due to retention; transrectal ultrasound is capable of determining the size of the prostate and to differentiate BPH from prostate cancer; cystourethroscopy is used to decide if there is outflow obstruction and to note any alterations in the bladder; IVP can be used to determine any effect on urinary structures particularly to visualize distended ureters; TRUS uses an instrument inserted into the rectum to send sound waves towards the prostate gland with recording of pictures that would indicate the presence of the tumor; CT scans and MRIs can outline the prostate gland in order to visualize the tumor; tissue biopsy provides conclusive evidence for type of malignant cells; cystometry is used to evaluate all aspects of bladder function and can diagnose prostatic obstruction.
Perform a sexuality assessment: monitor for concerns about sexual relations, worry about libido if disease progresses, concern about ability to have sex as disease progresses, and concern about urinary incontinence during sex.	Patients frequently have some concerns about sexual function, especially following surgical interventions.

Instruct patient to attempt to void every 2 to 3 hours and have patient double void: void, sit on toilet for 3 to 5 minutes, and then void again.	This will assist patient to empty bladder more completely, avoiding urinary retention and bladder distention.
Teach patient to palpate bladder to check for distention.	The patient can detect bladder distention and intervene prior to bladder fully distending and becoming painful, which may result in incontinence and dribbling.
Monitor post-void residual.	Helps to determine the degree of retention with each voiding.
Administer luteinizing hormone-releasing hormone agonists (LH-RH) such as Lupron® or Zoladex® as ordered and monitor for side effects; teach patient about annoying side effects and need for injections on a regular basis for an indefinite period of time.	LH-RH agonists can be given intramuscularly or subcutaneously, or Viadur® can be given through an implant; these medications are indicated for the treatment of advanced prostate cancer; they suppress androgen production in the testes and the effects are similar to those of surgical castration (orchiectomy). Side effects include hot flashes, loss of libido, and erectile dysfunction.
Administer androgen receptor agonists (flutamide, nilutamide) as ordered and monitor for side effects of gynecomastia (most common), nausea, vomiting, and diarrhea.	Used for advanced metastatic prostate cancer along with LH-RH agonists; blocks androgen receptors in the cancer cells; prostate cancers are generally androgen dependent for growth, leading to a reduction in the size of the prostate gland and improvement in urine flow.
Implement dietary strategies to control urinary retention and incontinence: avoid alcohol, give or increase zinc and vitamin E in diet, avoid over-the-counter decongestants or other anticholinergic or alpha-agonist medications.	Alcohol exacerbates retention; zinc and vitamin E help reduce nocturnal urinary symptoms; over-the-counter decongestants increase smooth muscle tone of the prostate, which increases urinary retention.
Limit intake of fluids after 6 p.m. and avoid consuming large amounts of fluid at one time.	Fluids after 6 p.m. increase the likelihood of nocturia; drinking large volumes of fluid at one time is more likely to cause retention.
Teach patient/family how to insert straight catheter to empty bladder of urine.	If urinary retention is persistent, the patient may require frequent catheterization. Patient/family will maintain independence if

(continues)

(continued)

INTERVENTIONS	RATIONALES
	they can learn how to safely and effectively insert catheters.
Teach the patient the signs and symptoms of UTI: fever, cloudy urine, foul-smelling urine, and hematuria (see nursing diagnosis "Risk for Infection").	UTI can occur due to retention of the urine in the bladder and subsequent backup or reflux into the ureters and kidney.
Teach the patient and family about disease process and possible options for treatment of prostate cancer: transurethral resection, open prostatectomy, orchiectomy, chemotherapy, and radiation (see nursing diagnoses "Impaired Urinary Elimination: Post-Operative," "Deficient Knowledge," and "Acute Pain").	Knowledge of the disease and its treatment allow the patient to make informed decisions.
Prepare for possible surgical or other invasive procedures according to orders or agency protocol.	Depending upon the stage of the disease and patient symptoms, prostatectomy may be indicated (see nursing diagnosis "Impaired Urinary Elimination: Post-Operative").

NIC *Urinary elimination management*
Urinary retention care

Evaluation

Determine the degree to which the outcomes have been achieved. The patient should report an improvement in symptoms of impaired urinary elimination. Urinary output is sufficient (200 cc each voiding), and bladder distention is absent. The patient will verbalize an understanding of all strategies needed to improve urine output.

Community/Home Care

At home, the patient will need to implement strategies to improve urinary output. A health care provider will need to teach the patient and significant other how to handle symptoms that could be annoying. It is crucial that the patient understands the concepts of urinary retention and bladder distention and is able to relieve this if at all possible. Encourage the patient to keep a record of intake and to make a conscious effort to refrain from drinking after 6 p.m. in order to avoid any nocturia or bladder

filling that would cause retention during the night. Alcohol and over-the-counter cough preparations can cause urinary retention, and the nurse must be implicit in his or her instructions to the patient to avoid these items. The patient at home needs to make a concerted effort to empty the bladder at regular intervals to avoid distention. Intake of fluids throughout the day is needed to maintain bladder tone and prevent urinary stasis. The patient should know how to catheterize himself to relieve retention/ distention and how to measure the output. However, because of the tumor growth in the prostate, the patient may encounter resistance when attempting catheterization and should be informed never to force the catheter, but instead to seek medical attention. Symptoms of urinary obstruction should be known to the patient so that if it occurs, immediate medical attention can be sought to avoid effects to the kidney parenchyma. Follow-up care is needed to assess the progression of the disease and to determine what interventions might be needed.

Documentation

Chart an assessment of the urinary system, including the AUA Symptom Score and any current complaints of altered urinary function. Intake and output should be documented with attention to amount voided with each voiding. If the patient has been catheterized for residual, document this in the patient notes, including amount obtained. Always include in the documentation the interventions implemented and the patient's response. If teaching has been done, document this along with the patient's ability to return demonstrate skills taught and verbalize understanding of information provided.

NURSING DIAGNOSIS 2

 ACUTE PAIN

Related to:

Presence of cancer

Obstruction of urinary elimination

Bladder spasm

Bone metastasis

Defining Characteristics:

Complaint of pain

Grimacing

Pain on urination

Surgical incision

Presence of drainage catheters

Goal:

The patient will state that pain is relieved.

Outcome Criteria

✔ The patient states that pain is decreased or relieved 1 hour after intervention and reports satisfaction with degree of pain control.

✔ The patient verbalizes methods to reduce pain.

NOC *Pain: Disruptive effects*
Pain level
Pain control

INTERVENTIONS	RATIONALES
Assess the patient's pain using a pain rating scale.	Provides a more objective assessment.
Assess or take history regarding time of onset, location, precipitating factors, relieving factors, effect on function, and complaints of pain in new locations.	These will assist in accurate diagnosis and treatment; new pain onset in bones may indicate metastasis; knowing how pain affects function will provide information needed to assist patient with home care needs.
Administer medications specific to the treatment of prostate cancer (androgen receptor agonists, LH-RH agonists, chemotherapeutic agents, etc.).	These medications act to decrease the growth of the pain-causing tumor.
Administer analgesics, as ordered (based on pain and disease severity); narcotics may be required in late disease and in the presence of metastasis.	Helps to decrease pain and discomfort and improve quality of life.
Give all medications on a regular dosing schedule rather than prn.	Provides better relief.
Teach relaxation techniques such as music therapy, massage, distraction, and meditation.	These techniques enhance the effect of analgesics and may decrease reliance on medications for complete relief.
For the post-operative patient, assess all drainage tubes for patency; tube insertion sites and surgical wounds for signs of infection such as purulent	Infections in wounds or at drainage sites can be an additional source of pain, drainage tubes that are kinked or obstructed can cause pain.
drainage; warmth, redness, or edema; implement strategies to prevent infection (see nursing diagnosis "Risk for Infection").	Careful assessment can detect problems early and prevent undue pain.
Post-operatively, implement strategies to decrease bladder spasms as ordered (see nursing diagnosis "Impaired Urinary Elimination: Post-Operative").	Bladder spasms can increase pain sensation at surgical site.
Assess the effectiveness of all interventions, especially medications.	Helps to determine if revisions to the treatment plan are required and to stay attuned to the patient's needs.

NIC *Simple relaxation therapy*
Analgesic administration
Pain management

Evaluation

Assess the degree to which the patient reports pain has been relieved by interventions. For persistent pain, the nurse should investigate additional measures to relieve pain. Determine if the patient is able to verbalize how to reduce pain.

Community/Home Care

The patient with prostatic cancer at home will require monitoring for pain control, especially in the later stages of the disease and if prostatectomy has been performed. Most people associate a diagnosis of cancer with pain, and this often causes anxiety regarding whether pain control can be achieved. The nurse will play a crucial role in pain management, especially as the disease progresses or in the presence of metastasis. These patients may require regular adjustments to the medication regimen to achieve control and a degree of quality of life, defined as being able to be alert and participating in "life" and "functional roles." A combination of pharmacological and non-pharmacological efforts should be recommended for use at home. The services of a visiting nurse should be helpful for patient and family as they attempt to adapt to and cope with the diagnosis and the presence of pain. It is crucial that the nurse be aware of cultural or religious practices that may affect the patient's perception and control of pain. Cultural and religious practices can serve as an adjunct to prescribed analgesics and provide the added benefit of psychosocial comfort for the patient. Later in the disease, the services of hospice may be sought to provide holistic care at home with attention to caring, comfort, and death with dignity (see nursing diagnosis "Ineffective Coping"). If the disease is cured with surgery or hormonal treatment, pain may not be an issue. Surgical incisions often cause some degree of pain for all patients and can be managed with simple oral narcotics. The patient needs to understand the need for rest and schedule rest periods throughout the day to restore the body, as fatigue can intensify perception of pain. Health care providers should follow up to determine if the pain prevents the patient from performing activities of daily living (ADLs). If it does, a change in regimen should be undertaken. The patient will need to understand the side effects of all medication and know what symptoms need to be reported to a health care provider. Because of the progressive nature of cancer, home care providers should be attuned to the possibility of frustration, depression, and altered body image in patients for whom a cure or long-term survival was not achieved with surgery or other therapies.

Documentation

Document all interventions implemented for pain control, including the non-pharmacological ones. Specific patient complaints relevant to pain should be included in the chart, including specific locations of pain, as there may be more than one source. Chart the patient's responses to therapies using a pain rating scale. If at any time a tolerable level of pain cannot be achieved, document this and chart revisions made in the plan of care. Include in the patient record the patient's verbalized satisfaction with pain control.

NURSING DIAGNOSIS 3

 DEFICIENT KNOWLEDGE

Related to:

No previous history of the disease/new onset of disease

Lack of information about the disease and its treatment: surgery, hormonal, radiation

Misinformation

Concern about sexual function

Impaired urinary function

Defining Characteristics:

Asks no questions

Has many questions/concerns

Hesitant or embarrassed to ask questions, state concerns

Defining Characteristics:

Many or no questions

Verbalizes a lack of knowledge/understanding

Goal:

The patient will understand prostate cancer and its treatment.

Outcome Criteria

✔ The patient and significant other verbalize a desire to learn necessary information.

✔ The patient verbalizes an understanding of prostate cancer treatment options (surgery, radiation, and hormonal therapy), including untoward effects of treatment and possible complications such as altered sexual function and urinary incontinence.

✔ The patient or family demonstrates how to care for indwelling urinary catheter (emptying, applying leg bag, cleansing, and proper positioning).

✔ The patient verbalizes an understanding of how to perform pelvic floor exercises.

✔ The patient verbalizes an understanding of pain management.

✔ The patient verbalizes an understanding of follow-up care required and expresses a willingness to comply.

NOC   *Knowledge: Disease process*
        Knowledge: Treatment regimen
        Compliance behavior

INTERVENTIONS	RATIONALES
Assess the patient's current knowledge and ability and readiness to learn.	The nurse needs to ascertain what the patient already knows and build on this; if the patient is not capable of learning or is not ready to learn, teaching will not be effective due to disinterest or inability to understand. The patient may not be ready to learn if in a state of denial or if extremely angry.

INTERVENTIONS	RATIONALES
Start with the simplest information and move to complex information.	Patients can understand simple concepts easily and then can build on those to understand concepts that are more complex.
Collaborate with physician to teach patient and significant others: — Disease process of prostate cancer, staging, and possible treatments (hormonal, surgical, radiation, chemotherapy) — Pain medications used to treat cancer pain including dosage, frequency, side effects, scheduling, and interactions with other medications; answer questions or concerns — Signs and symptoms that would indicate a need to seek health care (poor pain control, new onset of back, hip, or other bone pain, being unable to urinate, fresh bleeding, and chills and fever) — Strategies to prevent infections (urinary and wound) as well as signs and symptoms of UTI and wound infection (see nursing diagnosis "Risk for Infection")	Knowledge of disease, treatments required, and prevention of complications empower the patient to take control and be compliant; back pain is an early sign of cord compression due to metastasis to the spine; being unable to urinate is indicative of obstruction; fresh bleeding indicates hemorrhage; fever, and chills are indicative of infection.
Collaborate with physician and instruct patient regarding external beam radiation as ordered: — Method of action — Course/duration of treatment, usually five treatments each week for 6 to 8 weeks — Signs and symptoms of radiation side effects such as diarrhea, abdominal cramping, erectile dysfunction, dysuria, frequency, hesitancy, urgency, nocturia, fatigue, proctitis, and ulcers close to rectal area; teach that these problems may resolve 2 to 3 weeks after completion of therapy. — Skin changes to note include redness, sloughing, and tenderness	Radiation is common in the treatment of prostate cancer, especially for older men who may not be good surgical candidates. It can be offered as the only type of treatment or in conjunction with surgery. The radiated skin is sensitive, and ointments, powder, creams, rubbing, etc., may cause burning and skin sloughing, and interfere with radiation. The patient must know how to protect the skin from impairment; knowing what to expect in terms of radiation helps the patient to be more compliant and feel more in control.

INTERVENTIONS	RATIONALES
— Skin care: do not apply soap, ointments, creams, or powder to area; do not rub, scrub, or scratch the area; do not try to wash off markings — Wear loose-fitting clothes — Teach the patient about possible effects on sexuality, i.e. erectile dysfunction; inform patient that appearance of these problems may be delayed for months	
Teach patient and family about hormonal therapy and its effects: — Method of action — Specific pharmacological agents used for treatment (such as LH-RH agonists, flutamide) — Schedule for taking medications and side effects — Orchiectomy — Effect of medications and orchiectomy on sexual function/erectile dysfunction	Knowledge about medications and their effects will assist with compliance, and the patient can make informed decisions about therapy options. Knowing what to expect in terms of sexuality can help the patient cope or minimize frustrations with alterations in sexuality.
For patients who had prostatectomies teach — Care of indwelling catheter: prevention of infection by use of aseptic techniques and procedures according to agency protocol; signs and symptoms of UTI; proper use of leg bag if going home with indwelling catheter, including how to empty and cleanse and the need to empty the leg bag every 2 to 3 hours to prevent reflux of urine into bladder — Care of incision: perineal and abdominal: keep clean and dry, gently flushing perineal incision with warm water daily when discharged home and after each bowel movement and washing hands thoroughly before touching surgical incision; how to change dressing if required — No sex for 6 weeks — No heavy lifting or strenuous activity for 4 to 8 weeks	The patient needs to be prepared to care for himself; knowledge of what to expect helps the patient cope with untoward side effects and better equips him to take responsibility for managing the illness and engaging in self-care. Sex, strenuous activity, or lifting could disrupt incisional lines. Other interventions are aimed at preventing complications such as infections.

(continues)

(continued)

INTERVENTIONS	RATIONALES
— Showers, but not tub baths — Control of fatigue: balance of rest and activity; if receiving radiation therapy, naps may be needed	
Teach the patient to implement dietary strategies to prevent constipation and ensure adequate output and dilution of urine: — Consume 2000 to 3000 ml of fluid. — Increase fiber in diet and intake of prune juice or apple juice. — Teach to take stool softeners or laxatives as needed or prescribed.	Adequate fluid intake is necessary to keep urine diluted and prevent infection. Constipation can cause disruption of the surgical incision, and straining to defecate increases pain in patients who have had prostatectomies, especially perineal types.
For incontinence, teach Kegel exercises; instruct on use of pads with odor control substances.	Kegel exercises improve perineal muscle tone and may reduce incontinence; pads keep patient dry and promote hygiene.
Teach patient and family the need for follow-up care to have PSA levels done and for bone scans.	PSA levels give clues about response to treatment and progression of disease. Bone scans are done to identify bone metastasis.
Provide patient and family with information on hospice and other community service agencies such as the American Cancer Society.	These agencies can assist with educational literature, durable medical equipment, in-home care providers, support, and other services.
Assess the patient and family's understanding of all teaching by encouraging them to repeat information and ask questions as needed.	This allows the nurse to hear in the patient's own words what was taught and makes it easier to know what information may need to be reinforced.
Provide the patient with written materials that contain the information that was taught.	Allows for review and can be used as a reference later.
Establish that the patient has the resources required to be compliant, such as transportation to chemotherapy treatments and radiation therapy and finances to buy medications and supplies.	If needed resources such as finances and transportation to follow-up appointments are not available, the patient cannot be compliant; the nurse will need to make necessary referrals. This may be a real problem for patients from remote and rural areas, especially if family support is not available.

NIC　*Learning readiness enhancement*
Learning facilitation
Teaching: Procedure/treatment
Teaching: Psychomotor skill
Teaching: Disease process
Teaching: Prescribed medication

Evaluation

Evaluate the degree to which the patient has achieved the outcome criteria relevant to the teaching sessions. The patient should verbalize an understanding of content presented by repeating the information, particularly the disease process, treatments (radiation, chemotherapy, surgery), and medications. Determine if the patient is able to perform psychomotor skills such as emptying the drainage bag and applying a leg bag by having him demonstrate these procedures. Ask the patient whether he understands how to perform Kegel exercises and the rationale for their use. The patient demonstrates an understanding of pain control measures. The nurse must determine if the patient is capable of being compliant with the recommended regimen. If further teaching is required at time of discharge, the appropriate referrals should be made to continue education.

Community/Home Care

The patient and family will need to implement the medical regimen in the home setting over an extended period of time. The success of this implementation will depend upon the degree to which the patient has received adequate teaching and has subsequently understood and internalized it. In most instances, the patient will need to return to an outpatient facility or doctor's office for follow-up or radiation therapy. As indicated in the preceding teaching plan, there are many facets of care that the patient and family need to understand. The volume of information may prove overwhelming at first, and in almost all instances, a visiting nurse should be employed to assist and determine that the patient is able to employ the strategies outlined. The ability to care for incisions, drainage devices, and indwelling catheters should be reassessed once the patient is at home. Questions that the patient or family may have include what to empty the urine or other drainage into, how to empty in the commode without soiling self, how to cleanse the bag, and how to store the urinary drainage bag at home. The nurse can provide the patient with a urinal from the hospital to use for emptying contents of drainage bags. All supplies for catheter care or incisional care can be kept in the bedroom and stored in heavy plastic storage containers with lids purchased from most any retail store. These can be labeled according to their purpose. Patients may be hesitant to leave the home if the indwelling catheter is in place, but should be encouraged to do so if health permits in order to avoid social isolation. Using the leg bag when going out should be recommended as it fits snugly on the leg and is well hidden by clothing. Radiation therapy patients will need to be monitored for ability to care for skin properly and prevent further tissue destruction. Because the patient is seen on a regular basis for radiation, health care providers can determine if further teaching or reinforcement is required. Pain control is a big part of home care and will require frequent follow-up to ensure patient satisfaction. As uncured prostate cancer progresses, bone pain may become severe, causing the patient to limit activities, especially ambulation. At this point, the family and patient need to be supported in their efforts to obtain pain control or relief so that the patient can have a measure of quality of life. The nurse can assist the patient in the home by making note cards with instructions on them, especially for information such as signs and symptoms of infections, symptoms to notify a health care worker about, and how to perform Kegel exercises.

Documentation

Document the specific content taught and the titles of any printed documents given to the patient. Include in the chart the patient's degree of understanding of the content and the methods used to evaluate learning. The nurse should be sure to include specifically the patient's ability to perform psychomotor skills such as dressing changes, applying a leg bag, and care of indwelling catheters. Any areas that need to be reinforced should be documented to ensure appropriate follow-up. If family members are present for the teaching sessions, document this in the chart, and always document any referrals made.

NURSING DIAGNOSIS 4

RISK FOR INFECTION

Related to:

Surgical interventions

Enhanced opportunity for invasion by organisms

Urinary retention

Drainage devices

Defining Characteristics:

None

Goal:

The patient does not acquire an infection.

Outcome Criteria

✔ The patient will have a negative urine culture.

✔ The patient will report no pain on urination.

✔ The patient will be afebrile.

✔ Incisions will have no redness, warmth, or purulent drainage.

NOC *Infection severity*
Knowledge: Infection control

INTERVENTIONS	RATIONALES
Assess for signs and symptoms of UTI: frequency with voiding of small amounts, dysuria, fever, chills, costovertebral angle tenderness, flank tenderness on palpation, pyuria, and hematuria (if patient has had surgery, some hematuria may be present in the early post-operative period).	These are all symptoms of UTI and give clues to severity of the infection; costovertebral angle tenderness and flank tenderness are symptoms of pyelonephritis, indicating invasion of the renal tissue. Many of the symptoms that the patient with prostate cancer experiences are also indicators of urinary tract infection; knowing what symptoms the patient normally has can help distinguish between the two.
Obtain urine specimen for routine urinalysis and culture and sensitivity, and send to lab immediately.	Provides a definitive diagnosis and identifies the causative organism, which is needed for appropriate antibiotic therapy. A colony count of 10^3 organisms

(continues)

(continued)

INTERVENTIONS	RATIONALES
	per milliliter of urine constitutes a positive culture. Immediate transport to the lab is needed, for if urine is left at room temperature, bacterial count will double every 30 to 40 minutes; routine urinalysis will reveal the presence of casts, white blood cells (WBCs), and bacteria.
Assess any surgical wounds for drainage, redness, edema, or warmth, and drainage devices (Jackson Pratt, Penrose drains, etc.) for amount, color, and consistency of drainage. Note purulent drainage.	Helps to detect changes in the surgical site or in the drainage from drainage devices that may indicate infection.
Monitor results of laboratory tests and note abnormalities indicative of infection: positive urine culture, positive blood culture, positive culture from wound drainage, and elevated WBC count.	Cultures provide a positive identification of the causative organism for infection; WBC count provides further evidence for infection as elevations occur as a natural defense.
Monitor results of other diagnostic tests: serum creatinine, BUN, and IVP.	These tests give indications of any impaired renal function; IVP can demonstrate obstructed urine flow.
Take temperature every 4 hours and administer antipyretics, as ordered.	Monitors for elevations that may occur with UTI; give antipyretics to reduce fever and monitor response.
Observe urine noting amount, color, any blood, and odor.	Infected urine is usually cloudy, foul-smelling, and may contain small amounts of blood due to irritation, and amounts at each voiding may be small; monitor for improvement in response to treatment.
Administer antibiotics specific to culture and sensitivity, as ordered. Often the first choice antibiotic is trimethoprim-sulfamethoxazole (Bactrim).	Helps to decrease bacteria through bacteriocidal or bacteriostatic action.
Change dressings at surgical site and drainage tube sites, as ordered, using sterile technique.	Helps to decrease risk of introducing organisms into wounds; for patients with low midline incisions of a suprapubic prostatectomy, the dressing is easily soaked with urine, and a suprapubic tube through the incision will require meticulous

	care with frequent dressing changes; perineal resections have urinary leakage around the wound for several days after removal of the catheter, requiring frequent dressing changes; the wound is in close proximity to the rectum, also increasing the risk for infection.
Have the patient void every 2 hours when urinary catheters have been removed.	Helps to prevent stasis of urine and enhance emptying of bladder.
If indwelling catheter is present, maintain aseptic technique when handling, and perform perineal care every shift or according to agency protocol.	The indwelling catheter is a frequent source of infection, and maintaining aseptic technique in its care decreases risk for infection.
For the patient who has had a perineal resection, perform gentle flushing/rinsing of the perineal area with sterile normal saline daily and after each bowel movement.	The incisional area is close to the rectal area, and cleansing decreases bacteria count, thus reducing the risk for infection.
Increase fluids to at least 3 to 4 liters per day by mouth, if not contraindicated due to cardiac disease.	Helps to dilute urine and prevent irritation of the bladder.
Avoid liquids containing caffeine; include liquids such as cranberry juice or prune juice.	Caffeine is a bladder irritant and will aggravate symptoms; cranberry and prune juice will acidify urine, and bacteria generally do not flourish in acidic urine.
Offer a well-balanced diet that is rich in iron, vitamin C, and protein.	The body, especially the skin, requires these nutrients in adequate supply for tissue repair and healing.
Implement strategies to address impaired urinary elimination (see diagnoses "Urinary Retention").	Strategies to reduce bladder distention/retention can help prevent infection by preventing backflow of urine to ureters and decreases the possibility of bacteria growth in stagnant urine in the bladder.

NIC *Wound care*
Urinary elimination management
Medication management
Infection control
Surveillance
Infection protection

Evaluation

Assess the patient's status in regards to the urinary tract and surgical wound, noting any signs of infection. Evaluate the degree to which the outcome criteria have been met. The patient should have no evidence of urinary tract infection such as pain, frequency, urgency, fever, or chills. Wounds and drainage tube insertion sites should be free of warmth, redness (or other discoloration), and purulent drainage. Laboratory results indicate decreased WBCs and negative urine or wound drainage culture.

Community/Home Care

The patient with prostate cancer will remain at risk for UTIs and will need to implement measures to decrease that risk by preventing urinary retention if the prostate gland has not been removed (see nursing diagnosis "Urinary Retention"). Because the risk for upper UTI is great for the patient with urinary retention, prevention is important. If the patient has been treated surgically for prostate cancer and has been discharged home with an indwelling catheter, the risk for infection is even greater. An in-home nurse should be sure that the patient or a family member knows how to care for the catheter properly, and understands measures to prevent UTIs and signs and symptoms of infection (see nursing diagnosis "Risk for Infection"). At home, the patient may be prescribed prophylactic antibiotics, and the nurse should stress to the patient the need to take the medications until they are gone. At home, fluids will need to be encouraged to a level possibly above what the patient normally consumes. The patient and family devise a plan to ensure adequate intake. Water bottles filled with water or the patient's favorite non-caffeinated beverage can be used and made available to the patient to sip on throughout the day. Ones with measurements on the side can assist the patient to keep track of the amount consumed. For those patients who have had prostatectomies for prostate cancer, appropriate wound care should be taught to the family and patient. The patient at home will need to implement strategies to prevent infection, which includes how to keep the wound clean, how to change the dressing, how to assess the wound or urine for signs of infection, and how to recognize which symptoms warrant a return to the health care providers. Even though the patient and family may verbalize understanding of all content and return demonstrate psychomotor skills, when called upon to perform those same skills without the supervision or comfort level of having the nurse present, the patient may feel some degree of anxiety. Having a home nurse present for the first attempt is recommended to ensure that the patient or family is comfortable with the task. The role of nutrition in infection control, wound healing, and general health should be incorporated into teaching sessions with the patient. Be sure that the patient has financial means to purchase any required dressing supplies or antibiotics and to return to the health care provider for follow-up. When the patient is discharged, it is recommended that the nursing staff provide the patient with needed supplies for at least 24 hours.

Documentation

Chart the results of all assessments. Urinary elimination patterns should be documented, including any complaints of urgency, frequency, dysuria, and feelings of fullness or burning on urination. Also chart whether an indwelling urinary catheter is present and give a description of the urine noting color, amount, and whether there is hematuria. Assessments of the surgical incision should be documented, including color, temperature, and a description of any drainage. Patient complaints of pain are documented with follow-up assessment following interventions. Document all interventions that have been implemented to address the problem of risk for infection (urinary and wound), and the patient's response to treatment. Document administration of antibiotics and vital signs, especially temperature, in accordance with agency standards. If specimens are sent to the laboratory, note this in the patient's record.

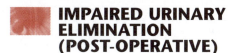

NURSING DIAGNOSIS 5

IMPAIRED URINARY ELIMINATION (POST-OPERATIVE)

Related to:

Surgical intervention for prostate cancer (prostatectomies)

Defining Characteristics:

Blood in urine

Bladder spasms

Presence of indwelling urinary catheter

Goal:

Urine output will be adequate.

Outcome Criteria

✔ Urine output will be ≥ 50 cc per hour post-operatively and return to normal color after 48 hours.

✔ Indwelling catheter will remain patent.

✔ The patient will have no symptoms of fluid overload due to bladder irrigation.

NOC *Urinary elimination*
Fluid balance

INTERVENTIONS	RATIONALES
Post-operatively assess for decreased urinary output, hemorrhage (decreased hemoglobin [Hgb] and hematocrit [Hct], tachycardia, hypotension), blood clots, and bladder spasms.	Bleeding and passage of clots following prostate surgery are more common during the first 24 hours, and the patient should be assessed frequently for early identification; clots can obstruct the drainage device; bladder spasms need to be treated to prevent pain and decreased output. Pink to red-colored urine is normal the day of surgery; very dark red may indicate increased venous bleeding or that the irrigant is not effective in diluting urine; bright red urine is caused by arterial bleeding and requires an increase in irrigant; occasional clots are normal, but frequent blood clots require an increase in irrigant to prevent occlusion of tube; clear to pink-colored urine after the first post-operative day is normal.
Following transurethral and retropubic resection of the prostate, maintain continuous bladder irrigation with normal saline to keep the output light pink or very pale yellow (diluted urine); for suprapubic resection of the prostate, maintain cystotomy tube or drain through incision; for perineal resection of the	Drainage tubes (Penrose, Jackson Pratts) drain fluid from the surgical site, and cystotomy tubes drain urine following suprapubic resection of the prostate tumor through the bladder. Following surgical interventions for prostate cancer, clots may develop and cause a blockage to the outflow of urine; this is more likely
prostate gland, maintain patency of perineal drains; maintain patency of indwelling 30 ml balloon catheter for all types of resection, noting the presence of any clots or frank bleeding. For patients on continuous bladder irrigations, increase irrigant, in accordance with agency protocol or as ordered, if clots or frank bleeding is noted.	during the first 24 to 48 hours. Continuous bladder irrigation maintains patency and flushes the bladder of any clots.
Accurately monitor intake and output every 1 to 2 hours, especially the amount of irrigant infused.	Careful calculation is required to determine that irrigant is not excessive and actual urine output is sufficient.
Teach the patient to refrain from trying to void around catheter.	The presence of a large balloon on the catheter creates a sensation of pressure and a need to void, but if the patient tries to void around the catheter, spasms will increase and may cause excruciating pain.
Give the patient medications for pain or bladder spasms as ordered (Ditropan®, opiates, belladonna).	Spasms can increase pain, and comfort of the patient should be a priority; they can occur with all types of resections, but are more frequent following transurethral and suprapubic resections.
Assess the patient for signs of water intoxication if on continuous bladder irrigation: confusion, restlessness, and decreased serum sodium levels. If present, slow irrigant and notify physician.	These symptoms occur as the irrigant is absorbed; early identification allows for initiation of treatment before serious neurological or cardiovascular complications occur.
For the patient without continuous bladder irrigation, irrigate indwelling catheter as ordered or according to agency protocol.	Helps to maintain patency of catheter by preventing obstruction from sediment or clots.
Encourage intake of 2 to 3 liters of fluid daily.	Helps to dilute urine and prevent bacteria growth.
Implement strategies to prevent UTI and wound infection (see nursing diagnosis "Risk for Infection").	Use of instrumentation such as indwelling catheters and breaks in skin due to surgical incisions predispose the patient to infection, as can urinary retention prior to surgery. Patients with perineal resections are susceptible to infection due to the close proximity of the

INTERVENTIONS	RATIONALES
	surgical incision to the rectum; patients with suprapubic resections are at high risk for incisional infections due to frequent soaking of the abdominal dressing with urine.
Remove catheter when ordered, and monitor output, color, and consistency of urine. Assess the patient for retention as well as dribbling following removal. Explain to the patient that he may perceive a sensation to void and with initial voiding may experience small amounts of blood in the urine, as well as some dribbling and some discomfort.	These symptoms occur as the bladder adapts to removal of the large ballooned catheter and attempts to recapture normal tone. The blood is generally due to irritation and not frank bleeding.
Teach patient Kegel exercises: voluntary tightening and relaxing of the perineal and gluteal muscles that support the bladder and urethra.	Helps restore tone and minimize incontinence; patients having transurethral, radical, and perineal resections are at higher risk for development of incontinence.
Administer stool softeners and implement dietary measures such as prune juice, fiber in diet, and fruits to address bowel elimination.	Patients undergoing open prostatectomies may experience constipation and pain with defecation. Interventions are required to prevent both. Perineal resections present a unique problem because the incision is in close proximity to the rectum; straining to evacuate the rectum will be painful.

NIC *Pelvic muscle exercise*
Bladder irrigation
Fluid monitoring
Urinary elimination management

Evaluation

Examine the extent to which the patient has achieved the outcome criteria. Urine output should be > 50 cc per hour, have no frank bleeding or clots, and gradually return to a normal color. The patient should have no signs or symptoms of water intoxication and report an absence of bladder spasms. In addition, the patient should have no indications of hemorrhage. All urinary drainage devices should remain patent.

Community/Home Care

The patient who has had surgery for prostate cancer will need follow-up care to ensure that urinary output and bladder function return to normal or to an optimum state. For some patients, discharge home is accomplished with the indwelling catheter still in place and for this group, the patient and a family member must be taught how to care for it, including emptying, proper positioning, measuring output, and appropriate perineal care (see nursing diagnosis "Deficient Knowledge"). A return demonstration of the techniques for emptying, attaching leg bags, and care of ports should be required. If the patient goes home without a catheter, he will need to monitor output to be sure that retention is not an issue. Rather than voiding directly in the toilet, the patient should be provided with a urinal and encouraged to use this to allow for measurement of urine with each voiding. Of concern for the patient following TURP and prostatectomy is the possibility of incontinence and altered sexual function. These are not likely to surface in the early post-operative period, but become apparent as the patient recuperates at home. During follow-up visits, the health care provider should establish the type of rapport and comfort level with the patient that would allow questioning of the patient regarding these two areas and institute necessary measures to address them. The patient needs to know which signs and symptoms necessitate immediate return to the health care provider (see nursing diagnosis "Deficient Knowledge").

Documentation

Document the findings from a thorough assessment regarding the urinary system. Include the presence of catheters and a description of the urine. Record the amount of urine and the amount of irrigant on the appropriate intake and output records according to agency protocol. The patient's subjective reports of any type are also charted. If the patient has pain or spasms, document specific complaints and interventions implemented to address them as well as the resolution of the complaint following interventions.

NURSING DIAGNOSIS 6

 INEFFECTIVE COPING

Related to:

Diagnosis of prostate cancer

Fear of dying

Poor prognosis

Alterations in sexuality

Alterations in urinary function: incontinence

Defining Characteristics:

Anger

Expressions of fear

Restlessness and anxiety

Crying

Expression of distress at potential loss

Goal:

Anxiety is decreased or alleviated.

Outcome Criteria

✔ The patient identifies one coping mechanism to be used.

✔ The patient verbalizes fears and concerns.

✔ The patient reports being less anxious and demonstrates no outward signs of anxiety such as restlessness or agitation.

NOC *Grief resolution*
Anxiety control
Comfort level
Coping

INTERVENTIONS	RATIONALES
Assess level of anxiety (mild, moderate, severe); have patient rate on a scale of 1 to 10 with 10 being the greatest.	Gives the nurse a better perception of extent of any anxiety.
Have the patient identify at least one way that he has coped with stressful or challenging situations in the past.	Past ways of successful coping can be used in new situations.
Recognize the role of culture in the patient's method of grieving and the verbalization of fears and concerns especially related to sexuality and urinary function.	Culture often dictates how a person grieves and handles concerns of a sensitive nature. The nurse must recognize this in order to support the patient in a successful grief process.
Encourage the patient to verbalize feelings, fears, concerns, and expressions of loss and or grief regarding the diagnosis of prostate cancer and the patient's prognosis, and support them as appropriate by answering questions, making referrals, and listening attentively.	Verbalizations of fears and feelings contribute to dealing with concerns; being attentive relays empathy to the patient; assisting the family to deal with the diagnosis and prognosis will enhance his ability to cope.
Engage the patient and family in open dialogue regarding options for treatments and care.	Discussion of care options early in the disease allows the patient to be more in control, giving him a sense of empowerment that may assist with coping with the disease.
Keep the patient informed of all that is going on, including information about diagnostic tests and therapeutic interventions.	The patient and family need to be informed in order to make decisions and to decrease anxiety. Knowledge also may give the patient a sense of being in control.
Seek spiritual consult, as needed or requested by the patient and/or family.	Meeting the patient's spiritual needs helps him to deal with fears through use of spiritual or religious rituals.
Provide the patient and family with information regarding advance directives and support decisions made.	Allows the patient and family the opportunity to plan for the patient's wishes in the event that he becomes incompetent to make his own decisions.
Engage the patient in honest dialogue regarding the effect treatment for prostate cancer has on sexuality and urinary functioning; referrals may need to be made to professional counselors in the area of sexuality.	If the patient can have questions answered honestly, he will be better equipped to move forward with coping.

NIC *Grief work facilitation*
Coping enhancement
Emotional support
Spiritual support

Evaluation

Evaluate the extent to which the outcome criteria have been achieved. The patient should be assessed for behaviors that would indicate adjustment to the diagnosis of prostate cancer. Determine if the patient has acceptable coping strategies that can be used during treatment for prostate cancer and during recovery. The patient should verbalize fears and concerns and be able to identify one way that he can cope with the diagnosis of prostate cancer. The extent to which the patient displays appropriate coping behaviors should be noted. If the patient is unable to talk about the diagnosis and communicate concerns, the nurse should explore further new interventions to assist the patient.

Community/Home Care

Nurses should assess which coping mechanisms work for the patient and encourage their use by the patient at home. Problems with coping and grieving may continue for a long period of time, and follow-up by a health care provider can detect ineffective coping. The family or significant others should be taught what is appropriate grieving and coping and what is not. Extreme self-isolation and depression should be noted and reported to a health care provider. For many patients and families, spiritual/religious rituals provide a means of coping with difficult, stressful situations. The patient's culture may dictate how he copes and grieves and with whom he shares this process. It is crucial that the nurse and family support the patient as needed to foster a healthy psychological state, and recognize that anger and denial are common. As the disease progresses, the patient may require new strategies for coping with the disease and the anticipated loss of life if a cure was not achieved through surgery. The patient may benefit from quiet periods of meditation during the day or the use of relaxation strategies such as quiet music, nature walks, or reading. Support to long-term caregivers will be important, as they too need to be supported in a grief process. Hospice can play an important role in the home situation through provision of counselors, chaplains, and in-home care providers. If questions should arise at home regarding the patient's health status or prescribed regimen, the patient should have a means of contact with a health care provider for answers.

Documentation

Document whether the patient is able to discuss feelings regarding a diagnosis of prostate cancer. Chart the patient's verbalizations as the patient states them and include in the record coping mechanisms utilized by the patient. The degree to which the patient has decreased anxiety should be documented in the patient record. A rating system provides an objective way to relay to others the extent of the anxiety. Document findings from an assessment of the patient's psychological state and whether there is depression, anger, crying, sadness, etc. Document any referrals to hospice or religious leaders.

CHAPTER 11.122

SEXUAL ASSAULT/RAPE-TRAUMA SYNDROME (ACUTE)

GENERAL INFORMATION

Sexual assault occurs when a victim is forced into a sexual act without consent. This can happen to members of either sex, although females are more frequently the victims. Frequently a weapon is used and the victim sees the event as life-threatening. Often there is a pattern of behavior following the assault known as rape-trauma syndrome typified by emotional discomfort and stress, in which a wide array of emotions may be displayed, including denial or disbelief, shock, guilt, blame, and extreme personal lifestyle disorganization. Victims of sexual assault may refuse to report the assault because of fear, social stigma, cultural beliefs, and discovery by loved ones. In addition to the immediate psychological trauma that accompanies sexual assault, physiological trauma may also be evident. Injuries due to physical trauma include injuries to cervical canal, groin, and vagina; injury to the throat if choking was employed; knife wounds; and blunt trauma due to use of fists or objects to beat the victim. The aftereffects of the assault may be short- or long-term. Some survivors of sexual assault suffer immeasurable damage to their mental health and require long-term support and treatment.

NURSING DIAGNOSIS 1

RAPE-TRAUMA SYNDROME (COMPOUND OR SILENT REACTION)

Related to:

Forced, violent, non-consensual sex

Forced attempted rape

Defining Characteristics:

Report of and description of event

Evidence of physical assault

Delay in seeking care

Physical trauma to various body parts

Vivid recollection of place, person, sounds, smells

Goal:

The patient's psychological state begins to heal.

Outcome Criteria

✔ The patient will return to normal level of functioning.

✔ The patient will identify coping mechanisms and use at least one.

✔ The patient will express feelings about the rape or attempted rape in an appropriate manner.

NOC *Abuse recovery: Emotional*
Abuse recovery: Sexual
Personal well-being
Coping

INTERVENTIONS	RATIONALES
Place the victim in a private, quiet place but do not leave the victim alone.	This provides the victim a "safe" place where stressors are minimized to the greatest extent possible. The patient should be afforded every opportunity to regain his or her dignity with a sense of security.
Assure the patient that he or she is in a safe place now.	The victim may feel that no place is safe. Reassurance will help the patient realize that he or she is safe.
Explain all procedures carefully and give the patient	This helps the patient understand what is happening

INTERVENTIONS	RATIONALES
opportunities to make choices whenever possible.	and feel that he or she has some control over the situation.
Utilize the services of a sexual assault nurse examiner (SANE), and whenever possible, have the same person who is obtaining the history also do the evidence collection (the SANE).	This provides continuity and is less intrusive; the SANE is qualified to obtain forensic evidence needed for prosecution but also to obtain a thorough history.
Evaluate the patient for injuries: scrapes, cuts, bruises, ecchymosis of genitalia or abdomen, vaginal discharge, and rectal bleeding/tears.	Often the victim of sexual assault has also been physically harmed.
Obtain a detailed history of the assault, including date and time of the assault, whether the perpetrator used a weapon, and whether the victim bathed, showered, douched, changed clothing, vomited, urinated, defecated, ate, or drank prior to coming to the hospital. Obtain past medical history.	Helps the nurse to know from where to collect evidence and to check for trauma.
Collect and preserve evidence (vaginal, rectal, or oral smears, and any other as ordered), and ensure appropriate procedures are followed: — Carefully label each specimen and place in a secured place, such as a safe or locked refrigerator. Only law enforcement officers or other authorized agents should transfer evidence to the crime labs. — Inform the patient that he or she has the right to refuse to report the crime. The caregiver, however, is obligated to report it. If the patient chooses not to speak with police, that is his or her right. — Assure the patient that evidence will not be turned over to law enforcement personnel unless consent is given by him or her. Suggest that evidence be collected and properly stored by the hospital authorities in the event that the patient changes his or her mind at a later date.	Helps to ensure integrity of evidence; smears (vaginal, rectal, oral, and other) for sperm can be a vital piece of evidence (motile sperm in vaginal fluid indicates that less than six hours have passed since intercourse).

INTERVENTIONS	RATIONALES
— Follow agency and law enforcement protocol.	
Assist with collection of laboratory specimens for: serum human chorionic gonadotrophin, vaginal smear for detection of sexually transmitted diseases (STDs), and specimen for HIV testing.	These tests are performed to determine a baseline of the patient's status for comparison later, in the event that pregnancy, STDs, or HIV occur.
Notify the family or significant other, with the victim's permission.	Helps to serve as a support network in time of crisis.
Encourage the patient to verbalize feelings and fears about the assault, such as fear of pregnancy or STDs resulting from the assault.	Verbalization is the first step towards healing and may assist the victim to begin using coping strategies.
Provide constant reassurance and empathy.	Helps to establish a trusting relationship and provide emotional support.
Plan discharge so that the patient goes to a protected environment either at home with someone or to a safe shelter.	Due to fear and emotional instability, the patient/victim should never feel unsafe or go home unattended following a sexual assault.
Refer the patient to an advocacy group.	Rape advocates can help the patient to determine his or her rights and obtain restraining order(s), can act as an advocate through the legal system, can provide psychological counseling and a "safe home," and can make referrals to professionals, health care agencies, and support groups.
Ascertain the patient's understanding of what has happened, of therapeutic interventions and evidence collection, of rights, and of pregnancy and STD prevention possibilities.	During times of crisis, it is often easy to misunderstand information presented. It is necessary to make sure the patient understands the events and the numerous requests being made.
Treat physical injuries, as ordered.	Physical injuries require treatment, but the main focus of intervention is on the patient's psychological state. If wounds are present and require cleansing, do so gently and speak to the patient before touching him or her. Following assault, the patient may startle with simple touching due to the shock of what has happened.

NIC   *Counseling*
      Rape-trauma treatment
      Calming technique
      Presence

Evaluation

The patient is able to talk about the experience with an advocate, law enforcement officer, or health care provider. The victim expresses feelings and concerns openly. At least one coping strategy has been identified by the patient and has been utilized to cope with the situation. Prior to exiting the health care system, the patient identifies resources for support.

Community/Home Care

Victims of sexual assault are rarely hospitalized unless physical trauma is serious or emotional stability is compromised. Discharge from the emergency room should be carefully orchestrated with the use of a multidisciplinary team. The victim should never be discharged home alone because of the fear of further harm but also because of the need for continued emotional support required to feel "safe." Effects of the rape or attempted rape may last for extended periods of time, and the victim needs to have available resources for counseling, advocacy, and legal services. Married victims may experience difficulty communicating with spouses following sexual assault and feel that they are to blame for what happened. Spouses may require some assistance in dealing with the incident as well, and in some instances may shun the victim, creating further mental anguish for the victim due to the loss of a loved one as a source of support in a troubling time. Family and significant others should be reminded that the patient has been a victim of a criminal act and that acts of rejection or blame leveled at the victim causes further emotional trauma and insult to self-esteem. Individual and/or family therapy may be the best option for assisting the patient to a return to normalcy. If criminal charges are brought against the perpetrator, the victim must also prepare for functioning in the legal system. Telephone numbers for hotlines such as rape crisis centers that offer immediate communications with a trained volunteer should be given to the patient for possible use. Follow-up care is required to monitor the progress of the victim towards healing or recovery and coping with the event.

Documentation

Chart the findings of a thorough physical exam performed at time of entry into the emergency room with a special note describing the patient's emotional state. This should include an examination for physical trauma as well as documentation of evidence obtained by the SANE. The disposition of all specimens obtained will need to be indicated in the patient record. The patient's description of the event should be documented in his or her own words. Referrals to social workers, advocacy groups, or housing organizations should be charted. All visitors to the victim should be documented, including law enforcement officers and family.

NURSING DIAGNOSIS 2

 ### INEFFECTIVE INDIVIDUAL COPING

Related to:
   Sexual trauma
   Violence

Defining Characteristics:
   Difficulty verbalizing traumatic event
   Expressions of fear
   Negative statements about self
   Crying

Goal:
   The patient is able to express feelings and to cope.

Outcome Criteria

✔ The patient identifies and uses one coping strategy.
✔ The patient verbalizes fears and concerns.

NOC   *Comfort level*
      Coping
      Abuse recovery: Sexual
      Fear level

INTERVENTIONS	RATIONALES
Assess patient for expressions of fear, anxiety, negative statements about self, and other displays of ineffective coping.	When patients have been victims of violent acts, the emotional response can vary greatly; the nurse needs to note specific expressions to establish a starting point for interventions. Often the victim has fears of additional violence, does not want to be alone, and may relive the event repeatedly in his or her mind.
Monitor for sexuality concerns about/fears of becoming pregnant and acquiring STDs and avoidance of sex with intimate partner; inform patient about HIV, STDs, and pregnancy testing.	Particularly when the perpetrator is unknown to the patient there may be constant fears related to the consequences of unsafe/unprotected sex, including unwanted pregnancy and STDs. Appropriate testing for baseline information for later comparison is done in the emergency room, and these procedures should be explained to the patient.
Keep the patient informed of all that is going on, including information about appropriate procedures for obtaining specimen samples and his or her legal rights as the victim of a violent crime.	Communicating what is going on in the emergency room helps to allay anxiety and fear.
Stay with the patient as needed or desired by the patient and allow other visitors as requested by the patient.	Provides emotional support and promotes a sense of comfort.
Encourage the patient to verbalize feelings regarding what has happened and to express any fears or concerns while listening attentively. The patient may require a professional consult to assist with expression of feelings.	Verbalization of feelings, fears, and concerns contributes to dealing with the sexual assault; being attentive relays empathy to the patient.
Explain legal proceedings to the patient.	Knowing what to expect may calm some of the patient's fears and prepares him or her to deal with the events that may follow being a victim of a sexual assault.
Ask the patient to identify all strategies that he or she has used in the past to cope with stressful events.	Strategies that have previously worked can be used as a starting point for coping with more serious stressful events, and can help the patient focus.
Control multiple sources of stimuli that can occur when numerous people need or want contact with the patient.	Overstimulation can worsen fear and anxiety.
Assist with the development of new skills and strategies for coping, including referral to a professional counselor.	When major stressors such as sexual assault occur, new strategies for coping may be required. These new strategies may be more sophisticated than those a generalist nurse is able to offer.
Encourage the family and/or significant other to verbalize honest feelings and seek appropriate resources for help coping with the event.	Verbalization of feelings by the family or significant other needs to occur if they are to be a source of support for the victim; some family members or significant others may blame the victim for what has happened; in the case of intimate partners, the intimate nature of sexual acts may cause them to reject the victim. Until these issues are resolved, they cannot be relied on to offer emotional support. At this point, consideration is given to seeking professional help for the victim and family/significant other.
Recognize the role of cultural and religious beliefs in a patient's method of coping with stressors and particularly sexual assault.	Culture often dictates how a person copes with stressors and particularly issues of a sexual nature.
Provide counseling referrals for the immediate time and for long-term assistance as well.	The effects of sexual assault on the emotional/mental state of the victim can be long-lasting, and the patient may need continued assistance with coping skills.
Seek spiritual consult as needed or requested by the patient and/or family.	Meeting spiritual needs of the patient helps the patient cope with fears through use of spiritual or religious rituals, and provides support.

NIC *Coping enhancement*
  Emotional support
  Spiritual support

Evaluation

Evaluate the extent to which the outcome criteria have been achieved. The patient should be assessed for appropriate coping skills/strategies that can be used to deal with the traumatic event. Concerns, fears, and feelings of being able to cope should be detected in the patient. The patient's ability to verbalize what has happened will be a beginning point for resolution of the traumatic event. If, however, the patient is unable to talk about what has happened, the nurse should explore further the need for new interventions to assist the patient.

Community/Home Care

Sexual assault victims must cope with the effects of sexual trauma for extended periods of time after being discharged from the emergency department. The patient should be encouraged to identify coping strategies that have been successful in the past and prompted to use them in this situation. Sexual assault is a significant violation of a person's being that has both physical and social ramifications. Coping with the physical injury is usually the simplest aspect of the assault, as healing of injuries will occur in most instances in a short period of time. However, it may be harder to achieve a complete recovery from the social aspect of being a victim of sexual assault. This is due in part to the social stigma that may be attached to sexual assault in some cultural contexts and the intimate nature of sex in society. The victim not only copes with being a victim of sexual assault but also the rejection that may occur from the victim's partner or family. Humiliation, blame, shame, and fear are all emotions that the patient will experience at home. Coupled with the perception of rejection by his or her significant other, the victim may avoid sex with his or her intimate partner. Other responses at home could possibly include nightmares, difficulty making decisions, memory loss, suicidal ideations, and alcohol abuse. Follow-up care will need to monitor for and intervene for this to prevent long-term permanent psychological scars. New strategies for dealing with stressors will probably be required. Coping through use of support from outside sources such as nurse therapists or professional counselors will be most helpful to the victim. For many patients, spiritual rituals may be a means of coping with difficult stressful situations. Once at home, the family or a health care provider will need to support the patient as needed to foster a healthy psychological state, recognizing that a wide array of feelings may be expressed. The patient can keep a diary in which to record feelings, especially when experiencing periods of depression or feelings of guilt and shame. If the perpetrator has been identified, and the patient has consented to proceeding with legal actions, coping strategies will need to be firmly in place and ready for recall and use. Court appearances are likely to be scheduled months or even years away from the actual event and the patient will be called upon to relive the event. At this time, old emotions and feelings of stress can resurface, dictating that the patient implement previously used coping strategies. Follow-up by a health care provider, social worker, or professional therapist is almost always necessary.

NURSING DIAGNOSIS 3

SITUATIONAL LOW SELF-ESTEEM

Related to:

Sexual assault

Defining Characteristics:

Expressed shame and guilt

Self-blame for sexual assault

Verbalizations of negative self-talk

Humiliation

Goal:

The patient returns to a positive self-esteem.

Outcome Criteria

✔ The patient will replace negative self-talk with positive self-talk.

✔ The patient will state that he or she is not to blame for sexual assault.

NOC *Abuse recovery: Sexual*
Self-esteem

INTERVENTIONS	RATIONALES
Assess the patient's self-esteem by noting any negative self-talk.	It is normal for victims of sexual assault to blame themselves and to start negative talk about themselves, even in areas not related to sexuality. The nurse needs to be attuned to these comments in order to intervene appropriately.

INTERVENTIONS	RATIONALES
Assess the patient's understanding of the sexual assault and what is now required to move forward.	The patient who is blaming him or herself or engaging in negative self-talk will need to be assisted in moving forward with life and establishing coping strategies that can start the healing process and enhance self-esteem, understanding that self-blame is not a warranted response.
Encourage verbalization of feelings (anger, dismay, concern, fear, etc.) and put the sexual assault into perspective of the victim's total life.	Recognition of own feelings helps the patient to deal with the event better and start the beginning of acceptance of what has happened; a review of life will assist the patient to identify the positive aspects of the self-esteem and not dwell on the negative events.
Be empathetic and nonjudgmental, listening attentively to the patient, and be aware of fears and concerns, avoiding blaming questions.	Listening to the patient will help to identify opportunities for further interventions. Because many patients experience self-blame, it is important that the health care provider remain nonjudgmental.
Help the patient identify personal strengths and mobilize coping strategies.	Discussions like this will help the patient to cope with the situation and enhance self-esteem.
Stay with the patient or have family or significant others present if appropriate.	A sexual assault victim should never be left alone due to fear of violence and concerns over mental health.
Refer to counseling, as needed.	Sexual assault is a major violation of a person's self-image. In order to cope with this effectively, professional counseling over an extended period of time may be required to return the victim to his or her usual state of self-esteem. Professional counselors can help the survivor and his or her family or significant other effectively deal with the problems that may occur as a result of the sexual assault.

NIC *Self-esteem enhancement*
Presence
Emotional support

Evaluation

The patient is able to verbalize feelings regarding his or her self-worth or self-esteem. The patient refrains from negative self-talk and replaces negative talk with positive comments regarding self, particularly in terms of blaming self for sexual assault. A positive outcome reveals that the patient talks about him or herself and identifies personal strengths that can be mobilized to assist with coping.

Community/Home Care

Situational low self-esteem can continue for a period of time of variable length. Usually the victim returns to the previous level of self-esteem with the assistance of supportive family or significant others, through counseling, or sometimes through reliance on religious or spiritual practices. Because of the profound effect that sexual assault can have on a person, continued monitoring of self-esteem should be undertaken to detect any abnormal or morbid responses to the event. The issue of self-esteem can be worsened if the significant other or intimate partner rejects the patient. For the victim, positive engagement in sexual activities may be problematic until self-esteem has been restored, and some healing from the traumatic assault has occurred. The nurse or other health care provider who sees the patient for follow-up will need to be alert to subtle hints that may indicate that the patient has not improved his or her self-esteem.

Documentation

Document the progress the victim has made towards meeting outcome criteria. A thorough assessment of the patient's psychological state should be charted, including specific statements made by the patient that indicate negative or positive self-esteem. If the nurse detects difficulties with coping, interacting with family/significant other, or verbalizations of reactions and feelings about the sexual assault, this should be included in the patient's chart. Any referrals to professional counseling should be documented.

CHAPTER 11.123

SYPHILIS

GENERAL INFORMATION

Syphilis is a sexually transmitted disease (STD) caused by the spirochete *Treponema pallidum*, which enters the body through mucous membranes or small breaks in the skin during sexual activity and has the potential to affect several body systems. The disease can also be transmitted through sharing of intravenous (IV) needles (IV drug users), as well as through contact with infected skin lesions. The incubation period for syphilis is approximately 3 weeks but can range from 10 to 90 days after the initial exposure. The *Treponema pallidum* organism is easily destroyed by washing with soap and water, drying, or heating. The primary stage of the disease lasts for approximately 3 to 8 weeks and is characterized by painless lesions (chancres) on the penis, vulva, vagina, rectum, mouth, and lips, and lymphadenopathy. Drainage from the lesions is highly contagious at this time. Untreated, the disease progresses to the secondary stage, which is characterized by systemic symptoms such as fever, hair loss, headache, sore throat, arthralgias, sores on the body, and rash. Secondary syphilis lasts for 2 to 4 years; the exudate from the lesions is highly contagious, and blood samples reveal the presence of the organism. The latent stage has no clinical signs and endures throughout life or until the disease progresses to the late stage. The disease is easily cured but if left untreated it will progress to late disease, which may appear from 3 to 20 years after initial infection. In late syphilis/tertiary syphilis, the lesions (called "gumma") proliferate and erupt on any area of the body. In the central nervous system syphilis can cause a variety of neurological deficits including sudden attacks of pain anywhere, paralysis, seizures, personality changes, and progressive motor ataxia (tabes dorsalis); musculoskeletal changes include joint instability and lack of coordination, which make ambulation difficult; and in the cardiovascular system, manifestations include aortic valve insufficiency and thoracic aneurysms.

If the disease progresses to the late stage, it is often terminal. The highest incidence of syphilis occurs in young adults from 10 to 30 years old. Men and women are equally affected. Congenital syphilis is also seen in neonates of infected/untreated mothers. In all 50 states of the United States, it is mandatory to report cases of syphilis to the local health department.

NURSING DIAGNOSIS 1

INFECTION*

Related to:

Invasion of body by *Treponema pallidum*

Defining Characteristics:

Genital chancre

Enlarged lymph nodes

Culture positive for *Treponema pallidum*

Skin rash on palms of hands and/or soles of feet

Alopecia

Arthralgias

Sore throat

Headache

Goal:

Infection will be resolved, and secondary or latent syphilis will be avoided.

Outcome Criteria

✔ The patient will have no lesions on genitalia.

✔ The patient will be afebrile.

✔ The patient will have no further symptoms such as sore throat, enlarged nodes, or headache.

NOC *Infection severity*

Community risk control:
Communicable disease

Knowledge: Infection control

INTERVENTIONS	RATIONALES
Monitor diagnostic studies: venereal disease research laboratory test (VDRL) and rapid plasma regain (RPR); fluorescent treponemal antibody absorption test (FTA-ABS) and immunofluorescent stains.	VDRL and RPR become positive 4 to 6 weeks after inoculation but are not specific to syphilis; FTA-ABS is specific for *Treponema pallidum* and is used to confirm the diagnosis following a positive VDRL test; immunofluorescent staining examines microscopically the fluid from lymph nodes or lesions to identify the causative organism.
Monitor the patient for clinical manifestations of the disease: enlarged lymph nodes; skin lesions on trunk, feet, hands; presence of lesions on genitalia or other mucous membranes; chancre on genitalia, cervix, anus, rectum, hands, lips, tongue, or pharynx.	These clinical signs are common indicators of the disease in the primary and secondary stages of the disease; assessment for these will add support to validation of disease while awaiting results of laboratory tests.
Administer antibiotics, as ordered, and monitor for side effects: benzathine penicillin G, usually 2.4 million units given intramuscularly in one dose for primary and secondary stages; in later stages or for re-infection, give three doses one week apart for a total of 7.2 million units or as ordered. For patients allergic to penicillin, an alternate antibiotic such as 100 mg of Vibramycin® (doxycycline) is given orally twice a day for 2 weeks. Side effects include skin rash (most common), anaphylaxis, pain at injection site, and nephrotoxicity. Observe patient for at least 30 minutes following administration to detect reactions.	These medications will resolve the infection through bacteriocidal and bacteriostatic activities and protect the health of the larger community by stopping transmission. Monitoring for side effects allows for dosage adjustment and prevention of complications.
For those patients taking oral agents, teach to complete the prescribed regimen of medications.	Failure to take all medications may result in inadequate resolution of the disease and increased risk for re-infection.
Cleanse lesions with warm soapy water or as prescribed.	Good hygiene is required, especially on the genitalia, to promote healing.
Conduct extensive teaching to patient regarding sexual practices.	It is crucial to teach the patient the importance of practicing safe sex in order to protect against STDs.
Notify local health department following positive laboratory results (VDRL, FTA-ABS), according to agency protocol or guidelines.	Public health law requires that syphilis be reported to the local health department.
Collaborate with other disciplines to protect the community by assisting with identification of sexual contacts and providing education for screening and treatment.	Identifying sexual contacts and providing treatment is crucial to halting the transmission of the disease and preventing the progression of the disease to the later stages.
Stress the need for abstinence during treatment of both patient and partners.	Sexual intercourse during treatment predisposes the patient to re-infection.
Inform the patient of the need to return to a health care facility as directed for follow-up testing.	Repeat testing is needed to ensure successful treatment of the disease.

NIC *Infection control*

Health screening

Communicable disease
management

Infection protection

Medication management

Evaluation

Health care workers that follow the patient in the community will undertake evaluation of this problem. Determine the extent to which the patient has achieved the expected outcome criteria. The patient should begin to have resolution of symptoms such as enlarged lymph nodes, sore throat, and, most importantly, lesions. The patient should verbalize an understanding of the medication treatment being implemented and particularly the need to abstain from sexual activity and to identify sexual contacts.

Community/Home Care

All patients with a diagnosis of syphilis will require some degree of follow-up and management by a public health program for prevention of communicable disease in keeping with the Centers for Disease Control and Prevention guidelines. The public health nurse or other health care provider should monitor the patient for resolution of symptoms of syphilis, particularly the dissipation of lesions and enlarged lymph nodes. The most critical aspect of community or home care is the prevention of transmission and the identification of sexual contacts. The nurse must be vigilant in this effort, recognizing that there may be more than one sexual partner. Cooperation of the patient is a must, but some patients may not work with public health workers due to the embarrassment or stigma of having a STD, as well as the possible loss of relationships. The patient needs to refrain from sexual activity during treatment and for 1 month following completion of treatment. At home, the patient needs to cleanse any lesions several times a day due to exudates, and warm soapy water should suffice. If lesions worsen, the patient should report to a health care provider immediately for re-evaluation. For those patients who must take oral antibiotics, public health workers/nurses will need to establish that the patient is taking all medications as prescribed by the physician and knows the importance of staying on the regimen for its duration. Effective teaching on disease stages, prevention of re-infection, safe-sex practices, and long-term effects of the disease is crucial for the patient (see nursing diagnosis "Deficient Knowledge").

Documentation

Document the findings from a comprehensive sexual history and physical assessment with special attention to any lesions (size, color, location, drainage). Include patient's specific complaints such as headaches, arthralgias, fatigue, pain, or nervous system involvement (ataxia, paralysis). Because it is difficult to know which stage of disease a patient is in at initial time of contact, always document the findings from a cardiovascular assessment. Always chart therapeutic interventions that have been implemented, especially antibiotic administration, and the patient's specific responses to those interventions. Results of testing for syphilis are documented according to agency protocol. All teaching and referrals are documented in the patient's record.

NURSING DIAGNOSIS 2

DEFICIENT KNOWLEDGE

Related to:

New diagnosis of syphilis

Insufficient knowledge of syphilis

Misconception regarding transmission

Safe-sex practices

Defining Characteristics:

Asks many questions

Asks no questions about health status

Verbalizes a lack of knowledge/understanding about syphilis

Goal:

The patient verbalizes an understanding of syphilis.

Outcome Criteria

✔ The patient verbalizes a desire to learn necessary information.

✔ The patient verbalizes a willingness to keep appointments and follow prescribed regimen.

✔ The patient demonstrates knowledge of the pathophysiology of syphilis and how to prevent transmission and reinfection.

✔ The patient demonstrates knowledge of safe-sex practices.

NOC *Risk control: Sexually transmitted disease*
    Knowledge: Disease process
    Knowledge: Treatment regimen
    Compliance behavior

INTERVENTIONS	RATIONALES
Assess the patient's current knowledge, ability and readiness to learn, and risk for noncompliance.	Teachings need to be tailored to the patient's ability and willingness to learn for maximum effectiveness; assessment of the patient for likelihood of noncompliance will allow the nurse to intervene early.
Create a quiet environment conducive to learning.	Environmental noise and distractions can prevent the learner from focusing on what is being taught.
Teach the learners the following information about syphilis: — Disease process of syphilis (causative organism, stages of	Knowledge of disease, medications, and prevention of transmission empowers the patient to take control and be

INTERVENTIONS	RATIONALES
the disease, clinical manifestations) — Prevention of transmission to others through abstinence from sexual activity until patient and all sexual partners are cured — Prescribed medications: (benzathine penicillin G, doxycycline), or others as ordered, including action and side effects (see nursing diagnosis "Infection"); if taking oral medications, include schedule, duration of therapy, and importance of adhering to the regimen as prescribed — Importance of returning for appointments for follow-up testing at 3 months and 6 months — Symptoms of progressive disease: neurological problems such as stiff neck, paresis, confusion, ataxia, paralysis, seizures; cardiovascular symptoms such as shortness of breath, changes in vital signs that may indicate valve insufficiency	compliant. Stressing the adherence to the regimen as prescribed will prevent re-infection. Identification of side effects will minimize anxiety if these untoward effects should occur. Abstinence is necessary in order to stop transmission.
Stress to the patient the need to identify sexual partners to the appropriate public health officials.	Sexual partners need to be treated; untreated partners can re-infect the patient and anyone else with whom they have intimate contact.
Teach the patient about safe-sex practices: use of condoms with all sexual intercourse, how to choose condoms, how to apply condoms, and where to obtain free condoms.	Condoms provide a barrier to invasive organisms but must be used properly.
Ask the patient to repeat information and ask questions as needed.	This allows the nurse to hear in the patient's own words what was taught and makes it easier to know what information may need to be reinforced.
Establish that the patient has the resources required to be compliant.	If needed resources such as finances, transportation, and psychosocial support are not available, the patient may be at risk for noncompliance.
Refer to appropriate disciplines as needed (social worker, public health nurse, etc.).	These disciplines can provide additional services to help the patient be compliant with prescribed regimen.
Give printed information covered in teaching session to the patient.	The patient may be more comfortable at home knowing that there is printed material for future reference.

NIC *Teaching: Disease process*
Teaching: Prescribed medication
Teaching: Safe sex
Learning readiness enhancement
Learning facilitation

Evaluation

Evaluate the degree to which the patient has achieved the expected outcomes. The patient verbalizes an understanding of the treatment of syphilis, including the prescribed antibiotics and their common side effects. The patient demonstrates knowledge of how to prevent transmission of syphilis to others, primarily through the practice of safe sex once the disease is cured. Health care workers should ascertain that the patient is able to identify which signs and symptoms would necessitate contact with a health care provider. The patient is able to repeat all information for the nurse and asks questions about the information that has been taught.

Community/Home Care

For patients with syphilis, care is provided on an outpatient basis, and the cornerstone of care is education about the disease and prevention of transmission to others. Because the treatment of syphilis for most patients consists of one intramuscular injection of medication, compliance with recommendations regarding sexual practices rather than the medication regimen is the most critical aspect of the patient's care. Successful control of the transmission of the disease will depend on the patient's understanding of the information provided in teaching sessions and the internal motivation to implement health-promoting behaviors such as safe-sex practices and identification of sexual partners. In addition to practicing safe sex, the patient will need to abstain from sex for approximately 1 month following treatment. For the patient on oral antibiotics, follow-up by a community health nurse is required to determine if medication administration is occurring and to check for signs and symptoms of side effects of medications. If it is determined that the patient is noncompliant, measures should be implemented to protect the public, such as identifying another person to administer the medications to the patient or having the patient travel to a clinic to be observed taking the medications. All patients will need reminders to return to a designated location for follow-up testing at 3 and 6 months. Most health care providers will probably recommend testing for other STDs (HIV testing is highly recommended for patients diagnosed with syphilis), and the patient needs to be aware of this and interested enough in his or her health to consent to this testing.

Documentation

Document the specific content taught and the titles of printed materials given to the patient. Chart the patient's understanding of the content and the methods used to evaluate learning. The nurse must clearly indicate areas that need to be reinforced. After the teaching session is complete, the nurse should assess to determine if the patient indicates a willingness to comply with health care recommendations, particularly safe sex and identification of sexual partners. For the patient who is taking penicillin or other antibiotics for the first time, document the patient's understanding of the medication and its side effects. If the teaching included a significant other, indicate this in the documentation. In addition, if referrals are made, these should be documented in the patient record.

CHAPTER 11.124

UTERINE/ENDOMETRIAL CANCER

GENERAL INFORMATION

Endometrial cancer occurs in the lining of the uterine wall, and most cases are adenocarcinomas that are stimulated to grow by estrogen. Risk factors for development of endometrial cancer include nulliparity, late menopause, use of tamoxifen, menses before 12 years of age, and estrogen replacement therapy. Adenocarcinoma of the endometrium grows slowly and is also slow to metastasize; as a result, there is a high cure rate (96 percent 5-year survival rate) with a hysterectomy when detected early. It is the most common cancer of the female reproductive tract in the United States, with an estimated 39,300 new cases each year and approximately 6600 deaths each year (American Cancer Society, 2004). The most common clinical manifestation seen early in the disease is abnormal painless vaginal bleeding. Later in the disease, other manifestations include cramping or pelvic pain, bleeding after sexual intercourse, and abdominal pressure. Endometrial cancer occurs most often in women over 50 years of age and more frequently in Caucasians than in African Americans; however, the mortality rate among African American women is twice that of Caucasian women.

NURSING DIAGNOSIS 1

 ANXIETY

Related to:

Unknown prognosis and outcome

Diagnosis of cancer

Uncertain stage of disease at time of diagnosis

Surgery

Defining Characteristics:

Expressions of fear

Restlessness

Verbalization of anxiety

Crying

Goal:

Anxiety is decreased or alleviated.

Outcome Criteria

✔ The patient identifies one coping mechanism to be used.

✔ The patient verbalizes fears and concerns.

✔ The patient reports being less anxious.

✔ The patient demonstrates no outward signs of anxiety such as restlessness or agitation.

NOC *Anxiety control*
Comfort level
Coping

INTERVENTIONS	RATIONALES
Assess level of anxiety (mild, moderate, severe); have patient rate on a scale of 1 to 10, with 10 being the greatest.	Gives the nurse a better perception of extent of the anxiety.
Have the patient identify at least one way that she has coped with stressful situations or anxiety in the past.	Past ways of successful coping can be used for new situations.
Encourage the patient to try relaxation techniques such as guided imagery, massage, music, and deep breathing to relieve anxiety.	These strategies can relax the patient and give her a feeling of mental comfort.
Recognize the role of culture in a patient's method of coping with illness and the acceptability of verbalizing fears and concerns.	Culture often dictates how a person copes, and the nurse must recognize this in order to support the patient in identifying successful coping strategies.

(continues)

(continued)

INTERVENTIONS	RATIONALES
Encourage the patient to verbalize feelings, fears, or concerns regarding the diagnosis of endometrial cancer and support her as appropriate by answering questions and making referrals while listening attentively.	Verbalization of fears contributes to dealing with concerns; being attentive relays empathy to the patient; assisting family members to deal with the diagnosis and prognosis will enhance their ability to cope with serious illness.
Engage patient and family in open dialogue regarding options for treatments and care.	Discussion of care options allows the patient to be more in control, giving her a sense of empowerment that may assist with coping with a diagnosis of uterine cancer.
Keep the patient informed of all that is happening, including information about diagnostic tests and planned therapeutic interventions using a calm, reassuring manner.	Communication in a reassuring, calm, and straightforward manner may help to relieve anxiety and gives the patient a sense of well-being.
Seek spiritual consult as needed or requested by the patient and/ or family.	Meeting spiritual needs of the patient helps the patient to deal with fears through use of spiritual or religious rituals.
Teach the patient regarding possible surgical intervention (hysterectomy with bilateral salpingectomy and oophorectomy).	This is the treatment of choice for endometrial cancer, and understanding the procedure can aid in the reduction of anxiety.

 NIC *Anxiety reduction*

  Coping enhancement

  Emotional support

  Spiritual support

Evaluation

Evaluate the extent to which the outcome criteria have been achieved. The patient should be assessed for behaviors that would indicate adjustment to the diagnosis of endometrial cancer. Even though a majority of endometrial cancers are cured with surgery, the patient may still grieve the loss of reproductive function required by surgery and suffer anxiety regarding the unknown. The patient should verbalize fears and concerns and be able to identify one way to cope with the diagnosis of cancer. The extent to which the patient displays appropriate coping

behaviors should be noted. If the patient is unable to talk about the diagnosis and communicate concerns, the nurse should explore further interventions to assist the patient.

Community/Home Care

Nurses should assess which coping mechanisms work for the patient and encourage their use by the patient at home. Even for those patients whose disease was detected early and treated surgically, problems with anxiety may continue for a long period of time. At least one follow-up visit by a health care provider should be initiated to assess for ineffective coping. The patient should be encouraged to identify coping strategies that have been successful in the past and prompted to use those regularly. Anxiety regarding prognosis usually continues and is more pronounced for those patients for whom the disease was detected late with some extension beyond the uterine cavity. For this group, coping through use of support from outside sources may be required. Monitor for extreme self-isolation and depression, reporting any symptoms to the physician. For many patients and families, spiritual/religious rituals provide a means of coping with difficult, stressful situations. The patient's culture may dictate how she copes and/or grieves and with whom she shares this process. It is crucial that the nurse and family support the patient as needed to foster a healthy psychological state, recognizing that anger and denial are common. Because a hysterectomy is the most common treatment procedure, health care providers should anticipate some anxiety and grieving related to the loss of reproductive organs. As the disease progresses, the patient may require new strategies for coping with the disease and the anticipated loss of life. The patient may benefit from quiet periods of meditation during the day. Support to long-term caregivers will be important, as they too need to be supported in a grief process. Hospice can play an important role in the home situation through provision of counselors, chaplains, and in-home care providers. If questions should arise at home regarding the patient's health status or prescribed regimen, the patient should have a means of contact with a health care provider for answers.

Documentation

The degree to which the patient has decreased anxiety should be documented in the patient record. A rating system provides an objective way to relay to others the extent of the anxiety. Document whether the patient is able to discuss feelings regarding the diagnosis of endometrial cancer. Chart the patient's verbalizations as she states them and include in the record coping mechanisms utilized by the patient. Document findings from an assessment of the patient's psychological state, including whether there is depression, anger, crying, sadness, etc. Document referrals to hospice or religious leaders.

NURSING DIAGNOSIS 2

 ## ACUTE PAIN

Related to:

Presence of tumor in pelvic cavity

Surgical intervention (hysterectomy)

Defining Characteristics:

Facial grimace

Complaints of pain in abdomen or pelvic area

Goal:

Pain control is achieved.

Outcome Criteria

✔ The patient will verbalize that pain is reduced or relieved 1 hour following interventions.

✔ The patient states satisfaction with pain control measures.

NOC *Pain level*

Pain control

Comfort level

Medication response

INTERVENTIONS	RATIONALES
Have the patient rate pain intensity using a pain rating scale.	Gives a more objective assessment of the pain intensity.
Administer analgesics as ordered.	Helps to provide pain relief and decrease anxiety.
Teach relaxation techniques and other distraction techniques such as guided imagery, deep breathing, and use of music.	Helps to enhance effects of pharmacological interventions.
Assess effectiveness of interventions to relieve pain.	Helps to determine whether interventions have been effective in relieving pain or if new strategies need to be employed.
Establish a quiet environment.	Helps to enhance effects of analgesics.
If abdominal hysterectomy has been performed, implement strategies to reduce post-operative pain, including splinting abdomen when moving (see nursing care plan "Hysterectomy").	Splinting supports incisional site and prevents stress on operative area.

NIC *Pain management*

Analgesic administration

Anxiety reduction

Evaluation

The patient is able to report that the pain has been relieved or alleviated following interventions. Based on pain rating scales, the patient's pain has decreased. The degree to which the patient is able to assist in the management of the pain through anxiety reduction and relaxation techniques is assessed.

Community/Home Care

Home care required for the management of pain will depend on the type of treatments implemented and the stage of the cancer. In patients with endometrial cancer who have been treated with a hysterectomy, the pain may be temporary, subsiding as the wound heals and requiring only mild analgesics for post-operative pain. However, for patients with late disease who are being treated with chemotherapy, radiation, or hormonal therapy, the problem will probably become more pronounced as the disease progresses, as these treatments only provide tumor shrinkage and slowing of growth. Initially, pain medications may be given by mouth to obtain satisfactory pain control. However, in the later stages pain control may require the services of hospice or a home nurse when more invasive means of administering narcotics may be needed for control. Ineffective in-home management of pain may cause undue emotional stress for the patient and family, necessitating hospitalization. Teaching the patient how to utilize non-pharmacological measures to enhance the effects of analgesics will be crucial to obtaining satisfactory outcomes. The patient can record her favorite soft music and use headphones to listen to it when in pain. Resting in an easy chair while listening to music should relax the patient and decrease the perception of pain. Assessing pain control is an important facet of follow-up care by the home health nurse, hospice, or other health care worker and should include the patient's ability to purchase prescribed analgesics.

Documentation

Include in the documentation all assessments made relevant to the reproductive system and pain control. Document in the patient's own words the description of the pain and rating of the level of pain. All interventions employed for pain control and the patient's responses are documented. All teaching should be indicated in the patient record with an indication of the patient's level of understanding.

NURSING DIAGNOSIS 3

 DEFICIENT KNOWLEDGE

Related to:

New onset of disease

Treatments required

Possible complex treatment protocol

Misunderstanding of information

Defining Characteristics:

Many or no questions

Verbalizes a lack of knowledge/understanding about endometrial cancer

Goal:

The patient will understand endometrial cancer and its treatment.

Outcome Criteria

✔ The patient verbalizes a desire to learn necessary information.

✔ The patient verbalizes an understanding of diagnostic procedures (endometrial biopsy).

✔ The patient verbalizes an understanding of endometrial cancer treatment options (surgery, radiation, chemotherapy), including untoward effects of treatment and possible complications.

✔ The patient verbalizes an understanding of pain management.

✔ The patient verbalizes an understanding of follow-up care required and expresses a willingness to comply.

NOC *Knowledge: Disease process*
Knowledge: Treatment regimen
Compliance behavior

INTERVENTIONS	RATIONALES
Assess the patient's current knowledge as well as ability and readiness to learn.	The nurse needs to ascertain what the patient already knows and build on this; if the patient is not capable of learning or is not ready to learn, teaching will not be effective due to disinterest or inability to understand. The patient may not be ready to learn if in a state of denial or if extremely angry.
Start with the simplest information and move to complex information.	Patients can understand simple concepts easily and then can build on those to understand concepts that are more complex.
Teach patient and significant others: — Diagnostic studies: endometrial biopsy — Disease process of endometrial cancer — Pain medications used to treat cancer pain, including dosage, frequency, side effects, scheduling, and interactions with other medications — Signs and symptoms that would indicate a need to seek health care	Knowledge of disease process and identification of complications empowers the patient to take control and be compliant; endometrial biopsy is performed under local anesthesia and involves excising a sample of tissue for pathological analysis.
Teach patient and family regarding post-operative hysterectomy care (see nursing care plan "Hysterectomy").	Total hysterectomy with bilateral oophorectomy and salpingectomy is often the first treatment implemented, especially in the absence of metastasis; the patient will need to know post-operative care requirements.
Instruct patient regarding internal radiation (for late disease not cured with a hysterectomy)	If the patient knows what to expect, anxiety can be reduced, and the patient will be better

INTERVENTIONS	RATIONALES
and assist with implementation as ordered. — Internal radiation: implants will be placed and remain in place for 24 to 72 hours. — Remain flat in bed on strict bedrest with head of bed elevated no more than 20 degrees. — Maintain urinary drainage device. — Cleanse bowel prior to start of treatment. — Use gauze packing to keep implants in place. — There is a possibility of uterine contractions and the need for analgesics. — Fluid intake should be 2500 ml. — Use radiation safety precautions for visitors/family. — Monitor for symptoms of radiation syndrome: nausea, vomiting, anorexia, and malaise. — Post-treatment: there may be foul-smelling vaginal discharge; douche at home to control odor; slight vaginal bleeding may continue for several months. — There may be a need for vaginal dilation due to stenosis. — Long-handled forceps are needed in case of dislodgement.	equipped to make decisions and more likely to comply.
Teach patient and family about external radiation (for late disease): — Method of action — Course/duration of treatment, usually five treatments each week for 4 to 6 weeks — Skin changes to note: redness/discoloration, sloughing, and tenderness — Skin care: no soap, ointments, lotions, creams, or powder applied to the area; no rubbing, scrubbing, or scratching the area; no washing off markings; avoid exposing the treated area to the sun during the treatment and for 1 year following treatments — Loose-fitting clothes; panties may need to be avoided due to risk of irritation	Radiation is used with uterine cancer when surgery is not an option or in the presence of metastasis, and the patient needs to be informed of what to expect. The radiated skin is sensitive, and ointments, creams, ultraviolet rays, rubbing, etc., may cause burning and skin sloughing and interfere with radiation. The patient must know how to protect the skin from impairment; knowing what to expect in terms of radiation helps the patient to be more compliant and feel more in control.
— Control of fatigue: importance of energy conservation; intake of high energy foods rich in vitamin C, protein, and iron; taking a nap each day especially after treatment	
Teach patient and family about chemotherapy (for late disease) and its effects: — Method of action — Specific agents used for treatment — Alopecia: assist the patient to plan for hair loss by investigating purchasing of wigs or having hair cut short and using hair for a specially made wig before alopecia; find a resource that could teach women how to prepare fashionable head wraps — Nausea/vomiting: teach to use anti-emetics before meals prophylactically; avoid foods with strong odors, and in the hospital setting have lids removed from trays outside the room (when lids are removed from food trays the smell is often overwhelming to the gastrointestinal [GI] system and causes nausea); attempt frequent small meals avoiding spicy foods — Care of access sites: prevent of infection by use of aseptic techniques and procedures according to agency protocol — Control of fatigue: balance rest and activity, and on chemotherapy days a designated nap time should be scheduled — Prevention of infection: chemotherapy causes a depression of white blood cells (WBCs), predisposing the patient to infection; avoid people with infections and large crowds; practice good hand hygiene; know WBC counts	Knowledge of what to expect helps the patient cope with untoward side effects and better equips her to take responsibility for managing the illness and engaging in self-care.
Teach the patient and family about hormonal therapy (Megace, tamoxifen) as required for advanced disease.	Hormonal therapy is used in advanced disease when the cancer is well differentiated.

(continues)

(continued)

INTERVENTIONS	RATIONALES
Provide the patient and family with information on hospice and other community service agencies such as American Cancer Society.	These agencies can provide psychological support as well as resources to the patient and family.
Assess the patient's and family's understanding of all teaching by encouraging them to repeat information and ask questions as needed.	This allows the nurse to hear in the patient's own words what was taught and makes it easier to know what information may need to be reinforced.
Establish that the patient has the resources required to be compliant.	If needed resources such as finances and transportation to follow-up appointments are not available, the patient cannot be compliant; nurse will need to make necessary referrals.

NIC   *Teaching: Procedure/treatment*

Learning readiness enhancement

Learning facilitation

Teaching: Disease process

Teaching: Prescribed medication

Evaluation

Evaluate the degree to which the patient has achieved the outcome criteria relevant to the teaching sessions. The patient should verbalize an understanding of the content presented by repeating the information, particularly the disease process, diagnostic procedures, type of surgical procedure (hysterectomy) required, radiation treatment process, chemotherapy, and medications for pain or nausea. The nurse must determine if the patient is capable of being compliant with the recommended regimen. If further teaching is required at time of discharge, the appropriate referrals should be made to continue education.

Community/Home Care

The patient will need to implement the prescribed regimen in the home setting; the amount of time that the patient will require visitation or follow-up

will depend on the type of treatment employed. For the patient treated with a hysterectomy alone, teaching regarding wound care and activity restrictions should be undertaken with reinforcement by a visiting nurse (see nursing care plan "Hysterectomy"). In addition, attention needs to be given to the patient's psychological state, particularly self-esteem, body image, and sexuality (see nursing care plan "Hysterectomy"). At home the patient will likely experience fatigue following any of the treatments, but this is especially true with radiation or chemotherapy treatments. The patient needs to schedule short, uninterrupted periods of rest during the day when at home. If chemotherapy is employed, hair loss, nausea, and vomiting may also occur as result of treatments. For the patient receiving chemotherapy, it is important to monitor weight if the patient is experiencing nausea and vomiting. Health care providers or dieticians can assist the patient to prepare a diet that is both nutritional and easy to digest. Encourage the patient to monitor food intake and to keep a food diary. Weekly weights are done at home so that trends in weight can be detected. Both of these can be shared with the nurse visiting in the home or with other health care providers at follow-up appointments. If the patient is receiving external radiation therapy, she will need to return to an outpatient facility. External radiation therapy patients will need to be monitored for ability to care for skin properly to prevent further tissue destruction. The patient treated with internal radiation will need to continue perineal hygiene for several weeks at home as the discharge may continue, requiring daily douches. Of critical importance at home for the woman who has had internal radiation is the likelihood of vaginal stenosis requiring dilation several times a week. If not performed, the vagina may become so stenosed that examination and sexual intercourse may become virtually impossible. Most sources recommend that if the woman has a sexual partner, dilation be achieved through regular sexual intercourse. Because the patient is seen on a regular basis for general follow-up, for post-operative care, for chemotherapy, or for radiation therapy, health care providers can determine if further teaching or reinforcement is required. Pain control following hysterectomy is achieved with mild narcotics such as Percocet®, but will be a bigger part of home care in the later stages of the disease if a cure was not effected with surgery and will require frequent follow-up to ensure patient satisfaction. Those health care workers providing follow-up care need to ensure that the family and patient understand that dependence on medication should not be a concern for the cancer patient and that comfort is the ultimate goal.

Documentation

Document the specific content taught and the titles of any printed documents given to the patient. Include in the chart the patient's degree of understanding of the content and the methods used to evaluate learning. An assessment of the patient's ability to be compliant with the regimen in terms of radiation, chemotherapy, or follow-up should be made in the chart with indicators of referrals made. Any areas that need to be reinforced should be documented to ensure appropriate follow-up. If family members are present for the teaching session, document this in the chart, and always document any referrals made.

UNIT 12

ENDOCRINE SYSTEM

CHAPTER 12.125

ADRENAL EXCESS: CUSHING'S SYNDROME

GENERAL INFORMATION

Adrenal excess (Cushing's syndrome) is a disorder of the adrenal gland in which there are excessive amounts of circulating corticosteroids, especially glucocorticoids. Primary Cushing's syndrome occurs because of a tumor (benign or malignant) of the adrenal gland with production of excessive cortisol that eventually suppresses the action of the pituitary gland's production of cortisol. Secondary Cushing's syndrome results from disorders of the pituitary (most often an adenoma) or hypothalamus that stimulate the release of excess amounts of adrenocorticotrophic hormone (ACTH) or increased ACTH caused by a disorder outside the adrenal gland such as a lung or pancreatic tumor. Iatrogenic Cushing's syndrome is attributed to the widespread long-term use of glucocorticoids for a variety of medical conditions, including chronic lung disease. Clinical manifestations are numerous, and include skin that is thin and easily bruised; a round moon appearance to the face; fat deposits on the abdomen; fat deposits under the skin of the clavicle referred to as "buffalo humps"; muscle wasting, especially noted on the legs; weakness; decreased libido; excessive facial hair; polyuria; polydipsia; hypertension; hypokalemia; and hypernatremia. The disorder occurs more often in women than men, and most often in women ages 20 to 40 years.

NURSING DIAGNOSIS 1

DEFICIENT KNOWLEDGE

Related to:

New onset of disease

No previous experience with Cushing's syndrome

Need for surgery or implementation of a complex regimen

Need for change in usual activities

Defining Characteristics:

Confusion and questions about therapeutic interventions

Asks many questions

Asks no questions

New experience with adrenal excess

Goal:

The patient verbalizes understanding of adrenal excess and its treatment.

Outcome Criteria

✔ The patient verbalizes an understanding of adrenal excess/Cushing's syndrome.

✔ The patient verbalizes an understanding of the surgery or medication requirements for adrenal excess.

✔ The patient verbalizes an understanding of the dietary requirements for adrenal excess.

✔ The patient verbalizes an understanding of interventions required to prevent injury.

✔ The patient is able to carry out the prescribed treatment plan.

NOC *Knowledge: Disease process*
Knowledge: Health behavior
Treatment behavior: Illness or injury

INTERVENTIONS	RATIONALES
Assess the readiness of the patient to learn (motivation, cognitive level, and physiological status).	The patient must be motivated to learn, have the capability to learn the content, and be free of distractions from learning such as pain and emotional distress.
Assess what the patient already knows.	The patient may have some knowledge about adrenal

INTERVENTIONS	RATIONALES
	excess, and teaching should begin with what the patient already knows.
Create a quiet environment conducive to learning.	Environmental noise can prevent the learner from focusing on what is being taught.
Teach the learners about the normal function of the adrenal glands and the pathophysiology of adrenal excess/Cushing's syndrome.	Understanding of normal function and pathophysiology will facilitate understanding of the rationale for therapeutic interventions, including medications.
Teach patient about medications: — Mitotane used in adrenal cancer suppresses action of adrenal cortex; ketoconazole or metyrapone inhibits cortisol synthesis by the adrenal cortex and is used in ectopic adrenal excess (tumors that cannot be surgically removed) — Action and expected outcomes (reduction in amount of circulating cortisol) — Side effects — Dosages	Knowledge of medications, treatment regimen, actions, why the medication is needed, dosages, and side effects will improve compliance.
Teach the patient about required diet: high potassium and low sodium.	The patient needs to ingest enough potassium in diet to prevent hypokalemia and limit sodium to prevent further fluid retention and elevations in blood pressure.
Teach the patient how to recognize infection.	Increased levels of glucocorticoids alter the immune system and the normal inflammatory response so that redness or heat may not be noted; a feeling of malaise may be the first indicator of infection, and usually the patient only has a low-grade fever in the presence of infection.
Teach the patient and family regarding prevention of injury (see nursing diagnosis "Risk for Injury").	The patient is at high risk for disruption of skin integrity due to thin fragile skin caused by excess cortisol; falls may occur due to electrolyte imbalances that cause weakness (hypokalemia, hypocalcemia); pathological fractures can occur due to increased absorption of calcium and demineralization of bones.
Review symptoms of abnormal response to treatment and signs that require prompt attention: adrenal deficit following treatment, wounds that do not heal, continued malaise, shortness of breath, increasing weakness especially in extremities, swelling over bony areas, or obvious poor alignment of an extremity (sign of fracture) accompanied by pain.	The patient needs to be able to identify symptoms that would encourage him or her to seek medical assistance; the patient needs to be aware of complications such as congestive heart failure due to water retention, poorly healing wound, signs of pathological fracture, signs of electrolyte imbalance, or adrenal deficit following treatment.
Teach patient about medical/surgical interventions: — Transsphenoidal resection of the pituitary gland or adrenalectomy — Pre-operative and post-operative care required: replacement of glucocorticoids for patients having a bilateral adrenalectomy, dressing changes, prevention of infection, as well as monitoring for Addisonian crisis and hypovolemic shock — Radiation therapy — Gradual lowering or discontinuing of glucocorticoid therapy, if this is the cause of Cushing's syndrome	The patient needs to be aware of all options for treatment and interventions to be performed after treatment by the patient.
Teach the patient to inform all other health care providers, such as dentists, podiatrists, cardiologists, etc., about adrenal excess/Cushing's syndrome.	These providers need to know this due to the increased risk of infection in wounds or following otherwise routine procedures.
Provide literature on obtaining a Medic-Alert bracelet.	In the event the patient is unconscious, caregivers will be able to identify possible causes and implement strategies for emergency care.
Evaluate the patient's understanding of all content covered by asking questions.	Helps to identify areas that require more teaching and to ensure that the patient has enough information to ensure compliance.
Give the patient written information on the disease, diet, and medications, including a schedule for administration.	Provides material for later reference, and for review.
Encourage regular appointments with physician.	Physician can monitor progress and medication response.

NIC *Teaching: Disease process*
Teaching: Individual
Teaching: Diet

Evaluation

The patient is able to repeat all information for the nurse and asks questions about adrenal excess and possible outcomes (positive and negative). Prior to discharge, the patient verbalizes an understanding of required medications and their administration and diet requirements (increased potassium, decreased sodium), and agrees to be compliant. The patient is able to state what adrenal excess is, and what causes it, and demonstrates an understanding of the interventions required (medications or surgery) and the need for lifelong therapy. The patient is able to state signs and symptoms that indicate an emergency and what is required if they occur. All paperwork required to obtain a Medic-Alert bracelet has been completed, and the patient agrees to wear it. The patient should know and be able to inform the nurse when health care assistance should be sought.

Community/Home Care

For patients who have adrenal excess, the therapeutic regimen could be implemented over a short period of time, or it could be a lifetime commitment. Teaching by the health care team should be thorough with opportunities for discussions. Knowledge needs are identified early in order to improve the likelihood that the patient will be prepared for self-care and self-monitoring once at home. The major components of the regimen are dietary and medications. The patient will need to implement strategies to decrease sodium in the diet and increase potassium (see nursing diagnosis "Excess Fluid Volume"). A consultation with the dietician is necessary to complete education on this aspect of home care. The patient will likely need to adjust his or her diet, and adaptation will be easier if the diet is palatable and is in keeping with the patient's usual food preferences and cultural or religious restrictions. For patients who have had removal of the pituitary gland or a resection of ectopic tumors, such as in the lung, a cure usually is effected with the surgery, but during the recovery period ACTH production is not sufficient for the body, and cortisol replacement is required for 6 to 24 months to allow for return of function of the adrenal glands. If the patient had a bilateral adrenalectomy, administration of replacement glucocorticoids and mineralocorticoids will be lifelong. The patient may tire of this regimen, but the nurse must make it clear to the patient that failure to comply will result in a crisis. The patient will need to develop methods of remembering to take the prescribed medications, especially if working outside the home, as at least one dose will usually be needed during working hours. The patient can place medications in a place where they will be noticeable, such as the kitchen or bathroom counter, as a daily reminder. The patient should have a clear plan for what to do if he or she is unable to take the medications, this may include injecting parenteral cortisone. For all patients having surgery for adrenal excess, teaching is needed to ensure that the patient can implement wound care and monitor for infection. Once at home, the patient may need further reinforcement and should have access to a health care provider to call for clarification; at this time the nurse or others can evaluate the patient's understanding of all content taught and ability and willingness to follow through. Follow-up with a health care provider focuses on assurance that no complications have occurred and that the patient has a clear understanding of how to manage all aspects of adrenal excess.

Documentation

Document all content taught and the patient's verbalization of understanding. Specific attention should be given to documentation of any specific concerns that the patient expresses. Include in the documentation the patient's willingness to comply with all recommendations made regarding the diet, post-operative care, administration of glucocorticoids and mineralocorticoids if a bilateral adrenalectomy was performed, and emergency care. Include the patient's demonstration of how to perform an injection of cortisone. Any area that requires further teaching should be clearly indicated in the record. Include in the record appointments that have been made for outpatient procedures as well. Chart any questions or concerns that the patient has verbalized. Always include the titles of any printed literature given to the patient for reinforcement.

NURSING DIAGNOSIS 2

 EXCESS FLUID VOLUME

Related to:

Hypernatremia

Excessive mineralocorticoids

Defining Characteristics:

Increased serum sodium above 145 mEq/L

Edema

Hypokalemia

Crackles in lungs

Elevated blood pressure

Goal:

No signs of fluid volume excess are noted and electrolyte balance is achieved.

Outcome Criteria

✔ The patient will lose excess fluid as demonstrated by weight loss.

✔ Sodium levels will return to normal range: 135–145 mEq/L.

✔ Potassium will return to normal range.

✔ Lungs will be clear to auscultation.

✔ The patient will have no edema.

NOC *Fluid balance*

Fluid overload severity

Electrolyte and acid/base balance

Vital signs

INTERVENTIONS	RATIONALES
Assess for signs of fluid volume excess, such as edema, hypertension, and crackles in lungs.	Clinical manifestations such as these must be detected early to initiate treatment and prevent complications.
Monitor vital signs every 4 hours.	Helps to detect abnormalities; blood pressure and pulse will be elevated with excess volume.
Monitor intake and output.	Helps to determine fluid balance.
Monitor laboratory results: cortisol, 24-hour urine for ketosteroids and 17-hydroxycorticosteroids, ACTH level, serum electrolytes, glucose, and computed tomography (CT) scan.	The cortisol levels will vary depending on the time of day but typically will show elevations at times other than the normal diurnal pattern; 24-hour urine tests measure free cortisol and androgens, and are increased in Cushing's disease/syndrome; electrolytes are measured to determine potassium or other electrolyte replacement needs; potassium levels are low and sodium is high in the person
	with Cushing's disease; glucose levels are elevated; CT scans and an MRI are used to locate sites of tumors.
Administer diuretics as ordered.	Decreases total body water and promotes excretion of sodium.
Weigh patient in similar clothes on the same scale at same time (before breakfast, after voiding) each day.	Helps to determine the response to diuretic therapy; weight is the best determinant of fluid loss or retention; 1 kg of weight loss = 1 liter of fluid loss. It is important to weigh the patient under similar conditions for accuracy.
Restrict intake of high-sodium foods, such as processed meats, seafood, canned foods, processed grains, dried fruit, spinach, celery, carrots, and snack foods.	Decreases serum sodium levels.
Restrict fluid intake to 1000–2000 ml/day; spread out fluid intake throughout the day, ensuring that fluids served with meals and taken with medications are included. Scheduling a certain amount for 8-hour intervals will help keep the patient compliant.	Helps to decrease total body water and decrease risk of congestive heart failure.
Administer potassium replacements as ordered.	The patient with Cushing's disease/syndrome has low potassium levels; efforts to correct fluid excess involve diuretics, which may further lower potassium levels, making it necessary to give supplements.
Encourage foods rich in potassium such as bananas, cantaloupe, raisins, and orange juice.	Increases potassium levels naturally.

NIC *Fluid monitoring*

Fluid management

Electrolyte management: Hypernatremia

Electrolyte management: Hypokalemia

Evaluation

Determine the extent to which the outcome criteria have been achieved. The patient should have a resolution of fluid volume excess as demonstrated by absence of edema and clear breath sounds. The patient's blood pressure and pulse are at baseline, and serum sodium and potassium levels are within normal range. The patient, when weighed, will demonstrate a weight loss indicative of fluid loss, and no edema will be present.

Community/Home Care

Ensure that patient at home understands the importance of monitoring fluid status. The patient should have a reliable scale that is calibrated and easily accessible. Weighing daily at home will allow the patient to monitor weight and notice subtle changes in fluid retention that may indicate a recurrence of the problem, especially during the early phase of the disorder while treatment is becoming effective. Patients should be informed to take note of clothing that becomes too tight in a short period of time, which is an indicator of fluid retention. The patient who has increased sodium levels with fluid volume excess needs to restrict sodium intake. At home, the patient needs to limit the intake of salt and sodium-rich foods. The patient should be taught how to read food labels for sodium content, as many people find it difficult to decipher labels. Provide the patient with a list of foods that are good sources of potassium and encourage the patient to include them in his or her daily diet, especially in the early days of treatment. Diet instructions for home should consider the patient's normal diet and any cultural or religious preferences and restrictions. Have the patient keep a log of food and fluid intake, as well as weights. Assist the patient to develop a schedule for taking prescribed diuretics that is mindful of his or her lifestyle and daily routines. Stress the need for follow-up care to assess sodium and potassium level as well as other electrolytes.

Documentation

Always document the extent to which the outcome criteria have been achieved. An assessment of fluid status that includes intake and output, blood pressure, pulse, weights, and breath sounds should be noted. Be sure that fluid restrictions are indicated in the record, with specifications for amounts to be administered each shift. Medications that are administered for excess fluid volume should be documented on the medication administration record; the amount of fluid the patient lost in response should be documented as well. Chart the patient's understanding of the therapies for eliminating fluid excess.

NURSING DIAGNOSIS 3

RISK FOR INJURY

Related to:

Muscle wasting

Loss of calcium from bones

Fragile, thin skin

Loss of protein from bone

Defining Characteristics:

None

Goal:

The patient will not sustain injury.

Outcome Criteria

✔ The patient will not bleed from skin.

✔ Skin will remain intact.

✔ No pathological fracture occurs.

✔ The patient will not fall.

NOC *Fall prevention behavior*
Risk control

INTERVENTIONS	RATIONALES
Assess the patient's risk for injury: calcium level, potassium level, and condition of skin.	Electrolyte imbalance may cause weakness, and decreased calcium predisposes the patient to pathological fracture; thin, fragile skin seen in Cushing's syndrome predisposes the patient to easy injury, even with minor trauma; elevated levels of cortisol also contribute to easy bruising and purpura.
Assess the environment for safety hazards.	Helps to determine adjustments that need to be made for safety.
Clear pathways of clutter such as rugs, furniture, or other objects.	Helps to prevent falls.
Assist the patient as needed with ambulation.	Prevents injury; electrolyte imbalances cause muscle weakness and fatigue, predisposing the patient to falls.
Encourage the patient to use assistive devices for ambulation and for getting in and out of tubs or showers.	Decreases risk for falls.

INTERVENTIONS	RATIONALES
Encourage the patient to wear shoes or non-skid slippers when out of bed ambulating.	Helps to reduce the risk of falls from slipping on floors, especially non-carpeted flooring.
Assess the patient for abnormal positions of extremities and pain in extremities with movement or bruising over a bony site.	Pathological fractures may occur with normal movement due to demineralization of bones, and these symptoms are indicators of a fracture.
If mobility is limited due to fatigue or weakness, encourage the patient to reposition self every 2 hours.	Frequent repositioning is needed to prevent breakdown of the fragile skin.
Protect skin from injury due to bumping into objects by having patient wear protective clothing and scan environment when ambulating.	The skin is thin and fragile and will bruise and lacerate easily; scanning the environment will prevent accidental bumps.
Cleanse any open areas with normal saline or other solution as ordered and apply a protective covering.	Helps to prevent infection and further injury.

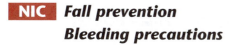 **NIC** *Fall prevention*
Bleeding precautions

Evaluation

No pathological fracture occurs, and the patient experiences no falls. Skin remains intact, no bleeding is noted, and bruising is minimal. The environment is enhanced for safety by removing clutter and providing lighted pathways.

Community/Home Care

Because the therapeutic effects of treatment for Cushing's syndrome may take an extended period of time to occur, the patient will need to implement practices to promote safety in the home. It is important that the patient understand the need to prevent injury and the alterations that contribute to the problem (increased cortisol, low potassium, loss of calcium). The patient and family should clear pathways of clutter by removing objects such as throw rugs, small tables, or decorative items from pathways. It is important that the family and patient be aware of the signs of pathological fractures and be aware they can occur with normal movement and not just with injuries such as falls; pathological fractures may not have the characteristic

severe pain except when movement is attempted. The skin poses a special problem because it is fragile, thin, and bruises easily. The patient should protect it from injury by wearing protective garments, especially over arms. Simple tasks such as working in the garden or doing household chores may end in bruises or skin tears if the patient is not careful. The patient should inspect the skin frequently for new skin tears or bruises that would allow for protection to the impaired areas. Dietary increases in potassium and calcium can help the problem by correcting electrolyte imbalances that cause weakness. The health care provider should assess the patient's functional ability and question the patient regarding falls or skin alterations.

Documentation

Chart the findings from an assessment of muscle strength and skin, noting any of the defining characteristics of Cushing's syndrome, such as bruising, purpura, muscle weakness, and thin skin. Chart teaching that has been done regarding prevention of pathological fractures, prevention of falls, and creation of a safe environment. Include in the documentation use of special devices or assistive devices for ambulation.

NURSING DIAGNOSIS 4

 DISTURBED BODY IMAGE

Related to:

Effects of increased cortisol

Excessive androgen

Altered fat metabolism

Defining Characteristics:

Fat deposits on abdomen/truncal obesity

Fat deposits in shoulders/buffalo hump

Thin, wasted legs

Increased facial hair

Thin head hair

Moon face

Goal:

The patient accepts the change in physical appearance and continues social activities and interpersonal relationships.

Outcome Criteria

✔ The patient states willingness to look at and touch the body.

✔ The patient does not verbalize negative feelings toward self.

✔ The patient verbalizes acceptance of body appearance.

✔ The patient verbalizes an understanding of causes of changes in appearance.

NOC *Body image*

INTERVENTIONS	RATIONALES
Assess the patient for characteristic changes of Cushing's syndrome: moon face, thin legs, truncal obesity, buffalo hump, thin skin, bruises, facial hair, and thinning head hair.	These changes typically cause an alteration in body image and self-esteem; the patient often perceives the changes negatively, evaluating self based on physical appearance.
Encourage the patient to communicate feelings regarding change in appearance, and assure the patient that his or her feelings are normal.	The patient should understand that his or her emotions are real and should be expected; talking about the changes may sometimes be the beginning of acceptance.
Identify the effects of the patient's culture or religion on body image.	A patient's culture and religion often help define his or her reactions to changes in body image and self-worth.
Monitor the patient for feelings about self, interpersonal relationships with family members and friends, withdrawal, social isolation, fear, anxiety, embarrassment by appearance, fear that appearance will be displeasing to loved ones, and desire to be alone.	Helps to detect early alterations in social functioning, prevent unhealthy behaviors, and intervene early through referral to counseling.
Inform the patient of the causes of the alterations in appearance and that the changes are temporary in most cases, with resolution occurring with treatment.	The patient may be fearful that the changes are permanent. Educating the patient on the prognosis may assist him or her to adapt to the changes and protect his or her body image. Cushing's syndrome changes may resolve when treatment becomes effective. In patients who have surgery (bilateral adrenalectomy), the changes may not completely resolve if
	the patient must be on permanent glucocorticoid replacement therapy, but they will not be as pronounced.
Discuss with the patient methods to disguise some of the changes with makeup, fashionable loose clothing, pants rather than skirts or dresses, and shaving head or wearing hairpieces for thinning head hair. An occupational therapist may be of assistance.	If the patient can implement simple strategies to disguise the alterations in physical appearance of the body, he or she may begin to cope with the change.
Encourage the patient to participate in at least one outside/public activity each week.	Prevents patient from isolating self from others; because of obvious changes in appearance, the patient may refrain from social interaction.
Offer reassurance, positive praise, and feedback on efforts.	The patient will feel better if others recognize his or her efforts, and will better adjust to the change.

NIC *Body image enhancement*
Emotional support
Socialization enhancement

Evaluation

The patient is able and willing to learn about the strategies to improve appearance, and implements suggestions. Determine if the patient is able to verbalize feelings regarding the changes in the body appearance and the perceived impact it will have on relationships, socialization, and role performance. Time is required for the patient to completely assimilate the change in body appearance into his or her self-perception. It is crucial that the nurse evaluates to what degree the patient is beginning to do this. Communication of feelings and concerns relevant to the change in appearance should be taken as a positive sign that progress towards meeting the outcome criteria is being made.

Community/Home Care

At home, continued monitoring of the patient's body image is needed. The health care provider who interacts with the patient during follow-up will need to be alert to subtle hints that may indicate that the patient has not completely adapted to the change in body appearance. For the patient with Cushing's syndrome, the change in appearance may be very noticeable, especially the round face and fat deposits. The patient may be anxious about having others, even a significant other, see him or her, and may refrain from socialization. Wearing clothing that can disguise some of the changes is encouraged, but one must consider the cost involved. Most women have some pants, and these can be worn in public instead of dresses or skirts that may reveal the thin legs. Because of the truncal obesity, new clothes may need to be purchased in any event. Stylish, flowing, loose-fitting garments for women can be obtained; for men, wearing shirts outside the pants may also disguise the fat deposits. Makeup can hide acne and cover changes in skin color or marks from shaving. Support from family, friends, and significant others makes acceptance of the changes easier. The patient needs to employ coping mechanisms that can help him or her deal with the changes. In some instances just knowing that the changes are likely temporary is enough to enhance coping. It is important that family or significant others encourage continued participation in outside activities and avoidance of self-imposed isolation. Open discussions regarding the changes and their accompanying frustrations are crucial to the patient's ability to maintain a positive body image. If the patient is an active member of a religious or civic organization, such venues may provide a good place to start social interaction, as the patient may have some sense of comfort with the people there and be more willing to attempt interactions.

Documentation

Chart any specific behaviors or verbalizations that may indicate an altered body image. Document a precise description of the physical change in appearance that is causing the disturbed body image. Include all interventions that have been employed to address this issue and the patient's responses. Note when and if the patient begins to verbalize feelings about the change in appearance. Document instruction regarding how to disguise the changes with makeup or clothing.

CHAPTER 12.126

ADRENAL INSUFFICIENCY: ADDISON'S DISEASE

GENERAL INFORMATION

Adrenal insufficiency, also known as adrenocortical insufficiency, Addison's disease (chronic adrenal insufficiency), or hypopituitarism by the adrenal gland, is a disorder characterized by the lack of production of glucocorticoids, mineralocorticoids, and androgens. There is a deficiency of cortisol and aldosterone as well. Primary adrenal insufficiency (Addison's disease) is caused by destruction of the adrenal cortex thought to result from an autoimmune response. In primary adrenal insufficiency, levels of adrenocorticotrophic hormone (ACTH) are increased due to a compensatory mechanism of the pituitary gland. Other disorders that contribute to the development of primary adrenal insufficiency include tuberculosis, septicemia, adrenalectomy, cancer, AIDS, hemorrhage or tumors of the adrenal gland, injury to the adrenal gland as a result of abdominal trauma, or fungal infections. Clinical manifestations of primary adrenal insufficiency include hyperpigmentation of the skin, hypotension (especially postural), fatigue, weight loss, nausea/vomiting, irritability, and fluid/electrolyte imbalances (hyponatremia, hyperkalemia, and hypochloremia), hypoglycemia, and extracellular dehydration. Onset is slow over a period of months, and at the time the diagnosis is confirmed, approximately 90 percent of function has been lost. Secondary adrenal insufficiency is usually the result of pituitary tumors, or any disorder that suppresses pituitary gland function, and the abrupt withdrawal of steroid therapy. In secondary adrenal insufficiency, there are low amounts of circulating cortisol and ACTH, but there is not a deficit of corticosteroids, and aldosterone levels are sufficient; thus the patient does not have the significant electrolyte imbalances or hyperpigmentation of the skin that are seen in primary adrenal insufficiency. Manifestations of secondary adrenal insufficiency include pallor, water retention, and mild hyponatremia. Addison's disease is seen more often in women and in persons under the age of 60 years. Addisonian crisis is an emergency situation that occurs when the patient with adrenal insufficiency requires increases in hormones of the adrenal gland due to major stressors such as infection, surgery, pregnancy, or emotional stress. It may also occur if glucocorticoid therapy is withdrawn abruptly and the pituitary gland and hypothalamus are unable to fulfill their function of increasing the amount of circulating glucocorticoid due to long-term suppression. In Addisonian crisis, the patient presents with any of the same symptoms of adrenal insufficiency, but these are more pronounced with significant hypotension, abdominal pain, high fever, pronounced weakness, and, if undetected, circulatory collapse with concomitant shock. Treatment is supportive with intravenous (IV) glucocorticoids and aggressive fluid administration.

NURSING DIAGNOSIS 1

INEFFECTIVE MANAGEMENT OF THERAPEUTIC REGIMEN

Related to:

Knowledge deficit related to adrenal insufficiency

Need for implementation of a complex regimen

Need for change in usual activities

Defining Characteristics:

Confusion and questions about therapeutic interventions

Asks many questions

Asks no questions

New experience with adrenal insufficiency

Goal:

The patient verbalizes understanding of adrenal insufficiency and its treatment.

Outcome Criteria

✔ The patient verbalizes an understanding of the disease: adrenal insufficiency.

✔ The patient verbalizes an understanding of the medication requirements for adrenal insufficiency.

✔ The patient verbalizes an understanding of the dietary requirements for adrenal insufficiency.

✔ The patient is able to state what to do in times of stress (physiological or emotional).

✔ The patient is able to carry out the prescribed treatment plan.

NOC *Knowledge: Disease process*
Knowledge: Health behavior
Treatment behavior: Illness
or injury

INTERVENTIONS	RATIONALES
Assess the readiness of the patient to learn (motivation, cognitive level, and physiological status).	The patient must be motivated to learn, have the capability to learn the content, and be free of distractions from learning such as anxiety and emotional distress.
Assess what the patient already knows.	The patient may have some knowledge about adrenal insufficiency, and teaching should begin with what the patient already knows.
Create a quiet environment conducive to learning.	Environmental noise can prevent the learner from focusing on what is being taught.
Teach the patient and family: — Normal function of the adrenal glands (secretion of glucocortoids, mineralocorticoids, androgens, role of adrenal glands and secretions in response to emotional and physiological stress) — Pathophysiology of adrenal insufficiency/Addison's disease	Understanding of normal function and pathophysiology will facilitate understanding of the rationale for therapeutic interventions including medications.
Teach patient about medications: glucocorticoids and mineralocorticoids: — Action and expected outcomes — Side effects — Dosages — Timing of dosages to mimic normal release: need two-thirds of glucocorticoid dose in the morning and one-third in afternoon (before 4 p.m.), and mineralocorticoids given in the evening (patients with secondary adrenal insufficiency do not require mineralocorticoids) — Taken with food or after meals to decrease gastrointestinal (GI) distress — Necessity of lifelong therapy — Need for additional medications in times of stress (psychological or physiological such as infection, trauma, and surgery) — How to inject cortisone — Importance of carrying an emergency supply of injectable cortisone with him or her	Knowledge of medications, treatment regimen, actions, need for medication, dosages, and side effects will improve compliance. Because the patient cannot produce cortisol when stressed, there is a need to adjust oral steroid agents to accommodate. Having injectable cortisone available is necessary in case the patient is unable to take medications orally. Taking medicine with food or after meals decreases GI distress.
Teach the patient about diet required: low potassium and high sodium.	The patient needs to ingest enough sodium in diet to prevent hyponatremia and limit potassium to avoid complications of hyperkalemia.
Teach the patient how to recognize infection.	Use of glucocorticoids alters the normal inflammatory response so that normal/usual indicators of infection may not be noted.
Teach the patient to inform all other health care providers, such as dentists, podiatrists, cardiologists, etc., about adrenal insufficiency.	These providers need this information to ensure safety of patient if performing procedures or prescribing medications.
Provide literature on how to obtain a Medic-Alert bracelet.	In the event patient is unconscious, caregivers will be able to identify possible causes and implement strategies for emergency care.
Encourage regular appointments with the physician.	The physician can monitor progress and medication response.
Review symptoms of abnormal response to treatment or worsening condition and signs	The patient should be able to identify symptoms that would require him or her to seek

(continues)

(continued)

INTERVENTIONS	RATIONALES
that require prompt attention: signs of adrenal excess or deficit, high fever, weight loss, or increasing weakness.	medical assistance. Any of these could be a symptom of Addisonian crisis.
Evaluate the patient's understanding of all content covered by asking questions.	Helps to identify areas that require more teaching and to ensure that the patient has enough information to comply.
Give the patient written information on diet, medications (including a schedule), use of the injectable cortisone, and the disease.	Provides material for reference at a later time, and for review.

NIC　*Teaching: Disease process*
Teaching: Individual
Teaching: Diet
Teaching: Psychomotor skill

Evaluation

The patient is able to repeat all information for the nurse, and asks questions about adrenal insufficiency and possible outcomes (positive and negative). Prior to discharge, the patient verbalizes an understanding of required medications and their administration and diet requirements (increased sodium, decreased potassium), and agrees to be compliant. The patient is able to state what adrenal insufficiency is and what causes it, as well as an understanding of the need for lifelong therapy. The patient is able to state what to do in an emergency and what is required in terms of stress situations, and agrees to comply. All paperwork required to obtain a Medic-Alert bracelet has been completed and the patient agrees to wear it. The patient should know and be able to inform the nurse when health care assistance should be sought.

Community/Home Care

For patients who have adrenal insufficiency, the therapeutic regimen is a lifetime commitment that will need to be continued in the home. Teaching by the health care team should be thorough and include opportunities for discussions. Knowledge needs are identified early in order to improve the likelihood that the patient will be prepared for

self-care and self-monitoring once at home. The major components of the regimen are dietary and medications. The patient will need to implement strategies to increase sodium in the diet and limit potassium (see nursing diagnosis "Deficient Fluid Volume"). A consultation with the dietician is necessary to complete education on this aspect of home care. The patient needs to verbalize to the nurse or dietician the names of foods that are high in potassium that should be eliminated from the diet. The patient will likely need to adjust his or her diet, and adaptation will be easier if the diet is palatable and in keeping with the patient's usual food preferences and cultural or religious restrictions. A list of foods that are acceptable and those to be avoided should be given to the patient following teaching sessions. Of greatest importance is to be sure that the patient has understood the teaching regarding medications. Administration of glucocorticoids and mineralocorticoids will be lifelong. The patient may tire of this regimen, but the nurse must make it clear to the patient that failure to comply will result in a crisis. The patient will need to develop methods of remembering to take the prescribed medications, especially if working outside the home, as at least one dose will usually be needed during working hours. Purchasing a cheap watch that alarms or beeps can be used as a reminder at work by setting it to alarm at the scheduled medication time. The patient can place medications in a noticeable place, such as the kitchen or bathroom counter, as a daily reminder. The patient should have a clear plan for what to do if he or she is unable to take the medications, which may include injecting parenteral cortisone. At home, the patient will need to implement assessment methods to detect signs of insufficiency to prevent a crisis. Once at home, the patient may need further reinforcement and should have access to a health care provider to call for clarification; at this time the nurse or other provider can evaluate the patient's understanding of all content taught and the patient's ability and willingness to follow through. Follow-up with a health care provider focuses on assurance that no complications have occurred and that the patient has a clear understanding of how to manage all aspects of adrenal insufficiency.

Documentation

Document all content taught and the patient's verbalization of understanding. Specific attention should be given to documentation of any specific concerns that the patient expresses. Included in the documentation is the patient's willingness to comply with all recommendations made regarding the diet, administration of glucocorticoids and mineralocorticoids, and emergency care. Include the patient's demonstration of how to perform an injection of cortisone. Any area that requires further teaching should be clearly indicated in the record. Chart any questions or concerns that the patient has verbalized. Always include the titles of any printed literature given to the patient for reinforcement. Referrals to the dietician are documented in the patient record.

NURSING DIAGNOSIS 2

 ### DEFICIENT FLUID VOLUME

Related to:

Cortisol insufficiency

Hyponatremia

Excess water secretion

Diarrhea

Vomiting

Defining Characteristics:

Tachycardia

Weakness, lethargy

Hypotension

Dry mucous membranes

Poor skin turgor

Hyperpigmentation of skin

Salt craving

Syncope

Severe electrolyte imbalance (hyponatremia and hyperkalemia)

Significantly decreased cortisol (> 5 mg/dl)

Decreased chlorides

Hypoglycemia

Increased hematocrit (Hct)

Increased blood urea nitrogen (BUN)

Sudden weight loss

Goal:

The patient's fluid volume and electrolyte imbalance are corrected.

Outcome Criteria

✔ Urine output is > 30 ml/hour.

✔ Hypotension resolves and blood pressure returns to baseline.

✔ Pulse rate is > 60 but < 100.

✔ The patient reports no craving for salt.

✔ Electrolytes (sodium, potassium, chloride) return to normal.

✔ Skin turgor is normal and mucous membranes are moist.

✔ No injury occurs.

NOC *Hydration*

Fluid balance

Electrolyte and acid/base balance

INTERVENTIONS	RATIONALES
Assess for signs of dehydration/ volume deficit: decreased blood pressure, increased pulse, dry mucous membranes, poor skin turgor and hyperpigmentation, and decreased urinary output.	An assessment is required to determine the degree of dehydration and to assist in planning interventions; ongoing assessment of these parameters is required to evaluate response to treatment. Reduced aldosterone secretion with accompanying deficits in mineralocorticoids causes water and electrolyte imbalances. Hyperpigmentation occurs due to uncontrolled release of ACTH, which stimulates the release of melanocyte stimulating hormone, causing a bronzing of the skin in Caucasian or lighter-skinned persons and a general darkening of the skin in darker-skinned people. This hyper-pigmented skin tends to be drier than normal skin with poorer turgor.
Monitor laboratory results: ACTH stimulation test, serum cortisol levels, urinary 17-hydroxycorticoid and 17-ketosteroids (17 KS), plasma ACTH, electrolytes, glucose, BUN, urine specific gravity, Hct, and arterial blood gases (ABGs).	ACTH stimulation test demonstrates an inability of the adrenal glands to raise cortisol levels when stimulated with ACTH; cortisol levels are decreased; urinary 17-hydroxycorticoids, which are metabolites of glucocorticoids,

(continues)

(continued)

INTERVENTIONS	RATIONALES
	and 17-ketosteroids, which are metabolites of adrenal androgens, are decreased. ACTH is increased in primary adrenal insufficiency and decreased in secondary adrenal insufficiency; in adrenal insufficiency, volume deficits and aldosterone deficiency alter many plasma components. Potassium levels are increased; sodium and chloride are decreased; glucose levels are decreased due to lack of glucocorticoids with subsequent decrease in glycogenesis and gluconeogenesis; BUN is elevated due to dehydration secondary to decreased glomerular filtration rate; urine specific gravity is increased due to hemoconcentration; elevated Hct is due to severe fluid loss; ABGs reveal metabolic acidosis due to reabsorption of hydrogen ions as a result of hyperkalemia. Monitoring these values can guide replacement therapy and determine the extent of disease.
Assess for symptoms of electrolyte imbalance: muscle weakness, dizziness/syncope, lethargy, extreme thirst, and salt cravings.	Low sodium levels impact functioning of nervous tissue, and increased potassium affects the ability of muscles to contract properly. The hyponatremia is severe enough in many instances to cause the patient to crave salt.
Maintain strict intake and output.	Helps to detect imbalances and monitor for restoration of hydration status.
Monitor cardiac status at least every 4 hours or as ordered: vital signs, electrocardiogram (EKG), and capillary refill.	Significant fluid deficits alter cardiac output due to decreases in circulating volume and subsequent decreases in perfusion. The patient may display signs of hypovolemic shock: tachycardia, hypotension, capillary refill > 2 seconds, sharp-peaked T waves and wide QRS complex due to hyperkalemia; temperature 103 to 104 degrees F; dizziness and syncope due to hypotension and electrolyte imbalances.
Monitor nutritional status: abdominal pain, nausea, vomiting, diarrhea, and weight loss.	The patient can lose both electrolytes and fluid through GI upsets, which are common. Abdominal pain may cause the patient not to take adequate amounts of fluid, and weight loss is common.
Establish IV access and initiate fluid replacement therapy as ordered, often with 5 percent dextrose in normal saline, as guided by degree of dehydration.	Adrenal insufficiency is characterized by dehydration, and if uncorrected, severe dehydration can cause acute adrenal insufficiency (Addisonian crisis). The saline helps replace lost sodium, and glucose is given to treat hypoglycemia.
Administer corticosteroids such as hydrocortisone and mineralocorticoids such as fludrocortisone as ordered, and monitor for side effects.	Replacement therapy is essential to correct the causative factor.
Administer anti-emetics and antidiarrheals.	Helps to decrease fluid and electrolyte losses from GI tract.
Encourage frequent, small meals.	Frequency of meals needs to increase to prevent hypoglycemia; large meals may not be tolerated due to nausea and vomiting.
Offer foods with high sodium content and low potassium.	Sodium loss is significant and needs to be replaced if possible through food; sodium is required by nervous tissue; eliminating potassium-rich foods from the diet can assist in lowering potassium levels.
Encourage oral intake of fluids, 3000 ml/day, that are potassium-poor and sodium-rich.	Helps to rehydrate patient and balance electrolytes; cortisol deficiency causes a loss of extracellular water and electrolytes.
Assist the patient with activities, especially ambulation or activities that require mental alertness.	The hypotension that accompanies adrenal insufficiency can cause severe orthostatic hypotension that could cause a patient to become dizzy and fall if unassisted. Low sodium levels interfere with nervous tissue function and cause the patient to be lethargic.
Weigh patient daily.	Helps to assess stabilization of nutritional status and to detect excessive fluid loss.

INTERVENTIONS	RATIONALES
Teach the patient information regarding replacement of fluids and electrolytes, and treating hypoglycemia.	Helps to enhance understanding of the disease and its treatment.

NIC *Fluid monitoring*

Hypovolemia management

Intravenous insertion

Intravenous therapy

Electrolyte management: Hyponatremia

Electrolyte management: Hyperkalemia

Evaluation

Assess the patient for return of normal fluid volume. The patient's blood pressure should return to baseline, and the pulse should be strong and regular. Skin should be warm, and color should return to the patient's normal appearance. Renal function should not be impaired, with an hourly output on the average of 30 ml/hour. Sodium, chloride, and potassium levels return to normal, and the patient has no symptoms of hypoglycemia. All other symptoms of fluid and electrolyte imbalance have been alleviated. The patient sustains no injury due to weakness or postural hypotension. Following fluid replacement, the patient should also be assessed for fluid overload that may occur in the elderly and those with chronic left ventricular disease due to the extremely rapid rate of administration for intravenous fluids.

Community/Home Care

Patients treated for deficient fluid volume secondary to adrenal insufficiency should have normal fluid status restored prior to discharge home. Patients with adrenal insufficiency need education regarding the prevention of dehydration and electrolyte imbalance through adequate intake and control of the adrenal insufficiency. The patient should be taught how to self-assess for dehydration by monitoring mucous membranes and skin turgor, as well as to be attuned to the amount of fluid consumed. Even though it is contradictory to most health practices, the patient should be encouraged to consume foods with sodium content to ensure that hyponatremia does not occur. Potassium-rich foods such as

bananas, orange juice, cantaloupes, etc., should be restricted until the patient returns for a follow-up appointment to verify that the potassium level is normal. The diet will also need to include foods that will raise the blood sugar level, but not concentrated sweets. A dietician is best suited to work with the patient and family in establishing appropriate menus that will meet all nutritional requirements. The patient will need a reference tool for use at home that lists the type of foods that supply the needed nutrients (sodium and glucose) and the type of foods to be restricted due to potassium content. This tool can be laminated to protect it from damage and posted on the refrigerator for easy reading. Having the patient create a sample menu following the education sessions will allow the dietician and nurse to determine further education goals. Measures to prevent dehydration at home can be simple, including having the patient keep liquids nearby in water bottles and sipping on them throughout the day. Crucial to home management is the schedule for taking the replacement hormones (see nursing diagnosis "Ineffective Management of Therapeutic Regimen"). The patient should always wear a Medic-Alert bracelet to alert health care workers of their needs in case of an emergency. Because of the combined effect of the fluid deficit, hypotension, and electrolyte imbalance, fatigue may be an issue at home, especially until the disease is controlled. Simply informing the patient to perform activities as tolerated and avoid driving or operating machinery until stamina/endurance is re-established is all that is needed to manage this. Because of the danger of postural hypotension, the patient should rise slowly from sitting or lying positions. When performing normal activities around the home that require bending or stooping to get objects, the patient should use the same precautions because when he or she returns to the upright position, dizziness can occur, predisposing the patient to injury. The patient may want to keep a log that records amount of food and liquid taken each day, medication administration, feelings of fatigue, if any, and assessments of hydration status. This information can then be shared with the health care provider at follow-up appointments that are required to monitor response to therapy.

Documentation

Document the extent to which the outcome criteria have been met. Findings from an assessment of hydration status are charted, including all findings such as blood pressure, pulse, temperature, intake/output, skin status, and mental status. Include any complaints of tiredness, lethargy or muscle weakness, or cramps. Document all interventions such as intravenous catheter insertion, fluids initiated (type, rate), type of diet ordered, and percentage of food consumed. Teaching regarding the therapeutic regimen is documented in the record. Replacement therapy medications administered are charted on the medication administration record according to agency guidelines. Be specific when charting patient responses to treatment so that other health care providers can clearly determine whether improvement has occurred.

NURSING DIAGNOSIS 3

DECREASED CARDIAC OUTPUT

Related to:

Addisonian crisis

Decreased cortisol levels, which may eventually lead to severe dehydration and hypovolemic shock

Increased need for glucocorticoids and mineralocorticoids due to stress

Defining Characteristics:

Decreased peripheral pulses

Severe hypotension

Mental status changes (restless, agitated, and anxious)

Urine output < 30 ml/hour

Decreased level of consciousness

Pale, cool, clammy skin

Poor skin turgor

Goal:

The patient's cardiac output is restored.

Outcome Criteria

✔ Blood pressure returns to baseline.

✔ The patient exhibits strong peripheral pulses.

✔ Pulse returns to baseline.

✔ The patient is not agitated or restless, and reports decreased anxiety.

✔ Urine output is > 30 ml/hr.

NOC *Circulatory status*
Tissue perfusion: Cardiac
Tissue perfusion: Peripheral
Tissue perfusion: Cerebral
Vital signs

INTERVENTIONS	RATIONALES
Complete a thorough cardiovascular assessment: cardiac rate, rhythm, capillary refill, and changes on EKG.	Helps to detect abnormalities and establish a baseline for evaluation of response to interventions. All of the above manifestations occur as a result of severe dehydration, lack of mineralocorticoids and glucocorticoids, and accompanying hypotension. EKG changes include sharp-peaked T waves and a wide QRS complex.
Assess for Addisonian crisis: pronounced hypotension, progressive weakness, severe abdominal or back pain, high fever, and signs of dehydration.	Addisonian crisis develops rapidly, and the patient needs to be aware of the first signs of a crisis; treatment is needed quickly to prevent shock. Sudden onset of severe hypotension is an indicator of crisis.
Place patient with trunk flat, head not higher than 10 degrees, and legs elevated 20 degrees.	This position increases venous return to the heart from the periphery, thereby adding more fluid to the circulating volume.
Give oxygen, as ordered.	Helps to maintain pO$_2$ at > 90 percent; due to hypoperfusion tissues may be hypoxic; this increases amount of oxygen available for gas exchange.
Assess blood pressure and pulse every 15 minutes.	Addisonian crisis patients have severe hypotension, and in some cases tachycardia is present. The patient's blood pressure and pulse are monitored to detect correction of crisis or progression to shock (a decreased blood pressure with narrowing pulse pressure; a rapid, weak, and thready pulse).
Assess peripheral pulses.	Due to hypotension and volume depletion, perfusion becomes impaired, leading to peripheral pulses that are weak, diminished, or absent, as the heart is unable

INTERVENTIONS	RATIONALES
	to maintain perfusion to extremities.
Assess skin temperature and color.	If the crisis progresses to shock, the perfusion to skin and periphery will be inadequate to maintain warmth or normal color, but as shock develops, the extremities assume the characteristic finding of being cool and clammy due to lack of perfusion.
Assess temperature at least every 4 hours; administer antipyretics as ordered; and document.	Patients with Addisonian crisis may experience hyperpyrexia (extreme elevation of temperature). Assessing temperature often will allow for early intervention. Antipyretics such as acetaminophen (Tylenol) are given to reduce the temperature.
Assess mental status: level of consciousness, confusion, agitation, and restlessness.	Changes in mental status indicate a decrease in cerebral tissue perfusion and an inability of the body's compensatory mechanism to provide adequate oxygenation to cerebral tissue; cerebral hypoxia due to hypovolemia and hypotension causes restlessness and agitation that can progress to confusion, then coma.
For Addisonian crisis, administer glucocorticoids IV, as well as IV fluids containing glucose, rapidly—often as much as 1000 ml over 30 minutes, as ordered (see nursing diagnosis "Deficient Fluid Volume"); determine the cause of the crisis.	Addisonian crisis responds to fluid replacement and glucocorticoids. Addisonian crisis occurs most often in undiagnosed people at times of stress (psychological or physiological: surgery, infection, trauma) or abrupt withdrawal of adrenocortical hormones. Glucocorticoids will cause peripheral vasoconstriction due to its effect on norepinephrine, and their replacement restores normal vasculature. Fluid volume deficit correction will enhance cardiac output by improving vascular volume.
Assess urinary output every hour.	Decreased urinary output (< 30 ml/hour) indicates decreased perfusion to kidneys and progression of Addisonian crisis to shock.
Assess respiratory status, noting adventitious breath sounds.	Decreased cardiac output leads to decreased perfusion to lungs, causing crackles and dyspnea.
Maintain bedrest.	Severe hyponatremia and hypotension increase the risk for injury and cause undue weakness of muscles. Bedrest is maintained until fluid volume, sodium levels, and blood pressure return to baseline.
Assist the patient with all activities, particularly ambulation, once acute crisis is controlled.	Orthostatic hypotension is a common problem in patients with Addison's disease, and the electrolyte imbalances contribute to the problem of possible injury due to muscle weakness.
Create a quiet environment free of stress.	The patient's ability to respond to stress is minimized due to lack of adrenal gland function.

NIC *Fluid management*
  Fluid monitoring
  Electrolyte management: Hyponatremia
  Shock prevention
  Shock management: Volume
  Vital signs monitoring

Evaluation

Note the degree to which outcome criteria have been achieved. The patient should demonstrate adequate cardiac output, improvement in abnormalities, and resolution of Addisonian crisis. Peripheral pulses should be present and skin, when touched, should be warm. If cardiac output is improved, perfusion to the kidneys should be adequate with the patient producing at least 30 ml of urine per hour on average. The pulse should be within the patient's baseline and should be strong and regular. Laboratory results reveal a normal glucose (possibly low normal) and improvement in electrolyte imbalance. There are no signs of dehydration evident. ABGs should return to normal or show compensation, and oxygen saturation should be > 90 percent.

Community/Home Care

Patients who have adrenal insufficiency or Addisonian crisis will implement strategies to prevent a recurrence of the crisis and decreased cardiac output.

There is little need for a visiting nurse to follow the patient, as the alteration is resolved rather quickly. The patient will need to be aware of stressors in his or her life that can increase the need for corticosteroids. The patient usually understands the impact that medical problems such as surgery or infection have on his or her health but often forgets about other stressors. Of particular note is any emotional/personal stress that can precipitate a crisis, especially if the patient has not taken medications as prescribed. The nurse can give the patient a list of situations or events that may require more medications, such as emotional upsets, losses, dental work, dental extractions or surgery, infections, and stressors at work. In addition, the patient should be aware of changes in health status that may signal adrenal insufficiency and the need for early interventions. These include progressive weakness, signs of hypoglycemia (headaches, feeling jittery, hunger, and diaphoresis), fever, and feeling dizzy when standing. Health care providers should help the patient to identify locations for free blood pressure checks. A local drug store or health department in the community may be the best choice, and the patient should record results in a log or on a card often found at the blood pressure monitor at drug stores. Even though the patient could purchase a wrist machine for self-monitoring, experience has proven that these are not reliable for accurate readings. If at any time the patient discovers drops in blood pressure or if the blood pressure is below set parameters, the patient should notify the health care provider. After a period of acute illness, the patient will need to know how to gradually increase activities at home with a balance of rest and activity. The patient will need to monitor his or her response to activity, noting any shortness of breath, increased respiratory rate, or increased pulse rate. Home care follow-up may be required for some patients, especially if they verbalize feelings of anxiety or lack of knowledge about the emergency situation that necessitated in-hospital care. For most patients, specific attention to decreased cardiac output caused by adrenal insufficiency is not required once fluid balance is restored and corticosteroids are administered. However, a follow-up appointment is needed to be sure that the patient has returned to his or her usual level of functioning with normal potassium, sodium, and glucose levels.

Documentation

Chart the results of all assessments made, particularly of the parameters relevant to adrenal gland function and the cardiac system. Initiation of IV fluids and administration of corticosteroids are documented on the medication administration record. All interventions should be documented in a timely fashion with the patient's specific response to each intervention. Chart blood pressure and pulse according to agency/unit protocol. Temperature should be taken at least every 4 hours (possibly more often) and documented to detect early trends towards hyperthermia. If antipyretics are given for fever, document this as well as a follow-up temperature. Always include the patient's psychological status: whether he or she appears anxious, restless, or fearful, and whether significant others are present.

CHAPTER 12.127

DIABETES INSIPIDUS (DI)

GENERAL INFORMATION

Diabetes insipidus (DI) is a disorder defined as a lack of antidiuretic hormone (ADH) secondary to dysfunction of the posterior pituitary gland. There are two basic types of DI, neurogenic and nephrogenic. Neurogenic (central) DI occurs as a result of the lack of production of ADH secondary to a disruption of the hypothalamus and the pituitary gland. Some causes of neurogenic DI include transsphenoidal resection of the anterior pituitary, posterior hypophysectomy, pituitary tumors, and head injuries. Nephrogenic DI is the result of a lack of response or sensitivity of the renal tubules to ADH caused by renal failure or a familial tendency. No matter the underlying cause, the patient with DI experiences pronounced polyuria of dilute urine (~ 12 to 20 L/day) and excessive thirst (polydipsia). If the fluid is not replaced, the patient may experience symptoms of hypovolemia and impaired cerebral function (due to hyperosmolality) such as hypotension, tachycardia, dry mucous membranes, dry skin with poor turgor, irritability, and mental dullness. Sleep may be disturbed due to the need to drink liquids almost constantly. The disorder can be permanent or transient.

NURSING DIAGNOSIS 1

DEFICIENT FLUID VOLUME

Related to:

Lack of adequate ADH

Loss of sensitivity of renal tubules to ADH

Defining Characteristics:

Polyuria

Polydipsia

Dry mucous membranes

Dry skin with poor turgor

Excessive output, output greater than intake

Hypernatremia

Hyperosmolality

Altered mental status

Goal:

Fluid balance will be restored.

Outcome Criteria

✔ The patient will have balanced intake and output.

✔ The patient will have a normal output (30 to 50 ml/hour).

✔ Skin and mucous membranes will be moist.

✔ The patient will verbalize an absence of thirst.

✔ Serum sodium level will be within normal range.

NOC *Hydration*

Fluid balance

Electrolyte and acid/base balance

INTERVENTIONS	RATIONALES
Assess for signs of dehydration/ volume deficit: decreased blood pressure, increased pulse, dry mucous membranes, poor skin turgor, excessive urinary output, and polydipsia.	An assessment is required to determine the degree of dehydration and to assist in planning interventions; ongoing assessment of these parameters is required to evaluate response to treatment. The lack of adequate ADH causes the patient to lose excessive volumes of water, upwards of 12 to 20 L per day; polydipsia occurs due to excessive loss of fluids, and the patient with DI usually desires cold liquids.
Weigh daily.	Weights are an accurate way to detect amount of fluid lost.

(continues)

(continued)

INTERVENTIONS	RATIONALES
Maintain strict intake and output.	Helps to detect imbalances and monitor for restoration of hydration status.
Monitor cardiac status at least every 4 hours or as ordered: blood pressure, pulse, capillary refill, and peripheral pulses.	Significant fluid deficits alter cardiac output due to decreases in circulating volume and subsequent decreases in perfusion. The patient may display signs of hypovolemic shock: tachycardia, hypotension, capillary refill > 2 seconds, dizziness, and syncope occur due to hypotension and electrolyte imbalances.
Monitor serum sodium, potassium, serum osmolality, and urine osmolality.	Sodium is usually elevated due to loss of excess fluid; potassium is decreased due to loss with excess output, serum osmolality is high, normal, or elevated, and urine osmolality is decreased.
Determine the patient's preferred fluids, obtain them, and encourage their intake as well as liberal intake of water; keep fluids chilled.	Due to the excessive amounts of water lost, the patient should be allowed to drink any preferred liquid; patients with DI prefer chilled or iced fluids.
If the patient is unable to drink adequate amounts, or if cerebral manifestations of hypernatremia or cardiac symptoms occur, establish IV access and initiate fluid replacement therapy, as ordered.	In neurogenic DI, the fluid loss may be so great that the patient is unable to compensate by drinking fluids; thus, IV fluids are required to prevent hypovolemic shock and further changes in mental functioning.
Administer medications such as desmopressin acetate (synthetic vasopressin), as ordered, and monitor for side effects.	Vasopressin exerts an antidiuretic effect. Side effects include elevated blood pressure and angina.
Administer medications such as chlorpropamide (Diabinese®) and clofibrate (Atromid-S®) as ordered and monitor for side effects.	These medications are used in neurogenic diabetes insipidus to stimulate release of endogenous ADH.
Assist the patient with activities, especially ambulation or activities that require mental alertness.	The hypotension that accompanies serious fluid deficits could cause a patient to become dizzy and fall if unassisted. High sodium levels cause mental status changes that also place the patient at risk for injury.

NIC   *Fluid management*
Fluid monitoring
Hypovolemia management
Intravenous insertion
Intravenous therapy

Evaluation

Assess the patient for return of normal fluid volume. The patient's blood pressure should return to baseline, and the pulse should be strong and regular. Skin should be warm, and color should return to the patient's normal status with good turgor. Output should gradually decrease and return to normal. Sodium and potassium levels return to normal, and the patient has no symptoms of electrolyte imbalance, such as muscle weakness and mental status changes. The patient sustains no injury due to weakness or postural hypotension. Following fluid replacement, the patient should also be assessed for fluid overload, which may occur in the elderly and those with chronic left ventricular disease.

Community/Home Care

Patients treated for deficient fluid volume secondary to DI should have normal fluid status restored prior to discharge home. Patients need education regarding the prevention of dehydration and electrolyte imbalance through adequate intake and control of the DI. The patient should be taught how to self-assess for dehydration by monitoring mucous membranes and skin turgor, as well as to be attuned to the amount of urine output. While the patient is learning about the disease, he or she should measure his or her output to get an accurate measurement of output. A measuring hat, like those in health care institutions, can be obtained from the health care provider or a medical supply store. This would provide the patient with a way to determine fluid intake requirements. Measures to prevent dehydration at home can be simple, including having the patient keep liquids nearby in water bottles and sipping on them throughout the day, or making a schedule for intake of a set amount of fluid at designated times. Medications that will be taken at home should be stored properly, and the patient should demonstrate proper administration of nasal medication if ordered. In addition, the patient needs to have written instructions for the dosing schedule that may need to be adjusted during the early days of treatment until urine volume is controlled. If the sodium levels remain high, the patient should restrict high-sodium foods in the diet at home as directed by the physician. The loss of potassium with the excess fluid loss necessitates the intake of potassium-rich foods, such as bananas, orange juice, and cantaloupes. A dietician is best suited to work with the patient and family in establishing appropriate menus that will meet all nutritional requirements. The patient will need a reference tool for use at home that lists the type foods that supply the needed nutrients (potassium) and the type of foods to be restricted due to sodium content. This tool can be laminated to protect it from damage and posted on the refrigerator for easy reading. Because of the combined effect of the fluid deficit, hypotension, and electrolyte imbalance, fatigue may be an issue at home, especially until the disease is controlled. This can be handled simply by informing the patient to perform activities as tolerated until stamina/endurance is re-established and suggesting restraint from driving or operating machinery. The patient may want to keep a log that records amount of food and liquid taken each day, urinary output, medication administration, feelings of fatigue, if any, and assessments of hydration status. This information can then be shared with the health care provider at follow-up appointments, which are required to monitor response to therapy.

Documentation

Document the extent to which the outcome criteria have been met. Findings from an assessment of hydration status are charted, including all assessment findings such as blood pressure, pulse, temperature, intake/output, skin status, and mental status. Include any complaints of tiredness, lethargy or muscle weakness, or cramps. Document all interventions, such as intravenous (IV) catheter insertion, fluids initiated (type, rate), and medication administration. It is crucial to document an accurate measure of output, including weight as well as amount of urine voided. Document instruction regarding the therapeutic regimen in the record. Be specific when charting patient responses to treatment so that other health care providers can clearly determine that improvement or deterioration has occurred.

 DEFICIENT KNOWLEDGE

Related to:

New onset of disease

No prior knowledge of diabetes insipidus

Defining Characteristics:

Confusion and questions about therapeutic interventions

Asks many questions

Asks no questions

Goal:

The patient verbalizes understanding of DI and its treatment.

Outcome Criteria

✔ The patient verbalizes an understanding of DI.

✔ The patient verbalizes an understanding of the medication requirements for DI.

✔ The patient verbalizes an understanding of the fluid intake requirements for DI.

✔ The patient is able to identify signs and symptoms of dehydration.

✔ The patient is able to carry out the prescribed treatment plan.

NOC *Knowledge: Disease process*
Knowledge: Health behavior
Treatment behavior: Illness or injury

INTERVENTIONS	RATIONALES
Assess the readiness of the patient to learn (motivation, cognitive level, and physiological status).	The patient must be motivated to learn, have the capability to learn the content, and be free of distractions from learning such as pain and emotional distress.
Assess what the patient already knows.	The patient may have some knowledge about DI, and teaching should begin with what the patient already knows.

(continues)

(continued)

INTERVENTIONS	RATIONALES
Create a quiet environment conducive to learning.	Environmental noise can prevent the learner from focusing on what is being taught.
Start with simple concepts first and move to complex concepts.	If the patient understands simple concepts, these can be used as a foundation to build on for more complex concepts.
Teach the learners about the pathophysiology of DI: — Role of ADH in maintaining fluid balance — Signs and symptoms of the disease: excessive urine output (polyuria) and excessive thirst (polydipsia) — Signs and symptoms of dehydration: dry skin, poor skin turgor, and dry mouth — Risk for injury due to hypotension and electrolyte imbalance that causes muscle weakness and general weakness	Understanding of normal function and pathophysiology will facilitate understanding of the rationale for therapeutic interventions. Instructing the patient on signs and symptoms of dehydration will allow the patient to note abnormalities and monitor for improvement or worsening.
Teach patient about the medication desmopressin (DDAVP), including: — Action: exerts antidiuretic effect — Expected outcomes: decreased urine output, decreased thirst — Side effects: angina, hypertension, overdose: water intoxication (headache, drowsiness), weight gain, decreased output — Administration technique: intranasally twice a day	Knowledge of medication actions, need for medication, dosages, and side effects will improve compliance. The patient needs to demonstrate how to instill intranasal medications correctly.
Teach patient about the need for aggressive fluid intake.	The patient needs to drink enough liquid to prevent dehydration and hypovolemic shock.
Teach the patient how to measure urinary output using a measuring hat.	The patient needs to be able to determine the amount of output per day to assess for improvement in the condition and to adjust intake accordingly.
Encourage regular appointments with physician.	The physician can monitor progress and medication response.
Review symptoms of abnormal response and signs that require	The patient needs to be able to identify symptomatology that
prompt attention: continued excessive urine output, pronounced thirst and weakness, or side effects of the medication.	would encourage him or her to seek medical assistance in a timely fashion to prevent serious complications of circulatory collapse.
Evaluate the patient's understanding of all content covered by asking questions.	Helps to identify areas that require more teaching and to ensure that the patient has enough information to ensure compliance.
Give the patient written information on medications and concise information on the disease.	Provides material for reference at a later time, and for review.

NIC   *Teaching: Disease process*
Teaching: Individual
Teaching: Prescribed medication
Teaching: Psychomotor skill

Evaluation

The patient is able to state what DI is and what causes it, and asks questions about DI and possible outcomes (positive and negative). Prior to discharge, the patient verbalizes an understanding of required medications (purpose, side effects) and their administration, fluid replacement needs, and dietary requirements (decreased sodium, increased potassium), and agrees to be compliant. Prior to exiting the health care agency, the patient demonstrates the proper technique for administering the medication intranasally. The patient knows and should be able to inform the nurse when health care assistance should be sought.

Community/Home Care

Major components of the regimen for controlling DI include monitoring output, assuring fluid replacement, and taking medications. The most important aspects include monitoring output and adjusting intake accordingly. The patient needs to obtain a measuring hat and place it in the home bathroom to measure urine output daily. A small notebook can be kept in the bathroom for recording the output, and the patient can also record the intake here for calculating the balance between the two. The patient should keep fluids readily available for intake throughout the day. Instruction by the health care team should be thorough, with opportunities for discussions. Knowledge needs are identified early in order to improve the likelihood that the patient will be prepared for self-care and self-monitoring once at home. Of greatest importance is to be sure that the patient has understood the instructions regarding medications and how to detect side effects that require immediate intervention. Once at home, the patient may need further reinforcement and should have access to a health care provider to call for clarification, at which time the nurse or other provider can evaluate the patient's understanding of all content taught and the patient's ability and willingness to follow through. Follow-up with a health care provider focuses on assurance that no complications have occurred and that the patient has a clear understanding of how to manage all aspects of DI.

Documentation

Document all content taught and the patient's verbalization of understanding. Specific attention should be given to documentation of any specific concerns that the patient expresses regarding the diagnosis and treatment of DI. Include the patient's demonstration of how to administer medications intranasally. Chart in the patient record his or her willingness to comply with all recommendations made regarding medications, fluid intake, and monitoring urine output. Any area that requires further teaching should be clearly indicated in the record. Always include the titles of any printed literature given to the patient for reinforcement. Include in the record appointments that have been made for follow-up and any referrals made.

CHAPTER 12.128

DIABETES MELLITUS

GENERAL INFORMATION

Diabetes mellitus is a disorder of endocrine function in which there is a relative lack of insulin or an absolute absence of insulin. Insulin is required for glucose (found in serum) to be transported into the cells. If glucose is not available to the cells, it remains in the circulating volume and fatty acids are used for energy in its place with resulting hyperglycemia and ketoacidosis. The disease is categorized into type 1, type 2, gestational, and other specific types (only type 1 and type 2 will be discussed in the care plan). Type 1 diabetes occurs due to an inability of the beta cells of the islets of Langerhans to secrete insulin and is thought to have an autoimmune basis, even though there are cases in which there is no evidence for autoimmune beta cell destruction. Type 1 diabetes has a peak onset in people younger than 30 years of age. In type 2 diabetes the beta cells produce insulin, but in most cases, not enough, and in addition there appears to be a resistance of the cells to insulin, which is affected by obesity, medications, and other factors. Type 2 diabetes is responsible for the majority of the cases of diabetes (approximately 90 percent), has a strong genetic predisposition, and occurs in the middle to later years. It has a gradual onset and the patient may have had the disorder for years prior to diagnosis. Classic findings in diabetes mellitus include polyuria, polydipsia, and polyphagia, often accompanied by weight loss and a general feeling of tiredness. In type 2 diabetes, the clinical findings are not usually as severe as in type 1 and the disease may go unrecognized by the patient with the diagnosis made as a result of a health care visit for some other reason, frequently for visual disturbances or continued complaints of being tired. Diabetes mellitus is the leading cause of nontraumatic amputations and the leading cause of new blindness in the United States. It is estimated that approximately 18.2 million persons in the United States have diabetes mellitus, with 13 million of those being diagnosed and another 5.2 million persons remain unaware that they have the disease. Diabetes mellitus is more prevalent in ethnic subgroups. The highest incidence is seen in Native American and Alaskan Natives, and African Americans having the second highest rate.

NURSING DIAGNOSIS 1

IMBALANCED NUTRITION: MORE THAN BODY REQUIREMENTS

Related to:

Excessive intake of foods containing glucose

Deficiency of insulin (not enough, or insulin that is not effective)

New onset diabetes

Stress

Illness

Defining Characteristics:

Elevated serum fasting glucose level (> 126 mg/dl)

Polyuria

Polydipsia

Polyphagia

Glycosuria/ketonuria

Warm, red skin

Fatigue

Metabolic acidosis

Goal:

Symptoms of diabetes mellitus are resolved.

Outcome Criteria

✔ Serum glucose returns to normal.

✔ The patient offers no complaints of increased urination.

✔ The patient offers no complaints of increased hunger.

✔ The patient offers no complaints of increased thirst.

✔ The patient is compliant with dietary and medication regimen.

NOC   *Nutritional intake: Nutrient intake*
Hydration
Blood glucose level

INTERVENTIONS	RATIONALES
Assess patient for signs and symptoms of diabetes mellitus/ hyperglycemia: polyuria, polydipsia, polyphagia, fatigue, smell of ketosis (sweet, musty, like moldy peaches) on breath, vomiting, abdominal distention, dry skin, poor skin turgor, and nausea.	The patient reports these symptoms due to the inability of the body to utilize glucose; glucose has an osmotic diuretic effect causing an increased output; because of the excessive output, the patient becomes thirsty; due to the lack of nutrients for metabolism and energy, hunger occurs, as does fatigue.
Monitor laboratory results: serum glucose, glycosylated hemoglobin, urine for ketones, and glucose.	Elevated glucose levels are expected; glycosylated hemoglobin measures the amount of glucose permanently bound to hemoglobin, and the level will reflect the average glucose level over 2–3 months; high levels indicate uncontrolled diabetes or glucose level; in the absence of available glucose for energy, fat is used, with ketones being the end product of fat metabolism; as the renal threshold for glucose is reached, the kidneys excrete both ketones and glucose in the urine.
Take a history relevant to risk behaviors and contributing factors for elevated glucose levels such as inappropriate diet, sedentary lifestyle, obesity, and familial history of type 2 diabetes mellitus.	Knowing this information will allow for better planning for needed interventions to address the knowledge needs for diabetes mellitus.
Refer patient to a diabetic educator and a dietician for teaching.	These experts can provide structured teaching on diabetes mellitus; the dietician needs to be involved in planning prescribed dietary interventions that consider activity level, body weight, risk for cardiovascular disease, glucose levels, and patient preferences.
Administer insulin as ordered, and begin teaching the patient to self-administer insulin (see nursing diagnosis "Deficient Knowledge").	Insulin reduces the blood glucose level by increasing peripheral glucose uptake, especially in skeletal and fat tissue; inhibits the breakdown of glycogen to glucose by the liver.
Administer oral antidiabetic agents as ordered (see nursing diagnosis "Deficient Knowledge").	Helps to lower glucose levels in type 2 diabetes mellitus, stimulates functioning beta cells to secrete insulin, and increases the sensitivity of peripheral insulin receptors to insulin.
Monitor the patient for signs of hypoglycemia: feeling nervous or jittery, diaphoresis, headache, and palpitations.	Especially in the early phase of diagnosis, the patient is prone to hypoglycemia due to overcorrection of the elevated blood glucose.
If hypoglycemia occurs, treat as ordered: if patient is alert, offer a fast-acting glucose source such as 4 to 6 ounces of orange juice, hard candy such as LifeSavers™ (approximately 6 to 8), or sweetened drinks. If the patient is lethargic, place highly sweetened substances such as honey, molasses, or syrup under the tongue for absorption; if unresponsive, administer glucagon or 50 percent dextrose as ordered or according to agency protocol, and give complex carbohydrates when the patient is alert.	The patient needs a quick source of glucose to resolve symptoms until complex dietary substances can be provided. Hypoglycemic episodes carry the added risk of neurological impairment as hypoglycemic states impair cerebral tissue oxygenation. Liquid substances such as molasses or honey can be absorbed through the vascular membranes of the oral cavity. Glucagon, which stimulates hepatic gluconeogenesis, is given intramuscularly (IM) or subcutaneously, and effects can be seen in 5 to 20 minutes. Fifty percent dextrose is given intravenously (IV) and has an almost immediate response.
Encourage intake of diet as developed by patient and dietician and as prescribed by physician with consideration for usual activity level, required nutrients, and timing and dose of medications.	Dietary modifications are one of the mainstays of treatment and control for diabetes mellitus. Common requirements include carbohydrates and monosaturated fats for 60 to 70 percent of diet, protein intake of 15 to 20 percent of diet, 10 percent of total kcal from saturated fats, 20 to 30 grams of fiber, and an overall limitation of concentrated sweets. The overall

(continues)

(continued)

INTERVENTIONS	RATIONALES
	goal of the diet is to supply adequate nutrients for the body, control blood glucose levels, improve overall health, keep lipids in normal range, and attempt to deter chronic complications.
Check glucose levels before meals and at bedtimes as ordered.	Helps to determine glucose levels before meals to decide if rapid-acting insulin is needed due to ingestion of additional glucose sources in meals.
Encourage patient to incorporate exercise into daily routine.	Exercise increases the uptake of glucose by muscles and in some instances decreases the amount of insulin required.
Teach the patient about the chronic complications of diabetes (diabetic retinopathy, peripheral neuropathy, renal disease, cardiovascular disease, and stroke).	The patient needs to be aware of these long-term complications in order to assess self for changes that may indicate problems, but also to enhance early treatment.

NIC   *Hyperglycemia management*
Hypoglycemia management
Medication administration
Nutritional counseling

Evaluation

The patient has a normal blood glucose level and glycosylated hemoglobin (Hgb) on return visits to the health care provider. The patient has no symptoms of hypoglycemia or hyperglycemia after initiation of interventions to treat diabetes mellitus. The patient agrees to be compliant with the prescribed diet, medication, or other interventions, and is able to implement them at home.

Community/Home Care

The patient with newly diagnosed diabetes mellitus must manage a therapeutic regimen that includes diet, activity, and medications. Patients diagnosed with diabetes mellitus should have glucose levels that are restored to normal or near normal. The patient will need to monitor glucose and hydration levels to ensure that they are stable. It is suggested that the patient review basic information regarding diabetes and how to prevent acute episodes of hypoglycemia or hyperglycemia. Included in the review should be diet, insulin or oral antidiabetic therapy, early signs of hyperglycemia, and signs of hypoglycemia. Having the patient make a chart that outlines the various complications such as hypoglycemia and hyperglycemia (early and late signs) can assist with review, and placing it in easy sight can serve as a reminder to review. In addition, the chart should include interventions that can be implemented at the first sign of either problem. The diet plays a vital role in the management of diabetes, and it is crucial that the recommended diet is palatable to the patient. It must not be so strict as to prevent the patient from being compliant because of the severe restrictions. Adherence to the diet is enhanced if the patient is an active participant in its development and if normal diet, food preferences, and cultural and religious restrictions are considered. Mealtimes will need to become more routinized rather than being taken "as desired." Acceptance of the dietary restrictions can be enhanced if other members of the family also partake of the same foods or very similar foods so that the patient does perceive his or her diet to be significantly different from diets of others. Eating out may be problematic, especially for new diabetics, because of the variance in restaurant menus and cooking methods. Having the patient make sample menus for meals within the recommendations using foods he or she likes can assist the dietician to assess the patient's ability to plan acceptable meals. If the patient is overweight, strategies to lose weight should be undertaken as part of the diet plan. The patient will probably be asked to check glucose levels using Accu-Chek frequently during the first few weeks following the diagnosis. Monitoring urinary output to detect unusual patterns of increased output will help the patient recognize problems early for prompt treatment. Home care should focus on prevention of episodes of diabetic ketoacidosis (DKA) or hypoglycemia. The educational requirements of newly diagnosed diabetics are enormous, and enrollment in a community program for diabetics or a diabetes clinic can enhance the patient's capability for reinforcement of teaching and for self-care. Care must address the prevention of long-term chronic complications such as renal disease, diabetic retinopathy, peripheral neuropathy, strokes, and heart attacks. Have the patient keep a daily journal of all aspects of daily care. By recording results of Accu-Chek, dietary intake, insulin administration (type, dose, time of injection), oral medications, complaints of any type, and physical activity, the patient and caregiver will be able to determine when alterations in the therapeutic interventions should be made. The health care provider may want the patient to return for a follow-up appointment to ensure that parameters such as glucose and glycosylated hemoglobin have returned to normal.

Documentation

In this situation, document initial assessment findings relevant to diabetes mellitus such as glucose, blood pressure, pulse, respirations, skin status (turgor, mucous membranes), polyuria, polyphagia, and polydipsia. It is important to document interventions at the time of performance to allow for better monitoring of responses. Medication administration (insulin, oral agents) should be documented in accordance with agency protocol. Be specific when charting patient responses to treatment so that other health care providers can clearly determine progress towards glucose control. Chart referrals to diabetic educators or dieticians and all teaching done. If the patient expresses concern or has questions regarding diet requirements or any aspect of the plan, chart these exactly as stated.

NURSING DIAGNOSIS 2

INEFFECTIVE MANAGEMENT OF THERAPEUTIC REGIMEN

Related to:

Knowledge deficit related to diabetes mellitus

Complexity of therapeutic regimen requirements

Newly diagnosed diabetes mellitus

Defining Characteristics:

Does not understand the regimen

Asks no questions

Has many questions/concerns

Shows no interest in learning about the disease

Goal:

The patient is able to control diabetes mellitus and verbalizes an understanding of diabetes mellitus and its management.

Outcome Criteria

✔ The patient verbalizes an understanding of diabetes mellitus.

✔ The patient verbalizes an understanding of the medication requirements (insulin or oral agents).

✔ The patient understands the role of diet in the therapeutic regimen.

✔ The patient understands the role of exercise in controlling the disease.

✔ The patient is able to correctly perform Accu-Cheks and insulin administration.

✔ The patient is able to identify chronic complications of diabetes (renal failure, retinopathy, peripheral neuropathy).

✔ The patient is able to carry out the prescribed treatment plan and has appropriate resources (human and financial).

NOC   *Knowledge: Disease process*
        Knowledge: Diabetes
             management

INTERVENTIONS	RATIONALES
Assess the readiness and ability of the patient to learn (motivation, cognitive level, physiological status); assess fine motor skills.	The patient must be motivated to learn, have the capability to learn the content, and be free of distractions from learning such as pain and emotional distress. Fine motor skills are needed to be able to perform Accu-Chek and insulin withdrawal and administration.
Assess what the patient already knows.	The patient may have some knowledge about diabetes mellitus, and teaching should begin with what the patient already knows.
Create a quiet environment conducive to learning.	Environmental noise can prevent the learner from focusing on what is being taught.
Start with simple concepts first and move to complex concepts.	If the patient understands simple concepts, these can be used as a foundation for presenting more complex concepts.
Teach the learners about the pathophysiology of diabetes mellitus: — Lack of adequate insulin to control blood glucose	Understanding of normal function and pathophysiology will facilitate understanding of the rationale for therapeutic interventions. Instructing the

(continues)

(continued)

INTERVENTIONS	RATIONALES
— Signs and symptoms of the disease: polyuria, polyphagia, polydipsia, malaise, blurred vision	patient on signs and symptoms of elevated glucose will allow the patient to note abnormalities and monitor for improvement or worsening.
Teach patient about hypoglycemia: — Causes: too much insulin, skipping meals, dieting, not adhering to schedule for meals and medication, strenuous exercise — Signs and symptoms: feeling jittery, tremors, diaphoresis, palpitations/fast heart rate — Treatment: take a quick-acting carbohydrate such as hard candy, fruit juice such as orange juice, sweetened sodas/drinks — Keep hard candy on person at all times	The patient needs to be able to identify hypoglycemia and understand the dangers of repeated episodes. Information allows the patient to implement strategies to raise blood sugar and reduce emergency room visits.
Teach the patient about hyperglycemia: — Causes: too much food, not enough medication, skipping medications, physiological or emotional stress, infections or surgery — Signs and symptoms: increased urination, hunger, blurred vision, dry mouth, thirst — Treatment: Accu-Chek to check glucose, administer insulin, and drink fluids	The patient needs to be able to identify signs of elevated blood glucose to initiate treatment early. In addition, if the patient understands what causes the glucose level to elevate even when he or she adheres to the regimen, he or she will be better equipped to avoid emergency situations.
Teach the patient about the role of exercise in glucose control: — Exercise lowers blood glucose by increasing the uptake of glucose by body muscles and improving insulin utilization. — Exercise should be done on a regular schedule. — Exercise is contraindicated during periods of hyperglycemia. — During the early period following diagnosis, have patient test glucose before, during (if possible), and after exercise.	Exercise is an insulin sensitizer and can assist in maintaining better glucose control. In addition, regular exercise lowers risk of cardiovascular disease, and diabetic patients are at higher risk for both strokes and heart attacks.
Teach patient about insulin, including — Action: insulin increases the uptake of glucose. — Types: rapid-acting: used for immediate action, given based on Accu-Chek or before meals for extra coverage, onset of action is 5 (Aspart) to 30 (regular) minutes dependent on the specific insulin, peak action is 0.75 to 3 hours, duration of action is 3 to 6 hours, can be given IV; intermediate-acting: used as the maintenance dose, onset of action is 1.5 to 2.4 hours, peak action is 4 to 12 hours, and duration of action is 22 to 24 hours; long-acting: used as a maintenance dose, onset of action is 1 to 4 hours, duration of action is 24 to 28 hours; combination insulin: used as the maintenance dose but contains both rapid acting and intermediate acting, onset of action is 0.2 to 0.5 hours, peak action is 1 to 6.5 hours, duration of action is 22 hours. — Explain that regular insulin is clear and longer-acting insulins are cloudy. — Expected outcomes include decreased blood glucose levels. — Side effects include local reactions at the site and hypoglycemic symptoms. — Administration: subcutaneous is at times ordered by physician, but usually before meals. — Sites include arms, thighs, or abdomen; abdominal area is preferred site because of a more consistent absorption rate; rotation of sites is recommended if using pork insulin; rotate within a site if using other types, making injection sites 1 inch apart. — Avoid use of thighs or legs immediately preceding exercise or if heat is to be applied. — Storage: insulin can be stored at room temperature for up to	The patient needs to be knowledgeable about all aspects of insulin administration; this will ensure compliance and prevent complications. Knowledge of medication action, need for the medication, dosages, and side effects will improve compliance. Exercise and heat increases the rate of absorption of insulin causing a more rapid onset of action and a faster peak time.

INTERVENTIONS	RATIONALES
30 days and if not used, discard. Keep unopened vials in refrigerator. — Keep insulin and administration supplies in his or her presence when traveling.	
Teach correct technique for administration of insulin injection: — Drawing up the correct dose of insulin — Selecting the correct site for administration, including rotation within an anatomical site — How to inject the medicine subcutaneously — Mixing two insulins in one syringe (put rapid-acting insulin into syringe first) — Disposal of syringe and needle	The patient will need to know how to draw up the medication, inject it into the correct site, and in some instances mix two types of insulin together. The patient needs dexterity for the procedure as well as visual acuity, and should be assessed for both.
Teach patient/family how to use an insulin pump.	The patient (with possible help from family members) will be able to become independent; the technique for insulin pumps are guided by manufacturer guidelines.
Teach the patient how to perform Accu-Cheks, the concept of sliding scales, and proper storage of Accu-Chek equipment, according to the manufacturer's instructions.	The patient will need to learn how to check blood sugars at designated intervals, but particularly during the time of trying to establish diabetic control. Glucose checks should be done before meals and prior to bedtime or at any time the patient feels symptomatic. Many physicians provide patients with a sliding scale schedule for insulin administration based on the results of Accu-Cheks.
Teach the patient regarding oral medications: — Sulfonylureas stimulate the pancreas to release more insulin (example: Amaryl®, Glucotrol®). — Meglitinides and d-phenylalanines, also called mealtime insulin secretagogues, stimulate pancreas to release more insulin (example: Prandin®, Starlix®). — Alpha-glucosidase inhibitors block glucose absorption in	Oral agents are used to treat type 2 diabetes and are effective in lowering glucose levels. The patient needs to know what type he or she is taking and when to take it to effect better control. Even though episodes of hypoglycemia are infrequent, they can occur.
the small intestines (example: Precose®). — Biguanides reduce blood glucose levels by reducing hepatic glucose production and by enhancing insulin sensitivity in muscle and fat cells (example: Glucophage®). — Thiazolidinediones increase insulin sensitivity, primarily in the peripheral tissue and reverse or partially reverse insulin resistance; decrease hepatic glucose output (example: Avandia®, Actos®). — Schedule for administration. — Side effects of medications include hypoglycemia on occasion, particularly in the elderly.	
Teach the patient how to check urine for glucose and ketones, and encourage him or her to do so if glucose is elevated.	This will help the patient with early detection of DKA.
Collaborate with the dietician to instruct the patient on the prescribed diet (see nursing diagnosis "Imbalanced Nutrition") and consider the patient's culture, religious restrictions, and preferences when developing the diet.	A prescribed diet is a major part of the regimen for diabetics; considering the patient's preferences and culture enhances compliance.
Teach the patient regarding proper foot care (see nursing diagnosis "Risk for Impaired Skin Integrity").	Diabetics are prone to infection and injury of the feet due to neurovascular changes and increased levels of glucose.
Teach the patient how to handle sickness of short duration: — Monitor glucose every 2 to 4 hours. — Test urine for ketones if glucose is over 240. — Continue to take oral agents or insulin unless otherwise directed by a health care provider. — Drink 8 to 12 ounces of sugar-free liquids every hour. — Continue meals if possible. — If unable to tolerate solid foods due to nausea or vomiting, consume liquids equal to the carbohydrate content of a meal. — Notify physician if unable to take any fluids or food by mouth.	Part of self-management is to take control of problems. The patient at home can manage illnesses of short duration with constant monitoring of the blood glucose level.

(continues)

(continued)

INTERVENTIONS	RATIONALES
Encourage the patient to have regular eye exams.	Diabetes is a leading cause of new blindness. Regular exams can provide early detection for diabetic retinopathy.
Encourage regular appointments with the health care provider.	Regular follow-up is required to monitor blood sugar and progress towards control and self-management, as well as for early detection of complications.
Refer the patient to a diabetes educator, dietician, and/or a diabetes clinic for structured teaching.	Experts in diabetes education can provide more formal instruction.
Evaluate the patient's understanding of all content covered by asking questions.	Helps to identify areas that require more teaching and to ensure that the patient has enough information to ensure compliance.
Give the patient written information on medications and concise information on the disease.	Provides material for reference at a later time, and for review.

NIC *Teaching: Disease process*
Teaching: Psychomotor skill
Teaching: Individual
Teaching: Prescribed medication
Teaching: Prescribed activity/exercise

Evaluation

The patient is able to discuss all information for the nurse and asks questions about all aspects of the therapeutic regimen for diabetes mellitus. The patient is able to state what diabetes mellitus is and what causes it, as well as the long-term complications. The patient verbalizes an understanding all aspects of the prescribed regimen including required medications (purpose, side effects), diet, and exercise, and demonstrates psychomotor skills of insulin administration and Accu-Cheks. Verbalization of signs and symptoms of hyperglycemia and hypoglycemia are given by the patient. The patient should be able to inform the nurse when health care assistance should be sought.

Community/Home Care

The regimen required in the home to control diabetes mellitus is complex and multifaceted. All patients receive information regarding the disease, diet, medication, exercise, and preventing complications. One of the most important aspects of the regimen includes taking the medication (oral or insulin) as prescribed each day and monitoring response through Accu-Chek. The patient and one other person should demonstrate how to inject insulin and perform Accu-Cheks. A nurse or diabetic educator should assess the patient's dexterity and visual acuity to determine that the patient can see the numbers on the syringe and the labeling on the medicine, and is able to manipulate the syringe well enough to draw up the medicine and inject it correctly. Good dexterity is also required for performing Accu-Cheks. Of particular concern are patients who have deformities from arthritis, neuropathy, and visual disorders such as glaucoma or cataracts. A solution may be to have someone else draw up daily insulin doses in syringes and leave in the refrigerator. However, this will not address insulin administration that may need to be given in response to Accu-Chek results. The patient needs to be able to identify the side effects of medications that require immediate intervention. Most of these symptoms represent hypoglycemia due to taking medication and not eating, or hyperglycemia caused by excessive eating or not taking medication. It is recommended that the patient keep the medication and syringes in the same place, and most patients choose the refrigerator. A small plastic storage box can be purchased at most retail stores. Keeping the insulin covered in the refrigerator will protect it from accidental spills from other substances in the refrigerator. Disposal of syringes and needles in the home should be discussed with the health care provider. In some instances, the patient is given or is asked to purchase appropriate hazardous waste containers, even though any puncture-proof heavy plastic container can be substituted. When filled, the container should be taped closed with duct tape or electrical tape prior to placing in the trash. Oral medications can be kept in any place where the patient can remember to take them, possibly the bathroom or the kitchen. The diet may pose the biggest challenge in the home for the patient. The dictician or diabetic educator is utilized to teach the patient about the prescribed diet and can assist the patient by preparing sample diets for the patient that utilize their preferred foods, considering any cultural and religious restrictions. A typed copy of the sample diet or meal plan can be laminated for protection and kept in the kitchen for quick reference. In addition, the patient needs to be able to read food labels and understand that foods labeled dietetic are not necessarily good nor are they calorie-free. Many may have few calories or carbohydrates but a higher fat content. There should be ample opportunity for the patient to ask questions regarding the diet and to receive reinforcements in diet education through diabetes nutrition classes or through in-home visits. Having the patient plan a sample set of menus for review by the dietician will demonstrate effectiveness of the teaching. A realistic plan for exercise should be implemented into the regimen; however, if the patient was not active prior to the diagnosis, it may be risky to include exercise as a part of the regimen when deciding on the medication dosage. Exercise goals need to be realistic based on the patient's preference for type of exercise, lifestyle, and motivation. It is unrealistic to expect the patient to remember all information presented; however, it is crucial that he or she understand the medication, diet, acute complications (hyperglycemia/hypoglycemia), and foot care (see nursing diagnosis "Risk for Impaired Skin Integrity"). Giving the patient written information to have as a reference when needed can reinforce instructions on sick-day rules and long-term complications. The patient may want to develop a schedule that includes time for medications, time for meals, and time of any exercise, and post it in a visible place. This may be especially true during the period immediately following diagnosis when the patient is still trying to adapt and establish a routine. The health care worker teaching the patient can develop a notebook that contains written information regarding different topics with each topic having a different color of paper and place it in a brightly colored folder or binder with a chart on the front to indicate which topic is on which color. Once at home, the patient may need further reinforcement and should have access to a health care provider to call for clarification or further teaching, at which time the nurse or others can evaluate the patient's understanding of all content taught and his or her ability and willingness to follow through. The nurse or social worker needs to be sure that the patient has the means to purchase the medications (insulin, oral agents) and the syringes as well as the supplies needed to perform the Accu-Cheks. Patients should be referred to special classes or diabetic clinics for continued education; however, this service may not be available in rural areas. Follow-up with a health care provider focuses on assurance that no complications have occurred and that the patient has a clear understanding of, an ability to, and a willingness to manage all aspects of diabetes mellitus.

Documentation

Document all content taught and the patient's verbalization of understanding. Specific attention should be given to documentation of any specific concerns that the patient expresses regarding the diagnosis of diabetes mellitus. Included in the documentation is the patient's report that he or she has a means to purchase the medication, supplies needed for injections, and a glucose monitor. Document the patient's ability to perform psychomotor skills of injection and Accu-Chek. He or she should express a willingness to comply with all prescribed interventions for treating and controlling diabetes. Any area that requires further teaching should be clearly indicated in the record. Include in the record appointments that have been made for follow-up or blood draws for laboratory tests. If the patient is referred to a diabetic clinic or diabetes classes, document this in the record. Always include the titles of any printed literature given to the patient for reinforcement.

NURSING DIAGNOSIS 3

RISK FOR IMPAIRED SKIN INTEGRITY

Related to:

Hyperglycemia

Peripheral neuropathy

Defining Characteristics:

None

Goal:

The patient's skin will remain intact.

Outcome Criteria

✔ The patient will have no undetected trauma to feet.

✔ The patient will verbalize an understanding of proper foot care.

✔ The patient will demonstrate proper foot care.

✔ The patient will have no areas of skin breakdown.

NOC *Sensory function: Cutaneous*
Tissue integrity: Skin and mucous
    membranes
Tissue perfusion: Peripheral

INTERVENTIONS	RATIONALES
Perform a complete assessment of all skin surfaces, with particular attention to the feet. Assess skin turgor, color, capillary refill, peripheral pulses, presence of any breaks, rashes, scaliness, corns, calluses, blisters, temperature of feet, and sensation in feet.	This is needed to establish a baseline and to identify any areas of potential problem. Diabetic patients are at high risk for skin impairment due to neuropathy and impaired peripheral circulation. Peripheral pulses may be diminished or absent, indicating a greater need for aggressive attention to preventing injury. A cool extremity indicates a lack of perfusion and places the extremity at high risk for complication. Calluses or corns rubbing in shoes can create skin impairments and should be addressed.
Assess nails of feet for thickness, excessive length, or fungal infections.	Many diabetic patients are prone to fungal infections making nails difficult to clip and nails become thick and long.
Refer patient to a qualified podiatrist for nail care.	A specialist should undertake foot care for diabetics especially clipping nails; accidental nicking of an area can lead to significant impairment.
On each visit, perform a foot inspection.	Helps to detect abnormalities and institute measures to prevent complications.
Have patient wear proper-fitting shoes that do not rub toes, heel, or side of foot, and suggest changing shoes during the day.	Ill-fitting shoes can cause blisters and corns that could lead to ulcerations; changing the shoes during the day prevents continuous pressure in one site that could be caused by the shoes.
Suggest that the patient be measured for proper-fitting shoes.	Measurement ensures correct sizing.
Teach patient to inspect feet daily, especially the bottoms of feet.	Helps to identify areas of concern and allows for prompt treatment; the bottoms of the feet often have some loss of sensation, and injury may go unnoticed.
Teach patient to wash feet daily with warm water, mild soap, and dry well, especially between toes, but to use gentle patting rather than rigorous rubbing.	Areas between the toes often remain moist following bathing and can become a good source for microorganism growth. Hot water and harsh deodorant soaps add to dryness.
Teach the patient to note changes in skin, and if dry scales/scaliness occurs, take fewer baths and lubricate skin with lanolin or other moisturizing agents. Avoid alcohol-based products.	Scaliness indicates lack of moisture; bathing with harsh soaps such as scented deodorant soaps can worsen the condition of the skin. Fewer baths will allow for return to normal; lanolin or moisturizers add moisture back to the skin.
Teach patient basic principles of preventing injury: — Wear shoes at all times. — Wear socks. — Before placing foot into shoe, check shoes for foreign objects. — Do not place feet on or close to heat sources such as space heaters or fireplaces. — Test temperature of water before bathing. — Do not use heating pads, hot water bottles, or electric blankets. — Wear protective clothing over arms if doing hazardous tasks outside such as trimming hedges, working in rose bushes, or walking in the woods. — Avoid crossing legs. — Avoid constrictive socks. — Avoid shoes with high, spiked heels. — Do not scratch minor lesions or insect bites.	All of these measures serve to protect the skin, especially the feet, from traumatic injury. Many patients have neuropathy that causes a decrease in the ability to sense injury. In addition, minor skin impairments can lead to significant impairment necessitating hospitalization or loss of limb due to rapid onset of infection.
Maintain good glucose control.	Elevated glucose levels predispose the patient to skin impairment and infection.
If the patient smokes, encourage him or her to stop.	Nicotine is a vasoconstrictor that further decreases peripheral circulation.
Teach the patient all suggested interventions listed and explain the pathophysiology of diabetes that causes the neuropathy and circulation disturbances that adds to skin impairment, especially in the feet.	Educating the patient on the pathophysiology and on what constitutes good foot care equips him or her with information needed to implement the practices in the home and will increase likelihood of compliance.

NIC *Teaching: Foot care*
Lower extremity monitoring
Skin surveillance

Evaluation

The patient experiences no ulcerations of skin, and feet are without areas of impairment. The patient is able to verbalize strategies that are needed to prevent injury to the feet and agrees to comply. The patient is able to demonstrate proper foot care of washing, drying, and inspection of the feet.

Community/Home Care

Implementation of strategies for foot care is undertaken in the home unless the patient is admitted for acute symptoms. At home, the patient must remember all the strategies suggested and make them a part of the daily routine. Inspection of the feet each day is the one most important aspect of in-home care. When the patient washes the feet and completes the drying process, he or she should sit in a comfortable position and, with the use of a mirror, inspect the feet. A handheld mirror that magnifies or a larger mirror standing on the floor can be used for this purpose. The key is that all aspects of the foot must be inspected, including the underside of the toes, and if the toes are curled, they must be uncurled for inspection. The patient needs to understand that even a simple stubbed toe can lead to amputation if peripheral circulation is impaired. Having the patient develop a "foot-skin status consciousness" is called for; simply put, the patient becomes so attuned to the status of the foot that assessment and inspection become a part of his or her consciousness. This includes having the ability to do quick assessments while changing shoes and noting the feel of the skin (dry, rough, scaly, lumps, etc.) and the temperature and color (redness, darkening, other discoloration) of the skin. Even though most people think of their homes as safe, for the diabetic there are many hazards that predispose him or her to foot injury. These include furniture placed close together that the patient is more likely to bump into, hidden objects in carpeting (such as used staples, straight pins), and even children's toys. For this reason, the patient should always wear shoes when walking around the house, especially in carpeted areas. The patient should also avoid socks or hose that are heavily dyed. Some stores and medical supply stores sell socks that are advertised particularly for "the diabetic." For the fashion-conscious woman, finding shoes that are suitable for the diabetic foot may prove to be a challenge, as high heels or narrow, constricting toes should be eliminated from the wardrobe due to their high risk for rubbing the foot and causing pressure in many areas. Many persons engage in self-trimming of toenails, but the diabetic patient should receive instruction about correct techniques from a health care provider. The provider must ascertain that the patient has the ability to afford a podiatrist along with other health care expenses; it may also be difficult to find a podiatrist in small rural towns. In addition to the attention to the foot, the patient should also institute measures to protect other areas as well. Activities such as gardening, working in the yard, or any other activity that carries the risk of nicking the skin or causing excoriations to the skin should be avoided, or the patient should take precautions against injury such as wearing long pants, long-sleeved shirts, and gloves. If despite all efforts at prevention, skin impairment, ulceration, or injury occurs, the patient should seek immediate health care attention and refrain from using home remedies.

Documentation

Document the findings from a thorough skin assessment, including in-depth assessment of the foot. Peripheral pulses, color, temperature, and sensation are specifically indicated being sure to indicate the quality of the pulses. The location of any areas at high risk for complication such as calluses, corns, blisters, or reddened areas are noted in the chart. Include in the chart teaching done with the patient regarding foot care to prevent complications. Chart the patient's verbalization of understanding, and if referrals are made to special classes or clinics related to foot care, include this as well.

NURSING DIAGNOSIS 4

ANXIETY

Related to:

New diagnosis of diabetes mellitus

Complexity of regimen to be implemented

Change in health status

Threat to lifestyle

Fear of unknown

Defining Characteristics:

> Anxiety and restlessness
>
> Distraction, decreased concentration
>
> Expressions of fear and concern

Goal:

> Anxiety is relieved.

Outcome Criteria

✔ The patient verbalizes that anxiety has been reduced.

✔ The patient has no physiological signs of anxiety (tachycardia, diaphoresis, restlessness).

✔ The patient or family/significant other asks appropriate questions about diabetes mellitus.

✔ The patient indicates an ability to cope with the new diagnosis and manage diabetes.

NOC   *Anxiety control*

   Acceptance: Health status

INTERVENTIONS	RATIONALES
Have patient rate anxiety on a numerical scale if he or she is able.	Allows for a more objective measure of anxiety level.
Assess the patient for physiological signs of anxiety such as tachycardia, nervousness, restlessness, and diaphoresis.	Moderate to severe anxiety often produces physiological symptoms due to a sympathetic nervous system response and will vary from patient to patient.
Implement strategies to manage diabetes mellitus (see nursing diagnoses "Ineffective Management of Therapeutic Regimen" and "Imbalanced Nutrition").	Implementing strategies to control the problems of diabetes mellitus will help to reduce anxiety level.
Reassure patient by teaching the patient and family about all aspects of the therapeutic regimen (diet, medication, checking glucose, foot care, exercise).	Knowing what to expect from the disease and how to treat it enhances compliance and gives the patient a sense of control.
Assess knowledge regarding chronic complications: renal disease, heart disease, sexual dysfunction, retinopathy, amputations, and neuropathy, and encourage patient to verbalize concerns about health status.	Verbalizing concerns can help patient deal with issues and avoid negative feelings. Often the patient has heard talk of chronic complications, and some of what has been heard may be misinformation. Giving
	factual information on treatment and prevention may decrease anxiety.
Assess patient's ability to manage the regimen in terms of motivation and financial resources.	Diabetes can be an expensive health problem, and if finances are lacking, this could cause anxiety for the patient. The patient may find the regimen overwhelming and not be motivated to follow through.
Discuss with the patient and encourage him or her to express the psychosocial impact the disease may have on lifestyle: occupational (absences, type of job, shift work), economic (insurance, cost of medications, doctors visits), and psychological impact (fear of disability, concern about sexual function, stress, no food for pleasure/restricted diet).	Diabetes has an impact on all aspects of a person's life, and requires major lifestyle changes, including in some cases change in occupation. Being frank and open with the patient regarding the impact the disease has on lifestyle helps the patient to recognize the possibilities and begin acceptance of the disease.
Assist patient with identification/development of coping mechanisms.	The patient needs support to cope with the new diagnosis, and new coping mechanisms may be needed to help reduce anxiety.
Refer the patient to support groups as needed.	Support groups can provide needed emotional support for the patient.
Include family or significant other in teaching sessions.	Family support enhances compliance.

NIC   *Anxiety reduction*

   Calming technique

   Emotional support

   Presence

Evaluation

The patient expresses that he or she is able to cope with the diagnosis of diabetes mellitus. Assess the patient for the extent to which anxiety is reduced or alleviated and that he or she feels comfortable. Assess the patient for physiological signs of anxiety such as increased pulse and sweating. During evaluation, be sure to inquire about the use of relaxation techniques and coping strategies. The patient will also need to report that he or she understands the disease process and all aspects of the prescribed regimen for diabetes mellitus that has changed his or her health status. The patient verbalizes a willingness to implement strategies to control the disease.

Community/Home Care

The patient will need to know how to control anxiety in the home setting. It is crucial that health care providers equip the patient with knowledge regarding the many facets of diabetes mellitus in order to make the patient feel in control of his or her health. Once the patient learns more about the various aspects of the suggested regimen (diet and medication), the anxiety may resolve. However, the patient may continue to be anxious with the thought that his or her life cannot be normal and that long-term complications will occur necessitating total changes in lifestyle and quality of life. For this reason, one of the most important interventions that needs to be carried out by the health care provider is to educate the patient regarding the disease and how to prevent some of the complications that the patient fears most. Because the early days of managing diabetes mellitus are challenging as the patient learns how to control the disease, it is important that the patient has identified coping strategies that can be effective in relieving anxiety, stress, and feelings of being overwhelmed. By ensuring that the patient understands the health care regimen and knows what to do if acute symptoms develop, the health care provider may prevent unnecessary concern and worry regarding health status. It is strongly recommended that community support groups be used by the patient if available, especially for newly diagnosed diabetics.

Documentation

Document the degree of anxiety experienced by the patient. Using some type of numerical rating scale similar to the pain scale will provide health care providers with a more objective measure of the degree of anxiety the patient is experiencing. Document any physiological or observable signs of anxiety such as restlessness, tachycardia, or diaphoresis. Interventions implemented to treat these should be documented along with subsequent assessments to determine their effectiveness. Document the type of coping mechanisms the patient uses successfully. Document content of all teaching done.

CHAPTER 12.129

DIABETIC KETOACIDOSIS (DKA)

GENERAL INFORMATION

Diabetic ketoacidosis (DKA) is an emergency situation of insulin insufficiency that can be caused by illness in which insulin requirements increase, by omitting a dose of insulin, or by not adhering to the prescribed diet. A lack of insulin causes an inability of cells/muscles to utilize glucose. Breakdown of fat occurs in an attempt to provide energy for metabolism that causes release of fatty acids. The body's homeostatic mechanism begins the process of gluconeogenesis and glycogenolysis. This results in added glucose in the circulation, which the body cannot use. The kidneys reach their threshold for glucose and glycosuria occurs, which serves as an osmotic diuretic causing the excessive secretion of water (dehydration). Free fatty acids continue to be produced with resulting ketone bodies that are acid products. The condition continues in the absence of insulin and exceeds the body's ability to secrete acids or maintain acid/base balance. Ions such as potassium exit the cells causing hyperkalemia. The disorder is characterized as one of acidosis, ketosis, hyperglycemia, and dehydration and if uncorrected, circulatory collapse and shock may occur. Clinical manifestations include a fruity odor to breath, Kussmaul's respirations, tachycardia with a weak pulse, warm dry skin, lethargy, dry mucous membranes, weakness, and decreased blood pressure. Laboratory tests reveal glucose levels ranging from 350 to 1500, ketonuria, and elevated potassium levels. The elderly may not present with classic symptoms, and in some instances the symptoms are masked by other diseases.

NURSING DIAGNOSIS 1

DEFICIENT FLUID VOLUME

Related to:
Severe hyperglycemic state
Osmotic diuresis

Defining Characteristics:
Serum glucose > 350 mg/dl
Elevated potassium levels
Ketones in urine
Fruity odor to breath
Kussmaul's respirations
Dry skin
Dry mucous membranes
Excessive urinary output
Hypotension
Elevated serum osmolality

Goal:
The patient's fluid volume deficit, glucose, and electrolyte imbalance is corrected.

Outcome Criteria

✔ The patient's skin and mucous membranes will be moist and skin will be resilient (when pinched skin returns to normal position in < 3 seconds).
✔ The glucose level will drop below 250.
✔ Urinary output will be at least 30 ml per hour.
✔ Potassium level will be within normal range.
✔ Serum osmolality will return to normal.
✔ The patient's vital signs will return to baseline (pulse will decrease, blood pressure will increase, and no Kussmaul's respirations).
✔ The patient's level of consciousness improves to baseline.

NOC *Blood glucose level*
Hydration
Fluid balance
Electrolyte and acid/base balance
Vital signs

INTERVENTIONS	RATIONALES
Assess for signs of severe dehydration and DKA: decreased blood pressure, increased pulse, dry mucous membranes, poor skin turgor, excessive urinary output followed by decreased urinary output, and Kussmaul's respirations.	Helps to determine the seriousness of the problem to guide treatment and to assess effectiveness of treatments. Blood pressure decreases and pulse increases due to loss of volume; skin turgor is poor due to lack of moisture due to excessive loss of fluid. Urinary output is excessive initially but decreases as a compensatory mechanism when circulating volume decreases. Kussmaul's respirations are common in DKA and there is a fruity odor to the breath due the presence of acetone.
Assess glucose level on admission and every hour until stable (decrease to 250 mg); monitor urine for ketones before, during, and after treatment.	Helps to determine the extent of the problem and to guide treatment. The glucose level on admission is usually > 350 mg/dl; urine is monitored for resolution of ketonuria following treatment.
Assess potassium, serum osmolality, and arterial blood gases (ABGs).	Helps to determine fluid and electrolyte replacement needs as well as the extent of the fluid deficit. Total body potassium levels are decreased due to the effects of osmotic diuresis, but serum potassium levels may be elevated due to exit of potassium from the cells. Serum osmolality will be elevated and ABGs reveal metabolic acidosis.
Initiate intravenous (IV) fluid replacement, as ordered.	Correction of fluid deficit is dependent on the severity of the disorder and physician preference. A common infusion is to give 500 ml of normal saline IV over 1 to 2 hours to correct extracellular fluid depletion and raise the blood pressure. The infusion is slowed when the patient's blood pressure begins to normalize and urine output is approximately 30 ml/hr. The solution is generally changed to 5 percent dextrose and half-normal saline when blood glucose drops to 250 mg/dl. Fluid replacement must be aggressive and immediate to

	prevent progression to coma and decreased cardiac output and perfusion secondary to severe serum osmolality.
Administer regular insulin: an IV bolus and then an IV infusion, as ordered based on results of serum glucose level.	IV insulin is required to adequately control blood glucose since subcutaneous uptake may be delayed or erratic in DKA; insulin should be given at a dose that will decrease serum glucose by 100 mg/dl per hour. The dosage of insulin should be calculated so that serum glucose will drop to 250 mg/dl. The return to this level may require upwards of 4 to 6 hours.
Monitor output every hour; insert indwelling urinary catheter if needed or ordered.	Helps to be able to assess output accurately and to detect return of glomerular function.
Monitor neurological status for abnormalities: headache, lethargy, and changing level of consciousness.	Severe dehydration causes dehydration of cerebral tissue cells and manifests itself in changes in mental status. DKA uncorrected can lead to coma.
Once glucose normalizes following insulin administration, administer potassium chloride as ordered until serum potassium level returns to normal.	The patient with DKA initially has an elevated potassium level as potassium leaves the cells during dehydration; however, the total body potassium is low due to losses with diuresis. The administration of insulin causes potassium to shift back into the cells with a subsequent low serum level that needs correction.
Administer sodium bicarbonate IV, as ordered.	If pH levels drop below 7.0, bicarbonate is needed to correct the acidosis.
Monitor for signs of overcorrection—fluid overload and signs of hypoglycemia—and if present, treat as ordered.	Aggressive treatment sometimes results in fluid overload (crackles in lungs) and hypoglycemia (decreased blood sugar, nervousness, and diaphoresis).
Once the patient is alert, administer a long-acting carbohydrate or a meal.	Helps to sustain blood glucose level and counteract effects of insulin.
Teach the family and patient about the pathophysiology and precipitating causes for DKA.	DKA can be prevented by adhering to the prescribed regimen, taking note of output trends (diuresis followed by decreased output), and monitoring for events that increase the need for insulin, such as infections.

NIC *Hyperglycemia management*

Hyperglycemia management

Acid/base management:
  Metabolic acidosis

Fluid monitoring

Fluid management

Electrolyte management:
  Hyperkalemia

Evaluation

Assess the patient for return of normal or near-normal glucose levels, normal fluid volume, and electrolyte balance. Vital sign monitoring reveals the absence of Kussmaul's respiration, an increase in blood pressure, and a decrease in pulse to the patient's baseline. Urine output will be at least 30 ml/hour, and urine has no ketones. Skin should be warm, and color should return to the patient's normal appearance. Serum osmolality and potassium levels should be within normal range.

Community/Home Care

Patients treated for DKA should have normal fluid status and glucose levels restored prior to discharge home. Once the patient is discharged, he or she will need to monitor glucose and hydration levels to ensure that they are stable. The patient should be able to identify the specific situation or event that caused the DKA (illness, infection, not taking medication, indulging in foods not allowed on diet, etc.) and institute measures for prevention. It is suggested that the patient review basic information about diabetes and how to prevent hyperglycemia. Included in the review should be the prescribed regimen for diet, insulin therapy, and early signs of hyperglycemia. Having the patient make a chart that outlines the various complications such as hypoglycemia and hyperglycemia (early and late signs) can assist with review, and placing it in easy sight can serve as a reminder to review. In addition, the chart can include interventions that can be implemented at the first sign of hyperglycemia. The patient who has experienced an episode of DKA should frequently check glucose levels using Accu-Chek during the first few days back at home. Monitoring urinary output to detect unusual patterns of increased output will help the patient recognize problems early for prompt treatment. Home care should focus on prevention of future episodes of

DKA. Newly diagnosed diabetics will need to learn how to manage the disease and hyperglycemia (see nursing care plan "Diabetes Mellitus"). Immediately following discharge from the hospital, a visiting nurse can visit to perform an assessment for fluid status and glucose, and if abnormalities are identified, they can be reported to the physician. The health care provider may want the patient to return for a follow-up appointment to ensure that parameters such as glucose and potassium have returned to normal.

Documentation

In this situation, document initial assessment findings such as glucose, blood pressure, pulse, respirations, skin status (turgor, mucous membranes), and mental status. It is important to document interventions at the time of performance to allow for better monitoring of responses. IV fluid administration should be documented along with insulin administration according to agency guidelines. Be sure to document the patient's intake and output every hour or as ordered. Document all other interventions such as indwelling catheter insertion, results of serum glucose, or results of Accu-Chek. Be specific when charting patient responses to treatment so that other health care providers can clearly determine improvement or deterioration in hydration, electrolyte balance, or glucose level.

NURSING DIAGNOSIS 2

DEFICIENT KNOWLEDGE

Related to:

  Anxiety

  Diabetic ketoacidosis (prevention)

Defining Characteristics:

  Verbalizes a lack of understanding about the cause of DKA

  Has many questions

  Has no questions

  Verbalizes misunderstanding

Goal:

  The patient verbalizes an understanding of diabetic ketoacidosis, its prevention, and its treatment.

Outcome Criteria

✔ The patient verbalizes a willingness and desire to learn the necessary information.

✔ The patient verbalizes an understanding of DKA.

✔ The patient verbalizes an understanding of dietary restrictions required.

✔ The patient verbalizes a willingness to be compliant with treatment recommendations.

NOC *Diabetes self-management*
Knowledge: Disease process
Knowledge: Health behavior
Treatment behavior: Illness or injury

INTERVENTIONS	RATIONALES
Assess readiness of client to learn (motivation, cognitive level, and physiological status).	The patient must be motivated to learn, have the capability to learn the content, and be free of distractions from learning such as anxiety and emotional distress.
Assess what the patient already knows.	The patient may have some knowledge about diabetic ketoacidosis, and teaching should begin with what the patient already knows.
Create an environment conducive to learning (quiet, no distractions, adequate time).	Environmental noise and distractions as well as a feeling of being rushed can prevent the learner from focusing on what is being taught.
Teach the learners about the normal function of the pancreas and the pathophysiology of DKA.	Understanding of normal function and pathophysiology assists the patient to understand the rationale for therapeutic interventions and prevention of DKA.
Teach the patient about causative factors for DKA: — Omission of insulin — Failure to comply with diabetic diet — Acute illness, especially infection — Psychological stress	If the patient understands causes of DKA, he or she is more likely to be compliant. Skipping insulin or reducing the dose makes glucose unavailable to the cells leading to increased new glucose production that cannot be used making hyperglycemia worse; ingesting foods not allowed on the diet or in large portions adds to
	hyperglycemia, as not enough insulin is available to make the glucose from the food available to the body; stress of infection or illness causes increased energy levels and resultant gluconeogenesis.
Teach the patient about signs and symptoms of DKA: malaise, excessive urination, headache, fruity odor to breath, rapid respirations, or thirst.	Being able to recognize the symptoms of DKA early can prevent a crisis that requires visits to emergency rooms or hospitalization.
Reinforce previous teaching or begin teaching about diet and medications required for control of diabetes (see nursing care plan "Diabetes Mellitus").	The patient must understand dietary requirements and insulin requirements to control glucose levels and prevent DKA.
Evaluate the patient's understanding of all content covered by asking questions.	Helps to identify areas that require more teaching and to ensure that the patient has enough information to ensure compliance.
Give the patient written information on DKA, treatment, diet, or medications.	Provides material for reference at a later time, and for review.

NIC *Teaching: Disease process*
Teaching: Individual
Teaching: Diet

Evaluation

The patient is able to repeat information for the nurse and asks questions about DKA and possible outcomes (positive and negative). The patient is able to state what DKA is and what causes it. Prior to discharge, the patient verbalizes an understanding of how to prevent DKA, treatment, proper insulin administration, and diet restrictions, and agrees to be compliant. The patient is able to identify the early signs of DKA and when health care assistance should be sought.

Community/Home Care

For patients who have diabetes mellitus and have experienced DKA, the therapeutic regimen will need to be continued in the home. Teaching by the health care team should be thorough, with opportunities for discussions. Knowledge needs are identified early in order to improve the likelihood that the patient will be prepared for self-care and self-monitoring once at home and to prevent a recurrence of DKA. If the patient is a newly diagnosed diabetic, some follow-up care in the home or with a diabetic educator should be made to ensure that the patient is progressing with self-management of the disease. The major components of the disease that the patient must acquire knowledge on are dietary causes, medication (insulin) causes, stress or illness causes, signs/symptoms, and treatment needed. The nurse needs to assess the technique for administering the insulin, especially in patients with visual impairments, as under-medication leading to DKA could be an inadvertent result of the patient's inability to measure the medication accurately. Some adaptations in procedure may be required for the elderly patient who may have visual disturbances, such as obtaining insulin syringes with larger numbers or obtaining a magnifying glass for use in measuring. During visits in the home, the nurse needs to evaluate once more the patient's understanding of all content taught and the patient's ability and willingness to follow through.

Documentation

Document all content taught and the patient's verbalization of understanding. Specific attention should be given to documentation of any specific concerns that the patient expresses. Include in the documentation the patient's willingness to comply with all recommendations made about the diet, administration of insulin, checking glucose levels, and seeking follow-up care. Any area that requires further teaching should be clearly indicated in the record. Chart any questions or concerns that the patient has verbalized. Always include the titles of any printed literature given to the patient for reinforcement.

CHAPTER 12.130

HYPERGLYCEMIC HYPEROSMOLAR NON-KETOTIC SYNDROME (HHNS)

GENERAL INFORMATION

Hyperglycemic hyperosmolar non-ketotic syndrome is a hyperglycemic emergency seen in type 2 diabetes mellitus that is characterized by blood sugar levels > 600 mg/dl, but in many cases, the glucose is as high as 1000 mg. In addition to the severe hyperglycemia (with serum glucose ranges of 600 to 2000 mg/ml) caused by insulin deficiency, HHNS is characterized by extreme dehydration, severe electrolyte imbalances, a decreased level of consciousness, an absence of serum ketones, and the absence of acidosis as is seen in diabetic ketoacidosis. HHNS has a slow onset over a period of days to weeks. It typically occurs in older persons, the chronically ill or debilitated, newly diagnosed or undiagnosed persons, and in the presence of another disease, usually an infection. Initially the patient has an elevated blood sugar with accompanying diuresis. The patient is unable to replace water lost or respond to the thirst mechanism, and as a result glomerular filtration rate decreases, which reduces the excretion of excess glucose that cannot be used by the cells. Counter-regulatory hormones signal the body to increase glucose production. As the cycle continues, fluid shifts from the intracellular space to the extracellular space with even more diuresis resulting in total body dehydration leading to compromised circulating volume leading to hypovolemic shock and eventually coma. The accumulation of glucose and sodium in the circulating volume causes the serum osmolality to rise above normal. HHNS may go undetected due to the patient's inability to respond with increased intake or to verbalize thirst. The hallmarks of the disease are the extremely elevated serum glucose and the absence of ketones. Other clinical manifestations are hypotension, increased body temperature, elevated BUN, electrolyte imbalance, increased serum osmolality, lethargy, dry skin and mucous membranes, poor skin turgor, and eventually coma. The mortality rate for HHNS is extremely high (reported ranges vary from 35 to 70 percent) due to the lack of recognition of the presence of the condition, treatment that is inadequate, or other complicating underlying conditions.

NURSING DIAGNOSIS 1

DEFICIENT FLUID VOLUME

Related to:

Severe hyperglycemic state

Inability to respond to thirst mechanisms

Massive diuresis

Defining Characteristics:

Dry skin

Dry mucous membranes

Serum glucose > 600 mg/dl

Hypotension

Electrolyte imbalance

Elevated serum osmolality

Elevated BUN

Goal:

The patient's fluid volume deficit and glucose and electrolyte imbalance are corrected.

Outcome Criteria

✔ The patient's skin and mucous membranes will be moist and skin will be resilient (when pinched skin returns to normal position in < 3 seconds).

✔ Serum sodium will be within normal range of 135 to 145 mEq/L.

✔ The glucose level will drop below 250.

✔ Urinary output will be at least 30 ml per hour.

✔ Serum osmolality will return to normal.

✔ The patient's vital signs will return to baseline (temperature will decrease, blood pressure will increase).

✔ The patient's level of consciousness improves to baseline.

NOC *Fluid balance*

Electrolyte and acid/base balance

Vital signs

INTERVENTIONS	RATIONALES
Assess for signs of severe dehydration: decreased blood pressure, increased pulse, dry mucous membranes, poor skin turgor, decreased urinary output, and elevated temperature.	Determines the seriousness of the problem, to guide treatment, and to assess effectiveness of treatments.
Insert indwelling urinary catheter and monitor output every hour.	Helps to be able to assess output accurately and to detect return of glomerular function.
Monitor sodium, potassium, and serum osmolality.	Helps to determine fluid and electrolyte replacement needs as well as the extent of the fluid deficit. Serum sodium will be increased due to hemoconcentration, potassium may be normal or low, and serum osmolality is elevated.
Monitor glucose level on admission and every hour until stable (decrease to 250 mg).	Guides treatment. The glucose is usually > 600 mg/dl.
Monitor for decreasing level of consciousness, lethargy, somnolence, and seizure activity.	Severe dehydration causes dehydration of cerebral tissue cells and manifests itself in changes in mental status. HHNS uncorrected can lead to coma.
Initiate aggressive fluid replacement intervention, as ordered. Initially, a common infusion is to give one liter of normal saline intravenously (IV) over the first hour, followed by a half-normal saline solution. In accordance with physician orders, slow the rate of the solution when the patient's blood pressure	Patients in true HHNS may have a fluid volume deficit of 9 to 12 liters. Fluid replacement must be aggressive and immediate to decrease serum osmolality quickly, as increased serum osmolality causes progressively severe decreasing levels of consciousness and compromises the cardiac system's ability to

begins to normalize and urine output is approximately 30 ml/hr; in most instances, the IV solution is changed to 5 percent dextrose and half-normal saline when blood glucose drops to 250 mg/dl.	maintain cardiac output and perfusion. As much as half of the required fluid may be given in the first 12 hours of treatment.
Administer potassium chloride as ordered until serum potassium level returns to normal.	With the severe dehydration comes a loss of potassium, which will lead to cardiac complications.
Administer small doses of insulin IV, as ordered.	Insulin is needed to decrease the extremely high glucose level and may be given at a dose that will decrease serum glucose by 100 mg/dl per hour until it reaches 250 mg/dl. In some cases, insulin will not be necessary because fluid replacement will correct/reduce serum glucose levels.
Encourage at least 3000 ml/day fluid intake if the patient is tolerating oral liquids, unless contraindicated.	Increases body fluids and restores fluid balance.
Treat the underlying cause.	Correcting the underlying cause, especially infections, can correct the HHNS.
Teach the family and patient about the pathophysiology and precipitating causes for HHNS.	HHNS can often be prevented by taking note of output trends (diuresis followed by decreased output), fluid intake, and monitoring for other diseases that cause HHNS such as infections and stroke/cerebrovascular accident (CVA).

NIC *Fluid monitoring*

Fluid management

Fluid and electrolyte management

Electrolyte management: Hypernatremia

Electrolyte management: Hypokalemia

Hyperglycemia management

Evaluation

Assess the patient for return of normal fluid volume. The patient's blood pressure and pulse should return to baseline. The pulse should be strong and regular, and at the patient's baseline or only slightly increased. Skin should be warm and color should return to the patient's normal appearance. There should be no signs of neurological involvement due to severe dehydration and sodium excess. Renal function should not be impaired, with an hourly output on the average of 30 ml/hour. Serum osmolality, BUN, sodium, potassium, and glucose levels should be within normal range.

Community/Home Care

Patients treated for deficient fluid volume secondary to HHNS should have normal fluid status restored prior to discharge home. Once the patient is discharged, he or she will need to continue to receive adequate amounts of fluid. Providing the patient or family with a list of drinks and foods that are appropriate will be helpful so that the patient has a handy reference. If the patient is able to drink fluids, encourage him or her to keep a water bottle filled with water at work or home to enhance the likelihood that he or she will drink adequate amounts of fluid. For patients who are chronically ill, debilitated, and unable to obtain fluids independently, the caregiver will need to establish a routine for administering fluids and monitoring output and glucose. This may include recording the intake and output in a log and determining imbalances; this can be taught by the nurse prior to discharge home. Monitoring the output in the early days of recovery can help the family and patient detect continued dehydration or stabilization of fluid balance as the output returns to normal. Some patients may not require any follow-up as this is an acute emergency situation; however, prevention of future episodes of HHNS must be undertaken. The patient may need close monitoring of the glucose level until the underlying cause has been corrected. If this is an infection, it should be stressed to the patient or caregiver to take all of the medications prescribed to assure resolution. Newly diagnosed type 2 diabetics will need to learn how to manage the disease and hyperglycemia (see nursing care plan "Diabetes Mellitus"). Patients who experience a severe loss of fluid often experience fatigue and weakness that will need to be addressed at home. This can be handled by informing the patient to perform activities as tolerated until stamina/endurance is re-established. Immediately following the patient's discharge from the hospital, a nurse can visit to perform an assessment for fluid status and glucose, and if abnormalities are identified,

they can be reported to the physician. Whether the patient is returning to the home or an extended care facility, an evaluation should be made to determine the patient's ability to respond to thirst signals or to get sufficient fluids to prevent dehydration. The health care provider may want the patient to return for a follow-up appointment to ensure that parameters such as sodium, glucose, BUN, potassium, and serum osmolality have returned to normal.

Documentation

In this situation, document initial assessment findings such as blood pressure, pulse, respirations, temperature, skin status (turgor, mucous membranes), and mental status. Be sure to document the patient's intake and output every hour until condition stabilizes and then every shift. Document all interventions such as insulin administration, intravenous catheter insertion, fluids initiated (type, rate), indwelling catheter insertion, urine output (amount, color), and dietary modifications such as sodium restrictions. Chart Accu-Cheks and any insulin given based on results. Be specific when charting patient responses to treatment so that other health care providers can clearly determine improvement or deterioration in hydration, electrolyte balance, or glucose level.

NURSING DIAGNOSIS 2

 DECREASED CARDIAC OUTPUT

Related to:

　　Severe fluid deficit

Defining Characteristics:

　　Hypotension

　　Tachycardia

　　Decreased oxygen saturation

　　Skin cool to touch

　　Peripheral cyanosis

　　Urinary output < 30 ml/hour

　　Diminished peripheral pulses

　　Delayed capillary refill > 2 seconds

　　Decreased level of consciousness

Goal:

　　The patient's cardiac output returns to normal.

Outcome Criteria

✔ The patient's blood pressure and pulse return to baseline.

✔ The patient's level of consciousness improves and returns to baseline.

✔ Urinary output is > 30 ml per hour.

✔ The patient's skin is warm and dry.

✔ Capillary refill is < 2 seconds.

NOC *Circulatory status*
Tissue perfusion: Cardiac
Tissue perfusion: Peripheral
Tissue perfusion: Cerebral
Cardiac pump effectiveness
Vital signs

INTERVENTIONS	RATIONALES
Assess vital signs, particularly blood pressure and pulse, as ordered, but at least every 4 hours.	Changes in blood pressure and pulse give indicators of patient status. In severe fluid loss, a decreased blood pressure with narrowing pulse pressure may be noted; the pulse may be rapid, weak, and thready.
Assess neck veins.	Absence of visible neck veins when the patient is supine indicates decreased circulating volume.
Assess urinary output.	Decreased urinary output (< 30 ml/hour) indicates decreased perfusion to kidneys secondary to deficient fluid volume.
Assess skin temperature and color.	If severe dehydration as is seen in HHNS goes unchecked, perfusion to skin and periphery is inadequate to maintain warmth or normal color.
Assess peripheral pulses.	If cardiac output starts to decrease due to loss of volume, peripheral pulses become weak, diminished, or absent, as the heart is unable to maintain perfusion to extremities.
Assess mental status: level of consciousness, lethargy, somnolence, and impending coma.	Changes in mental status indicate a decrease in cerebral tissue perfusion and an inability of the body's compensatory

mechanism to provide adequate oxygenation to cerebral tissue.

Assess cardio-respiratory status, noting adventitious breath sounds, oxygen saturation, and complaints of chest pain.	Decreased cardiac output leads to decreased perfusion to lungs causing crackles and dyspnea; loss of fluid volume can create a decreased ability to perfuse tissues resulting in lowered oxygen saturation. In decreased cardiac output, activity causes increased demands for oxygenated blood; however, when the heart attempts to increase its output the demand for oxygen cannot be supplied, resulting in chest pain.
Implement strategies to correct the fluid loss and hyperglycemia and restore intravascular volume as ordered (see nursing diagnosis "Deficient Fluid Volume").	Replacing intravascular volume is needed to improve cardiac output.
Maintain bedrest during acute treatment phase.	Helps to decrease the workload of the heart.

NIC *Cardiac care*
Fluid management
Fluid monitoring
Vital signs monitoring

Evaluation

Note the degree to which outcome criteria have been achieved. The patient should demonstrate adequate cardiac output or improvement in abnormalities. Peripheral pulses should be present, and skin, when touched, should be warm. If cardiac output is improved, perfusion to the kidneys should be adequate, with the patient producing at least 30 ml of urine per hour on average. The pulse should be within the patient's baseline and should be strong and regular. Oxygen saturation should be > 90 percent. The patient demonstrates adequate cerebral tissue perfusion as demonstrated by correction of lethargy and the patient's return to his or her usual mental state or level of consciousness.

Community/Home Care

Patients who have experienced HHNS should have no lingering effects of the disorder, particularly related to cardiac output, at time of discharge.

However, they may experience some degree of fatigue due to the severity of the disorder in terms of the electrolyte imbalance and dehydration. They or their family members will need to know how to gradually increase activities when at home with a balance of rest and activity. Response to activity should be monitored noting any chest pain, shortness of breath, increased respiratory rate, or increased pulse rate. Having a comfortable chair readily available for rest periods is suggested, as is having scheduled rest periods. It is important that the patient, family, or other caregiver remain cognizant of how much output occurs during a day and what signs indicate dehydration. This will help prevent future excessive fluid loss that could lead to decreased cardiac output. At home, caregivers need to make a conscious effort to give the patient adequate amounts of fluid to prevent dehydration. For most patients, once the problem has been identified as HHNS and the underlying cause has been treated, cardiac output is re-established with restoration of adequate fluid balance. For those patients with disease processes such as CVA (stroke) as the causative factor, more aggressive treatments are required, and follow-up may center on treating the offending disease to prevent a recurrence. Visitation in the home may be recommended for some patients, especially if they verbalize feelings of anxiety or lack of knowledge about the emergency situation (HHNS) that necessitated in-hospital care. A follow-up appointment is needed to be sure that the patient has returned to a normal level of functioning.

Documentation

Chart the results of all assessments made, particularly of the respiratory and cardiac systems and hydration status. Document intake/output, blood pressure, pulse, and results of Accu-Cheks, according to agency protocol. Include in the record any patient complaints made relevant to the cardiac system exactly as the patient states it. If chest pain occurs, document what the patient was doing at the time of pain and how it was relieved. Medications and intravenous fluids are charted on the medication administration record and in accordance with agency guidelines. All other interventions should be documented in a timely fashion with the patient's specific response to each intervention. Always include in the patient's record his or her psychological status—whether the patient appears anxious, restless, or fearful, and whether significant others are present.

CHAPTER 12.131

HYPERTHYROIDISM

GENERAL INFORMATION

Hyperthyroidism is a disorder in which levels of thyroid hormone are elevated; its causes include autoimmune reactions (Graves's disease); thyroid tumors (toxic multinodular goiter); thyroid stimulating hormone (TSH) secreting pituitary tumors, or thyroiditis; and excessive thyroid hormone (TH) replacement. Regardless of the cause, the result is increased levels of TH that increases metabolic rate, increases the activity of the sympathetic nervous system, and increases the metabolism of protein, fat, and carbohydrate. Clinical manifestations of hyperthyroidism include weight loss, increased appetite, intolerance to heat, increased heart rate, elevated temperature, tiredness/malaise, exophthalmos, and goiter. Graves's disease, the most common form of hyperthyroidism, occurs most often in women 20 to 40 years of age. Thyroid storm, also known as hyperthyroid crisis, usually occurs in undiagnosed or untreated hyperthyroidism at times of significant metabolic stress due to trauma, infection, diabetic ketoacidosis, and surgery. Thyroid storm is a life-threatening emergency characterized by pronounced signs of increased metabolic rate, including tachycardia, hyperthermia, dysrhythmias, decrease in mental status, hypertension, abdominal pains, tremors, and tachypnea. The body is unable to sustain itself in this hypermetabolic state, and treatment must occur quickly (ideally within two hours of onset), as the patient becomes severely exhausted and develops heart failure that progresses to cardiac arrest. The mortality rate from uncorrected or delayed correction of thyroid storm can range from 20 to 60 percent.

NURSING DIAGNOSIS 1

DECREASED CARDIAC OUTPUT

Related to:

Hypermetabolism resulting from hyperthyroid state

Severely increased myocardial workload

Dysrhythmias

Increased sensitivity to catecholamines

Defining Characteristics:

Tachycardia

Hypertension

Diaphoresis

Decreased level of consciousness

Diminished or absent peripheral pulses

Prolonged capillary refill (> 2 seconds)

Complaint of chest pain and palpitations

Fever

Goal:

Cardiac output will be restored.

Outcome Criteria

✔ Pulse rate is between 60 and 100.

✔ Skin is warm and dry.

✔ Perfusion is restored, as demonstrated by absence of peripheral cyanosis, and capillary refill is < 2 seconds.

✔ Urinary output is > 30 ml/hour average.

✔ Blood pressure returns to patient's baseline.

NOC *Circulatory status*
Cardiac pump effectiveness
Vital signs

INTERVENTIONS	RATIONALES
Assess vital signs, particularly blood pressure and pulse, as ordered, but at least every 4 hours.	Changes in blood pressure and pulse give indicators of patient status. In states of hyperthyroidism, systolic hypertension may be noted, pulse is rapid, and temperature is elevated.

INTERVENTIONS	RATIONALES
Assess for cardiac compromise, including edema, neck vein distention, palpitations, chest pain, and crackles.	Helps to determine effects of elevated thyroid levels on the cardiac system; increased TH causes an increased metabolic rate, which in turn causes the tissues to require more oxygen and blood flow, placing more demands on the heart.
Monitor results of diagnostic tests: TSH, free T4, T3, thyroid uptake of radioactive iodine (RAIU), serum thyroglobulin, and thyroid autoantibody (TA) tests.	TSH is suppressed, free T4 will be elevated, T3 will be elevated, RAIU will demonstrate increased uptake of iodine, RAIU can also be used to examine the size of the thyroid, serum thyroglobulin will be elevated in hyperthyroidism, and TA are elevated in Graves's disease.
Keep the environment cool.	Patients with hyperthyroidism have intolerance to heat and need a cool environment.
Create a quiet and calm environment.	Stressors and stimulating environments increase catecholamines, which in turn increase the workload of the heart and further increase the metabolic demands.
Administer thioamide medications (Propylthiouracil®, Tapazole®), as ordered, to reduce hyperthyroidism.	These medications inhibit the synthesis of TH and prevent T4 to T3 conversion. Note that the effect is not instantaneous.
Administer potassium iodide agents (SSKI), as ordered.	These medications stop the synthesis and release of TH; they also shrink the thyroid gland and are used pre-operatively to reduce the vascularity of the gland.
Administer beta blockers (Inderal®), as ordered.	Helps to decrease cardiovascular effects; used to control tachydysrhythmias and muscle tremors; decreases heart rate and work of the myocardium.
Assist with radioactive iodine treatments, as ordered.	Radioactive iodine destroys thyroid gland cells. The patient may receive from one to several treatments. The first dose can demonstrate some immediate effects, but the maximum effect may take place in one to three months.
Administer antipyretics, as ordered, and keep the patient's room cool; remove covers from bed, and provide cooling blanket if necessary.	Fever will increase metabolic demands, further decreasing cardiac output.
Avoid aspirin products.	Aspirin increases free TH levels.
Consider use of sedatives.	Sedatives reduce metabolic demands, reduce the work of the myocardium, and cause muscle relaxation and rest.
Prepare the patient for surgical procedure, as ordered.	When hyperthyroidism cannot be controlled, removal of 80 percent of the thyroid gland may be the therapeutic intervention of choice.
Limit physical exercise; encourage rest.	Physical activity increases metabolic demands and puts further demand on the heart; the patient is usually fatigued.
Assess mental status, including anxiety and agitation.	Patients with hyperthyroidism experience anxiety, restlessness, and agitation due to increased metabolic rate and stimulation.
Encourage the use of calming relaxation techniques such as guided imagery, deep breathing, music, and meditation.	Helps to decrease stimuli, stressors, and anxiety that can increase cardiac workload.
Assess respiratory status, noting adventitious breath sounds and oxygen saturation.	With increased metabolic rates, the cardiac system may not be able to sustain cardiac output sufficiently to meet perfusion needs of the lungs, causing crackles and dyspnea.
Administer supplemental oxygen, as ordered.	Helps to ensure maximum oxygenation and to compensate for excessive oxygen consumption.
Monitor the patient for signs of thyroid crisis/storm, including pronounced symptoms of hyperthyroidism such as elevated temperature, systolic hypertension, tachycardia, diarrhea, and tremors progressing to delirium or psychosis, and treat as ordered (give beta blockers, place in quiet room, give intravenous fluids, and keep the patient cool).	Thyroid storm is an emergency that requires immediate attention; monitoring for this allows for prompt treatment.

NIC *Cardiac care*
Vital signs monitoring

Evaluation

Note the degree to which outcome criteria have been achieved and the patient's symptoms of hyperthyroidism are improving. The patient should demonstrate adequate cardiac output or improvement in abnormalities. The pulse and blood pressure should be within the patient's baseline, and the pulse should be strong and regular. Temperature returns to normal, and the patient verbalizes being comfortable with environmental temperature. Peripheral pulses should be present, and skin should be warm to the touch. The patient has indicators of decreased metabolic rate, such as decreased anxiety and restlessness. Oxygen saturation should be > 90 percent.

Community/Home Care

Patients with hyperthyroidism will need to continue therapies in the home. Of critical importance is continued implementation of strategies to decrease the production of TH and meet the metabolic demands of the body. The patient will need to understand how to take medications for hyperthyroidism, especially if surgery has not been undertaken, and understand that he or she will need these medications for the rest of his or her life. Placing medications in a noticeable place can help the patient to remember to take the medication daily. Because of the length of time required for medication effectiveness, the patient will need to be aware of worsening symptoms of thyroid excess. Interventions in the home include weighing self, taking pulse, and being aware of feelings of anxiety/being jittery and excessive fatigue. If these symptoms do not gradually improve, the patient should contact the health care provider to be sure that the symptoms do not indicate thyroid crisis. Keeping a log of pulse rates, weights, and any other complaints can help the patient notice patterns in resolution of the disease or worsening. For many patients, there will be a need to adapt the temperature of the home due to heat intolerance, at least until treatment is effective. This is especially true in the summer months, and particularly in hot, humid climates. Air conditioning makes this task easier, but in some instances the temperature required for comfort may be uncomfortable for other family members, and compromises or solutions will

need to be developed. Even though most people assume that all homes are air conditioned, this is not necessarily true. For those homes without air conditioning, fans can be of limited assistance; however, window fans can be very effective at night. The patient will need to adjust clothing and linens, and seek out other methods of cooling, such as using a wet towel or washcloth to dampen forehead, face, arms, or underarms periodically. Early in the disease, prior to effective treatment, diaphoresis is common, and the patient may need to change clothes several times during the day and bed linens at night. For most patients, once the hyperthyroidism is controlled, the symptoms will gradually resolve, and cardiac output restored. However, follow-up is required to determine the status of the disease through laboratory tests and symptoms.

Documentation

Chart the results of all assessments made, particularly symptoms of hyperthyroidism and of the cardiac system. Document blood pressure and pulse according to agency protocol. Include in the record any patient complaints made relevant to thyroid symptoms and the cardiac system exactly as the patient states them. Chart the administration of medications for treatment of hyperthyroidism and measures taken to prepare the patient for radiation therapy or surgery. All interventions should be documented in a timely fashion with the patient's specific response to the intervention. Always include in the patient's record his or her psychological status: whether he or she appears anxious, jittery, or restless.

NURSING DIAGNOSIS 2

 IMBALANCED NUTRITION: LESS THAN BODY REQUIREMENTS

Related to:

Severely increased metabolic demands

Hypermotility of gastrointestinal (GI) tract

Vomiting

Diarrhea

Defining Characteristics:

Weight loss

Increased fatigue

Decreased albumin

Decreased transferrin

Goal:

The patient's dietary intake is sufficient to meet metabolic needs.

Outcome Criteria

✔ The patient's weight remains stable at baseline.

✔ The patient consumes at least 3000 to 5000 calories.

✔ Serum transferrin and albumin return to normal.

NOC *Nutritional status*
Nutritional status: Energy

INTERVENTIONS	RATIONALES
Complete a nutritional assessment and monitor for usual dietary intake, weight loss, vomiting, insatiable appetite, severe thirst, nausea, decreased albumin, and decreased transferrin.	Helps to establish a baseline of nutritional status; the patient with hyperthyroidism often eats extensively without weight gain in an effort to supply enough nutrients for the increased metabolic rate; as many as 5000 calories may be required. Decreased albumin and transferrin indicate protein deficiency that needs to be corrected to ensure enough protein for energy.
Weigh daily and record.	Helps to assess accurately for weight loss.
Assess for activity tolerance: monitor for ability to perform activity, signs of muscle wasting, extreme fatigue, and generalized weakness.	Because of inadequate nutrient intake to meet metabolic demands, the patient may feel fatigued/tired and unable to perform usual activities.
In cooperation with the dietician, arrange for frequent (at least 6 small), high-calorie, high-carbohydrate, high-protein meals and snacks. Determine the patient's likes and dislikes, as well as any religious or cultural restrictions.	A high-calorie intake (as high as 5000 calories) is essential while metabolic needs are high; frequent meals with snacks provide an easier way to get enough nutrients; the patient will consume foods that he or she likes and that are part of his or her usual diet.
Administer vitamins, as ordered.	Helps to meet the body's vitamin requirements.
Administer glucose supplements, as ordered.	Glucose can be used as a calorie/energy source, but monitor the patient for hyperglycemia.
Administer insulin, as ordered.	Small amounts of insulin are used to control increased serum glucose levels.
Administer medications for control of nausea, vomiting, or diarrhea.	Loss of nutrients through emesis and stools can add to fatigue and worsen nutritional status.
Encourage periods of alternating rest and activity; assist patient as tolerated.	The patient may require rest periods to decrease metabolic rate and nutrient needs.
Collaborate with the dietician to teach the patient regarding dietary requirements for hyperthyroidism.	The patient will require a special diet until the hyperthyroidism is controlled and needs to know how to prepare a diet to meet caloric requirements.

NIC *Nutritional monitoring*
Nutritional management

Evaluation

The patient's nutritional status is stable, as demonstrated by stabilization of weight with no weight loss. The patient verbalizes an interest in eating and understands the need for increased amounts of food and nutrients due to the hypermetabolic state. No further weight loss occurs, and the patient consumes adequate calories through frequent small meals and snacks that are high in protein and carbohydrates. The patient reports a gradual return of energy.

Community/Home Care

The patient must continue to give attention to nutrition and the need for increased intake, which may double his or her usual intake, in order to meet metabolic demands. A dietary consultation is crucial in assisting the patient to calculate the amount of food needed to consume adequate calories for metabolic demands. Giving the patient a list of foods that can provide good sources of the required nutrients will be helpful. Frequent small meals and snacks are continued to increase the likelihood that the patient can ingest enough nutrients to meet calorie requirements. With this in mind, the patient and family will need to remember the signs and symptoms of hyperglycemia, as large doses of carbohydrates and increased calories may elevate glucose levels. A diet rich in protein is also needed for energy levels, but for vegetarians good non-meat sources of protein need to be identified. Significant others or family members can play an active role in implementing strategies to improve nutrition by preparing meals and snacks that are palatable and encouraging the patient to ingest them. A handy reference guide can be created that includes categories of foods with their calorie counts. Supplemental drinks can improve nutritional status by significantly increasing calories, and could include commercial products on the market (Boost, Ensure), as well as homemade types such as milkshakes or fresh fruit smoothies. However, the patient may need to experiment with which ones are satisfying. The patient may need to remain on multivitamins and other nutritional supplements until the hyperthyroidism is controlled. Teach the patient to monitor nutrition/intake by keeping a log of what, when, and how much he or she eats. Even though the patient may not want to weigh every day, weighing at least every other day is a good way to keep track of weight loss or stabilization. This information can be shared with the health care provider at each follow-up visit to provide data for revision in prescribed therapeutic interventions.

Documentation

Chart the results of a nutritional assessment that includes a history of usual intake. Document vital signs and intake and output at least every shift or every 8 hours and chart weights daily according to agency protocol. Include in the chart the amount of food the patient consumes at each meal and what, if any, supplements or between-meal snacks are taken by the patient. For patients taking nutritional supplements (vitamins, liquid supplements, etc.), chart this in the patient's medication record. Always include in the record any referrals made, especially to the dietician. If the patient verbalizes concerns regarding diet requirements, chart this in the record.

NURSING DIAGNOSIS 3

RISK FOR INJURY

Related to:

Thyroidectomy

Accidental removal of parathyroid glands

Exophthalmus

Defining Characteristics:

None

Goal:

The patient will have no injuries due to thyroid surgery or hyperthyroidism.

Outcome Criteria

✔ The patient will have no corneal injury.

✔ The patient will have no hemorrhage from surgical site.

✔ The patient will maintain patent airway.

✔ Hoarseness will resolve following thyroidectomy, and voice tone will be normal.

✔ The patient will have no signs of tetany.

✔ The patient verbalizes an understanding of all possible complications of surgery.

NOC   *Respiratory status: Airway patency*

       Electrolyte and acid/base balance

       Blood loss severity

       Risk control: Visual impairment

INTERVENTIONS	RATIONALES
Assess the patient for exophthalmos and visual changes.	About a third of patients with Graves's disease have bulging eyes (exophthalmos) caused by fat deposits in the orbit and inflammation. Other changes include diplopia and difficulty focusing.
Protect the eye from injury: wear eye shields, use artificial tears, tape eye shut at night, and elevate the head of the bed when the patient is sleeping.	If the eye is protruding, there is risk for corneal abrasion and drying. Artificial tears prevent excess dryness of the eye that could become irritating; wearing a shield protects from injury and risk of infection; and taping the lid closed at night prevents injury and drying during sleep. Elevation of the head of bed promotes drainage from the area surrounding the eye.
Assess for signs and symptoms of hypocalcemia following thyroidectomy: serious neuromuscular dysfunction that may be indicative of tetany (tonic muscular spasms), paresthesias (numbness and	During thyroidectomy, there is a risk for accidental injury or removal of the parathyroid gland resulting in hypocalcemia. A serum calcium level should be obtained as well.

INTERVENTIONS	RATIONALES
tingling around the mouth and in the hands and feet), muscle spasms of the face and extremities, hyperactivity of reflexes, laryngospasm, and seizures. If present, notify physician and administer calcium preparations intravenously (IV), as ordered.	
Post-operatively, assess for hemorrhage by checking behind the neck and shoulders for bleeding from the incision; check for edema of the neck area.	Because of the location of the incision, bleeding will drain behind the neck or down onto the back of the shoulder and not necessarily saturate the dressing; edema in the neck may indicate bleeding from the site.
Assess the patient for hoarseness and loss of voice post-operatively.	Because of the close proximity of the larynx and laryngeal nerve to the thyroid gland, the risk for damage during surgery is high. Hoarseness is expected for a short period of time, but complete loss of voice and persistent hoarseness are signs of complications.
Teach the patient about eye care, assessment for hypocalcemia, assessment for hemorrhage, and worsening of hoarseness.	The patient will need to implement eye care and assessments in the home environment.

NIC   *Bleeding reduction: Wound*
Electrolyte management:
   Hypocalcemia
Surveillance

Evaluation

Determine that the outcome criteria have been met. The patient has experienced no injuries or problems due to exophthalmos or hypocalcemia. The cornea is protected, and no abrasion or excessive drying occurs. Hoarseness has dissipated, and the patient's voice has returned to normal. No hemorrhage occurs post-operatively, and the patient can verbalize an understanding of all potential complications.

Community/Home Care

The patient with hyperthyroidism receives a majority of care in the home, and hospital stays for surgery are short. The patient needs to be equipped to assess him or herself for complications such as

loss of voice and hemorrhage. The patient can relieve discomfort of throat soreness by simple gargles or analgesic lozenges. If hoarseness persists for longer than a week, the health care provider should be notified for follow-up. Monitoring for hemorrhage is simple, as the bulky neck dressings of the immediate post-operative period will be replaced with a small, simple dressing. The patient can feel the drainage from bleeding trickling down the neck. Standing in front of the mirror will allow the patient to inspect the surgical site daily. To avoid irritation, the patient should avoid clothes, such as turtleneck sweaters, that cover the surgical site. Tetany is more likely following discharge (1 to 7 days post-operatively), making it necessary for the patient to monitor him or herself for signs such as twitching of muscles, tingling of toes, fingers, and lips, and tremors. For the patient with exophthalmos, eye care is needed at home to prevent visual disturbances and permanent damage to the cornea that is prone to dryness. The patient needs to learn how to administer eye drops and instill artificial tears into eyes as prescribed. A patch over the eye protects it from drying or injury during the night if the eye does not close completely. If any problems develop, the patient should contact the health care provider for immediate attention.

Documentation

Document all assessments performed to detect problems following surgery for hyperthyroidism, as well as assessments for exophthalmos. Chart complaints the patient verbalizes regarding corneal dryness or inability to close eye. Status of the incisional site is documented along with assessments regarding signs and symptoms of hypocalcemia. All interventions employed to detect or treat problems are documented along with the patient's responses. All teaching regarding post-operative care and care of the eyes is documented.

NURSING DIAGNOSIS 4

 RISK FOR INEFFECTIVE AIRWAY CLEARANCE

Related to:

   Laryngeal spasms

   Edema of neck

   Hemorrhage

Defining Characteristics:

None

Goal:

The patient's airway is patent.

Outcome Criteria

✔ The patient's breath sounds will be present and clear bilaterally.

✔ The patient will have no cyanosis.

✔ The patient will have normal respirations without stridor, wheezing, nasal flaring, or dyspnea.

✔ The patient will have no edema in neck at surgical site.

NOC *Respiratory status: Airway patency*
        Respiratory status: Ventilation

INTERVENTIONS	RATIONALES
Assess respiratory status: respiratory rate, rhythm, depth, note changes in respiratory rate (tachypnea), oxygen saturation, dyspnea; monitor for specific indicators of obstructed patient airway such as swallowing blood, cyanosis, retractions, use of accessory muscles, stridor, and wheezing.	Due to surgical intervention, laryngospasm and edema in the neck may occur. Absence of breath sounds and abnormal breathing patterns such as retractions, stridor, and flaring of nostrils indicate a significant decline in respiratory status and airway patency; if parathyroid glands have been accidentally damaged, hypocalcemia can occur, which could lead to laryngeal spasms, causing symptoms of occluded airway; assessments are needed to establish baseline and monitor response to interventions.
Assess neck for edema and ask patient about feeling of tightness.	Edema in the neck could be an indicator of bleeding from the surgical site that could occlude the airway by compressing the trachea; a feeling of tightness indicates an accumulation of drainage or blood in the neck. The risk for bleeding is high due to the vascularity of the thyroid gland.
Monitor arterial blood gases (ABGs) and oxygen saturation, as ordered.	Helps to assess respiratory status.
Provide humidified oxygen, as ordered, to maintain oxygen saturation at > 90 percent.	Oxygen may be ordered in the early hours post-operatively to ensure oxygenation to tissues.
Place patient in high Fowler's position with head elevated.	Prevents edema in surgical site and maximizes chest excursion and subsequent movement of air.
Following thyroidectomy, keep a tracheostomy tray at bedside.	Tracheostomy tray may be needed for emergency use in case of occlusion of airway.
Have suction equipment available at bedside.	Blood that may occlude the airway can be removed via suctioning.
Monitor patient for signs of aspiration of blood into lungs: abnormal breath sounds, fever, and increased secretions.	When foreign substances are in the airway, particles may be aspirated into lungs and may cause aspiration pneumonia; detects early symptoms that may require further treatment.
If signs of occluded airway occur, assist with the establishment of an open airway by use of airway adjuncts, endotracheal intubation or surgical airway, as ordered.	The use of appropriate airway adjuncts or endotracheal intubation to open and protect the airway, or the surgical creation of an airway (via cricothyrotomy or tracheostomy) to bypass an obstruction may be necessary.
Assess for damage to laryngeal nerve following thyroid surgery; note persistent soreness and loss of voice.	Damage to the laryngeal nerve can cause spasms of the vocal cord.
Assess the patient with a goiter for gradually closing airway and implement measures to assist with emergency creation of an airway.	The goiter can be so large as to occlude the airway.

NIC *Airway management*
        Respiratory monitoring

Evaluation

Assess the patient to determine the extent to which the outcome criteria have been met. Assessments of the respiratory system should reveal that acute symptoms of airway obstruction have not occurred. The patient's airway should be clear, the patient should be able to speak in a normal tone, and the patient should be breathing easy. Breath sounds should be present and even though there may be some discomfort with respirations; no respiratory distress should be noted. ABGs and oxygen saturation should indicate adequate oxygenation, and there should be no cyanosis.

Community/Home Care

For the patient who is at high risk for airway obstruction due to goiter or thyroidectomy, in-home care may not be required except as it relates to follow-up relevant to the hyperthyroidism rather than respiratory issues. The patient can enhance comfort of the throat by using lozenges or gargling with a saline solution at home every 2 to 4 hours. Care of the surgical incision following thyroidectomy is minimal, and in most instances the incision is left open to air or covered with a clean dressing that the patient can easily apply. The patient who has a goiter should see gradual improvement in his or her ability to breathe as the hyperthyroidism is controlled. By the time of discharge, edema in the surgical site should have subsided, and the dangers of bleeding into the airway should have been eliminated. However, the patient and family should still be aware of the signs and symptoms of airway obstruction and what to do in the event that they should occur once at home. Written information can be given to the patient outlining the signs and symptoms of obstruction.

Documentation

Document a comprehensive respiratory assessment, including an assessment of the surgical site and voice. Of particular note should be complaints of hoarseness, sore throat, breath sounds, color, oxygenation status, respiratory rate, respiratory depth, and any nonverbal signs that the patient is having difficulty breathing. Chart the patient's description of how the throat feels, such as a "tight feeling," or "something trickling." Include in the patient record interventions carried out to prevent airway obstruction, such as positioning, and the patient's responses. Note specifically changes in breath sounds in response to interventions and the patient's emotional state. Vital signs should be documented according to agency protocol. Always include in the documentation the patient's progress towards achievement of the stated outcome criteria.

CHAPTER 12.132

HYPOTHYROIDISM

GENERAL INFORMATION

Hypothyroidism is a condition of the thyroid gland where there is inadequate thyroid hormone (TH), which results in a slowing of the metabolic rate of the body. When there is insufficient TH, the gland is stimulated to compensate for the low levels by attempting to increase production. Because of this stimulation, the gland enlarges, and a goiter may form. The causes of hypothyroidism are varied but include Hashimoto's thyroiditis (the most common cause of primary hypothyroidism), a congenital defect in the thyroid gland, treatment for hyperthyroidism (removal, irradiation, medications) that destroys or removes thyroid tissue, and pituitary gland disorders that cause a thyroid-stimulating hormone (TSH) deficiency or iodine deficiency. All body systems are affected, and the early signs of disease have an insidious onset, are vague, or are wrongly attributed to other more common causes, and thus often go undetected. Clinical manifestations include intolerance to cold, lethargy, fatigue, weakness, constipation, bradycardia, hypotension, hair loss, dry skin, periorbital edema, alterations in libido, changes in menses, and a goiter. Later in the disease, the patient may develop a characteristic finding of myxedema that is the accumulation of non-pitting edema in body tissues, giving a puffy appearance to the face. For the most part, hypothyroidism affects women between the ages of 30 and 60 years. Myxedema coma is a very rare but highly lethal complication of hypothyroidism in which the symptoms of hypothyroidism become more pronounced due to an increased metabolic stressor such as surgery, trauma, infection, congestive heart failure, general anesthesia, sudden exposure to cold temperatures, the use of medications such as sedatives, narcotics, or antidepressants, and psychological stress. The patient suffers from severe hypothermia and eventually lapses into a coma. Mortality rates range from 30 to 80 percent. Myxedema coma usually occurs in those patients who have suffered from chronic hypothyroidism and is most commonly seen in the elderly in the cold winter months. Therapeutic intervention must be aggressive, and should be directed towards the catalytic disease or event.

NURSING DIAGNOSIS 1

 IMBALANCED NUTRITION: MORE THAN BODY REQUIREMENTS

Related to:

Slowed metabolic rate

Defining Characteristics:

Weight gain

Dry, brittle fingernails

Constipation

Decreased activity level

Decreased bowel sounds

No change in usual diet

Goal:

The patient's nutritional status will be maintained.

Outcome Criteria

✔ The patient will not gain weight.

✔ The patient will verbalize an understanding of required dietary restrictions.

✔ The patient will consume 2000 ml of fluid per day.

NOC *Nutritional status: Nutrient intake*

Weight: Body mass

Nutritional status: Food and fluid intake

INTERVENTIONS	RATIONALES
Gather a diet and weight history, including common abnormalities of constipation, weight gain, edematous tongue, abdominal distention, decreased bowel sounds, paralytic ileus, and dry, brittle fingernails; determine dietary habits and intake, methods of food preparation, meal schedule, favorite foods to consume, 24-hour dietary recall, and calorie count.	These pieces of data give evidence for the extent of the problem and provide a starting point for intervention. Health care providers need to know this baseline information about the patient in order to tailor a plan that is individualized to the patient.
Ascertain likes and dislikes, and assist the patient in making healthy dietary choices based on the food pyramid.	Even though the patient's weight gain is caused by a medical disorder, it is important to help the patient retain a sense of control and confidence while feeling a sense of support; the patient needs to understand how to eat healthily and prevent weight gain.
Weigh patient on first encounter and monitor weekly.	The first weight establishes a baseline to use for evaluation of the success of interventions; weekly weights monitor progress towards weight stabilization.
Assess patient for usual activity level.	Because of the fatigue caused by the decreased metabolic rate, many patients with hypothyroidism have a sedentary lifestyle with limited or no physical exercise that adds to the weight gain.
Encourage the patient to implement the following general strategies for better nutrition: — Eat a low-fat, low-cholesterol, reduced calorie diet. — To the extent possible, plan all meals in advance to avoid last-minute rushed meals that are likely to be high in calories and less nutritious. — Have set meal times and do not skip meals. — Learn to bake, broil, grill, or steam food. — Avoid snacking throughout the day, but have scheduled nutritious snacks. — Cut up fresh fruit or raw vegetables and place in sealable plastic food storage bags for easy access.	These strategies help control unhealthy nutritional habits by changing eating behaviors. The patient with hypothyroidism requires fewer calories, fat, or cholesterol due to the decreased metabolic rate. Having healthy snacks readily available assists the patient to make the right choice. Increased fluids and raw fruits and vegetables prevent constipation that is common in hypothyroidism.
— Avoid highly concentrated sweets. — Drink 6 to 8 glasses of water each day. — Avoid sweetened beverages.	
Arrange a consultation with a dietician for planning the reducing diet.	This type of diet can enhance weight loss and the dietician is best prepared to assess the patient's nutritional status and develop a plan of action for weight loss or stabilization.
Administer thyroid replacement medications such as levothyroxine as ordered	Helps to raise the level of TH, which will increase the patient's metabolic rate and assist in correcting the cause for imbalanced nutrition.
Increase fiber in the diet.	Helps to prevent constipation caused by decreased gastrointestinal (GI) motility.
Offer stool softeners or laxatives as needed.	Helps to prevent and treat constipation.
Reinforce instruction by the dietician and teach patient and family members or significant other about the need for adequate nutrition for proper body functioning; provide with sample menus.	Knowledge will enhance the patient's ability to implement suggested strategies to improve nutritional status.

NIC *Weight reduction assistance*
Nutritional counseling
Nutritional monitoring

Evaluation

Determine the degree to which the patient has achieved the stated outcome criteria. The patient should verbalize an understanding of the need for acceptable nutritional behaviors to avoid excessive weight gain secondary to hypothyroidism. The patient verbalizes an understanding of new behaviors required for healthy nutrition and verbalizes a willingness to comply. Following implementation of the stated strategies, the patient's weight will be stable without further weight gain.

Community/Home Care

The patient with hypothyroidism should seek to stabilize weight by giving attention to two areas: healthy eating and exercise. Education by a dietician is the best source of information regarding what is acceptable to eat and what to avoid. Even though calories must be limited for the hypothyroidism patient, enough food needs to be consumed to meet nutrient requirements of the body. For many patients, following simple rules of good nutrition when they do eat and incorporating exercise into the daily routine will assist in halting weight gain. The patient will need to be sure that healthy snacks are readily available and that snack foods such as potato chips, cookies, sodas, and candy are not purchased. Fresh fruit and vegetables can be pre-sliced and placed in sandwich bags in the refrigerator, making a readily accessible snack. When buying groceries, the patient should make a list and stick to it rather than picking up tempting items that have no nutritional value but are high in calories and fat. Exercise may be the biggest challenge because of the fatigue and weakness that accompany the disease. The patient needs to identify activities that are acceptable. Simple exercises such as short walks, riding a stationary bicycle, and simple aerobics can be a starting point for incorporating exercise into a routine. If the patient has small handheld weights, he or she can hold these and lift arms above head while sitting around the home. Most experts recommend 20 to 30 minutes of exercise on most days but at least 3 to 4 times a week. During hypothyroidism treatment, continued monitoring of the patient's weight is needed to be sure that weight gain is not continuing, and that eating behaviors have improved.

Documentation

Chart the patient's weight according to agency protocol. Include in the patient record the findings from a comprehensive dietary history and nutritional assessment, specifically noting the patient's weight. Of particular importance is the patient's 24-hour dietary recall and his or her usual dietary habits. Include in the record the percentage of meals consumed and the patient's understanding of the need for dietary restrictions to avoid weight gain. All interventions are documented in the record along with whether the patient has achieved the stated outcomes. Chart all teaching done and referrals for follow-up.

NURSING DIAGNOSIS 2

DECREASED CARDIAC OUTPUT

Related to:

Thyroid hormone deficit

Defining Characteristics:

Bradycardia

Hypotension

Lethargy

Decreased thyroid hormone levels

Goal:

Cardiac output will be maintained.

Outcome Criteria

✔ Blood pressure will return to patient's baseline.

✔ Pulse will return to patient's baseline or be > 60.

✔ Peripheral pulses will be strong.

✔ Skin will be warm and dry.

NOC *Circulatory status*
Cardiac pump effectiveness
Vital signs

INTERVENTIONS	RATIONALES
Assess vital signs, particularly blood pressure and pulse, as ordered but at least every 4 hours.	Changes in blood pressure and pulse give indicators to patient status. In states of hypothyroidism, hypotension may be noted, the pulse is slowed, and the temperature is decreased.
Assess other indices of cardiac output: peripheral pulses, skin color and temperature, and periorbital edema.	Diminished peripheral pulses may be an indication of decreased perfusion that often accompanies hypotension and bradycardia. Dry, scaly skin and cool, pale skin are indicators of decreased perfusion. Periorbital edema is a common finding in hypothyroidism.
Monitor results of diagnostic tests: TSH, T4, T3, thyroid uptake of radioactive iodine (RAIU), serum thyroglobulin, and thyroid autoantibody (TA) test.	TSH is increased in primary hypothyroidism, T4 will be decreased, T3 will be decreased, RAIU will demonstrate decreased uptake of iodine, RAIU can also be used to examine the size of the thyroid, and TA is normal.
Begin replacement therapy by administering synthetic thyroid hormones (levothyroxine	Replaces natural THs that are not being produced or are not being produced in adequate

INTERVENTIONS	RATIONALES
[Synthroid®, Levothroid®]), as ordered. Give medications at the same time each day, in the morning 1 hour before or 2 hours after eating, and monitor for side effects.	amounts; side effects include insomnia and signs of hyperthyroidism (palpitations, weight loss, diaphoresis, fidgetiness).
Implement strategies to keep the patient warm: control environment, keeping it warm as desired by patient; apply blankets; encourage warm clothing; offer warm fluids.	The patient with hypothyroidism has intolerance for cold.
Monitor for decreased tolerance for physical activity: weakness, tiredness, fatigue, muscle cramps, joint aches, and joint stiffness.	Fatigue and intolerance to activity are common due to the slowed metabolic rate; bradycardia adds to the problem due to the decreased cardiac output and subsequent decrease in oxygenation of tissues needed for muscle function. The patient may report difficulty "getting going" in the morning.
Schedule rest periods and quiet times, and schedule activities in clusters, assisting the patient as needed.	Helps to provide maximum rest and energy conservation and to decrease the workload of the heart. Any activity that causes palpitations, chest pain, or dizziness should be discontinued, and the physician should be notified.
Perform a respiratory assessment: monitor for respiratory rate, depth, hypoventilation, and crackles.	Abnormal breath sounds (crackles) and increased respiratory rate may indicate fluid overload secondary to decreased cardiac output or beginning of myxedema coma.
Monitor urine output and electrolytes.	In hypothyroidism, there may be decreased blood flow to the kidneys as a result of bradycardia and decreased cardiac output resulting in decreased water excretion and hyponatremia.
Monitor the patient for signs of myxedema coma: pronounced symptoms of hypothyroidism such as severe hypothermia, hypotension, bradycardia, hyponatremia, hypoglycemia, and progression to coma; notify physician and treat as ordered.	Myxedema is a life-threatening emergency that is caused by trauma, infection, stress, central nervous system (CNS) depressants such as sedatives, extremely cold temperatures, and failure to take thyroid replacement hormones.

NIC *Cardiac care*
Vital signs monitoring

Evaluation

Note the degree to which outcome criteria have been achieved and the patient's symptoms of hypothyroidism are improving. The patient should demonstrate adequate cardiac output or improvement in abnormalities. The pulse and blood pressure should be within the patient's baseline, and the pulse should be strong and regular. Temperature returns to normal, and the patient verbalizes being comfortable with environmental temperature. Peripheral pulses should be present, and skin should be warm to the touch. The patient has indicators of increased metabolic rate, including a report of improved activity tolerance.

Community/Home Care

Patients with hypothyroidism will need to continue therapies in the home to prevent complications of decreased cardiac output and prevent myxedema coma. Of critical importance is continued implementation of strategies to increase levels of TH. The patient will need to understand how to take the medication (levothyroxine) for hypothyroidism and understand that it will be required for life. Keeping it in a noticeable place can help the patient to remember to take the medication daily. Because of the length of time required for medication effectiveness, the patient needs to be aware of worsening symptoms of thyroid deficiency that may occur until the medication reaches a therapeutic serum level. Interventions in the home include weighing self, taking pulse, and being aware of feelings of excessive fatigue and lethargy. The patient needs to know how to take his or her pulse to detect worsening of bradycardia and a local drugstore or grocery store can be used for blood pressure checks. Keeping a log of pulse rates, weights, and any other complaints can help the patient notice patterns in resolution of the disease or worsening. For many patients, there will be a need to adapt the temperature of the home due to cold intolerance, at least until treatment is effective. This is especially true in the winter months and particularly in extremely cold climates. Unfortunately, in some instances when extra heat is needed by the patient, the temperature required for comfort may be uncomfortable for other family members and compromises or solutions will need to be developed. The patient may need to obtain extra blankets for the bed and dress in layers to retain heat. For most patients, once the hypothyroidism is controlled the symptoms will gradually resolve, and cardiac output will be restored. If symptoms of hypothyroidism do not gradually improve, the patient should contact the health care provider to be sure that this is not a precursor to myxedema coma. In any event, follow-up is required to determine the status of the disease through laboratory tests and symptoms review.

Documentation

Chart the results of all assessments made, particularly symptoms of hypothyroidism and of the cardiac system. Document blood pressure and pulse according to agency protocol. Include in the record any patient complaints made relevant to thyroid symptoms and the cardiac system in the patient's own words. Chart the administration of medications for treatment of hypothyroidism. All other interventions should be documented in a timely fashion with the patient's specific response to the intervention.

NURSING DIAGNOSIS 3

DEFICIENT KNOWLEDGE

Related to:

New onset of hypothyroidism

Lack of information about the disease and its treatment

Misinformation

Defining Characteristics:

Asks no questions

Has many questions/concerns

Shows no interest in learning about the disease

Goal:

The patient verbalizes understanding of hypothyroidism and its treatment.

Outcome Criteria

✔ The patient verbalizes an understanding of hypothyroidism.

✔ The patient verbalizes an understanding of the medication requirements.

✔ The patient is able to identify signs and symptoms of complications.

✔ The patient is able to carry out the prescribed treatment plan.

NOC *Knowledge: Disease process*
Knowledge: Health behavior
Treatment behavior: Illness or injury

INTERVENTIONS	RATIONALES
Assess the readiness of the patient to learn (motivation, cognitive level, and physiological status).	The patient must be motivated to learn, have the capability to learn the content, and be free of distractions from learning such as pain and emotional distress.
Assess what the patient already knows.	The patient may have some knowledge about hypothyroidism, and teaching should begin with what the patient already knows.
Create a quiet environment conducive to learning.	Environmental noise can prevent the learner from focusing on what is being taught.
Start with simple concepts first and move to complex concepts.	If the patient understands simple concepts, these can be used as a foundation to build on for further concepts that are more complex.
Teach the learners about the pathophysiology of hypothyroidism: — Role of TH in regulating metabolic rate — Signs and symptoms of the disease: weight gain, intolerance to cold, constipation, fatigue, weakness, slowed pulse, decreased blood pressure, and facial edema, especially around eyes — Signs and symptoms of myxedema: worsening of symptoms, pronounced lethargy, slow speech, severe hypothermia	Understanding of normal function and pathophysiology will facilitate understanding of the rationale for therapeutic interventions. Teach the patient signs and symptoms of myxedema will allow the patient to note abnormalities and monitor for improvement or worsening so that myxedema can be prevented.
Teach patient about medication levothyroxine/Synthroid, including: — Action: replacement of TH — Expected outcomes: improvement of symptoms with increased energy levels, increased pulse, and blood	Knowledge of medication actions, need for the medication, dosages, and side effects will improve compliance.

INTERVENTIONS	RATIONALES
pressure to normal, normal body temperature, resolution of edema, stabilization of weight — Side effects: insomnia (most common); signs of excessive thyroid hormone, including increased pulse, weight loss, palpitations, angina, hypertension, feeling jittery — Administration: by mouth once a day in the morning before breakfast or 2 hours after	
Encourage regular appointments with a physician.	The physician will monitor progress and medication response to decide if revisions are needed.
Review with the patient symptoms of abnormal response and signs that require prompt attention: continued excessive fatigue, intolerance to cold, bradycardia, neurological changes, periorbital edema, or side effects of the medication.	The patient needs to be able to identify symptoms that would require him or her to seek medical assistance.
Evaluate the patient's understanding of all content covered by asking questions.	Helps to identify areas that require more teaching and to ensure that the patient has enough information to comply.
Give the patient written information on medications and concise information on the disease.	Provides material for reference at a later time, and for review.

NIC *Teaching: Disease process*
Teaching: Individual
Teaching: Prescribed medication

Evaluation

The patient is able to repeat information for the nurse and asks questions about hypothyroidism and possible outcomes (positive and negative). The patient is able to state what hypothyroidism is and what causes it. Prior to discharge, the patient verbalizes an understanding of required medications (purpose, side effects, administration), and agrees to be compliant. In addition, the patient is able to describe myxedema. The patient should know and be able to inform the nurse when health care assistance should be sought.

Community/Home Care

Hypothyroidism can be controlled in the home environment through administration of thyroid replacement hormones. If teaching has been effective, the patient will have very few requirements for in-home care. Teaching by the health care team should be thorough with opportunities for discussions. Of greatest importance is to be sure that the patient has understood the teaching regarding daily medications, how to monitor response through noting improvement of symptoms, and how to detect side effects that require immediate intervention. Most of these side effects will be symptoms of hyperthyroidism such as increased pulse, feeling jittery, and weight loss in the presence of increased intake. The patient also needs to be aware of the signs of worsening of hypothyroidism, such as changes in mental status, further slowing of the pulse, and excessive fatigue, that may signal the beginning or progression to myxedema coma. If this occurs after treatment has begun, it is usually due to stressors or the patient's lack of medication. The nurse or social worker needs to be sure that the patient has the means to purchase the medications, as control of the disease depends upon taking the synthetic hormone. Once at home, the patient may need further reinforcement and should have access to a health care provider to call for clarification, at which time the nurse or others can evaluate the patient's understanding of all content taught and ability and willingness to follow through. Follow-up with a health care provider focuses on laboratory tests to evaluate thyroid function, assurance that no complications have occurred, and the patient's clear understanding of how to manage all aspects of hypothyroidism.

Documentation

Document all content taught and the patient's verbalization of understanding. Specific attention should be given to documentation of any specific concerns that the patient expresses regarding the diagnosis of hypothyroidism. Included in the documentation is the patient's report that he or she has a means to purchase the medication and his or her willingness to comply with all recommendations made regarding medications and follow-up care. Any area that requires further teaching should be clearly indicated in the record. Include in the record appointments that have been made for follow-up or blood draws for laboratory tests. Always include the titles of any printed literature given to the patient for reinforcement.

CHAPTER 12.133

SYNDROME OF INAPPROPRIATE ANTIDIURETIC HORMONE (SIADH)

GENERAL INFORMATION

Syndrome of inappropriate antidiuretic hormone (SIADH) is a disorder of the posterior pituitary gland in which there is an excessive secretion of antidiuretic hormone with resulting free water retention and hypo-osmolality. Aldosterone is suppressed, the kidneys stop reabsorption of sodium, and fluid moves into the cells causing an increased intracellular volume. Most cases of SIADH occur secondary to the production of antidiuretic hormone ADH by small cell cancers of the lung. Other causes of the disorder include medications such as sulfonylurea chlorpropamide. Clinical manifestations mimic those of hyponatremia and in the early phase include weight gain, muscle weakness, irritability, nausea, or vomiting. In later disease, symptoms include worsening neurological symptoms, such as lethargy, headache, decreased deep tendon reflexes, and progression to coma, accompanied by a low serum sodium level, decreased osmolality, and increased sodium in urine.

NURSING DIAGNOSIS 1

EXCESS FLUID VOLUME

Related to:

Impaired pituitary function

Ectopic production of ADH by cancerous cells

Defining Characteristics:

Decreased serum sodium levels

Increased urinary sodium

Decreased osmolality

Headache

Irritability

Muscle weakness

Decreased deep tendon reflexes

Weight gain

Nausea

Malaise

Goal:

Fluid and electrolyte balance will be restored.

Outcome Criteria

✔ Sodium levels will return to normal.

✔ Sodium content in urine will return to normal.

✔ The patient will offer no complaints of muscle weakness.

✔ The patient's neurological status will return to baseline (no irritability, disorientation, lethargy, or headache).

NOC *Fluid balance*
Fluid overload severity
Electrolyte and acid/base balance
Vital signs

INTERVENTIONS	RATIONALES
Assess for signs of hyponatremia: malaise, muscle weakness, nausea/vomiting, irritability, disorientation, headache, lethargy, and decreased deep tendon reflexes.	Clinical manifestations such as these must be detected early to initiate treatment and prevent complications. Confusion, irritability, headache, and vomiting may be indicators of increased intracranial pressure due to cerebral edema.
Assess breath and heart sounds.	In the presence of fluid excess, crackles may be auscultated in the lungs and a third heart sound may be heard due to congestion.

INTERVENTIONS	RATIONALES
Monitor vital signs.	Blood pressure and pulse will be elevated with excess volume. A slow, bounding pulse and an elevated blood pressure may indicate increased intracranial pressure.
Monitor intake and output.	Helps to determine fluid balance and whether water retention persists.
Monitor laboratory results: serum and urine sodium, serum osmolality, and specific gravity.	Determines sodium or other electrolyte replacement needs and fluid restrictions. In the presence of fluid volume excess of SIADH, there may not be a true sodium deficit, but the low sodium instead results from dilution. Serum osmolality is decreased, and urine osmolality is increased.
Weigh patient daily at same time (before breakfast, after voiding) on the same scale, with the patient wearing similar clothes each time.	Weight is the best determinant of fluid retention; 1 kg of weight gained = 1 L of fluid gained. It is important to weigh the patient under similar conditions for accuracy. Patients with SIADH may retain large amounts of water each day.
Restrict fluid intake to 500 to 800 ml/day; distribute fluid intake throughout the day, ensuring that fluids served with meals and needed for medications are included. Scheduling a certain amount at 8-hour intervals will help keep the patient compliant.	Helps to decrease total body water and decrease risk of increased intracranial pressure development.
Administer loop diuretics (with concurrent electrolyte replacement), as ordered.	Decreases total body water and corrects electrolyte imbalance. Loop diuretics induce isotonic diuresis and fluid volume loss that will raise the serum concentration of sodium.
If the sodium deficit is severe, < 120 mEq/L, initiate hypertonic intravenous (IV) sodium solutions as ordered, and monitor sodium levels every 1 to 2 hours.	Solutions containing sodium are required immediately to prevent or correct central nervous system symptoms caused by severe hyponatremia. The infusion is maintained until the serum sodium is elevated to 125 mEq.
Administer medications demeclocycline or lithium carbonate, as ordered.	These medications block the action of ADH on the renal tubules.

NIC   *Fluid monitoring*
Fluid management
Hypervolemia management
Electrolyte management: Hyponatremia

Evaluation

Determine the extent to which the outcome criteria have been achieved. The patient's blood pressure and pulse are at baseline, and serum and urine sodium levels are within normal range. The patient, when weighed, will demonstrate a weight loss indicative of fluid loss. There are no signs of neurological impairment due to the low sodium level or increased fluid in the cerebral tissue.

Community/Home Care

Ensure that the patient at home understands the importance of monitoring fluid status. The patient should have a reliable scale that is calibrated and easily accessible. Weighing daily at home will allow the patient to notice subtle changes in fluid retention that may indicate a recurrence of the problem. Patients should be informed to take note of areas of the body that may develop pads of fluid, such as the area over the sternum. The patient who has decreased sodium levels due to SIADH may need to continue fluid restrictions at home for a period of time. Making a planned schedule for fluid intake helps the patient to stay on target. Ice chips may be helpful in relieving thirst, but the patient must count these as intake just as water. Keeping attuned to intake and output by calculating the balance at the end of the day will help the patient with early recognition of fluid retention. The patient will need to monitor weight at least weekly and record this in a log or journal to carry to the health care provider. Any weight gain that is unexplained should be reported, as this may be a sign of fluid retention. If the patient develops headaches or lethargy, these should be reported immediately, as they may indicate cerebral edema. In some instances, the patient may be asked to increase the sodium in the diet for a short period of time. Instruction of the patient should include which foods are adequate in sodium and how to read food labels for sodium content. Diet instructions for the patient at home will consider his or her normal diet and any cultural or religious preferences and restrictions. Assist the patient to develop a schedule for taking prescribed diuretics that is mindful of his or her lifestyle and daily routines. Stress the need for follow-up care to assess sodium levels.

Documentation

Always document the extent to which the outcome criteria have been achieved. An assessment of fluid status should be noted that includes intake and output, blood pressure, pulse, weights, and breath sounds. Indicate in the record any neurological signs and symptoms that occur and interventions employed to address them. Medications that are administered for excess fluid volume should be documented on the medication administration record, and the nurse's notes should indicate the amount of fluid the patient lost in response. Any teaching done or referrals made are charted according to agency protocol. Chart the patient's understanding of the therapies for eliminating fluid excess.

NURSING DIAGNOSIS 2

INEFFECTIVE TISSUE PERFUSION: CEREBRAL

Related to:

>   Swelling of cerebral cells
>   Increased pressure in cranial vault

Defining Characteristics:

>   Altered levels of consciousness
>   Headache
>   Lethargy
>   Confusion
>   Seizures
>   Decreased deep tendon reflexes
>   Nausea/vomiting
>   Serum sodium level is < 135 mEq/L

Goal:

>   The patient will return to usual state of cerebral functioning.

Outcome Criteria

✔ The patient will be alert and oriented.
✔ The patient will have no seizures.
✔ The patient will be free of headaches.
✔ Lethargy will resolve.

NOC *Neurological status:*
        Consciousness
    Tissue perfusion: Cerebral

INTERVENTIONS	RATIONALES
Perform a neurological assessment to detect abnormalities: headache, lethargy, muscle weakness, decreased deep tendon reflexes, confusion, personality changes, muscle twitching, hyperreflexia, seizures, decreasing level of consciousness, and nausea/vomiting.	These are common findings with decreased sodium levels, cerebral edema, and increased intracellular fluid volume; patients with neurological manifestations related to hyponatremia may be at increased risk for injury and seizures.
Assess serum sodium.	Hyponatremia places the patient at risk for seizures due to excitability of cerebral tissue.
Maintain bed in low position with side rails elevated.	Helps to decrease the risk of falls if the patient becomes confused or is lethargic; decreases fall distance should the patient fall out of bed.
Implement seizure precautions, notify the physician immediately if seizures occur, and treat seizures as ordered (see nursing care plan "Seizures").	If sodium levels are uncorrected and continue to drop to levels at or below 120 mEq/L, seizures are likely. The patient needs to be protected from injury.
Place call bell within easy reach.	Facilitates communication from patient to nurse.
Implement strategies to correct sodium deficits; administer IV fluids containing sodium, and give dietary sodium as ordered.	Helps to correct the underlying cause (see nursing diagnosis "Excess Fluid Volume").
Implement fluid restriction, as ordered.	Helps to decrease symptoms of cerebral edema.
Provide a quiet environment.	A calm and quiet environment reduces stimuli that could excite the central nervous system.

NIC *Electrolyte management:*
        Hyponatremia
    Surveillance
    Risk identification
    Neurologic monitoring
    Seizure precautions
    Cerebral edema management

Evaluation

Determine that the outcome criteria have been met. The patient has no symptoms of impaired cerebral function such as headaches or lethargy. The patient should be protected from injuries that might result from altered neurological function. If a seizure occurs, the patient should be protected and sustain no injury.

Community/Home Care

When discharged home, the patient's ineffective cerebral perfusion and risk for injury have already been resolved, as the sodium levels should have returned to normal or close to normal ranges. No special in-home care is required unless the sodium level drops again. However, the patient will need to continue interventions to maintain sodium levels at a normal range and control SIADH (see nursing diagnosis "Excess Fluid Volume"). Maintaining adequate cerebral function involves restricting fluid at home as well and monitoring for fluid retention. The patient can keep a log of fluid intake in order to be sure that fluid intake is not excessive. Diet instructions regarding sodium intake should be clear to the patient and take into consideration cultural/religious practices and the patient's usual dietary preferences. The patient should be able to identify the signs and symptoms of cerebral edema or central nervous system disturbances that are attributed to hyponatremia, and if these are noted, a health care provider should be contacted.

Documentation

Chart results of an assessment of the neurological/musculoskeletal system, noting the presence of any abnormalities such as decreased deep tendon reflexes, headaches, changes in level of consciousness, and muscle weakness. Document all interventions implemented to treat any problems that occur and to treat the low sodium levels. All medications and IV fluids administered are charted according to agency protocol. If seizures occur, document a description of the seizure, duration, and patient status following the seizure, including mental status (alert, lethargic) and vital signs.

UNIT 13

PSYCHOSOCIAL SYSTEM

CHAPTER 13.134

ALCOHOL: ACUTE INTOXICATION/ OVERDOSE

GENERAL INFORMATION

Acute alcohol intoxication or alcohol overdose may constitute a medical emergency and may be life-threatening. It is the most frequently seen type of intoxication in the hospital setting. In the body, alcohol acts as a central nervous system (CNS) depressant. Each ounce of liquor, glass of wine, or 12-ounce beer raises the blood alcohol level by 15 to 25 mg/dl. Alcohol levels in excess of 0.5 percent can cause coma, respiratory depression, peripheral collapse, and death. The clinical manifestations of acute alcohol intoxication vary from patient to patient but include lethargy, respiratory depression with Cheyne-Stokes respiration, vomiting, and hypoglycemia. Acute alcohol intoxication may be a first-time event or a return to alcohol after a period of abstinence. Acute ingestion of excessive amounts of alcohol will cause severe metabolic acidosis, coma, and death if not corrected. When alcohol intoxication is suspected, it is essential to rule out other causes of the patient's symptoms (such as diabetic ketoacidosis, overdose of another substance, or head trauma). A frequent complication of patients who are intoxicated is aspiration of emesis.

NURSING DIAGNOSIS 1

 POISONING

Related to:

Acute ingestion of large amounts of alcohol

Defining Characteristics:

Elevated blood alcohol level

Hypotension or systolic hypertension

Dysrhythmias

Cheyne-Stokes respirations

Headache

Tachypnea

Decreased level of consciousness (lethargy, drowsiness, coma)

Arterial blood gases (ABG) (pH < 7.2 with highly decreased bicarbonate levels)

Goal:

The patient's signs of poisoning/intoxication are alleviated.

Outcome Criteria

✔ The patient is alert, and respirations are unlabored and < 24.

✔ Blood alcohol level returns to normal.

✔ Serum pH returns to normal.

✔ Blood pressure, pulse, and respirations return to patient's baseline.

NOC *Risk control: Alcohol use*
Personal safety behavior

INTERVENTIONS	RATIONALES
Monitor laboratory/diagnostic tests: blood alcohol level, serum glucose, serum electrolytes (especially magnesium and potassium levels), toxicology screen for the presence of other medications/drugs, liver function studies, electrocardiogram (EKG), pulse oximetry, and ABGs.	Blood alcohol level will be elevated, generally > 0.5 percent; when blood alcohol levels are measured, it is important to remember that peak levels are reached a half hour to three hours after the last drink, depending upon whether or not the patient has also eaten food; glucose is low due to poor food intake with substitution of alcohol for food; magnesium and potassium are low; low magnesium predisposes the

INTERVENTIONS	RATIONALES
	patient to seizure, and low potassium predisposes the patient to cardiac dysrhythmias; toxicology screens rule out other drugs as the cause of symptoms; liver function studies (liver enzymes) give indicators of impaired liver function due to chronic use of alcohol; EKG will show dysrhythmias; pulse oximetry gives evidence of effectiveness of respirations in maintaining oxygen saturation in tissues; and ABGs may reveal metabolic acidosis.
Complete a thorough cardiac assessment, including blood pressure, pulse, and peripheral pulses.	Alcohol intoxication causes systolic hypertension, tachycardia, dysrhythmias, and weak, thready peripheral pulses. Frequent monitoring is required to detect cardiac dysfunction and to intervene early to prevent complications such as peripheral cardiovascular collapse.
Assess neurological status, including level of consciousness, motor activity, speech, gait, tremors, and orientation. Monitor particularly for the presence of slowed thinking, slurred speech, agitation, nystagmus, seizures, headache, and decreased sensory awareness.	Elevated alcohol levels cause CNS system depression that manifests itself with any combination of these symptoms. Depending upon the patient's tolerance for alcohol, the blood alcohol level that produces CNS depression varies from person to person. Continued monitoring is needed to detect improvement or worsening.
Establish intravenous (IV) access and administer IV fluids as ordered.	Provides hydration and dilutes alcohol in circulating volume.
Administer sodium bicarbonate, as ordered.	Helps to correct severe acidosis. Must be used with great caution because it may cause alkalosis when fluid replacement and electrolyte balance are regained.
Administer IV thiamine, as ordered.	Many patients presenting for alcohol intoxication are chronic alcoholics who are at risk for developing Wernicke's encephalopathy secondary to decreased thiamine levels; this disorder is difficult to distinguish from acute intoxication, so thiamine is given as a precaution.

Administer 50 percent glucose IV or other glucose solutions, as ordered.	Hypoglycemia is common in patients with alcohol intoxication due to poor food intake and needs to be reversed. Many symptoms of hypoglycemia mimic those of intoxication. Treatment of hypoglycemia allows better assessment of the effects of alcohol on the nervous system.
Give magnesium (IV or intramuscularly [IM]), as ordered.	Helps to restore magnesium levels and decrease risk for seizures and impaired reflexes.
Anticipate the use of renal dialysis and assist as needed when the pH reaches 7.1.	When serum pH < 7.1, a life-threatening condition exists that must be immediately corrected.
Give ipecac as ordered.	If alcohol was consumed within the past 1 to 2 hours, it may be possible to remove some of the alcohol via emesis. (Note: this intervention is only appropriate if the patient is conscious.)
Perform gastric lavage if necessary and as ordered.	Removes alcohol from stomach.
Once the patient is awake, take a history on last drink, amount ingested, type ingested, and history of blackouts. Investigate use of an assessment tool such as the CAGE test or Michigan Alcoholism Screening Test.	Provides clues to the extent of the drinking and whether this is a one-time occurrence or an issue of dependency. Using these tools (which can be found in most psychiatric texts) provides an objective way to do alcohol screening.
Monitor for withdrawal symptoms, and implement interventions as ordered or required (see nursing care plan "Alcohol Withdrawal").	Once the acute intoxication phase is resolved, the patient is still at risk for experiencing withdrawal symptoms.
When the patient is conscious or alert, educate the patient and family about the acute toxic effects and long-term complications of alcohol abuse.	Education of the patient and family about alcohol abuse is needed to enhance the possibility that the patient will be motivated to seek assistance.

NIC   *Surveillance: Safety*
Fluid/electrolyte management
Acid/base management:
   Metabolic acidosis
Acid/base monitoring

Evaluation

Determine whether the patient has achieved the stated outcomes. The patient is awake and alert. The patient's pH level should return to normal following treatment, and acid/base balance should be achieved. Magnesium levels are normal following treatment, and the patient has no problems with reflexes and no seizure activity. Vital signs indicate a return of the blood pressure, pulse, and respirations to the patient's baseline.

Community/Home Care

Following successful treatment of the acute episodes, attention is given to monitoring for withdrawal (see nursing care plan "Alcohol Withdrawal"). When returning home, the patient who has been treated for alcohol intoxication must realize the seriousness of alcohol abuse. If chronic dependency is an issue, the patient should be referred to a long-term treatment program or to community programs such as Alcoholics Anonymous. The nurse has a professional responsibility to refer the patient to social service agencies who can assist with this effort. If alcohol use is continued, the risk for repeat episodes of alcohol poisoning/intoxication are possible, with the risk of serious complications, even death. Educating the patient and family about the effects of alcohol is needed to motivate the patient to refrain from excessive alcohol use.

Documentation

Document whether the patient has achieved the stated outcome criteria. Include in the patient record findings from respiratory, cardiovascular, and neurological assessments with specific attention to symptoms of impaired CNS function. Interventions should be charted with indications of the patient's responses to those interventions. If the patient does not improve, document revisions to the plan of care. Document all referrals made for assistance in withdrawing from alcohol, as well as the patient's indication of willingness to comply with recommended treatment.

NURSING DIAGNOSIS 2

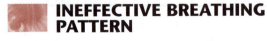

INEFFECTIVE BREATHING PATTERN

Related to:
Respiratory depression

Elevated blood alcohol levels
CNS depression

Defining Characteristics:
Cheyne-Stokes respirations
Tachypnea
Use of accessory muscles of respiration
ABGs

Goal:
The patient's respirations are regular.

Outcome Criteria

✔ The patient's respirations are unlabored and < 28.
✔ The patient has no Cheyne-Stokes respirations.
✔ The patient's ABGs will return to baseline.

NOC *Respiratory status: Ventilation*
Respiratory status: Gas exchange
Vital signs

INTERVENTIONS	RATIONALES
Assess respiratory status by noting respiratory rate, depth, chest expansion, rhythm, breath sounds, ABGs, pulse oximetry, and skin color, and note any of the following abnormalities: — Increased respiratory rate — Cheyne-Stokes respirations — Severe dyspnea that has progressively worsened — Cyanosis (nailbeds, lips) — Decreased oxygen saturation — Use of accessory muscles of respiration	Any of these abnormalities would indicate a compromised respiratory status and indicate progression of poisoning; acute alcohol intoxication causes a respiratory depression secondary to CNS depression; these assessments also establish a baseline for future comparisons.
Place patient in high Fowler's position, or position for easy respiration.	Helps to maximize thoracic cavity space, decrease pressure from diaphragm and abdominal organs, and facilitate the use of accessory muscles.
Provide humidified, low-flow (2 liters/min) oxygen, as ordered.	Provides supplemental oxygen to improve oxygenation.
Monitor laboratory results: blood alcohol level, pulse oximetry (oxygen saturation), ABGs, toxicology screen for other medications/drugs, and urine for ketones.	Blood alcohol levels will help to determine the extent of intoxication and evaluate response to treatment. Toxicology screens will rule out other possibilities for alterations

INTERVENTIONS	RATIONALES
	in respiratory status. Pulse oximetry and ABGs provide evidence to support the diagnosis of ineffective breathing pattern and may yield decreased levels of oxygen and poor oxygen saturation. Variations in acid/base balance may be noted, including respiratory alkalosis caused by the increased elimination of carbon dioxide via hyperventilation; the patient may have metabolic acidosis and/or alcoholic ketoacidosis due to use of fat for energy in the presence of malnutrition.
Establish IV access and administer IV fluids as ordered.	Provides a means to administer emergency medications and to improve hydration state; fluids dilute alcohol and assist in reversing the respiratory depressant effects of the alcohol poisoning.

NIC *Respiratory monitoring*
      Oxygen therapy
      Positioning

Evaluation

The patient should show indications that breathing patterns have returned to baseline and are effective in meeting the body's need for oxygen. The rate should return to baseline, preferably between 12 to 24 breaths per minute, and be unlabored. Cheyne-Stokes respirations or tachypnea should be resolved. The return of ABGs and pulse oximetry to the patient's baseline or to within normal range should be expected.

Community/Home Care

Prior to discharge, immediate needs of the patient who has experienced acute alcohol intoxication have been resolved. In most cases, breathing patterns and respiratory function have been returned to normal, and no home care is indicated for respiratory problems. However, prior to discharge to the home setting, attention is diverted to psychosocial needs and evaluations are made to determine whether the patient uses alcohol as a coping mechanism or whether this was a one-time occurrence. If alcohol is being abused, professional counseling is needed in the form of treatment programs or counseling (see nursing diagnosis "Ineffective Health Maintenance" and nursing care plan "Alcohol Withdrawal"). Follow-up care should focus on treatment of the patient's alcohol abuse, if applicable.

Documentation

Chart the results of a comprehensive assessment of the respiratory systems. Note respiratory rate, rhythm (Cheyne-Stokes or normal), chest expansion, use of any accessory muscles, breath sounds, and results of ABGs and pulse oximetry. Include in the patient's chart all interventions employed to address ineffective breathing pattern (oxygen, positioning) and the patient's responses to the interventions that would indicate the problem has been resolved. Document whether the outcome criteria have been met, and if the patient's breathing is no better, indicate how the plan has been revised.

NURSING DIAGNOSIS 3

  RISK FOR ASPIRATION

Related to:
    Decreased level of consciousness
    Inability to spontaneously clear secretions
    Vomiting
    High likelihood of emesis

Defining Characteristics:
    None

Goal:
    The patient does not aspirate gastric contents.

Outcome Criteria

✔ The patient has no signs of aspiration (coughing, labored breathing).

✔ The patient maintains a patent airway.

✔ The patient has an oxygen saturation > 90 percent.

✔ Breath sounds are clear.

NOC *Respiratory status: Airway patency*
      Respiratory status: Ventilation

INTERVENTIONS	RATIONALES
Elevate head of bed.	Helps to reduce risk of aspiration.
Assess respiratory status: breath sounds, respiratory rate, oxygen saturation, and ABGs.	Establishes a baseline and monitors response to interventions.
Monitor patient for signs of aspiration: coughing, vomiting of gastric contents, and cyanosis.	Airway may obstruct without the patient being able to notify health care worker due to CNS depression.
Determine if the patient has taken any medications, especially disulfiram (Antabuse®) or metronidazole (Flagyl®).	Alcohol could potentiate the effect of certain medications. Disulfiram, given in alcohol detoxification programs, may cause severe nausea and vomiting, diaphoresis, headache, tachycardia, tachypnea, hypotension, and lowered level of consciousness. Flagyl can cause disulfiram-like reaction when mixed with alcohol.
Give anti-emetics, as ordered.	Helps to reduce risk of vomiting, which would predispose the patient to aspiration.
Keep suction equipment at bedside and ready for immediate use; suction as needed.	Alcohol's sedative effect decreases the natural cough reflex that would occur if the patient vomits; decreased levels of consciousness and relaxation of the oropharyngeal muscles add to the risk of aspiration.
If the patient vomits, turn him or her to a side-lying position with head of bed slightly elevated.	In the event of vomiting and possible aspiration, the patient needs to be in a position that allows for drainage of emesis from oral cavity and that prevents aspiration into trachea.
If patient vomits, maintain patent airway and prepare airway adjuncts.	The patient with a high blood alcohol level is at an increased risk for aspiration, which can cause airway obstruction due to CNS depression and loss of gag reflex.
Monitor for signs and symptoms of respiratory infection: fever, rales, increased mucous production, elevated white blood cell (WBC) count, and chest x-ray reports.	Aspiration often leads to pneumonia; early detection provides for prompt treatment.

NIC *Aspiration precautions*
Airway management
Respiratory monitoring
Oxygen therapy

Evaluation

Assess the client to determine the extent to which the outcome criteria have been met. The patient's airway should be clear, and the patient should be able to cough with expectoration of secretions. Nausea and vomiting are controlled, and the risk for aspiration has been decreased. Breath sounds should be clear, and there should be no cyanosis. Oxygen saturation should be > 90 percent, and blood gases should be within normal range. If criteria have not been met, determine whether expected outcomes were realistic or whether more time is needed for achievement. If more time is needed, note the degree of progress the patient is making towards meeting the goals.

Community/Home Care

Once the patient has been treated for acute intoxication, the risk for ineffective airway clearance and risk for aspiration should no longer exist. No specific care will be required for this problem, but attention is given to educating the patient on the effects of alcohol misuse.

Documentation

Document a comprehensive respiratory assessment. Include in the patient record all interventions carried out for the patient and the patient's responses. Note specifically whether the patient has a gag reflex, the presence of vomiting, secretions, and whether the patient has required suctioning. A description of any emesis suctioned is recorded in the patient's chart, with the amount being documented on the intake and output record according to agency protocol. If the patient is alert and able to participate in expectorating emesis, document this in the chart. Vital signs should be documented according to agency protocol.

NURSING DIAGNOSIS 4

 RISK FOR INJURY

Related to:

General CNS depression

Impaired judgment

Lowered response reflexes

Decreased level of consciousness

Ataxic gait

Poor judgment

Impaired vision

Inability to sense/avoid danger

Defining Characteristics:

None

Goal:

The patient is in a safe environment and sustains no injury.

Outcome Criteria

✔ The patient does not fall during hospitalization.

✔ The patient is not injured as a result of seizures.

✔ The patient does not traumatically remove tubes or lines.

NOC *Fall prevention behavior*
Personal safety behavior
Seizure control
Risk control

INTERVENTIONS	RATIONALES
Place the patient in quiet, protected area; lower bed; pad side-rails.	Patients who have a high blood alcohol level can neither sense nor avoid danger and may endanger themselves. In addition, they are at a high risk for seizures due in part to decreased magnesium levels. A quiet room is needed to decrease stimuli, which increase agitation.
Speak in calm, authoritative manner.	Establishing control of situation will encourage patient compliance in lieu of his or her inability to control own actions.
Administer diazepam (Valium), as ordered.	Controls seizure activity if present.
Administer dextrose 50 percent and thiamine 100 mg, as ordered.	Helps to prevent Wernicke-Korsakoff syndrome (encephalopathy and psychosis that is alcohol-induced due to severe vitamin deficiency).

When patient is alert and able, assist with activities, particularly ambulation.	The patient who has been intoxicated or is currently intoxicated has ataxia, altered sensory awareness, and impaired reflexes.
Keep call bell within easy reach, and answer promptly.	Helps to prevent the patient from attempting to get out of bed or attend to own needs, which would predispose him or her to falls.
When the patient is awake, orient him or her to reality frequently but do not attempt to argue with the patient; try reality orientation; recognize the patient's feelings of fear; and repeat that the patient is in a safe place. Involve the patient in activities based in reality, such as listening to music.	Argumentative approaches increase agitation; talking about the real environment and assuring the patient that he or she is safe is the best approach. Alcohol interferes with perception of reality; patients who have been intoxicated experience short-term memory loss and may not realize where they are once intoxication starts to abate; the patient may also be frightened.
Monitor patient for belligerence or potential for violence.	As the patient emerges from intoxication, disorientation and fear may cause the patient to become severely agitated or violent.
Monitor for seizures and implement seizure precautions: keep bed in low position, keep suction and oral airway at bedside, pad side rails, and keep rails up. If seizures occur, implement strategies for safety: remain with patient, maintain airway, and monitor neurological status.	These interventions allow the nurse to provide for patient safety by anticipating complications and being prepared to treat as required. Maintaining a patent airway is required in the event of a seizure, as the patient's tongue is a frequent cause of blocked airways.

NIC *Substance use treatment:*
Alcohol withdrawal
Surveillance
Seizure precautions
Environmental management
Fall prevention

Evaluation

The patient should remain safe, as evidenced by the fact that the patient does not fall and no injury has occurred. The patient has not removed any treatment devices, and strategies to ensure that a safe environment is maintained are implemented. If awake and alert, the patient can verbalize an understanding of the measures implemented to keep him or herself and others safe. Increasing agitation or threats to others should be reported, and the plan of care will need to reflect interventions that have been implemented to address such occurrences.

Community/Home Care

Whether the patient remains at risk for injury following discharge from the health care system will depend on the patient's ability to cease intake of alcohol. Some of the later symptoms of withdrawal may become evident after discharge if the patient stops taking prescribed medication or resumes heavy drinking and then stops. The best method for addressing this problem would be to work with the patient and other health care disciplines to locate alcohol treatment programs that will provide long-term assistance to the patient. Family members need to be aware of the signs of intoxication as well as withdrawal in each stage so that they will understand when to seek health care. The patient needs to establish acceptable coping strategies to use in stressful situations and have a means of seeking support. There is the probability that the patient will discontinue prescribed medications that have been ordered for the treatment of alcohol withdrawal. A key point for patient and family to know is that the abrupt discontinuance of some medicines such as Serax® can precipitate withdrawal symptoms such as seizures, tremors, and confusion. If these occur, the patient will remain at risk for injury, particularly falling. At home, the family members or significant other must be cognizant of the risk for injury by vehicle use if the patient is impaired. Efforts should be made to prevent the operation of vehicles if the patient has been drinking. Follow-up through an outpatient clinic or with a home-visiting organization is required to ensure that the patient is able to implement recommendations for successful withdrawal or cessation of alcohol use.

Documentation

Chart the findings from a complete neurological assessment with specific attention to the continued presence of intoxication or signs of withdrawal such as tremors, impaired gait, and disorientation. If seizures occur, document the duration, treatment, and specific patient behaviors during and after the seizure. Any injuries are recorded in the notes, and appropriate incident reports are completed and filed. All interventions implemented to prevent injury are documented, and the patient's responses to interventions are always included in the patient record. Initiation of medications such as Serax is charted according to agency protocol for medication administration.

NURSING DIAGNOSIS 5

 INEFFECTIVE INDIVIDUAL COPING

Related to:

Loss of control

Fear of withdrawal symptoms

Lack of a support system

Defining Characteristics:

Expressions of fear and anxiety

Expressed worry about ability to cope

Verbalization of alcohol abuse as a coping strategy

Chronic alcohol abuse

Patient/family denial

Failure to understand that chronic alcohol use is a serious disorder

Goal:

The patient is able to express feelings and ability to cope.

Outcome Criteria

✔ The patient identifies and uses one acceptable coping strategy.

✔ The patient verbalizes fears and concerns.

✔ The patient expresses a willingness to seek assistance for alcohol abuse.

NOC *Comfort level*

Coping

Health-seeking behavior

INTERVENTIONS	RATIONALES
Assess patient for expressions of fear, anxiety, negative self-statements, and other indicators of ineffective coping.	When patients experience alcohol overdose, the emotional response can vary greatly; the nurse needs to note specific expressions to establish a starting point for interventions.
Encourage the patient to verbalize feelings about current status and what has happened to cause hospitalization and any fears or concerns. Listen attentively and be nonjudgmental in approach.	Verbalization of feelings, fears, and concerns contributes to dealing with the issue of alcohol use; being attentive relays empathy to patient.
Obtain complete history of alcohol abuse, asking how often the patient drinks, how much he or she drinks, and for how long he or she has been drinking; assess the patient's level of alcohol use or abuse as a coping strategy by using screening tools such as the CAGE questionnaire, Michigan Alcoholism Screening Test, or a drug abuse screening test.	The patient may have suddenly found him or herself unable to cope due to a particular stressor; measurement tools offer a more objective measure of determining alcohol use or dependence and are easy to use.
Assist patient with relaxation techniques: deep breathing, mental imagery, meditation, music therapy, and spirituality.	Relaxation techniques can help to reduce anxiety and assist patient to be open to learning and adapting new coping skills.
Keep the patient informed of all that is going on, explaining about symptoms that are occurring and necessary interventions.	Communicating what is going on helps to allay anxiety and fear.
Stay with the patient during acute withdrawal symptoms and allow other visitors, as requested by the patient.	Helps to provide emotional support and promote a sense of comfort.
Ask the patient to identify all strategies other than alcohol that he or she has used in the past to cope with stressful events.	Strategies other than alcohol that have previously worked can be used as a starting point for coping with more serious stressful events, and can help the patient focus.
Assist with the development of new skills and strategies for coping, including referral to a professional counselor or to Alcoholics Anonymous.	During withdrawal, new strategies for coping may be required for patients who abuse alchohol. These new strategies need to be more sophisticated than those a generalist nurse is able to offer.
Provide reassurance and encouragement for efforts to stop drinking.	Encouragement and reassurance help to provide patient with "energy" to succeed.
Encourage patient/family to directly confront addiction/seek assistance.	Acknowledgement of addiction is the first step to recovery. Co-dependency must be discouraged.
Assist the patient in identifying those factors that trigger the need for alcohol, such as family problems, financial problems, and problems at work; when the triggers are identified, encourage the patient to seek psychosocial support.	Identifying the root cause of the drinking problem allows the patient to begin to develop new methods of coping and reduces the risk of return to alcohol.
Recognize the role of cultural and religious beliefs in a patient's method of coping with stressors, particularly alcohol abuse, and inquire about these.	Culture often dictates how a person copes with stressors, particularly issues that have a negative social stigma.
Provide counseling referrals for the immediate time and for long-term assistance as well. Assistance through Alcoholics Anonymous, rehabilitation programs, and support groups may be helpful.	Excessive use of alcohol may be a symptom of a greater psychosocial need and may represent the patient's only method of coping with life events; the patient may need continued assistance with coping skills.
Seek spiritual consult as needed or requested by the patient and/or family.	Meeting the patient's spiritual needs helps him or her cope with fears through use of spiritual or religious rituals; provides support.
Set limits on the patient's behavior and monitor interaction with health care team.	Patients who abuse alcohol often display manipulative behavior and are unable to establish limits.

NIC *Counseling*
Coping enhancement
Emotional support
Spiritual support

Evaluation

Evaluate the extent to which the outcome criteria have been achieved. The patient should be assessed for appropriate coping skills/strategies that can be used to deal with life stressors and should identify at least one acceptable coping strategy. Concerns, fears, and feelings of being able to cope should be detected in the patient. The patient should report that he or she will try to stop using alcohol and seek appropriate assistance. An ability to verbalize the nature of the alcohol problem will be a starting point for developing new coping strategies. If, however, the patient is unable to admit to using alcohol as a way of coping and express a desire to use other coping strategies, the nurse should explore further the need for new interventions to assist the patient.

Community/Home Care

A major factor in achieving positive outcomes following alcohol intoxication and subsequent withdrawal is education on the effects of alcohol on the body. Often the patient is unaware of the long-term complications that can occur when alcohol is abused. Successful treatment of alcohol intoxication should have as an end result the patient's enrollment in some program that can assist the patient to discontinue alcohol use, especially when the patient uses alcohol as a coping strategy. If the alcohol intoxication was the result of a one-time binge, in-home care may be minimal, but some attention is still given to the possibility that the patient used alcohol as a coping mechanism. Thorough assessment of the patient should be made to ascertain whether further counseling is required. The availability of social supports in the community or at home is required to help the patient comply with recommendations for refraining from alcohol use. Community programs such as Alcoholics Anonymous can provide support for the transition from abuse to abstinence. The provider who follows up with the patient once acute alcohol intoxication is resolved and withdrawal is complete should assist the patient to learn and use an alternative method of coping with stressors. Nurses, counselors, or other providers should help the patient to identify areas that may be contributing to the perceived need to drink, such as interpersonal relationships, work

environment, or home environment. Recognition of problem areas is the first step the patient must make towards taking charge of his or her life and implementing more appropriate strategies for coping. Successful control of alcohol intake will depend on the patient's understanding of the information provided in teaching sessions and the internal motivation to implement health-promoting behaviors. Many patients who go through withdrawal will return to excessive use of alcohol if not equipped to deal with simple day-to-day stressors in an appropriate manner. Having the support of others enhances the patient's sense of well-being. Education on alcohol abuse and symptoms of withdrawal should be given to patient and family with recommendations for continuing health care (see nursing care plan "Alcohol Withdrawal"). Follow-up with social workers, counselors, or other health care workers is needed to ensure that the patient is not experiencing new or continued difficulties with alcohol.

Documentation

Document an assessment of the patient's emotional state, including the subjective symptoms of anxiety and physiological signs of anxiety (pacing, restlessness) and complaints of fear. Any verbalizations regarding coping strategies previously used should be included in the chart. Document whether the patient has met the outcome criteria, especially the identification of new coping strategies to replace alcohol use. If referrals are made, include these in the patient chart. Document if the patient indicates a willingness to comply with health care recommendations, particularly attendance at Alcoholics Anonymous (AA) meetings and follow-up health care examinations. In addition, any referrals that are made should be documented in the patient record.

CHAPTER 13.135

ALCOHOL WITHDRAWAL

Alcohol withdrawal occurs when a chronic alcohol user ceases alcohol intake either voluntarily or involuntarily. Onset varies from patient to patient but in general begins 10 to 12 hours after the last drink. Because the body is accustomed to the presence of alcohol, this withdrawal produces physiological symptoms that in some instances may be life-threatening. It is essential to assess a patient's alcohol intake history to determine if a patient is at risk for alcohol withdrawal so that severe symptomatology can be prevented. The symptoms vary but generally can be classified into three categories: minor, major, or life-threatening. The minor symptoms (also referred to by some as "the shakes") include restlessness, anxiety, sleep difficulties, mild tremors, increased pulse, increased blood pressure, and sweating. This stage of withdrawal may appear as early as 3 hours or as late as 36 hours after the last drink. Major symptoms (also referred to by some as the stage of "acute hallucinations") include hallucinations, worsening tremors that lead to delirium tremors, tachycardia (pulse > 100), pronounced sweating, elevated blood pressure with a diastolic reading > 100, and seizures. This stage may occur at any point following the onset of tremors, and alcoholic seizures typically occur 12 to 48 hours after the last drink. The life-threatening symptoms (also referred to by some as the stage of "delirium tremens") include disorientation, inability to recognize familiar items or people, delusions, severe agitation, hallucinations, excessive diaphoresis, and seizures. This stage usually occurs 24 to 72 hours after the last drink and may last for 3 to 5 days. This phase of alcohol withdrawal is considered a medical emergency and requires hospitalization. Medical interventions for the patient experiencing alcohol withdrawal should include a thorough evaluation for other medical problems such as liver disease and malnutrition.

NURSING DIAGNOSIS 1

DISTURBED SENSORY PERCEPTION (VISUAL, AUDITORY, KINESTHETIC)

Related to:

Acute alcohol withdrawal

Defining Characteristics:

Impaired judgment

Impulsive actions

Agitation

Irritability

Confusion/disorientation

Hallucinations (visual and auditory)

Muscle tremors

Decreased level of consciousness

Seizures

Tachycardia

Hypertension

Goal:

The patient is not injured.

The patient's sensory alterations are alleviated.

Outcome Criteria

✔ The patient's withdrawal symptoms resolve within 1 week.

✔ The patient verbalizes an improvement in symptoms.

✔ The patient sustains no injuries due to changes in sensory perception or seizures.

✔ The patient discusses safety measures.

✔ The patient can set personal limits that will assure safety.

NOC *Seizure control*
Personal safety behavior
Fall prevention behavior
Vital signs

INTERVENTIONS	RATIONALES
Place the patient in a quiet environment and remain with patient; control multiple sources of stimuli in the environment.	Patient should not be left alone during acute symptoms due to risk of injury; overstimulation can worsen withdrawal symptoms, especially agitation.
Assess vital signs every 15 minutes during acute withdrawal symptoms, monitoring for rises in pulse above 100 and diastolic blood pressure above 100.	During acute withdrawal, temperature, pulse, and blood pressure, especially diastolic pressure, increase. Vital signs can provide indicators of response to treatment. Monitoring allows for early intervention to prevent or treat serious complications such as dysrhythmias and further sensory compromise.
Monitor blood alcohol levels.	The blood alcohol level is predictive of the type of central nervous system (CNS) disturbances seen. In most locales legal intoxication is 100 mg/dl (0.10 percent). The motor vehicle administration in most states set the legal limit for driving at 0.08 percent. The patient who is withdrawing may also be acutely intoxicated (see nursing care plan "Acute Alcohol Intoxication"). A goal of treatment is to reduce the blood alcohol level to < 100 mg, which usually requires 6 to 10 hours. However, for some patients, when a blood alcohol level drops 100 mg/dl below their "normal" blood alcohol level, withdrawal will begin to occur.
Monitor for signs and symptoms of alcohol withdrawal (see "General Information") and assess orientation frequently. To detect fine tremors hold patient's hands. If withdrawal symptoms are present, stay with patient.	Helps to detect progression of the withdrawal and response to interventions. Assessment data can guide treatment.
Monitor electrolyte levels with particular attention to magnesium level.	Allows for early detection of electrolyte imbalances that predispose the patient to seizure. Electrolyte imbalances are common due to poor dietary habits.
Avoid quick movements towards the patient or unsanctioned touching without warning.	Quick movements may startle the patient, which could amplify withdrawal symptoms.
Administer benzodiazepines (Serax), as ordered.	Alcohol withdrawal occurs approximately 10 to 12 hours after a chronic alcohol user has stopped drinking. Benzodiazepines are used to control symptoms of alcohol withdrawal but are not given until the blood alcohol level is < 0.10 percent. Withdrawal causes adrenergic excess that produces hypermetabolism.
Administer magnesium sulfate, as ordered, in response to laboratory results.	Helps to correct magnesium imbalance. Chronic alcoholism is the most common cause of hypomagnesia; low levels of magnesium cause excess neuromuscular excitability and tremors in a patient who is already at risk for tremors due to the effects of alcohol withdrawal. This heightened state of the neuromuscular system creates a physiological environment that predisposes the patient to seizures.
Use cooling measures to reduce fever (e.g., cooling blanket, cool compresses).	Do not use acetaminophen or salicylates because of the high risk of underlying liver disease or gastrointestinal (GI) bleeding.
Monitor for seizures and implement seizure precautions: keep patient in low position, keep suction and oral airway at bedside, pad side rails, and keep rails up. If seizures occur, implement strategies for safety: remain with patient, maintain airway, and monitor neurological status.	These interventions allow the nurse to provide for patient safety by anticipating complications and being prepared to treat as required. Maintaining a patent airway is required in the event of a seizure, as the patient's tongue is a frequent cause of blocked airways.
Orient to reality but do not attempt to argue with patient who is experiencing delusions and hallucinations; try reality orientation; do not focus on the	Argumentative approaches that downplay what the patient perceives to be reality increases agitation; talking about the real environment and assuring the

INTERVENTIONS	RATIONALES
content of the hallucination but recognize the patient's feelings of fear, and repeat that the patient is in a safe place. Involve patient in activities based in reality such as listening to music.	patient that he or she is safe is the best approach.
Assist the patient with activities of daily living (ADLs), as needed.	The patient may need assistance because of tremors, lethargy, or disorientation due to the effects of alcohol, and will need support until the symptoms of withdrawal abate.

NIC **Substance use treatment: Alcohol withdrawal**

Surveillance

Seizure precautions

Environmental management

Fall prevention

Hallucination management

Vital signs monitoring

Evaluation

The patient should remain safe as evidenced by no injury in general and none if seizures have occurred. Strategies to ensure that a safe environment is maintained are implemented. The patient has a decrease in or elimination of withdrawal symptoms following interventions. If alert and awake, the patient can verbalize an understanding of the measures implemented to keep him or her and others safe. Increasing agitation or threats to others should be reported, and the plan of care will need to reflect interventions that have been implemented to address such situations.

Community/Home Care

Whether the patient remains at risk for injury following discharge from the health care system will depend on the patient's ability to cease intake of alcohol. Significant others or family members will need to have information on what to do if the patient experiences seizures or has hallucinations. Both of these may occur once the patient is at home, and may be frightening for those around him or her. Written instructions on how to respond and how to create a safe environment should be given to the patient and his or her family. Some of the later symptoms of withdrawal may become evident after discharge if the patient stops taking prescribed medication or resumes heavy drinking and then stops. The best method for addressing this problem would be to work with the patient and other health care disciplines to locate alcohol treatment programs that will provide long-term assistance to the patient. Family members need to be aware of the signs of withdrawal at each stage so that they will understand when to seek health care. The patient needs to establish acceptable coping strategies to use in stressful situations and have a means of seeking support. There is the probability that the patient will discontinue prescribed medications that have been ordered for the treatment of alcohol withdrawal. A key point for patient and family to know is that the abrupt discontinuance of medications used to treat withdrawal symptoms, such as Serax, can precipitate withdrawal symptoms such as seizures, tremors, and confusion. Follow-up through an outpatient clinic or with a home-visiting organization is required to ensure that the patient is able to implement recommendations for successful withdrawal or cessation of alcohol use.

Documentation

Chart the findings from a complete neurological assessment with specific attention to the presence of signs of withdrawal such as tremors, impaired gait, orientation, and behaviors that indicate the presence of hallucinations. All interventions to treat disturbed sensory perception/risk for injury and the patient's responses to interventions are always included in the patient record. If the patient is unable to perform ADLs, document this in the chart. Strategies to create a safe environment (such as padding bed rails, applying restraints, keeping side rails up at all times) are charted. Because of the specific changes in the pulse and blood pressure, documentation of vital signs in a timely fashion is important for care decisions. Vital signs should be documented according to agency protocol and may be included in the notes as well as on the graphic sheets. Any injuries are recorded in the notes, and appropriate incident reports are completed and filed. When medications such as Serax are begun, this is charted according to agency protocol for medication administration.

NURSING DIAGNOSIS 2

INEFFECTIVE INDIVIDUAL COPING

Related to:

Loss of control

Fear of withdrawal symptoms

Lack of a support system

Defining Characteristics:

Expressions of fear and anxiety

Expressed worry about ability to cope

Verbalization of alcohol abuse as a coping strategy

Report of significant stressors

Goal:

The patient is able to express feelings and ability to cope.

Outcome Criteria

✔ The patient identifies and uses one acceptable coping strategy.

✔ The patient verbalizes fears and concerns.

✔ The patient expresses a willingness to seek assistance for alcohol abuse.

NOC *Comfort level*

Coping

Health-seeking behavior

INTERVENTIONS	RATIONALES
Assess the patient for expressions of fear, anxiety, negative self-statements, and other indicators of ineffective coping.	When patients experience alcohol withdrawal, the emotional response can vary greatly; the nurse needs to note specific expressions to establish a starting point for interventions.
Encourage the patient to verbalize feelings regarding current status and what has happened to cause hospitalization or a visit to any other health care facility and any fears or concerns. Listen attentively and be nonjudgmental in approach.	Verbalization of feelings, fears, and concerns contributes to dealing with the issue of alcohol use; being attentive relays empathy to the patient.
Assess the patient's level of alcohol use or abuse as a coping strategy by using screening tools such as the CAGE questionnaire and the Michigan Alcoholism Screening Test.	These tools offer a more objective measure of determining alcohol use or dependence and are easy to use. The Michigan Alcoholism Screening Test can be found on the Internet, and other tools can be found in psychiatric nursing journals.
Assist patient with relaxation techniques: deep breathing, mental imagery, meditation, music therapy, and spirituality.	Relaxation techniques can help to reduce anxiety and assist the patient to be open to learning and adapting new coping skills.
Keep the patient informed of all that is going on, explaining about symptoms that are occurring and necessary interventions.	Communicating to the patient what is going on helps to allay his or her anxiety and fear.
Stay with the patient during acute withdrawal symptoms and allow other visitors, as requested by the patient.	Helps to provide emotional support and promote a sense of comfort. Withdrawal symptoms may be frightening to the patient.
Ask the patient to identify all strategies other than alcohol that he or she has used in the past to cope with stressful events.	Strategies other than alcohol that have previously worked can be used as a starting point for coping with more serious stressful events, and can help the patient focus.
Assist with the development of new skills and strategies for coping, including referral to a professional counselor or Alcoholics Anonymous (AA).	Patients who abuse alcohol may require new strategies for coping during times of withdrawal. These new strategies may be more sophisticated than those a generalist nurse is able to offer.
Provide reassurance and encouragement for efforts to stop drinking.	Encouragement and reassurance help to provide patient with "energy" to succeed.
Encourage the patient/family to directly confront addiction and seek assistance; obtain educational literature for the family and provide factual information regarding alcohol abuse or dependency.	Acknowledgement of addiction is the first step to recovery. Co-dependency must be discouraged. Information regarding alcoholism or alcohol abuse may be helpful for the family. The nurse can find information to use in educational endeavors with the family from the National Institute on Alcohol Abuse and Alcoholism (www.niaaa.nih.gov).
Assist the patient in identifying those factors that trigger the	When the triggers are identified, encourage the patient to seek

INTERVENTIONS	RATIONALES
need for alcohol, such as family problems, financial problems, or problems at work.	psychosocial support to reduce risk of return to alcohol.
Recognize the role of cultural and religious beliefs in a patient's method of coping with stressors and particularly alcohol abuse or alcoholism.	Culture often dictates how a person copes with stressors and particularly issues that have a negative social stigma.
Provide counseling referrals for the immediate time but for long-term assistance as well.	Excessive use of alcohol may be a symptom of a greater psychosocial need of the patient and represents the patient's only method of coping with life events; the patient may need continued assistance with coping skills.
Seek spiritual consult as needed or requested by the patient and/or family.	Meeting the patient's spiritual needs helps him or her to cope with fears through the use of spiritual or religious rituals for coping; provides support.
Set limits on patient behavior and interaction with health care team.	Patients who abuse alcohol often display manipulative behavior and are unable to establish limits.

NIC   *Counseling*
       Coping enhancement
       Emotional support
       Spiritual support

Evaluation

Evaluate the extent to which the outcome criteria have been achieved. The patient should be assessed for appropriate coping skills/strategies that can be used to deal with life stressors. The nurse assesses to what degree the patient is able to express concerns, fears, and feelings. The patient's recognition that he or she needs help and the ability to verbalize the nature of the alcohol problem will be a starting point for developing new coping strategies. If, however, the patient is unable to admit to using alcohol as a way of coping and express a desire to use other coping strategies, the nurse should explore further the need for new interventions to assist the patient.

Community/Home Care

The patient who has experienced alcohol withdrawal should be encouraged to identify other coping strategies that have been successful in the past and prompted to use them at home. The patient should be able to communicate fears and feelings about withdrawal/hospitalization. Many patients who go through withdrawal will return to excessive use of alcohol if not equipped to deal with simple day-to-day stressors in an appropriate manner. For this reason, health care providers should encourage the patient to attend some type of group meeting such as AA or see a professional counselor who can work with the patient on developing coping strategies. Coping through use of support from significant others will be vital to a positive outcome because they can be available for listening when the patient becomes tempted to return to alcohol. In remote rural areas where no AA groups meet, local clergy may be a source of counseling services. Having the support of others enhances the patient's sense of well-being. Follow-up with a social worker, counselor, or other health care worker is needed to ensure that the patient is not experiencing new or continued difficulties with alcohol.

Documentation

Document an assessment of the patient's emotional state including the subjective symptoms and physiological signs of anxiety (pacing, restlessness) and complaints of fear. Any verbalizations regarding coping strategies previously used should be included in the chart. Document whether the patient has met the outcome criteria, especially the identification of new coping strategies to replace alcohol use. Referrals for counseling or recommendations for attending AA should be included in the patient chart.

NURSING DIAGNOSIS 3

 DEFICIENT KNOWLEDGE

Related to:

   Chronic alcohol abuse

   Lack of support from family/friends

   Lack of information about the disease and its treatment and prevention

   Misinformation

   Denial

   Failure to understand that chronic alcohol use is a serious disorder

Defining Characteristics:

Previous attempts to withdraw from alcohol

Expresses concern about ability to comply

Asks no questions

Has many questions/concerns

Noncompliance

No interest in learning about the alcohol abuse

Goal:

The patient verbalizes an understanding of alcohol abuse.

Outcome Criteria

✔ The patient verbalizes a desire to learn necessary information.

✔ The patient verbalizes a willingness to keep appointments and follow prescribed regimen.

✔ The patient demonstrates knowledge of the effects of alcohol on the body.

✔ The patient demonstrates knowledge of treatment for alcohol withdrawal and alcoholism.

NOC *Knowledge: Disease process*
Knowledge: Treatment regimen
Compliance behavior

INTERVENTIONS	RATIONALES
Assess the patient's current knowledge, ability to learn, readiness to learn, and risk for noncompliance.	Teachings need to be tailored to the patient's ability and willingness to learn for maximum effectiveness; assessment of the patient for likelihood of noncompliance will allow the nurse to intervene early.
Create a quiet environment conducive to learning.	Environmental noise and distractions can prevent the learner from focusing on what is being taught.
Teach incrementally, going from simple to complex.	The patient can understand the simplest concepts more easily, and then the teacher can build on these. Small amounts of information are easier to understand.
Teach the learners the following information about alcohol:	Knowledge of alcohol and its effects on the body,
— Alcohol withdrawal: minor symptoms, major symptoms, life-threatening symptoms (see nursing diagnosis "Disturbed Sensory Perception") — Prescribed medications, (Serax or others as ordered): action and side effects, schedule, duration of therapy, and importance of adhering to the regimen for the duration as prescribed — Long-term effects of alcohol use — Importance of complying with follow-up appointments with treatment or support groups — Locations and meeting times of local AA meetings	medications, and support available empowers the patients to take control and be compliant. Stressing the adherence to the regimen as prescribed will prevent a relapse and re-hospitalization.
Ask the patient to repeat information and ask questions as needed.	This allows the nurse to hear in the patient's own words what was taught and makes it easier to know what information may need to be reinforced.
Establish that the patient has the resources required to be compliant, particularly psychosocial support.	If needed resources such as finances, transportation, and psychosocial support are not available, the patient may have difficulty being compliant. In times of stress, the presence of psychosocial support can prevent a relapse or binge drinking.
Refer to appropriate disciplines as needed for assistance in the treatment of alcohol abuse (social worker, home health nurse, etc.).	These disciplines can provide additional services to help the patient be compliant with the prescribed regimen and get help for withdrawal.
Give printed material to patient on information covered in teaching session.	The patient may be more comfortable at home knowing that there is printed material for future reference.

NIC *Teaching: Disease process*
Teaching: Prescribed medication
Learning readiness enhancement
Learning facilitation
Counseling

Evaluation

Evaluate the degree to which the patient has achieved the expected outcomes. The patient verbalizes an understanding of the treatment of alcohol withdrawal, including the prescribed medications and their common side effects. The patient is able to identify the signs of withdrawal from alcohol and understands when to seek health care. When asked, the patient can identify available community resources to assist with treatment of alcohol abuse. Health care workers should ascertain that the patient is willing to comply with the prescribed treatment plan. The patient is able to repeat all information for the nurse and asks questions about the information that has been taught.

Community/Home Care

A major factor in achieving positive outcomes following alcohol withdrawal is education on the effects of alcohol on the body. Often the patient is unaware of the long-term complications that can occur when alcohol is abused. Successful teaching should have as an end result the patient's enrollment in some program that can assist him or her to discontinue alcohol use, especially when the patient uses alcohol as a coping strategy. The availability of social supports in the community or at home is required to help the patient comply with recommendations for refraining from alcohol use. Community programs such as AA can provide support for the transition from abuse to abstinence. In some areas, there are hotlines or mentors assigned through alcohol treatment centers that the patient may be able to call when he or she senses things getting out of control and fears a relapse. The provider who follows the patient once acute alcohol withdrawal is complete should assist the patient to learn and use an alternative method of coping with stressors. Nurses, counselors, or other providers should help the patient to identify areas of his or her life that may be contributing to the perceived need to drink. This could be interpersonal relationships, work environment, or home environment. The patient's recognition of problem areas is the first step towards taking charge of his or her life and implementing strategies for coping that are more appropriate. Successful control of alcohol intake will depend on the patient's understanding of the information provided in teaching sessions and the internal motivation to implement health-promoting behaviors.

Documentation

Include in the patient's chart the specific content taught and the titles of printed materials given to the patient. Chart the patient's understanding of

the content and the methods used to evaluate learning. The nurse must clearly indicate areas that need to be reinforced. After the teaching session is complete, the nurse should assess to determine if the patient indicates a willingness to comply with health care recommendations, particularly attendance at AA meetings, enrollment in treatment programs, and follow-up health care examinations. For the patient who is taking medication to control withdrawal symptoms, document the patient's understanding of the medication and its side effects. If the teaching included a significant other, indicate this in the documentation. In addition, referrals made should be documented in the patient record.

NURSING DIAGNOSIS 4

IMBALANCED NUTRITION: LESS THAN BODY REQUIREMENTS

Related to:

    Decreased appetite

    Alcohol abuse

Defining Characteristics:

    Reports of decreased appetite

    Loss of weight

    Verbalizes no interest in food, only in alchohol

    Decreased albumin, thiamine, iron, folic acid, and electrolyte levels

Goal:

    Adequate dietary/fluid intake is maintained.

Outcome Criteria

✔ The patient verbalizes an understanding of the importance of adequate nutrition.

✔ The patient does not lose weight.

✔ The patient reports an increase in appetite and consumption of > 50 percent of food served.

✔ The patient's laboratory results are within normal limits (albumin, iron, thiamine, electrolytes, and folic acid levels).

NOC *Nutritional status: Food and
               fluid intake*

         Nutritional status: Nutrient intake

INTERVENTIONS	RATIONALES
Conduct a fluid and nutritional assessment, including assessing for nausea, vomiting, poor skin turgor, dry, pale mucous membranes, diarrhea, dietary intake, fluid intake and output, and poor dietary habits.	Patients who use alcohol excessively often have poor dietary practices that lead to imbalanced nutrition. When patients are experiencing withdrawal, nausea and vomiting are common effects. (Do not give the patient anti-emetics because they will lower the threshold for seizures.)
Monitor for the presence of liver disease: ascites, enlarged liver, gastric distention, abdominal tenderness, and liver function studies.	Patients who have abused alcohol or who are addicted to alcohol often develop liver damage as a long-term complication. Ascites and abdominal distention cause the patient to feel full early before consuming adequate nutrients. Liver enzymes (ALT, AST) will be elevated. The symptoms above are indicators of liver abnormalities.
Assess laboratory results: albumin, iron, electrolytes, folic acid, thiamine level, and ammonia.	In the presence of liver disease, the albumin level is decreased as the liver is unable to synthesize albumin; the liver stores iron and thiamine, and is responsible for removal of ammonia. Iron, folic acid, and electrolytes decrease as nutritional intake decreases. Patients with low magnesium levels are more likely to experience seizures; early detection and treatment of low levels can prevent seizure.
Weigh patient and monitor weight daily or weekly.	Establishes a baseline for comparison and for early detection of any significant weight loss.
Monitor intake and output; document according to agency protocol.	Helps to detect inadequate fluid intake. Adequate hydration is needed for function and removal of alcohol from the bloodstream.
Encourage the patient to take increased nutrients as ordered (small meals with between-meal snacks).	Promotes adequate intake of food; for patients with decreased appetite, a small meal is more likely to be ingested and seen as desirable.
Give nutritional supplements as ordered, by mouth, intramuscularly (IM), or intravenously (IV): folic acid, thiamine, and multivitamins.	Helps to supplement nutrient intake; patients with liver disease often have some degree of malnutrition and need these nutrients; thiamine deficiency is a common disorder in alcoholic

	patients that can lead to Wernicke's encephalopathy.
Provide diet instructions to the patient, explaining the effect of alcohol on nutritional status.	The patient needs accurate information regarding nutrition; knowing the rationales for nutritional interventions enhances compliance.

NIC *Nutritional monitoring*
        Nutritional management

Evaluation

The patient's nutritional status is stable as demonstrated by the laboratory values (iron, electrolytes, thiamine, folate, etc.). The patient verbalizes an interest in eating and understands the effect of alcohol on nutrition. Weight loss is minimized and the patient consumes regular meals.

Community/Home Care

Once acute symptoms of alcohol withdrawal are alleviated, the patient must begin to address the impact that alcohol has on his or her life. One of the areas requiring attention at home is nutrition. Many patients who drink excessively suffer from some degree of malnutrition that needs attention. Significant others play a role in implementing strategies to improve nutrition by preparing meals and encouraging the patient to ingest them. The patient is more likely to have proper nutrition when supported by family and friends. Follow-up providers should assess the patient for weight loss and monitor laboratory results for improvement. The patient may need to remain on multivitamins, folic acid, and thiamine for an extended period of time. Cessation of alcohol intake is crucial to achieving and maintaining adequate nutrition; thus, any efforts at improving nutrition should also include treatment for alcohol abuse.

Documentation

Chart the results of a nutritional assessment and diet history. Document the strategies implemented to improve the patient's nutritional status, such as double portions or frequent small meals. Always monitor the amount of food consumed at each meal and any complaints (such as nausea, vomiting, or abdominal pain) the patient may have. Weigh the patient and record the weight according to agency guidelines. All medications given to treat nutritional deficits are documented on the medication administration record according to agency guidelines.

CHAPTER 13.136

ANOREXIA NERVOSA

GENERAL INFORMATION

Anorexia nervosa is a disorder seen primarily in adolescents. Patients with anorexia nervosa are usually females who have serious body image fixations and who are fearful of becoming obese. In an effort to prevent the perceived obesity, persons with anorexia nervosa attempt to starve themselves while simultaneously engaging in excessive exercise. There is no one cause for the disorder, but risk factors include hormonal imbalances and pressure by family members or other significant others such as peers to be small. Some patients also engage in purge activities to rid themselves of ingested food, including inducing vomiting, taking laxatives, and using of diuretics if able to obtain them.

NURSING DIAGNOSIS 1

 IMBALANCED NUTRITION: LESS THAN BODY REQUIREMENTS

Related to:

Insufficient food intake

Vomiting

Defining Characteristics:

Serum electrolyte imbalance

Hypoglycemia

Elevated serum uric acid levels

Excessive weight loss

Weight less than normal for height and body build (< 85 percent of normal)

Cardiac dysrhythmias

Hypotension

Not eating meals

Poor skin turgor

Muscle wasting

Goal:

The patient verbalizes understanding of dietary needs and the importance of caloric intake.

The patient demonstrates proper dietary intake.

Outcome Criteria

✔ The patient's weight increases and weight is closer to normal.

✔ The patient verbalizes a need for intake of more nutrients.

✔ The patient consumes 50 percent of needed calories.

NOC **_Nutritional status: Nutrient intake_**
Weight: Body mass
Nutritional status: Food and fluid intake

INTERVENTIONS	RATIONALES
Perform an assessment and gather a diet and weight history, including dietary habits and intake, 24-hour dietary recall, calorie count, marked body weight loss (> 25 percent without physical illness), obsession with calories and fat content of food, binge eating, refusal to eat/fasting, lack of hunger, urinary and fecal output, vomiting (self-induced) (may be bloody from forced emesis), history of weight gain/weight loss, worries about gaining weight, and use of laxatives and diuretics.	These pieces of data give evidence for the diagnosis and provide a starting point for intervention. Health care providers need to know baseline information on the patient. Many patients who have anorexia nervosa take laxatives and force vomiting as a way to lose weight.
Monitor for cardiovascular symptoms: tachycardia or bradycardia, hypotension,	Electrolyte imbalances can cause alterations in cardiac tissue function, which may create

(continues)

(continued)

INTERVENTIONS	RATIONALES
mild hypothermia, dysrhythmias, poor skin turgor, and complaints of being cold.	dysrhythmias and problems with pacing; decreased circulating volume can cause a decrease in pressure that manifests in hypotension. Poor intake and decreased fluids also decrease perfusion to tissue/skin, which causes a drop in body temperature (hypothermia and complaints of being cold).
Monitor serum electrolytes, blood glucose, potassium levels, arterial blood gases (ABGs), blood urea nitrogen (BUN), creatinine, and protein.	Hypokalemia occurs due to vomiting and decreased intake, which results in acidosis; azotemia with increased BUN and creatinine occurs due to decreased circulating volume, causing decreased renal perfusion, which alters excretion of waste products; hypoglycemia is present due to decreased intake of food and fluid; protein levels, especially albumin, may fall due to decreased or absence of intake of protein foods.
Monitor for reports of excess exercise and if present, set limits on amount of time to be spent exercising.	Patients with anorexia nervosa often exercise extensively in an effort to lose more weight.
Weigh patient on first encounter and monitor weekly.	The first weight establishes a baseline to use for evaluation of the success of interventions; weekly weights monitor progress.
Consult with dietician, as ordered.	The dietician is better prepared to assess the patient's nutritional status and develop a plan of action.
Ascertain likes and dislikes, and assist the patient in making dietary choices.	It is important to help the patient retain a sense of control and confidence while feeling a sense of support.
Provide nutrition as ordered and possibly arrange for smaller, more frequent meals and snacks.	Adequate nutrition is needed to prevent starvation, and smaller meals appear less overwhelming. A prolonged period of minimal food intake may have caused gastric size to be reduced, and larger meals may not be tolerated.
Encourage intake of fluids, especially those rich in electrolytes;	Helps to restore fluid and electrolyte imbalance and

in the case of severe electrolyte imbalance, intravenous (IV) fluids may be needed.	prevent cardiac dysrhythmias.
Provide close supervision.	Close supervision is essential to monitor the patient's eating habits. This will prevent the patient from going into private places to induce vomiting or hide/dispose of food.
Administer tube feedings and other dietary intake assistive devices/techniques, as ordered.	It is essential to provide needed calories and nutrients when a patient will not eat.
Consider administering cyproheptadine (Periactin®), as ordered.	Cyproheptadine/Periactin is an appetite stimulant.
Teach the patient and family members or significant other about the need for adequate nutrition for proper body functioning, and provide them with sample menus.	Knowledge will enhance the patient's ability to implement suggested strategies to improve nutritional status.
Collaborate with a physician to arrange for counseling for the disorder.	Anorexia nervosa is considered a psychological disorder that requires therapy.

NIC *Eating disorders management*
Fluid and electrolyte management
Nutritional counseling
Nutritional monitoring
Weight gain assistance

Evaluation

Determine the degree to which the patient has achieved the stated outcome criteria. The patient should verbalize an understanding of the need for acceptable nutritional behaviors. Following implementation of the stated strategies, the patient will not lose weight and will consume 50 percent of meals served and increase this amount daily. The patient is able to express a desire to gain weight and refrain from purging activities.

Community/Home Care

The person who experiences anorexia nervosa will require continued monitoring at home to be sure that nutrition is sufficient to meet metabolic demands. Many patients will require professional counseling to assist them to cope with their fears and concerns regarding weight. Attention should be given to the possibility that there are psychological issues or family processes that are contributing to the disorder. Because self-esteem and body image are disturbed, the patient will need to continue to work on these issues with the counselor to move forward in accepting his or her body and self. Family members can play a vital role in the patient's achievement of goals. Through encouraging healthy eating habits and monitoring dietary intake, family members can demonstrate their support, and those responsible for food preparation or purchase can consult with the patient to prepare foods at mealtime that the patient finds appealing or desirable. Parents will need to be mindful of how much the patient eats and whether the patient disappears immediately following meals, which could be an indicator that the patient is leaving meals to go to a selected place to start purging activities. Nutritious snacks that the patient is likely to eat should be purchased. Taking the patient to the grocery store to assist with food purchases may be helpful. The patient will need to focus on consuming enough nutrients to prevent weight loss and electrolyte imbalance. Family members will also need to monitor the amount of time the patient spends in exercise and attempt to set limits on both the amount and the intensity of exercise. Treatment may last for a long period of time, and relapse is a possibility. Family members or a significant other will need to offer acceptance and support in the patient's effort to cope with this disorder but also closely monitor the patient's nutritional habits.

Documentation

Chart the patient's weight according to agency protocol. Include in the patient record the findings from a comprehensive dietary history and nutritional assessment. Of particular importance are the patient's 24-hour dietary recall and usual dietary habits. Specifically document the amount of food consumed at each meal and any snacks or drinks taken between meals. Document reports of abnormal weight loss, vomiting, or use of laxatives to lose weight. Any report of psychological problems or family dysfunction should be included. All interventions are documented in the record along with whether the patient has achieved the stated outcomes.

NURSING DIAGNOSIS 2

DISTURBED BODY IMAGE

Related to:

Feelings of being overweight

Fear of obesity

Dysfunctional family

Defining Characteristics:

States that he or she is obese

Verbalizing concerns about being obese

Personal loss of control

Negative feelings about self

Indifferent toward caregivers/family

Uses denial frequently

States that he or she feels bad, embarrassed, ashamed

Unable to make a decision; always defers to others

Goal:

The patient develops a positive body image and self-esteem.

Outcome Criteria

✔ The patient is able to establish realistic body-weight goals.

✔ The patient states one positive aspect of body and self.

✔ The patient verbalizes that self is liked and makes no negative statements regarding self.

✔ The patient verbalizes satisfaction with body appearance.

NOC *Body image*
      Self-esteem
      Weight: Body mass

INTERVENTIONS	RATIONALES
Monitor the patient for expressions such as fear of being overweight, worry over others' acceptance, feelings about self/ relationships, and fear of loss of	For the patient with anorexia nervosa, acceptance by peers and others is important, and fears about appearance are common.

(continues)

(continued)

INTERVENTIONS	RATIONALES
love of others if he or she gains weight.	
Monitor for expressions of self-value/interpersonal relationships: feelings about self; low self-esteem; inability to communicate well with family/friends; withdrawal from social contact; statements about being overweight, unattractive, or unpopular; or fear/anxiety.	Helps to detect alterations in social functioning, to prevent unhealthy behaviors, and to intervene early through referral to counseling. The patient with anorexia nervosa often suffers from low self-esteem, and because of feelings of having an unacceptable appearance, may shun social contacts. Recognition of this helps the health care provider begin planning for intervention.
Encourage the patient to communicate feelings about physical appearance and talk to the patient about body appearances and how body may have changed.	Open dialogue about body appearance helps the patient to start accepting his or her body.
Listen attentively to the patient and be aware of fears and concerns. Also look for misinterpretations or misunderstandings.	Listening to the patient will help you identify opportunities for teaching.
Help the patient identify personal strengths and mobilize coping strategies.	Discussions like this will help the patient to cope with the situation.
Help the patient to set realistic goals for food intake and weight control.	Setting small, achievable goals will help the patient to see rewards from his or her efforts; achieving small outcomes/goals instills hope in the patient at times when he or she may be experiencing negative thoughts about self.
Arrange for psychosocial counseling, as ordered or required.	Helps to provide psychological evaluation and assistance to help the patient accept his or her body appearance and incorporate it into a positive self-image.
Identify the effects of the patient's culture or religion on perception of self-concept and body image.	A patient's culture and religion often help define body image and self-worth.

NIC   *Body image enhancement*
Emotional support
Self-esteem enhancement
Role enhancement

Evaluation

The patient is able to express concerns about body appearance. It is crucial that the nurse evaluate to what degree the patient is beginning to accept his or her weight. Assess for verbalizations that would indicate that the patient is beginning to assimilate weight into his or her self-perception, such as asking appropriate questions related to nutrition or the recommended dietary requirements. Communication of feelings and concerns relevant to weight and the need to consume more food for metabolic demands should be taken as a positive sign that progress is being made towards meeting outcome criteria. Determine whether the patient is able to openly discuss feelings with family or significant other.

Community/Home Care

At home, continued monitoring of the patient's perception of body image and self-esteem is needed. The perceived negative appearance of the body may present a challenge to be mastered for the patient. For patients with anorexia nervosa, the notion of being overweight may cause mental anguish and grief, especially in a society that values being thin, as demonstrated by media portrayals. These presentations make an impression on young people, and assistance is required to create a feeling of acceptance of the body as it is by finding positive attributes and strengths. Counselors will need to continue to work with the patient until he or she has garnered enough self-confidence and elevated his or her self-esteem to the point that he or she feel goods about him or herself. Family members, friends, and significant others must provide support to the patient with anorexia nervosa, assisting him or her to take in enough nutrients to maintain health and weight (see nursing diagnosis "Imbalanced Nutrition: Less than Body Requirements"), but also by making positive statements about body appearance. Because most anorexia nervosa patients are treated on an outpatient basis in the absence of medical complications, other psychosocial issues such as depression and ineffective coping may not be evident to the health care provider unless time is spent taking a thorough psychological history. The nurse or other health care provider who sees the patient for follow-up will need to be alert to subtle hints that may indicate that the patient is not making progress towards conquering the eating disorder and has not completely accepted his or her weight. Open discussions regarding disturbed body image and interventions to prevent social isolation and withdrawal should continue with the patient.

Documentation

Chart any specific behaviors or verbalizations that may indicate a lowered self-esteem or altered body image. Note when and if the patient begins to verbalize positive statements regarding weight. In addition to a thorough assessment of the patient's psychological state, include all interventions that have been employed to address this issue, and the patient's responses. Include referrals to counselors in the patient record.

CHAPTER 13.137

BULIMIA NERVOSA

GENERAL INFORMATION

Bulimia nervosa is an eating disorder characterized by binge eating followed by purging activities to rid the body of ingested food. Binge eating involves ingesting large amounts of food within a short period of time. The purging is accomplished by taking emetics, laxatives, or diuretics, or by manually inducing vomiting with a finger. Persons engaging in these activities usually do so secretly in the afternoon and evening. Clinical manifestations in addition to binging and vomiting are not always noticed but include normal or stable weight, erosion of tooth enamel, and irritation of the throat and esophagus from frequent vomiting. In some cases, electrolyte imbalances, especially hypokalemia, are noted because of the fluid loss from laxatives and vomiting. Bulimia is twice as common as anorexia nervosa and is seen most often in female adolescents aged 15 to 24 years. Frequently patients with bulimia nervosa have other psychological needs and suffer from depression.

NURSING DIAGNOSIS 1

IMBALANCED NUTRITION: MORE THAN BODY REQUIREMENTS

Related to:

Intake of more food than required for metabolic needs

Defining Characteristics:

Serum electrolyte imbalance

Hypokalemia

Binge eating

Weight gain or stable weight

Evidence of fluid imbalance: poor skin turgor, dry skin

Cardiac dysrhythmias

Hypotension

Erosion of tooth enamel

Throat irritation

Goal:

The patient verbalizes understanding of dietary needs and the importance of caloric intake.

The patient demonstrates proper dietary intake.

Outcome Criteria

✔ The patient's weight is stable or normal for height.

✔ The patient verbalizes a need to refrain from binge eating.

✔ The patient verbalizes an understanding of the dangers of purge activities with the use of laxatives, emetics, manually-induced vomiting, and diuretics, and expresses a commitment to stop.

✔ Electrolytes will be normal, particularly potassium.

NOC *Nutritional status: Nutrient intake*
Weight: Body mass
Nutritional status: Food and fluid intake

INTERVENTIONS	RATIONALES
Gather a diet and weight history and note the following: dietary habits and intake; 24-hour dietary recall; calorie count; weight gain; binge eating; urinary and fecal output; vomiting (self-induced), which may be bloody from forced emesis; history of weight gain/weight loss; and use of laxatives and diuretics.	These pieces of data give evidence for the diagnosis and provide a starting point for intervention. Health care providers need to know baseline information on the patient. Many patients who have bulimia take laxatives and force vomiting as a way to purge ingested food.

INTERVENTIONS	RATIONALES
Monitor for cardiovascular symptoms: tachycardia or bradycardia, hypotension, dysrhythmias, and poor skin turgor.	Electrolyte imbalances (especially hypokalemia) can cause alterations in cardiac tissue function, which may create dysrhythmias and problems with pacing; decreased circulating volume can cause a decrease in pressure that manifests in hypotension.
Monitor serum electrolytes, potassium levels, arterial blood gases (ABGs), blood urea nitrogen (BUN), and creatinine.	Hypokalemia occurs due to vomiting and decreased intake, which may result in acidosis; azotemia with increased BUN and creatinine occurs due to decreased circulating volume causing decreased renal perfusion, which alters excretion of waste products.
Refer the patient to professional counselor, psychologist, or psychiatrist.	Patients with bulimia often have other psychological needs and require professional assistance in order to overcome the disorder.
Weigh patient on first encounter and monitor weekly.	The first weight establishes a baseline to use for evaluation of the success of interventions; weekly weights monitor progress.
Consult with a dietician as needed or ordered.	A dietician can assess the patient's nutritional status and develop a plan of action.
Ascertain the patient's likes and dislikes, and assist the patient in making healthy dietary choices based on the food pyramid.	It is important to help the patient retain a sense of control and confidence while feeling a sense of support; the patient needs to understand healthy diets.
Provide nutrition, as ordered, and possibly arrange for smaller, more frequent meals and snacks.	Adequate nutrition is needed to prevent electrolyte imbalances; smaller meals appear less overwhelming. Periods of purging may have caused serious electrolyte imbalances and inadequate absorption of nutrients, leading to poor nutritional status.
Encourage intake of fluids, especially those rich in electrolytes; in the case of severe electrolyte imbalance, intravenous (IV) fluids may be needed.	Helps to restore fluid and electrolyte imbalance and prevent cardiac dysrhythmias.
Provide close supervision following meals.	Close supervision is essential to monitor the patient's eating

INTERVENTIONS (cont.)	RATIONALES (cont.)
	habits. This will prevent the patient from going into private places to induce vomiting or hide food.
Administer tube feedings and other dietary intake assistive devices/techniques as ordered.	It is essential to provide needed calories and nutrients when a patient induces vomiting or other means of elimination.
Reinforce teaching from dietician and teach the patient and family members or significant other about the need for adequate nutrition for proper body functioning; provide sample menus.	Knowledge will enhance the patient's ability to implement suggested strategies to improve nutritional status.
Examine the oral cavity of the patient to note eroded tooth enamel and erosion of throat; if needed arrange for a dental consult.	Because of the frequent vomiting, the tooth enamel erodes and the throat becomes irritated. A dental consult may be needed to repair the teeth.

NIC *Eating disorders management*
Fluid and electrolyte management
Nutritional counseling
Nutritional monitoring

Evaluation

Determine the degree to which the patient has achieved the stated outcome criteria. The patient should verbalize an understanding of the need for acceptable nutritional behaviors and should indicate a desire to stop binging and purging activities. In addition, the patient is able to verbalize the effects of purging on the metabolic state of the body. Following implementation of the stated strategies, the patient's weight will be stable and normal for his or her height. Electrolyte imbalances will be corrected.

Community/Home Care

The person who experiences bulimia nervosa will require continued monitoring at home to be sure that nutrition is sufficient to meet metabolic demands. Attention should be given to the possibility that there are psychological issues or family processes that are contributing to the disorder. For this reason, many patients will require professional counseling to assist them to cope with their fears and concerns regarding eating. In all eating disorders, there is some degree of low self-esteem and disturbed body image; thus, the patient will need to continue to work on this with the counselor to move forward in accepting body and self. Family members can play a vital role in the patient's achievement of goals by encouraging healthy eating habits and monitoring dietary intake. The patient will need to focus on retaining enough food to prevent weight loss and electrolyte imbalance. Education for home care also includes providing the patient with information on how to eat healthily without gaining weight. Open discussions about the dangers of binge eating and then purging should occur between the patient and the family or significant others. In the early stages of treatment, when the patient has not recognized that there is an eating disorder, someone may need to supervise the patient closely after meals to prevent him or her from inducing vomiting. Those who are close to the patient should observe the environment closely, noting the presence of medications that are used for purge activities such as laxatives, emetics, and diuretics. Treatment may last for a long period of time, and relapse is a possibility. Family member or significant others will need to offer acceptance and support in the patient's effort to cope with this disorder.

Documentation

Chart the patient's weight according to agency protocol. Include in the patient record the findings from a comprehensive dietary history and nutritional assessment. Chart weights and percentage of food consumed according to agency protocol. Of particular importance are the patient's 24-hour dietary recall and usual dietary habits. Reports of binge eating, vomiting, and the use of laxatives or diuretics to rid the body of food should be documented. Any report of psychological problems or family dysfunction should be included. All interventions are documented in the record along with whether the patient has achieved the stated outcomes.

NURSING DIAGNOSIS 2

DEFICIENT FLUID VOLUME

Related to:

   Excessive use of laxatives and diuretics

   Self-induced vomiting

Defining Characteristics:

   Electrolyte imbalance

   Changes in vital signs (increased pulse, decreased blood pressure)

   Poor skin turgor

   Dry mucous membranes

   Increased hematocrit (Hct) and hemoglobin (Hgb)

Goal:

   Fluid and electrolyte balance is normal.

Outcome Criteria

✔ The patient will have good skin turgor (when pinched, skin will return to normal position in < 2 seconds).

✔ The patient will have normal electrolyte levels.

✔ The patient will have moist mucous membranes.

✔ The patient's skin will be warm and dry.

✔ The patient's blood pressure and pulse will return to baseline.

✔ The patient will verbalize an understanding of fluid and electrolytes and express a willingness to refrain from purging activities.

NOC *Fluid balance*

INTERVENTIONS	RATIONALES
Assess fluid status by examining blood pressure, pulse, skin turgor, skin temperature, skin color, and urinary output.	Skin turgor will be poor (decreased elasticity) for the patient with fluid deficit; cool skin that is pale or that has decreased color indicates poor perfusion. Decreased urinary output is noted when decreased volume causes decreased perfusion. Noting these can give clues to treatment and response.
Take a history from the patient regarding episodes of vomiting, excessive urination, or excessive bowel movements (noting consistency), as well as number and amount of any laxatives, diuretics, or emetics taken.	Patients with bulimia take medications to purge body of food. These agents rob the body of fluid and electrolytes. Knowing the amount taken and results can give clues to extent of deficits.
Monitor results of laboratory results: Hct, BUN, creatinine, and electrolytes (especially potassium).	Hct fluctuates in response to fluid status; severe absolute loss of fluid from the circulating volume would produce a decrease in Hct

INTERVENTIONS	RATIONALES
	with further drops during fluid replacement due to hemodilution; BUN and electrolytes would give indicators of renal function; BUN may be elevated initially, but decrease later due to hemodilution of fluid replacement.
Monitor cardiac status: blood pressure and pulse (quality and rate).	Blood pressure decreases and pulse elevates when fluid status decreases; electrolyte imbalances, particularly potassium, cause alterations in cardiac function.
If fluid deficit is severe, establish intravenous (IV) access and administer IV fluids rapidly, as ordered.	Restoring fluid to the intravascular space is needed to improve fluid status, especially if the patient is unwilling to consume large amounts of fluid in the presence of severe deficit and electrolyte imbalance. Fluid needs are dictated by patient parameters.
Implement strict intake and output.	Helps to accurately assess adequacy of fluid intake.
Provide the patient with information on effects of fluid and electrolyte deficits on the body, complications that could occur, and how to correct imbalances.	Having factual information regarding fluid and electrolytes helps the patient understand the importance of maintaining fluid and electrolyte balance and the dangers of purging activities, and may motivate the patient to be compliant with recommendations.
Strongly discourage the use of laxatives, emetics, or diuretics.	Continued use of these agents for purging will counteract the effects of oral and IV fluid replacement.

NIC   *Fluid management*
        Fluid monitoring
        Hypovolemia management
        Intravenous insertion

Evaluation

Assess the patient for return of normal fluid and electrolyte balance. The patient's skin should be warm and dry, and return to patient's baseline color. Blood pressure and pulse return to baseline or are only slightly outside the range. Hct and Hgb are normal, and mucous membranes are moist. The patient is able to verbalize why fluids are needed and the dangers of electrolyte imbalances, and expresses a willingness to refrain from purging activities.

Community/Home Care

Patients who have problems with fluid volume deficit have fluid status restored prior to returning home. At home, the patient may not require any follow-up with respect to fluid status, as this is an acute situation that for the most part has no long-term implications. However, for some bulimia patients, fluid imbalance will occur again if they continue to use laxatives, diuretics, and vomiting as a method to purge themselves. Close observation in the home by family or significant others will be required for some period of time. Prevention of hospitalization for this problem is a goal, but it may not be achieved until the patient identifies the underlying causes of the eating disorder and receives treatment for this (see nursing diagnoses ("Disturbed Body Image" and "Imbalanced Nutrition"). A professional counselor can assist in this area, as can an advanced practice nurse. Family members may monitor the patient for signs of fluid and electrolyte imbalances that may indicate continued problems with losing electrolytes and fluids due to purging. Several indicators to note are undue fatigue, muscle cramping, and complaints of sore throat that would indicate frequent vomiting. If these are noted, or if the patient complains of mouth dryness or dry skin, encourage the intake of electrolyte-containing fluids. The health care provider may want the patient to return for a follow-up appointment to ensure that parameters such as Hgb, Hct, electrolytes, and BUN have returned to baseline, and fluid status has been maintained.

Documentation

Document findings from a comprehensive assessment with attention to blood pressure, pulse, and skin (color, temperature, and turgor). Document all output, including stool, emesis, and urine. Interventions implemented to correct fluid deficits (type and amount of fluid consumed or infused) are to be included in the patient chart, with documentation of the patient's response to the intervention. Always document whether the patient met the stated outcome criteria.

NURSING DIAGNOSIS 3

 ## DISTURBED BODY IMAGE

Related to:

Abnormal perception of self

Fear of obesity

Dysfunctional family

Depression

Defining Characteristics:

Fear of becoming obese

Personal loss of control

Negative feelings about self

Indifferent toward caregivers/family

Uses denial frequently

Statements about feeling bad, embarrassed, ashamed

Goal:

The patient develops a positive body image and self-esteem.

Outcome Criteria

✔ The patient is able to establish realistic nutritional goals.

✔ The patient states one positive aspect of body and self.

✔ The patient verbalizes that self is liked.

✔ The patient verbalizes satisfaction with body appearance.

✔ The patient makes no negative statements regarding self.

NOC *Body image*
      Self-esteem

INTERVENTIONS	RATIONALES
Monitor for fear of being overweight, worry over others' acceptance, feelings about self/ relationships, and fear of loss of love of others if gains weight.	For the patient with bulimia, acceptance by peers and others is important, and fears about appearance are common.
Monitor for expressions of self-value/interpersonal relationships: expressions of feelings about self, low self-esteem, inability to communicate well with family/ friends, withdrawal from social contact, statements about being overweight, unattractive, or unpopular.	The patient with bulimia often suffers from low self-esteem and has feelings of having an unacceptable appearance. He or she may actually shun social contact because of fear of having purging activities discovered. Recognition of this helps the health care provider begin planning for intervention.
Encourage the patient to communicate feelings about physical appearance and talk to the patient about body appearances and how body may have changed.	Open dialogue about body appearance helps the patient to start accepting his or her body and may promote changes in behavior.
Listen attentively to the patient and be aware of fears and concerns. Also look for misinterpretations or misunderstandings.	Listening to the patient will help you identify opportunities for teaching.
Help the patient identify personal strengths and mobilize coping strategies.	In order to move forward in resolving bulimia, the patient must identify ways to cope with stressors or own feelings of despair regarding eating disorders; using strengths to overcome weaknesses is a first step.
Help patient to set realistic goals, such as "I will eat 50 percent of a meal and retain it."	Setting small, achievable goals will help the patient to see rewards from his or her efforts; achieving small outcomes/goals instills hope in the patient at times when he or she may be experiencing negative thoughts about self.
Arrange for psychological counseling.	Helps to provide psychological evaluation and assistance to help the patient identify the root cause of the abnormal eating behaviors and incorporate it into a positive self-image.
Identify the effects of the patient's culture or religion on his or her self-concept and body image.	A patient's culture and religion often help define reactions to changes in body image and self-worth.

NIC *Body image enhancement*
      Emotional support
      Self-esteem enhancement
      Role enhancement

Evaluation

The patient is able to express that a problem exists with nutritional practices. It is crucial that the nurse evaluate to what degree the patient is beginning to accept that binge and purging behaviors are detrimental to his or her well-being. Assess for verbalizations that would indicate that the patient is beginning to assimilate positive dietary habits into his or her daily routine and is asking appropriate questions related to nutrition or the recommended dietary requirements. Communication of feelings and concerns relevant to weight and the need to consume more food for metabolic demands should be taken as a positive sign that progress is being made towards meeting outcome criteria. Determine whether the patient is able to discuss feelings openly with family members or significant others.

Community/Home Care

At home, continued monitoring of the patient's body image and self-esteem is needed. Health care workers will need to continue to investigate the reason for the patient engaging in binge eating and purging. For some, it may be a perceived negative appearance of the body. Bulimia generally represents another psychological problem that needs to be addressed by a professional counselor. Frequently, the patient suffers from depression, and if so, needs to be treated in order to move forward with establishing healthy nutritional habits. Counselors provide assistance to the patient in creating a feeling of acceptance of the person and the body as it is and by identifying positive attributes and strengths to build upon. Counselors will need to continue to work with the patient until the patient has garnered enough self-confidence and elevated his or her self esteem to the point that he or she feels good about him or herself. Finding the right counselor who can establish a good rapport with the patient may be a challenge, and this type of service may be limited in rural areas. Family members, friends, and significant others must provide support to the patient with bulimia by assisting him or her to take in enough nutrients to maintain health and weight but also by making positive statements about the patient's bodily appearance. Because most bulimia patients are treated on an outpatient basis in the absence of medical complications, other psychosocial issues such as ineffective coping may not be evident to the health care provider unless time is spent taking a thorough psychological history. The nurse or other health care provider who sees the patient for follow-up will need to be alert to subtle hints that may indicate that the patient is not making progress towards conquering the eating disorder. Open discussions regarding this disturbed body image and interventions to prevent social isolation and withdrawal should continue with the patient.

Documentation

Chart any specific behaviors or verbalizations that may indicate a lowered self-esteem or altered body image. In addition to a thorough assessment of the patient's psychological state, include all interventions that have been employed to address this issue and the patient's responses. Note when and if the patient begins to verbalize positive statements about him or herself. Referrals to counselors are included in the patient record.

CHAPTER 13.138

ABUSE: DOMESTIC

GENERAL INFORMATION

Domestic abuse occurs as a threat to the well-being of another person by a domestic partner. The abuse can occur as physical abuse, sexual abuse, or emotional abuse, with violence often occurring. In most cases, domestic violence is abuse of a woman by her male partner, with some sources estimating that 95 percent of the victims of domestic abuse are women. Violence against men by their female partners also exists, but does not occur as frequently. Domestic abuse/violence happens in gay and lesbian relationships but is not seen frequently. Victims of domestic abuse are often made to feel responsible, disempowered, alone, and without recourse or help. Often there are threats to the children in the relationship, rendering the victims powerless and unable to leave the situation. Despite some myths to the contrary, domestic violence can and does occur at all socioeconomic levels, cultural groups, and religious denominations. Domestic violence (especially against women) has risen to epidemic proportions, and the CDC estimates that nearly 5.3 million intimate partner victimizations occur yearly in the United States in women older than 18 years of age, with 2 million injuries and approximately 1300 deaths. In addition, countless others are psychologically abused. There are no specific manifestations of abuse, but generally the victim denies the abuse even when physical trauma is obvious and injuries are inconsistent with the story of how injuries occurred, attempts to hide the abuse through self-isolation, avoids eye contact, verbalizes that she or he has nowhere else to go, is self-blaming, expresses fear for her or his life, and has evidence of prior physical abuse such as old, healed injuries.

NURSING DIAGNOSIS 1

POST-TRAUMA RESPONSE

Related to:

Domestic violence

Defining Characteristics:

Reports history of previous domestic abuse

Fear of additional injury or death

Anger

Embarrassment

Fear of identifying injurer

Low self-esteem/self-blame

Revenge

Goal:

The patient requests legal, social, and psychological assistance.

Outcome Criteria

✔ The patient admits that the current situation is dangerous.

✔ The patient seeks assistance in finding a safer environment.

✔ The patient returns to a safe environment.

✔ The patient verbalizes feelings.

✔ The patient states one strategy to ensure safety.

✔ The patient identifies one community resource available for assistance.

✔ The patient feels empowered to make a decision— at least, the first decision to leave the abuse environment.

NOC ***Abuse recovery: Emotional***
Abuse recovery: Physical
Coping
Abuse recovery status
Abuse protection
Abuse: Cessation

INTERVENTIONS	RATIONALES
Place the patient in a private, quiet place but do not leave the victim alone.	This provides the victim a "safe" place where stressors are minimized to the greatest extent possible.
Reassure patient that she or he is safe.	The patient must know that abuse/neglect will not occur in present location and that she or he is safe.
Assess for or assist with assessment for signs of physical trauma/injuries (recent and historical): — Assess for injury: rib fractures (splinting of ribs with inspiration/expiration); strangle marks; bruises on back, chest, or arms; injuries in specific patterns made with hands or objects; difficulty breathing; lack of movement in any extremity; pain on movement of extremity; or abdominal and chest contusions. — Take history: severe headache, double vision, dizziness, agitation, and confusion. — Assess for pain, especially with inspiration and in pelvic area.	Persons who have been abused may have a variety of injuries, and offer a multitude of psychosocial/interactional responses that indicate fear. A thorough examination and a history from the client is the first step in validating the abuse. If sexual assault has occurred, follow through with appropriate protocols and interventions (see nursing care plan "Sexual Assault"). Pictures may need to be taken of obvious injuries such as bruises, scratch marks, or lacerations.
Note results of x-rays and computed tomography (CT) scans for abnormalities: skull abnormalities, rib fractures, old healed fractures, and arm and wrist fractures.	X-rays confirm current injuries and demonstrate old injuries that are healing or healed; provide the nurse with information to assist in planning care.
Treat injuries as ordered by physician.	Injuries need to be taken care of to make the patient feel protected and to prevent complications from injuries such as fractures.
Encourage the patient to tell you what happened without the partner present.	If the patient is willing to discuss abuse and abusers, legal interventions may occur faster and for a more permanent time; the abuser will be brought to justice. If the abuser is present, the patient will not talk.
Interview the victim using recall questions and the SAFE mnemonic: — S = Do you feel **safe** at home with your partner? Should we be concerned for your safety?	These questions focus the interview and are open-ended, allowing the victim to give details in her or his own words rather than being lead by the question. This makes the information richer/

— A = Are there times when you have felt **afraid** at home? Threatened with harm? Physically harmed?
— F = Do you have **friends** who know you have been hurt? **Family?** Do you think you can tell them? Can they help?
— E = Do you have an **emergency** plan? A safe place for you and your children to go? Would you be in danger if you went home now? Do you need help finding a safe place? Would you like to talk to someone about an emergency plan?

more meaningful. (The SAFE mnemonic is taken from Delmar's Electronic Care Plan Maker.)

Encourage patient to express emotions.	Feelings of fear, concern, and anger are real. Expression of them is the first step to effective, empowering decision-making.
Inform the patient that she or he has legal rights, and encourage the patient to seek legal and social help.	When violence has occurred in the home, the potential for recurrence is great. Encourage the patient to seek assistance and protection from both social and law enforcement agencies.
Arrange for social and/or legal consult, if desired.	Domestic violence must be reported to the appropriate legal authorities. Encourage the patient to report the event and to seek legal and social assistance; professionals with intervention skills in domestic violence situations can offer alternatives where the patient feels there is an adequate support system that will enable him or her to leave the current domestic arrangement. Social workers are needed to assist with proper inquiry into the abuse and to make alternate living arrangements.
Refer the patient for professional psychological counseling.	The patient may need help in identifying coping strategies and beginning to deal with domestic violence.
Encourage the patient to explore what to do about the situation.	Many victims of abuse do not believe that they can change the situation and need assistance in exploring options.

(continues)

(continued)

INTERVENTIONS	RATIONALES
Assist the patient in determining what support systems are available.	The patient may need support systems to help deal with the current situation by providing emotional support or shelter.
Carefully document findings.	These may be used in legal actions and must be concise and complete.
Report abuse to proper authorities according to agency protocol.	Experts in the area of domestic abuse will intervene on behalf of the patient's safety and well-being.
Provide gentle care and reassuring words.	Helps to reestablish the patient's trust and confidence; encourage social interaction and trust.
If the patient has been seen in the emergency room, encourage physicians to admit the patient.	Allows for further observation and investigation.

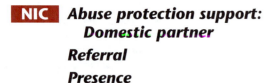 **Abuse protection support: Domestic partner**

Referral

Presence

Evaluation

Determine if the patient has achieved the stated outcomes. If the patient is able, she or he should report feeling safe. There will be no injury to the patient, or if the patient has been injured, the injuries are healing. Referrals to social services or legal authorities result in appropriate actions being taken to protect the patient and arrange for care needs once exiting the health care system. The patient is aware of community resources available for assistance and is assured of a safe place to go.

Community/Home Care

For the patient who has been a victim of domestic abuse and has entered the health care system, the health care system will need to investigate ways to prevent subsequent episodes of abuse. Investigations by social services, legal authorities, counselors, or health care workers should focus on why the abuse has occurred. In some instances the causative factor cannot be identified by the victim or those working with the patient. Community resources that provide services for abused partners should be identified by social services. The family or those involved may need

referrals for multiple needs, including counseling. Many victims leave home under the threat of imminent danger and physical trauma and are without money, identification, credit cards, or other vital possessions. If the victim needs to return to the home to obtain these items and personal supplies, social services should arrange for an escort to go to the home with the patient for safety. Give the patient a list of vital items to obtain, such as birth certificate, social security card, drivers license, passport, any legal documents such as restraining orders or custody papers, children's school records, banking statements or checkbook, cash, credit cards, bankcards, keys, medications, and cell phone. In many instances, the domestic abuse victim will need to find alternative living arrangements to protect her or him, and in some instances, her or his children, from harm. Work through social services to obtain information for the patient about safe houses and shelters. Discussions related to the legal ramifications of the abuse are required. For patients that return home to the same environment, formal, timely, and frequent follow-up with the victim should be attempted. It is recommended that professional counseling with experts in domestic abuse be undertaken with the purpose of empowering the victim. Physical injuries should be monitored to ensure that healing has occurred without complications.

Documentation

Chart the findings from a thorough physical assessment, noting the specific location of any injuries. If the patient complains of pain, document the location, intensity, relief measures taken, and the patient's responses. All interventions taken to treat the injuries should be charted. Include in the record the patient's overall mental state, being sure not to inject personal judgmental statements. Document whether the patient has met the stated outcome criteria, and if not, chart the necessary revisions in the plan of care. In cases of domestic abuse chart, any referrals made to social services as well as any visits from legal authorities. If documenting information verbalized to the nurse by the patient, state it verbatim.

NURSING DIAGNOSIS 2

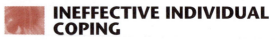 **INEFFECTIVE INDIVIDUAL COPING**

Related to:

Domestic abuse

Violence

Defining Characteristics:

   Expressions of fear

   Fear of returning home

   Negative statements regarding self

   Crying

Goal:

   The patient demonstrates effective coping.

Outcome Criteria

✔ The patient identifies and uses one coping strategy.

✔ The patient verbalizes fears and concerns.

NOC *Coping*

INTERVENTIONS	RATIONALES
Assess the patient for expressions of fear, anxiety, negative self-statements, and other displays.	When patients have been victims of domestic violence, the emotional response can vary greatly; the nurse needs to note specific expressions to establish a starting point for interventions. Often the victim has fears of additional violence and does not want to be alone, and may relive the event repeatedly in her or his mind.
Stay with the patient and allow other visitors only as requested by the patient.	Helps to provide emotional support and promote a sense of comfort.
Encourage the patient to verbalize feelings regarding what has happened and to express any fears or concerns; listen attentively. The patient may require a professional consult to assist with expression of feelings.	Verbalization of feelings, fears, and concerns contributes to dealing with the abuse; being attentive relays empathy to the patient.
Explain legal proceedings to the patient.	Knowing what to expect may calm some of the patient's fears and prepares him or her to deal with the events that may follow being a victim of domestic violence.
Ask the patient to identify all strategies that worked in the past to cope with stressful events.	Strategies that have previously worked can be used as a starting point for coping with more serious stressful events, and can help the patient focus.
Control multiple sources of stimuli that can occur when numerous	Overstimulation can worsen fear and anxiety.

people need or want contact with the patient.	
Assist with the development of new skills and strategies for coping, including referral to a professional counselor.	When major stressors such as domestic abuse occur, new strategies for coping may be required. These new strategies may be more sophisticated than those a generalist nurse is able to offer.
Encourage the family to verbalize honest feelings and seek appropriate resources for helping them to cope with the situation, especially if there are serious physical injuries to the victim.	Verbalization of feelings by family members needs to occur if they are to be a source of support for the victim; some family or significant others may blame the victim for what has happened. Until these issues are resolved, they cannot be relied on to offer emotional support. At this point, consideration is given to seeking professional help for the victim.
Recognize the role of cultural and religious beliefs in a patient's method of coping with stressors and particularly domestic abuse.	Culture and religion often dictate how a person copes with stressors, particularly issues of a sensitive nature.
Provide counseling referrals for the immediate time, but for long-term assistance as well.	The effects of domestic abuse on the emotional/mental state of the victim can be long-lasting and the patient may need continued assistance with coping skills.
Seek spiritual consult as needed or requested by the patient and/or family.	Meeting the patient's spiritual needs helps him or her cope with fears through use of spiritual or religious rituals, and provides support.
Ask the patient to state how she or he plans to cope following exit from the health care system, and where she or he will find support and assistance.	Helps to ensure that the patient has a plan.
Give the patient telephone numbers of the domestic violence hotline or other community resources that can assist including support groups.	Equips the patient with information to use in order to enhance coping skills.

NIC   *Coping enhancement*
     Emotional support
     Spiritual support

Evaluation

Evaluate the extent to which the outcome criteria have been achieved. The patient should be assessed for appropriate coping skills/strategies that can be used to deal with the current situation and the past history of trauma from domestic abuse. Concerns, fears, and feelings of being able to cope should be detected in the patient. The patient's ability to verbalize what has happened will be a beginning point for resolution and moving on to take action. If, however, the patient is unable to talk about what has happened, the nurse should explore further the need for new interventions to assist the patient in developing coping skills.

Community/Home Care

Victims must cope with the effects of domestic abuse or violence for extended periods of time when discharged from the emergency department. The patient should be encouraged to identify coping strategies that have been successful in the past and prompted to use them in this situation. Domestic abuse is a significant violation that has physical, emotional, and psychosocial ramifications. Coping with the physical injury may be easier for the patient to handle, as healing of injuries will usually occur in a short period of time. Recovery from the psychological trauma of abuse by someone the victim trusted or loved will require a different type of skill. It is crucial that the victim is equipped with a variety of coping strategies to use to adapt to the current situation. This is particularly true if the victim has been unable to return home and is living in shelters or safe houses with others. The ability to cope with separation from the partner will be difficult, and the victim will need community resources such as counseling, support groups, and even legal services. Especially when alone, the victim may feel humiliation, self-blame, shame, and fear. When this occurs, the victim will need to utilize hotlines, support persons, or other ways to cope. Keeping a journal is a good way to express feelings, and helps to reduce tension; sharing these later with a counselor helps in the emotional healing process. Follow-up care will need to monitor and intervene for this to prevent long-term, permanent psychological scars. New strategies for dealing with stressors will probably be required for a major crisis such as domestic violence, especially if the victim is moving forward with major life changes. Coping through use of support from outside sources such as nurse therapists or professional counselors will be most helpful to the victim. For many patients, spiritual rituals may be a means of coping with difficult, stressful situations. Once at home, the nurse and family will need to support the patient as needed to foster a healthy psychological state, recognizing that a wide array of feelings may be expressed. If the victim is proceeding with legal actions, court appearances are likely to be scheduled months or even years away from the actual event, and the patient will be called upon to relive the domestic abuse. At this time, old emotions and feelings of stress can resurface, dictating that the patient implement previously used coping strategies. Follow-up by some entity, a health care provider, social worker, or professional therapist, is recommended.

NURSING DIAGNOSIS 3

SITUATIONAL LOW SELF-ESTEEM

Related to:

Domestic abuse

Defining Characteristics:

Expressed shame and guilt

Self-blame

Denies physical abuse, but presents with unexplained injuries

Explains injuries in embarrassed or evasive manner

Denial of abuse situation

Verbalizations of negative self-talk

Humiliation

Verbalization of no control over situation

Expressions of powerlessness/hopelessness

Goal:

The patient returns to a positive self-esteem.

Outcome Criteria

✔ The patient will replace negative self-talk with positive self-talk.

✔ The patient will state that she or he is not to blame for the domestic violence.

✔ The patient will state one strategy to use to remedy the situation.

✔ The patient is discharged to a safe environment.

✔ The patient states a willingness to seek assistance.

NOC   *Abuse recovery: Emotional*
     Self-esteem
     Hope
     Personal autonomy

INTERVENTIONS	RATIONALES
Assess the patient's self-esteem by noting any negative talk regarding self.	It is normal for victims of domestic abuse to blame her or himself and to start to talk negatively about her or himself, even in areas not related to the abuse. The nurse needs to be attuned to these comments in order to intervene appropriately.
Assess the patient's understanding of domestic abuse and violence and what is now required to prevent a recurrence and move forward.	The patient who is blaming her or himself or having negative self-talk will need to be assisted in moving forward with life and establishing coping strategies that can start the healing process and enhance self-esteem, understanding that self-blame is not a warranted response.
Encourage verbalization of feelings (anger, dismay, concern, fear, etc.), allow the patient to talk about self and verbalize feelings about the abuse, and put the domestic abuse into perspective of the victim's total life.	Recognition of own feelings helps the patient to deal with the situation better and start acceptance of what has happened; a review of life will assist the patient to identify the positive aspects of the self-esteem and not dwell on the negative events; having an attentive listener allows the patient the opportunity to talk about what has happened freely and is the start of healing.
Be empathetic and nonjudgmental; listen attentively to the patient and be aware of fears and concerns, avoiding blaming questions.	Listening to the patient will help to identify opportunities for further interventions. Because many patients experience self-blame, it is important that the health care provider remain nonjudgmental.
Help patient identify personal strengths and mobilize coping strategies (see nursing diagnosis "Ineffective Individual Coping").	Discussions like this will help the patient to cope with the situation and enhance self-esteem.
Stay with the patient or have the family or significant others present if appropriate.	A domestic abuse victim should never be left alone due to fear of further violence and concerns over mental health.
Collaborate with physician or social worker to arrange for counseling and participation in support groups as needed.	Domestic abuse/violence is a major violation of a person's perception of her or himself. In order to cope with this effectively, professional counseling over an extended period of time may be required to return the victim to her or his usual state of self-esteem. Professional counselors can help the victim and her or his family or significant other effectively deal with the problems that may occur as a result of the abuse.
Encourage the patient to keep a diary and to record positive aspects of her or himself and of her or his life.	Helps the patient to focus on the positive and feelings of worth that should enhance rebuilding of self-esteem.

NIC   *Self-esteem enhancement*
     Presence
     Emotional support

Evaluation

The patient is able to verbalize feelings regarding self-worth or self-esteem. The patient refrains from negative self-talk and replaces negative talk with positive comments regarding self, particularly in terms of blaming self for the acts of domestic abuse/violence. A positive outcome reveals that the patient talks about her or himself and identifies personal strengths that can be mobilized to assist with coping. The patient is protected and eventually placed in a safe environment and indicates a willingness to accept assistance offered that may change the situation. The patient should verbalize feeling less powerless and more in control.

Community/Home Care

Situational low self-esteem can continue for a varied period of time. The victim can return to her or his previous level of self-esteem with the assistance of supportive family or significant others, through counseling, or sometimes through reliance on religious or spiritual practices. Because of the profound effect that abuse can have on a person, continued monitoring of self-esteem should be undertaken to detect any abnormal or morbid responses. The issue of self-esteem can be worsened if the victim does not identify positive aspects of her or his life and engage in social activities that reinforce the positive. For the victim, restoration of self-esteem may occur after a stressful period in which she or he doubted her or his self-worth. Participation in counseling and support groups may be needed to assist the patient to move towards total healing following domestic abuse/violence. Powerlessness may continue to be a problem once the patient leaves the health care system if she or he returns to her or his previous living arrangements. As the patient moves toward a feeling of comfort with the overall situation, the feeling of helplessness and powerlessness will be resolved or improved. Follow-up may be more appropriate for a social worker after referral to community agencies for services regarding safe housing, finances, etc. If children are involved, the victim must take control of her or his life while simultaneously engaging in activities to protect children and assist with her or his psychological well-being. The nurse or other health care provider who sees the patient for follow-up will need to be alert to subtle hints that may indicate that the patient has not improved her or his self-esteem.

Documentation

Document the progress the victim has made towards meeting outcome criteria. A thorough assessment of the patient's psychological state should be charted, including specific statements made by the patient that are indicators of negative or positive self-esteem. Include any verbalizations by the patient that indicate a state of powerlessness such as "I can't do anything about it," "that's just the way it is," or self-negating statements. If the nurse detects difficulties with coping, difficulties interacting with family members/significant other, or verbalizations of reactions and feelings about the domestic abuse, this should be included in the patient's chart. All referrals should be documented.

CHAPTER 13.139

ELDER ABUSE OR NEGLECT

GENERAL INFORMATION

Abuse and/or neglect of the elderly have become increasingly recognized as a problem in American society. Two landmark papers on the topic published by the House of Representatives House Select Committee on Aging (Elder Abuse: Examination of a Hidden Problem, 1981 and Elder Abuse: A Decade of Shame and Inaction, 1990) propelled the issue into prominence beginning in 1981. Far too often, the elderly are abused by their family members, guardians, or caregivers, and are fearful of reporting the abuse. Elderly persons may not discuss or report the abuse/neglect because they are physically unable or because they are ashamed or afraid. Health care workers should be suspicious of abuse and neglect when the patient presents with signs and/or symptoms that are poorly correlated with the history of events that has been given. Be suspicious when there are unexplained bruises, when the patient has had repeated falls, or when there are bruises or fractures in various states of healing. A classic sign of abuse is when the patient withdraws if a person enters the room or if he/she is touched. The nurse's primary responsibilities are to identify that the patient has been abused, to provide care to the patient, to ensure that the patient is safe, and to prevent further incidents. In addition, nurses are required to report such incidents or suspected incidents, to document findings carefully, and to be prepared to testify on behalf of the elder in the legal system.

NURSING DIAGNOSIS 1

 INJURY/RISK FOR INJURY*

Related to:

Evidence of previous injury

Neglect by abusive, neglectful, irresponsible person(s)

Caregiver role strain

Defining Characteristics:

Physical injuries

Psychosocial abuse

Physical and psychosocial neglect

Withdrawal from contact

Reports being abused

Unexplained weight loss

Poor hygiene

Skin breakdown

Goal:

The patient will be safe and injury-free.

Outcome Criteria

✔ The patient sustains no new injuries.

✔ The patient's injuries will heal without complications.

✔ The patient will verbalize an understanding of care required.

✔ Proper authorities are arranging for a safe place, proper care, and legal action.

NOC *Abuse protection*
Physical injury severity
Abuse cessation

INTERVENTIONS	RATIONALES
Reassure patient that he or she is safe.	The patient must know that abuse/neglect will not occur at the present location and that he or she is safe.
Assess and monitor for injuries (recent and historical). — Assess for injury: rib fractures (splinting of ribs with inspiration/expiration); strangle	Elders who have been abused may have a variety of injuries and offer a multitude of psychosocial/interactional responses that indicate fear.

(continues)

(continued)

INTERVENTIONS	RATIONALES
marks; bruises on back, chest, or arms; injuries in specific patterns made with hands or objects; difficulty breathing; lack of movement in any extremity; pain with movement of extremity; burns (especially cigarette, splash, and chemical); and abdominal and chest contusions.	A thorough examination and a history is the first step in validating the abuse. Neglect and sexual assault are also types of abuse that can lead to medical problems.
— Assess for signs of neglect: emaciation; dehydration/dry mucous membranes; poor skin turgor; weight loss or weight less than proportionate for age/body size; hunger (has not eaten or had anything to drink in days); thirst; anorexia; poor hygiene/smell of concentrated urine; presence of wet/soiled linen; clothing that appears to have not been changed in a long time; missing patches of hair; and skin breakdown on buttocks, perineum, heels, elbows, sacrum, or any other skin surface area.	
— Assess for indicators of abuse: fetal position; withdraws upon presence, touch, or voice; withdraws when caregiver enters the room, talks, or touches; does not want to talk with anyone.	
— Take history: severe headache, double vision, dizziness, agitation, and confusion.	
— Signs of sexual assault, vaginal tears, bruises, and presence of semen.	
Check x-rays for abnormalities: skull abnormalities, rib fractures, old, healed fractures, and arm and wrist fractures.	X-rays confirm current injuries and also demonstrate old injuries that are healing or healed.
Monitor for extremely passive behavior when in presence of caregiver.	This behavior could indicate a history of compliance with caregiver due to fear.
Treat injuries as ordered by physician.	Injuries need to be taken care of to make the patient feel protected and to prevent

	complications from injuries such as fractures.
Provide gentle care and reassuring words.	Helps to re-establish the patient's trust and confidence in a caregiver; encourages social interaction and trust.
Provide basic personal care if patient is in poor hygienic state.	Often when a patient is abused, caregivers also neglect basic personal care.
Provide nutritious food/meal and fluids if the patient reports being hungry or looks emaciated.	Emaciation and complaints of hunger are sometimes seen in patients who are neglected and abused.
After establishing some degree of rapport with the patient, encourage him or her to tell you what happened.	If patient is willing to discuss abuse and abusers, legal interventions may occur faster and for a more permanent time; abuser will be brought to justice. The patient is more likely to talk to the nurse if he or she has developed a relationship through provision of other care and treatment first.
If the patient is seen in the emergency room, encourage physicians to admit the patient.	Allows for further observation and investigation.
If caregiver is present, talk to him or her in a private place to determine if he or she is capable of providing care or if he or she is experiencing caregiver role strain, and refer as needed.	The caregiver may feel burdened financially, emotionally, and physically as a result of the caregiving role and may need intervention for assistance. Role strain and stress are risk factors for abuse. Time away from the patient may be needed.
Carefully document findings.	These may be used in legal actions and must be concise and complete.
Report abuse/neglect to proper authorities according to agency protocol.	Experts in the area of elder abuse and neglect will intervene on behalf of the patient's safety and well-being.
Refer to social services.	Social workers are needed to assist with proper inquiry into the abuse and with making alternate living arrangements.

NIC   *Abuse protection: Elder*
Referral
Respite care
Presence

Evaluation

Determine whether the patient has achieved the stated outcomes. If the patient is able, he or she should report feeling safe. There will be no injury to the patient, or, if the patient has been injured, the injuries are healing and no new injuries have occurred. Referrals to social services or legal authorities result in appropriate actions being taken to protect the patient and arrangements being made for care needs once the patient exits the health care system.

Community/Home Care

For the patient who has been a victim of elder abuse, the health care system will need to investigate ways to prevent subsequent episodes of abuse. Investigations by social services, counselors, or health care workers should focus on why the abuse has occurred. In some instances, the causative factor is caregiver role strain that results from caring for a loved one; role strain may worsen as the physical demands of care increase, especially incontinence. Community resources such as home health aides, volunteer visitors, or sitters who can assist with the care of the patient can be identified by social services. The family or those involved need referrals for respite care and, in some instances, counseling. In rural areas there may be no avenues for respite care, and social services in this case, should work with the caregiver to establish other means of providing relief, such as engaging other family members in the care at set times. For serious cases of physical abuse, the patient will need to be placed in alternative living arrangements to protect him or her from harm. Preparing the patient for placement at nursing homes, foster homes, or assisted living facilities may be difficult, and those involved in the process should ensure that the patient is well informed and understands the need for such an arrangement. If patients are not cognitively impaired, discussions related to the legal ramifications of the abuse are required. For patients that return home to the same environment, formal, timely, and frequent follow-up with the patient and family is required to protect the elder. Patients should understand how to activate the 911 system in case of subsequent abuse. Physical injuries should be monitored to ensure that healing has occurred without complications.

Documentation

Chart the findings from a thorough physical assessment, specifically noting any injuries. Record the patient's verbalizations of what happened and any other complaints exactly as stated. If the patient complains of pain, document the location, intensity, relief measures taken, and the patient's responses. All interventions taken to treat the injuries should be charted. Include in the record the patient's overall mental state, being sure not to inject personal judgmental statements. Document whether the patient has met the stated outcome criteria, and if not, chart the necessary revisions in the plan of care. In cases of elder abuse, chart any referrals made to social services as well as any visits from legal authorities.

NURSING DIAGNOSIS 2

 POWERLESSNESS

Related to:

> Verbalization of no control over situation
> Being elderly
> Inability to defend self
> Lack of understanding of why abuse happened
> Self-care deficit

Defining Characteristics:

> Crying
> Withdrawal
> Expression of hopelessness, powerlessness

Goal:

> The patient will express a sense of control.

Outcome Criteria

✔ The patient will make one decision.

✔ The patient is discharged to a safe environment.

✔ The patient states a willingness to seek assistance (if cognitively capable).

✔ The patient will have a legal guardian appointed if he or she is not competent.

NOC *Hope*

Personal autonomy

Participation in health care decisions

INTERVENTIONS	RATIONALES
Assess the patient's mental status.	Helps to establish a baseline for the patient's mental health and effects of abuse.
Allow the patient to talk about self and verbalize feelings about the abuse (see nursing diagnosis "Injury/Risk for Injury").	Having an attentive listener allows the patient the opportunity to talk about what has happened freely and is the start of healing.
Provide for continuity of care through assignment of consistent caregiver.	The patient may be fearful and anxious about all caregivers and the consistency of the provider gives the patient a feeling of comfort and decreases fear.
Assure the patient that he or she is safe and encourage him or her to make decisions regarding care.	Gives the patient a sense of control.
Ask the patient to describe relationship with family and significant others.	The nature of relationships with significant others will give clues to why the patient feels powerless and assist the nurse in planning interventions; many patients who are powerless are in dependent relationships without the opportunity to make decisions.
Arrange for social service consultation.	The social worker can assess the situation and make arrangements for a safer environment.
Arrange for consultation to review the patient's legal rights.	The patient should be informed of rights and available protection and of legal course of action.
Inform proper authorities of suspected abuse, according to agency protocol.	Helps to ensure patient protection, to assess situation and institute legal action where appropriate, and to ensure that patient has competent legal guardian who has the patient's best interest in mind.

NIC   *Self-responsibility facilitation*
Decision-making support
Emotional support
Presence

Evaluation

Assess the degree to which the patient has met the stated outcome criteria. The patient is protected and eventually placed in a safe environment. While in the care of others, the patient exerts some control over his or her situation by making decisions regarding his or her care and indicates that he or she is willing to accept assistance offered that may change the situation. The patient should verbalize that he or she feels less powerlessness and is in control.

Community/Home Care

Powerlessness may continue to be a problem once the patient leaves the health care system if he or she returns to the previous living arrangements. A home health nurse as well as social services will need to be involved in home care to monitor the patient's mental state and risk for future abuse. Powerlessness may be short term if the patient is placed in alternative living arrangements where he or she can be a more participatory player in decisions regarding his or her care and where he or she feels safe. Discussions with the patient and family prior to discharge should center on how to enhance decision making and create a sense of control for the patient rather than maintaining the totally dependent relationship. As the patient moves toward a feeling of comfort with the overall situation, the feeling of helplessness and powerlessness will be resolved or improved.

Documentation

Document the extent to which the outcome criteria have been achieved. Include any verbalizations by the patient that indicates a state of powerlessness such as "I can't do anything about it," "That's just the way it is," or self-negating statements. Chart all interventions that have been employed to address the issue of powerlessness, including empathetic listening and spending time with the patient. Indicate in the patient record where the patient is going at time of discharge and any concerns the patient may express about living arrangements. Referrals to social services or legal authorities are included in the chart.

CHAPTER 13.140

GRIEF

GENERAL INFORMATION

Grief is an emotional state caused by the actual or anticipated loss of a significant person, object, body part, body function, or relationship. The level of loss may vary: losing a friend because he or she is moving away, permanent loss resulting from death, amputation of a body part, or loss of employment. The way a person grieves is influenced by a variety of factors including culture, religion, age, past experiences, and social support. At the end of a period of time (that may range from a few months to a few years), the individual begins to restructure his or her life and adjust to a life without the lost object or person. While theorists have attempted to categorize distinct stages of the grieving process, responses to grief remain highly individualized and variable. In anticipatory grief, the loss is a potential one, e.g., through terminal illness (including the patient's own death), a critical illness, or injury in which the outcome is uncertain, or the loss of a limb through surgery. The person (or family) begins to grieve before the loss event occurs. This type of grief can help the patient or family better adjust to the final loss when it takes place. In some situations though, the grief may not be expressed appropriately, and thus may become dysfunctional. Oftentimes, an individual or family may deny the loss (or possible loss) and fail to display the appropriate emotional response. Because of this, the individual or family members cannot move forward to restructuring their lives without the lost object, relationship, or person.

NURSING DIAGNOSIS 1

 ANTICIPATORY GRIEVING

Related to:

Anticipated loss

News of a terminal disease

Critical illness or injury in which the outcome is uncertain

Defining Characteristics:

Grief that occurs before an actual loss occurs

Anger

Expressions of fear

Restlessness and anxiety

Crying

Expresses distress at potential loss

Goal:

The patient expresses grief.

Outcome Criteria

✔ The patient identifies one coping mechanism to be used.

✔ The patient verbalizes fears and concerns.

✔ The patient reports being less anxious.

✔ The patient demonstrates no outward signs of anxiety such as restlessness or agitation.

✔ The patient discusses feelings regarding anticipated loss.

NOC *Grief resolution*
Anxiety control
Comfort level
Coping

INTERVENTIONS	RATIONALES
Examine the family/significant other and patient in relation to meaning of loss, available support systems, interpersonal relationships, usual coping style, and previous experience with loss or death.	Provides information on the patient's resources and what the loss may mean for the patient, as well as giving clues to how the patient may deal with loss.

(continues)

(continued)

INTERVENTIONS	RATIONALES
Establish a trusting relationship with patient and family and communicate openly and reassuringly.	Communication in a reassuring, calm, and straightforward manner may help to relieve anxiety and fear.
Stay with patient as possible and allow family to visit.	Helps to provide emotional support and promote a sense of comfort.
Encourage the patient to verbalize fears, concerns, and expressions of grief, and listen attentively; avoid use of phrases such as "everything will be okay" and "don't cry."	Verbalization of fears contributes to dealing with concerns; being attentive relays empathy to the patient; use of these phrases minimizes the patient's feelings and avoids explanations of the loss. This may impede successful communication.
Provide a private place for the patient and family.	Grieving is a private process for most people; the patient and family members need a private, comfortable environment where grieving can occur.
Do not give false reassurance. Be realistic.	Giving false reassurance is not fair to the patient, as he or she cannot psychologically begin grieving if clinging to a false hope.
Help the patient create a plan for action.	A plan will assist the patient in taking the next step, which is usually very difficult.
Control multiple sources of stimuli that could cause sensory overload.	Over-stimulation can worsen anxiety and fear.
Seek spiritual consult as needed or requested by the patient and or family.	Meeting spiritual needs of the patient helps the patient to deal with fears through use of spiritual or religious rituals.
Recognize the role of culture in the patient's method of grieving and the verbalization of fears and concerns.	Culture often dictates how a person grieves, and the nurse must recognize this in order to support the patient in a successful grief process.
Engage the patient and family in open dialogue regarding options for treatment and care.	During the final stages of life, the patient and family may not be able to care for the patient alone; discussion of care options allows the patient to be more in control and gives him or her a sense of empowerment that may assist in coping with the loss.

For losses that are not life threatening, discuss with the patient changes that will occur secondary to the loss (i.e., loss of leg, loss of breast, loss of childbearing function, loss of sight, etc.).

Helping the patient to talk about the loss and its impact on life will help the patient to start coping with the loss.

NIC *Presence*
Grief work facilitation
Coping enhancement
Emotional support
Spiritual support

Evaluation

Evaluate the extent to which the outcome criteria have been achieved. The patient should be assessed for behaviors that would indicate appropriate responses to the anticipated or actual loss and should have no indicators of anxiety such as agitation. The patient should verbalize fears and concerns and be able to identify one way to cope with loss and grief. The extent to which the patient displays appropriate coping behaviors should be noted. If the patient is unable to talk about the loss and communicate concerns, the nurse should explore further interventions to assist the patient.

Community/Home Care

Nurses should assess which coping mechanisms work for the patient and encourage their use by the patient at home. Problems with grieving may continue for a long period of time, and follow-up by a health care provider can detect ineffective coping. The nurse should discuss with the patient and family appropriate responses to loss and grieving, as well as acceptable coping strategies. Extreme self-isolation and depression should be noted and reported to a health care provider. Those involved in the care of the patient or who are the patient's support network will need to encourage the patient to engage in some of his or her usual activities if health permits. Even simple activities such as taking a ride or going to church can help alleviate simple depression. For many patients and families, spiritual/religious rituals provide a means of coping with difficult, stressful situations, particularly during grieving. The patient's culture may dictate how he or she grieves and with whom he or she shares this process. The culturally competent nurse will question the patient and family regarding their approach to grieving and support the family and patient's methods. It is crucial that the nurse and family provide support to the patient as needed to foster a healthy psychological state, recognizing that anger and denial are common. The person may benefit from quiet periods of meditation during the day. If grieving is caused by a terminal illness, support to long-term caregivers will be important, as they too need to be supported in a grief process. Follow-up with a health care provider or counselor is important for persons who grieve to ensure that progression towards restructuring of their life has begun.

Documentation

The degree to which the patient has achieved the outcome criteria should be documented in the patient record. Document findings from an assessment of the patient's psychological state, whether there is depression, anger, crying, sadness, etc. The patient's verbalization of fears, concerns, and grieving should be documented specifically as the patient states them. Coping strategies that have been employed by the patient are included in the record. Document referrals to social workers, hospice, or religious leaders.

NURSING DIAGNOSIS 2

DYSFUNCTIONAL GRIEVING

Related to:

Loss (actual or anticipatory)

Defining Characteristics:

Sustained denial

Inability to grieve

Unwillingness to acknowledge or accept the loss

Goal:

The patient begins to go through the phases of functional grieving.

Outcome Criteria

✔ The patient verbalizes that a loss has occurred or will occur.

✔ The patient is able to talk about the loss/anticipated loss.

✔ The patient will recognize that grieving is normal.

NOC *Psychosocial adjustment:*
        Life change
     Coping
     Family: Coping
     Grief resolution

INTERVENTIONS	RATIONALES
Allow the patient and family the opportunity to talk and practice attentive listening.	It may help the patient to first vent before actually being able to deal with the loss.
Be direct in getting the patient and family to focus on reality.	Let the patient know in a firm but caring manner the reality of the situation.
Encourage significant others to grieve with the patient and to be supportive of the patient.	The patient should know that it is okay to grieve in the presence of family/friends.
Help the patient to identify/ explore the reason for the avoidance/denial; be attentive and kind, but firm.	The patient must recognize that he or she is in denial before moving on to acceptance of the loss; helping the patient to identify reasons for avoidance reconfirms the reality of the situation.
Solicit the help of others (family, friends, health care professionals) to support expressions of grief.	A consistent approach by those who are caring and knowledgeable may help the patient to begin to grieve.

NIC *Grief work facilitation*
     Presence
     Active listening
     Coping enhancement

Evaluation

Positive outcomes have been achieved when the patient demonstrates beginning evidence of recognizing that a loss has occurred or will occur. The patient is able to talk about the loss with professionals or family members. In addition, the patient expresses feelings and realizes that grieving is normal.

Community/Home Care

The patient or family who has experienced a loss but is having difficulty recognizing the loss will need follow-up to ensure that eventual validation of the loss occurs. Failure to respond appropriately to a loss can lead to morbid grief reactions that have far reaching consequences for the patient/family. Morbid reactions may include continued progressive social isolation with alteration in interpersonal relationships, imagined health symptoms, agitation, depression, and in some instances, hostility. If a person does not grieve a loss, for example, impending death or even divorce, attention may not be given to life work such as business decisions and planning for family. Professional counselors may be needed when the patient is at home to continue to work with the patient on recognition and resolution of the loss. A supportive family network or significant other plays a key role in this issue since these people will be with the patient for extended periods of time and in a position to make astute observations that may indicate a need for aggressive therapy.

NURSING DIAGNOSIS 3

SPIRITUAL DISTRESS

Related to:

Loss (challenge to belief system)

Terminal illness

Lack of choice

Lack of control over the situation

Lack of any positive finding that may offer hope

Defining Characteristics:

Expresses doubt or despair regarding personal beliefs

States that he or she no longer believes in a higher being

States inability to continue with personal belief system

Requests presence of a religious professional

Expressions of hopelessness

Appears to be giving up

Passive behavior

Isolation/withdrawal

Goal:

The patient uses spiritual beliefs as a coping strategy.

Outcome Criteria

✔ The patient or family describes their spiritual or religious belief system.

✔ The patient states that he or she will utilize his or her belief systems to cope with loss.

✔ The patient verbalizes a desire to practice his or her religious and spiritual rituals.

✔ The patient is able to identify choices.

✔ The patient is able to participate in creating a plan of action.

NOC *Hope*
Spiritual health

INTERVENTIONS	RATIONALES
Gain an understanding of the patient's belief system and respect what he or she believes.	As a caregiver, it is important to remain non-judgmental, supportive, and understanding of the patient's beliefs.
Assist the patient with goal setting that is realistic and attainable.	Setting goals that are too high can cause a sense of hopelessness.
Offer the patient an opportunity for spiritual counseling/visit; arrange for a visit by clergy or spiritual advisor of his or her choice. Permit the patient to practice spiritual beliefs without judgment; allow patient to engage in prayers or rituals.	When hope is lost, religion or spirituality may provide comfort or rekindle hope, and may provide comfort when there are no concrete answers, possibly providing a source of support that the health care provider is unable to offer.
Provide spiritual/religious music, literature, or television of the patient's choice, if acceptable to the patient.	These may be used as methods of relaxation and enhancement of spiritual well-being.
Seek to obtain religious articles the patient requires with assistance from other disciplines such as social workers.	The patient's ability to practice religious or spiritual rituals may be dependent on having particular items. Activities such as reading from holy books is often comforting.
Encourage the patient to verbalize feelings; be empathetic and listen attentively.	Verbalization is the first step to accepting life changes. The patient needs to know that the nurse is available to listen and is genuinely concerned about his or her spiritual health.
Encourage the patient without false reassurance.	When someone feels hopeless, he or she will miss opportunities to recognize positive events, goals, etc.

INTERVENTIONS	RATIONALES
Offer accurate, complete, and current information, and allow time for questions.	The patient may have incorrect or incomplete information or may have come to incorrect conclusions.
Assist the patient to recognize the importance of the loss and how to incorporate the loss into his or her life.	Recognition of the loss and its significance will help the patient adapt to the loss successfully.

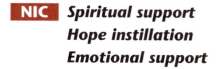

NIC *Spiritual support*
Hope instillation
Emotional support

Evaluation

Determine whether the outcome criteria have been met. The patient describes and discusses religious or spiritual beliefs with health care providers. The patient recognizes his or her own religious beliefs and spirituality as sources of comfort and as a strategy for coping. Observations of the patient utilizing religious or spiritual articles and rituals that are important to him or her indicates successful achievement of outcomes. The patient's ability to make choices and ask questions about what is going on around him or her is a sign of realistic hope.

Community/Home Care

Depending upon the nature of the loss, the risk for spiritual distress will continue to be a concern as the patient or family attempts to adjust to the loss. Religious leaders can serve as counselors and persons of support to the patient and family for extended periods of time. These leaders can also assist the patient to find meaning in life through engagement in serious conversations of religion and spirituality. Often patients experiencing losses do not want to discuss their feelings with family members or health care workers but feel that spiritual/religious leaders are better prepared for this task, and confidentiality is ensured. For many patients, leaders from their own religious affiliation can address this need, but in other instances, referrals may need to be made at the patient's request. Maintaining hope and spiritual well-being reduces anxiety and allows the patient to focus on positive aspects of life. In instances of terminal illness or illnesses that limit the patient's ability to be mobile, some means of providing transportation to religious services should be identified if desired. Many churches have transportation vans that can accommodate wheelchairs, and this should be investigated. Arranging for communion or other rituals in the home at appropriate times is another means of maintaining religious or spiritual practices that the patient or family may find comforting. Simple methods of finding peace that can meet the spirituality needs include meditation, taking nature walks, listening to soothing music, or talking to counselors.

Documentation

Chart any specific patient verbalization of religious or spiritual needs and findings from an assessment of the patient's emotional state. Document all interventions implemented to address spiritual distress, including visits by clergy or other spiritual leaders. Include the patient's use of religious items and observations of performance of religious rituals. If referrals are made to chaplains or other spiritual leaders, document the referral and any subsequent visits in the chart. Also document the patient's behavior before and after any visits.

CHAPTER 13.141

OVERDOSE (AND/OR POISONING)

Overdose occurs when a person intakes a toxic or near-lethal dose of a substance that significantly alters normal physiological function and places the person at risk for death. There are endless numbers of substances and medications that can cause an intentional or unintentional overdose. Patients who experience an overdose present with a varied array of clinical manifestations dependent on the substance ingested but most present with some impairment of respiratory function. In all poisonings or overdoses, the caregiver should try to obtain the following information simultaneously while beginning therapeutic interventions:

— Is the toxic substance(s) known?
— How is the toxic substance absorbed (ingested, injected, inhaled, absorbed through the skin or tissue)?
— How and where is the toxic substance catabolized?
— How is the toxic substance excreted?
— How can levels of the toxic substance be measured?
— What was the rate of administration of the toxic substance?
— How long ago was the toxic substance ingested?

It is essential to determine the substance's half-life, time to peak, and pharmacokinetics. The priorities in poisoning and/or overdose are to maintain the airway and ensure adequate ventilation and circulation to remove the toxic substance and to prevent further absorption of the substance. Poison centers are usually the best source of the most up-to-date information on any given substance. The local, state, or regional poison center will assist the caregiver by providing the most current information about the toxic substance and will provide information regarding the most current standards of care.

NURSING DIAGNOSIS 1

RISK FOR POISONING

Related to:

Presence of toxic substance in body

Ingestion of toxic substance (drug)

Defining Characteristics:

None

Goal:

The patient's risk of poisoning/toxicity is reduced.

Outcome Criteria

✔ The patient will have no signs of drug toxicity.

✔ The patient will have vital signs within normal/baseline range.

✔ The patient will have indicators of hemodynamic stability (renal function, respiratory status, cardiovascular status, and neurological status).

NOC *Risk control: Drug use*
Personal safety behavior

INTERVENTIONS	RATIONALES
Monitor laboratory and diagnostic tests: complete blood count (CBC), serum electrolytes, urine toxicology screen, serum toxicology screen, and others as ordered, depending upon suspected or known drug of abuse or specific signs and symptoms.	These tests provide information on hemodynamic state and effect of drug on vital organs. Toxicology screens help identify the substances ingested and provide information on amount of specific drugs in the body, which provides information on extent of the problem.
Perform a respiratory assessment: respiratory rate, rhythm, depth; pulse oximetry, and arterial blood gases (ABGs).	Many substances legal and illegal alter the respiratory system, particularly causing respiratory depression; a good

INTERVENTIONS	RATIONALES
	assessment is required to determine abnormalities or establish baselines.
Perform a cardiovascular assessment: blood pressure (low to high), pulse (from bradycardia to tachycardia), dysrhythmias, and electrocardiogram (EKG) changes.	Many legal and illegal substances have the potential to alter the cardiovascular system. The abnormalities vary widely depending upon the substance and amount ingested; the health care provider needs this information to determine specific effects and establish baselines.
Perform a neurological assessment: level of consciousness, motor activity, reflexes, tremors, seizures, hypo- or hypersthesia, and pain.	Helps to determine the effect if any on neurological functioning; many substances can depress or excite the central nervous system.
Perform a gastrointestinal (GI)/ genitourinary (GU) assessment: urinary output, bowel activity, abdominal pain, dietary/ fluid intake, and loss of appetite/anorexia.	Many substances that are taken in overdose situations affect kidney function and gastrointestinal performance. Assessments establish a baseline and gives clues to functioning.
Administer dextrose 50 percent intravenous (IV), as ordered.	Helps to prevent cerebral glucose deficit.
Administer naloxone (Narcan®) IV, as ordered.	Helps to reverse effects of opioids and relieve respiratory depression.
Administer thiamine intramuscularly (IM), as ordered.	Helps to prevent Wernicke-Korsakoff syndrome due to lack of vitamin B in the presence of high-dose glucose in chronic alcohol abuse if alcohol intoxication is suspected.
Administer specific antidote for ingested substance, as ordered.	If a substance has a specific antidote, it should be given as soon as possible to reverse adverse effects and prevent acute poisoning.
Induce emesis, as ordered, by administering syrup of ipecac. (Emesis is induced when a stomach lining irritant is introduced that stimulates the emetic center in the medulla.)	Emesis is a useful intervention to remove gastric contents in certain patients with certain types of ingestion. Emesis should not be induced if: (1) the patient has an altered mental state; (2) it can be predicted that airway compromise will occur rapidly due to central nervous system depression; (3) seizure activity is present or likely to occur; (4) the toxic substance is

	an acid or an alkali that can cause more damage when vomited; (5) the toxic substance is a petroleum distillate that can "creep" into the trachea during emesis; (6) the substance is an aliphatic hydrocarbon; (7) the patient has a history of cardiac disease, seizure disorder, or is pregnant; or (8) the patient is already bradycardic (and the vagal reflex that is stimulated during vomiting will further reduce heart rate). Continue giving the patient liquids as ordered and ensure that the patient vomits until stomach contents are clear.
Perform gastric lavage, as ordered, via a large bore nasogastric (NG) tube (usually 36 to 40 French in an adult). Consider sending a sample of gastric aspirate to the lab for analysis if the toxic substance is unknown.	Gastric lavage is done when there is a possibility that the toxic substance can readily be removed from the stomach. If the patient is unconscious, place him or her in a left lateral decubitus (swimmer's) position to avoid aspiration. Lavage should be done with a warmed normal saline solution at 200 ml per rinse in an adult or as ordered. Repeat the lavage until the fluid return is clear. Be sure to provide oral hygiene once the procedure has been completed and the tube has been removed.
Administer activated charcoal, as ordered. (Agents not well absorbed or bound by charcoal are acids, alkalis, cyanide, ethanol, ferrous sulfate, lithium, and methanol).	Activated charcoal is given by mouth or orogastric tube. It absorbs and binds many toxic substances. Tricyclic antidepressants, theophylline, digoxin, phenytoin, phenobarbital, carbamazepine, and products that have sustained-release properties may require multiple doses of activated charcoal.
Administer cathartics (magnesium, sulfate, magnesium citrate, sodium citrate, sorbitol), as ordered.	Cathartics are used to enhance secretion of poisons. Do not administer cathartics in the absence of bowel sounds.
Whole bowel irrigation, as ordered, with stimulants such as Golytely® and/or large volumes of fluids.	Whole bowel irrigation is used to cleanse the entire lower GI tract. It has proven to be useful for those substances that are not absorbed/bound by activated

(continues)

(continued)

INTERVENTIONS	RATIONALES
	charcoal, such as lithium, iron, lead, and zinc.
Arrange for renal dialysis, as ordered.	Certain toxic substances, such as digitalis or acetylsalicylic acid, methyl alcohol, ethylene, and diethylene glycol are most expeditiously removed via renal dialysis, especially in the presence of renal failure or severe metabolic acidosis.
Monitor the patient's response to interventions.	Helps to determine effectiveness and whether the plan of care requires revision.
Teach the patient and family the signs and symptoms of poisoning relevant to the substance that has been ingested.	The patient needs to be aware of signs of poisoning in order to seek appropriate health care assistance. Recognizing the dangers of ingesting harmful substances in dangerous amounts may cause the patient to seek help for the problem.

NIC *Surveillance: Safety*
Vital signs monitoring

Evaluation

Determine whether the patient has achieved the outcome criteria as stated. The patient should demonstrate no signs or symptoms of overdose or toxicity, and all assessments of system function are normal. All vital signs have returned to the patient's baseline. The patient understands that substances were intended to be taken in a certain dose and others not to be taken internally at all, and the seriousness of overdose and poisoning. If the overdose was an intentional suicide attempt, the patient expresses a willingness to seek appropriate help (see nursing care plan "Suicide: Attempt/Ideation").

Community/Home Care

Whether the patient remains at risk for poisoning following contact with the health care system will depend on his or her ability to recognize the seriousness of an overdose. The patient needs to be aware of the signs and symptoms of poisoning in order to seek early treatment and avoid serious complications. The best method for addressing the problem of risk for poisoning would be to work with the patient and other health care disciplines to determine how and why the overdose occurred. If it is determined that this was an intentional act in an attempt to commit suicide, the patient will need to attend individual or group counseling sessions to help provide assistance with dealing with the current situation. Follow-up with the patient and family is needed to monitor the patient's progress with developing healthy behaviors, and if needed, cessation of substance abuse (a frequent cause of overdose) and maintenance of self-esteem. The patient needs to establish acceptable coping strategies to use in stressful situations of life including work and family and have a means of seeking support. Follow-up through an outpatient clinic or with a home-visiting organization is required to ensure that the patient is able to implement recommendations for successful management of life.

Documentation

Chart the findings from an assessment of the neurological, cardiovascular, respiratory, and GI/GU systems, with specific attention to the presence of signs and symptoms of poisoning. Because of the variable changes with the different substances, documentation of even small changes in the vital signs in a timely fashion is important for care decisions. These should be documented according to agency protocol and may be included in the notes as well as on the graphic sheets. Any subjective reports of signs or symptoms or complaints are recorded in the notes as the patient states them. All interventions to prevent or treat poisoning and the patient's response to interventions are always included in the patient record. When medications are initiated to treat specific symptoms this is charted according to agency protocol for medication administration.

NURSING DIAGNOSIS 2

 INEFFECTIVE BREATHING PATTERN

Related to:

Respiratory depression

Presence of toxic levels of substances in the blood

Central nervous system (CNS) depression

Defining Characteristics:

Cheyne-Stokes respirations

Tachypnea

Use of accessory muscles of respiration

Abnormal blood gases (ABGs)

Goal:

The patient's respirations are effective in maintaining gas exchange.

Outcome Criteria

✔ The patients respirations are unlabored and < 28.

✔ The patient's ABGs will return to baseline.

NOC *Respiratory status: Ventilation*
Respiratory status: Gas exchange
Vital signs

INTERVENTIONS	RATIONALES
Assess respiratory system by noting respiratory rate, depth, chest expansion, rhythm, breath sounds, ABGs, pulse oximetry, and skin color, and note any of the following abnormalities: increased respiratory rate, Cheyne-Stokes respirations, severe dyspnea that has progressively worsened, cyanosis (nailbeds, lips), and use of accessory muscles of respiration.	Any of these abnormalities would indicate status of the respiratory system and progression of poisoning; many substances when taken in amounts that are toxic cause respiratory depression secondary to CNS depression; also establishes a baseline for future comparisons.
Place patient in high Fowler's position, or position for easy respiration.	Helps to maximize thoracic cavity space, decrease pressure from diaphragm and abdominal organs, and facilitate use of accessory muscles.
Provide humidified, low-flow (2 liters/min) oxygen, as ordered.	Helps to provide some supplemental oxygen to improve oxygenation.
Monitor laboratory results: blood alcohol, pulse oximetry, ABGs, toxicology screen for other medications/drugs, and urine for ketones.	Serum toxicology screens will help to determine the extent of the overdose and evaluate response to treatment. Pulse oximetry and ABGs provide evidence to support the diagnosis of ineffective breathing pattern and may yield decreased levels of oxygen and poor oxygen saturation. Variations in acid/base balance
	may be noted including respiratory alkalosis caused by the increased elimination of carbon dioxide via hyperventilation.
Establish IV access and administer IV fluids, as ordered.	Provides a means to administer emergency medications and to improve hydration status. In addition, increased circulatory volume may dilute the ingested or injected substances.
If respiratory assessment reveals deterioration, assist with mechanical ventilation.	Severe respiratory depression and progressive deterioration in respiratory status necessitate ventilatory assistance.

NIC *Respiratory monitoring*
Oxygen therapy
Positioning

Evaluation

The patient should show indications that his or her breathing pattern has returned to baseline and is effective in meeting the body's need for oxygen. The rate should return to baseline, preferably between 12 to 24 breaths per minute, and be unlabored. Cheyne-Stokes respirations or tachypnea should be resolved. The return of ABGs and pulse oximetry to the patient's baseline or to within normal range should be expected.

Community/Home Care

For the patient who experienced an overdose, immediate needs have been resolved prior to discharge. In most cases, breathing patterns and respiratory function have returned to normal, and no home care is indicated specifically. However, prior to discharge to the home setting, attention is diverted to psychosocial needs, with evaluations made to determine whether the patient's overdose was a suicide attempt and/or a coping mechanism, or whether this was a one-time accidental occurrence. If substances such as alcohol or illegal drugs are being abused, professional counseling is needed in the form of treatment programs or counseling (see nursing care plans "Alcohol Withdrawal" and "Substance Abuse"). Follow-up care should focus on treatment of the patient's most pressing psychosocial problems.

Documentation

Chart the results of a comprehensive assessment of the respiratory systems. Note respiratory rate, rhythm (Cheyne-Stokes or normal), chest expansion, use of any accessory muscles, breath sounds, and results of ABGs and pulse oximetry. Include in the patient's chart all interventions employed to address ineffective breathing pattern (oxygen, positioning) and the patient's responses to the interventions that would indicate the problem has been resolved. Document whether the outcome criteria have been met, and if the patient's breathing is no better, indicate how the plan has been revised.

NURSING DIAGNOSIS 3

INEFFECTIVE AIRWAY CLEARANCE

Related to:

Decreased level of consciousness

Inability to spontaneously clear secretions

High likelihood of emesis

Defining Characteristics:

Vomiting

Respiratory depression

Decreased oxygen levels

Labored respirations

Goal:

The patient maintains effective, open airway.

Outcome Criteria

✔ The patient has oxygen saturation > 90 percent.

✔ The patient's breath sounds are clear.

✔ The patient does not aspirate gastric contents.

NOC *Respiratory status: Airway patency*
Respiratory status: Ventilation

INTERVENTIONS	RATIONALES
Observe the patient carefully for the need for airway adjuncts.	The patient who has experienced an overdose of any substance is at an increased risk for airway obstruction due to aspiration of stomach contents secondary to
	CNS depression; airway adjuncts will protect the airway.
Elevate head of bed.	Helps to reduce risk of aspiration by keeping stomach contents in the stomach by gravity.
Assess respiratory status: breath sounds, respiratory rate, presence of cyanosis, wheezing, oxygen saturation, and ABGs.	Helps to establish baseline, to detect unobserved aspiration, and to monitor response to interventions; cyanosis indicates decreased oxygenation, crackles may be present due to the presence of foreign substances in the lungs, and wheezing occurs due to narrowed airways.
Monitor patient for signs of aspiration: coughing, vomiting of gastric contents, and cyanosis.	Airway may obstruct without the patient being able to notify health care worker due to CNS depression.
Try to determine what type substances the patient has taken.	Helps to determine the most appropriate mode of treatment and ascertain if emesis is likely or even dangerous. Aspiration occurs frequently when overdose patients vomit. Emesis can further erode the esophagus depending on the substance.
Administer humidified oxygen, as ordered.	Improves oxygenation and reduce risk of hypoxia due to CNS depression.
Give anti-emetics as ordered.	Reduces risk of vomiting, which would predispose the patient to aspiration.
Monitor for signs and symptoms of respiratory infection: fever, rales, increased mucous production, elevated white blood cell (WBC) count, and chest x-ray reports.	Aspiration pneumonia may occur; early detection is needed to initiate treatment early and prevent complications.
Keep suction equipment at bedside and ready for immediate use; suction as needed.	The sedative effect of many drugs decreases the natural cough reflex that would occur if the patient vomits; decreased levels of consciousness and relaxation of the oropharyngeal muscles add to the risk of aspiration. Suctioning is needed to clear the airway.

NIC *Aspiration precautions*
Airway management
Respiratory monitoring
Oxygen therapy

Evaluation

Assess the client to determine the extent to which the outcome criteria have been met. The patient's airway should be clear, and the patient should be able to cough with expectoration of secretions. Nausea and vomiting are controlled, and the risk for aspiration has been decreased. Breath sounds should be clear, and there should be no cyanosis. Oxygen saturation should be > 90 percent, and blood gases should be within normal range. If criteria have not been met, determine if expected outcomes were realistic or maybe needs more time for achievement. In this case, note the degree of progress the patient is making towards meeting the goals.

Community/Home Care

Once the patient has been treated for the acute symptoms of overdose, the risk for ineffective airway clearance and risk for aspiration should no longer exist. No specific care will be required for this problem, but attention is given to educating the patient on the effects of overdose of the identified substance. The care provider should investigate the need for professional counseling. Family members at home will need to face the reality of the dilemma of overdose and not trivialize it, which would prevent the patient from receiving assistance for psychological problems.

Documentation

Document a comprehensive respiratory assessment. Include in the patient record all interventions carried out for the patient and the patient's responses, with medications documented on the medication administration record. Note specifically the presence of vomiting, secretions, and whether the patient has needed suctioning. Document a description of any emesis or suctioned secretions. If the patient is alert and able to participate in expectorating emesis, document this in the chart. Vital signs should be documented according to agency protocol. Any teaching initiated should be charted with a clear indication of what was taught and to whom.

NURSING DIAGNOSIS 4

INEFFECTIVE INDIVIDUAL COPING

Related to:

Loss of control

Lack of a support system

Depression

Feelings of worthlessness

Suicidal ideations

Stress

Defining Characteristics:

Expressions of fear and anxiety

Expressed worry about ability to cope

Verbalization of substance abuse as a coping strategy

Patient/family denial

Intentional overdose

Goal:

The patient is able to express feelings and ability to cope.

The patient is referred to the appropriate caregivers for follow-up, discharge, and immediate and long-range planning.

Outcome Criteria

✔ The patient identifies and uses one acceptable coping strategy.

✔ The patient verbalizes fears and concerns.

✔ The patient expresses a willingness to seek assistance for life problems (depression, stress, substance abuse, etc.).

NOC *Comfort level*
Coping
Health-seeking behavior

INTERVENTIONS	RATIONALES
Assess patient for expressions of fear, anxiety, negative self-statements, and other indicators of ineffective coping.	When patients experience an overdose, the emotional response can vary greatly; the nurse needs to note specific expressions to establish a starting point for interventions.
Encourage the patient to verbalize feelings regarding current status and what has happened to cause hospitalization, and any fears or concerns. Listen attentively and be nonjudgmental in approach.	Verbalization of feelings, fears, and concerns contributes to dealing with the issue of overdose; being attentive relays empathy to the patient.

(continues)

(continued)

INTERVENTIONS	RATIONALES
Obtain complete history of the overdose event: What was taken? When? How much? Is it a substance the patient is abusing?	The answers to these questions provide background information on the event and clues to the extent of the problem. The patient may have suddenly found him or herself unable to cope due to a particular stressor.
Assist the patient with relaxation techniques: deep breathing, mental imagery, meditation, music therapy, and spiritual practices.	Relaxation techniques can help to reduce anxiety and assist the patient to be open to learning and developing new coping skills.
Keep the patient informed of all that is going on, explaining about symptoms that are occurring and necessary interventions.	Communicating what is going on helps to allay anxiety and fear.
Stay with the patient during any acute symptoms and allow other visitors as requested by the patient.	Helps to provide emotional support and promote a sense of comfort.
Ask the patient to identify all strategies that have been used in the past to cope with stressful events.	Strategies that have previously worked can be used as a starting point for coping with more serious stressful events, and can help the patient focus.
Arrange for psychosocial/ psychiatric consult for counseling.	It is important to assess the psychosocial situation and assess for potential for suicide; to plan for the appropriate contracts between the patient and health care worker and family members; and to ensure that the appropriate follow-up care is arranged.
Assist with the development of new skills and strategies for coping.	For patients who have overdosed, new strategies for coping are required and may include physical activity such as working out at a gym, talking to a religious leader, writing in a journal, using a hotline, etc. If new strategies are not in place, the patient may once again overdose when future stressors appear with a different outcome (death). The new strategies may need to be more sophisticated than those a generalist nurse is able to offer.
Encourage patient/family to directly confront the overdose behavior and seek assistance.	Acknowledgement of a problem is the first step to resolution. Denial of the fact that the patient has overdosed leads to co-dependency.
Assist the patient in identifying those factors that triggered the need to take enough of a substance large enough for an overdose, such as family problems, financial problems, or problems at work.	When the triggers are identified, encourage the patient to seek psychosocial support to reduce risk of a subsequent overdose.
Recognize the role of cultural and religious beliefs in a patient's method of coping with stressors.	Culture often dictates how a person copes with stressors and needs to be incorporated into the plan of care.
If the overdose is one of alcohol or illegal drugs, offer assistance through Alcoholics Anonymous (AA) or drug rehabilitation support groups.	Excessive use of alcohol or drugs may be a symptom of greater psychosocial need and represent the patient's only method of coping with life events; and the patient may need continued assistance with coping skills.
Seek religious or spiritual consult as needed or requested by the patient and or family.	Meeting the patient's spiritual needs helps the patient cope with fears through use of spiritual or religious rituals; provides support.
Set limits on the patient's behavior, and monitor interaction with health care team.	Patients who abuse substances often display manipulative behavior and are unable to establish limits.

NIC *Counseling*
Coping enhancement
Emotional support
Spiritual support

Evaluation

Evaluate the extent to which the outcome criteria have been achieved. The patient should be assessed for appropriate coping skills/strategies that can be used to deal with life stressors. Concerns, fears, and feelings of being able to cope should be detected in the patient. The patient's ability to verbalize the nature of his or her problems will be a starting point for developing new coping strategies. If, however, the patient is unable to admit to abusing substances or overdosing as a way of coping and expresses a desire to use other coping strategies, the nurse should explore further the need for new interventions to assist the patient, such as psychiatric evaluation.

Community/Home Care

A major factor in achieving positive outcomes following an overdose is education on the effects of the substance used for an overdose on the body. Often the patient is unaware of the untoward long-term complications that can occur when one overdoses. Successful teaching should have as an end result the patient's enrollment in some program that can assist the patient to discontinue alcohol or substance abuse, if this is the issue. Community programs such as AA or drug rehabilitation programs can provide support for the transition from overdose and abuse to abstinence. The availability of social supports in the community or at home is required to help the patient comply with recommendations for refraining from improper use of any substance. The provider that follows the patient once acute symptoms of overdose are resolved should assist the patient to learn and use an alternative method of coping with stressors. Nurses, counselors, or other providers should help the patient to identify areas of his or her life that may be contributing to a perceived need to use substances inappropriately, such as interpersonal relationships, work environment, or home environment. Recognition of problem areas is the first step towards taking charge of life and implementing strategies for coping that are more appropriate. Having the support of others enhances the patient's sense of well-being. Follow-up with social workers, counselors, or other health care workers is needed to ensure that the patient is not experiencing new or continued difficulties with coping.

Documentation

Document an assessment of the patient's emotional state including the subjective symptoms and physiological signs of anxiety (pacing, restlessness) and complaints of fear or being out of control. Any verbalizations regarding coping strategies previously used should be included in the chart. Document whether the patient has met the outcome criteria, especially the identification of new coping strategies. If referrals are made, include these in the patient chart. Document if the patient indicates a willingness to comply with health care recommendations, particularly attendance at counseling sessions or community programs. For the patient who may be prescribed medication for depression, document his or her understanding of the medication and its side effects.

CHAPTER 13.142

SUBSTANCE ABUSE

GENERAL INFORMATION

Substance abuse is a maladaptive pattern of use of substances (pharmacological or alcohol) that leads to impairment or distress. The patient demonstrates one of the following behaviors within a 12-month time frame: inability to carry out responsibilities of work, school, or home; uses drugs in situations when it is hazardous to do so; repeated legal problems related to substance use; and continued uses of the substance even though the drug use has caused social problems or made existing problems worse. Numerous pharmacological agents are abused. Some may be over-the-counter, some prescription, and some illegal. Regardless of the chemical composition of the drug, the patient is taking the drug for recreational purposes, in excess of prescribed dosages, or simply to experiment. The person who abuses drugs may have physical problems, psychological problems, or behavioral problems, and may report numerous reasons for abuse of the substance. The key to successful treatment of the problem is to identify the reason for the abuse. Each person is different and will respond to attempts at addressing or treating the abuse based on their developmental stage, culture/ethnicity, personality, and experiences. For this reason, health care providers must remember that all efforts at treatment must be highly individualized considering all of these factors. Substance abuse occurs across all age groups, socioeconomic strata, educational levels, and ethnic groups, and presents with a variety of psychological and possible physiological manifestations.

NURSING DIAGNOSIS 1

INEFFECTIVE INDIVIDUAL COPING

Related to:

Substance abuse

Low self-esteem

Stressors in life

Lack of coping strategies

Defining Characteristics:

Expressions of fear and anxiety

Expressed worry about ability to cope

Verbalization of substance abuse as a coping strategy

Denial

Previous attempts to detoxify

Unwillingness to accept responsibility for own actions

Reports inability to handle stressful situations

Goal:

The patient is able to express feelings and ability to cope.

Outcome Criteria

✔ The patient identifies and uses one acceptable coping strategy.

✔ The patient verbalizes fears and concerns.

✔ The patient expresses a desire for assistance and willingness to seek assistance for substance abuse.

✔ The patient recognizes personal responsibility for drug abuse.

NOC *Comfort level*

Coping

Health-seeking behavior

INTERVENTIONS	RATIONALES
Caringly confront patient with reality of drug abuse.	Denial is a major focus of drug abusers. Caring confrontation may cause the patient to look at the situation.

INTERVENTIONS	RATIONALES
Continue reassuring, caring, nonjudgmental attitude toward the patient to establish your honesty and directness.	Letting the patient know that you care and that you are not passing judgment on him or her can help develop a trusting relationship that is needed in order to assist the patient.
Encourage the patient to accept reality and praise the patient when he or she begins to discuss issues openly.	Anyone who is having difficulty accepting reality will need much positive feedback to continue with efforts.
Set limits and be firm.	Let the patient know that you are there to help, but only under certain conditions.
Assess patient for expressions of fear, anxiety, negative self-statements, and other indicators of ineffective coping.	When patients experience substance abuse, the emotional response can vary greatly; the nurse needs to note specific expressions to establish a starting point for interventions.
Encourage the patient to verbalize feelings regarding status and what has happened to cause hospitalization/institutionalization and any fears or concerns. Listen attentively and be nonjudgmental in approach.	Verbalization of feelings, fears, and concerns contributes to dealing with the issue of substance abuse. Attentiveness relays empathy to the patient.
Assess the patient's level of substance use or abuse as a coping strategy, including types of substances abused, how long substance has been abused, routes of administration, amount taken, what triggered abuse, etc. Use screening tools where available.	A thorough history of the abuse is required for effective treatment and establishes the seriousness of the problem. Keep in mind that the patient may not provide accurate information and may minimize the problem in terms of amount of substance used and length of time that substance has been used. Established tools offer a more objective measure of determining dependence and are easy to use.
Assist the patient with relaxation techniques: deep breathing, mental imagery, meditation, music therapy, and spirituality.	Relaxation techniques can help to reduce anxiety and assist patient to be open to learning and adapting new coping skills.
Keep the patient informed of all that is going on, explaining about symptoms that are occurring and necessary interventions.	Communicating what is going on helps to allay anxiety and fear.
Stay with the patient during acute withdrawal symptoms.	Helps to provide emotional support and promote a sense of comfort.
Ask the patient to identify all strategies other than substance abuse used in the past to cope with stressful events.	Strategies other than substance abuse that have previously worked can be used as a starting point for coping with serious stressful events, and can help the patient focus.
Assist with the development of new skills and strategies for coping, including referral to a professional counselor or help groups such as 12-step programs.	For patients who are substance abusers, new strategies for coping may be required during times of withdrawal. These new strategies may be more sophisticated than those a generalist nurse is able to offer.
Provide reassurance and encouragement for efforts to stop substance abuse.	Encouragement and reassurance help to provide patient with "energy" to succeed. Health care providers should remember that the patient may not be successful on first attempts to give up substance abuse.
Encourage the patient and family to confront addiction directly.	Acknowledgement of addiction is the first step to recovery. Co-dependency must be discouraged. The health care provider must reject the patient's efforts to blame others.
Assist patient in identifying those factors that trigger the need for substances, for example, family problems, financial problems, or problems at work.	When the triggers are identified, encourage the patient to seek psychosocial support to reduce risk of return to substance abuse.
Recognize the role of cultural and religious beliefs in a patient's method of coping with stressors and particularly substance abuse.	Culture often dictates how a person copes with stressors and particularly issues that have a negative social stigma.
Provide counseling referrals for the immediate time but for long-term assistance as well.	Substance abuse may be a symptom of a greater psychosocial need and may represent the patient's only method of coping with life events; the patient may need continued assistance with coping skills.
Seek spiritual consult as needed or requested by the patient and or family.	Meeting spiritual needs of the patient helps the patient cope with fears through use of spiritual or religious rituals for coping; provides support.
Set limits on patients behavior and interaction with health care team.	Patients who are substance abusers often display manipulative behavior and are unable to establish limits.

NIC *Substance use treatment*
Counseling
Support system enhancement
Coping enhancement
Emotional support
Spiritual support

Evaluation

Evaluate the extent to which the outcome criteria have been achieved. The patient should be assessed for appropriate coping skills/strategies that can be used to deal with life stressors. Concerns, fears, and feelings are expressed, and a sense of being able to cope should be detected in the patient. The patient's ability to verbalize the nature of the substance abuse problem will be a beginning point for developing new coping strategies. If, however, the patient is unable to admit to substance abuse as a way of coping and express a desire to use other coping strategies, the nurse should explore further the need for new interventions to assist the patient.

Community/Home Care

The patient who has experienced substance abuse should be encouraged to identify other coping strategies that have been successful in the past and prompted to use them at home. The patient should be able to communicate fears and feelings about withdrawal/hospitalization. Many patients who go through withdrawal will return to substance abuse if not equipped to deal with simple day-to-day stressors in an appropriate manner. For this reason, health care providers should encourage the patient to attend some type of group meeting such as Alcoholics Anonymous (AA) or to see a professional counselor who can work with the patient on developing coping strategies. Coping through use of support from significant others will be vital to a positive outcome because these supporters can be available for listening when the patient becomes tempted to return to substance abuse habits. Efforts at stopping substance abuse can only be successful if the patient can find other ways to cope that are socially desirable. Other avenues of dealing with stressors such as those found in the workplace or home include exercising, relaxation, engaging in physical labor around the house, gardening, using hotlines, and undergoing spiritual consultation. In some instances, the patient will need to refrain from fraternizing with previous acquaintances or associates who may still be engaged in substance-abuse behaviors. In remote rural areas where no AA groups or other support groups meet, local clergy may be a source of counseling services. Having the support of others enhances the patient's sense of well-being. Follow-up with social workers, counselors, or other health care workers is needed to ensure that the patient is not experiencing new or continued difficulties with substance abuse.

Documentation

Include in the patient's record the information obtained by the health care providers relevant to abuse history. Document an assessment of the patient's emotional state including the subjective symptoms of anxiety and physiological signs of anxiety (pacing, restlessness) and complaints of fear. Any verbalizations regarding coping strategies previously used should be included in the chart. Document whether the patient has met the outcome criteria, especially the identification of new coping strategies to replace substance abuse. Document the patient's willingness to be compliant with counseling recommendations and treatment programs. If referrals are made, include these in the patient's chart.

NURSING DIAGNOSIS 2

 RISK FOR POISONING

Related to:

Ingestion of toxic substance

Ingestion of large dosage of substance being abused

Inability to clear substance from body

Defining Characteristics:

None

Goal:

The patient's risk of poisoning/toxicity is reduced.

Outcome Criteria

✔ The patient will have no signs of drug toxicity.

✔ The patient will have vital signs within normal/ baseline range.

✔ The patient will have indications of hemodynamic stability (renal function, respiratory status, cardiovascular status, and neurological status).

Risk control: Drug use
Personal safety behavior

INTERVENTIONS	RATIONALES
Monitor laboratory and diagnostic tests: complete blood count (CBC), serum electrolytes, urine toxicology screen, serum toxicology screen, and others as ordered, depending upon suspected or known drug of abuse or specific signs and symptoms.	These tests provide information on hemodynamic state and effect of drug on vital organs; toxicology screens provide information on amount of specific drugs in the body, which alerts health care providers to the extent of the problem.
Perform a respiratory assessment: monitor respiratory rate, rhythm, depth; pulse oximetry; and arterial blood gases (ABGs).	Many substances, legal and illegal, alter the respiratory system, particularly causing respiratory depression; a good assessment is required to determine abnormalities or establish baselines.
Perform a cardiovascular assessment: blood pressure (low to high), pulse (from bradycardia to tachycardia), dysrhythmias, and electrocardiogram (EKG) changes.	Many substances that are abused, especially illegal drugs, have the potential to alter the cardiovascular system. The abnormalities vary widely dependent upon the substance; the health care provider needs this information to determine specific effects and establish baselines.
Perform a neurological assessment: level of consciousness, motor activity, reflexes, tremors, seizures, hypo- or hyperesthesia, and pain.	Helps to determine the effect if any on neurological functioning; many substances can depress or excite the central nervous system (CNS).
Perform a gastrointestinal (GI)/ genitourinary (GU) assessment: urinary output, bowel activity, abdominal pain, dietary/fluid intake, and appetite/anorexia.	Many substances that are abused affect kidney function and GI performance as well as alter appetite, and often the patient replaces diet intake with drugs.
Administer specific antidote for ingested drug, as ordered, if an overdose is suspected.	If a drug of abuse has a specific antidote, it should be given as soon as possible.
If an overdose is suspected, perform gastric lavage, as ordered.	Helps to remove undigested substances and to prevent further absorption of the drug and poisoning.
Administer activated charcoal, as ordered.	If the abuse has led to overdose or near overdose, charcoal is given to bind certain chemicals.

Monitor the patient's response to interventions.	Helps to determine effectiveness and whether the plan of care requires revision.
Teach the patient and family the signs and symptoms of poisoning relevant to the substance that has been abused.	The patient needs to be aware of signs of poisoning in order to seek appropriate health care assistance. Recognizing the dangers of substance abuse in terms of effects on vital organs may cause the patient to seek help for the problem of substance abuse.

Substance use treatment:
Drug withdrawal
Substance use treatment
Surveillance: Safety
Vital signs monitoring

Evaluation

Determine whether the patient has achieved the outcome criteria as stated. The patient demonstrates no signs or symptoms of drug toxicity, and all assessments of system function are normal. All vital signs have returned to the patient's baseline. The patient is aware of the role of substance abuse in causing poisoning and expresses a willingness to seek appropriate help with substance abuse problem.

Community/Home Care

Whether the patient remains at risk for poisoning following contact with the health care system will depend on the patient's ability to cease substance abuse. The patient needs to be aware of the signs and symptoms of poisoning in order to seek early treatment and avoid serious complications. The best method for addressing the problem of risk for poisoning would be to work with the patient and other health care disciplines to locate substance abuse treatment programs that will provide long-term assistance to the patient. Follow-up with the patient and family is needed to monitor the patient's progress with cessation of the substance abuse and maintenance of self-esteem. The patient needs to establish acceptable coping strategies to use in stressful situations of life including work and family and have a means of seeking support. There is a high probability that the patient will discontinue treatment and counseling that has been recommended for substance abuse and then return to a life of substance abuse. A key point for patient and family to know is that the abrupt discontinuance of some medications prescribed to treat withdrawal from certain substances can precipitate withdrawal symptoms such as seizures, tremors, and confusion. Follow-up through an outpatient clinic or with a home-visiting organization is required to ensure that the patient is able to implement recommendations for successful cessation of substance abuse.

Documentation

Chart the findings from an assessment of neurological, cardiovascular, respiratory, and GI/GU systems, with specific attention to the presence of signs and symptoms of poisoning. Because of the variable changes with the different substances, documentation of even small changes in the vital signs in a timely fashion is important for care decisions. They should be documented according to agency protocol and may be included in the notes as well as on the graphic sheets. Any subjective reports of signs or symptoms or complaints are recorded in the notes as the patient states them. All interventions carried out to reduce the risk of poisoning, to monitor for poisoning, or to treat poisoning, and the patient's responses to these interventions are always included in the patient record. When medications are initiated to treat possible withdrawal symptoms, this is charted according to agency protocol for medication administration.

NURSING DIAGNOSIS 3

SITUATIONAL LOW SELF-ESTEEM

Related to:

Use of drug(s) of abuse

Ineffective coping

Weak ego

Lack of life skills

Lack of family or support group

Defining Characteristics:

Expressed shame and guilt

Lack of or poor problem solving ability

Unkempt physical appearance

Verbalizations of negative self-talk

Verbalization of no control over situation

Expressions of powerlessness/hopelessness

Goal:

The patient returns to a positive self-esteem.

Outcome Criteria

✔ The patient will replace negative self-talk with positive self-talk.

✔ The patient will state one positive thing about him or herself.

✔ The patient identifies leisure activities that are healthy and productive.

✔ The patient will state one strategy to use to remedy the situation.

✔ The patient states a willingness to seek assistance for substance abuse problem.

NOC   *Self-esteem*
Social interaction skills

INTERVENTIONS	RATIONALES
Assess the patient's self-esteem by noting any negative talk regarding self.	People who are substance abusers often have little positive to say of themselves and may start negative talk about themselves even in areas not related to substance abuse. The nurse needs to be attuned to these comments in order to intervene appropriately.
Assess the patient's understanding of substance abuse and what is required to stop the abuse and move forward.	The patient will need to understand the definition and mechanism of substance abuse and will need to be assisted in moving forward with life and establishment of coping strategies that can enhance self-esteem.
Encourage patient to share thoughts; be nonjudgmental and be a good listener; encourage verbalization of feelings about substance abuse and allow patient to talk about self and his or her overall life.	If the patient feels that there is someone who cares and who is concerned, he or she may begin to speak about issues that have brought about the drug abuse situation. Acknowledging the reality of the situation will help the patient assume responsibility for his or her actions. A review of life will assist the patient to identify the positive aspects of the self-esteem and not dwell on the negative events.

INTERVENTIONS	RATIONALES
Be empathetic and non-judgmental, listening attentively to the patient, and be aware of concerns.	Listening to the patient will help to identify opportunities for further interventions. Because of the stigma attached to substance abuse, it is important that the health care provider remain nonjudgmental.
Discuss ways drugs have made the situation worse instead of better.	Drugs are used as an excuse to not face reality. Sometimes when this is heard by the patient, amazing movement toward recovery may occur.
Help the patient identify personal strengths and mobilize coping strategies (see nursing diagnosis "Ineffective Individual Coping").	Discussions like this will help the patient to cope with the situation and enhance self-esteem.
Collaborate with physician to provide referral for counseling as needed and arrange for support group participation.	Peer acceptance is crucial for the patient. Participation in a support group will direct attention away from self. Substance abuse is often characterized by dependency, and in order to successfully cope with this and return to a usual state of self-esteem, professional counseling over an extended period of time may be required.
Encourage the patient to keep a diary and to record positive aspects of him or herself and his or her life.	Helps the patient to focus on the positive and on feelings of self-worth that should enhance rebuilding of self-esteem.
Have the patient identify one social activity that he or she can participate in that will help demonstrate a positive self and return the patient to a normal state of social interaction.	Patients who are substance abusers may isolate themselves from normal social activities and family for fear of discovery of the abuse; this further decreases self-esteem.
Help the patient to identify what role religion or culture plays in his or her perception of self as it relates to self-esteem.	Culture and religion often influence how one perceives self, especially when one is engaging in undesirable behaviors such as substance abuse. Recognizing this can help the patient and nurse plan activities to address the issue.

NIC *Self-esteem enhancement*
Presence
Emotional support
Socialization enhancement

Evaluation

The patient is able to verbalize feelings regarding self-worth or self-esteem. The patient refrains from negative self-talk and replaces negative talk with positive comments regarding self. A positive outcome reveals that the patient talks about him or herself and identifies personal strengths that can be mobilized to assist with coping. The patient verbalizes a need for professional help to enhance self-esteem and end substance abuse. The patient should verbalize that he or she feels able to deal with the substance abuse and is in control of his or her life.

Community/Home Care

Situational low self-esteem can continue for a varied period of time. The patient can return to his or her previous level of self-esteem with the assistance of supportive family or significant others, through counseling, or sometimes through reliance on religious or spiritual practices. Because of the profound effect that substance abuse may have on a person and his or her family, continued monitoring of the self-esteem should be undertaken to detect any abnormal or morbid responses. The issue of self-esteem can be worsened if the person stops the substance abuse but has no way of coping with stressors in his or her life. Once in the home environment or community, the person may be tempted to return to a life of substance abuse when interacting with friends. If the person does not identify positive aspects of his or her life and engage in social activities that reinforce the positive, remaining free of substance abuse may be difficult, recidivism occurs, and a vicious cycle of low self-esteem begins. Restoration of self-esteem may occur only after a number of stressful periods in which the patient doubts his or her self-worth but is able to move forward by participation in counseling and support groups. The patient will need specific information on treatment programs that are available to him or her in terms of geographic region, financial resources, and time. Follow-up with a social worker may be more appropriate after referral to community agencies for these services. The nurse or other health care provider who sees the patient for follow-up will need to be alert to subtle hints that may indicate that the patient has not improved his or her self-esteem and has returned to negative lifestyles.

Documentation

Document the progress the patient has made towards meeting outcome criteria. A thorough assessment of the patient's psychological state should be charted, including specific statements made by the patient that indicate negative or positive self-esteem. Include any verbalizations by the patient that indicate a state of powerlessness such as "I can't do anything about it," "that's just the way it is," or self-negating statements. If the nurse detects difficulties with coping, interacting with family/significant other, or verbalizations of reactions and feelings about the substance abuse, this should be included in the patient's chart. All referrals should be documented.

NURSING DIAGNOSIS 4

INEFFECTIVE HEALTH MAINTENANCE

Related to:

Lack of motivation

Ineffective coping

Altered social interaction/communication skills

Drug abuse

Lack of knowledge

Lack of availability of assistance for drug problem

Defining Characteristics:

Failed efforts for cessation of substance abuse

Verbalizations of inability to manage health issues

Verbalizations of drug abuse problem

Goal:

The patient will verbalize a willingness to change habits.

Outcome Criteria

✔ The patient states the effect that substance abuse has on health.

✔ The patient will report a willingness to comply with health recommendations.

✔ The patient will enroll in a substance abuse cessation program.

NOC *Adherence behavior*
   Knowledge: Treatment regimen

Health-seeking behaviors
Knowledge: Substance use control

INTERVENTIONS	RATIONALES
Take a history of the drug abuse problem: how often used, how much used, triggering factors, past experiences with attempting cessation, and type of substances abused.	A history will give the nurse a place to begin with planning care to enhance health maintenance.
Assess the patient's understanding regarding substance abuse, seriousness of the problem and the dangers it brings, and the family's understanding of the patient's abuse problem.	This will provide a starting point for education on the dangers of substance abuse and the type of interventions required.
Assess the patient's current financial status, including employment status and work habits.	Many patients who are substance abusers have financial difficulties due in part to using finances to support the habit of substance abuse and because of absences from work due to abuse or termination from employment. Resources for health promotion may not be available.
Assess for other health problems or issues such as nutritional status, dental health, or hypertension.	Often basic health may be neglected due to substance abuse, and any contact with a health care provider is an opportunity to initiate change in health behaviors.
Encourage the patient to identify those people who have influence on his or her life and then assist family and patient to begin to identify enabling behaviors.	Family and friends may engage in enabling activities that prevent the patient from stopping substance abuse. The family may not be aware of enabling behaviors or may not know how to avoid the enabling behaviors.
Teach the patient about substance abuse, including — Review of the definition of substance abuse and dependence — Use of substance abuse as a coping strategy — Ability of substance abuse to alter perception of reality — Substance abuse becomes a priority that prevents one from recognizing the other important aspects of life and giving attention to health care needs	The patient and family need to know detailed factual information about substance abuse and its treatment, and should be aware of the dangers of substance abuse so that informed decisions can be made regarding treatment.

INTERVENTIONS	RATIONALES

— Types of treatment programs available

— Drugs used to treat substance abuse

— The effect of substance abuse on all body systems and the resulting negative health states such as changes in blood pressure and pulse, EKG changes, decreased appetite and taste, altered motor responses

Portray an expectation that the patient will comply with recommendations for treatment of substance abuse problem.	Substance abuse, if left untreated, will continue to affect the patient's entire life; attending treatment programs is an indicator of the patient's recognition of the problem.
Collaborate with the social worker to identify treatment programs that are available to the patient and within his or her means to pay.	Treatment programs must be accessible and affordable to enhance compliance.
Encourage and praise small progressive steps towards cessation.	Praise will do much to give the patient the courage to continue.
Monitor for noncompliance with treatment regimen through questioning and drug screens (urine and serum), as ordered.	Helps to determine if the patient is remaining drug-free, and if not, to intervene to get the patient back on target with therapeutic regimen.
Have the patient establish healthy leisure activities to replace substance abuse.	It is more difficult to abstain from substance abuse during recovery if there are no leisure or diversional activities to engage in when the person is tempted to relapse.

NIC *Substance use treatment*
Financial resource assistance
Counseling

Evaluation

The patient has met all outcome criteria. The patient and family are able to discuss what substance abuse is and how it is treated. Effects that substance abuse has on overall health are verbalized, and the patient reports a desire to practice health-promoting behaviors. Following contact with the health care system, the patient verbalizes a willingness to enroll in a substance abuse treatment program.

Community/Home Care

Effective health maintenance for the person involved in substance abuse will continue to be a problem for an extended period of time with subsequent difficulty maintaining a healthy state. Often the abused substances take a priority in the scheme of life to the detriment of other issues. Efforts to engage in healthy behaviors may be met with disdain from the person's circle of friends who remain abusers. It is crucial that the patient has developed strategies that enable him or her to be firm and remain focused on rehabilitation. However, if the patient is not motivated to change his or her health habits and stop the substance abuse, any action by family and health care providers will probably be in vain, for the patient has to be ready for life changes. Outlets for expressions of feelings and relief of stress need to be in place so that when they are needed the patient can use them readily rather than using the abused substance. Suggested methods to recommend to the patient include exercising, community service, sports, civic or religious activities, meditation, art therapy, music therapy, or more family time. The support of the family and significant others is vital to the patient's ability to successfully complete treatment programs. Friends, family, and significant others need to support the patient as he or she tries to overcome substance abuse. The patient needs to be educated on what substance abuse is and the effect it has on health in general. Factual information can be shared verbally and in written form with periods for questions and answers that allow the patient to ascertain exactly what is required for treatment. The most successful means for cessation of substance abuse is enrollment in a structured treatment program that can be inpatient or outpatient. However, many sources recommend that the patient seek inpatient treatment in order to avoid contact with acquaintances who may still be abusers and who tempt the patient during times of vulnerability. Maintaining health as it relates to substance abuse places responsibility on self to engage in health-promoting behaviors. There will be times when the patient needs encouragement and conversation. Hotlines and community support groups can play a role here to provide support and encouragement when the patient is tempted with relapse.

Documentation

Document whether the patient has met the outcome criteria. Chart the results of a complete history of the substance abuse including the substance or substances abused, the length of time the abuse has been going on, prior experience with treatment efforts, etc. Also include the results of a health history and physical examination to detect physiological alterations in health status. The patient's verbalization of any information regarding substance abuse is documented in his or her own words. Teaching is documented, including specific content taught, learners present, and evaluation of understanding. Any referrals made are documented, with pertinent information regarding treatment programs offered to the patient. If urine and serum toxicology screens are done, document the results as required by the agency.

CHAPTER 13.143

SUICIDE: ATTEMPTED/IDEATION

GENERAL INFORMATION

Suicide ideation occurs when a person is thinking about committing suicide. An attempted suicide is when the patient has actually made an attempt to take his or her life. There are numerous risk factors for suicide, including mental illness, alcohol and substance abuse, family history of suicide, previous suicide attempt, major life losses, serious physical illness, and hopelessness, to name a few. There is an increase in suicides in the fall and spring, and suicide attempts are usually successful if the patient has a well-thought-out plan and a weapon. One of the keys to therapeutic intervention in suicide ideation is to determine if the patient has an actual plan and the means to carry out that plan. Suicide is a serious problem in the United States and is the eighth leading cause of death among adults and the third leading cause of death among people aged 15 to 24 years old. Each year in the United States, more than 30,000 people successfully commit suicide. The number of known unsuccessful suicide attempts is staggering, reaching more than a million. In light of these statistics, all suicide attempts must be considered serious. Females attempt suicide more than males; however, males are more successful.

NURSING DIAGNOSIS 1

 RISK FOR SUICIDE

Related to:

Psychiatric illness

Depression

Panic

Hopelessness

Debilitating illness

Terminal illness

Loss of loved one

Divorce

Serious financial problems

Self-esteem disturbance

Defining Characteristics:

Has suicidal ideations with a plan

Attempts suicide

Discusses suicide with others

Expresses despair

Verbalizes that "don't want to live anymore"

Goal:

The patient's risk for self-directed violence is reduced, and suicide is avoided.

Outcome Criteria

✔ The patient verbalizes a feeling of self-worth.

✔ The patient states one way to cope with life.

✔ The patient verbalizes a willingness to attend counseling.

✔ The patient expresses feelings.

NOC *Impulse self-control*
Personal well-being
Suicide self-restraint

INTERVENTIONS	RATIONALES
Take suicide precautions; directly observe the patient via closed camera in a special room or check at least every 15 minutes, if hospitalized.	Suicide precautions include removing all objects from the room that could possibly be harmful to the patient, ensuring that the patient is not left alone, and restraining a patient (physically or chemically) to reduce the possibility of harm to him or herself.

(continues)

(continued)

INTERVENTIONS	RATIONALES
Isolate the patient from others, but place him or her in a room close to the nursing station.	The patient will need a private space that is safe for both the patient and caregiver.
Take a history and assess the patient's risk for completing suicide by asking the following questions: — Have you ever attempted suicide or thought about suicide before? — Do you feel like hurting yourself? — Has anyone in your immediate family committed suicide? — Do you have a plan, and if, so what is it?	Positive responses to these questions indicate a high probability that the threat is serious. If the person has a developed plan, this indicates serious contemplation of suicide.
Identify risk factors for suicide, such as suicidal statements, feeling of extreme happiness, giving personal items away, and history of previous suicide attempts.	These are all predispositions for suicide. When patients are contemplating suicide, they often become happy or euphoric and give away personal items to significant others. Identifying or recognizing these actions can allow for intervention.
Encourage the patient to verbalize feelings.	Helps to begin the process of self-healing and decrease suicidal thoughts.
Consult with a professional psychiatric nurse-counselor.	Specifically trained persons are needed to talk to the patient about reasons for suicide ideation.
Practice presence with the patient.	Often the patient may need someone empathetic, nonjudgmental, and willing to listen, and at times someone to just be present without requiring conversation. Presence may promote a sense of comfort for the patient.
Administer antidepressants, as ordered.	Helps to provide mental rest and to suppress thoughts of personal destruction, panic, anxiety, and hopelessness.
Reevaluate the patient's mental status.	The patient's mental status may change from moment to moment. Be particularly cognizant of a sudden mood change to happy and euphoric, which may indicate that the patient has a suicide plan.
Be sure that the patient takes all medication.	Helps to prevent the possibility of hoarding medications to use later in a suicide attempt.
Develop a written contract for the patient that asks the patient not to harm self.	Helps the patient to assume a sense of responsibility for what happens and portrays a sense of caring from the nurse.

NIC *Suicide prevention*
Behavior management: Self-harm
Crisis intervention
Patient contracting

Evaluation

The patient is kept safe. The patient is able to verbalize feelings with nurses and counselors. Verbalization about self and suicide ideations occurs. The patient discusses intent to refrain from hurting self.

Community/Home Care

In the home environment, the focus is on maintaining a safe environment for the patient with suicide ideation or failed suicide. Any firearms are hidden or locked away where the person cannot locate them, or ammunition is removed from the home. It is difficult to remove all dangerous items since many regular household items, such as kitchen knives, bed sheets, cleaning agents, etc., can be used for suicide. Medications should be locked and hidden away as well, since many agents that are harmless in normal doses can be lethal in large doses. Family and friends will need to be vigilant in their efforts to monitor the patient's actions and whereabouts. All patients who have attempted suicide need structured counseling in order to work through the situation. The nurse or counselor may want to also use a written contract with the patient. The patient should be encouraged to call counselors or to use hotlines in times of crisis when suicidal thoughts occur. Counseling may need to be undertaken on a daily basis until the immediate crisis is over and the patient has more control, and to enhance feelings of self-worth. There is still a stigma attached to suicide; as a result, the family may try hard to conceal the patient's problems, and in the effort isolate the patient more. Close friends and family need to know about the suicide attempt so that if the patient hints at suicide in the future, such statements will be taken seriously. Those around the patient at home should never downplay the patient's comments regarding suicide and should be attuned to subtle hints of suicide, including self-negating comments. All those close to the patient should try to ensure that the patient follows through with all counseling appointments. In instances of teenagers, family as well as individual counseling may be needed.

Documentation

Document comments the patient makes exactly as stated, especially expressed thoughts of suicide. All interventions are charted, including simple sitting with the patient and just talking. All referrals are documented, as are visits by psychiatric specialists or counselors. If wounds are present, document the location along with an assessment of the injury. Medications that are initiated are documented according to agency guidelines for medication administration.

NURSING DIAGNOSIS 2

INEFFECTIVE INDIVIDUAL COPING

Related to:

Low self-esteem

Stressors in life

Lack of coping strategies

Defining Characteristics:

Expresses fear and anxiety

Situational crisis

Expresses worry about ability to cope

Verbalizes suicide ideation

Attempts suicide

Reports inability to handle stressful situations

Goal:

The patient is able to express feelings and to cope.

Outcome Criteria

✔ The patient identifies and uses one acceptable coping strategy.

✔ The patient verbalizes fears and concerns.

✔ The patient expresses a desire for assistance and willingness to seek assistance for suicide ideation or attempt.

✔ The patient accepts personal responsibility for suicide attempt and ideation.

NOC *Suicide self-restraint*
         Coping
         Health-seeking behavior

INTERVENTIONS	RATIONALES
Caringly confront patient with reality of suicide ideation or attempt.	Denial of the seriousness of the problem may be present. Caring confrontation may force the patient to look at the situation.
Assess the patient for causative factors of suicide, such as life stressors.	Identification of stressors or causes of suicide ideation or attempt is the first step towards problem solving.
Assess the patient's available coping strategies and help to identify new ones.	The patient needs to identify how he or she usually copes; new methods of coping may be required during a crisis.
Assess the patient for expressions of fear, anxiety, negative self-statements, and other indicators of ineffective coping.	The emotional response following a suicide attempt can vary greatly; the nurse needs to note specific expressions to establish a starting point for interventions.
Continue reassuring, caring, nonjudgmental attitude toward patient to establish your honesty and directness.	This lets the patient know that you care and that you are not passing judgment on him or her. This can help develop a trusting relationship.
Encourage the patient to verbalize feelings regarding the current situation and assist in identifying those factors that triggered the thoughts of suicide, such as family problems, financial problems, problems at work, or a loss. Listen attentively and be nonjudgmental in approach.	Verbalization of feelings, fears, and concerns contributes to dealing with the issue of suicide. When the triggers are identified, encourage the patient to seek psychosocial support to reduce risk of suicide attempts or ideation. Being attentive relays empathy to the patient.
Assist the patient with relaxation techniques: deep breathing, mental imagery, meditation, music therapy, and spirituality.	Relaxation techniques can help to reduce anxiety and assist the patient to be open to learning and adapting new coping skills.
Assist with the development of new skills and strategies for	For patients who attempt suicide or have suicide ideations,

(continues)

(continued)

INTERVENTIONS	RATIONALES
coping, including referral to a professional counselor or support groups.	new strategies for coping are required during times of stress, as previous coping strategies were ineffective. These new strategies may be more sophisticated than those a generalist nurse is able to offer.
Provide reassurance and encouragement for efforts to deal with suicide ideations/attempts.	Encouragement and reassurance help to provide the patient with "energy" to succeed.
Recognize the role of cultural and religious beliefs in a patient's method of coping with stressors and particularly in how suicide is viewed.	Culture often dictates how a person copes with stressors, and many religions have specific views on suicide.
Provide counseling referrals for the immediate time and for long-term assistance as well.	Suicide ideation or attempts may be a symptom of a greater psychosocial need of the patient and may represent the patient's only method of coping with life events; the patient may need continued assistance with coping skills.
Seek spiritual consult as needed or requested by the patient and/or family.	Meeting the patient's spiritual needs helps him or her cope with fears through use of spiritual or religious rituals for coping; provides support.

NIC   *Counseling*

Support system enhancement

Coping enhancement

Emotional support

Spiritual support

Evaluation

Evaluate the extent to which the outcome criteria have been achieved. The patient should be assessed for appropriate coping skills/strategies that can be used to deal with life stressors. Feelings of being able to cope are expressed by the patient. The patient's ability to verbalize the nature of the suicide attempt/ideation will be a starting point for developing new coping strategies. If, however, the patient is unable to identify why he or she has considered suicide as a way of coping and does not express a desire to use other coping strategies, the nurse should explore further the need for new interventions to assist the patient.

Community/Home Care

The patient who has attempted or considered suicide must be encouraged to identify new coping strategies and prompted to use them at home. The patient should be able to communicate fears and feelings about his or her life. Many patients who have attempted suicide will try again if not equipped to deal with problems once out of the health care system. Patients need to be able to deal with simple day-to-day stressors in an appropriate manner. For this reason, health care providers should encourage the patient to attend some type of counseling session that can work with the patient on developing coping strategies. Coping through use of support from family members and significant others will be vital to a positive outcome because they can be available for listening when the patient becomes tempted to try suicide again. Efforts at resolving the suicide ideation or attempt can only be successful if the patient can find other ways to cope that are socially desirable. Other avenues of dealing with stressors include exercising, relaxation, engaging in physical labor around the house, gardening, using hotlines, and receiving spiritual consultation. In some areas, particularly rural areas, local clergy may be a source of counseling services if no counselors trained to work with suicide attempts are available. Having the support of others enhances the patient's sense of well-being. Follow-up with social workers, counselors, or other health care workers is needed to ensure that the patient is not experiencing new or continued difficulties with managing his or her life.

Documentation

Include in the patient's record the information obtained by the health care providers relevant to the patient's ability to cope and issues related to suicide. Document an assessment of the patient's emotional state, including subjective symptoms and physiological signs of anxiety (pacing, restlessness) and verbalizations that indicate ineffective coping. Include in the patient record whether the patient has met the outcome criteria, especially the identification of new coping strategies. Document the patient's willingness to be compliant with counseling recommendations and treatment programs. If referrals are made, include these in the patient chart.

NURSING DIAGNOSIS 3

HOPELESSNESS

Related to:

Loss

Stressful stimuli

Reason for suicide attempt

Defining Characteristics:

Expresses hopelessness and despair

Expresses a feeling of lacking meaning in life

Has impaired interpersonal relationships

Perceives an impossible situation

Goal:

The patient will state that hopelessness is lessening.

Outcome Criteria

✔ The patient begins to identify those issues that have created the feeling of hopelessness.

✔ The patient begins to problem-solve to identify alternatives to deal with emotions.

✔ The patient verbalizes concerns about life to a professional nurse or counselor.

✔ The patient makes one positive statement about life.

✔ The patient expresses spiritual beliefs and practices.

NOC *Hope*

Coping

Spiritual health

INTERVENTIONS	RATIONALES
Develop a supportive relationship with the patient by expressing concern, a wish to help, and a sense of hope.	The caregiver must be able to assess how serious the patient is about the suicide attempt and the level of hopelessness the patient feels.
Provide a nonjudgmental atmosphere where the patient feels comfortable/safe verbalizing his or her thoughts.	The beginnings of a therapeutic relationship are based on nonjudgmental environments.
Encourage the patient to talk about the events that lead to the suicide decision.	Sometimes simply reliving or reviewing the events verbally will help the patient to identify the irrational thought processes being used.
Help the patient to begin to problem-solve to find healthy alternatives for coping with problems.	If the patient can identify ways to problem-solve, suicide will usually not be the only alternative.
Encourage the patient to participate in valued interpersonal relationships.	Helps to promote psychological well-being and comfort.
Have the patient write down positive aspects of life.	Focuses the patient on identifying reasons to live and self-worth.
Have patient identify any religious or spiritual practices that can be useful in coping with life. Provide privacy or an environment that is conducive to carrying out religious practices.	Many religions have programs or even rituals that help to raise self-esteem or self-worth; spirituality is self-defined but allows the patient to relax and find meaning in life.
Arrange for a consult with a minister or other religious representative, as requested by the patient.	Clergy may be a source of comfort for the patient during a crisis.
Arrange for a psychiatric evaluation and consultation (with a psychiatric clinical nurse specialist or psychiatrist).	Professional help is imperative to assess the suicide risk and to create a plan for therapeutic interventions.
Monitor for progress towards alleviation of hopelessness and spiritual distress.	Helps to determine effectiveness of interventions.

NIC *Hope instillation*

Counseling

Evaluation

The patient begins to have expressions that indicate hope. Through counseling and talking with professionals, the patient is able to begin identification of ways to deal with problems and emotions. Positive verbalizations regarding self-worth and life occur. Following reflection and possible visits from religious or spiritual representatives, the patient is able to participate in religious practices and attempt problem solving.

Community/Home Care

The patient's feelings of hopelessness should be lessened once he or she exits the health care system, but full recovery in this area will require time. The patient needs to be supported in decision making, and family members must allow this to occur. Being able to make decisions gives the patient a sense of control and allows him or her to carry out his or her role responsibility. At home, the patient should have an intact social support network in place who can serve as active, nonjudgmental listeners for the patient when he or she is stressed. Ideally, these people would have been involved in counseling sessions with the patient and aware of appropriate responses when the patient makes negative statements. The patient should continue on at least a weekly basis to do a life review in which he or she documents the positive things in his or her life, possibly listing the good things that had happened during the week. For any problem or negative thought that he or she experiences, the patient should record how he or she deals with it. This information can be used as a way of verbalizing concerns and as a diary of sorts to share with a counselor that may give indications of progress towards eliminating hopelessness. The patient should be encouraged to engage in any religious or spiritual practices that he or she feels are important in his or her life; for these often provide strength for "getting through" and having "hope for tomorrow." An in-home nurse may not be needed, but the patient will need to participate in individual counseling, and in some instances group sessions as well. Follow-up care will assess whether the patient feels better and can see a positive life in the future.

Documentation

Chart whether the patient has met the outcome criteria. Always chart an assessment of the patient's psychological state. Include in the patient record any statements made by the patient in his or her own words. If the patient participates in counseling or has visits from religious leaders, document this in the record. Avoid interjecting opinion into the patient's record.

REFERENCES

Adams, M., Josephson, D., and Holland, L. (2005). *Pharmacology for nurses: A pathophysiologic approach.* Upper Saddle River, NJ: Pearson Prentice Hall.

American Cancer Society. (2005). *Cancer Facts & Figures—2005.* Atlanta: Author.

American Heart Association. (2004). *Heart Disease and Stroke Statistics—2004 Update.* Dallas: Author.

Black, J. and Hawks, J. (2005). *Medical-surgical nursing: Clinical management for positive outcomes.* St. Louis: Elsevier Saunders.

Carpenito-Moyet, L. (2004). *Nursing diagnosis: Application to clinical practice.* (10th ed). Philadelphia: J.B. Lippincott.

Lehne, R. (2004), *Pharmacology for nursing care.* (5th ed). St. Louis: Saunders.

Lemone, P., and Burke, K. (2004). *Medical surgical nursing: Critical thinking in client care.* (3rd ed). Upper Saddle River, NJ: Pearson Prentice Hall.

Lewis, S., Heitkemper, M., and Dirksen, S. (2004). *Medical-surgical nursing: Assessment and management of clinical problems.* (6th ed). St. Louis: Mosby.

McCloskey Dochterman, J., and Bulechek, G. (2004). *Nursing interventions classification (NIC).* (4th ed). St. Louis: Mosby.

Moorhead, S., Johnson, M., and Maas, M. (2004). *Nursing outcomes classification (NOC).* (3rd ed). St. Louis: Mosby.

NANDA International. (2005). *Nursing Diagnoses: Definitions & Classifications 2005–2006.* Philadelphia: Author.

National Heart, Lung, and Blood Institute. (2004). *The seventh report of the Joint National Committee on prevention, detection, evaluation, and treatment of high blood pressure.* Bethesda: National Institutes of Health.

Pagana, K. and Pagana, T. (2005). *Mosby's diagnostic and laboratory test reference.* (7th ed.) St. Louis: Elsevier Mosby.

Phipps, W., Monahan, F., Sands, J., Marek, J., and Neighbors, M. (2003). *Medical surgical nursing: Health and illness perspectives.* (7th ed). St. Louis: Mosby.

APPENDIX A

NANDA NURSING DIAGNOSES 2005–2006

Activity Intolerance
Risk for Activity Intolerance
Impaired Adjustment
Ineffective Airway Clearance
Latex Allergy Response
Risk for Latex Allergy Response
Anxiety
Death Anxiety
Risk for Aspiration
Risk for Impaired Parent/Infant/Child Attachment
Autonomic Dysreflexia
Risk for Autonomic Dysreflexia
Disturbed Body Image
Risk for Imbalanced Body Temperature
Bowel Incontinence
Effective Breastfeeding
Ineffective Breastfeeding
Interrupted Breastfeeding
Ineffective Breathing Pattern
Decreased Cardiac Output
Caregiver Role Strain
Risk for Caregiver Role Strain
Impaired Verbal Communication
Readiness for Enhanced Communication
Decisional Conflict (Specify)
Parental Role Conflict
Acute Confusion
Chronic Confusion
Constipation
Perceived Constipation
Risk for Constipation
Defensive Coping
Ineffective Coping
Readiness for Enhanced Coping
Ineffective Community Coping
Readiness for Enhanced Community Coping
Compromised Family Coping
Disabled Family Coping
Readiness for Enhanced Family Coping
Risk for Sudden Infant Death Syndrome
Ineffective Denial
Impaired Dentition
Risk for Delayed Development
Diarrhea
Risk for Disuse Syndrome

Deficient Diversional Activity
Energy Field Disturbance
Impaired Environmental Interpretation Syndrome
Adult Failure to Thrive
Risk for Falls
Dysfunctional Family Processes: Alcoholism
Interrupted Family Processes
Readiness for Enhanced Family Processes
Fatigue
Fear
Readiness for Enhanced Fluid Balance
Deficient Fluid Volume
Excess Fluid Volume
Risk for Deficient Fluid Volume
Risk for Imbalanced Fluid Volume
Impaired Gas Exchange
Anticipatory Grieving
Dysfunctional Grieving
Risk for Dysfunctional Grieving
Delayed Growth and Development
Risk for Disproportionate Growth
Ineffective Health Maintenance
Health-Seeking Behaviors (Specify)
Impaired Home Maintenance
Hopelessness
Hyperthermia
Hypothermia
Disturbed Personal Identity
Functional Urinary Incontinence
Reflex Urinary Incontinence
Stress Urinary Incontinence
Total Urinary Incontinence
Urge Urinary Incontinence
Risk for Urge Urinary Incontinence
Disorganized Infant Behavior
Risk for Disorganized Infant Behavior
Readiness for Enhanced Organized Infant Behavior
Ineffective Infant Feeding Pattern
Risk for Infection
Risk for Injury
Risk for Perioperative-Positioning Injury
Decreased Intracranial Adaptive Capacity
Deficient Knowledge
Readiness for Enhanced Knowledge (Specify)
Risk for Loneliness

Impaired **M**emory
Impaired Bed **M**obility
Impaired Physical **M**obility
Impaired Wheelchair **M**obility
Nausea
Unilateral **N**eglect
Noncompliance
Imbalanced **N**utrition: Less than Body Requirements
Imbalanced **N**utrition: More than Body Requirements
Readiness for Enhanced **N**utrition
Risk for Imbalanced **N**utrition:
　　More than Body Requirements
Impaired **O**ral Mucous Membrane
Acute **P**ain
Chronic **P**ain
Readiness for Enhanced **P**arenting
Impaired **P**arenting
Risk for Impaired **P**arenting
Risk for **P**eripheral Neurovascular Dysfunction
Risk for **P**oisoning
Post-Trauma Syndrome
Risk for **P**ost-Trauma Syndrome
Powerlessness
Risk for **P**owerlessness
Ineffective **P**rotection
Rape-Trauma Syndrome
Rape-Trauma Syndrome: Compound Reaction
Rape-Trauma Syndrome: Silent Reaction
Impaired **R**eligiosity
Readiness for Enhanced **R**eligiosity
Risk for Impaired **R**eligiosity
Relocation Stress Syndrome
Risk for **R**elocation Stress Syndrome
Ineffective **R**ole Performance
Sedentary Life Style
Bathing/Hygiene **S**elf-Care Deficit
Dressing/Grooming **S**elf-Care Deficit
Feeding **S**elf-Care Deficit
Toileting **S**elf-Care Deficit
Readiness for Enhanced **S**elf-Concept
Chronic Low **S**elf-Esteem
Situational Low **S**elf-Esteem
Risk for Situational Low **S**elf-Esteem
Self-Mutilation
Risk for **S**elf-Mutilation

Disturbed **S**ensory Perception
　　(Specify: Visual, Auditory, Kinesthetic,
　　Gustatory, Tactile, Olfactory)
Sexual Dysfunction
Ineffective **S**exuality Patterns
Impaired **S**kin Integrity
Risk for Impaired **S**kin Integrity
Sleep Deprivation
Disturbed **S**leep Pattern
Readiness for Enhanced **S**leep
Impaired **S**ocial Interaction
Social Isolation
Chronic **S**orrow
Spiritual Distress
Risk for **S**piritual Distress
Readiness for Enhanced **S**piritual Well-Being
Risk for **S**uffocation
Risk for **S**uicide
Delayed **S**urgical Recovery
Impaired **S**wallowing
Effective **T**herapeutic Regimen Management
Ineffective **T**herapeutic Regimen Management
Readiness for Enhanced Management
　　of **T**herapeutic Regimen
Ineffective Community **T**herapeutic
　　Regimen Management
Ineffective Family **T**herapeutic
　　Regimen Management
Ineffective **T**hermoregulation
Disturbed **T**hought Processes
Impaired **T**issue Integrity
Ineffective **T**issue Perfusion (Specify Type:
　　Renal, Cerebral, Cardiopulmonary,
　　Gastrointestinal, Peripheral)
Impaired **T**ransfer Ability
Risk for **T**rauma
Impaired **U**rinary Elimination
Readiness for Enhanced **U**rinary Elimination
Urinary Retention
Impaired Spontaneous **V**entilation
Dysfunctional **V**entilatory Weaning Response
Risk for Other-Directed **V**iolence
Risk for Self-Directed **V**iolence
Impaired **W**alking
Wandering

APPENDIX B

NURSING OUTCOMES CLASSIFICATIONS (NOC)

Abuse Cessation
Abuse Protection
Abuse Recovery Status
Abuse Recovery: Emotional
Abuse Recovery: Financial
Abuse Recovery: Physical
Abuse Recovery: Sexual
Abusive Behavior Self-Restraint
Acceptance: Health Status
Activity Tolerance
Adaptation to Physical Disability
Adherence Behavior
Aggression Self-Control
Allergic Response: Localized
Allergic Response: Systemic
Ambulation
Ambulation: Wheelchair
Anxiety Level
Anxiety Self-Control
Appetite
Aspiration Prevention
Asthma Self-Management

Balance
Blood Coagulation
Blood-Glucose Level
Blood Loss Severity
Blood Transfusion Reaction
Body Image
Body Mechanics Performance
Body Positioning: Self-Initiated
Bone Healing
Bowel Continence
Bowel Elimination
Breastfeeding Establishment: Infant
Breastfeeding Establishment: Maternal
Breastfeeding: Maintenance
Breastfeeding: Weaning

Cardiac Disease Self-Management
Cardiac Pump Effectiveness
Caregiver Adaptation to Patient Institutionalization
Caregiver Emotional Health

Caregiver Home Care Readiness
Caregiver Lifestyle Disruption
Caregiver-Patient Relationship
Caregiver Performance: Direct Care
Caregiver Performance: Indirect Care
Caregiver Physical Health
Caregiver Stressors
Caregiver Well-Being
Caregiving Endurance Potential
Child Adaptation to Hospitalization
Child Development: 1 Month
Child Development: 2 Months
Child Development: 4 Months
Child Development: 6 Months
Child Development: 12 Months
Child Development: 2 Years
Child Development: 3 Years
Child Development: 4 Years
Child Development: Middle Childhood
Child Development: Adolescence
Circulation Status
Client Satisfaction: Access to Care Resources
Client Satisfaction: Caring
Client Satisfaction: Communication
Client Satisfaction: Continuity of Care
Client Satisfaction: Cultural Needs Fulfillment
Client Satisfaction: Functional Assistance
Client Satisfaction: Physical Care
Client Satisfaction: Physical Environment
Client Satisfaction: Protection of Rights
Client Satisfaction: Psychological Care
Client Satisfaction: Safety
Client Satisfaction: Symptom Control
Client Satisfaction: Teaching
Client Satisfaction: Technical Aspects of Care
Cognition
Cognitive Orientation
Comfort Level
Comfortable Death
Communication
Communication: Expressive
Communication: Receptive
Community Competence

Community Disaster Readiness
Community Health Status
Community Health Status: Immunity
Community Risk Control: Chronic Disease
Community Risk Control: Communicable
Community Risk Control: Lead Exposure
Community Risk Control: Violence
Community Violence Level
Compliance Behavior
Concentration
Coordinated Movement
Coping

Decision Making
Depression Level
Depression Self-Control
Diabetes Self-Management
Dignified Life Closure
Discharge Readiness: Independent Living
Discharge Readiness: Supported Living
Distorted Thought Self-Control

Electrolyte and Acid/Base Balance
Endurance
Energy Conservation

Fall Prevention Behavior
Falls Occurrence
Family Coping
Family Functioning
Family Health Status
Family Integrity
Family Normalization
Family Participation in Professional Care
Family Physical Environment
Family Resiliency
Family Social Climate
Family Support During Treatment
Fear Level
Fear Level: Child
Fear Self-Control
Fetal Status: Antepartum
Fetal Status: Intrapartum
Fluid Balance
Fluid Overload Severity

Grief Resolution
Growth

Health Beliefs
Health Beliefs: Perceived Ability to Perform
Health Beliefs: Perceived Control
Health Beliefs: Perceived Resources
Health Beliefs: Perceived Threat
Health Orientation
Health-Promoting Behavior

Health-Seeking Behavior
Hearing Compensation Behavior
Hemodialysis Access
Hope
Hydration
Hyperactivity Level

Identity
Immobility Consequences: Physiological
Immobility Consequences: Psycho-Cognitive
Immune Hypersensitivity Response
Immune Status
Immunization Behavior
Impulse Self-Control
Infection Severity
Infection Severity: Newborn
Information Processing

Joint Movement: Ankle
Joint Movement: Elbow
Joint Movement: Fingers
Joint Movement: Hip
Joint Movement: Knee
Joint Movement: Neck
Joint Movement: Passive
Joint Movement: Shoulder
Joint Movement: Spine
Joint Movement: Wrist

Kidney Function
Knowledge: Body Mechanics
Knowledge: Breastfeeding
Knowledge: Cardiac Disease Management
Knowledge: Child Physical Safety
Knowledge: Conception Prevention
Knowledge: Diabetes Management
Knowledge: Diet
Knowledge: Disease Process
Knowledge: Energy Conservation
Knowledge: Fall Prevention
Knowledge: Fertility Promotion
Knowledge: Health Behavior
Knowledge: Health Promotion
Knowledge: Health Resources
Knowledge: Illness Care
Knowledge: Infant Care
Knowledge: Infection Control
Knowledge: Labor and Delivery
Knowledge: Medication
Knowledge: Ostomy Care
Knowledge: Parenting
Knowledge: Personal Safety
Knowledge: Postpartum Maternal Health
Knowledge: Preconception Maternal Health
Knowledge: Pregnancy
Knowledge: Prescribed Activity

Knowledge: Sexual Functioning
Knowledge: Substance Abuse Control
Knowledge: Treatment Procedure(s)
Knowledge: Treatment Regimen

Leisure Participation
Loneliness Severity

Maternal Status: Antepartum
Maternal Status: Intrapartum
Maternal Status: Postpartum
Mechanical Ventilation Response: Adult
Mechanical Ventilation Weaning Response: Adult
Medication Response
Memory
Mobility
Mood Equilibrium
Motivation

Nausea & Vomiting Control
Nausea & Vomiting: Disruptive Effects
Nausea & Vomiting Severity
Neglect Cessation
Neglect Recovery
Neurological Status
Neurological Status: Autonomic
Neurological Status: Central Motor Control
Neurological Status: Consciousness
Neurological Status: Cranial Sensory/Motor Function
Neurological Status: Spinal Sensory/Motor Function
Newborn Adaptation
Nutritional Status
Nutritional Status: Biochemical Measures
Nutritional Status: Energy
Nutritional Status: Food and Fluid Intake
Nutritional Status: Nutrient Intake

Oral Health
Ostomy Self-Care

Pain: Adverse Psychological Response
Pain Control
Pain: Disruptive Effects
Pain Level
Parent-Infant Attachment
Parenting: Adolescent Physical Safety
Parenting: Early/Middle Childhood Physical Safety
Parenting: Infant/Toddler Physical Safety
Parenting Performance
Parenting: Psychosocial Safety
Participation in Health Care Decisions
Personal Autonomy
Personal Health Status
Personal Safety Behavior
Personal Well-Being
Physical Aging

Physical Fitness
Physical Injury Severity
Physical Maturation: Female
Physical Maturation: Male
Play Participation
Post Procedure Recovery Status
Prenatal Health Behavior
Preterm Infant Organization
Psychomotor Energy
Psychosocial Adjustment: Life Change

Quality of Life

Respiratory Status: Airway Patency
Respiratory Status: Gas Exchange
Respiratory Status: Ventilation
Rest
Risk Control
Risk Control: Alcohol Use
Risk Control: Cancer
Risk Control: Cardiovascular Health
Risk Control: Drug Use
Risk Control: Hearing Impairment
Risk Control: Sexually Transmitted Diseases
Risk Control: Tobacco Use
Risk Control: Unintended Pregnancy
Risk Control: Visual Impairment
Risk Detection
Role Performance

Safe Home Environment
Seizure Control
Self-Care Status
Self-Care: Activities of Daily Living (ADL)
Self-Care: Bathing
Self-Care: Dressing
Self-Care: Eating
Self-Care: Hygiene
Self-Care: Instrumental Activities of Daily Living
Self-Care: Nonparenteral Medication
Self-Care: Oral Hygiene
Self-Care: Parenteral Medication
Self-Care: Toileting
Self-Direction of Care
Self-Esteem
Self-Mutilation Restraint
Sensory Function Status
Sensory Function: Cutaneous
Sensory Function: Hearing
Sensory Function: Proprioception
Sensory Function: Taste and Smell
Sensory Function: Vision
Sexual Functioning
Sexual Identity
Skeletal Function
Sleep

Social Interaction Skills
Social Involvement
Social Support
Spiritual Health
Stress Level
Student Health Status
Substance Addiction Consequences
Suffering Severity
Suicide Self-Restraint
Swallowing Status
Swallowing Status: Esophageal Phase
Swallowing Status: Oral Phrase
Swallowing Status: Pharyngeal Phase
Symptom Control
Symptom Severity
Symptom Severity: Perimenopause
Symptom Severity: Premenstrual Syndrome (PMS)
Systemic Toxin Clearance: Dialysis

Thermoregulation
Thermoregulation: Neonate

Tissue Integrity: Skin and Mucous
    Membranes
Tissue Perfusion: Abdominal Organs
Tissue Perfusion: Cardiac
Tissue Perfusion: Cerebral
Tissue Perfusion: Peripheral
Tissue Perfusion: Pulmonary
Transfer Performance
Treatment Behavior: Illness or Injury

Urinary Continence
Urinary Elimination

Vision Compensation Behavior
Vital Signs

Weight: Body Mass
Weight Control
Will to Live
Wound Healing: Primary Intention
Wound Healing: Primary Intention

Reprinted from Moorhead, S., Johnson, M., & Maas, M., *Nursing Outcomes Classifications,* 3rd edition, © 2004. Copyright 2004, with permission from Elsevier Science.

APPENDIX C

NURSING INTERVENTIONS CLASSIFICATIONS (NIC)

Abuse Protection Support
Abuse Protection Support: Child
Abuse Protection Support: Domestic Partner
Abuse Protection Support: Elder
Abuse Protection Support: Religious
Acid/Base Management
Acid/Base Management: Metabolic Acidosis
Acid/Base Management: Metabolic Alkalosis
Acid/Base Management: Respiratory Acidosis
Acid/Base Management: Respiratory Alkalosis
Acid/Base Monitoring
Active Listening
Activity Therapy
Acupressure
Admission Care
Airway Insertion And Stabilization
Airway Management
Airway Suctioning
Allergy Management
Amnioinfusion
Amputation Care
Analgesic Administration
Analgesic Administration: Intraspinal
Anaphylaxis Management
Anesthesia Administration
Anger Control Assistance
Animal-Assisted Therapy
Anticipatory Guidance
Anxiety Reduction
Area Restriction
Aromatherapy
Art Therapy
Artificial Airway Management
Aspiration Precautions
Assertiveness Training
Asthma Management
Attachment Promotion
Autogenic Training
Autotransfusion

Bathing
Bed Rest Care
Bedside Laboratory Testing

Behavior Management
Behavior Management: Overactivity/ Inattention
Behavior Management: Self-Harm
Behavior Management: Sexual
Behavior Modification
Behavior Modification: Social Skills
Bibliotherapy
Biofeedback
Bioterrorism Preparedness
Birthing
Bladder Irrigation
Bleeding Precautions
Bleeding Reduction
Bleeding Reduction: Antepartum Uterus
Bleeding Reduction: Gastrointestinal
Bleeding Reduction: Nasal
Bleeding Reduction: Postpartum Uterus
Bleeding Reduction: Wound
Blood Products Administration
Body Image Enhancement
Body Mechanics Promotion
Bottle Feeding
Bowel Incontinence Care
Bowel Incontinence Care: Encopresis
Bowel Irrigation
Bowel Management
Bowel Training
Breast Examination
Breastfeeding Assistance

Calming Technique
Capillary Blood Sample
Cardiac Care
Cardiac Care: Acute
Cardiac Care: Rehabilitative
Cardiac Precautions
Caregiver Support
Care Management
Cast Care: Maintenance
Cast Care, Wet
Cerebral Edema Management
Cerebral Perfusion Promotion

Cesarean Section Care
Chemical Restraint
Chemotherapy Management
Chest Physiotherapy
Childbirth Preparation
Circulatory Care: Arterial Insufficiency
Circulatory Care: Mechanical Assistive Device
Circulatory Care: Venous Insufficiency
Circulatory Precautions
Circumcision Care
Code Management
Cognitive Restructuring
Cognitive Stimulation
Communicable Disease Management
Communication Enhancement: Hearing Deficit
Communication Enhancement: Speech Deficit
Communication Enhancement: Visual Deficit
Community Disaster Preparedness
Community Health Development
Complex Relationship Building
Conflict Mediation
Constipation/Impaction Management
Consultation
Contact Lens Care
Controlled Substance Checking
Coping Enhancement
Cost Containment
Cough Enhancement
Counseling
Crisis Intervention
Critical Path Development
Culture Brokerage
Cutaneous Stimulation

Decision-Making Support
Delegation
Delirium Management
Delusion Management
Dementia Management
Dementia Management: Bathing
Deposition/Testimony
Developmental Care
Developmental Enhancement: Adolescent
Developmental Enhancement: Child
Dialysis Access Maintenance
Diarrhea Management
Diet Staging
Discharge Planning
Distraction
Documentation
Dressing
Dying Care
Dysreflexia Management
Dysrhythmia Management

Ear Care
Eating Disorders Management

Electroconvulsive Therapy (ECT) Management
Electrolyte Management
Electrolyte Management: Hypercalcemia
Electrolyte Management: Hyperkalemia
Electrolyte Management: Hypermagnesemia
Electrolyte Management: Hypernatremia
Electrolyte Management: Hyperphosphatemia
Electrolyte Management: Hypocalcemia
Electrolyte Management: Hypokalemia
Electrolyte Management: Hypomagnesemia
Electrolyte Management: Hyponatremia
Electrolyte Management: Hypophosphatemia
Electrolyte Monitoring
Electronic Fetal Monitoring: Antepartum
Electronic Fetal Monitoring: Intrapartum
Elopement Precautions
Embolus Care: Peripheral
Embolus Care: Pulmonary
Embolus Precautions
Emergency Care
Emergency Cart Checking
Emotional Support
Endotracheal Extubation
Energy Management
Enteral Tube Feeding
Environmental Management
Environmental Management: Attachment Process
Environmental Management: Comfort
Environmental Management: Community
Environmental Management: Home Preparation
Environmental Management: Safety
Environmental Management: Violence Prevention
Environmental Management: Worker Safety
Environmental Risk Protection
Examination Assistance
Exercise Promotion
Exercise Promotion: Strength Training
Exercise Promotion: Stretching
Exercise Therapy: Ambulation
Exercise Therapy: Balance
Exercise Therapy: Joint Mobility
Exercise Therapy: Muscle Control
Eye Care

Fall Prevention
Family Integrity Promotion
Family Integrity Promotion: Childbearing Family
Family Involvement Promotion
Family Mobilization
Family Planning: Contraception
Family Planning: Infertility
Family Planning: Unplanned Pregnancy
Family Presence Facilitation
Family Process Maintenance
Family Support
Family Therapy
Feeding

Fertility Preservation
Fever Treatment
Financial Resource Assistance
Fire-Setting Precautions
First Aid
Fiscal Resource Management
Flatulence Reduction
Fluid/Electrolyte Management
Fluid Management
Fluid Monitoring
Fluid Resuscitation
Foot Care
Forgiveness Facilitation

Gastrointestinal Intubation
Genetic Counseling
Grief Work Facilitation
Grief Work Facilitation: Perinatal Death
Guilt Work Facilitation

Hair Care
Hallucination Management
Health Care Information Exchange
Health Education
Health Policy Monitoring
Health Screening
Health System Guidance
Heat/Cold Application
Heat Exposure Treatment
Hemodialysis Therapy
Hemodynamic Regulation
Hemofiltration Therapy
Hemorrhage Control
High-Risk Pregnancy Care
Home Maintenance Assistance
Hope Instillation
Hormone Replacement Therapy
Humor
Hyperglycemia Management
Hypervolemia Management
Hypnosis
Hypoglycemia Management
Hypothermia Treatment
Hypovolemia Management

Immunization/Vaccination Administration
Impulse Control Training
Incident Reporting
Incision Site Care
Infant Care
Infection Control
Infection Control: Intraoperative
Infection Protection
Insurance Authorization
Intracranial Pressure (ICP) Monitoring

Intrapartal Care
Intrapartal Care: High-Risk Delivery
Intravenous (IV) Insertion
Intravenous (IV) Therapy
Invasive Hemodynamic Monitoring

Kangaroo Care

Labor Induction
Labor Suppression
Laboratory Data Interpretation
Lactation Counseling
Lactation Suppression
Laser Precautions
Latex Precautions
Learning Facilitation
Learning Readiness Enhancement
Leech Therapy
Limit Setting
Lower Extremity Monitoring

Malignant Hyperthermia Precautions
Mechanical Ventilation
Mechanical Ventilatory Weaning
Medication Administration
Medication Administration: Ear
Medication Administration: Enteral
Medication Administration: Eye
Medication Administration: Inhalation
Medication Administration: Interpleural
Medication Administration: Intradermal
Medication Administration: Intramuscular (IM)
Medication Administration: Intraosseous
Medication Administration: Intraspinal
Medication Administration: Intravenous (IV)
Medication Administration: Nasal
Medication Administration: Oral
Medication Administration: Rectal
Medication Administration: Skin
Medication Administration: Subcutaneous
Medication Administration: Vaginal
Medication Administration: Ventricular Reservoir
Medication Management
Medication Prescribing
Meditation Facilitation
Memory Training
Milieu Therapy
Mood Management
Multidisciplinary Care Conference
Music Therapy
Mutual Goal Setting

Nail Care
Nausea Management
Neurologic Monitoring

Newborn Care
Newborn Monitoring
Nonnutritive Sucking
Normalization Promotion
Nutrition Management
Nutrition Therapy
Nutritional Counseling
Nutritional Monitoring

Oral Health Maintenance
Oral Health Promotion
Oral Health Restoration
Order Transcription
Organ Procurement
Ostomy Care
Oxygen Therapy

Pain Management
Parent Education: Adolescent
Parent Education: Childrearing Family
Parent Education: Infant
Parenting Promotion
Pass Facilitation
Patient Contracting
Patient-Controlled Analgesia (PCA)
  Assistance
Patient Rights Protection
Peer Review
Pelvic Muscle Exercise
Perineal Care
Peripheral Sensation Management
Peripherally Inserted Central (PIC)
  Catheter Care
Peritoneal Dialysis Therapy
Pessary Management
Phlebotomy: Arterial Blood Sample
Phlebotomy: Blood Unit Acquisition
Phlebotomy: Cannulated Vessel
Phlebotomy: Venous Blood Sample
Phototherapy: Mood/Sleep Regulation
Phototherapy: Neonate
Physical Restraint
Physician Support
Pneumatic Tourniquet Precautions
Positioning
Positioning: Intraoperative
Positioning: Neurologic
Positioning: Wheelchair
Postanesthesia Care
Postmortem Care
Postpartal Care
Preceptor: Employee
Preceptor: Student
Preconception Counseling
Pregnancy Termination Care

Premenstrual Syndrome (PMS)
  Management
Prenatal Care
Preoperative Coordination
Preparatory Sensory Information
Presence
Pressure Management
Pressure Ulcer Care
Pressure Ulcer Prevention
Product Evaluation
Program Development
Progressive Muscle Relaxation
Prompted Voiding
Prosthesis Care
Pruritus Management

Quality Monitoring

Radiation Therapy Management
Rape-Trauma Treatment
Reality Orientation
Recreation Therapy
Rectal Prolapse Management
Referral
Religious Addiction Prevention
Religious Ritual Enhancement
Relocation Stress Reduction
Reminiscence Therapy
Reproductive Technology Management
Research Data Collection
Resiliency Promotion
Respiratory Monitoring
Respite Care
Resuscitation
Resuscitation: Fetus
Resuscitation: Neonate
Risk Identification
Risk Identification: Childbearing Family
Risk Identification: Genetic
Role Enhancement

Seclusion
Security Enhancement
Sedation Management
Seizure Management
Seizure Precautions
Self-Awareness Enhancement
Self-Care Assistance
Self-Care Assistance: Bathing/Hygiene
Self-Care Assistance: Dressing/Grooming
Self-Care Assistance: Feeding
Self-Care Assistance: IADL
Self-Care Assistance: Toileting
Self-Care Assistance: Transfer
Self-Esteem Enhancement

Self-Hypnosis Facilitation
Self-Modification Assistance
Self-Responsibility Facilitation
Sexual Counseling
Shift Report
Shock Management
Shock Management: Cardiac
Shock Management: Vasogenic
Shock Management: Volume
Shock Prevention
Sibling Support
Simple Guided Imagery
Simple Massage
Simple Relaxation Therapy
Skin Care: Donor Site
Skin Care: Graft Site
Skin Care: Topical Treatments
Skin Surveillance
Sleep Enhancement
Smoking Cessation Assistance
Socialization Enhancement
Specimen Management
Spiritual Growth Facilitation
Spiritual Support
Splinting
Sports-Injury Prevention: Youth
Staff Development
Staff Supervision
Subarachnoid Hemorrhage Precautions
Substance Use Prevention
Substance Use Treatment
Substance Use Treatment: Alcohol Withdrawal
Substance Use Treatment: Drug Withdrawal
Substance Use Treatment: Overdose
Suicide Prevention
Supply Management
Support Group
Support System Enhancement
Surgical Assistance
Surgical Precautions
Surgical Preparation
Surveillance
Surveillance: Community
Surveillance: Late Pregnancy
Surveillance: Remote Electronic
Surveillance: Safety
Sustenance Support
Suturing
Swallowing Therapy

Teaching: Disease Process
Teaching: Foot Care
Teaching: Group
Teaching: Individual
Teaching: Infant Nutrition

Teaching: Infant Safety
Teaching: Infant Stimulation
Teaching: Preoperative
Teaching: Prescribed Activity/Exercise
Teaching: Prescribed Diet
Teaching: Prescribed Medication
Teaching: Procedure/Treatment
Teaching: Psychomotor Skill
Teaching: Safe Sex
Teaching: Sexuality
Teaching: Toddler Nutrition
Teaching: Toddler Safety
Teaching: Toilet Training
Technology Management
Telephone Consultation
Telephone Follow-Up
Temperature Regulation
Temperature Regulation: Intraoperative
Temporary Pacemaker Management
Therapeutic Play
Therapeutic Touch
Therapy Group
Total Parenteral Nutrition (TPN) Administration
Touch
Traction/Immobilization Care
Transcutaneous Electrical Nerve Stimulation (TENS)
Transport
Trauma Therapy: Child
Triage: Disaster
Triage: Emergency Center
Triage: Telephone
Truth Telling
Tube Care
Tube Care: Chest
Tube Care: Gastrointestinal
Tube Care: Umbilical Line
Tube Care: Urinary
Tube Care: Ventriculostomy/ Lumbar Drain

Ultrasonography: Limited Obstetric
Unilateral Neglect Management
Urinary Bladder Training
Urinary Catheterization
Urinary Catheterization: Intermittent
Urinary Elimination Management
Urinary Habit Training
Urinary Incontinence Care
Urinary Incontinence Care: Enuresis
Urinary Retention Care

Values Clarification
Vehicle Safety Promotion

Venous Access Device (VAD)
  Maintenance
Ventilation Assistance
Visitation Facilitation
Vital Signs Monitoring
Vomiting Management

Weight Gain Assistance
Weight Management
Weight Reduction Assistance
Wound Care
Wound Care: Closed Drainage
Wound Irrigation

APPENDIX D

ABBREVIATIONS

AAA	abdominal aortic aneurysm		CNS	central nervous system
ABGs	arterial blood gases		COPD	chronic obstructive pulmonary disease
ACE	angiotensin-converting enzyme		CPP	cerebral perfusion pressure
ACTH	adrenocorticotrophic hormone		CRF	chronic renal failure
ADH	antidiuretic hormone		CSF	cerebral spinal fluid
ADLs	activities of daily living		CVA	cerebrovascular accident
AIDS	acquired immunodeficiency syndrome		CVP	central venous pressure
ALS	Amyotrophic lateral sclerosis		CVVD/ CVVHD	continuous veno-venous hemodialysis
ALT	alanine aminotransferase (also SGPT)		DI	diabetes insipidus
ANA	antinuclear antibody		DIC	disseminated intravascular coagulation
APTT	activated partial thromboplastin time		DHT	dihydrotestosterone
A-P	anterior-posterior		DKA	diabetic ketoacidosis
ARF	acute renal failure		DM	diabetes mellitus
AST	aspartate aminotransferase (also SGOT)		DVT	deep vein thrombosis
ATP	adenosine triphosphate		ECG/EKG	electrocardiogram
AUA	American Urological Association		EEG	electroencephalogram
BMI	body mass index		ELISA	enzyme-linked immunosorbent assay
BPH	benign prostatic hypertrophy/ hyperplasia		ESR	erythrocyte sedimentation rate
BSA	body surface area		ET	endotracheal
BUN	blood urea nitrogen		EGD	esophagogastroduodenoscopy
CABG	coronary artery bypass graft		EIA	enzyme immunoassay
CAD	coronary artery disease		ERCP	endoscopic retrograde cholangiopancreatography
cAMP	cyclic adenosine monophosphate		FEV	forced expiratory volume
CAP	community-acquired pneumonia		FIO$_2$	fraction of inspired oxygen
CBC	complete blood count		GGTP	gamma-glutamyl transpeptidase
CBI	continuous bladder irrigation		GI	gastrointestinal
CDC	Centers for Disease Control and Prevention		GU	genitourinary
CEA	carcinoembryonic antigen		HAP	hospital-acquired pneumonia
CHF	congestive heart failure		HAART	highly active antiretroviral therapy
CIN	cervical intraepithelial neoplasia		Hct	hematocrit
CK-MB	creatine kinase-MB			

Hgb	hemoglobin
HHNS	hyperglycemic hyperosmolar non-ketotic syndrome
HIV	human immunodeficiency virus
HPV	human papillomavirus
IABP	intraaortic balloon pump
IBD	inflammatory bowel disease
ICP	intracranial pressure
Ig	immune globulin
IM	intramuscular
INR	international normalized ratio
IOP	intraocular pressure
IS	incentive spirometry
ITP	idiopathic thrombocytopenia
IUD	intrauterine device
IV	intravenous
IVP	intravenous pyelogram
JP	Jackson Pratt
JVD	jugular vein distention
LDH	lactate dehydrogenase
LH-RH	luteinizing hormone-releasing hormone
LOC	level of consciousness
LUQ	left upper quadrant
LVF	left ventricular failure
MAP	mean arterial pressure
MI	myocardial infarction
MRI	magnetic resonance imaging
MS	multiple sclerosis
NIC	nursing interventions classification
NOC	nursing outcomes classification
NSAIDs	non-steroidal anti-inflammatory drugs
NSTEMI	non-ST segment elevation myocardial infarction
OA	osteoarthritis
O_2Sat	oxygen saturation
PAWP	pulmonary artery wedge pressure
PCA	patient-controlled analgesia
pO_2	arterial oxygen pressure
pCO_2	arterial carbon dioxide pressure
PE	pulmonary embolus
PEFR	peak expiratory flow rate

PEEP	positive end expiratory pressure
PET	positron emission tomography
PO	by mouth
PIC	peripherally inserted central catheter
PID	pelvic inflammatory disease
PPD	purified protein derivative
PSA	prostate-specific antigen
Pt/PT	prothrombin time
PTH	parathyroid hormone
Ptt/PTT	partial thromboplastin time
PVC	premature ventricular contraction
RA	rheumatoid arthritis
RBC	red blood cells
ROM	range of motion
RUQ	right upper quadrant
RVF	right ventricular failure
SANE	sexual assault nurse examiner
SCI	spinal cord injury
SIADH	syndrome of inappropriate antidiuretic hormone
SIMV	synchronized intermittent mandatory ventilation
SLE	systemic lupus erythematosus
SPA	salt-poor albumin
STD	sexually transmitted disease
STEMI	ST segment elevation myocardial infarction
SVR	systemic vascular resistance
TCDB	turn, cough, deep breathe
TENS	transcutaneous electrical nerve stimulation
TEP	transesophageal puncture
TH	thyroid hormone
TIBC	total iron-binding capacity
tPA	tissue plasminogen activator
TPN	total parenteral nutrition
TRAM	transverse rectus abdominis musculocutaneous
TSH	thyroid-stimulating hormone
TURP	transurethral resection of the prostate
UTI	urinary tract infection
VDRL	venereal disease research laboratories
V/Q	ventilation/perfusion ratio

INDEX

Note: **Bold** type indicates main entries which are nursing diagnoses.

IMPORTANT! READ CAREFULLY: This End User License Agreement ("Agreement") sets forth the conditions by which Thomson Delmar Learning, a division of Thomson Learning Inc. ("Thomson") will make electronic access to the Thomson Delmar Learning-owned licensed content and associated media, software, documentation, printed materials, and electronic documentation contained in this package and/or made available to you via this product (the "Licensed Content"), available to you (the "End User"). BY CLICKING THE "I ACCEPT" BUTTON AND/OR OPENING THIS PACKAGE, YOU ACKNOWLEDGE THAT YOU HAVE READ ALL OF THE TERMS AND CONDITIONS, AND THAT YOU AGREE TO BE BOUND BY ITS TERMS, CONDITIONS, AND ALL APPLICABLE LAWS AND REGULATIONS GOVERNING THE USE OF THE LICENSED CONTENT.

1.0 SCOPE OF LICENSE

1.1 <u>Licensed Content</u>. The Licensed Content may contain portions of modifiable content ("Modifiable Content") and content which may not be modified or otherwise altered by the End User ("Non-Modifiable Content"). For purposes of this Agreement, Modifiable Content and Non-Modifiable Content may be collectively referred to herein as the "Licensed Content." All Licensed Content shall be considered Non-Modifiable Content, unless such Licensed Content is presented to the End User in a modifiable format and it is clearly indicated that modification of the Licensed Content is permitted.

1.2 Subject to the End User's compliance with the terms and conditions of this Agreement, Thomson Delmar Learning hereby grants the End User, a nontransferable, nonexclusive, limited right to access and view a single copy of the Licensed Content on a single personal computer system for noncommercial, internal, personal use only. The End User shall not (i) reproduce, copy, modify (except in the case of Modifiable Content), distribute, display, transfer, sublicense, prepare derivative work(s) based on, sell, exchange, barter or transfer, rent, lease, loan, resell, or in any other manner exploit the Licensed Content; (ii) remove, obscure, or alter any notice of Thomson Delmar Learning's intellectual property rights present on or in the Licensed Content, including, but not limited to, copyright, trademark, and/or patent notices; or (iii) disassemble, decompile, translate, reverse engineer, or otherwise reduce the Licensed Content.

2.0 TERMINATION

2.1 Thomson Delmar Learning may at any time (without prejudice to its other rights or remedies) immediately terminate this Agreement and/or suspend access to some or all of the Licensed Content, in the event that the End User does not comply with any of the terms and conditions of this Agreement. In the event of such termination by Thomson Delmar Learning, the End User shall immediately return any and all copies of the Licensed Content to Thomson Delmar Learning.

3.0 PROPRIETARY RIGHTS

3.1 The End User acknowledges that Thomson Delmar Learning owns all rights, title and interest, including, but not limited to all copyright rights therein, in and to the Licensed Content, and that the End User shall not take any action inconsistent with such ownership. The Licensed Content is protected by U.S., Canadian and other applicable copyright laws and by international treaties, including the Berne Convention and the Universal Copyright Convention. Nothing contained in this Agreement shall be construed as granting the End User any ownership rights in or to the Licensed Content.

3.2 Thomson Delmar Learning reserves the right at any time to withdraw from the Licensed Content any item or part of an item for which it no longer retains the right to publish, or which it has reasonable grounds to believe infringes copyright or is defamatory, unlawful, or otherwise objectionable.

4.0 PROTECTION AND SECURITY

4.1 The End User shall use its best efforts and take all reasonable steps to safeguard its copy of the Licensed Content to ensure that no unauthorized reproduction, publication, disclosure, modification, or distribution of the Licensed Content, in whole or in part, is made. To the extent that the End User becomes aware of any such unauthorized use of the Licensed Content, the End User shall immediately notify Thomson Delmar Learning. Notification of such violations may be made by sending an e-mail to delmarhelp@thomson.com.

5.0 MISUSE OF THE LICENSED PRODUCT

5.1 In the event that the End User uses the Licensed Content in violation of this Agreement, Thomson Delmar Learning shall have the option of electing liquidated damages, which shall include all profits generated by the End User's use of the Licensed Content plus interest computed at the maximum rate permitted by law and all legal fees and other expenses incurred by Thomson Delmar Learning in enforcing its rights, plus penalties.

6.0 FEDERAL GOVERNMENT CLIENTS

6.1 Except as expressly authorized by Thomson Delmar Learning, Federal Government clients obtain only the rights specified in this Agreement and no other rights. The Government acknowledges that (i) all software and related documentation incorporated in the Licensed Content is existing commercial computer software within the meaning of FAR 27.405(b)(2); and (2) all other data delivered in whatever form, is limited rights data within the meaning of FAR 27.401. The restrictions in this section are acceptable as consistent with the Government's need for software and other data under this Agreement.

7.0 DISCLAIMER OF WARRANTIES AND LIABILITIES

7.1 Although Thomson Delmar Learning believes the Licensed Content to be reliable, Thomson Delmar Learning does not guarantee or warrant (i) any information or materials contained in or produced by the Licensed Content, (ii) the accuracy, completeness or reliability of the Licensed Content, or (iii) that the Licensed Content is free from errors or other material defects. THE LICENSED PRODUCT IS PROVIDED "AS IS," WITHOUT ANY WARRANTY OF ANY KIND AND THOMSON DELMAR LEARNING DISCLAIMS ANY AND ALL WARRANTIES, EXPRESSED OR IMPLIED, INCLUDING, WITHOUT LIMITATION, WARRANTIES OF MERCHANTABILITY OR FITNESS OR A PARTICULAR PURPOSE. IN NO EVENT SHALL THOMSON DELMAR LEARNING BE LIABLE FOR: INDIRECT, SPECIAL, PUNITIVE OR CONSEQUENTIAL DAMAGES INCLUDING FOR LOST PROFITS, LOST DATA, OR OTHERWISE. IN NO EVENT SHALL THOMSON DELMAR LEARNING'S

AGGREGATE LIABILITY HEREUNDER, WHETHER ARISING IN CONTRACT, TORT, STRICT LIABILITY OR OTHERWISE, EXCEED THE AMOUNT OF FEES PAID BY THE END USER HEREUNDER FOR THE LICENSE OF THE LICENSED CONTENT.

8.0 GENERAL

8.1 Entire Agreement. This Agreement shall constitute the entire Agreement between the Parties and supercedes all prior Agreements and understandings oral or written relating to the subject matter hereof.

8.2 Enhancements/Modifications of Licensed Content. From time to time, and in Thomson Delmar Learning's sole discretion, Thomson Delmar Learning may advise the End User of updates, upgrades, enhancements and/or improvements to the Licensed Content, and may permit the End User to access and use, subject to the terms and conditions of this Agreement, such modifications, upon payment of prices as may be established by Thomson Delmar Learning.

8.3 No Export. The End User shall use the Licensed Content solely in the United States and shall not transfer or export, directly or indirectly, the Licensed Content outside the United States.

8.4 Severability. If any provision of this Agreement is invalid, illegal, or unenforceable under any applicable statute or rule of law, the provision shall be deemed omitted to the extent that it is invalid, illegal, or unenforceable. In such a case, the remainder of the Agreement shall be construed in a manner as to give greatest effect to the original intention of the parties hereto.

8.5 Waiver. The waiver of any right or failure of either party to exercise in any respect any right provided in this Agreement in any instance shall not be deemed to be a waiver of such right in the future or a waiver of any other right under this Agreement.

8.6 Choice of Law/Venue. This Agreement shall be interpreted, construed, and governed by and in accordance with the laws of the State of New York, applicable to contracts executed and to be wholly preformed therein, without regard to its principles governing conflicts of law. Each party agrees that any proceeding arising out of or relating to this Agreement or the breach or threatened breach of this Agreement may be commenced and prosecuted in a court in the State and County of New York. Each party consents and submits to the nonexclusive personal jurisdiction of any court in the State and County of New York in respect of any such proceeding.

8.7 Acknowledgment. By opening this package and/or by accessing the Licensed Content on this Web site, THE END USER ACKNOWLEDGES THAT IT HAS READ THIS AGREEMENT, UNDERSTANDS IT, AND AGREES TO BE BOUND BY ITS TERMS AND CONDITIONS. IF YOU DO NOT ACCEPT THESE TERMS AND CONDITIONS, YOU MUST NOT ACCESS THE LICENSED CONTENT AND RETURN THE LICENSED PRODUCT TO DELMAR LEARNING (WITHIN 30 CALENDAR DAYS OF THE END USER'S PURCHASE) WITH PROOF OF PAYMENT ACCEPTABLE TO THOMSON DELMAR LEARNING, FOR A CREDIT OR A REFUND. Should the End User have any questions/comments regarding this Agreement, please contact Thomson Delmar Learning at delmarhelp@thomson.com.

SYSTEM REQUIREMENTS

The CD-ROM version will be developed to run on client systems with the following minimum configuration:

- Operating System: Microsoft Windows 98 SE, Windows 2000, Windows XP
- Processor: Pentium PC 120 MHz or higher
- RAM: 64 MB of RAM or better
- Free Drive Space: 25 MB free disk space
- CD-ROM Drive necessary for installation only
- Internet Connection Speed: 56K or better in order to view web links provided in program but is not required.
- Screen Resolution: 800 × 600 pixels or better
- Color Depth: 16-bit color (thousands of colors) or 24-bit color (millions of colors)
- Sound card: N/A

SET UP INSTRUCTIONS FOR CARE PLANS SOFTWARE

1. Double click My Computer
2. Double click the Control Panel icon
3. Double click Add/Remove Programs
4. Click the Install button and follow the on screen prompts from there.